Pigmented Ethnic Skin and Imported Dermatoses

Constantin E. Orfanos
Christos C. Zouboulis
Chalid Assaf
Editors

Pigmented Ethnic Skin and Imported Dermatoses

A Text-Atlas

Springer

Editors
Constantin E. Orfanos
The Free University of Berlin
Medical School Charité
Berlin
Germany

Chalid Assaf
Department of Dermatology and Venereology
HELIOS Klinikum Krefeld
Krefeld
Nordrhein-Westfalen
Germany

Christos C. Zouboulis
Departments of Dermatology, Venereology, Allergology and Immunology, Dessau Medical Center
Brandenburg Medical School Theodor Fontane
Dessau
Saxony-Anhalt
Germany

ISBN 978-3-030-09888-9 ISBN 978-3-319-69422-1 (eBook)
https://doi.org/10.1007/978-3-319-69422-1

Printed on acid-free paper

This Springer imprint is published by the registered company Springer Nature Switzerland AG
The registered company address is: Gewerbestrasse 11, 6330 Cham, Switzerland

Preface

The clinical presentation of skin diseases varies greatly depending on age, body area, the structure of the skin region involved and the impact of environmental influences such as temperature, humidity and exposure to UV light. In skin of colour, particularly in heavily pigmented ethnic populations, diagnosis of skin disease requires particular knowledge and experience of the attending dermatologist. Also the probability for any physician to be challenged by seen dermatoses in patients with pigmented skin or in travellers with white skin imported from hot climate zones has markedly increased during the last decade due to vivid tourism, increased migration and ongoing globalisation. Thus, it appeared to us timely to elaborate and improve the knowledge on dermatoses in pigmented skin among physicians not only in areas where these disorders originally occur but also in geographic regions they only rarely occurred in the past and remained often late recognised.

A most important educational instrument in dermatology is clinical photography. The contributing authors and the editors of this volume focussed their attention to carefully select representative clinical pictures of high educational value, based on their own long-term clinical and diagnostic experiences with patients of diverse ethnic background. This Text-Atlas of *Diseases in Pigmented Ethnic Skin and Imported Dermatoses* is divided into several comprehensive chapters covering a large spectrum of dermatological disorders in pigmented skin, presenting a brief introduction on their epidemiology and pathogenesis with emphasis on the peculiarities of their clinical pictures and possible management.

Our sincere hope is that this book will help the readers, both in developing and in developed countries, to get familiar with the diagnosis of such entities and facilitate their management. We would like this book to join all those who offer their medical services to patients with pigmented skin in solving any of their doubts and provide proper care. Finally, we truly hope that the Text-Atlas will become useful not only to our colleagues dermatologists but also to physicians of other disciplines who are interested in skin diseases. We are deeply grateful to all those who have contributed in this endeavour.

Berlin, Germany — Constantin E. Orfanos
Dessau, Germany — Christos C. Zouboulis
Krefeld, Germany — Chalid Assaf

Contents

Contributors

Marwa Abdallah, M.D. Department of Dermatology and Venereology, Ain Shams University, Cairo, Egypt

Shaden Abdelhadi, MD, FAAD, FEADV, FESPD Department of Dermatology and Allergy, Sheikh Khalifa Medical City, Abu Dhabi, UAE

Department of Dermatology, University Medical Center Brussels (UZ Brussels), The Free University of Brussels (VUB), Brussels, Belgium

Medhat Abdelmalek, M.D. Consultant Dermatologist and Venereologist, Amman, Jordan

Mohamed Badawy Abdel-Naser, M.D. Department of Dermatology and Venereology, Ain Shams University, Cairo, Egypt

Erkan Alpsoy, M.D. Department of Dermatology and Venereology, Akdeniz University School of Medicine, Antalya, Turkey

Alice U. Amani, M.D. Service de Dermatologie, Centre Hospitalier Universitaire, Kigali, Rwanda

Karalikkattil T. Ashique, M.D., MBBS, DDVL Department of Dermatology, Kims Alshifa Hospital, Perinthalmanna, Kerala, India

Chalid Assaf, M.D. Department of Dermatology and Venereology, HELIOS Klinikum Krefeld, Krefeld, Germany

Emilio Berti, M.D. Department of Pathophysiology and Transplantation, Università degli Studi di Milano, I.R.C.C.S. Foundation, Cà Granda Ospedale Maggiore Policlinico, Milan, Italy

Evelina Buinsauskaitė, Ph.D. Dermatovenereologist, Kaunas, Lithuania

Leah A. Cardwell, M.D. Department of Dermatology, Wake Forest University School of Medicine, Winston-Salem, NC, USA

Peter B. Chansky, B.A. Corporal Michael J. Crescenz Veterans Affairs Medical Center, Philadelphia, PA, USA

Department of Dermatology, Perelman School of Medicine, University of Pennsylvania, Philadelphia, PA, USA

Baraka M. Chaula, M.D. Dermatology Unit, Department of Internal Medicine, Mbeya Zonal Referral Hospital, Mbeya, Tanzania

Karlijn Clarysse, M.D. Department of Dermatology, Universitair Ziekenhuis Brussel, Vrije Universiteit Brussel, Brussels, Belgium

Anupam Das, Ph.D. Department of Dermatology, KPC Medical College and Hospital, Kolkata, West Bengal, India

Federica Dassoni, M.D. Ospedale Alessandro Manzoni, Lecco, Italy

Ncoza C. Dlova, M.B., Ch.B., F.C.Derm., Ph.D. Department of Dermatology, Nelson R Mandela School of Medicine, University of KwaZulu-Natal, Durban, South Africa

Moetaz El-Domyati, M.D. Department of Dermatology, STDs and Andrology, Al-Minya University, Al-Minya, Egypt

Steven R. Feldman, M.D., Ph.D. Department of Dermatology, Wake Forest University School of Medicine, Winston-Salem, NC, USA

Alireza Firooz, M.D. Center for Research and Training in Skin Diseases and Leprosy, Tehran University of Medical Sciences, Tehran, Iran

Mankul Goyal, M.D. Delhi Dermatology Group, Kubba Clinic, New Delhi, India

Somesh Gupta, M.D., DNB, MNAMS Department of Dermatology and Venereology, All India Institute of Medical Sciences, New Delhi, India

Vishal Gupta, MBBS, M.D. Department of Dermatology and Venereology, All India Institute of Medical Sciences, New Delhi, India

Jan Gutermuth, M.D. Department of Dermatology, Universitair Ziekenhuis, Vrije Universiteit Brussel, Brussels, Belgium

Anwar Al Hammadi, M.D., F.R.C.P.C., F.A.A.D. Department of Dermatology, Dubai Medical Center, Dubai, UAE

Achim Hoerauf, M.D. Institut für Med. Mikrobiologie, Immunologie und Parasitologie, Deutsches Zentrum für Infektionsforschung, Universitätsklinikum Bonn, Bonn, Germany

Sam T. Hwang, M.D., Ph.D. Department of Dermatology, University of California Davis School of Medicine, Sacramento, CA, USA

Lila Izadi Firouzabadi, M.D. Center for Research and Training in Skin Diseases and Leprosy, Tehran University of Medical Sciences, Tehran, Iran

Mansour Nassiri Kashani, M.D. Center for Research and Training in Skin Diseases and Leprosy, Tehran University of Medical Sciences, Tehran, Iran

Chelsea Kesty, BS. Department of Dermatology, Wake Forest University School of Medicine, Winston-Salem, NC, USA

Ali Khamesipour, BSc, MSPH, Ph.D Center for Research and Training in Skin Diseases and Leprosy, Tehran University of Medical Sciences, Tehran, Iran

Abdul-Ghani Kibbi, M.D., F.A.C.P. Department of Dermatology, American University of Beirut Medical Center, Beirut, Lebanon

Nour Kibbi, M.D. Department of Dermatology, Yale University, New Haven, CT, USA

Coleen Kivlahan, M.D., M.S.P.H. Department of Family and Community Medicine, Primary Care Services, UCSF School of Medicine, San Francisco, CA, USA

Emily K. Kozera, M.D. Department of Dermatology, St. George Hospital, University of South Wales, Sydney, NSW, Australia

Raj Kubba, M.D., FAAD Delhi Dermatology Group, Kubba Clinic, New Delhi, India

Amy McMichael, M.D. Department of Dermatology, Wake Forest University School of Medicine, Winston-Salem, NC, USA

Lavanya Mittal, B.A. Corporal Michael J. Crescenz Veterans Affairs Medical Center, Philadelphia, PA, USA

Department of Dermatology, Perelman School of Medicine, University of Pennsylvania, Philadelphia, PA, USA

Zamambo N.C. Mkhize, MB, ChB, FC Derm, PhD Department of Dermatology, Edendale Hospital Pietermaritzburg, Nelson R Mandela School of Medicine, University of KwaZulu-Natal, Durban, South Africa

Noha H. Moftah, M.D. Department of Dermatology, STD's and Andrology, Al-Minya University, Al-Minya, Egypt

Mourad Mokni, M.D. Service der Dermatologie, Hopital La Rapta, Tunis, Tunisia

Peter Mugisha, M.D. Department of Dermatology, Mbarara University of Science and Technology, Mbarara, Uganda

Dédée F. Murrell, M.A., B.M.B.Ch., M.D., F.A.C.D. Department of Dermatology, St. George Hospital, University of South Wales, Sydney, NSW, Australia

Bernard Naafs, M.D., Ph.D. Stichting Global Dermatology, Munnekeburen, Netherlands

Pietro Nenoff, M.D. Laboratory for Medical Microbiology, Mölbis, Germany

Adebola Ogunbiyi, M.D. Department of Medicine, University of Ibadan, Oyo, Nigeria

Emeka O. Okoro, M.D. Dermatology Unit, Department of Medicine, Federal Medical Centre, Keffi, Nigeria

Constantin E. Orfanos, M.D. The Free University of Berlin, Medical School Charité, Berlin, Germany

Valeska Padovese, M.D. Genito-Urinary Clinic, Mater Dei Hospital, Ministry of Health, Msida, Malta

Jaheersha Pakran, M.D. Department of Dermatology, Hatta Hospital and Rashi Hospital, Dubai Health Authority, Dubai, UAE

Joachim Richter Institut für Tropenmedizin und Internationale Gesundheit, Charité—Universitätsmedizin Berlin, Campus Virchow-Klinikum, Berlin, Germany

Luisa Carlotta Rossi, M.D. Department of Pathophysiology and Transplantation, Università degli Studi di Milano, I.R.C.C.S. Foundation, Cà Granda Ospedale Maggiore Policlinico, Milan, Italy

Zbigniew Ruszczak, Ph.D., F.A.A.D., F.E.A.D.V. Department of Dermatology and Allergy, Institute of Medicine, Sheikh Khalifa Medical City, Abu Dhabi, UAE

Lesley Ann Saketkoo, M.D., M.P.H. Tulane University School of Medicine, Tulane Lung Center, Clinical Immunology, Allergy and Rheumatology, Pulmonary Diseases, Critical Care and Environmental Medicine, New Orleans Scleroderma and Sarcoidosis Patient Care and Research Center, New Orleans, LA, USA

Lee Shapiro, M.D. Division of Rheumatology, Albany Medical College, Albany, NY, USA

Mohammad Shizarpour, M.D. Center for Research and Training in Skin Diseases and Leprosy, Tehran University of Medical Sciences, Tehran, Iran

Virginia D. Steen, M.D. Department of Medicine, Georgetown University Medical Center, Pasquerilla Healthcare Center, Washington, DC, USA

Cord Sunderkötter, Prof Dr. Department of Dermatology, Martin-Luther-University of Halle Wittenberg, Halle, Germany

Department of Dermatology and Venerology, Universitätsklinikum Münster, Münster, Germany

Mohamed Taha, Ph.D., Prof. Department of Microbiology, Zagazig University, Cairo, Egypt

Luis Torezan, M.D., Ph.D. Laser and Nonmelanoma Skin Cancer Divisions, Hospital das Clínicas, University of Sao Paulo Medical School, São Paulo, Brazil

Stefano Veraldi, M.D., Ph.D. Department of Pathophysiology and Transplantation, Università degli Studi di Milano, I.R.C.C.S. Foundation, Cà Granda Ospedale Maggiore Policlinico, Milan, Italy

Shyam B. Verma, MBBS, DVD, FAAD, FRCP Nirvana Skin Clinic, Vadodara, Gujarat, India

Sawko W. Wassilew, Prof Dr. Centre of Dermatology, Krefeld, Germany

Victoria P. Werth, M.D. Department of Dermatology, Perelman Center for Advanced Medicine, Philadelphia, PA, USA

Uwe Wollina, Prof Dr. Department of Dermatology and Allergology, Hospital Dresden-Friedrichstadt, Teaching Hospital of the Technical University of Dresden, Dresden, Germany

Anes Yang, BMed, MD, MPH, MSc Department of Dermatology, St. George Hospital, University of South Wales, Sydney, NSW, Australia

Egemen Yildiz Department of Dermatology, University of California Davis School of Medicine, Sacramento, CA, USA

Adel Botros Zaghloul, M.D. Cairo Skin Clinik, VD Hospital, Cairo, Egypt

Christos C. Zouboulis, Prof Dr. Departments of Dermatology, Venereology, Allergology and Immunology, Dessau Medical Center, Brandenburg Medical School Theodor Fontane, Dessau, Germany

Diseases in Pigmented Skin: An Introduction

1

Constantin E. Orfanos

The majority of the global population has non-Caucasian skin. In ethnic populations who live in hot climate zones, the skin appears colored; it is heavily pigmented or even black. The genetic background of such differences has been under-investigated; it now comes into focus following various international projects. The molecular genetics underlying the diversity of pigmentation in humans is complex and fascinating [1, 2]. In addition to the differences in skin, hair, and eye color, there are variations among ethnic groups in body mass, height, disease susceptibility, and also in their response to drugs.

Skin diseases arise in heavily pigmented skin to a large extent based on the environmental and climatic conditions in semi-urban and rural areas of hot climate zones, the savannas, forests, and lakes. If the average temperature increases by 2 °C, as is observed today in the southern hemisphere, the amount of precipitation is also reduced, resulting in extremely dry regions. Observations in the Sahel zone, p.e. in Somalia, Sudan, Chad, Niger, and Mauritania, indicate that changes of the frequency and duration of drought periods also cause changes in the socioeconomic and health conditions of their inhabitants. Changes related to the well-known greenhouse effect lead to further increase of the average global temperatures and to an increase of the rates of infections and infestations already common in the tropics by creating expanded habitats to pathogenic agents and favorable conditions for skin diseases.

Diseases developing in ethnic populations with pigmented ethnic skin include common dermatological entities such as contact dermatitis, atopic eczema, psoriasis, lichen, urticaria, bullous and various other immune dermatoses, scalp and hair disorders, etc., well described in white-skinned Caucasians. However, the prevalence, clinical picture, and course of these conditions may differ in patients with heavily pigmented skin, based on the geographic circumstances, the particular cultural and hygienic standards, and the genetic, nutritional, and other factors prevailing in their home countries. Needless to say, erythema as a visible marker of inflammation is masked in heavily pigmented or black skin. In addition, there are skin disorders common in the tropics that are being imported to developed countries by travelers and refugees such as deep fungal or sexual transmitted infections, cutaneous leishmaniasis, leprosy, schistosomiasis, onchocerciasis, filariasis, larva migrans, and other infestation. Thus, diagnosis and management often cause difficulties for the practicing physicians and health workers.

There is a dramatic increase of the number of tourists, businessmen, immigrants, and other individuals traveling around the world. Millions of tourists return to their home countries after having traveled in the rural tropics; around 3.4 million individuals with pigmented skin migrated into the EU only in 2013. An estimated number of 33.5 million live in the EU today but are not born in any of the EU countries [3]. An analysis of the complete data of thousands of diseased German travelers returning from Latin America, Africa, or Asia and several hundred diseased immigrants, originating from the same regions, revealed that the most frequent findings assessed in these groups were gastrointestinal illness with diarrhea as a leading symptom (38%), fever as a marker of disease (29%), and skin disorders (22%) [4]. In December 2015 the United Nations declared 2017 as the International Year of Sustainable Tourism for Development, to be a boost for economic growth. One should therefore expect that more of travel-related dermatoses will be seen in future by western physicians.

In addition, there are an increasing number of immigrants and refugees with pigmented or black skin from countries with socioeconomic problems moving across borders. Especially children are at risk to develop pyodermas and fungal, viral, or parasitic skin diseases; in a considerable number of cases, scabies is diagnosed [5]. Arthropod bites, cutaneous larva migrans, and skin or soft tissue infections

C. E. Orfanos
The Free University of Berlin, Medical School Charité, Berlin, Germany
e-mail: corfanos@t-online.de

C. E. Orfanos et al. (eds.), *Pigmented Ethnic Skin and Imported Dermatoses*, https://doi.org/10.1007/978-3-319-69422-1_1

were the most common dermatologic diagnoses to returning Canadian tourists and immigrants in Canada [6]. Pruritic, arthropod-reactive dermatitis, fever conditions of various severity and types are not rare. The influx of large immigrant populations on the demographic profile in western countries is considerable. In a recent study, eczematous dermatitis, alopecia, melasma, ringworm, scabies, HSV infections, keratosis pilaris, and skin xerosis were found significantly more frequent among immigrants than in an indigenous European population [7]. Around 5–10% of the visits in large skin departments in Europe are now assumed to be done by travelers and/or immigrants. Thus, tropical diseases and parasites from tropical and subtropical parts of the globe are now seen in developed countries of the northern hemisphere; rare diseases from the South are encountered in the North.

There is an increased need for all physicians to deal with these issues. Most of the individuals affected ask for and need medical services and require clear diagnosis and proper treatment. Especially the frequency of infections involving the skin is increasing due to intercontinental exchange with emerging markets in hot climate zones and traveling to remote areas for business, holidays, or pleasure. A growing number of people are in need for health promotion, mental health services, and fair policy planning [8].

This book is designed to improve awareness and contribute in aiding the international medical community to diagnose and register skin diseases in pigmented skin, understand any differences, highlight their particular reactive profiles, and provide information on their appearance, course, and treatment. The quality of health services and the number of physicians in countries of greatest need in hot climate zones are generally low, also due to an ongoing large-scale emigration [9]. In 2013 the American Medical Association identified 11,787 active physicians of sub-Saharan origin representing barely 1.3% of the 2013 US physician workforce but exceeding the total number of physicians reported by WHO in 34 sub-Saharan countries (n = 11,519) [10]. Rural health conditions and those of poverty define the spectrum of skin diseases in developing countries [11, 12], and disruption of sanitation during migration enforces the appearance of skin disease; a reemergence of migration-associated neglected infections is registered among asylum seekers [13]. The health workers in the West should be made familiar with the clinical presentation and characteristics of diseases in dark-skinned individuals and be encouraged to provide the medical services needed. Major clinical manifestations and schedules for management are presented in this book, as a basic guide to assist those who are likely inexperienced with such entities and facilitate management by physicians who are used to diagnose and treat dermatoses only in white Caucasian skin.

Several colleagues from around the world, most of those permanently based in hot climate zones or having collected long-term experiences in developing countries, have shared their particular knowledge and have contributed to enrich this volume with their personal expertise. We are deeply indebted to all coauthors and to the numerous centers, hospitals, and pioneer institutions which allowed the assessment of local patients. Lecturing in these regions and also participating in patient's management over the years in offices and hospitals [14], it has been possible to see and clinically document a series of skin diseases in highly pigmented and black-skinned patients. Some of these observations are shown for educational reasons in this volume. Hopefully, the numerous illustrations included will be helpful for better knowledge of the clinical presentations and better understanding of these conditions and their course in pigmented skin. All valuable contributions are thankfully recognized.

References

1. Huang T, Shu Y, Cai YD. Genetic differences among ethnic groups. BMC Genomics. 2015;16:1093.
2. Sturm RA. Molecular genetics of human pigmentation diversity. Forensic Sci Int Genet. 2007;1:105–1.
3. Eurostat Statistics, May 2015.
4. Herbinger KH, Alberer M, Berens-Riha N, et al. Spectrum of imported infectious diseases: a comparative prevalence study of 16,817 German travelers and 977 immigrants from the tropics and subtropics. Am J Trop Med Hyg. 2016;94:757–66.
5. Katsarou A, Armenaka M, Kosmadaki M, et al. Skin diseases in Greek and immigrant children in Athens. Int J Dermatol. 2012;51:173–37.
6. Stevens MS, Geduld J, Libman M, et al. Dermatoses among returned Canadian travellers and immigrants: surveillance report based on Can Trav Net data, 2009–2012. CMA J Open. 2015;3:E119–26.
7. Albares MP, Belinchón I, Ramos JM, et al. Epidemiologic study of skin diseases among immigrants in Alicante, Spain. Actas Dermosifiliogr. 2012;103:214–22.
8. Padovese V, Egidi AM, Melillo Fenech T, et al. Migration and determinants of health: clinical epidemiological characteristics of migrants in Malta (2010–11). J Public Health (Oxf). 2014;36:368–74.
9. Ogilvie L, Mill JE, Astle B, et al. The exodus of health professionals from sub-Saharan Africa: balancing human rights and societal needs in the twenty-first century. Nurs Inq. 2007;14:114–24.
10. Tankwanchi AB, Vermund SH, Perkins DD. Monitoring Sub-Saharan African physician migration and recruitment post-adoption of the WHO code of practice: temporal and geographic patterns in the United States. PLoS One. 2015;10:e0124734.
11. Naafs B, Padovese V. Rural dermatology in the tropics. Clin Dermatol. 2009;27:252–70.
12. Accorsi S, Barnabas GA, Farese P, et al. Skin disorders and disease profile of poverty: analysis of medical records in Tigray, northern Ethiopia, 2005–2007. Trans R Soc Trop Med Hyg. 2009;103:469–75.
13. Bloch-Infanger C, Bättig V, Kremo J, et al. Increasing prevalence of infectious diseases in asylum seekers at a tertiary care hospital in Switzerland. PLoS One. 2017;12:e0179537.
14. Orfanos CE. Dermatology in East Africa—the Regional Dermatology Training Centre (RDTC) in Moshi, Tanzania. Akt Dermatol. 2006;32:136–41. https://doi.org/10.1055/s-2006-925042.

2 Contact Dermatitis in Skin of Color

Zbigniew Ruszczak and Shaden Abdelhadi

Contact dermatitis, also known as contact eczema, is an adverse skin reaction after contact exposure to a foreign agent, caused either by its irritant (*irritant contact dermatitis*, ICD) or its allergenic property (*allergic contact dermatitis*, ACD). The clinical appearance of the lesions depends on the skin region involved and the duration of the exposure; it may be papular, urticaria-like, vesicular, or bullous, presented on an erythematous background. In dark pigmented or black skin, erythema is less recognizable, and the lesions are often hypo- or hyperpigmented; after repeated or persisting exposure eczematization occurs, and chronic pruritus often results in lichenification. In specific areas of the body such as the eyelids, penis, and scrotum, contact dermatitis can be presented as erythematous edema rather than papules or vesicles. Lesions can be provoked or aggravated by exposure to sun or UV light, resulting in a phototoxic or photoallergic reaction. The skin response also depends on the particular properties of the agent, the nature and duration of the contact, and the individual susceptibility of the patient.

Z. Ruszczak (✉)
Consultant Dermatology, Pediatric Dermatology and Allergy, Head of Arab Board Dermatology Residency Program, Chair, Division of Dermatology and Allergy
Director of Arab Board Dermatology Residency Program, Sheikh Khalifa Medical City, Abu Dhabi, UAE

S. Abdelhadi
Consultant Dermatology and Pediatric Dermatology, Department of Dermatology and Allergy, Sheikh Khalifa Medical City, Abu Dhabi, UAE

Department of Dermatology, University Medical Center Brussels (UZ Brussels), The Free University of Brussels (VUB), Brussels, Belgium

2.1 Potential of Skin of Color for Adverse Contact Reactions

The color of the skin and texture of the hair are the most apparent phenotypes to differentiate ethnic populations, and notable differences are seen in skin diseases and their clinical presentation based on the skin type [1]. Ethnic differences in skin function occur and may be responsible for differences in skin reactivity under physiologic and pathologic conditions including mechanisms of irritation, sensitization, and drug absorption [2]. Besides the different number and activity of the melanocytes and epidermal distribution of melanin functional parameters such as epidermal permeability, structure and size of dermal fibroblasts, etc. may differ in skin of color. The two most significant features having a direct impact of the development of ICD/ACD are homeostasis of the skin barrier and the potential of transcutaneous penetration [2]. Studies demonstrated that highly pigmented skin is generally more impervious than Caucasian and that the skin barrier function, which governs the absorption of external substances, appears superior in dark-skinned individuals showing decreased penetration. However, if the epidermis in black individuals was tape-stripped prior to application of the test substance, the difference between black and white skin was less significant. Other studies found slightly decreased absorption of contact allergens in skin types III and IV but increased absorption in Asian skin. The transepidermal water loss (TEWL) was significantly increased in patients with dark pigmented skin and in Asians compared with Caucasians, although patients with less pigmented skin had a tendency to stronger skin barrier dysfunction and longer recovery time [3, 4].

The overall results remained conflicting in part; however, there are differences between black and white skin during the development of irritant contact dermatitis, supporting the opinion that individuals with black skin are more resistant to irritants [5]. Irritation and TEWL after chemical exposure to sodium lauryl sulfate showed a different reac-

C. E. Orfanos et al. (eds.), *Pigmented Ethnic Skin and Imported Dermatoses*, https://doi.org/10.1007/978-3-319-69422-1_2

tion pattern in black-skinned persons and Hispanics who developed stronger irritant reactions than Caucasians [6, 7]. In patch testing no significant differences were found in earlier studies, although patients with black skin differed in their response to specific allergens [8]; statistically significant differences were documented particularly in the sensitization rate for *p*-phenylenediamine in black skin compared with white skin [9]. In a recent study black-skinned persons reacted more frequently not only to *p*-phenylenediamine (7.0% vs. 4.4%) but also to bacitracin (11.6% vs. 8.3%), mercaptobenzothiazole (2.7% vs. 1.8%), thiuram (6.2% vs. 4.3%), and mercapto mix (1.9% vs. 0.8%) [10]. Nevertheless, these results may indeed be related to differences in allergen exposure rather than determined by ethnicity [11].

Clinically, acute contact dermatitis presenting eczematous reaction with oozing and vesiculation seems to be more common in whites, whereas, reactions with hyper- or hypopigmentation often occur in black skin and early lichenification is most common. Hypopigmentations after exposure to phenolic detergents such as amylphenols, *p*-butyl, and monobenzylether of hydroquinone are well known. Hyperpigmentation occurs more often in dark skin individuals after contact with irritants and may be aggravated by prolonged or inappropriate use of hydroquinone, leading to ochronosis. In dark skin with acne, keratolytics and other chemicals used for management also cause hyperpigmentations.

2.2 Epidemiology

The prevalence of contact dermatitis is high in all geographic areas including the hot climate zones. Irritant contact dermatitis represents approximately 80% of all rashes seen in the UK and the USA [12], often due to local toxicity of chemicals, alkalis, acids, various solvents, detergents, etc. The prevalence of contact dermatitis was estimated to be between 1.5 and 5.4%, being the third most common reason for dermatology consultations [13]. The North American Contact Dermatitis Group found that 69% of all patients examined by patch testing confirmed ACD, while 15.4% had irritant reactions [14]; there was no difference in the response to common allergens between individuals with fairer and darker skin. The most common contact allergen within both groups was nickel; however, the dark-skinned population showed higher incidence of sensitivity to *p*-phenylenediamine and nickel than the Caucasian population.

In white Europeans, at least one positive allergic reaction was found in 40% of all individuals tested, and women were more often sensitized than men (50.2% vs. 29.9%); the frequency of the overall contact sensitization for the general adult population was estimated 28.0%, whereby 11.4% were positive for fragrance mix, 9.9% for nickel, and 3.2% for a topical mercury-containing compound, formerly used as an antiseptic (thimerosal) [15]. In another study a rising sensitization to topical corticosteroids was postulated [16]. Among the German population, 1.9–4.5 million individuals were reported sensitized to nickel and 1.4–3.4 million to fragrance mix [17]. Increasing role of plants and pesticide-related dermatoses were recently described with unusual clinical pictures mimicking urticaria, erythema multiforme, ashy dermatosis, parakeratosis variegata, porphyria cutanea tarda, and other disorders [18]. In farmers chronically exposed to the sun in hot climate zones, such lesions may be lichenified and resemble chronic actinic dermatitis. Plant and pesticide allergens should be included in patch test series applied for the evaluation of patients with suspected photoallergy [19].

In Asian countries cooks dealing with specific vegetables or fish often develop contact allergy to the products they deal with, i.e., parsley, onion, different types of capsicum, or tomato. Thai patients are frequently allergic to potassium dichromate, nickel sulfate, fragrances, and cobalt chloride. In China, *p*-phenylenediamine (used for hair dyes), nickel, mercury, fragrances, and rubber chemicals were the most common allergens; the main localization of an allergic eczema was hands and feet. Among Indian, Pakistani, and Bangladeshi populations in England with skin types IV and V, no statistical differences were found between this group and white Europeans, with slightly fewer patients from the Indian subcontinent showing a positive allergy skin test reaction [1]. In India, an estimated 2–10% of the population is likely to develop contact dermatitis, especially hand eczema, which is the most frequent occupational disease in the country. It comprises 9–35% of all occupational diseases and >80% of cases with occupational contact dermatitis. Using an Indian standard series for patch testing, chromate (28%); nickel (25%); vegetables (12%); medicaments (7%); *Parthenium hysterophorus,* a flowering plant of the aster family (6%); soap and detergents (5%) were most common allergens [20]. In another study *Parthenium*, colophony, fragrance mix, and PPD were detected, with *Parthenium* and perfume mix being the most common photoallergens in Indian patients with dermatitis in sun-exposed areas [21].

In Africa, a prevalence of 34.3% occupational hand dermatitis in a predominantly young group of female hairdressers was registered in Nigeria and was considered low in comparison with other countries. This was linked to a higher level of education on precautions and prevention of ACD among professionals [22]. Nickel was the most frequent sensitizer in Nigeria's construction workers, with an incidence of 12.3%, similar to 11% in North America. Recently, a cushion bush endemic in Australia (*Leucophyta brownii*) belonging to the Compositae family (*Asteraceae*) has become a popular pot and container plant. The plant produces sesquiterpene lactones such as pseudoivalin, calocephalin, and tomentosin which are known as strong sensitizers [23].

In Saudi Arabia patients with allergic skin diseases were the largest group in attendance in a referral hospital (65.2%), with allergic contact dermatitis (48.82%) and urticaria (10.5%) being the most common diagnosis [24]. Since the Compositae family is widely present in North African countries and the Middle East, both irritant and phytoallergic reactions including airborne allergies to such plants are seen in these geographic areas, also causing asthma symptoms. In our own studies on the contribution of aeroallergens for the development or aggravation of ACD and asthma in the United Arab Emirates, we found that in over 32% of the cases house dust mites were triggering allergic symptoms, followed by various other agents including grass subtypes (7%), mostly Bermuda grass. Compositae plants were found to be allergenic in only 2% of the cases.

2.3 Pathogenesis

Allergic contact dermatitis begins with a sensitization phase when haptens, usually small molecules, penetrate through the epidermal barrier and induce specific responses by activating Th1/Th2 lymphocytes [25]. Recently, the Th17 cells effector role has been postulated in the pathogenesis of ACD, followed by IL-17 and IL-22 upregulation, showing that IL-17 expression levels were significantly elevated in skin but not in serum of ACD patients as compared with healthy controls; it seems that IL-17 may mediate AD-related immune dysregulation by amplifying the inflammatory response [26]. After exposure, activated T-cells primed in skin draining lymph nodes and express skin homing molecules thus allowing effector memory cells to invade into the skin and control tissue response. The sensitization phase usually lasts for 10–15 days and may be asymptomatic. Repeated contact of sensitized individuals with the specific allergen leads to elicitation phase with the full picture of ACD, representing the delayed inflammatory response characteristics. The agents causing ACD can be found in personal skin care products, topical medications, jewelry, home remedies, herbs and spices, plants, as well as substances which come into contact with skin during traditional or religious cultural practices and professional activities, directly or through contact with other individuals (i.e., *consort contact dermatitis*).

2.4 Instances and Agents Causing ICD/ACD

(a) *Common health and cultural practices*

Health customs including skin care and cultural practices are playing an important role in the development of both ICD and ACD in ethnic groups.

Extensive hygiene perceptions even in populations with adequate availability of soap and water are one of the main causes of irritant or allergic contact dermatitis in patients with skin of color. The wide use of body creams and sanitizers, especially hand sanitizers, gels, and wet wipes, and the use of sanitizing soaps, etc. may cause ACD (Figs. 2.1 and 2.2); diaper contact dermatitis in babies and hand eczema in adolescents and adults are common examples (Fig. 2.3). Scrubs and extensive skin exfoliative cleaning procedures and tools (i.e., Moroccan bath, hammam gloves, scrubs for skin care, massage gloves, pumice stones) markedly impair the skin barrier function. They may increase the frequency and severity of skin reactions to sanitizers mostly containing ingredients such as carbomer, ethyl alcohol, triethanolamine, isopropyl myristate and fragrances, or to other products applied thereafter.

Skin care products and hair gels commonly used in Mediterranean, Arabic, African, and Indian populations contain not only metal salts or plant-derived artificial pigments as coloring agents but also surfactants and preservatives such as sodium lauryl sulfate which are known to be potent irritants. Hairstyling substances, often in regular use, contain agents such as lanolin and isopropyl myristate that can cause both irritant and allergic contact dermatitis [27].

Practices such as coin rubbing, cupping, moxibustion, etc. are popular in Asia as alternative medicine measures performed to improve blood circulation in the soft tissue and may lead to the development of contact dermatitis. The rubbing is performed by scraping the skin with items such as a coin, comb, spoon, or the edge of a jar cap. Moxibustion is a practice of traditional Chinese medicine, now modified and used in several countries, performed by lighting incense-like plant materials and applying them on certain acupuncture points of the skin [28]. Contact dermatitis, severe irritations and burns may result, and physicians who may not be aware of these cultural practices can confuse their effects as signs of physical abuse [29].

Capsaicin contact or generalized dermatitis caused by chili peppers is seen in Hispanic populations. Chili pep-

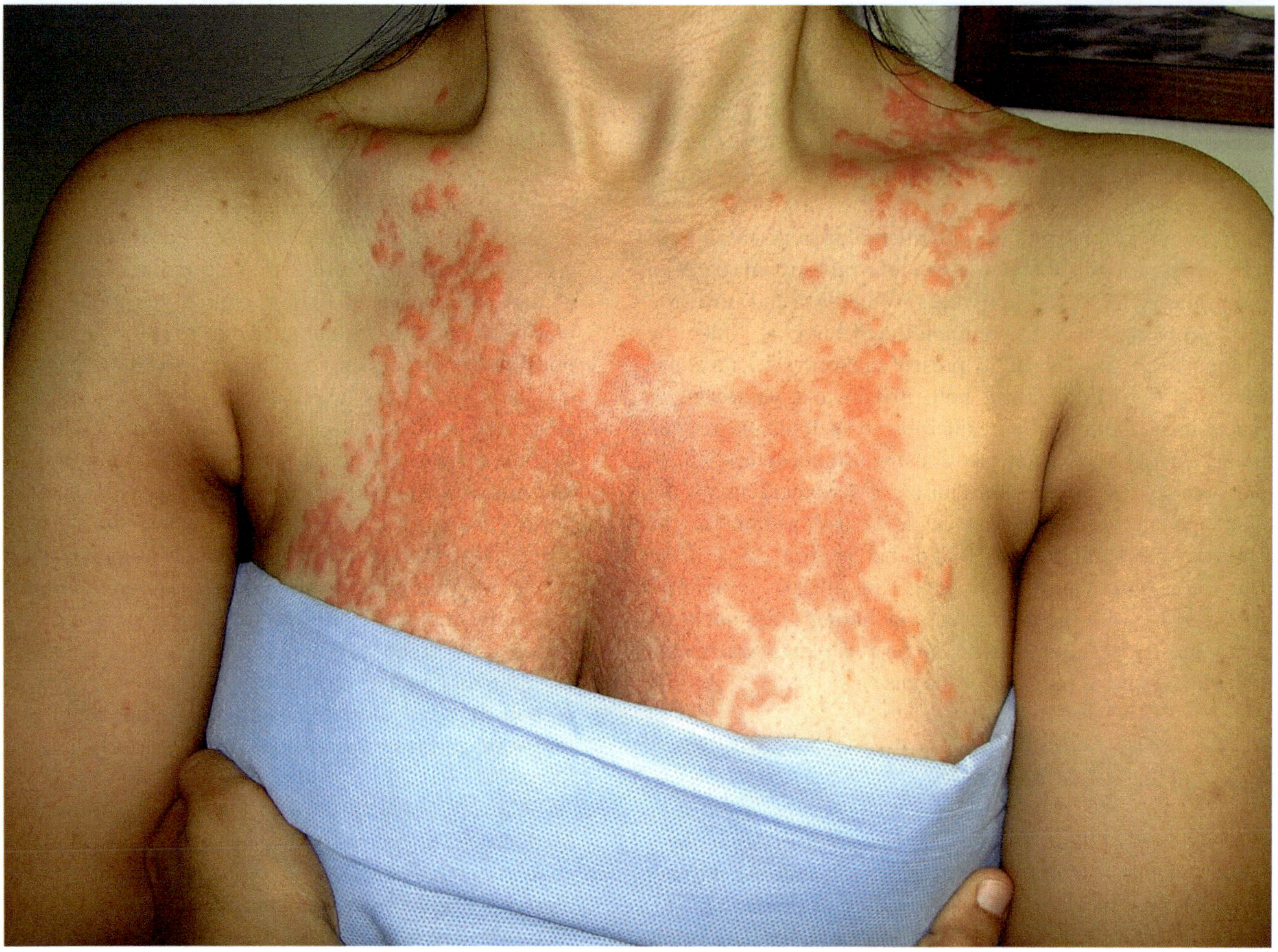

Fig. 2.1 Acute allergic contact dermatitis to a skin care product, possibly a chamomile-containing cosmetic body cream

pers are commonly used as a condiment in the Hispanic diet schedules. When they are handled barehanded, chili peppers often cause erythema and burning pain [30].

(b) *Textiles and leather*

Chemicals containing heavy metals are often used for coloring textile materials. In a recent study, high amounts of Al, Fe, and Zn were found in cotton undergarments; nylon undergarments had high levels of Cr, Cu, and Al, while polyester fabrics contained higher levels of Ni and Fe, if compared to cotton or nylon tissues. There is considerable hazard of using colored underwear since in all tested fabrics from manufacturing countries including China, India, and Egypt, high concentrations of metals were detected [31]. Black garments had high level of Fe and Cr; blue colors of Cu; brown colors, Fe and Cu; green, Cu and slightly less Fe; pink garments, Al; purple garments, Al and Cu; and red garments, Cr, Zn, and Al. Higher concentrations of metals may lead to systemic absorption and contribute to their development as long-term sensitizers, especially if such undergarments are used in neonates and children. Also chemicals making the cloths less likely to wrinkle or shrink, i.e., dimethyl dihydroxyethyleneurea, may cause ACD especially in areas when the clothing has close contact with the skin. The same reaction can be seen to other textile softeners and fragrances added at the end of the washing process to make the cloths soft and nice smelling.

Many individuals with dark pigmented skin live in countries in which the use of natural leather sandals without socks is not only a tradition but also a practical way to deal with climate challenges and to practice daily rituals. Such persons often develop ACD to chem-

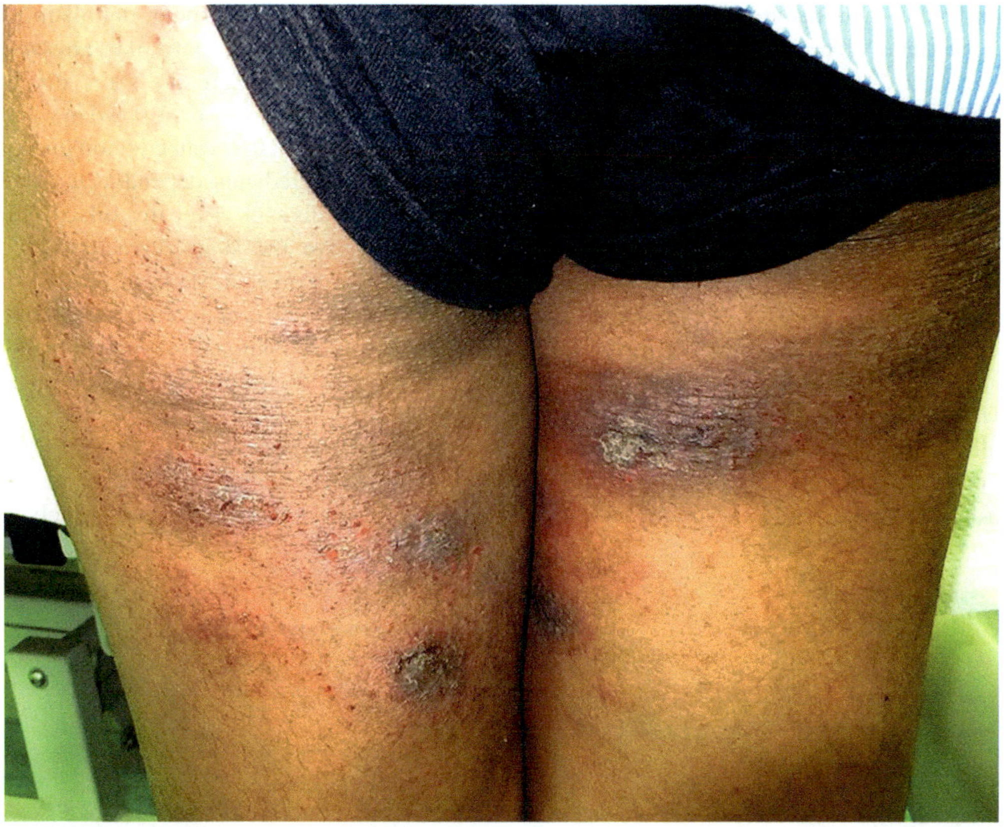

Fig. 2.2 *Contact dermatitis* caused by a toilet sanitizer in an 11-years-old school girl

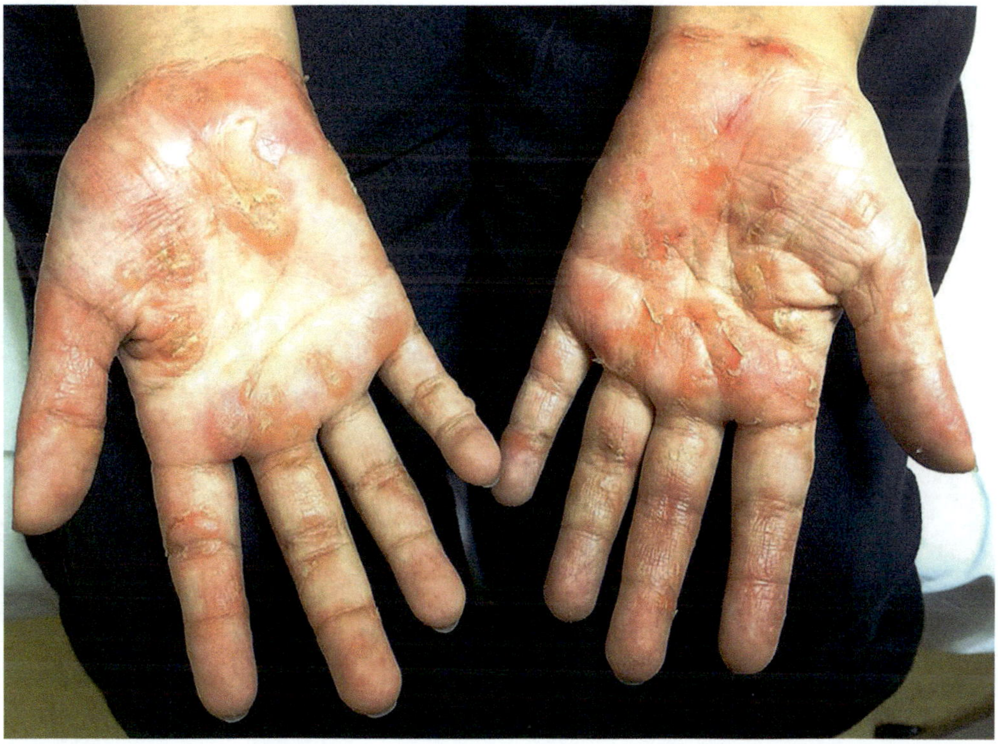

Fig. 2.3 Long-standing hand eczema in both palms (impetiginized)

icals used in leather manufacturing, especially formaldehydes, potassium dichromate, and leather dyes (Fig. 2.4).

(c) *Dyes: Henna and p-phenylenediamine*

Henna is the Arabic name of *Lawsonia inermis*, a flowering plant of which the fruits are small brown capsules. It is also known as *hina*, the *henna tree*, *mignonette tree*, or the *Egyptian privet*. Commonly, the term "henna" also refers to the dye prepared for temporary body art. Historically, henna is known since antiquity; it is frequently used today in the Arabian Peninsula, the Indian subcontinent, and the East and parts of North Africa to dye skin, hair, and fingernails, as well as natural fabrics including silk, wool, and leather [32]. The coloring agent was traditionally made from the rests of *Lawsonia* leaves and fruits found in the feces of the dromedary which inhabits the areas. Whole, unbroken henna leaves will not stain the skin until the *lawsone* molecules are extracted. To prepare the stain, dry henna leaves are mashed into a paste or a powder which is then mixed with liquids such as water, lemon juice, strong black tea, or other ingredients depending on the local tradition. Essential oils such as the tree oil, cajeput oil, or lavender oil improve the stain characteristics. Original henna stains are orange, but darken over a few days to a reddish brown color. To turn the color into black and enhance the durability of skin coloration, natural earth oil or its derivatives are often added to the henna paste ("black henna").

Today, *p-phenylenediamine* (PPD) is regularly used in "black henna" causing irritant and allergic reactions. PPD is an organic compound widely used as an artifi-

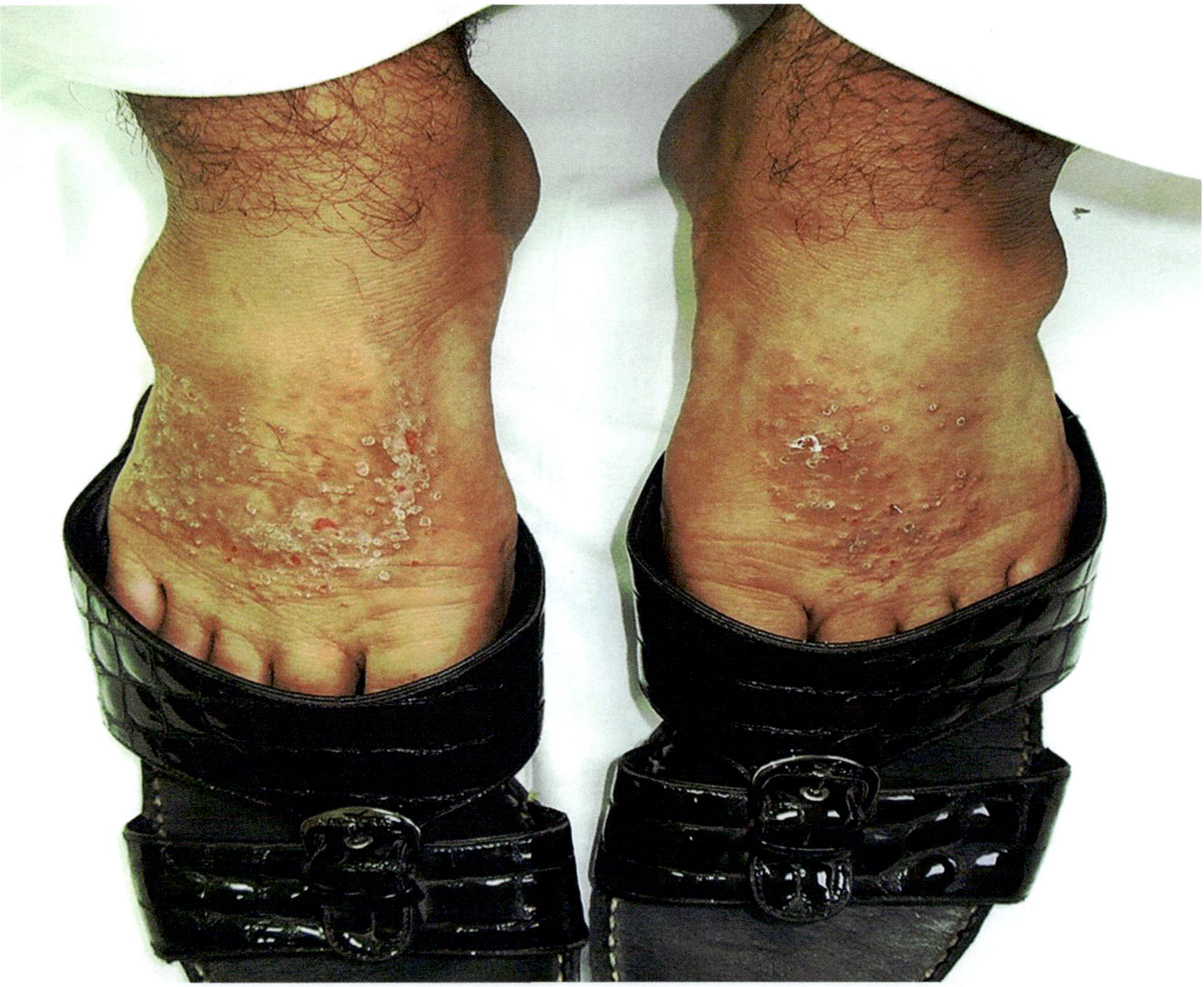

Fig. 2.4 *Eczematous contact dermatitis* caused by chemicals in black leather sandals

cial dye. It can darken via air oxidation and is used as a component of engineering polymers and composites and ingredient in hair dyes, mascaras, natural hair-bounding devices, and several other cosmetic products to turn the color to black-brown as a substitute for natural henna. Black henna is used in ceremonial skin decorations and deserves special attention as a most potent skin irritant and contact allergen [32, 33]. Brown or black substitutes of the natural henna may lead to PPD-sensitization with local blistering, hyperpigmentation or scarring, corresponding to the shape of the ornament (Figs. 2.5 and 2.6); it may also cause extensive and long-standing rashes. The compound may cross-react with other chemicals such as thiazide diuretics or anti-diabetic drugs.

Muslim men often use henna for dying their scalp hair and particularly their beards. This is considered *sunnah*, a commendable tradition of Prophet Muhammad. Furthermore, a *hadith* holds that Muslim women should dye their nails with henna to demonstrate femininity; several women in the Middle East continue today to apply henna to their finger- and toenails, hands, feet, and arms usually with highly artistic ornaments. Henna (*mehndi*) is also widely used in India for skin decoration. In the world regions where henna grows naturally, various communities (Jews, Muslims, Sikhs, Hindus, Zoroastrians, and Christians) are using henna to celebrate marriages and weddings, adoring the bride and often also the groom. Traditionally, girls and women of all ages decorate their skin for family celebrations and local and national events; henna is applied symbolizing luck, joy, and beauty, regarded as *barakah* (blessings). In males who dye their hair or beard with black henna, sensitivity reactions with hyperpigmentation may be seen (Figs. 2.7 and 2.8).

Studies have shown higher rates of sensitive responses to PPD in skin of color (Fig. 2.9); PPD-sensitive patients may have differences in their ability to acetylate *N*-acetyltransferase 1 and 2, thus resulting in higher or lower PPD-sensitivity [9]. PPD may also show systemic cross-sensitization with other compounds that contain an amine group in their benzene ring in *p*-position, i.e., *p*-aminobenzoic acid, sulfonamides, sulfonylureas, *p*-toluenediamine sulfate, azo dyes, benzocaine, tetracaine, procaine, and *p*-aminosalicylic acid. PPD-allergic individuals have higher risk of concurrent sensitivity to other chemically related hair dyes as well as clothing dyes [33]. PPD patch test-positive patients showed an increasing likelihood of cross-reactions to *N*-isopropyl-*N′*-phenyl-*p*-phenylenediamine, caine mix, and disperse yellow 3.

(d) *Occupational causes*
Occupation plays an important role in the development of ICD and ACD in populations with dark skin, also because preventive measures are often neglected. Increased sensitization to *p*-phenylenediamine is often detected in hairdressers in all geographical zones. Working as a hairdresser is associated with a prevalence of contact dermatitis ranging from 16.4% in larger cohort studies that included a clinical examination to 80% in smaller, questionnaire-based studies [34]. There are a series of agents in hair products that may sensitize both the women treated and/or the hairdresser [35]. Construction workers often develop ACD to chromate or other metals; in workers of the chemical industry, toxic vapors may cause severe irritant dermatitis (Figs. 2.10 and 2.11). In Brazil allergic contact dermatitis is the most prevalent occupational dermatitis, and the commonest etiological agent was chromium (13.9%) [36]. ACD to chromates and PPD (used as black leather stain) as well as formaldehydes are also common among individuals using specific personal protective equipment, leather gloves or shoes. Latex allergens are common within physicians and healthcare care workers using latex gloves. Interestingly, latex is cross-reacting with some citrus fruits, i.e., banana, kiwi, avocado, or chestnut.

(e) *Airborne contact dermatitis*
Allergens that are airborne and come in contact with the skin can result in different type of reactions including ACD. Contact dermatitis to ragweed in the USA and mimosa, mesquite, or various types of grasses in the Middle East is most commonly presented on the face. Prolonged exposure to such airborne contact allergens leads to chronic skin reactions, dryness, lichenification, and often secondary infection mostly located on face, neck, arms, and legs. The most common agents are the above mentioned plants as well as Compositae allergens, natural resins, woods, plastics, glue, rubbers, and both pesticides and insecticides, the latter being included into the list of occupational allergens in farmers and forest workers [18].

(f) *Iatrogenic causes*
Some of the most common substances causing irritant or allergic contact dermatitis are topical antiseptics, topical nonsteroidal anti-inflammatory drugs, colors and fragrances in cosmeceuticals, wound dressings, or certain antibiotics. In many Mediterranean, Middle East, or Asian countries, toothpaste is a popular home remedy for treatment of superficial burns since it often contains menthol and invokes a cooling effect drying out the burn surface. However, topical application of toothpaste can also provoke unexpected skin reactions.

Intentional induction of mild, tolerable contact dermatitis occurs in cases the reaction is part of treatment: Topical immune-modulating application of diphenyl-

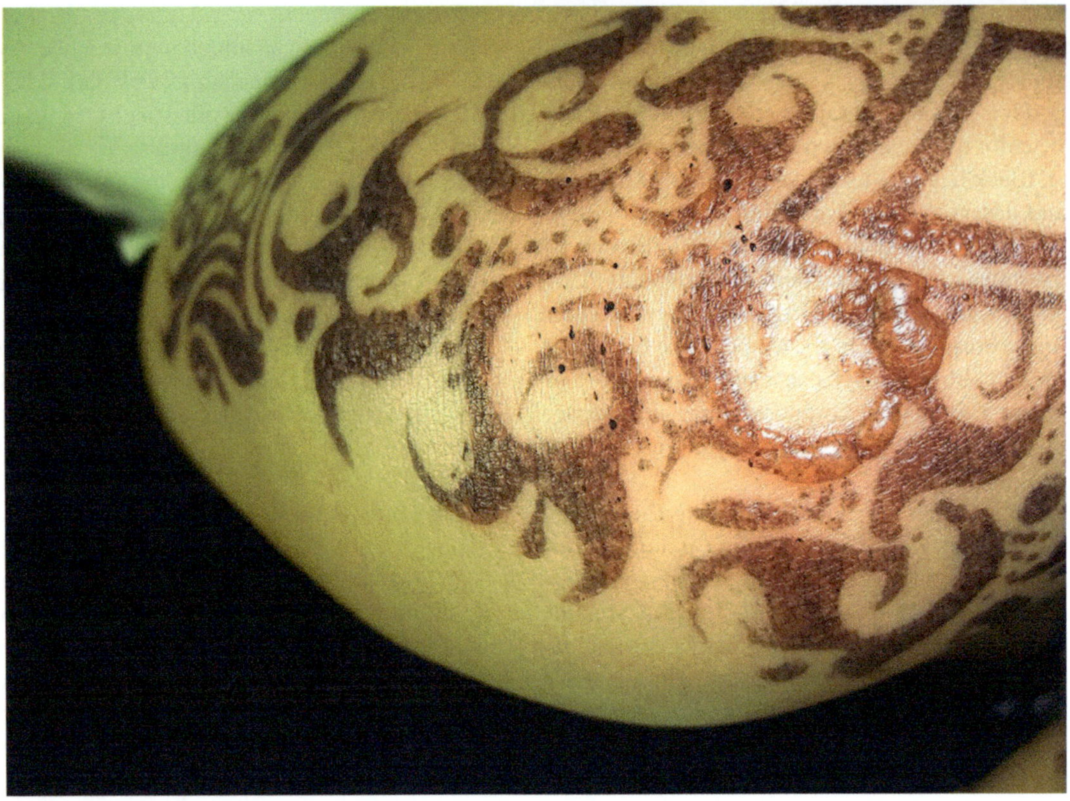

Fig. 2.5 Bullous skin reaction to brown henna body art, Emirati style

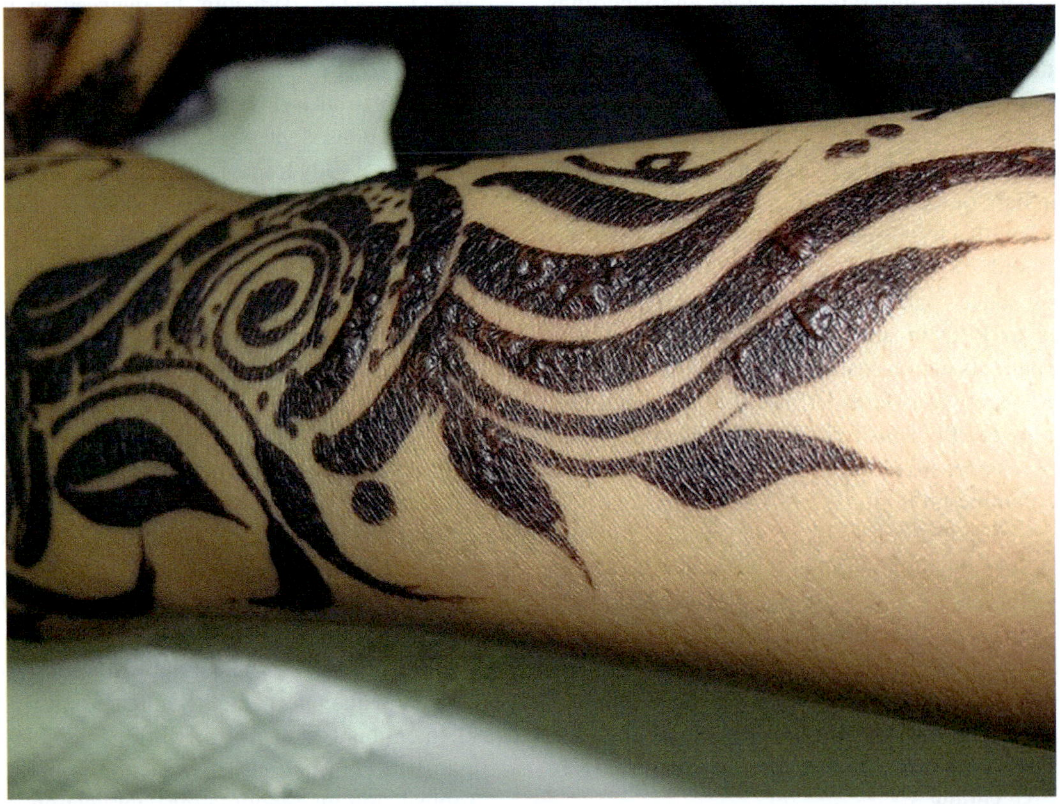

Fig. 2.6 Vesiculobullous skin reaction to black henna (containing *p*-phenylenediamine)

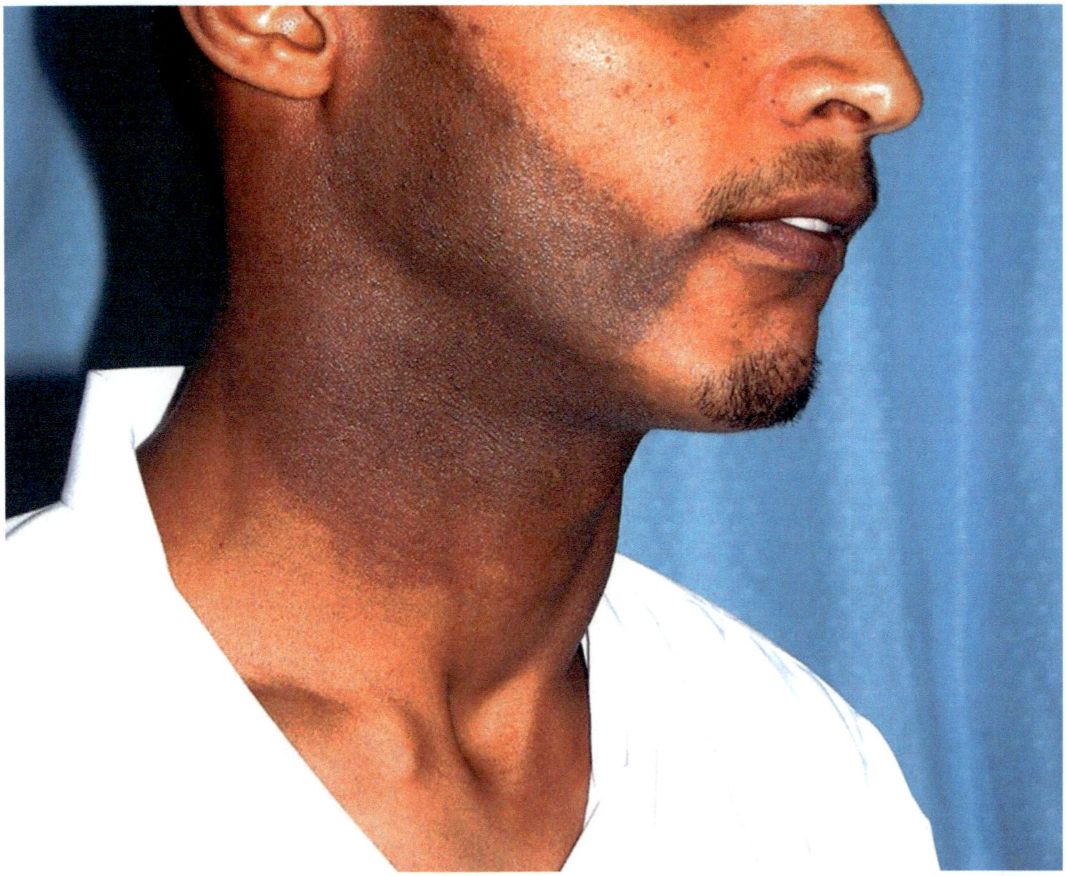

Fig. 2.7 *Hyperpigmented contact dermatitis* on the face after coloring birth and scalp hair with black henna

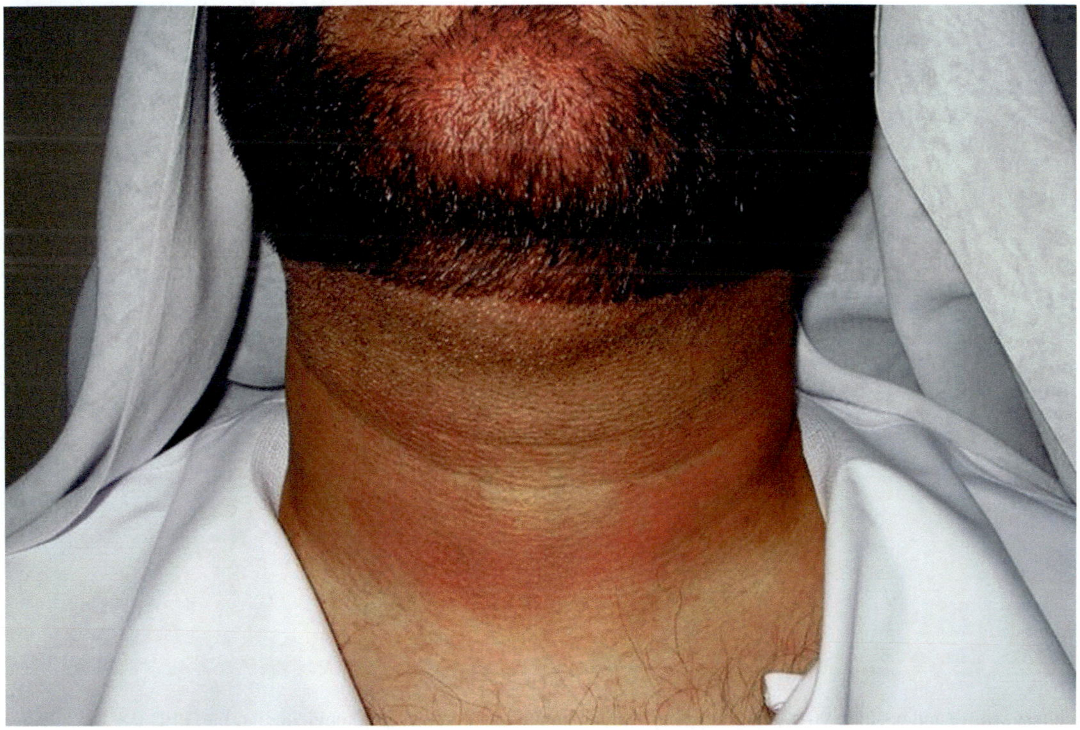

Fig. 2.8 *Hyperpigmented contact dermatitis* of the neck after coloring the beard with black henna

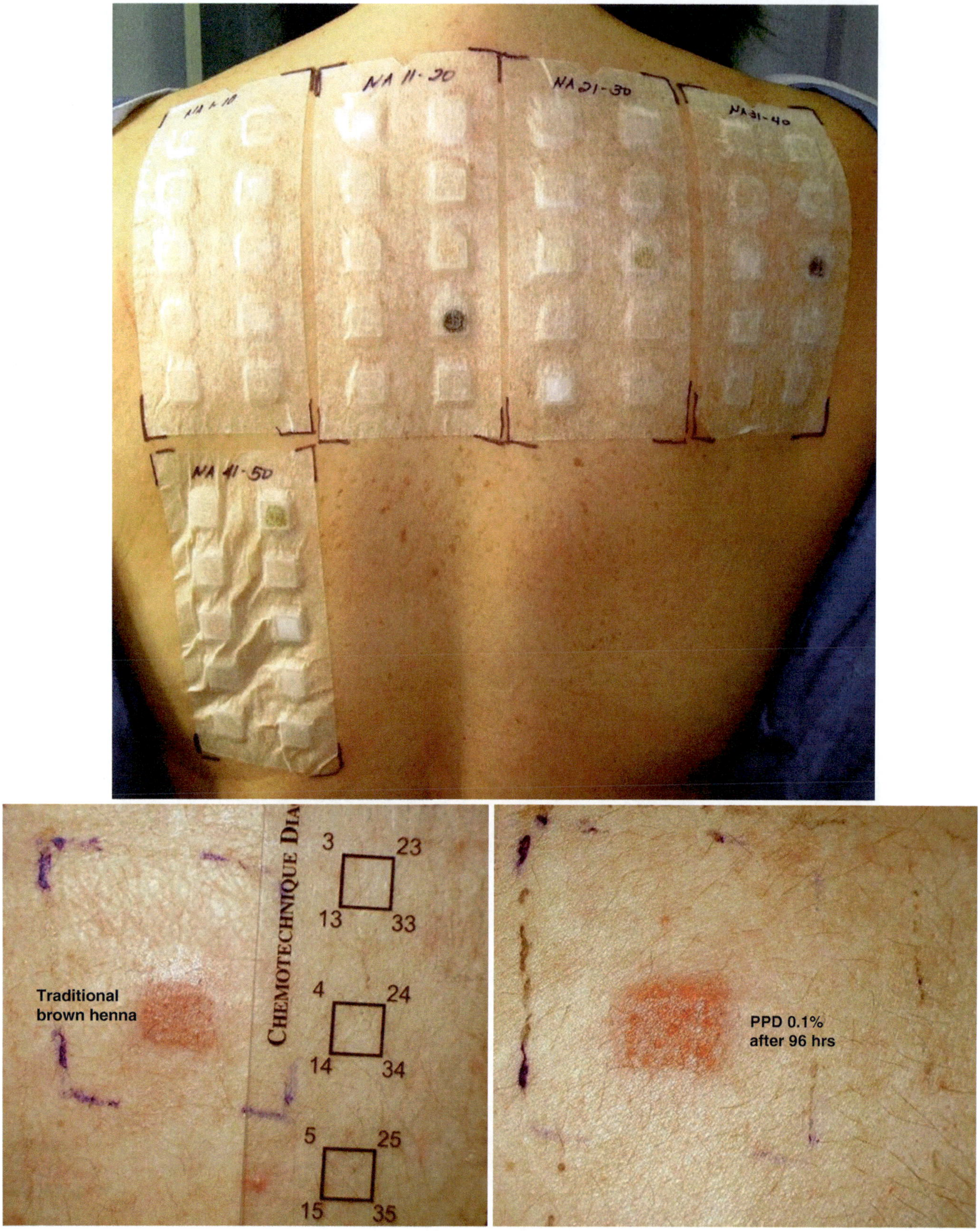

Fig. 2.9 Patch test setting and positive 96 h-reactions to brown henna and black henna (*p*-phenylenediamine, PPD 0.1%)

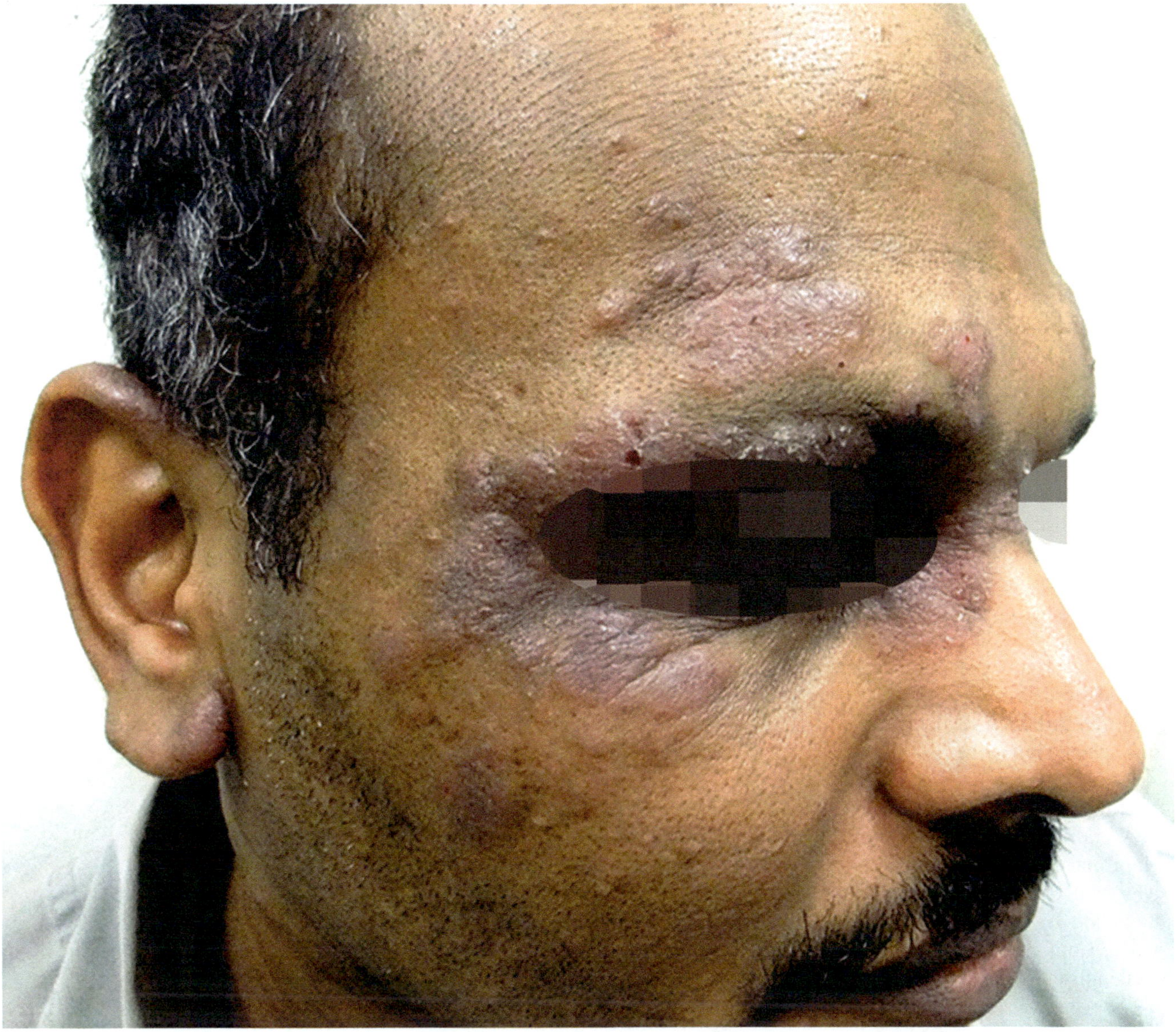

Fig. 2.10 Chronic *occupational contact dermatitis to cobalt and nickel* (lichenified; metal worker)

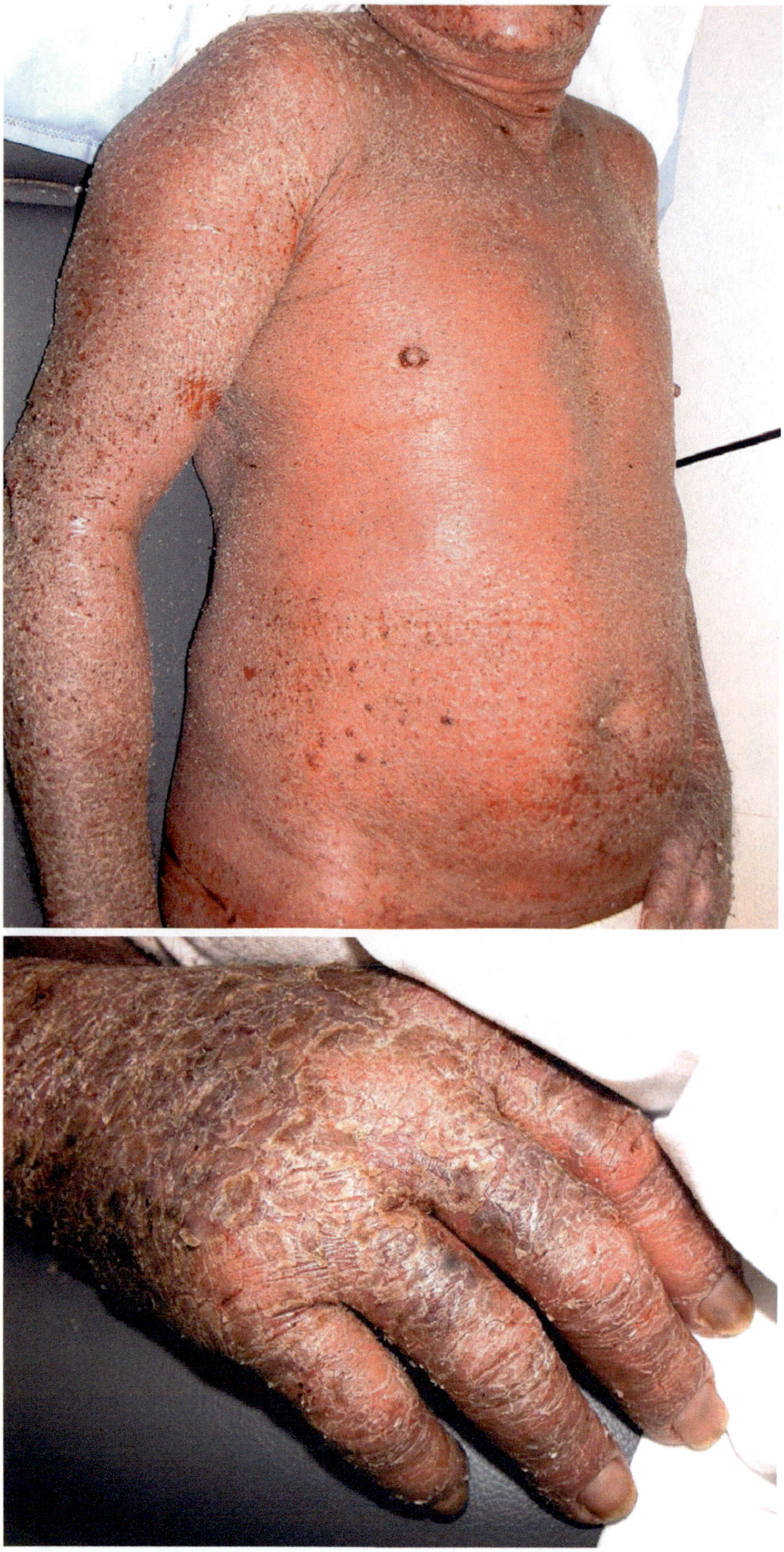

Fig. 2.11 Acute *erythrodermic occupational contact dermatitis* (industry worker; chemical vapors)

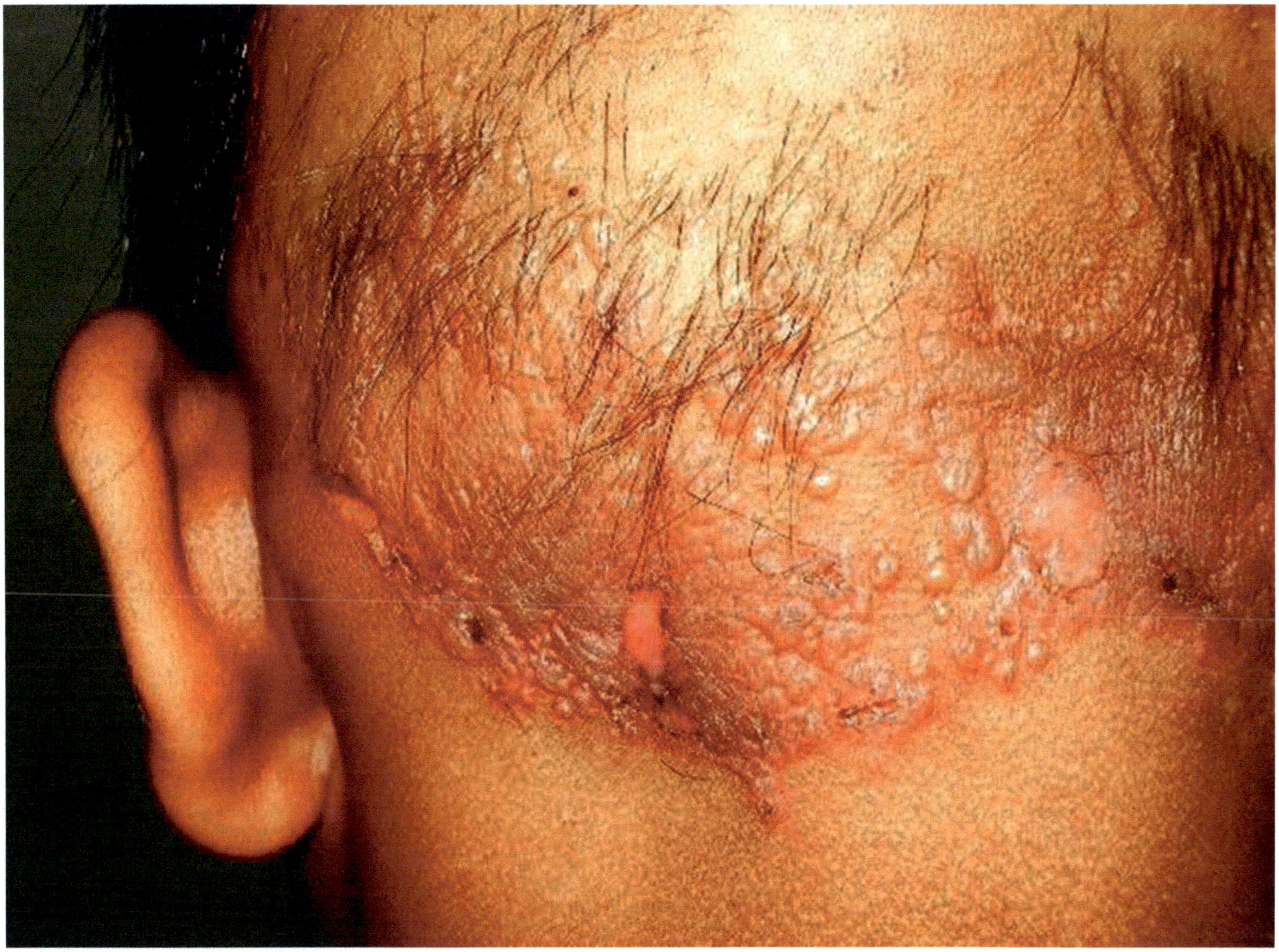

Fig. 2.12 Severe *irritant contact dermatitis* caused by DPCP treatment in alopecia areata

cyclopropenone (DPCP), squaric acid, or anthralin in alopecia areata may be seen as an intentionally induced ICD (Fig. 2.12). As a rule, beneficial effect is expected when an adequate level of local irritation/sensitization to the agent is achieved.

2.5 Differentiation ICD vs. ACD

Skin patch testing is a major tool to support or confirm the diagnosis of allergic contact dermatitis, exclude irritant reactions and guide the physician. In the Middle East, *p*-phenylenediamine, potassium dichromate, formaldehyde, fragrances, and preservatives in cosmetics were found the most common contact allergens, whereas in the USA, nickel sulfate, balsam of Peru, fragrances, quaterium-15, and neomycin sulfate are at the leading positions [13]. There is a lack of established patch test series designated specifically for non-Caucasians, but one can customize patch test series to the regional needs by using additional single allergens. In addition to standardized series, suspected products used by the patient may be added and evaluated. Skin patch testing will offer exact analysis and optimize the detection of any causing agent in sophisticated products, such as in fragrance allergy in Thailand [37].

If the application of a standardized patch test procedure is not possible or practicable, a *repeated open application test* (ROAT) should be considered, whereby the patient applies the suspected product on a predefined location twice a day for a period of 1–2 weeks; a common location for such tests is the flexor forearm. ROAT, however, often cannot distinguish between different ingredients contained in the product [6].

In hot climate zones, heat and humidity prevail, and skin patch testing becomes a challenge both for the dermatologist and the patient; occlusive procedures with sticky tapes may cause considerable discomfort, correct application is mandatory (Fig. 2.9). Also the tape fixed test chambers may get displaced because of sweating making the test reading difficult. This is also the case with waterproofed or water-resistant self-adhesive chamber sets [38].

When using the patch test, special attention needs to be given to sensitive patients and others with suspicion of strong sensitization, since the procedure may not only lead to flair-up of a preexisting eczema but also to development of severe reactions in the patch test field, occasionally with skin discoloration and scarring. In sensitive patients, the standard concentration of the test probes needs to be lowered and eventually gradually increased. Any test should be performed in caution; if severe reactions are expected, the tests should be placed in an area to be easily early removed and the reaction field treated.

2.6 Management

Omitting the suspected or detected and by patch testing confirmed allergen is an indispensable precondition for management of ICD and ACD. Once the allergen has been identified, written information about the agent with all international coding, synonyms, possible cross-allergens, and names of the most popular products should be issued and given to the patient. He/she should be also informed about alternatives available for use and the possibility of developing additional allergies in the future. Both the American and European Academies of Dermatology are providing comprehensive information and educational material. Also contact dermatitis societies and manufacturers of allergy skin tests are providing the necessary information. The patients should be also instructed to read the labels of the products, be aware of potential allergens, and stay updated on the nature of ingredients, i.e., in long-time used cosmetics, since the manufacturer may change product components. Additionally, components of a marketed product may differ in geographic areas not only between countries but also within the same country.

After withdrawal of possible allergen(s), the medical management of ACD focuses on anti-inflammatory topical medication to clear the dermatitis. Strict avoidance of the allergen or cross-reacting products is necessary to prevent relapses. Mild emollients and low potency corticosteroids are the mainstay for topical treatment for both ICD and ACD to be applied over a few days or a week; creams containing calcineurin inhibitors (tacrolimus or pimecrolimus) are potential alternatives, and an oral antihistamine may be added in case of intense pruritus to comfort the patient. A short course of systemic corticosteroids may be considered in cases with severe bullous reactions or generalized involvement.

Conclusions

The variety of allergenic substances and allergic reactions is universal, due to global exchange, trade of goods and products, and expansion of the Western lifestyle. Contact sensitization to chemicals has become a significant public health problem. In many parts of the world more than 20% of the adult population is suffering from contact allergy. Individuals with skin of color seem to differ from Caucasians in their skin sensitivity, reactivity to contact allergens and clinical presentation of allergic reactions. Although some research has been undertaken to improve our knowledge on ethnic skin, significant work remains to be done to assure proper diagnosis and management in non-Caucasian populations. In the Western world, nickel sulfate is the most prevalent allergen. In Africa, Asia, and in the Middle East, dyes, fragrances, and preservatives are the most common, whereas the role of airborne allergens in the development of ACD seems to be underestimated. Patch testing remains the gold standard for diagnosis. Quality control of patch testing procedures and region-customized patch test series would be helpful to assure adequate diagnosis and patient education in hot climate zones.

References

1. Zaidi Z. Skin of colour: characteristics and diseases. J Pak Med Assoc. 2017;67:292–9.
2. Berardesca E, Maibach H. Racial differences in skin pathophysiology. J Am Acad Dermatol. 1996;34:667–72.
3. Kompaore F, Marty JP, Dupont C. In vivo evaluation of the stratum corneum barrier function in blacks, Caucasians and Asians with two noninvasive methods. Skin Pharmacol. 1993;6:200–7.
4. Reed JT, Ghadially R, Elias PM. Skin type, but neither race of gender, influence epidermal permeability barrier function. Arch Dermatol. 1995;131:1134–8.
5. Hicks SP, Swindells KJ, Middelkamp-Hup MA, et al. Confocal histopathology of irritant contact dermatitis in vivo and the impact of skin color (black vs white). J Am Acad Dermatol. 2003;48: 727–34.
6. Berardesca E, Maibach HI. Racial differences in sodium-lauryl-sulphate induced cutaneous irritation: black and white. Contact Dermatitis. 1988;18:65–70.
7. Berardesca E, Maibach HI. Sodium-lauryl-sulphate-induced cutaneous irritation. Comparison of white and Hispanic subjects. Contact Dermatitis. 1988;19:136–40.
8. Kligman AM, Epstein W. Updating the maximization test for identifying contact allergens. Contact Dermatitis. 1975;1:231–9.
9. Dickel H, Taylor JS, Evey P, et al. Comparison of patch test results with a standard series among white and black racial groups. Am J Contact Dermat. 2001;12:77–82.
10. Deleo VA, Alexis A, Warshaw EM, et al. The Association of Race/Ethnicity and patch test results: North American Contact Dermatitis Group, 1998-2006. Dermatitis. 2016;27:288–92.
11. Berardesca E, Maibach H. Ethnic skin: overview of structure and function. J Am Acad Dermatol. 2003;48(S1):39–42.
12. National Health Services (NHS) Choices. Contact dermatitis. 2014. www.nhs.us/conditions/eczema-(contact-Dermatitis)/pages/introductionn.aspx.
13. Taylor JS, Amado A. Contact dermatitis and related conditions; August 2010 www.clevelandclinicmed.com/medicalpubs/diseasemanagement/dermatology/contact-dermatitis-and-related-conditions.
14. Pratt MD, Belsito DV, DeLeo DA, et al. North American contact dermatitis group patch test results, 2001-2002 study period. Dermatitis. 2004;15:176–83.
15. Schäfer T, Böhler E, Ruhdorfer S, et al. Epidemiology of contact allergy in adults. Allergy. 2001;56:1192–6.

16. Kot M, Bogaczewicz J, Kręcisz B, et al. Contact hypersensitivity to European baseline series and corticosteroid series haptens in a population of adult patients with contact eczema. Acta Dermatovenerol Croat. 2016;24:29–36.
17. Schnuch A, Uter W, Geier J, et al. Epidemiology of contact allergy: an estimation of morbidity employing the clinical epidemiology and drug-utilization research (CE-DUR) approach. Contact Dermatitis. 2002;47:32–9.
18. Spiewak R. Pesticides as a cause of occupational skin diseases in farmers. Ann Agric Environ Med. 2001;8:1–5.
19. Mark KA, Brancaccio RR, Soter NA, et al. Allergic contact and photoallergic contact dermatitis to plant and pesticide allergens. Arch Dermatol. 1999;135:67–70.
20. Trehan A, Singh K, Kanodia S, et al. Contact hypersensitivity and hand eczema–a study with Indian standard series of allergens. MedPulse. 2014;1:304–9.
21. Sharma VK, Bhari N, Wadhwani AR, et al. Photo-patch and patch tests in patients with dermatitis over the photo-exposed areas: a study of 101 cases from a tertiary care centre in India. Australas J Dermatol. 2016. https://doi.org/10.1111/ajd.12504.
22. Douglas KE, Ofure Agbi J, Akpovienehe O, et al. Occupational hand dermatitis among hair dressers in a semi-urban community in Rivers State, South-South Nigeria. Nigerian Health J. 2013;13:125–30.
23. Paulsen E, Hyldgaard MG, Andersen KE, et al. Allergenic sesquiterpene lactones from cushion bush (*Leucophyta brownii*): new and old sensitizers in a shrub-turned-a-pot plant. Contact Dermatitis. 2017. https://doi.org/10.1111/cod.12757.
24. Shahzad M, Alzolibani AA, Al Robaee AA, et al. Patients seen at the Dermatology ambulatory office in a tertiary care center in Qassim region, Saudi Arabia. Int J Health Sci. 2013;7:130–5.
25. Lachapelle JM. The spectrum of diseases for which patch testing is recommended. In: Lachapelle JM, Maibach HI, editors. Patch testing and prick testing. Berlin: Springer; 2009. p. 7–32.
26. Tan Q, Yang H, Liu E, et al. Establishing a role for interleukin-17 in atopic dermatitis-related skin inflammation. J Cutan Med Surg. 2017;21(4):308–15. https://doi.org/10.1177/1203475417697651.
27. Halder RM, Nootheti PK. Ethnic skin disorders overview. J Am Acad Dermatol. 2003;48:143–8.
28. Turner RN, Low RH. The principles and practice of moxibustion. Wellingborough: Thorsons Publishers; 1992.
29. Look KM, Look RM. Skin scarping, cupping, and moxibustion that may mimic physical abuse. J Forensic Sci. 1997;42:103–5.
30. Jurado-Palomo J, Moreno-Ancillo A, Bobolea ID, et al. Epidemiology of contact dermatitis. www.intechopen.com. https://doi.org/10.5772/26828.
31. Nguyen T, Saleh MA. Exposure of women to trace elements through the skin by direct contact with underwear clothing. J Environ Health Sci. 2016;52:1–6. https://doi.org/10.1080/10934529.2016.1221212
32. Berih A, Berhanu A. Allergic dermatitis – black henna (para-phenylenediamine) use among the East African patient population in a general practice setting. Aust Fam Physician. 2014;43:383–5.
33. Mukkanna KS, Stone NM, Ingram JR. Para-phenylenediamine allergy: current perspectives on diagnosis and management. J Asthma Allergy. 2017;10:9–15.
34. Khumalo NP, Jessop S, Ehrlich R. Prevalence of cutaneous adverse effects of hairdressing: a systematic review. Arch Dermatol. 2006;142:377–83.
35. Stallings A, Sood A. Hair-care practices in African American women: potential for allergic contact dermatitis. Semin Cutan Med Surg. 2016;35:207–10.
36. Plombom GY, Oliveira MS, Tabushi FL, et al. Epidemiological analysis of occupational dermatitis notified in Brazil in the period 2007 to 2012. An Bras Dermatol. 2016;91:732–73.
37. Vejanurug P, Tresukosol P, Sajjachareonpong P, et al. Fragrance allergy could be missed without patch testing with 26 individual fragrance allergens. Contact Dermatitis. 2016;74:230–5.
38. Goh CL. Patch tests in the tropics. Berlin: Springer; 2014. p. 143–7.

Atopic Dermatitis in Skin of Color

3

Zamambo N. C. Mkhize and Ncoza C. Dlova

Atopic dermatitis (AD) is a common inflammatory skin disease which occurs worldwide. It is a chronic relapsing eczematous skin disorder associated with xerosis and pruritus. AD is widespread in industrialized countries with an overall prevalence of 10–20% among school children from the USA and parts of Europe. The countries in South Europe and the African continent show lower prevalence; however, it is a growing clinical problem in sub-Saharan Africa. In West Africa and other parts of the continent, the incidence of AD is considered to involve around 5% of the population, and this rate is still rising. Atopic dermatitis can occur at any age but usually develops in childhood. Its acute phase occurs during infancy and has a predilection for the face and extensors. As the children grow older, the skin lesions become chronic and lichenified, usually involving the flexural areas. There is often an association of AD with a personal or family history of atopy, e.g., asthma, allergic conjunctivitis, and allergic rhinitis.

3.1 Epidemiology

The varying prevalence of AD suggests that there are multiple environmental risk factors that occur in different regions of the globe, including climate [1], residence in an urban area [2], water hardness and increased water exposure [3], early-life infectious exposures [4], diet, obesity [5, 6] and skin care practices [7]. Many of these risk factors differentially impact some sociodemographic groups, e.g., those with higher consumption of Western diet, obesity, and less early-life vaccination in African-Americans than in Caucasians. Lower water quality is more likely in areas of poverty and lower socioeconomic status [8]. It is possible that ethnic differences with respect to the above risk factors contribute to regional disparities in AD. In addition, black-skinned individuals had lower levels of skin ceramides than Asians and Caucasians [9] and higher levels of transepidermal water loss than Caucasians [10, 11]. The prevalence of atopic dermatitis in African-American children is significantly higher than in Caucasians [12]. However, the severity of AD was found in multivariate analyses significantly associated with lower household income, but not with ethnicity [13].

3.2 Pathogenesis

There is a genetic link with AD although a clear mode of inheritance has not been established. The chromosomal regions 3q21 and 5q31 have been linked with high serum IgE levels as well as with the presence of skin lesions, associated with impaired barrier function and consecutive xerosis. In particular, baseline measurements of transepidermal water loss were found significantly higher in Asians and black-skinned individuals as compared to white Caucasians, suggesting that black skin is more susceptible to xerosis [14] and more sensitive to irritants than white skin [15]. Low levels of ceramides also contribute to dryness of the skin in AD; the disrupted epidermal barrier causes high susceptibility to irritants, microbial and other allergens, and environmental factors. Irritants in AD include harsh detergents and soaps, synthetic fabrics, as well fragrances, and most frequent allergens are dust mites, pollen, animal dander, and molds. Food allergies occur primarily in children younger than 2 years, the most common food allergens are cow's milk, eggs, peanuts, soya, and wheat.

Z. N. C. Mkhize
Department of Dermatology, Edendale Hospital Pietermaritzburg, Nelson R Mandela School of Medicine, University of KwaZulu-Natal, Durban, South Africa

N. C. Dlova (✉)
Department of Dermatology, Nelson R Mandela School of Medicine, University of KwaZulu-Natal, Durban, South Africa
e-mail: Dlovan@ukzn.ac.za

C. E. Orfanos et al. (eds.), *Pigmented Ethnic Skin and Imported Dermatoses*, https://doi.org/10.1007/978-3-319-69422-1_3

Staphylococcus aureus frequently colonizes eczematous skin and can also act as a super antigen bypassing antigen-presenting cells to directly activate T cells resulting in the induction of a Th2-dominant immune response in skin. Staphylococci are also implicated in causing secondary impetigo in AD; in addition, AD patients are predisposed to both herpes simplex and pox virus infections leading to eczema herpeticum and molluscum contagiosum, respectively.

Another player in the pathogenesis of AD is *filaggrin* (FLG) which is broken down into a natural moisturizing factor in stratum corneum playing an integral role in skin barrier function [16]. Mutations of FLG gene lead to deficiency of this factor [17] resulting in xerosis [18]. Multiple FLG mutations have been identified, shown to be a risk factor for AD [19]. FLG mutations were detected in 27.5% of white-skinned and only in 5.8% of African-American children with AD [20]. A follow-up study demonstrated common loss of function mutations of the FLG2 gene in African-Americans, not present in patients with European ancestry. Children with FLG2 loss of function mutations were less likely to be symptom free over time [21]. A study of 18 African-American children with AD and ichthyosis vulgaris and 17 African-American non-atopic controls found that only 22.2% of those with AD and 5.9% of the controls were heterozygous for FLG null mutations [22]. Taken together, these studies suggest that FLG2 may play an important role in AD in African-Americans but that one or more factors other than filaggrin mutations are responsible for AD in African-Americans and other patient subsets.

3.3 Clinical Picture

There are three classical stages of atopic dermatitis seen in early infancy, in children and in adults, each of which may show an *acute*, *subacute*, and *chronic skin reaction pattern*.

The *acute stage* usually predominates in the infantile form; the lesions are eczematous, exudative with edematous papules and plaques, often excoriated and intensely pruritic. Vesicles, oozing, and serous crusting are seen within affected areas (Fig. 3.1).

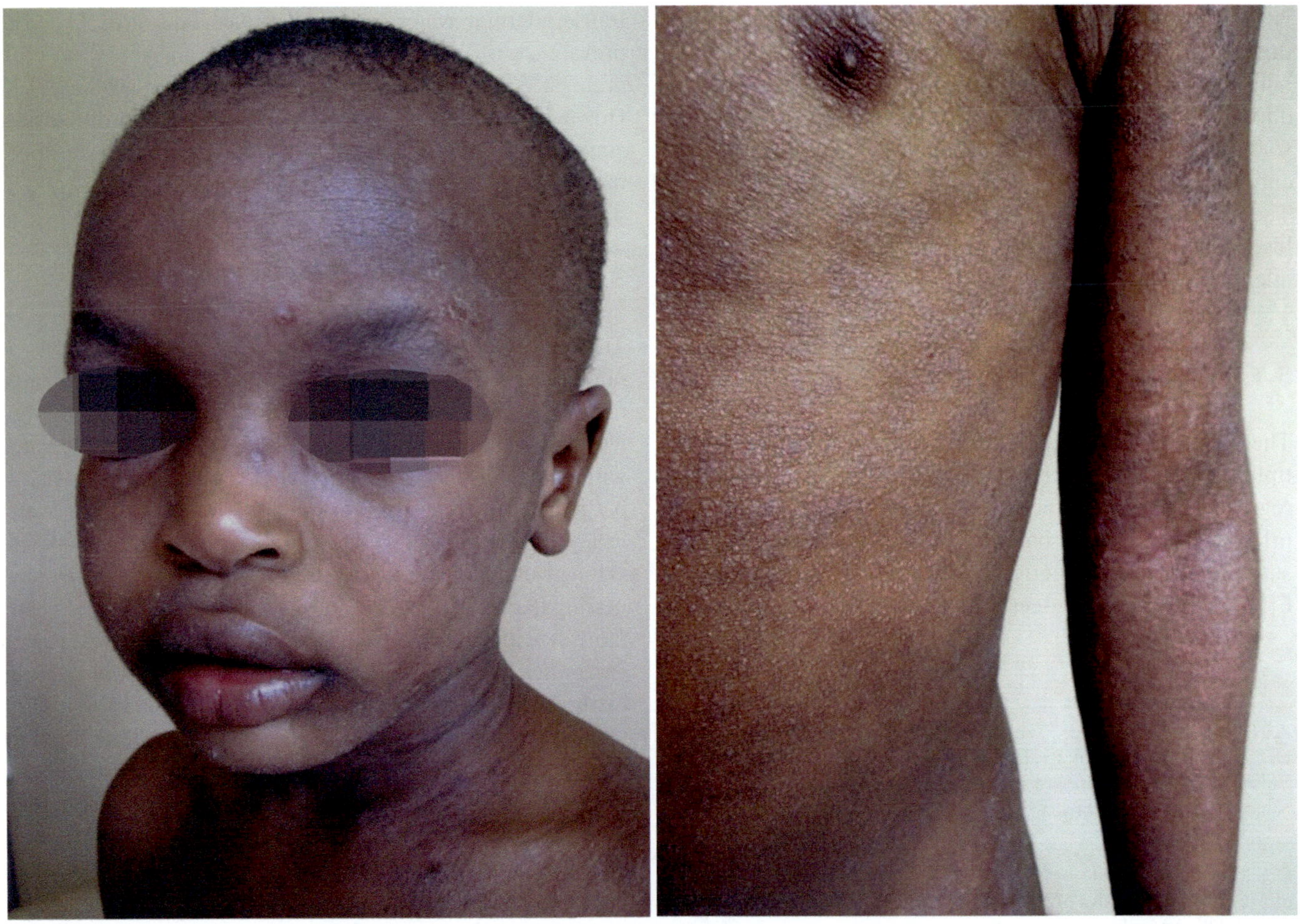

Fig. 3.1 *Atopic dermatitis*, early eczematous stage in childhood

In the *subacute stage*, erythematous papules and plaques are seen, with scaling and excoriations as secondary changes and beginning of lichenification. Staphylococcal impetigo may concomitantly appear as a complication (Fig. 3.2).

The final *chronic stage* is characterized by thickened, hyperkeratotic, and lichenified plaques with transient prurigo nodules. The disease may occasionally progress to erythroderma and/or to prurigo nodularis (Figs. 3.3, 3.4 and 3.5).

Pruritus is present regardless of the stage. In infants and young children, lesions are usually seen on the face, scalp, and extensor surfaces of the extremities and may be follicular; the diaper area is usually spared. As the child grows older, they tend to favor the flexural areas, the antecubital and popliteal fossae and posterior neck. In adults eczema is seen predominantly in a flexural distribution. For establishing the diagnosis, there are major and minor criteria, among them history of atopy, recurrent episodes of eczema with pruritus, xerosis, keratosis pilaris, Dennie-Morgan line, palmoplantar linearity, and presence of prurigo nodules.

The classical presentations of AD are essentially the same across all ethnic groups. However, there are a number of distinguishing features that occur more commonly in some populations than in others. In African black skin erythema often appears as a hyperpigmented or violaceous macule. A study in Nigeria documented that 54.1% of the patients had lichenoid lesions and 70.3% had a perifollicular, micropapular rash, on the extensor aspects of the joints [23]. Keloid formation may follow the chronic prurigo stage, and rashes of *follicular eczema* are sometimes seen on the trunk of dark-skinned African patients with AD, and this does not occur in white skin. When the lesions of AD resolve, they cause persistent dyschromia or pigmentary alterations resulting in either post-inflammatory hyperpigmentation or leukoderma which is always more pronounced in patients with darker skin phototypes [12]. These phenotypic differences may delay the diagnosis and treatment and allow for more severe disease to develop (Figs. 3.6 and 3.7).

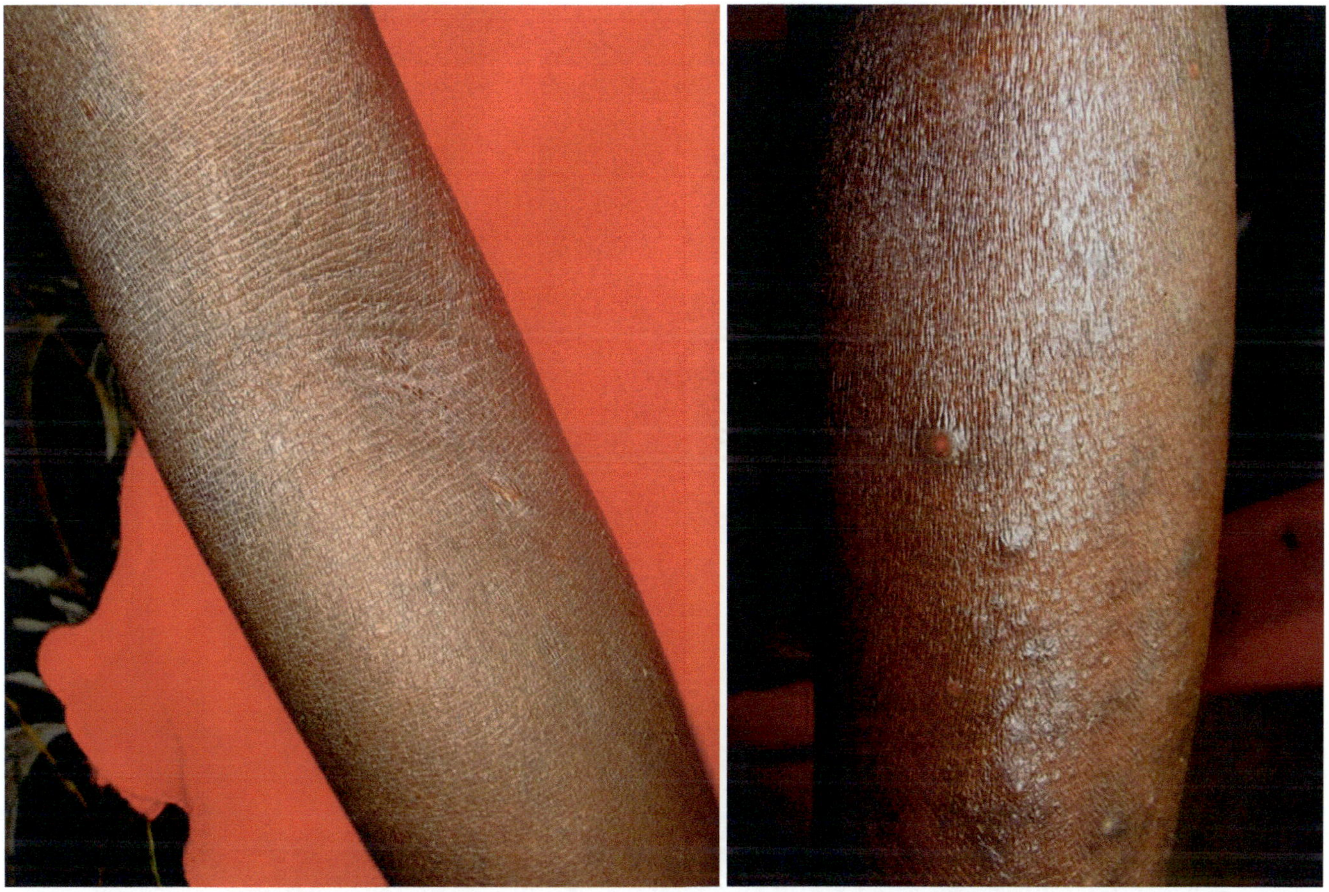

Fig. 3.2 Subacute stage of *atopic dermatitis* with flexural lichenification, perifollicular inflammatory reaction, and prurigo-like nodules in skin of color

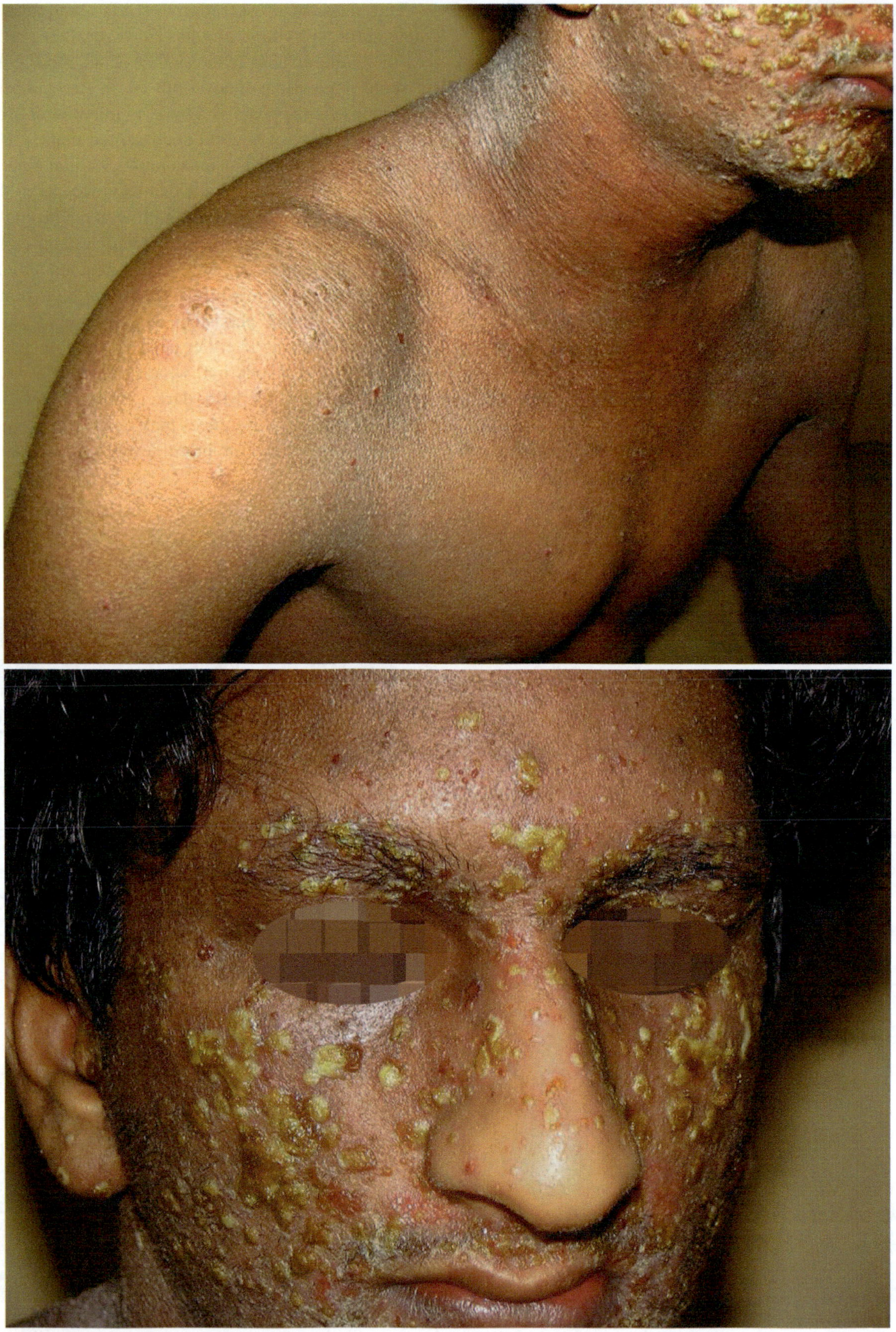

Fig. 3.3 Generalized, *chronic erythrodermic AD* with severe staphylococcal impetigo in face

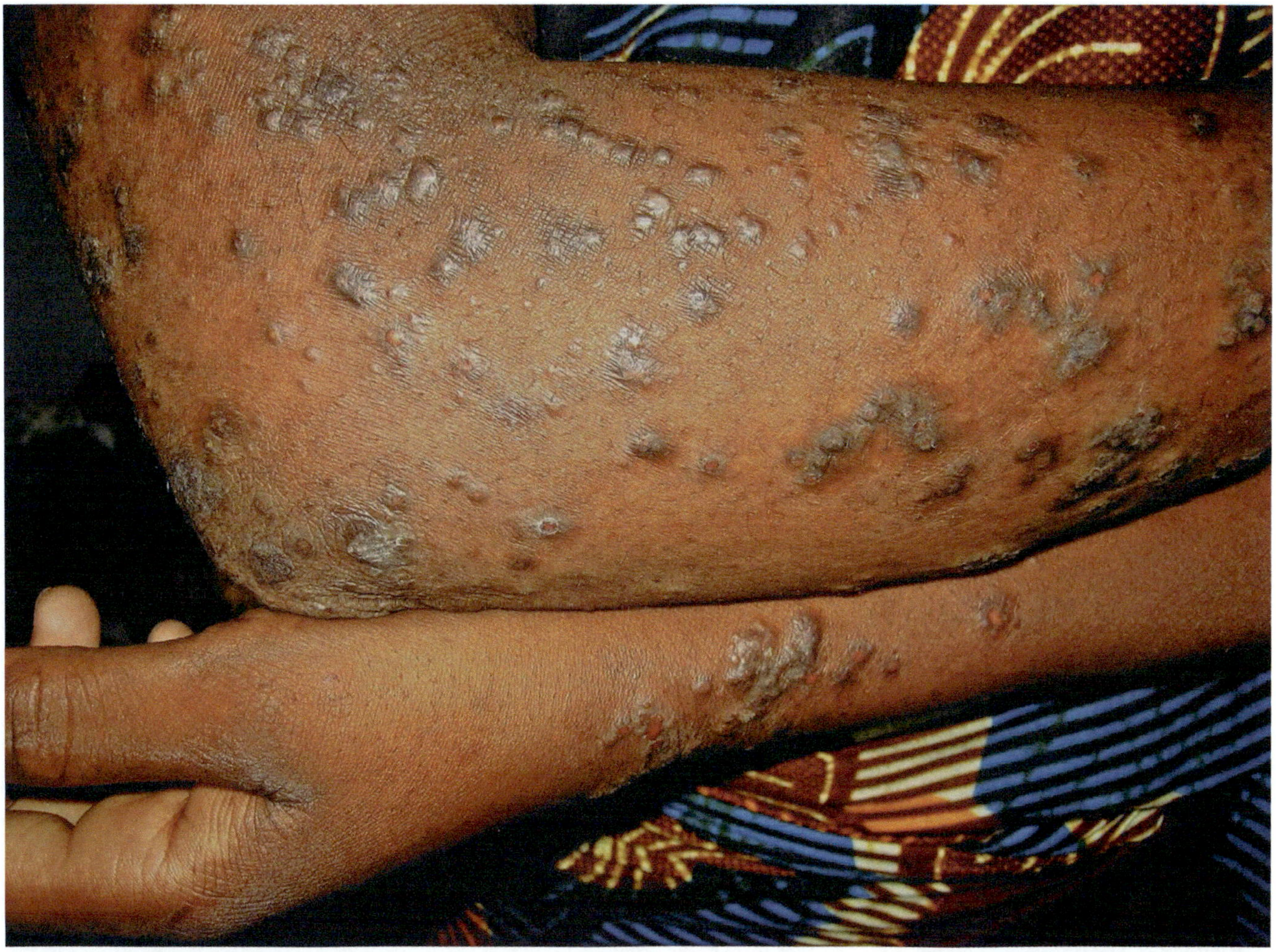

Fig. 3.4 *Chronic stage of AD* with extensive keloidal prurigo

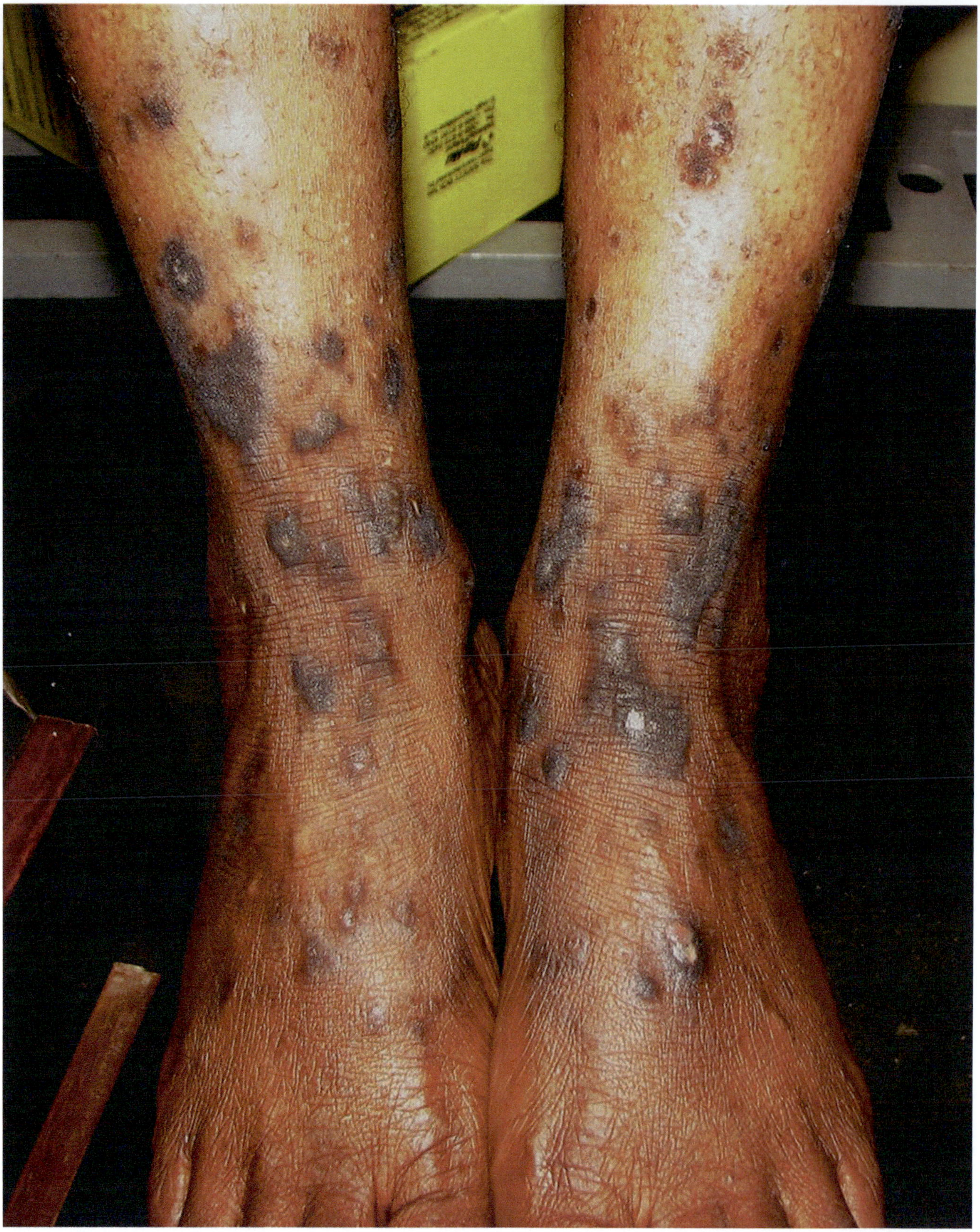

Fig. 3.5 Chronic atopic prurigo with transformation into prurigo nodularis

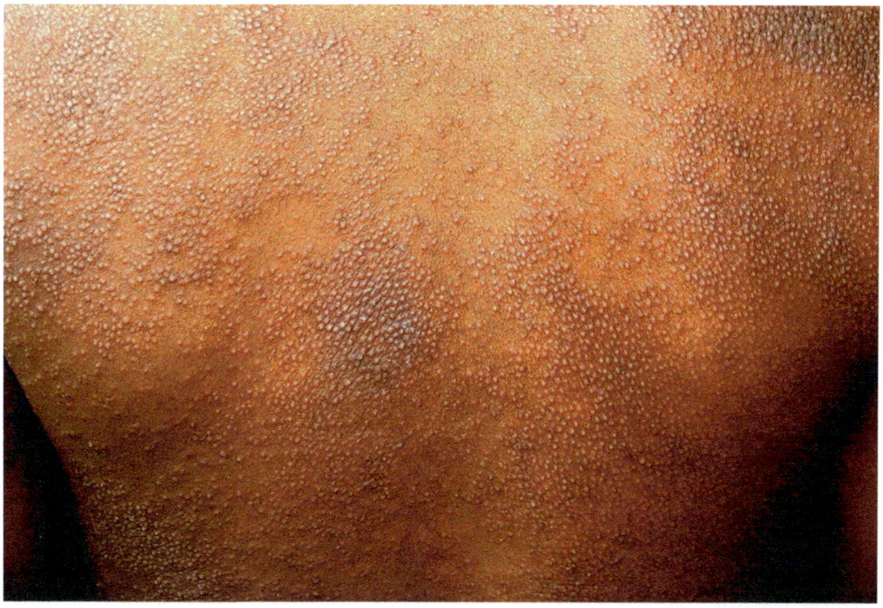

Fig. 3.6 Follicular eczematous rush on the trunk in an atopic patient (irritant dermatitis after local application of ointments of unknown composition)

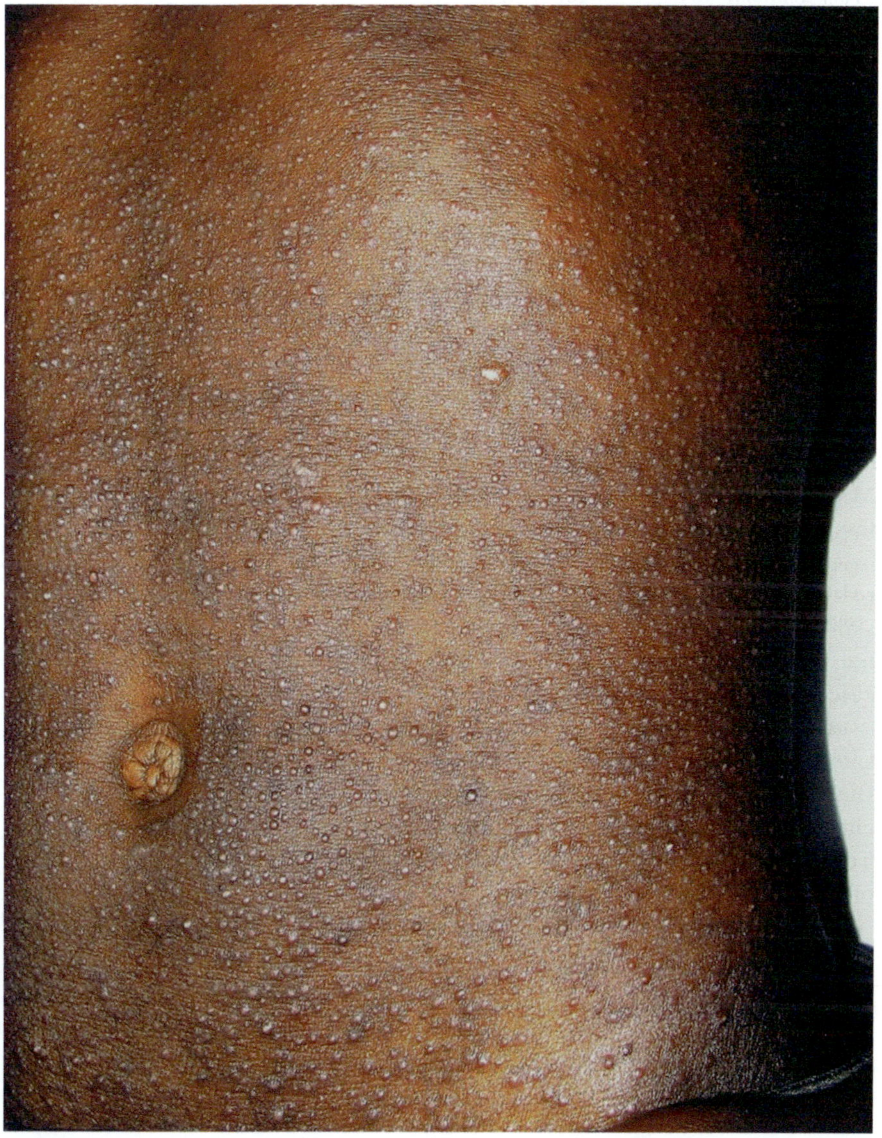

Fig. 3.7 *Follicular eczema*; 16-year-old boy (Uganda)

3.4 Course

In more than 50% of AD patients, the disease begins during infancy. It is a chronic condition with relapses and exacerbations which can also be seasonal, but the majority of patients report improvement as they grow older. It is difficult to assess how many cases progress to the adult form of the disease, but data may suggest that up to 40% of patients with childhood eczema have persistent or recurrent AD as adults.

3.5 Management

As a basic rule, the patients should be advised to avoid all type of possible skin irritants and allergens. They should bath less often, avoid hot water with harsh soaps and detergents, and opt for bath substitutes, e.g., glycerin-based soaps. Emollients must be applied soon after bathing to lock in moisture. *Topical moisturizers* are recommended to combat xerosis; alternatively agents such as petrolatum and mineral oils may be used to retard transepidermal loss of water. Liberal and frequent application of emollients is recommended also as prevention [7], together with oral sedating or non-sedating *antihistamines* to break the itch-scratch cycle and improve patients' quality of life. Extensive guidelines for care of AD are available [24, 25].

Topical corticosteroids are used in both adults and children and are the mainstay of anti-inflammatory management. For acute flares, daily use of topical steroids is recommended until the inflammatory lesions are significantly improved. After obtaining control, the goal is to prolong the period until the next flare by appropriate use of emollients. Low-potency preparations, e.g., 1% hydrocortisone, are recommended. Medium-potency steroids, e.g., betamethasone valerate and mometasone furoate, can be used for lesions on the trunk. More potent topical steroids should be avoided or tapered to less potent preparations.

Calcineurin inhibitors have the benefit of not carrying risk for cutaneous atrophy. They may be used at sensitive skin sites such as the face and the skin folds, topical tacrolimus ointment (0.03 and 0.1%) for moderate to severe disease, and pimecrolimus cream 1% for mild eczema.

Antimicrobials and antiseptics are frequently required, since atopic individuals are predisposed to skin infections. Bleach baths in conjunction with intranasal topical mupirocin can be used to eradicate colonization of staphylococci. They are preferred to topical antibiotics as there is less risk of resistance and contact dermatitis.

Phototherapies such as PUVA and narrowband UVB can be used alone or in combination with emollients and topical steroids [26]. No definitive recommendation can be made to differentiate between different forms of phototherapy in regard to efficacy. The use of light management may decrease the need for topical corticosteroids.

Systemic treatments of AD are usually reserved for severe, acute flares [27]. *Corticosteroids* should be generally avoided because the risks outweigh the benefits. Immunosuppressives such as oral *cyclosporine* (3–6 mg/kg/day) is effective, but renal toxicity, hypertension, and increased risk for malignancy limit its use. *Azathioprine* is also efficacious (1–3 mg/kg/day), tapered or discontinued after clearance. Concomitant phototherapy is not advised because of increased risk of DNA damage and possible UV-induced carcinogenicity. *Methotrexate*, 2.5–25 mg/week depending on patient's age and weight, is also effective; liver functions should be monitored as well as full blood counts. *Mycophenolate mofetil* (25–50 mg/kg/day) can also be used. After all systemic therapies, laboratory monitoring is important before and during treatment.

Conclusions

Atopic dermatitis is a rising health problem in developing countries in African countries and their populations. Black skin seems to be more susceptible to dryness due to high transepidermal water loss and increased sensitivity to irritants and allergens leading to eczema. Post-inflammatory hyperpigmentation or leukoderma is a serious concern for dark-skinned patients, and clinicians should make an attempt to address it, as it affects the patient's quality of life. The socioeconomic conditions may play an additional role and explain the increasing prevalence. There is a need to support educational interventions together with programs for prevention and schedules for management adjusted to the environmental circumstances in hot climate zones.

References

1. Silverberg JI, Hanifin J, Simpson EL. Climatic factors are associated with childhood eczema prevalence in the United States. J Invest Dermatol. 2013;133:1752–9.
2. Shaw TE, Currie GP. Eczema prevalence in the United States. J Invest Dermatol. 2011;131:67–73.
3. Chaumont A, Voisin C, Sardella A, et al. Interactions between domestic water hardness, infant swimming and atopy in the development of childhood eczema. Environ Res. 2012;116:52–7.
4. Silverberg JI, Horowitz KB, Kleiman E, et al. Association between varicella zoster virus infection and atopic dermatitis in early and late childhood. J Allergy Clin Immunol. 2010;126:300–5.
5. Silverberg JI, Simpson EL. Association between obesity and eczema prevalence, severity and poorer health in US adolescents. Dermatitis. 2014;25:172–81.
6. Zhang A, Silverberg JI. Association of atopic dermatitis with being overweight and obese; a systematic review and metaanalysis. J Am Acad Dermatol. 2015;72:606–16.
7. Simpson EL, Chalmers JR, Hanifin JM, et al. Emollient enhancement of the skin barrier from birth offers effective atopic dermatitis prevention. J Allergy Clin Immunol. 2014;134:818–23.

8. Subbaraman R, Shitole S, Shitole T, et al. The social ecology of water in a Mumbai slum: failures in water quality, quantity and reliability. BMC Public Health. 2013;13:173.
9. Jungersted JM, Hogh JK, Hellgren LI, et al. Ethnicity and stratum corneum ceramides. Br J Dermatol. 2010;163:1169–73.
10. Wesley NO, Maibach HI. Racial (ethnic) differences in skin properties; the objective data. Am J Clin Dermatol. 2003;4:843–60.
11. Proksch E, Folster-Holst R, Bräutigam M, et al. Role of epidermal barrier in atopic dermatitis. J Dtsch Dermatol Ges. 2009;7: 899–910.
12. Vachiramon V, They HL, Thompson AE, et al. Atopic dermatitis in African American children: addressing unmet needs of a common disease. Pediatr Dermatol. 2012;29:395–402.
13. Silverberg JI, Simpson EL. Associations of childhood eczema severity: a US population-based study. Dermatitis. 2014;25:107–14.
14. Wilson D, Berardesca E, Maibach HI. In vivo transepidermal water loss: differences between black and white skin. Br J Dermatol. 1988;119:647–52.
15. Kompaore F, Marty JP, Dupont C. In vivo evaluation of the stratum corner barrier function in blacks, Caucasians and Asians with two non-invasive methods. Skin Pharmacol. 1993;6:200–7.
16. McDaniel MK, Walfogel J. Racial and ethnic differences in the management of childhood asthma in the United States. J Asthma. 2012;49:785–91.
17. Kezic S, Kemperman PM, Koster ES, et al. Loss-of-function stations in the filaggrin gene lead to reduced level of natural moisturizing factor in the stratum corneum. J Invest Dermatol. 2008;128:2117–9.
18. O'Regan GM, Sandilands A, McLean WH, et al. Filaggrin in atopic dermatitis. J Allergy Clin Immunol. 2009;124(suppl 2):R2–6.
19. Weidinger S, O'Sullivan M, Illig T, et al. Filaggrin mutations, atopic eczema, hay fever, and asthma in children. J Allergy Clin Immunol. 2008;121:1203–9.
20. Margolis DJ, Apter AJ, Gupta J, et al. The persistence of atopic dermatitis and filaggrin in a US longitudinal cohort. J Allergy Clin Immunol. 2012;130:912–7.
21. Margolis DJ, Gupta J, Apter AJ, et al. Filaggrin-2 variation is associated with more persistent atopic dermatitis in African American subjects. J Allergy Clin Immunol. 2014;133:784–9.
22. Polcari I, Becker L, Stein SL. Filaggrin gene mutations in African Americans with both ichthyosis vulgaris and atopic dermatitis. Pediatr Dermatol. 2014;31:489–92.
23. Nnoruka EN. Current epidemiology of atopic dermatitis in southeastern Nigeria. Int J Dermatol. 2002;43:739–44.
24. Echenfield LF, Tom WL, Chamlin SL, et al. Guidelines of care for the management of atopic dermatitis: Section 1. J Am Acad Dermatol. 2014;70:338–51.
25. Sudbury R, Davis DM, Cohen DE, et al. Guidelines of care for the management of atopic dermatitis: Section 3. J Am Acad Dermatol. 2014;71:327–49.
26. Garritsen FM, Brouwer MW, Limpens J, et al. Photo(chemo) therapy in the management of atopic dermatitis. Br J Dermatol. 2014;170:501–13.
27. Roekevisch E, Spuls PI, Kuester D, et al. Efficacy and safety of systemic treatments for moderate to severe atopic dermatitis. J Allergy Clin Immunol. 2014;133:429–38.

Bacterial Infections

4

Stefano Veraldi, Luisa Carlotta Rossi, and Emilio Berti

Impetigo is a bacterial superficial infection of the skin. It is the most frequent bacterial dermatitis in infancy. In Western countries, it occurs mainly in preschool children, particularly during the summer. The disease is contagious: it is not rare to observe minor epidemics in kindergartens.

4.1 Epidemiology

Impetigo is very common in Sub-Saharan Africa. Epidemiological-clinical surveys were carried out in several countries: Ethiopia [1–5], Mali [6–9], Sierra Leone [10], Ghana [11–13], Togo [14], Nigeria [15–19], Gabon [13], Rwanda [13], Uganda [20], Tanzania [21–23], Malawi [24] and South Africa [25]. In 2 studies carried out in Mali in 1995 [6] and in Nigeria in 2010 [17], respectively, impetigo was the most frequent skin disease. In another study, impetigo represented 42.2% of all skin diseases observed in health centres in Bamako, Mali [7]. Finally, impetigo was the leading infectious skin disease in a hospital in Ibadan, Nigeria, 13.4% of all hospitalized children [18].

S. Veraldi (✉) · L. C. Rossi · E. Berti
Department of Pathophysiology and Transplantation, Università degli Studi di Milano, I.R.C.C.S. Foundation, Cà Granda Ospedale Maggiore Policlinico, Milan, Italy
e-mail: stefano.veraldi@unimi.it; luisa.rossi@unimi.it; emilio.berti@unimi.it

4.2 Pathogenesis

Impetigo is caused by staphylococcus and/or streptococcus species. The transmission is mainly by direct person-to-person contact. Predisposing factors are hot-humid-rainy climate [21, 24], low socio-economic level [5, 13, 18, 21], household crowding [5], poor household and/or individual hygiene [5, 6, 21, 24]. Personal factors (congenital or acquired abnormalities in humoral or cellular immunity, malnutrition, poor hygiene, presence of debilitating diseases, previous or concomitant systemic therapies with antibiotics, corticosteroids, immunosuppressives or antitumorals) are also important [26].

The term impetigo actually consists of two distinct entities from the aetiopathogenetic and clinical points of view: the *non-bullous*, also called impetigo contagiosa, vulgaris or pustular, and the *bullous impetigo* [26].

The *non-bullous impetigo* is caused by staphylococci or streptococci or both. In the past, in Western countries, streptococcal aetiology was more frequent. Group A β-haemolytic streptococci (*Streptococcus pyogenes*) were usually isolated, less frequently groups B, C, D and G [26]. However, in Ghana, non-group A streptococci were frequently isolated: 82% of the lesions were caused by group G streptococci and 18% by group C [11, 12]. *Corynebacterium diphtheriae* is also responsible for cases of impetigo in Tanzania [21, 27]. In Western countries, staphylococcal infections are currently more frequent (65–75% of cases). In a study carried out in Togo in 2011, 30 out of 84 (35.7%) *Staphylococcus aureus* isolated strains were methicillin-resistant [14].

The bullous impetigo is always caused by *Staphylococcus aureus*. The latter produces exotoxins with lytic and exfoliative properties. These toxins induce a detachment of keratinocytes of the granular layer of the epidermis, with consequent development of vesicles and blisters [26]. Impetigo can also develop on a pre-existing skin disease characterized by more or less severe pruritus and scratching: atopic dermatitis and

C. E. Orfanos et al. (eds.), *Pigmented Ethnic Skin and Imported Dermatoses*, https://doi.org/10.1007/978-3-319-69422-1_4

other allergic diseases [14, 22], chickenpox, pediculosis [10], scabies [15, 21, 22] and arthropod stings and bites [21]. In these cases the terms secondary impetigo or impetiginization are often used. In a survey carried out in Togo, secondary impetigo was observed in 20% of patients (eczema in 8.9% and mycoses in 3.3% of cases) [14]. However, impetigo on head lice was very rare in Sierra Leone [10].

4.3 Clinical Picture

Non-bullous impetigo is at first characterized by one or more round vesicles, small in size, containing a clear fluid and surrounded by an erythematous halo. These vesicles can rupture, resulting in erosions, or may remain intact; however, the fluid becomes purulent, with formation of pustules (Fig. 4.1). Subsequently, both erosions and pustules dry up and become crusts: these are yellowish in colour, surrounded by an erythematous halo and poorly adherent. Their removal shows an underlying erythematous-erosive, moist and red in colour surface. Uncovered areas are characteristically affected, particularly the nose, cheeks, lips and chin; covered areas can be involved by self-inoculation [26].

Bullous impetigo presents with isolated vesicles and/or blisters which may be widespread on the face, trunk and skin folds. These lesions are round, sometimes large (a few cm in diameter), flaccid, containing initially a clear fluid which becomes frankly purulent, surrounded by very mild or no erythema. The removal of the roof reveals moist erosions that may develop into flat ulcers which eventually become yellowish-brown crusts [26] (Fig. 4.2). This clinical picture is superimposable to that on pigmented skin. However, erythema is less visible and characterized by a grey colour rather than red.

Hot-humid climates and delayed diagnosis and treatment can facilitate the development of ulcerative lesions, usually caused by *Staphylococcus aureus* or group A β–haemolytic streptococcus [27–29].

Both varieties of impetigo are asymptomatic or accompanied by mild pruritus. General health is good. Only in chronic and/or diffuse infections fever may be occasionally registered. Lymphangitis and regional lymphadenitis are also rare

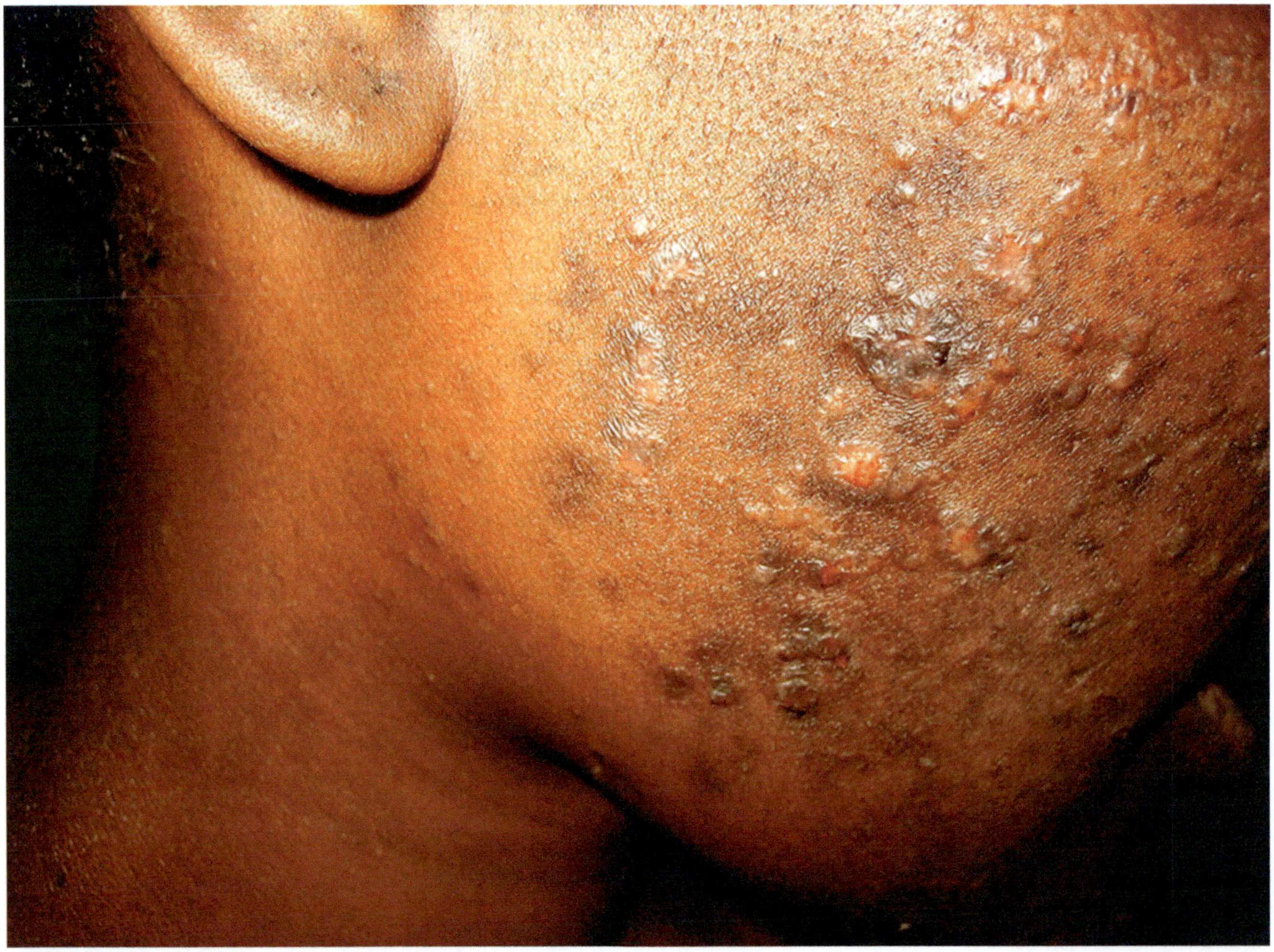

Fig. 4.1 Relapsing impetigo on the face (non-bullous type) in a 16-year-old male

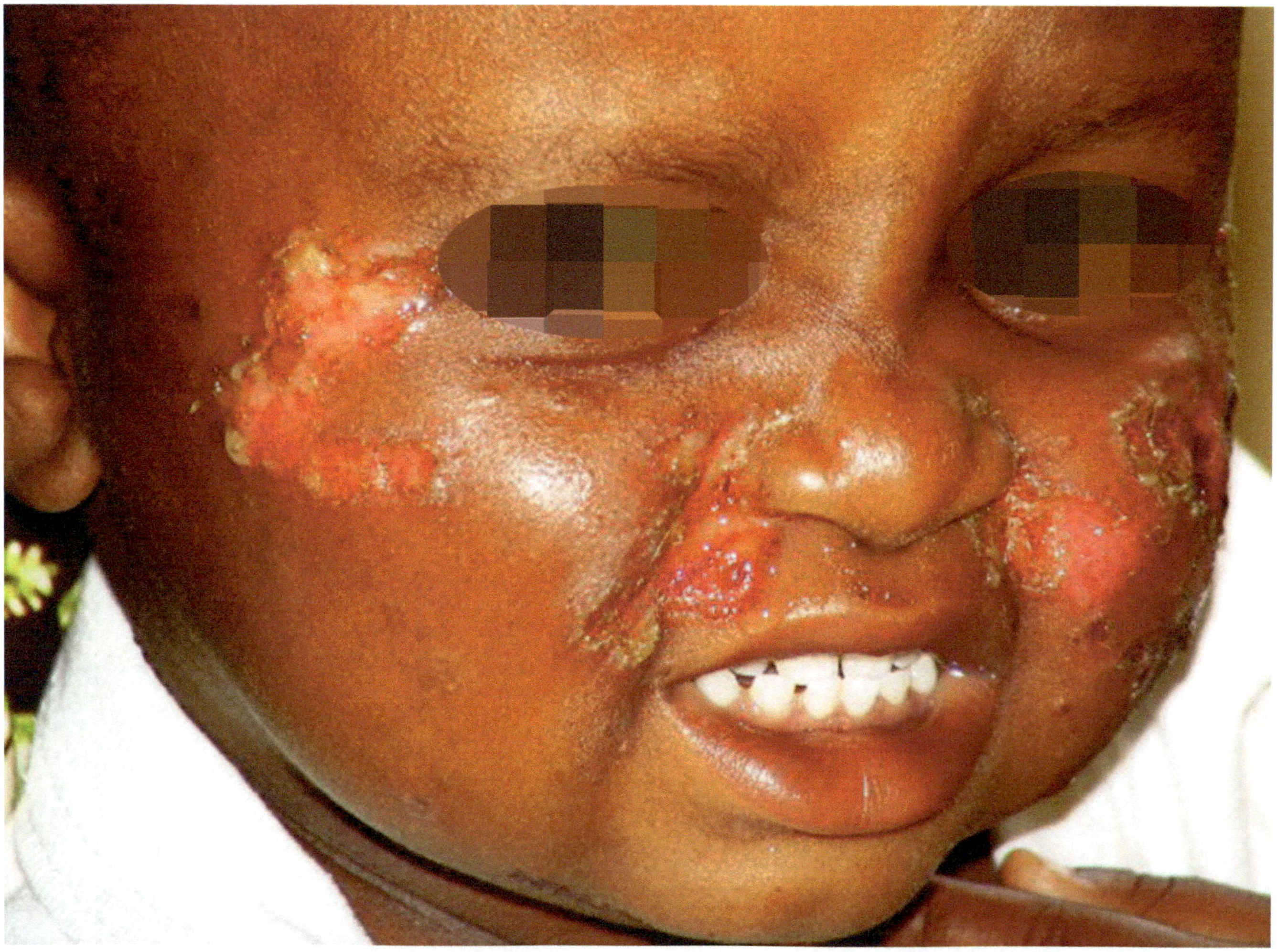

Fig. 4.2 Widely spread bullous impetigo on the face of a 2-year-old child, flatly ulcerated and progressive

[26]. Both varieties of impetigo can also resolve spontaneously within some weeks; with adequate management the duration usually is 5–7 days. The disease heals without leaving scars; on pigmented skin, hyperpigmentation can persist indefinitely [26]. Glomerulonephritis is currently rare in Western countries; however, it was common and severe in Ethiopia [1] and Nigeria [15]. Glomerulonephritis usually occurs 3–4 weeks (up to 7 weeks) after the appearance of the skin lesions and is at first characterized by proteinuria and microhaematuria [26]. Recurrences are possible if bacterial foci are not adequately eradicated in the patient, in his/her family and in the community.

4.4 Diagnosis

Diagnosis of impetigo is clinical. Bacteriological examination of the fluid or the pus removed from a vesicle, blister, or pustule and then Gram-stained allows the observation of both extracellular and intracellular (particularly in the cytoplasm of neutrophils) Gram-positive cocci, which are arranged in bunches or chains. The same modality of collection may be followed for bacterial culture and antibiogram [26].

Laboratory abnormalities are rare and non-specific: mild leukocytosis with neutrophilia and increase in inflammatory tests (erythrocyte sedimentation rate, C-reactive protein, α1-acid glycoprotein) [26]. Three to four weeks after cure, it is helpful to perform urinalysis to exclude a post-streptococcal glomerulonephritis.

Clinical diagnosis of impetigo is usually easy. However, it may sometimes enter in differential diagnosis with herpes simplex (small grouped vesicles on an erythematous base, which always recur at the same sites); irritant and allergic contact dermatitis (tiny vesicles on an erythematous base, accompanied by more or less severe pruritus); dermatitis herpetiformis (papular-vesicular lesions at typical sites (shoulders, elbows, lumbosacral region, buttocks, knees) accompanied by severe pruritus); and tinea corporis (erythematous-vesicular borders and scaling in the centre of the lesion) [26].

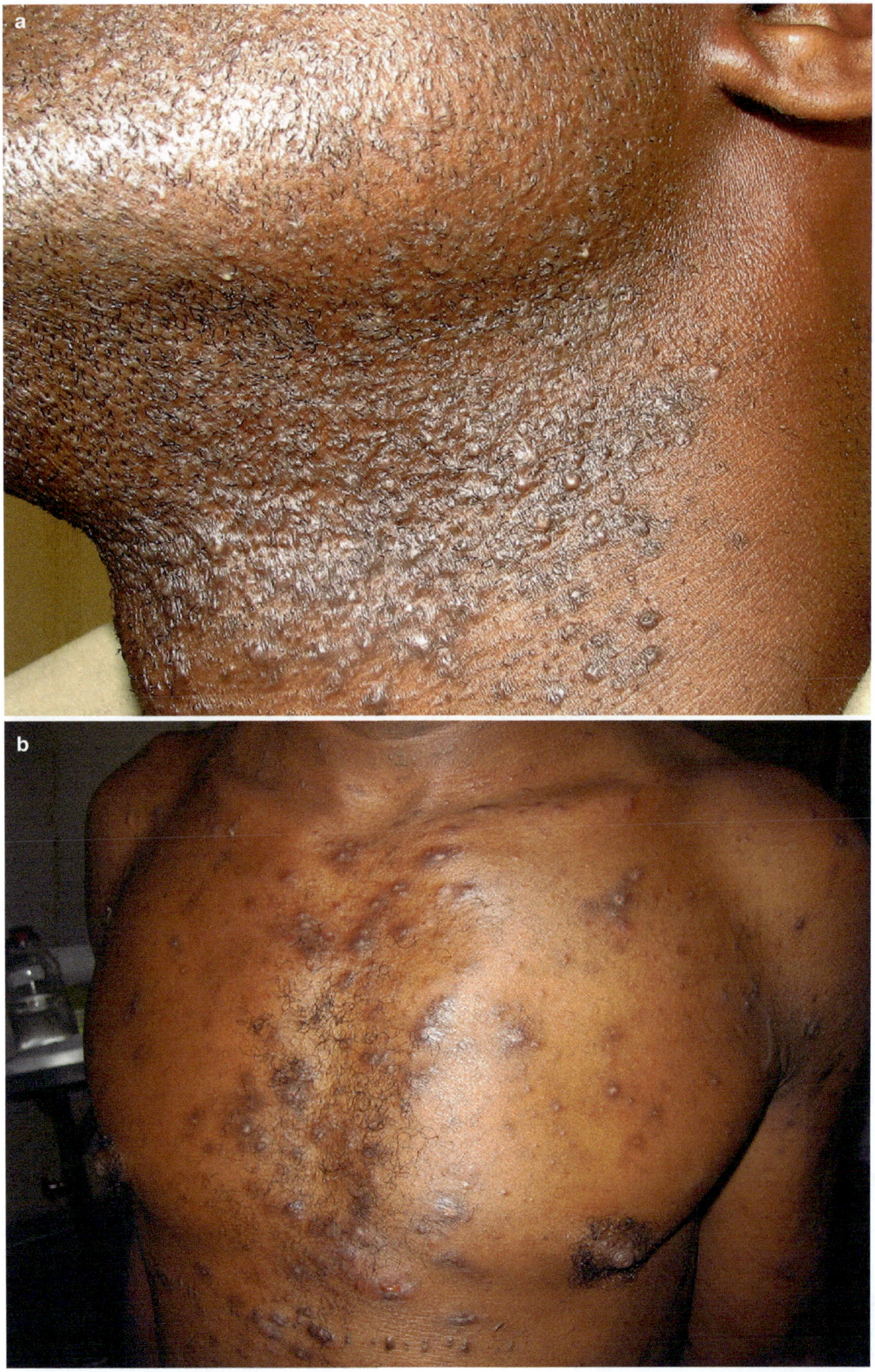

Fig. 4.3 (**a**) Folliculitis of the beard; (**b**) peri- and pseudo-folliculitis on the trunk in Tanzanian males

Other superficial and adnexal bacterial infections, such as folliculitis and perifolliculitis (Fig. 4.3), deep abscesses, erysipelas (Fig. 4.4), cellulitis, necrotizing fasciitis and ecthyma, do not present significant epidemiological and/or clinical differences on pigmented skin in comparison with fair skin. In tropical and subtropical geographic areas, bacterial superinfections of different dermatoses are rather common (Fig. 4.5).

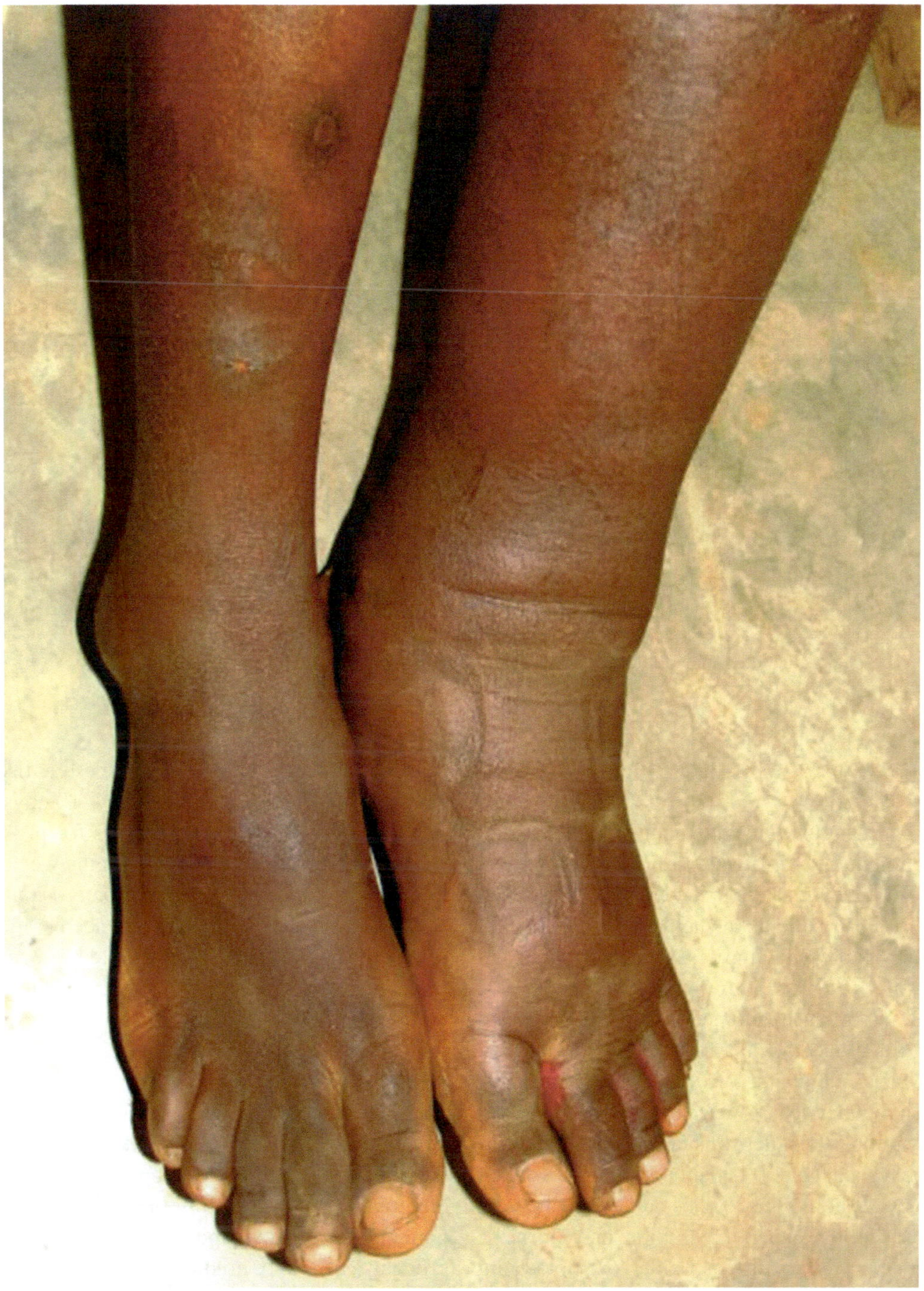

Fig. 4.4 Post-erysipelas subacute lymphedema of the left leg (DD: filariasis)

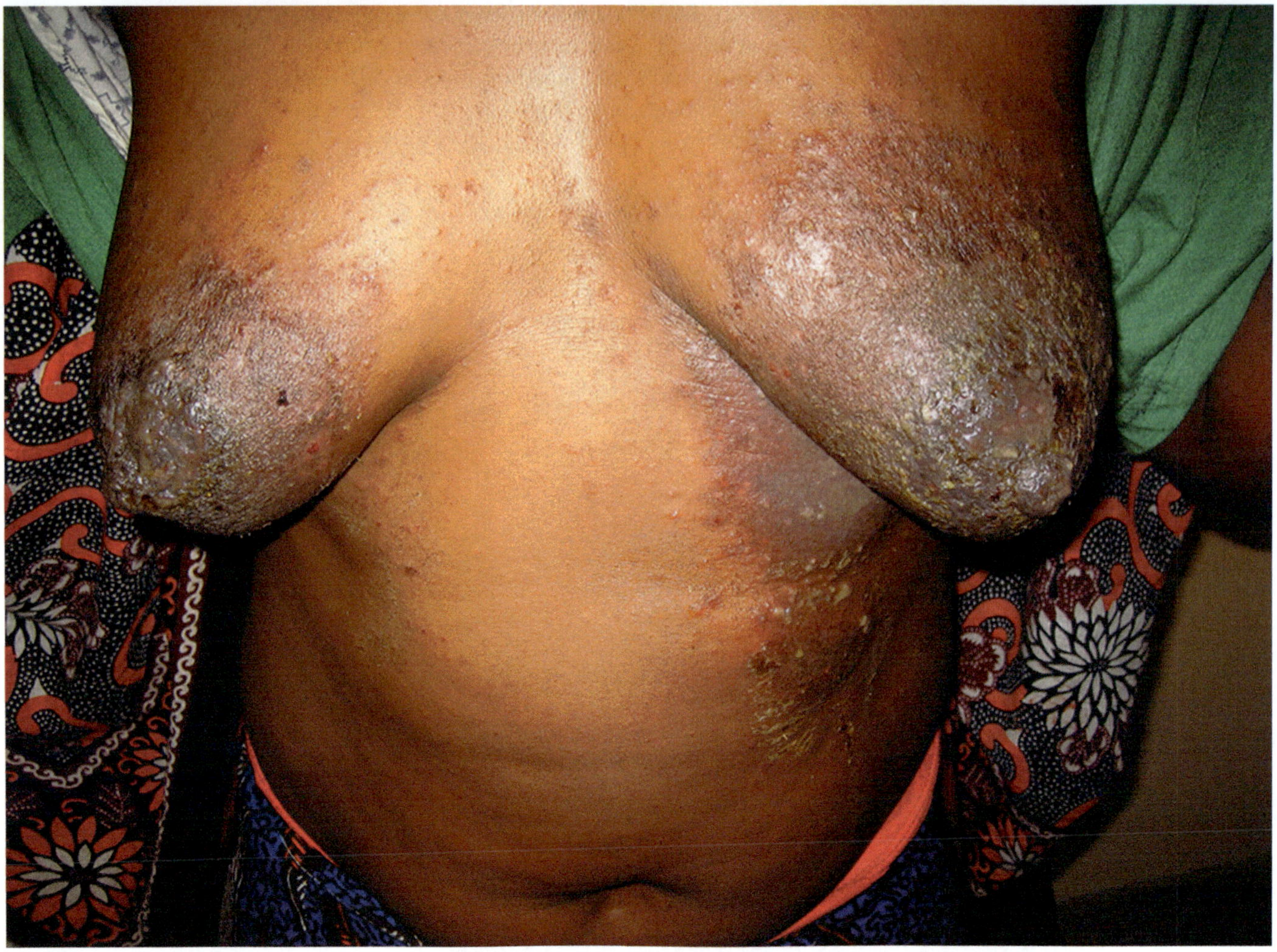

Fig. 4.5 Staphylococcal superinfection of bilateral perimammilary eczema in a 24-year-old breastfeeding female

4.5 Management

Early diagnosis and adequate management limit the extension of the infection and its diffusion within the family and the community. Treatment must be preceded or accompanied by careful search in the patient, his/her family and his/her contacts for any possible infective reservoir. For staphylococci, reservoirs are nostrils, auditory canal and skin folds (axillae, inguinal, interglutaeal and perineal folds); for streptococci, they are pharynx, tonsils, auditory canal and skin folds [26–29]. During the course of the disease, the patient should use personal underwear, towels and bedsheets.

It is necessary to open vesicles, blisters and pustules with the tip of a scalpel or a needle. It is then helpful to wash and disinfect the erosive lesions. This can be achieved with several cleansers/antiseptics: benzoyl peroxide or chlorhexidine digluconate or hydrogen peroxide or potassium permanganate (it is toxic by oral route; maximum caution must be taken by the patient; its use on the face must be avoided) and urea peroxide. All these antiseptics should be used two to three times a day for 7–10 days. These antiseptics may be also used as cleansers for prevention of recurrences (two to three cleanings or baths/week) [26]. However, the last Cochrane review on impetigo, published in 2012, stated that there is a lack of evidence for the benefit of antiseptics [30]. Therefore, they should be considered as a complementary treatment. In the same Cochrane review, a total number of 68 trials, based on 5.578 evaluable patients, reporting on 50 different treatments, including placebo, were considered as clinically and statistically evaluable [30]. Topical antibiotics showed better cure rates than placebo in 6 studies on 575 patients [30]. There is evidence that topical fusidic acid and mupirocin are equally, or more, effective than oral antibiotics [30]. In 4 studies on 440 patients, fusidic acid and mupirocin showed to be of similar efficacy [30]. In 10 studies on 581 patients, topical mupirocin was shown to be slightly superior to oral erythromycin [30]. Furthermore, penicillin was inferior to erythromycin in 2 studies on 79 patients and cloxacillin in 2 studies on 166 patients [30]. In a study carried out in Mali, amoxicillin showed to be efficacious and safe [9]. In our personal clinical experience, also gentamicin sulphate is effective in bullous impetigo; furthermore, it is very well tolerated, and resistance is rare, in spite of the fact that this drug was marketed many years ago [2].

Topical antibiotics should not be used for more than 14 days, with the aim of minimizing the possibility of development of resistant strains, particularly staphylococci [26].

References

1. Axemo P, Freij L, Hadgu P, et al. Streptococcal types in impetigo and acute glomerulonephritis among children in Addis Ababa. Scand J Infect Dis. 1976;8:161–4.
2. Dagnew MB, Günther E. Epidemiology of communicable skin diseases in school children of a rural area in North Ethiopia. Dermatol Monatsschr. 1990;176:219–23.
3. Dagnew MB, Erwin G. Epidemiology of common transmissible skin diseases among primary school children in north-west Ethiopia. Trop Geogr Med. 1991;43:152–5.
4. Tewodros W, Muhe L, Daniel E, et al. A one-year study of streptococcal infections and their complications among Ethiopian children. Epidemiol Infect. 1992;109:211–5.
5. Accorsi S, Barnabas GA, Farese P, et al. Skin disorders and disease profile of poverty: analysis of medical records in Tigray, northern Ethiopia, 2005–2007. Trans R Soc Trop Med Hyg. 2009;103:469–75.
6. Mahé A, Prual A, Konaté M, et al. Skin diseases of children in Mali: a public health problem. Trans R Soc Trop Med Hyg. 1995;89:467–70.
7. Mahé A, N'Diaye HT, Bobin P. The proportion of medical consultations motivated by skin diseases in the health centers of Bamako (Republic of Mali). Int J Dermatol. 1997;36:185–6.
8. Mahé A, Cissé IA, Faye O, et al. Skin diseases in Bamako (Mali). Int J Dermatol. 1998;37:673–6.
9. Faye O, Hay RJ, Diawara I, et al. Oral amoxicillin vs. oral erythromycin in the treatment of pyoderma in Bamako, Mali: an open randomized trial. Int J Dermatol. 2007;46(Suppl 2):19–22.
10. Gbakima AA, Lebbie AR. The head louse in Sierra Leone: an epidemiological study among school children, in the Njala area. West Afr J Med. 1992;11:165–71.
11. Belcher DW, Afoakwa SN, Osei-Tutu E, et al. Non-group A streptococci in Ghanaian patients with pyoderma. Lancet. 1975;2:1032.
12. Belcher DW, Afoakwa SN, Osei-Tutu E, et al. Endemic pyoderma in Ghana: a survey in rural villages. Trans R Soc Trop Med Hyg. 1977;71:204–9.
13. Hogewoning A, Amoah A, Bouwes Bavinck JN, et al. Skin diseases among schoolchildren in Ghana, Gabon, and Rwanda. Int J Dermatol. 2013;52:589–600.
14. Kombaté K, Dagnra AY, Saka B, et al. Prevalence of methicillin-resistant *Staphylococcus aureus* in community-acquired skin infections in Lomé, Togo. Med Trop. 2011;71:68–70.
15. Whittle HC, Abdullahi MT, Fakunle F, et al. Scabies, pyoderma and nephritis in Zaria, Nigeria. A clinical and epidemiological study. Trans R Soc Trop Med Hyg. 1973;67:349–63.
16. Ogunbiyi AO, Daramola OOM, Alese OO. Prevalence of skin diseases in Ibadan, Nigeria. Int J Dermatol. 2004;43:31–6.
17. Emodi IJ, Ikefuna AN, Uchendu U, et al. Skin diseases among children attending the out patient clinic of the University of Nigeria teaching hospital, Enug. Afr Health Sci. 2010;10:362–6.
18. Okafor OO, Akinbami FO, Orimadegun AE, et al. Prevalence of dermatological lesions in hospitalized children at the University College Hospital, Ibadan, Nigeria. Niger J Clin Pract. 2011;14:287–92.
19. Kalu EI, Wagbatsoma V, Ogbaini-Emovon E, et al. Age and sex prevalence of infectious dermatoses among primary school children in a rural South-Eastern Nigerian community. Pan Afr Med J. 2015;20:182.
20. Nsanzumuhire H, Taplin D, Lansdell L. Pyoderma among Ugandan children. East Afr Med J. 1972;49:84–8.
21. Masawe AE, Nsanzumuhire H, Mhalu F. Bacterial skin infections in preschool and school children in coastal Tanzania. Arch Dermatol. 1975;111:1312–6.
22. Masawe AE, Nsanzumuhire H. Scabies and other skin diseases in pre-school children in Ujamaa villages in Tanzania. Trop Geogr Med. 1975;27:288–94.
23. Ferié J, Dinkela A, Mbata M. Skin disorders among school children in rural Tanzania and an assessment of therapeutic needs. Trop Doct. 2006;36:219–21.
24. Kristensen JK. Scabies and pyoderma in Lilongwe, Malawi. Prevalence and seasonal fluctuation. Int J Dermatol. 1991;30:699–702.
25. Kakande B, Gumedze F, Hlela C, et al. Focus on the top ten diagnoses could reduce pediatric dermatology referrals. Pediatr Dermatol. 2016;33:99–102.
26. Veraldi S, Çuka E, Gaiani F. Impetigo. In: Katsambas AD, Lotti T, Dessinioti C, D'Erme AM, editors. European handbook of dermatological treatments. 3rd ed. Berlin: Springer; 2015. p. 443–6.
27. Zeegelaar JE. Ulcerating pyodermas. In: Faber WR, Hay RJ, Naafs B, editors. Imported skin diseases. 2nd ed. Oxford: Wiley-Blackwell; 2013. p. 107–13.
28. Rollier R, Rollier M, Vivas M. Recurrent and slow, serpiginous and ulcerous pyodermitis. Bull Soc Fr Dermatol Syphiligr. 1968;75:853–6.
29. Veraldi S, Leigheb G, Morrone A. Atlas of dermatological diseases on dark skin. Turin: Medical Communications; 2007. p. 27–31.
30. Koning S, van der Sande R, Verhagen AP, et al. Interventions for impetigo. Cochrane Database Syst Rev. 2012;1:CD003261.

5 Superficial Fungal Infections

Mohamed Taha and Adel Botros Zaghloul

Fungal infections of the skin and nails are the most common and widespread group of all mycoses; they affect more than 20–25% of the world's population [1]. The incidence of cutaneous mycoses continues to increase, particularly in tropical countries because of the heat and humidity, whereas the prevalence of the causative species of fungi involved has shifted or changed due to migration and changes in socioeconomic status and lifestyle [2]. People with colored skin, especially deeply pigmented or black-skinned populations, show high frequency of superficial mycosis, which may reach up to 41.9% of all dermatoses seen, as has been reported from West Africa [3]; they are frequently registered also in tourists and travelers. The clinical pictures can be subdivided into infections that induce minimal or no inflammatory response, e.g., pityriasis versicolor, tinea nigra, or piedra, and those that induce cutaneous inflammation such as cutaneous candidosis and tinea.

5.1 Pityriasis Versicolor

Pityriasis versicolor (PV) is a superficial fungal infection seen worldwide, with high prevalence observed in hot and humid climates. It affects young adults 20–45 years old, but it is not uncommon also among the children and elderly. There is evidence indicating higher prevalence of PV in males due to increased sebaceous activity [4]. There are conflicting findings on the prevalence of PV in different ethnic populations; in some reports predilection for dark-skinned individuals is registered [5].

PV is caused by different species of genus *Malassezia*, revised into seven, *M. globosa*, *M. restricta*, *M. obtusa*, *M. sympodialis*, *M. furfur*, *M. slooffiae*, and *M. pachydermatis*, as a part of the normal flora of the skin. These are all lipophilic yeasts except *M. pachydermatis*. Although *M. globosa* is considered as the dominant causative agent of PV in many parts of the world [6, 7], several studies revealed that *M. sympodialis* and *M. furfur* are most predominant [8–10].

Clinically, PV is characterized by the presence of fine scaly patches or macules which may be hyper- or hypopigmented; they are usually asymptomatic, and only few patients complain of itching (Fig. 5.1). Most of them are located on the upper part of the trunk, neck, axillae, and arms, although they may be also found on unusual sites such as the lower extremities and face. PV is clinically diagnosed, confirmed through the presence of yeast cells and hyphae in scales taken from lesions after KOH preparation ("spaghetti and meatballs"). Culture is of no need for routine laboratory diagnosis; however, it can be done on media as SDA with olive oil or Dixon's medium with addition of chloramphenicol 0.005 and cycloheximide 0.05, then incubating at 31 °C for 10 days.

Topical azoles (ketoconazole, clotrimazole, or miconazole), ciclopirox, and terbinafine are effective in limited PV lesions. Only in widespread, often recurrent cases systemic therapies with ketoconazole 200 mg/day for 10 days, fluconazole 150 mg/week for 3 weeks, or itraconazole 200 mg/day for 7 days may be warranted. As prophylaxis itraconazole 2× 200 mg once per month is recommended [11, 12].

5.2 Superficial Candidosis

Superficial cutaneous candidosis (candidiasis) includes infections caused by different species of genus *Candida* clinically manifested as *intertrigo*, *diaper dermatitis*,

M. Taha (✉)
Department of Microbiology, Zagazig University, Zagazig, Egypt

A. B. Zaghloul
Cairo Skin Clinic, VD Hospital, Cairo, Egypt

C. E. Orfanos et al. (eds.), *Pigmented Ethnic Skin and Imported Dermatoses*, https://doi.org/10.1007/978-3-319-69422-1_5

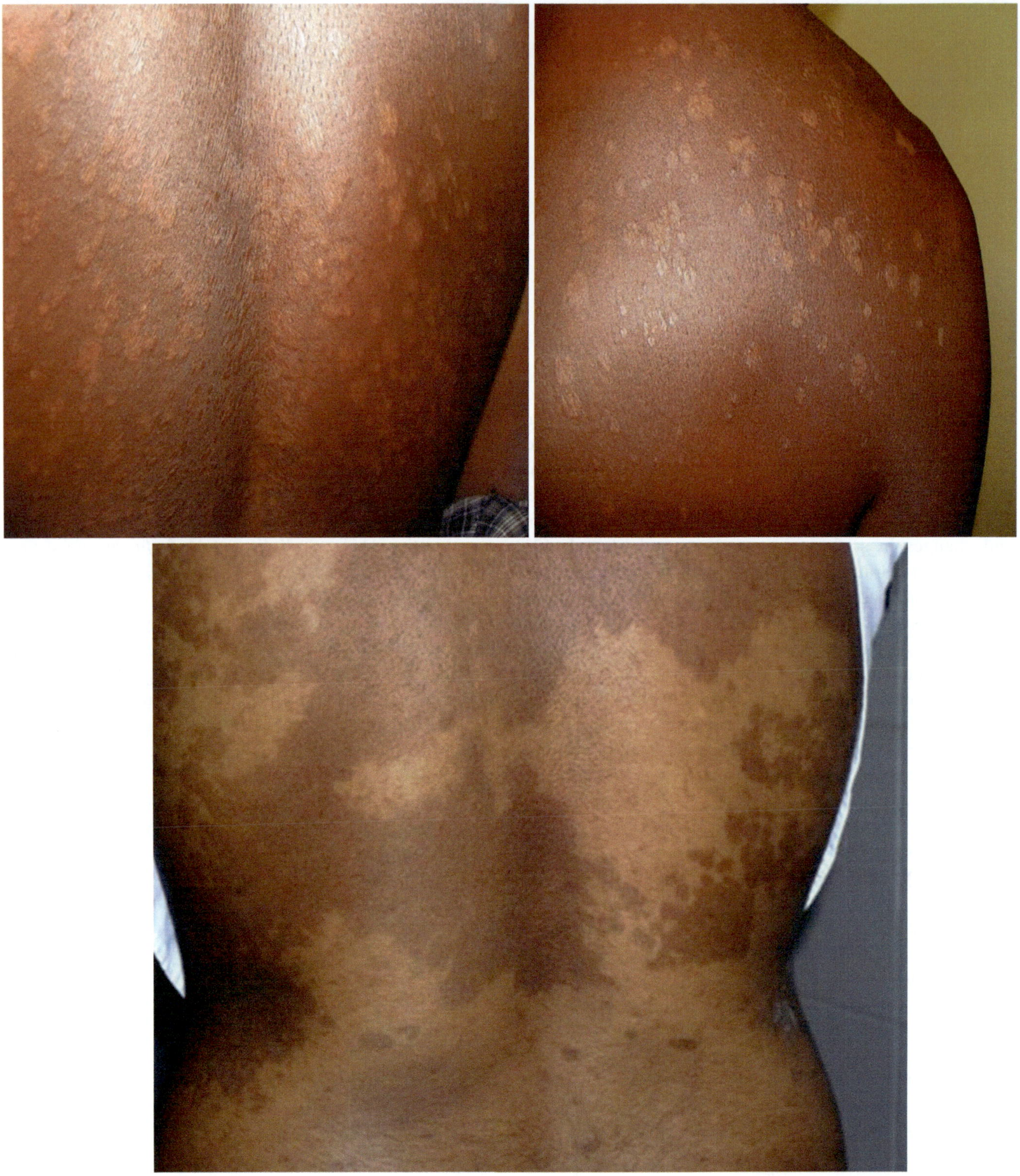

Fig. 5.1 Clinical types of *pityriasis versicolor*: Small hypochromic macules (up) and large hyperchromatic patches on the trunk of young adults

interdigital candidosis, and *candidal paronychia*. The yeast is found on the human skin or mucosa; the infection originates from the patient's own flora, seen in all age groups, often in neonates and the elderly [13]. The most common causative agent is *Candida albicans*; also *C. tropicalis, C. parapsilosis, and C. glabrata* can be considered in a few instances as a cause. Clinical disease starts when alteration of the host's immune response occurs and the saprophytic dimorphic yeast switches to the pathogenic mycelia form [14]. Mycological diagnosis is done by direct examination after KOH preparations which show blastoconidia and pseudohyphae and through cultures on SDA. *Candida albicans* is characterized by creamy pasty and smooth colonies on SDA, green colonies on chromogenic candida agar (CCA), and the presence of chlamydoconidia on cornmeal agar. Differentiation between *C. albicans* and non-albicans species can be done by growth on CCA, commercial kits such as API and Rap-ID, or by molecular methods, PCR [15] or MALDI-TOF [16].

Candida intertrigo starts as an erythematous pruritic rash with vesiculopustules, which may rupture and cause maceration and fissuring. The area involved has a scalloped border with white rim consisting of necrotic epidermis surrounding the erythematous macerated lesion. Satellite lesions are often found. The disease develops at moist skin of the submammary folds and the perigenital region, spreading out into the inner thigh area (Fig. 5.2). It occurs most frequently in adipose and diabetic patients and those confined to bed. *Diaper dermatitis* is clinically manifested as erythematous, eczematous patches affecting the gluteal, inguinal, perianal, and genital areas. In severe cases papules, erosions, and rarely ulcers may occur. *Interdigital candidosis*, *candidal paronychia*, and *onychomycosis* are also common. Chronic candidal paronychia shows erythema and swelling of the nail folds and brownish discoloration of the nail plate.

For treatment nystatin, azoles, and ciclopirox are usually used topically. Nystatin, fluconazole, and itraconazole are also administered orally for severe recalcitrant cases. The topical combination of an antimycotic or antiseptic compound with a moderate-strength topical corticosteroid is a good choice in inflammatory intertriginous yeast infections [17].

5.3 Tinea (Dermatophytosis)

Tinea (ringworm) is a superficial fungal infection of the skin, hair, and/or nails caused by dermatophytes, classified in *tinea capitis*, *corporis*, *manum*, *cruris*, *pedis*, and *unguium*. The predominant dermatophytes vary with the geographic area; most species are found worldwide, while some others are geographically restricted such as *T. yaoundi* and *T. soudanense* in Africa and *T. concentricum* in Western Pacific and Malaysia. Today, five or six species account for most dermatophytoses globally [18]. Their distribution is influenced by the changing patterns of migration, growth of tourism, and socioeconomic conditions. Significant changes of the dermatophyte spectrum were observed especially in *tinea capitis*: increased incidence of *T. tonsurans* in Southwest and East of the USA, reaching up to 60–91% due to immigration from Latin America; disappearance of *M. audouinii* and *T. schoenleinii* from Central Europe; as well as strongly increased prevalence of *M. canis* in Germany and West Europe [19, 20]. *M. canis* followed by *T. violaceum* and *T. tonsurans* were found to be predominant in China [21]. Increase of *M. canis* and *T. violaceum* is found in the Middle East [22]. *T. violaceum* is still the commonest cause of tinea capitis in India, Southeast Asia, and some regions of Africa (Ethiopia) [23] and in South America (Brazil). Generally, there is a predominance of anthropophilic dermatophytes with *T. rubrum* on the top [24] with the exception of a few countries.

Tinea capitis may be found as a noninflammatory form presenting round demarcated scaly patches with hair loss showing short stubble of broken hairs, caused by *Microsporum* species (Fig. 5.3). Scattered irregular patches of alopecia with indistinct borders show black dots when the hairs break off at the level of scalp leaving stubs (Fig. 5.4a). This form is caused by *T. tonsurans*, *T. violaceum*, and *T. soudanense*. Advanced infection with *M. canis* and *T. verrucosum* with strong host response showing boggy, purulent plaques with abscess formation has been called *kerion*. Some patients with kerion may develop extensive lymphadenopathy [25]. *Favus* is the most severe, inflammatory form of tinea capitis usually caused by *T. schoenleinii* (Fig. 5.4b). It presents as thick, yellow crusts composed of hyphae and skin debris (scutula) which may cover large areas of scalp. In chronic infections scarring alopecia often develops.

Tinea corporis involves the trunk, legs, and arms characterized by annular scaly lesions; also arcuate, gyrate, or circinate shapes may occur (Fig. 5.5a, b). Scales may be lessened or absent if topical corticosteroids were used (tinea incognito). Lesions can also be vesicular, granulomatous, or verrucous in appearance. Associated symptoms include pruritus and burning. Clinical variants of tinea corporis include *tinea profunda* and *tinea imbricate*; sometimes hypermelanotic lesions are seen in pigmented skin (Figs. 5.6 and 5.7). The first results from an excessive inflammatory response to a dermatophyte, corresponding to a kerion on the scalp, may have granulomatous or verrucous appearance, whereas the second is a rare form caused by *T. concentricum* presenting as large, concentric, scaly lesions resembling erythema gyratum repens [26]. Widespread, generalized tinea is observed in immune-compromised patients.

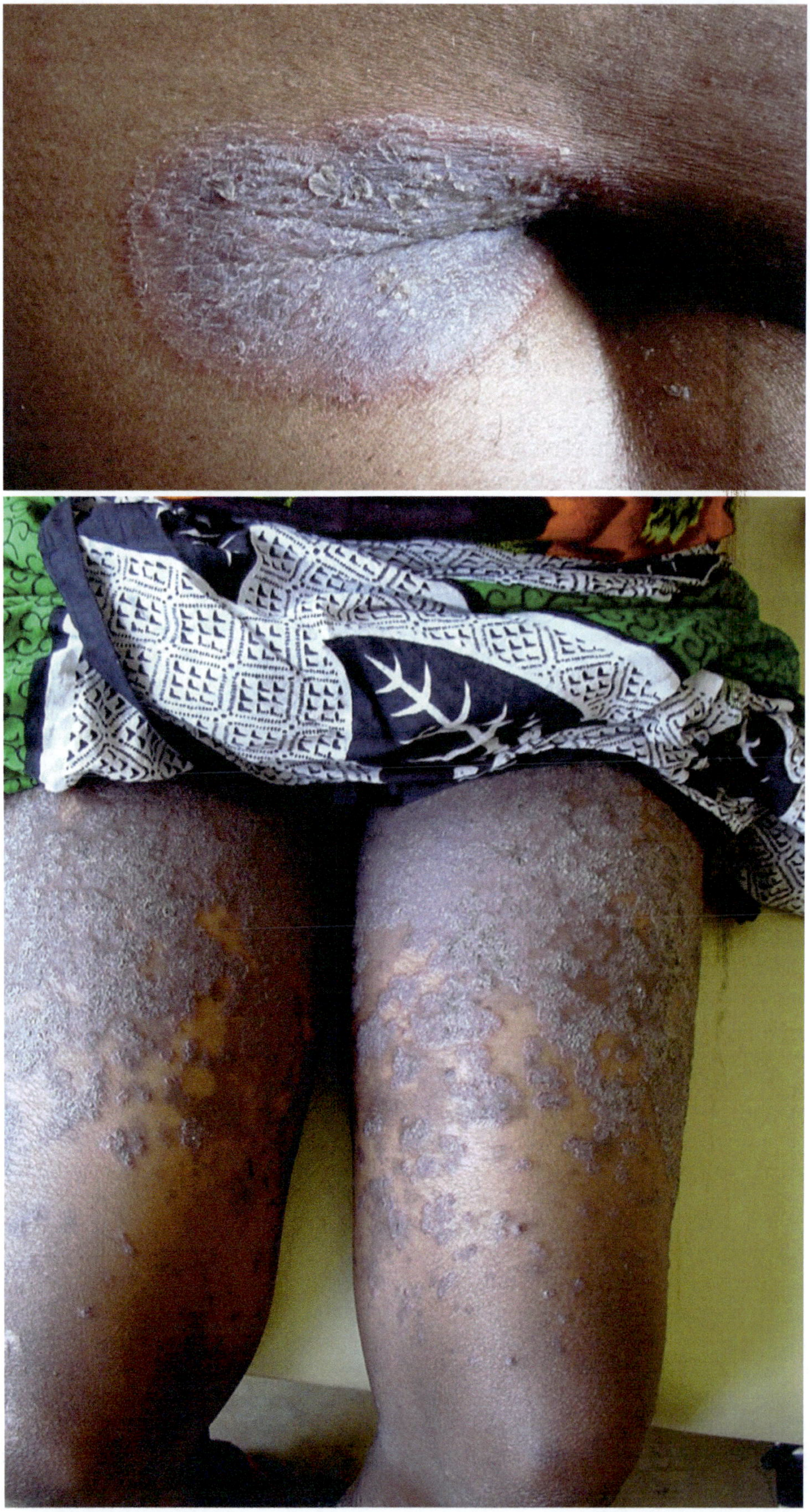

Fig. 5.2 *Candidosis*: Intertrigo type and widespread cutaneous dissemination in a young female (Uganda)

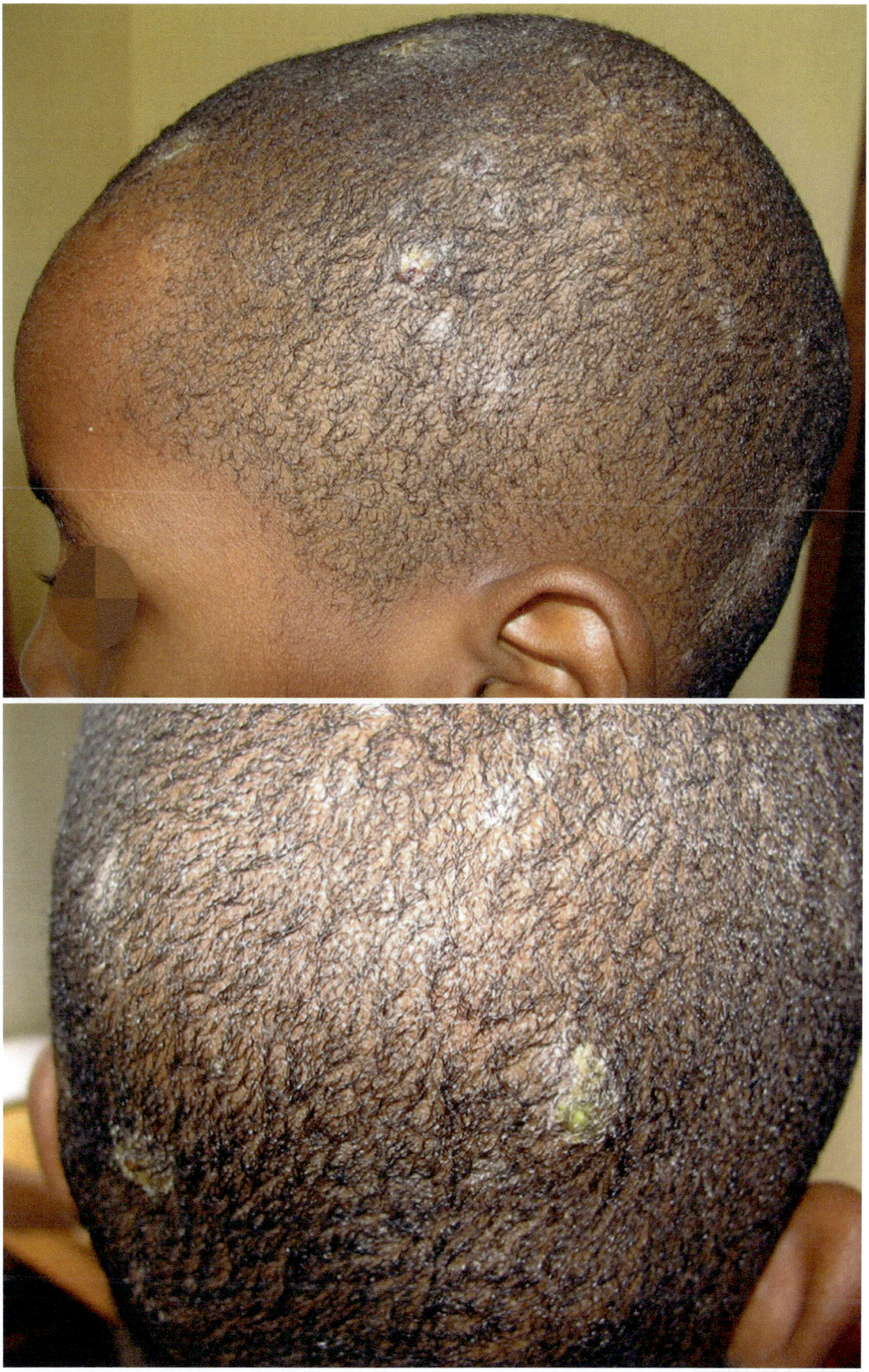

Fig. 5.3 Typical scaly patches of *tinea capitis* (*M. canis*) in young school boys in Tanzania

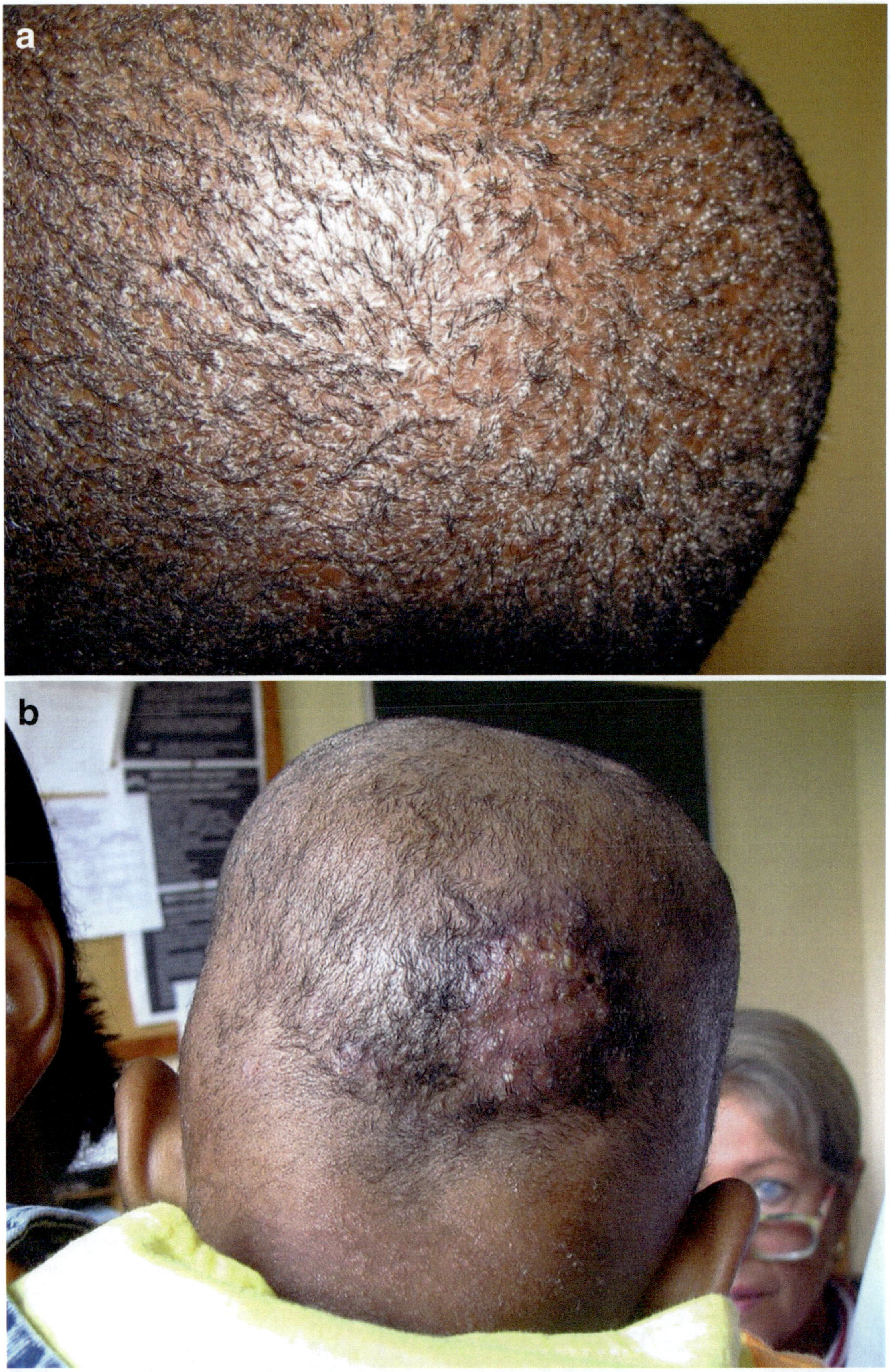

Fig. 5.4 *Tinea capitis.* (**a**). Diffuse fine scaling of the scalp with atrophic scarring alopecia; (**b**). Favus-like inflammatory lesion in a 6-month-old baby (possibly *T. schoenleinii*)

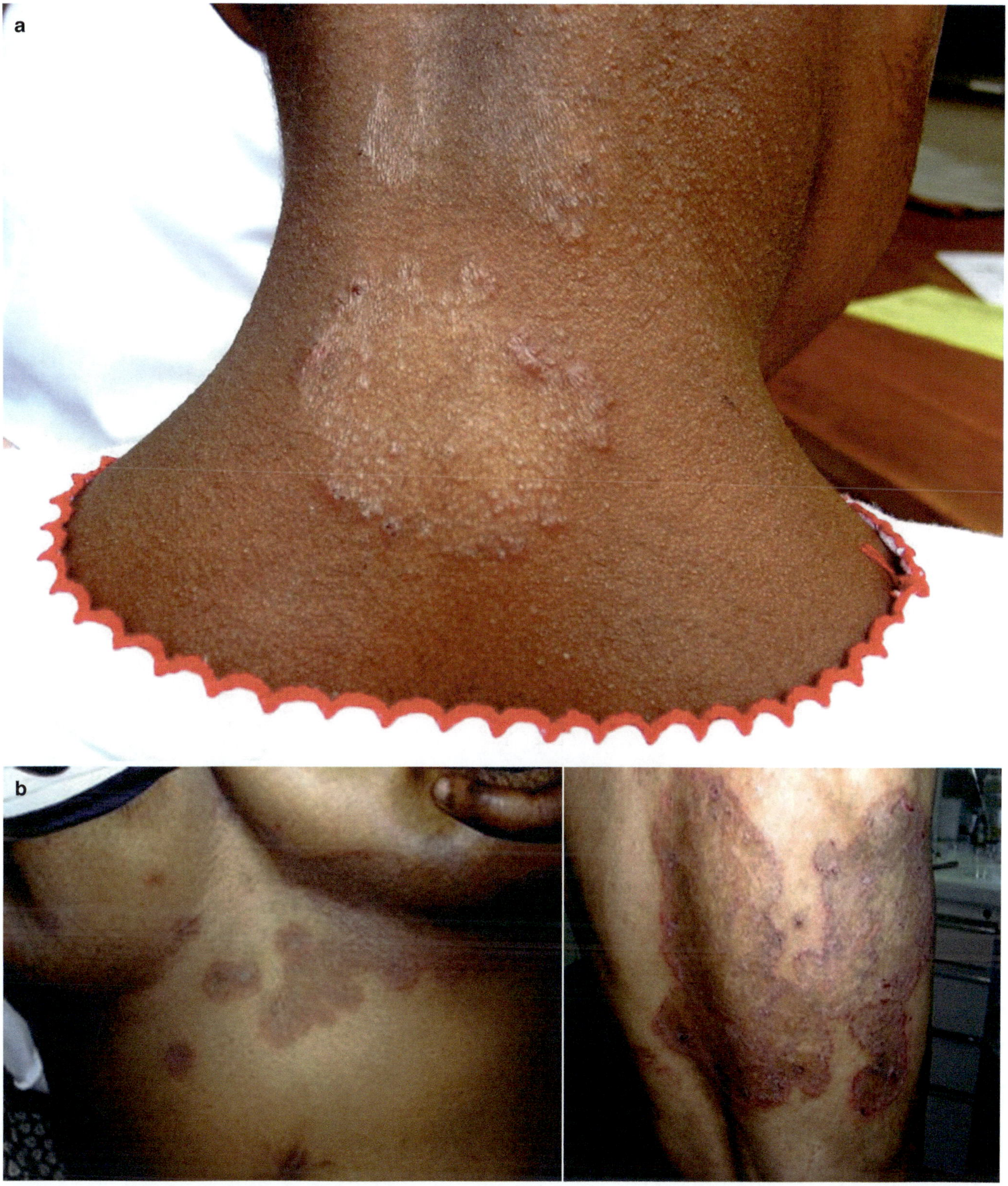

Fig. 5.5 *Tinea corporis:* (**a**). Lesion on the neck in a young school girl, *T. rubrum* (Tanzania); (**b**). Submammary *tinea corporis*, *M. canis* (Egypt); (**c**). *Tinea corporis* on the trunk, *T. rubrum* (Egypt)

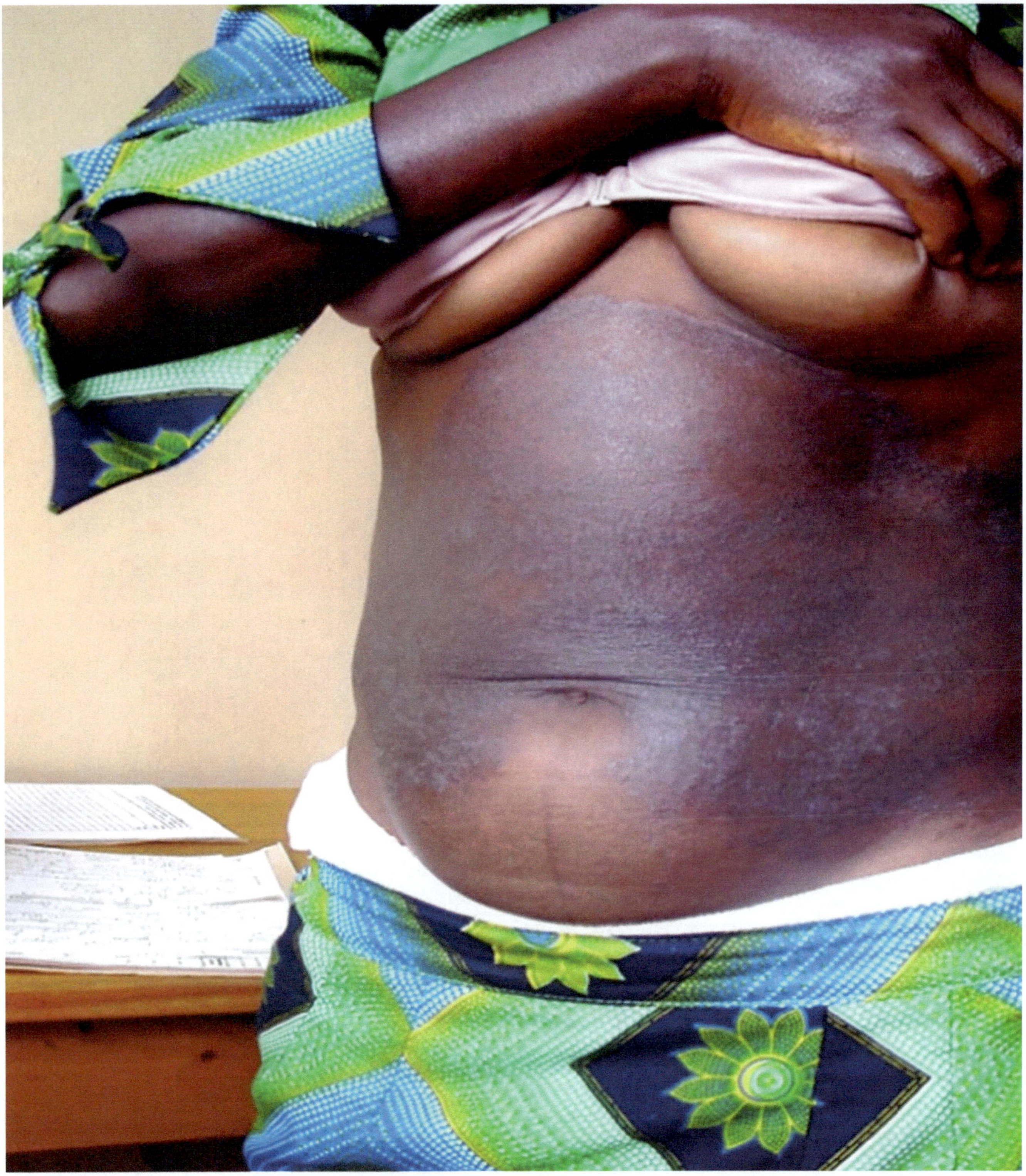

Fig. 5.6 Hypemelanotic *tinea corporis* (most likely *T. violaceum* or *T. soudanense*) in a young female (Uganda)

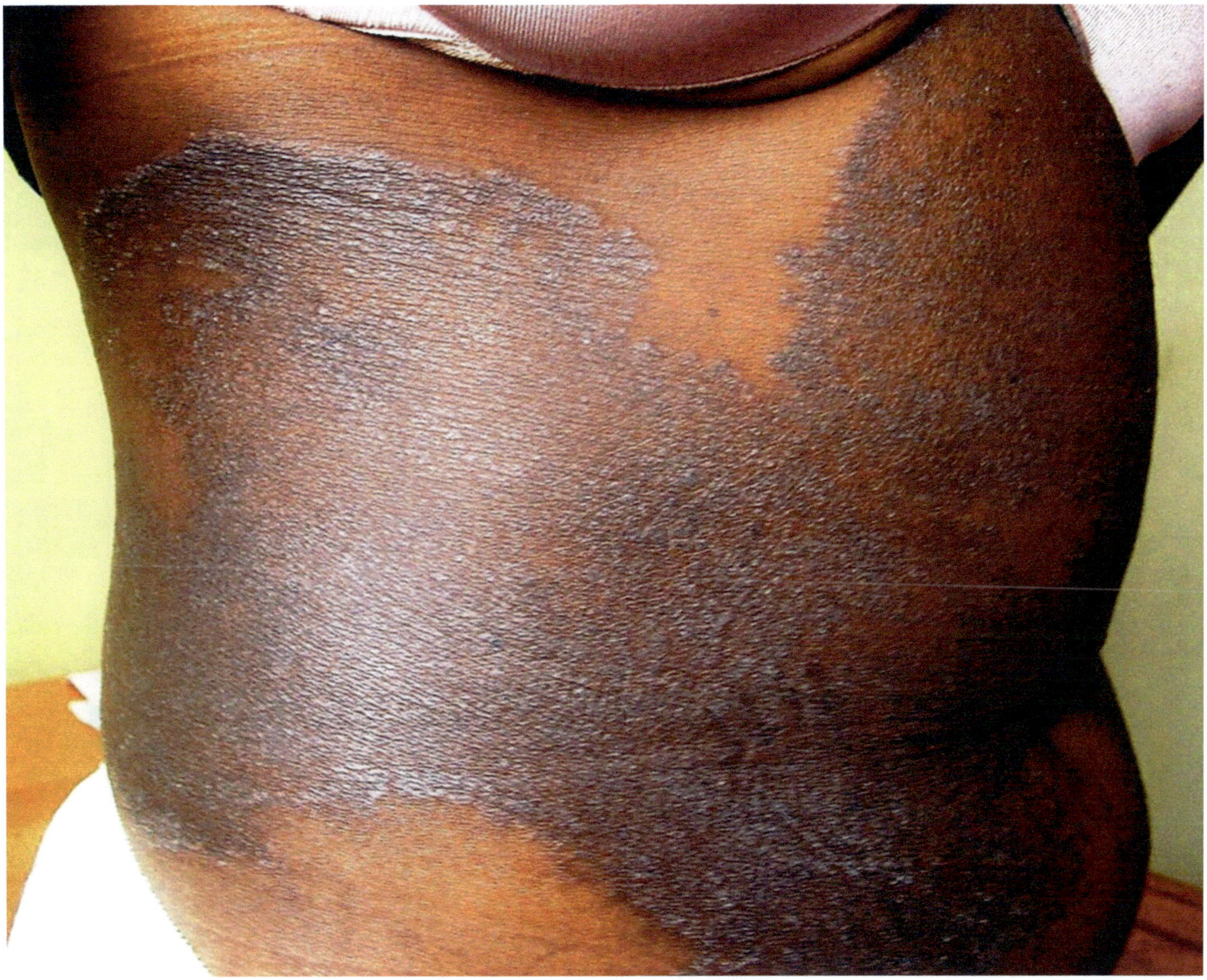

Fig. 5.7 Hypermelanotic *tinea corporis* (unidentified agent)

Tinea manum involves the palms and interdigital spaces caused by *T. rubrum*, *T. mentagrophytes*, and *E. floccosum*. Non-dermatophyte fungi, *Scytalidium dimidiatum* and *S. hyalinum*, can also cause the disease which is usually unilateral, noninflammatory, and showing diffuse hyperkeratosis. The differentiation of the individual agent is well possible in in vitro cultures (Fig. 5.8).

Tinea barbae is typically caused by the zoophilic *T. mentagrophytes* var. *mentagrophytes*, *T. verrucosum*, and *M. canis*. Due to the zoophilic organisms and the large number of terminal hair follicles in the affected area, the clinical presentation tends to be severe, with intense inflammation and multiple follicular pustules. Abscesses, sinus tracts, bacterial superinfection, and even a kerion-like lesion may develop. Noninflammatory forms caused by *T. violaceum* and *T. rubrum* resembling tinea corporis are also known.

Tinea cruris is an infection of the inguinal region, in particular the inner aspects of the upper thighs and crural folds, with extension on the abdomen and buttocks in more severe cases. While occurring worldwide in men and women, it is more common in tropical environment, caused

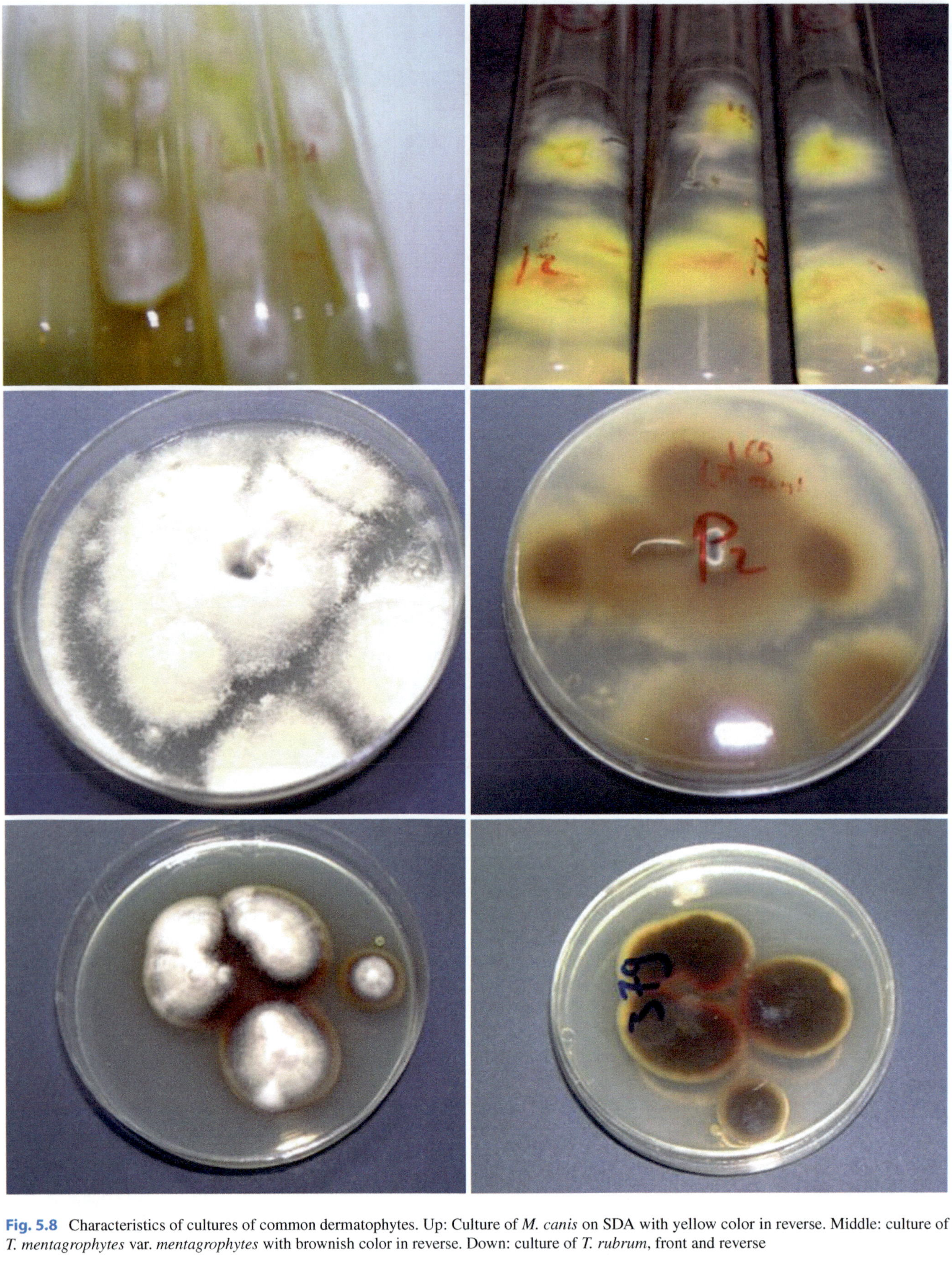

Fig. 5.8 Characteristics of cultures of common dermatophytes. Up: Culture of *M. canis* on SDA with yellow color in reverse. Middle: culture of *T. mentagrophytes* var. *mentagrophytes* with brownish color in reverse. Down: culture of *T. rubrum*, front and reverse

by *T. rubrum*, *T. mentagrophytes*, and *E. floccosum*. Characteristic lesions are sharply demarcated with a raised erythematous scaly advancing borders, often with containing vesicles or pustules. Beginning as circinate in shape, the lesion may become serpiginous, remain unilateral, or become bilateral and symmetric *tinea pedis*. The feet are a common location for dermatophyte infection in adults, affecting both sexes. The lack of sebaceous glands and the moist environment created by wearing occlusive shoes are contributing factors. It may involve the entire plantar surface covered with fine white scaling, sometimes vesicles and pustules, or be limited in the interdigital spaces, characterized by oozing, maceration, and fissuring (Fig. 5.9a) (Table 5.1).

Treatment of dermatophyte infections depends on the clinical type and the age of the patient. Topical antifungal preparations such as Whitfield ointment, sulfur in creams, and Castellani solution are still used in some developing countries for their low cost, but azoles, allylamine, terbinafine, and ciclopirox are being gradually introduced. Systemic management is needed in tinea capitis, chronic tinea corporis, tinea pedis, and others which do not respond to topical treatment. Particular care is to be taken for management in children [27, 28].

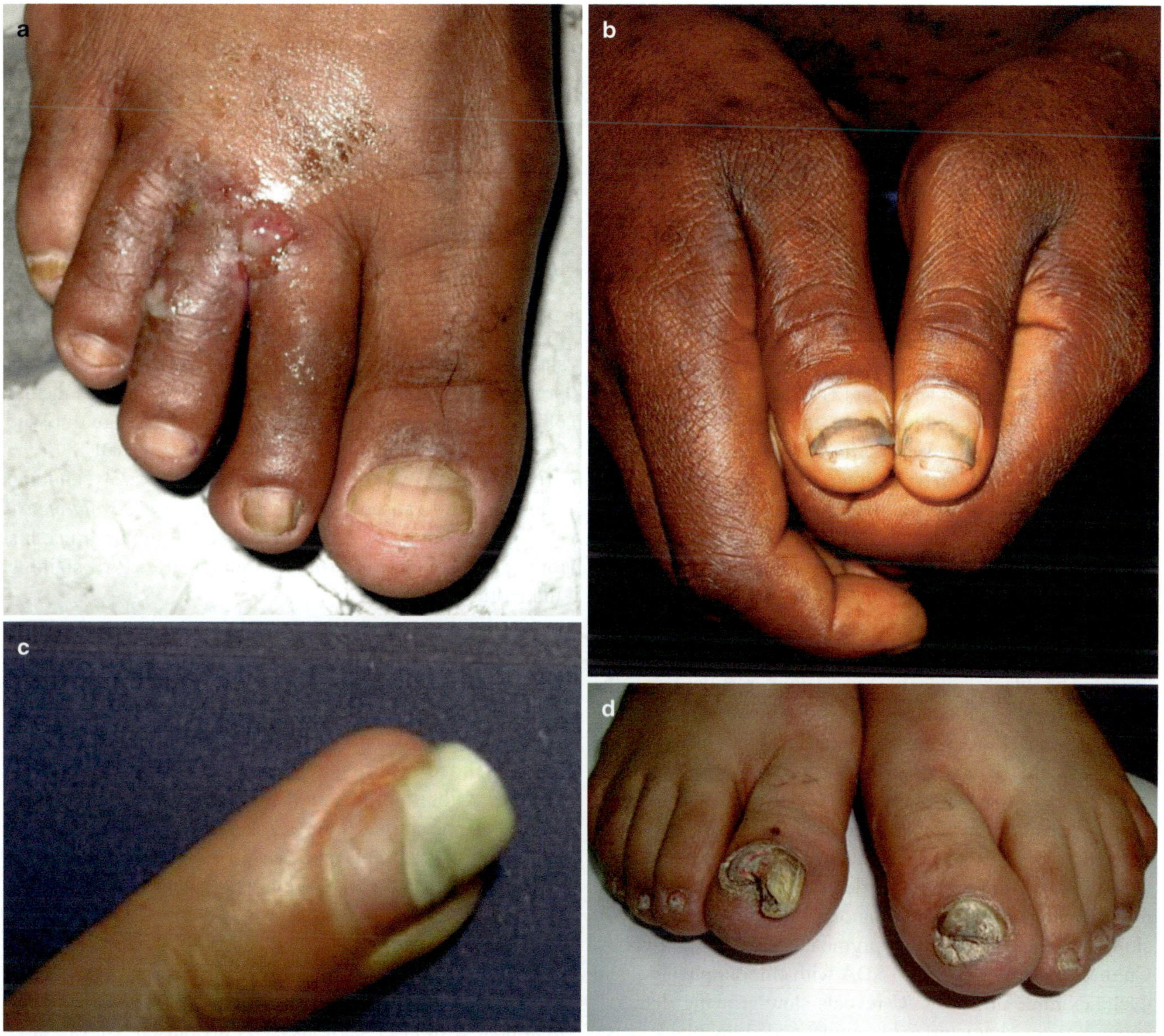

Fig. 5.9 (**a**). *Tinea interdigitalis*, superinfected; (**b**). *Proximal subungual onychomycosis* (PSO); (**c**). *Distal lateral subungual onychomycosis* (DLSO); (**d**). *Total dystrophic onychomycosis* (TDO)

Table 5.1 Treatment of tinea

Clinical type	Topical	Systemic
Tinea capitis	Shampoo as adjunct management	Griseofulvin (ultra-micronized suspension), 10 mg/kg/day for 6–12 weeks Terbinafine suspension, 7 mg/kg/day, for 6 weeks Fluconazole, 8 mg/kg once a week, for 8 weeks Itraconazole, 5 mg/kg/day, for 6 weeks
Tinea corporis/ tinea cruris	Azoles 2% 1×/day for 1–2 weeks Terbinafine 1–2×/day for1–4 weeks Ciclopirox 2×/day for 4 weeks	Terbinafine, 250 mg/day, for 2–4 weeks Fluconazole, 150 mg once/week, for 2–4 weeks Itraconazole, 200 mg/day, for 1 week
Tinea pedis/ tinea manum	Azoles 2% 1×/day for 6 weeks Terbinafine 1% 1×/day for 6 weeks Ciclopirox 0.77% 2×/day for 1 week	Terbinafine, 250 mg/day, for 2 weeks Fluconazole, 150 mg once a week, for 2–4 weeks Itraconazole, 200 mg 2×/day, for 1 week

5.4 Tinea Nigra

Tinea nigra is an uncommon superficial fungal infection of the stratum corneum caused by *Hortaea werneckii*, in rare instances by *Stenella araguata*, having a predilection for tropical and subtropical regions. Most reports originate from Latin America [29, 30] and Asia [31]. The disease may present as an imported condition from endemic regions to temperate climate zones, usually affecting children and young adults [32, 33]. *H. werneckii* belongs to the order *Capnodiales* in *Ascomycota* and is a halotolerant and halophilic fungus with its natural habitat in hot climate zones, in areas containing high concentration of salt as beach soil, salt pans, and seawater [34]. *Hortaea* has the ability to survive in high salinity and low pH; it thrives on the skin by production of polysaccharides and feeds by assimilation of decomposed lipids. The black color of the lesions results from the accumulation of melanin-like granules in the fungus. Clinically, the lesions are characterized by light brown to black macules which gradually transform into non-scaly patches. The affected areas lack erythema or induration; they usually occur on the palm or soles and may reach 1–5 cm in diameter. Most cases are unilateral. Using dermatoscope, wispy brown strands or pigmented spicules are recognizable and differentiate it from melanoma. KOH preparations of skin scrapings reveal dark pigmented branching hyphae. Culture of skin scrapings on SDA with chloramphenicol and cycloheximide at 25–28 °C reveals slow-growing dematiaceous isolates characterized by moist and shiny black yeast-like that turns to moldy phase with greenish black color. Microscopically, brown septated hyphae and conidia with transverse septa are seen. Dermoscopy may be useful for diagnosis [35].

Treatment is usually done using keratolytic agents such as urea, salicylic acid, and Whitfield ointment, but topical azoles such as miconazole and ketoconazole, terbinafine, or ciclopirox are preferred over several weeks [36]. Most oral antifungal drugs are not effective.

5.5 Onychomycosis

Onychomycosis represents 30% of superficial mycosis and 50% of all nail disorders, with increasing incidence in the elderly. It is caused by dermatophytes such as *T. rubrum* and *T. mentagrophytes*, by yeasts especially *C. albicans* and *C. parapsilosis*, and rarely by non-dermatophyte molds [37–39]. While dermatophytes are the most common agents in temperate countries, non-dermatophytes predominate in hot climate zones. The site and pattern of invasion lead to different clinical types: one may clinically classify [40] a *distal lateral subungual onychomycosis* (DLSO), a *superficial white onychomycosis* (SWO), a *proximal subungual onychomycosis* (PSO), the *endonyx* type, and a *total dystrophic onychomycosis* (TDO; see Fig. 5.9b–d). DLSO is the most common type, characterized by yellowish brown discoloration of the nail plate with onycholysis and subungual hyperkeratosis; PSO is rare and appears as onycholysis showing white to creamy or yellow crumply patches on the proximal part of the nail surface, while TDO affects the nail plate and often also the surrounding periungual tissue. Candidal onychomycosis mostly presents the DLSO type. Mixed types of onychomycosis may occur. Rarely, endonyx infections are caused by *T. violaceum* and *T. soudanense*. Diagnosis is done by conventional KOH preparations, histological examination of nail clippings after PAS staining, and cultures.

Onychomycosis may represent an independent and important predictor for development of diabetic foot syndrome and foot ulcer [40] and is difficult to cure due to the high rate of recurrences [41]. Topical treatment is sufficient for infected nail plates, while oral management is recommended for adequate cure when the nail matrix is affected. Other factors, such as the number of the affected toenails/fingernails, their size, multi-morbidity of the patient, drug interactions, as well as the pathogen agent involved, are also considered. The selection of the antifungal drug depends on the fungus isolated, especially in infections caused by non-dermatophytes (see Table 5.2) [42, 43].

The combination of topical and/or systemic antimycotic treatment with laser sessions (0.65 ms pulsed Nd:Yag laser, two to three sessions every 3 weeks) is a frequently used regimen, despite the absence of valid supporting study data.

5.6 Piedra

Piedra is a nonaggressive fungal infection characterized by nodular lesions formed around the hair shaft [44]. *White piedra* occurs more frequently in regions of tropical and mild climates such as in South America, the Middle East, India, Southeast Asia, Africa, parts of Japan, Europe, and Southeast USA. Causative agents are species of *Trichosporon*, a yeast widely distributed in nature, possibly also a part of normal flora of the human skin and nail. White piedra nodules can be seen by the naked eye usually localized in the distal part of the hair shaft and be easily detached. Between the nodules is the hair shaft, normal; no broken hairs are seen. The nodules can affect scalp hair, beard, moustache, and also pubic hairs [45]. In children the disease is more prevalent in the scalp hair [46]. Examination of infected hairs with 10% KOH shows the fungal elements as rounded arthrospores. Culture can be done by inoculating affected hair on Sabouraud's dextrose agar (SDA) and incubating for 7 days at 30 °C. The yeast appears as creamy rough and heaped with wrinkled surface colonies (Fig. 5.10). Individuals with black skin were

Table 5.2 Topical and systemic treatment of onychomycosis

Management	Fingernails	Toenails
Topical: Ciclopirox 8%	Once daily for 24 weeks	Once daily for 48 weeks
Topical: Amorolfine 5%	Once or twice weekly for 24 weeks	Once or twice for 36–48 weeks
Systemic: Fluconazole	150 mg/week for more than 6 months	150 mg weekly for more than 6 months
Systemic: Itraconazole	Pulse management: 200 mg twice/day for 1 week /month (2–3 pulses)	Pulse management, 200 mg/day for 12 weeks or 4–6 pulses
Systemic: Terbinafine	250 mg/day for 6 weeks	250 mg/day for 12 weeks

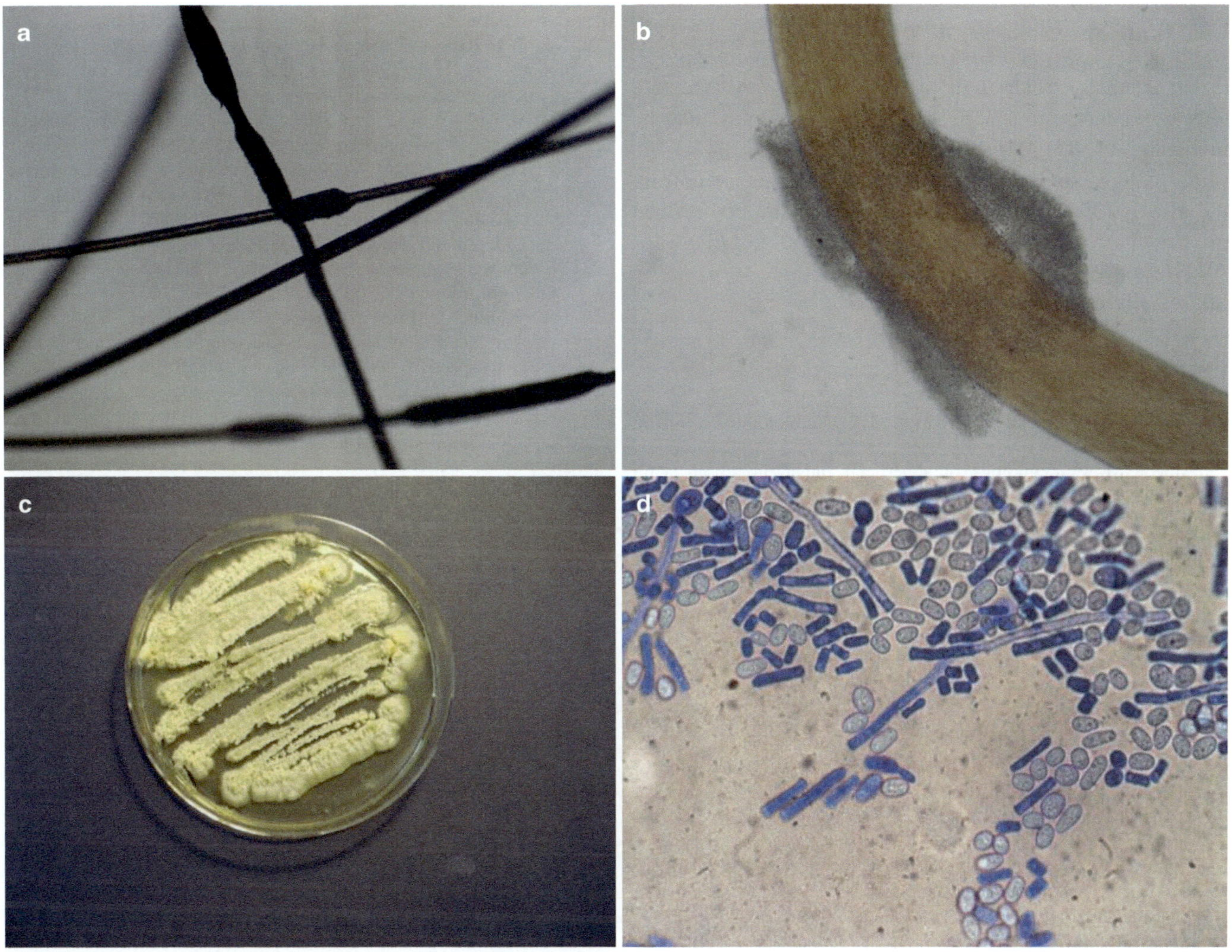

Fig. 5.10 *White piedra*: (**a**) nodules with different lengths; (**b**) nodules surrounding the hair shaft; (**c**) *Trichosporon* spp. colonies on SDA; (**d**) microscopic characters of *Trichosporon* spp. isolated from white piedra

found to be more frequently affected, preferably males 18–35 years old [46]. Best treatment is to shave the hair along with washing with 2% ketoconazole shampoo once a week for 3 months. A combination of an oral azole antifungal for 1 month together with topical treatment for 2–3 months may be also effective.

Black piedra is caused by an ascomycetous dematiaceous fungus, *Piedra hortae* [44]. It is prevalent in tropical countries, especially in South America and Southeast Asia. Due to world travel, it may occur sporadically in other regions. Adults tend to be significantly more often affected than children, without preference of gender. The fungus is keratolytic and forms its ascostroma within the nodules. KOH preparations of nodules show colored hyphae with arthroconidia, while mature nodules show banana-shaped asci with elongated ascospores. Culture of nodules on Sabouraud's medium containing cycloheximide reveals slow growth of compact brown-black colonies with brown thick-walled septated hyphae, chlamydoconidia, asci, and ascospores. On clinical examination the affected hairs generally show four to eight small dark brown and hard nodules strongly cemented to the hair shaft. Scalp hair is the most often affected, although beard, moustache, and pubic hairs may also be involved [44, 47]. Mixed black and white piedra in the same patient has been observed [48]. Shaving or cutting the affected hair and washing by azole shampoos proved to be ineffective; oral terbinafine 250 mg/day for 3–6 weeks was found successful [49].

References

1. Havlickova B, Cziaka C, Friedrich M. Epidemiological trends in skin mycoses worldwide. Mycoses. 2008;51:412–5.
2. Ameen M. Epidemiology of superficial fungal infections. Clin Dermatol. 2010;28:197–201.
3. Bari AU, Khan MB. Pattern of skin diseases in black Africans of Sierra Leone, West Africa. J Clin Diagn Res. 2007;5:361–8.
4. Heidrich D, Daboit TC, Stopiglla CD, et al. Sixteen years of pityriasis versicolor in metropolitan area of Porto Alegre, Southern Brazil. Rev Inst Med Trop Sao Paulo. 2015;57:277–80.
5. Kallini JR, Raiz F, Klachemoune A. Tinea versicolor in dark-skinned individuals. Int J Dermatol. 2014;53:137–41.
6. Crespo-Erchiga V, Ojeda Marios A, Vera Casano A, et al. *Malassezia globosa* as the causative agent of pityriasis versicolor. Br J Dermatol. 2000;143:799–804.
7. Gaitanis G, Velegraki A, Alexopoulos EC, et al. Distribution of *Malassezia species* in pityriasis versicolor and seborrhoeic dermatitis in Greece. Typing of the major pityriasis versicolor isolate *M. globosa*. Br J Dermatol. 2006;154:854–9.
8. Gupta AK, Kohli Y, Faergemann J, et al. Epidemiology of *Malassezia* yeasts associated with pityriasis versicolor in Ontario, Canada. Med Mycol. 2001;39:199–206.
9. Ghahfarokhi MS, Abyaneh MR. Rapid identification of Malassezia furfur from other Malassezia species. A major causative agent of pityriasis versicolor. Iran J Med Sci. 2004;29:36–9.
10. Khafagy A, El Fangary M, Shahin M, et al. Identification of *Malassezia* species isolated from pityriasis versicolor patients. Egypt J Dermatol Vener. 2006;26:9–14.
11. Velegraki A, Cafarchia C, Gaitanis G, et al. *Malassezia* infections in humans and animals: pathophysiology, detection, and treatment. PLoS Pathog. 2015;11:e1004523.
12. Mayser PA, Preuss J. Pityriasis versicolor: Aktuelles zu einer alten Erkrankung. Hautarzt. 2012;63:359–67.
13. Martin ES, Elwski BE. Cutaneous fungal infections in the elderly. Clin Geriatr Med. 2002;18:59–75.
14. Mayer FL, Wilson D, Hube B. *Candida albicans* pathogenicity mechanisms. Virulence. 2013;4:119–28.
15. Cornet M, Sendid B, Fradin C, et al. Molecular identification of closely related *Candida* species using two ribosomal intergenic spacer fingerprinting methods. J Mol Diagn. 2011;13:12–22.
16. Stevenson LG, Drake SK, Shea YR, et al. Evaluation of matrix-assisted laser desorption/ionization-time of flight mass spectrometry (MALDI-TOF) for identification of clinically important yeast species. J Clin Microbiol. 2010;48:3482–6.
17. Nenoff P, Krüger C, Paasch U, et al. Mycology—an update part 3: dermatomycosis: topical and systemic therapy. J Dtsch Dermatol Ges. 2015;13:387–410.
18. Ali R. Ecology and epidemiology of dermatophyte infections. J Am Acad Dermatol. 1994;31:S21–5.
19. Seebacher C, Bouchara JP, Mignon B. Updates on the epidemiology of dermatophytes. Mycopathologia. 2008;166:335–52.
20. Nenoff P, Kruger C, Ginter-Hanselmayer C, et al. Mycology—an update, Part 1: dermatomycosis: causative agents, epidemiology and pathogenesis. J Dtsch Dermatol Ges. 2014;12:764–77.
21. Zhu M, Li L, Wang J, et al. Tinea capitis in Southeastern China: a 16-year survey. Mycopathologia. 2010;169:235–9.
22. El Fangary M, Saudy W, Nabil T, et al. Prevalence of dermatophytes, yeasts, non dermatophyte moulds isolated from skin, hair, and nail fungal infections in the 6th October City-Giza Egypt. Egypt J Dermatol Venerol. 2011;31:5–10.
23. WildemanualY, Lekassu R, Chryssanthou E, et al. Prevalence of tinea capitis in Ethiopian school children. Mycoses. 2005;48:137–41.
24. Faure-Cognet O, Fricker-Hidalgo H, Pelloux H, et al. Superficial fungal infections in a French teaching hospital in Grenoble area: retrospective study on 5470 samples from 2001 to 2011. Mycopathologia. 2016;181:59–66.
25. Seebacher C, Abeck D, Brasch J, et al. Tinea capitis. J Dtsch Dermatol Ges. 2006;12:1085–91.
26. Bonifaz A, Archer-Dubon A, Saul A. Tinea imbricata or Tokelau. Int J Dermatol. 2004;43:506–10.
27. Dias MF, Quaresma-Santos MV, Bernardes-Filho F, et al. Update on therapy for superficial mycoses. An Bras Dermatol. 2013;88:764–74.
28. Chen X, Jiang X, Yang M et al. Systemic antifungal therapy for tinea capitis in children. Cochrane Database Syst Rev. 2016;(5):CD004685.
29. Severo LC, Bassanesi MC, Londero AT. Tinea nigra: report of four cases observed in Rio Grande do Sul (Brazil) and a review of Brazilian literature. Mycopathologia. 1994;126:157–62.
30. Perez C, Colella MT, Olaizola C, et al. Tinea nigra: report of twelve cases in Venezuela. Mycopathologia. 2005;160:235–8.
31. Uezato H, Gushi M, Hagiwara K, et al. A case of tinea nigra palmaris in Okinawa, Japan. J Dermatol. 2006;33:23–9.
32. Rezusta A, Gilaberte Y, Betran A, et al. Tinea nigra: a rare imported infection. J Eur Acad Dermatol Venereol. 2010;24:89–91.
33. Pegas JR, Crado PR, Lucena SK. Tinea nigra: report of two cases in infants. Pediatr Dermatol. 2003;20:315–7.
34. Elsayed A, Mowafy AM, Soliman HM, et al. Characterization of new strains of *Hortaea werneckii* isolated from salt marshes of Egypt. J Basic Appl Sci. 2016;3:350–6.

35. Maia Abinader MV, Cavalh Maron CM, Araújo LO, et al. Tinea nigra dermoscopy: a useful assessment. J Am Acad Dermatol. 2016;74:121–2.
36. Bonifaz A, Badali H, de Hoog GS, et al. Tinea nigra by *Hortaea werneckii*, a report of 22 cases from Mexico. Stud Mycol. 2008;61:77–82.
37. Summerbell RC, Cooper E, Bunn U, et al. Onychomycosis: a critical study of techniques and criteria for confirming the etiologic significance of non dermatophytes. Med Mycol. 2005;43:39–59.
38. Nenoff P, Ginter-Hanselmayer G, Tietz HJ. Fungal nail infections—an update: part I—prevalence, epidemiology, predisposing conditions and differential diagnosis. Hautarzt. 2012;63:30–8.
39. Martínez-Herrera EO, Arroyo-Camarena S, Tejada-García DL, et al. Onychomycosis due to opportunistic moulds. An Bras Dermatol. 2015;90:334–7.
40. Baran R, Hay RJ, Tosti A, et al. A new classification of onychomycosis. Br J Dermatol. 1998;139:567–71.
41. Gupta AK, Scher RK. Management of onychomycosis an North American perspective. Dermatol Ther. 1997;3:58–65.
42. Roberts DT, Taylor WD, Boyle J. Guidelines for treatment of onychomycosis. Br J Dermatol. 2003;48:402–10.
43. Gupta AK, Simpson FC. New therapeutic options for onychomycosis. Expert Opin Pharmacother. 2012;13:1131–42.
44. Cortes A, Orfanos CE. Piedra. In: Orfanos CE, Happle R, editors. Hair and hair diseases. Heidelberg: Springer; 1999. p. 745–9.
45. Kalter DC, Tachen JA, Cernoch PL, et al. Genital piedra: epidemiology, microbiology and therapy. J Am Acad Dermatol. 1986;14:982–93.
46. Rios X, Rojas RF, Hincapi ML. Eight white piedra pediatric cases. Rev Assoc Colomb Dermatol. 2012;20:175–80.
47. Combra CE, Santos RV. Black piedra among the Zoró Indians from Amazônia (Brazil). Mycopathologia. 1989;107:57–60.
48. Khatu SS, Poojary SA, Nagpur NG. Nodules on the hair: a rare case of mixed piedra. Int J Trichol. 2013;5:220–3.
49. Gip L. Black piedra: the first case treated with terbinafine (Lamisil). Br J Dermatol. 1994;130:26–8.

6 Subcutaneous and Deep Fungus Infections

Pietro Nenoff, Mohamed Taha, and Peter Mugisha

Moulds and yeasts, so-called dimorphic fungi, cause a number of cutaneous infections. Transmission takes place via inoculation of the agents as a result of injury, e.g. following barefoot walking in semiarid to arid areas, or through haematogenous spread, mostly from the lung. Examples for inoculation mycoses are mycetomas caused by various fungi and bacteria, chromoblastomycoses due to melanized or brown-pigmented fungi and sporotrichosis due to *Sporothrix schenckii*, a ubiquitous occurring dimorphic fungus. Secondary cutaneous involvement after haematogenous transmission occurs in blastomycosis, coccidioidomycosis, cryptococcosis and histoplasmosis, frequently in immunosuppressed patients.

Subcutaneous or deep fungal infections of the skin are considered diseases of the poor, as a part of the increasing number of neglected conditions in hot climate zones, which affect people living under low-level socioeconomic conditions and hygienic standards.

6.1 Mycetoma

Mycetoma (also called Madura foot) is a chronic putrid, nodular, sinus-forming infection of the subcutaneous tissue predominantly on the feet; it represents a chronic inflammation with the development of painless granulomas growing to form tumour-like masses. Destruction of deep tissues, such as muscles, bones, joints and rarely tendons, may result. The causative agents of *actinomycetomas* are bacteria, whereas *eumycetomas* are caused by various moulds. In rare cases mixed bacterial and fungal infections may occur. Eumycetomas and actinomycetomas are an infection of the poor carrying not only medical significance; they are frequently a medical and social challenge [1]. In distinct rural areas of Africa, but also in Asia (India) and Middle America (Mexico), mycetomas lead to socioeconomic consequences involving the affected patients, their families and the societies in general [2]. Mycetoma has been added by the WHO to its list of neglected tropical disease priorities [3].

6.1.1 Epidemiology

Barefoot-walking populations in India and in tropical countries of Africa may be affected by moulds and develop mycetomas. In the western part of the African continent, in Senegal and Sierra Leone, the infection is endemic; also Sudan is considered a mycetoma homeland. The African countries with endemic incidence are summarized as "trans-African mycetoma belt," the geographic region between Senegal and Sudan extending between the 15° and 30° North latitude, dry areas with sparse rainfall (50–1000 mm/year). There is an associate to distinct species of fungi and actinomycetes in the environment, depending on the amount of rainfall, temperature and humidity. In addition, mycetomas occur in the central and northern parts of South America, in French Guiana, in Guatemala and in Mexico [4]. Rarely, cases of mycetoma were reported in Bulgaria and Romania due to *Scedosporium apiospermum* and *Madurella mycetomatis*. In the USA *Scedosporium boydii* represents the most frequent pathogen. Overall, eumycetomas occur in tropical and subtropical climate zones, whereas actinomycetomas are more frequently seen in North Africa, e.g. in Morocco and Tunisia.

P. Nenoff (✉)
Laboratory for Medical Microbiology, Mölbis, Germany
e-mail: nenoff@mykologie-experten.de; Pietro.nenoff@gmx.de

M. Taha
Department of Microbiology, Zagazig University, Cairo, Egypt

P. Mugisha
Department of Dermatology, Mbarara University of Science and Technology, Mbarara, Uganda

C. E. Orfanos et al. (eds.), *Pigmented Ethnic Skin and Imported Dermatoses*, https://doi.org/10.1007/978-3-319-69422-1_6

6.1.2 Pathogenesis

The most common causative agent of eumycetoma is *Madurella mycetomatis*; actinomycetomas are caused by actinomycetes belonging to the genera *Actinomyces*, *Nocardia* and *Streptomyces* species. The agents are introduced by small traumas, usually through thorns into the subcutaneous tissue of barefoot-walking people. Distinctive for both eumycetoma and actinomycetoma is the formation of microcolonies of the organisms in the vital tissue, seen on their surface as 0.3–1 mm grains. Black, red, white (pale) or yellow grains are easily visible under the light microscope, also with naked eye in some cases, depending on the type of the causative agent [3] (see Table 6.1).

6.1.3 Clinical Picture

After inoculation of the mould, a painless tumour-like subcutaneous swelling occurs, spreading into the skin and the underlying deep tissues, finally leading to destruction of muscles, tendons and bones. The time course of the overall development takes a period of months or years. First symptoms are localized at the affected lower extremities, mostly the feet, where nodule and hard subcutaneous plaques are palpable. The superficial nodules often have multiple sinuses producing serosanguineous discharge, either spontaneously or following pressure.

Mycetomas affect mostly healthy, young adult males, although no age is exempted. The general condition of the patient remains unaffected; fever is rare. Although the lesions are generally found on the lower extremities (80%), mostly on the soles and the foot arches (Fig. 6.1), other localizations such as the scalp, shoulders, neck, arms, and hands may be also affected, especially in endemic areas (Fig. 6.2). In Togo, West Africa, 19 out of 30 patients suffered from a mycetoma of the feet; further affected body sites were the trunk, the head (scalp) and the arms. In India, actinomycetomas due to *Nocardia asteroides* have been described also affecting the neck, breast, back, buttocks, elbows, palms, groins, vulva, thighs and knee. The clinical picture of the two types of mycetoma is similar. Initial subcutaneous nodules occur in both (Fig. 6.3). In malnutrition and other illnesses in the tropics associated with immunodeficiency (HIV infection, leishmaniasis, repeated courses of malaria), fast proliferation of the microorganisms may occur; in late stages the limbs show bizarre deformations, leading to disablement, joint ankylosis, fibrosis, pain and limb atrophy.

For differential, other infections such as pseudomycetoma caused by dermatophytes, chromomycosis, hyalohyphomycosis etc. have to be considered. Botryomycosis represents a mycetoma-like infection of the skin due to staphylococci and/or streptococci and might also develop in individuals living in Europe and North America. Also, noninfectious conditions such as podoconiosis, malignant tumours of the soft tissue or bones and Kaposi's sarcoma may mimic mycetoma.

Madurella mycetomatis may be cultured in vitro for diagnostic purposes (Fig. 6.4); the formation of grains is a distinctive clinical feature [5], and their examination from the discharge may be helpful for diagnosis of tumour-like giant mycetomas occasionally seen (Fig. 6.5). Deep punch biopsies show epithelioid cell granulomas together with microcolonies or grains and druses, e.g. conglomerates of septated and branched, radially arranged broad hyphae, sometimes with vacuole formation. The grains show round, sometimes oval, or kidney-like configurations. In case of suspected actinomycetoma, Gram staining should be done.

Table 6.1 Colour of eumycetoma grains dependent from the species of the causative mould

Grains	Infective agents
Dark and black	*Madurella mycetomatis, Madurella grisea, Exophiala jeanselmei, Medicopsis romeroi, Leptosphaeria senegalensis, Leptosphaeria tompkinsii, Curvularia lunata*
Pale or unstained	*Pseudallescheria boydii, Acremonium* spp., *Fusarium* spp., *Neotestudina rosatii, Aspergillus nidulans, Aspergillus flavus, Microsporum ferrugineum, Microsporum audouinii, Microsporum langeronii*
White	*Scedosporium apiospermum*
Yellow-brown	*Nocardia brasiliensis, Nocardia caviae, Actinomadura madurae, Streptomyces somaliensis*
Yellow	*Pleurostomophora ochracea*

6.1.4 Management

Management comprises the application of systemic antibacterial agents for *actinomycetoma* and of antifungals in combination with surgical procedures for *eumycetoma*. If systemic antifungal treatment is not available or affordable, painless mycetomas progress to limb destruction and force amputation. Late stages can be complicated by secondary infections resulting in bacteraemia and septicaemia with lethal consequences.

For *eumycetomas* itraconazole 2 × 200 mg/day is recommended over 1–1½ year; terbinafine 250–500 mg/day may be an alternative. Experiences with posaconazole and vori-

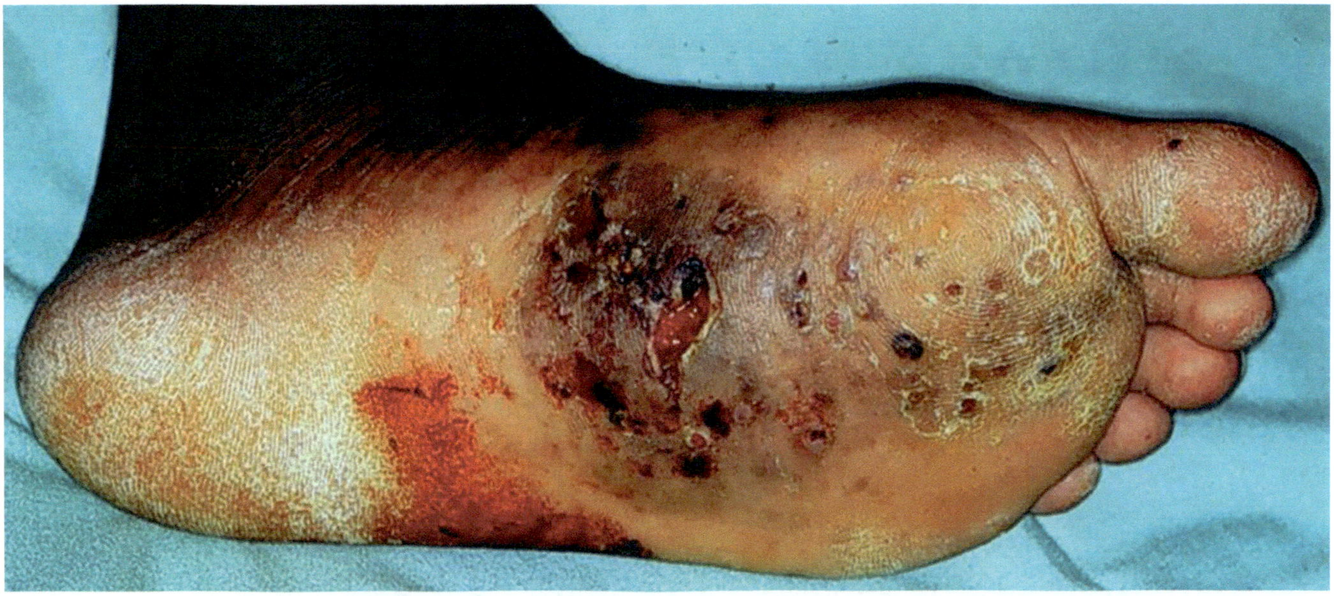

Fig. 6.1 A 17-year-old refugee from Senegal: *Eumycetoma* of the foot, showing hard nodules with multiple sinuses producing serosanguineous discharge. Nodules and grains at the instep

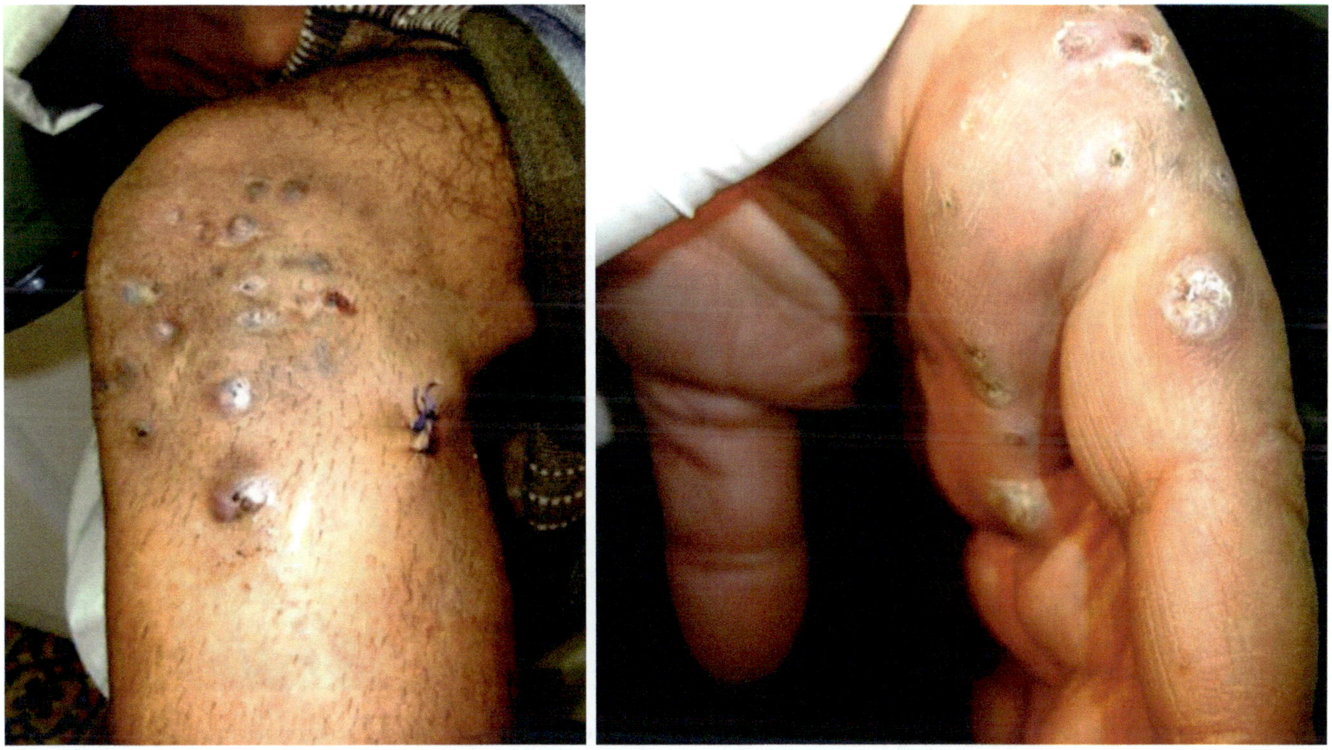

Fig. 6.2 Left: *Eumycetoma* of knee with multiple nodules in a patient from Yemen; right: multiple and firm nodules on the hand

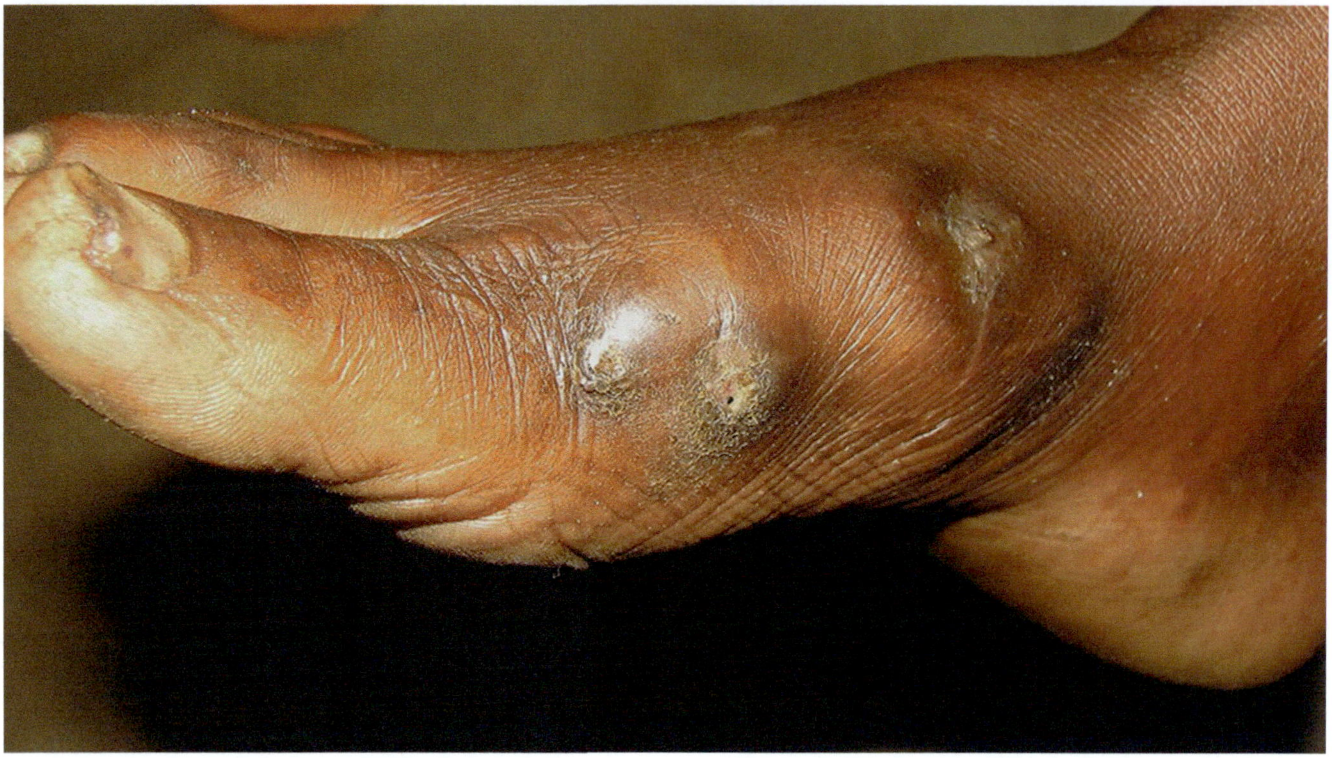

Fig. 6.3 Subcutaneous nodules of *mycetoma* on the dorsum pedis. A 20-year-old male in Tanzania

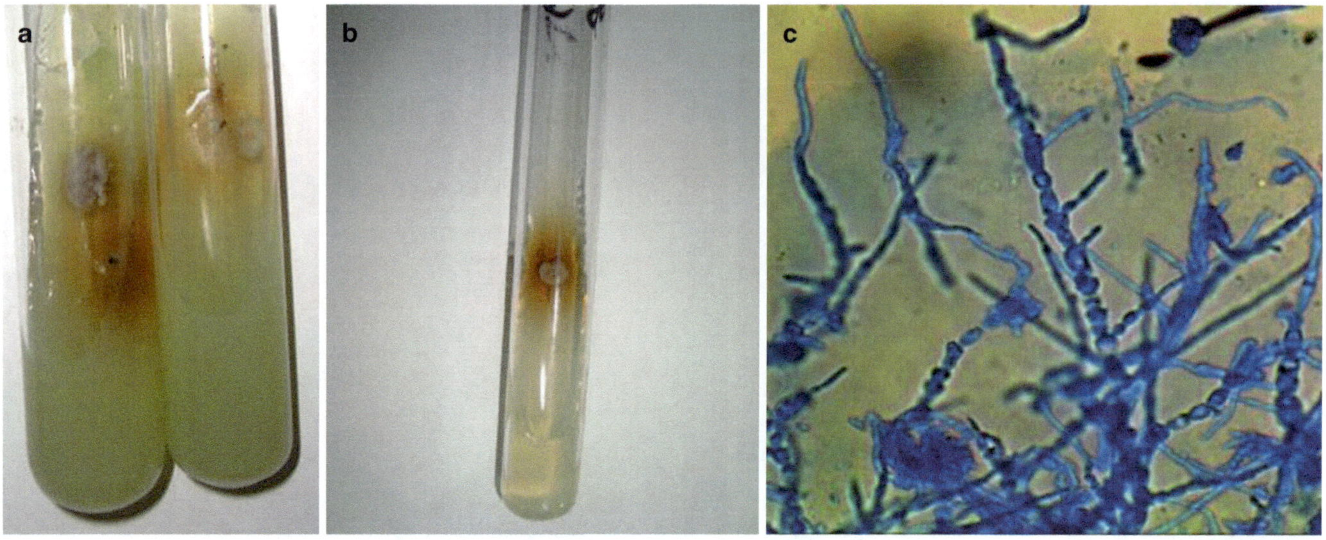

Fig. 6.4 (**a**–**c**) *Madurella mycetomatis*. (**a**) Primary culture from granules on Sabouraud's dextrose agar (Dermasel) showing diffuse brown pigment and grey to light brown thallus; (**b**) colonies on potato dextrose medium developing brown pigment; (**c**) microscopic picture showing hyphae and chlamydoconidia

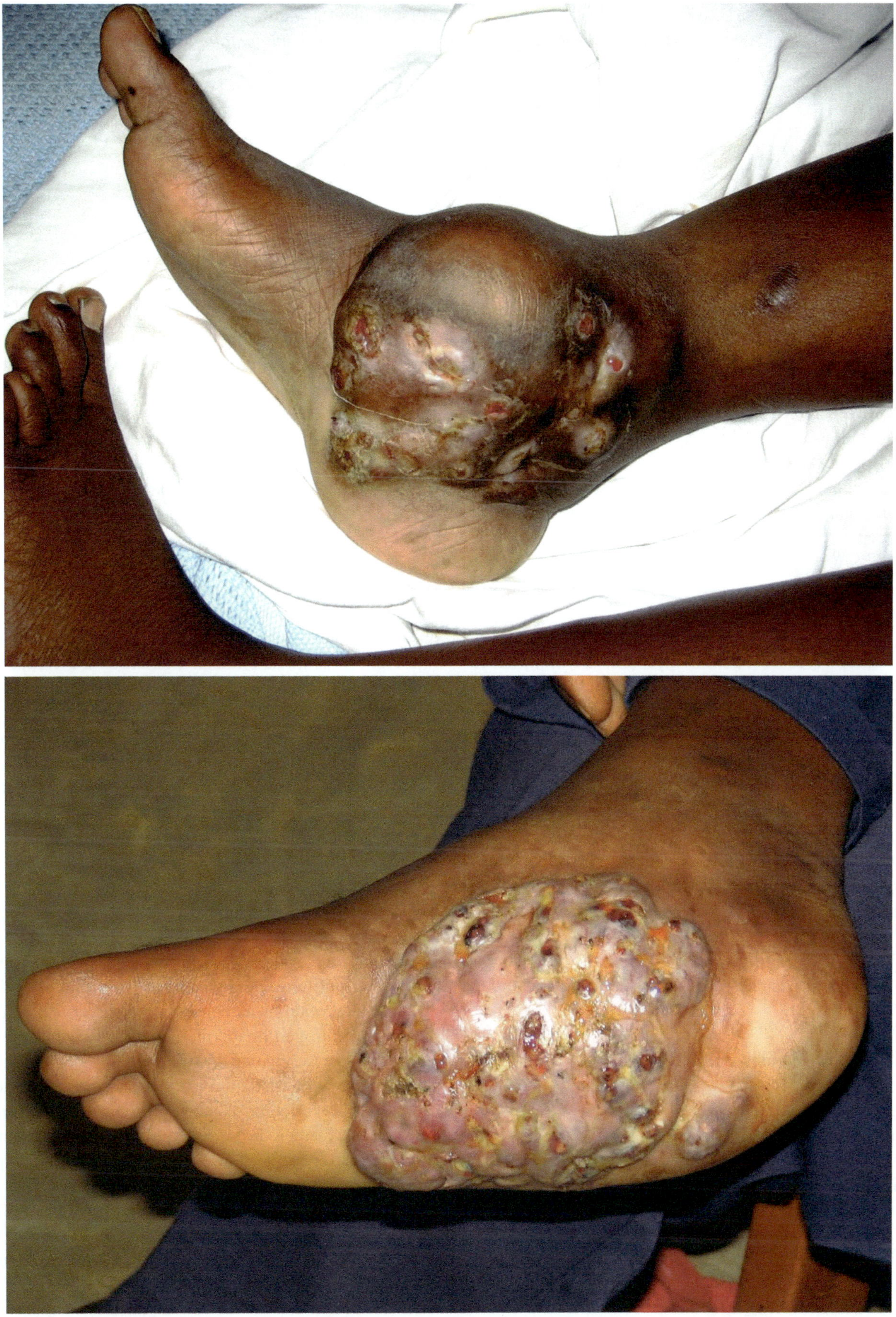

Fig. 6.5 *Giant mycetomas* with exophytic growth and serosanguineous discharge on the feet of young males (Kilimanjaro District, Tanzania). Black grains are seen on the surface

Table 6.2 Treatment of actinomycetomas

	Antimicrobial management
Actinomadura madurae	Streptomycin sulphate 1 g/day + dapsone 100–200 mg/day
Nocardia spp. *Streptomyces somaliensis* *Actimomyces pelletieri*	Trimethroprim-sulfamethoxazole 80/400 to 160/800 mg/day + dapsone 100–200 mg/day
Pronounced, widely spread actinomycetoma	Trimethroprim-sulfamethoxazole 80/400 to 160/800 mg/day + dapsone 100–200 mg/day over several months until clearing + amikacin i.v. 15 mg/kg bw/day, 3–5 pulses every 2–3 w

conazole are limited. Large tumourous eumycetomas often show delayed response to antifungals and should be removed surgically. Also *actinomycetomas* respond with delay to treatment (see Table 6.2). Overall recurrences are common and amputations unavoidable.

As a prophylaxis, walking barefoot in highly endemic countries should be avoided whenever simple shoes are available and affordable. Early wound disinfection is mandatory.

6.2 Chromoblastomycosis

Chromoblastomycosis or chromomycosis is a chronic subcutaneous fungal infection of the skin generally presented in form of verrucous or vegetating lesions on uncovered areas caused by melanized or brown-pigmented fungi of the order *Chaetothyriales* [6]. The disease occurs worldwide, although endemic areas are concentrated in the tropics and subtropics with higher prevalences in Latin America (Brazil and Venezuela), in Central America and in Africa. Cases were also seen in other countries, e.g. India, China, Japan, Sri Lanka, Malaysia and Australia. Affected patients are usually outdoor labourers, farmers or individuals routinely not wearing shoes, with history of inoculation of plant thorns or wood splinters. Most cases of chromoblastomycosis occur among males aged 30–60 years. There is no ethnic predisposition.

6.2.1 Pathogenesis

A large number of melanized (dematiaceous) fungi have been associated with chromoblastomycosis. The most common pathogen is *Fonsecaea pedrosoi* which is considered as the primary etiological agent worldwide, found in 80% of the total set of strains [7]. Pathogenesis depends on the conversion of hyphae into the muriform phase (sclerotia) with more melanin content. *F. pedrosoi* is saprophytic in nature, living in soil and plant debris. It was isolated from thorns of the tropical plant *Mimosa pudica*. The second most frequently isolated agent is *Cladophialophora carrionii*, geographically found in dry, desert regions in Latin America and Africa, isolated from cactus plants. Other less common pathogens include *Phialophora verrucosa* [8], *Rhinocladiella aquaspersa* and *Exophiala jeanselmei*, *spinifera* and *dermatitidis*.

6.2.2 Clinical Picture

Chromoblastomycosis is a benign, chronic skin infection believed to originate in traumatic inoculation of the causative agents, primarily involving the arms and legs. Papules of different sizes expand over several months to evolve into several types of skin lesions leading to polymorphic appearances. Hyperkeratotic nodules with verrucous surface and tumour-like masses are seen together with plaque-like lesions of various shapes and sizes, reddish to violaceous in colour (Fig. 6.6); regressional hypopigmented scarring areas may develop spontaneously or after therapies (Fig. 6.7). On their surface there are usually black dots of fungal cells and necrotic tissue, leading to ulcerations and scarring. Haematogenous or lymphogenous spread may lead to metastatic lesions and secondary bacterial infection to lymphatic obstruction and elephantiasis.

Diagnosis is made clinically, based on the characteristic features of the infection. Direct microscopy with KOH scrapings collected from crusts or black dots to detect the muriform phase of the fungus and cultures may be helpful to identify the *F. pedrosoi* as the causative agent (Fig. 6.8). Dematiaceous isolates are obtained after 10–15 days of incubation. Molecular identification based on PCR methods is suitable for identification of *F. pedrosoi* strains.

6.2.3 Management

Treatment of chromoblastomycosis consists of long-term courses of antifungal chemotherapy often combined with physical interventions as conventional surgery, cryosurgery with liquid nitrogen or thermotherapies. Itraconazole 200–400 mg/day or terbinafine 250–500 mg/day, respectively, for about 1 year will be required for clearing. Also, other triazoles such as voriconazole and posaconazole are seemingly more potent in their in vitro activity against the agents of chromoblastomycosis; however, only a few therapeutic experiences exist, and the higher cost makes their use unfavourable in many endemic areas. A case of extensive and severe chromoblastomycosis with therapeutic failure under first choice antifungals and good response to voriconazole has been recently reported [9].

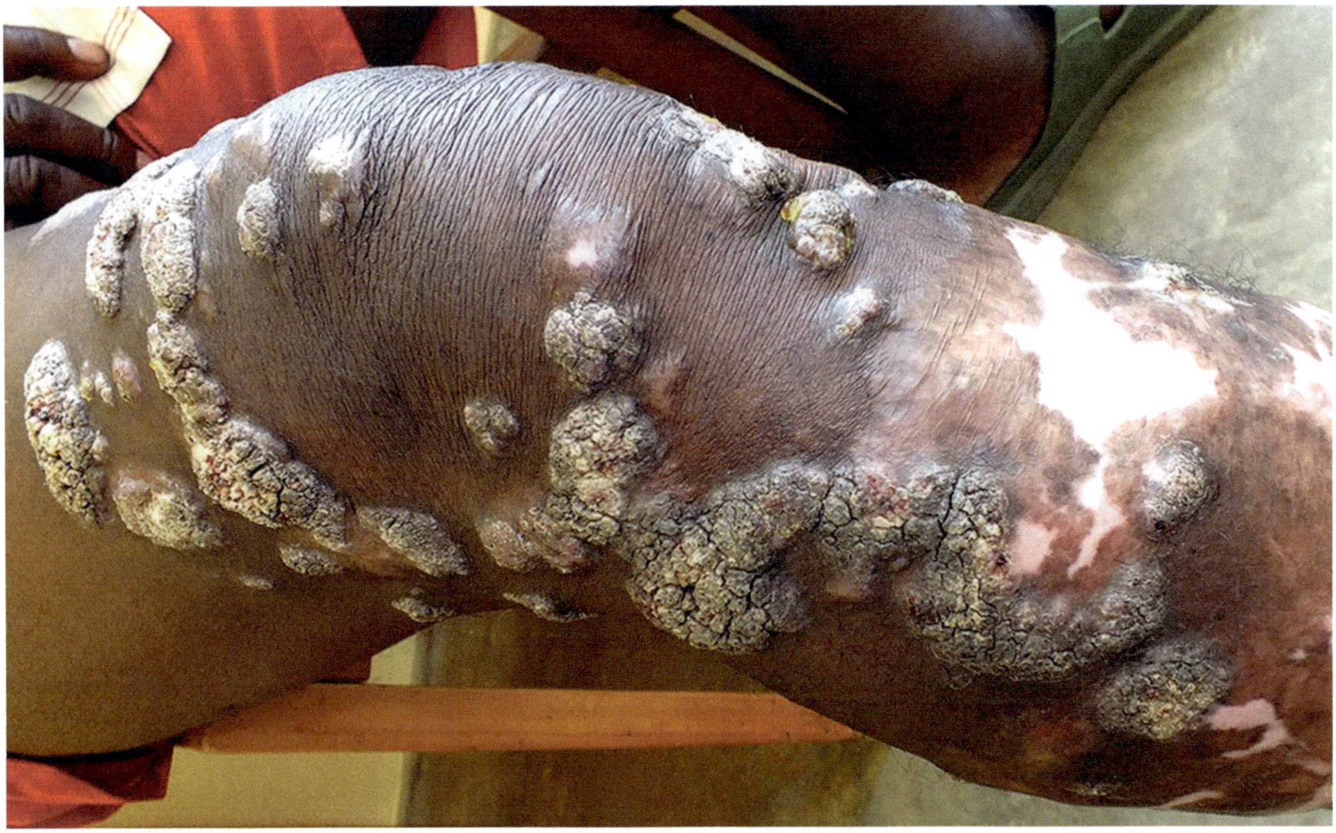

Fig. 6.6 *Chromoblastomycosis* of the right leg in a 64-year-old Tanzanian farmworker, showing subcutaneous nodules with verrucous surface. Hypopigmented scars are results of an intermittent antifungal treatment phase. RDTC Moshi, Tanzania; courtesy Prof. H. Grossmann

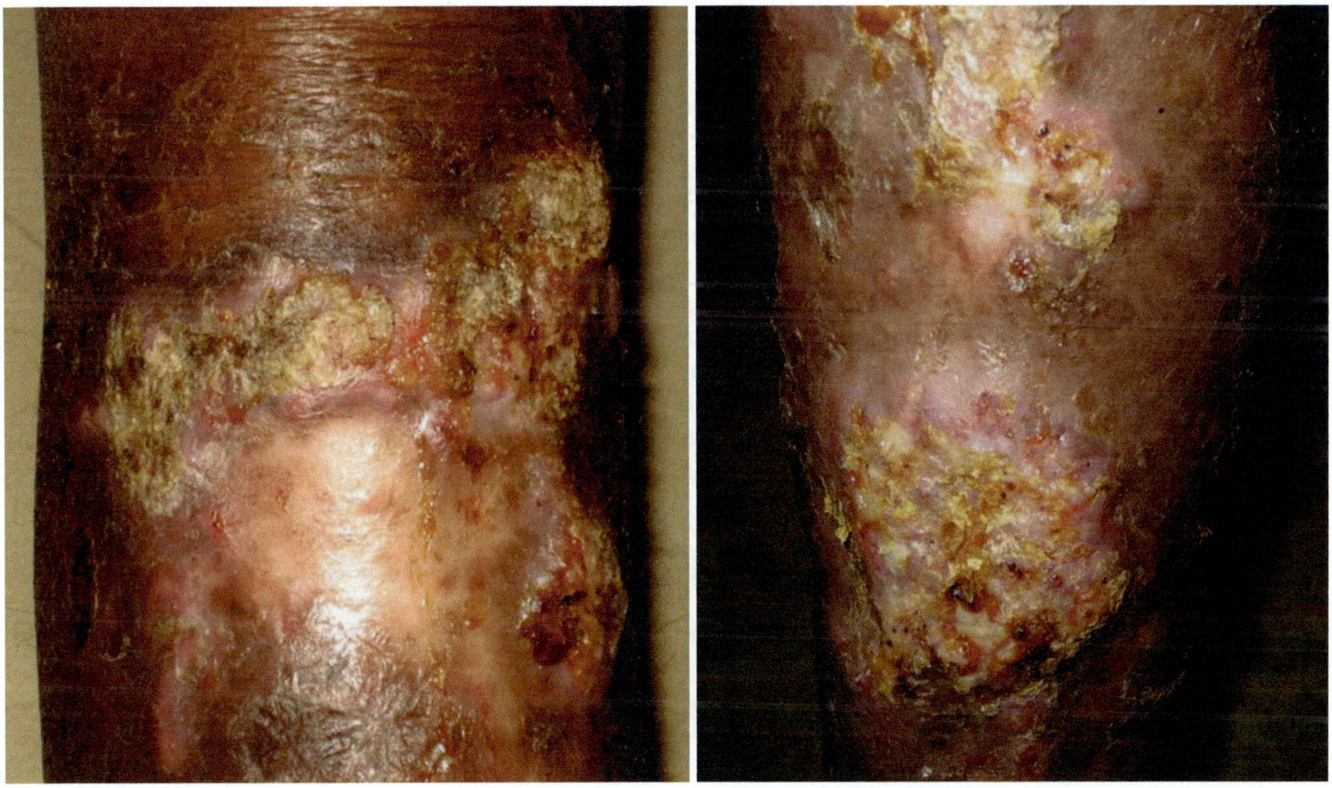

Fig. 6.7 Lesions of *chromoblastomycosis* with scarring under treatment with itraconazole over several months

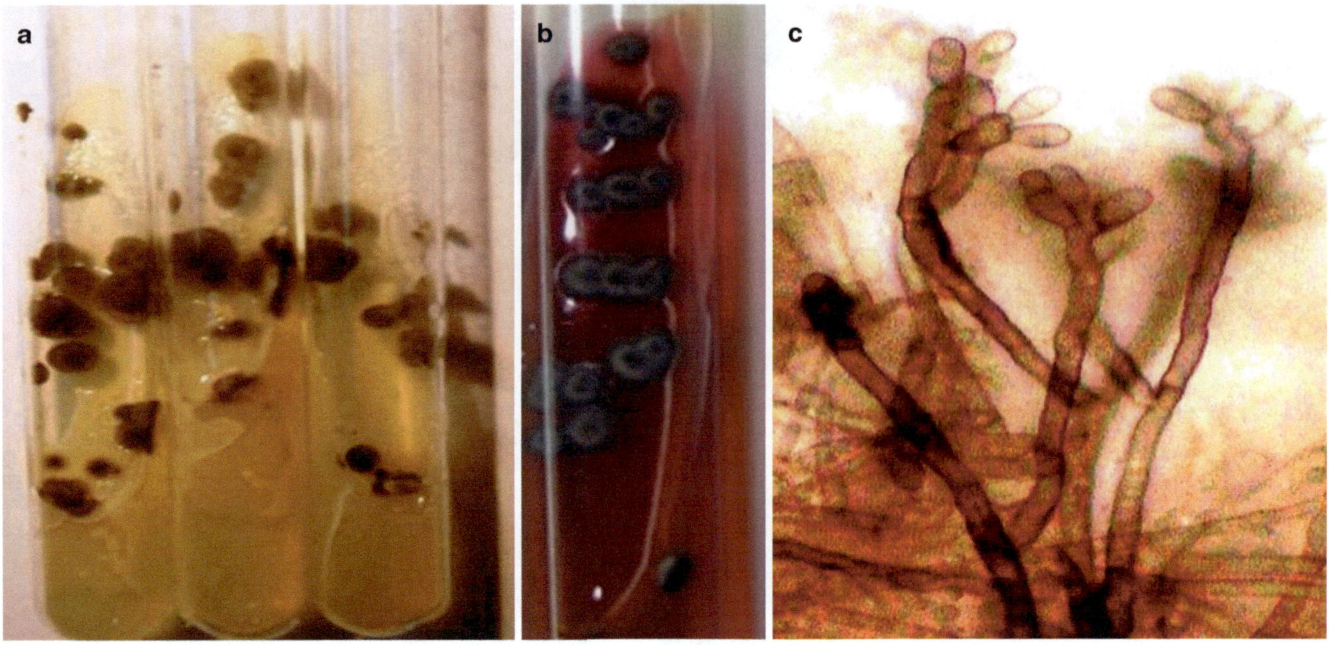

Fig. 6.8 *Fonsecaea pedrosoi.* (**a**) Colonies with greenish black thallus on Sabouraud's dextrose agar; (**b**) On dermatophyte test medium (DTM), the fungus grows with black thallus; the colour of the agar changes to red; (**c**) *Rhinocladiella*-like conidiation with 1–2 cell conidia is microscopically seen

6.3 Sporotrichosis

Sporotrichosis is a traumatic fungal infection with *Sporothrix schenckii* following thorn injuries of the skin, hands and/or arms or injuries of the lower extremities if walking barefoot, showing lymphogenic spread and distribution. Characteristically, the condition has been also called "rose gardener's disease" in the Anglo-American literature. Other body sites are rarely affected [10]. Infected animals (dogs, cats, horses, rats, pigs, armadillos, birds and reptiles) may also serve as a pathogen reservoir for human infection following scratching or biting [11].

Despite the fact that the fungus *Sporothrix schenckii* is ubiquitously found in nature in nearly all parts of the world, most sporotrichosis appears in tropical and subtropical countries. There are no studies concerning the exact incidence; each case represents a single infection reported as a rare event, most of them in the USA, India and Japan [12].

6.3.1 Pathogenesis

Causative agent of sporotrichosis is the dimorphic *Sporothrix schenckii*, an ubiquitous saprophytic fungus found on plants and in soil [12]. Currently, nine confirmed cases of cutaneous sporotrichosis were identified in the Northern territory of Australia. Patients were occupational or recreational gardeners, with each reporting exposure to mulching hay, originating from a single farm. Interestingly, the implicated hay had been stored over the monsoon season and had been affected by rain [13]. Six different species within the genus *Sporothrix* are known: *S. schenckii sensu stricto*, *S. brasiliensis*, *S. globosa*, *S. mexicana* and *S. albicans*. The dimorphic fungus *S. schenckii* develops tough, white yellowish, later on dark brown colonies with few aerial mycelium and submersed growing mycelium; thin septated hyphae are observed. Conidiogenous cells arise from hyphae and form conidia in groups on small clustered denticles.

6.3.2 Clinical Picture

At the port of entrance, slowly growing painless red, later on ulcerated putrid papules and crusted nodules develop along the lymphatics, indicating lymphangitis as a subcutaneously palpable hard and gnarled strand (Fig. 6.9). Rarely, haematogenous spread occurs in disseminated cutaneous sporotrichosis as a result of autoinoculation. Extracutaneous lesions and systemic infections are rare complications. For differential diagnosis other granulomatous inflammatory reactions, such as atypical mycobacteriosis, skin tuberculosis and cutaneous leishmaniasis, should be considered. For cultivation common growth media can be used with native tissue taken as a punch from the wound (Fig. 6.10). Biopsies show a granulomatous inflammatory reaction; in PAS and Grocott-Gomori stains, both cigar-shaped yeast cells and asteroid bodies may be detected.

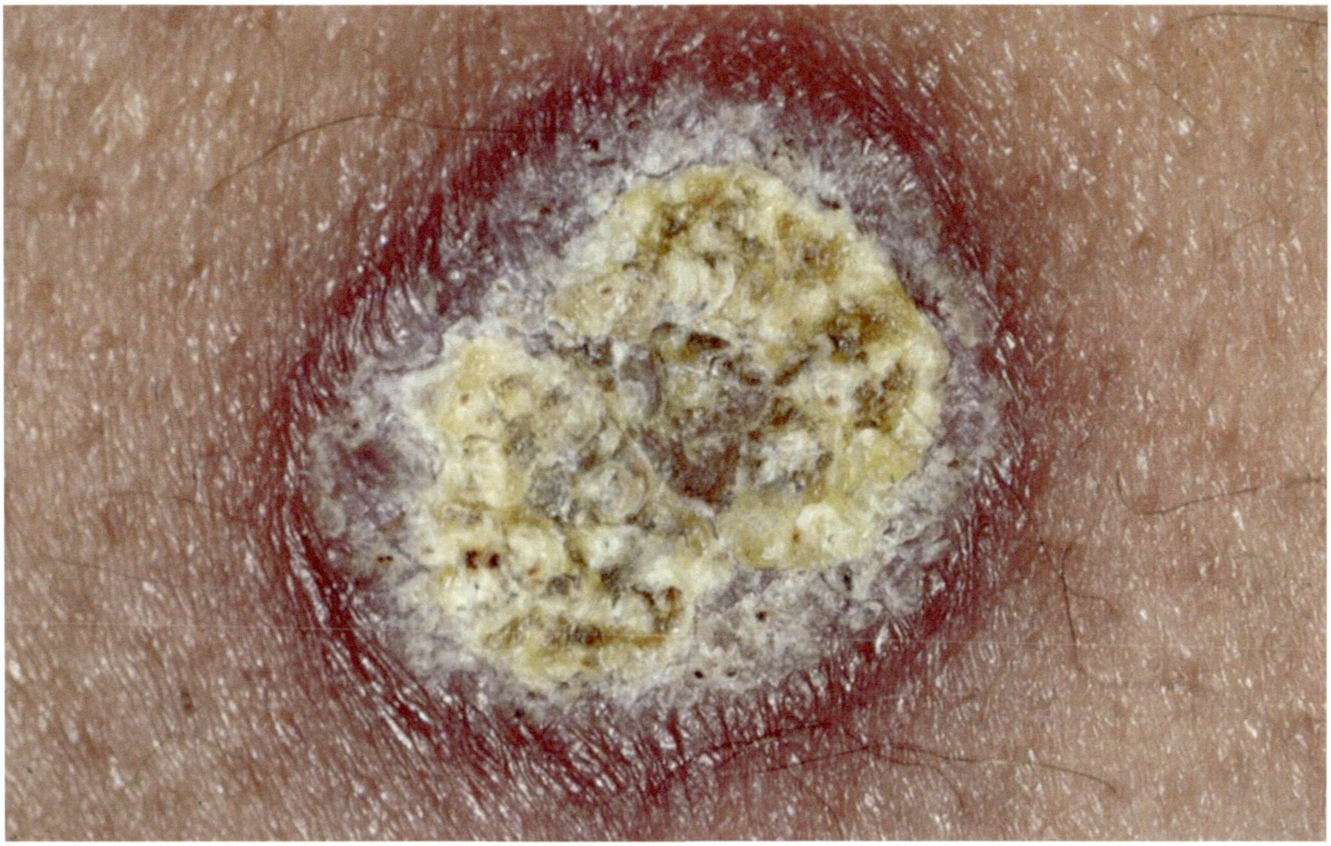

Fig. 6.9 Crusted lesion of *cutaneous sporotrichosis* after treatment with itraconazole. The patient had developed ulcerated nodules and palpable lymphangitis after a holiday trip to the Amazonas Delta in Brazil

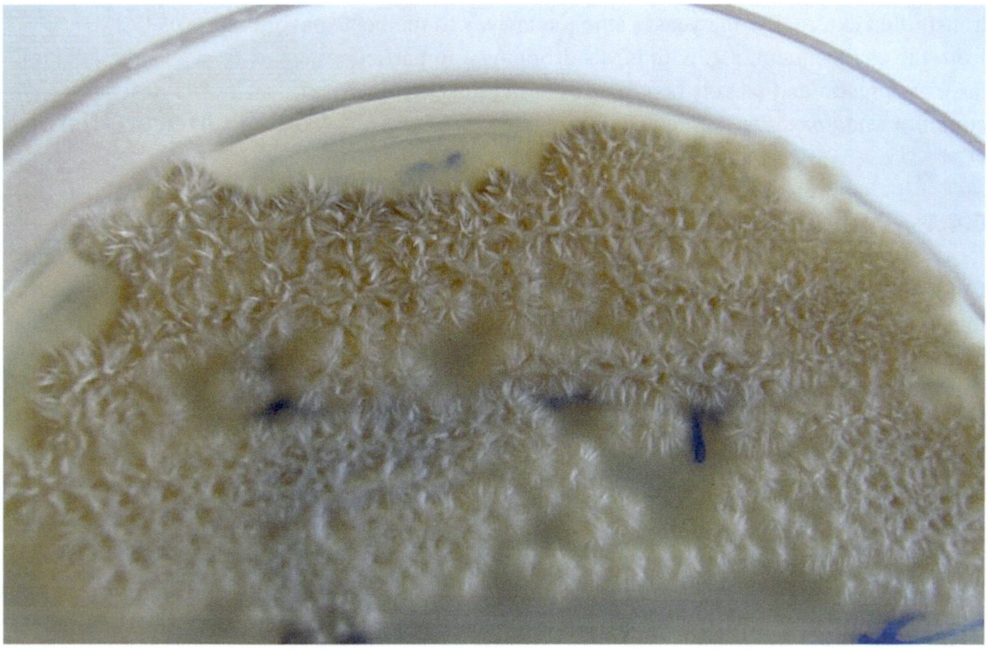

Fig. 6.10 Tough, white yellowish, later on dark brown colonies of *Sporothrix schenckii*

6.3.3 Management

Potassium iodide given orally in saturated solutions remains a first-line choice for treatment of uncomplicated cutaneous sporotrichosis in countries with poor resources [14]; initial dose is 0.5–1.0 mL 3×/day.

Itraconazole 100–200 mg/day is the current drug of choice in all forms of cutaneous and lymphangitic sporotrichosis, given for months to avoid relapses [15, 16]. Fluconazole can be also used in circumscribed cutaneous sporotrichosis at a dosage of 150 mg 1×/week. Fluconazole seems not be sufficient in lymphocutaneous sporotrichoid spread infections due to *S. schenckii*. Terbinafine at dosages of 500–1000 mg/day for 12–24 weeks was successfully administered in uncomplicated cutaneous sporotrichosis. Further options for managing are thermotherapy, cryotherapy with liquid nitrogen and photodynamic management with methylene blue. In disseminated infections and CNS involvement, amphotericin B should be considered.

6.4 Cutaneous Cryptococcosis

The capsulated yeasts *Cryptococcus neoformans* and *Cryptococcus gattii* are the two pathogenic species within the genus. *C. neoformans* occurs in animals, e. g. in the nasal cavity of koalas; its natural habitat has the yeast in hollow tree trunks. *C. gattii* causes infections in the tropics, e. g. in Central Africa, Australia, California, Central America and also South Europe. The occurrence of *C. gattii* in association with Eucalyptus trees is well known. Cryptococcoses are transmitted externally; the yeast pathogen arrives to the host from the environment, e.g. with bird's droppings, in particular from pigeon and parrots residues. Soil and dust also can contain *C. neoformans* yeast cells.

6.4.1 Pathogenesis

Cutaneous cryptococcosis usually affects immunocompromised HIV-infected patients; HIV-associated cryptococcosis is an AIDS-defining infection (see Chap. 37). Recipients of solid organ transplants are also at risk to develop cutaneous cryptococcosis [17]. Human cryptococcosis is caused by *C. neoformans* (capsule serotypes A, D and AD) and *C. gattii* (serotypes B and C). Characteristic are the mucous, bright colonies [18].

6.4.2 Clinical Picture

Haematogenous spread of the cryptococcus infection affects the central nervous system, in most cases as a result of a subclinical pulmonary cryptococcosis; in immunosuppressed patients meningoencephalitis is a serious, often lethal complication. Cryptococcosis of the skin develops predominantly as a secondary infection following haematogenous spread [19], often involving the face (Fig. 6.11). Cutaneous disseminated cryptococcosis presents skin-coloured nodules on the face, the arms and upper trunk, often umbilicated and mimicking mollusca (Fig. 6.12). In some cases also plaque-like lesions with ulceration and crusts as an aggressive cellulitis are found [20], with accompanying lymphadenitis. Rarely, primary cutaneous cryptococcosis may develop as a result of inoculation of the yeast from the environment.

From swabs taken from ulcerated skin lesions, cream-coloured to yellow brown, glossy, very slimy colonies grow on Sabouraud's dextrose agar. On *Guizotia abyssinica* creatinine agar (so-called Staib agar), brown-stained colonies are indicating *C. neoformans* (Fig. 6.13). Histology shows in PAS stain small yeast cells with unipolar budding.

6.4.3 Management

Initial management of cutaneous cryptococcosis comprises amphotericin B plus 5-fluorcytosin [21], combined with oral fluconazole. Monotherapy with fluconazole should be continued over several months [20]. Itraconazole represents the second-line antifungal drug in cryptococcosis. Echinocandins are not effective. After successful management, lifelong intake of fluconazole is recommended to avoid relapses [22].

6.5 African Histoplasmosis

African histoplasmosis is a rare infection caused by the dimorphic fungus *Histoplasma capsulatum var. duboisii* which is endemic in Central and West Africa, most likely also in South Africa and the island of Madagascar. A natural reservoir of the organism has been discovered in a bat cave in Nigeria with asymptomatic infections in its surroundings [23, 24]. An indigenous case has been recently reported from Kerala, India [25]. African histoplasmosis is established as an AIDS-defining infection in HIV-infected immunocompromised patients; it may occasionally occur combined with cryptococcosis. Infections of immunocompetent individuals were also registered in Senegal and Burkina Faso [26, 27]. An imported case was reported from France [28]. Severe lung histoplasmosis was detected in a Swiss tourist after having visited a cave in a trunk of a tree with colonies of bats in Uganda [29]. The port of entry of the infectious organism is unknown. There is a lack of awareness about

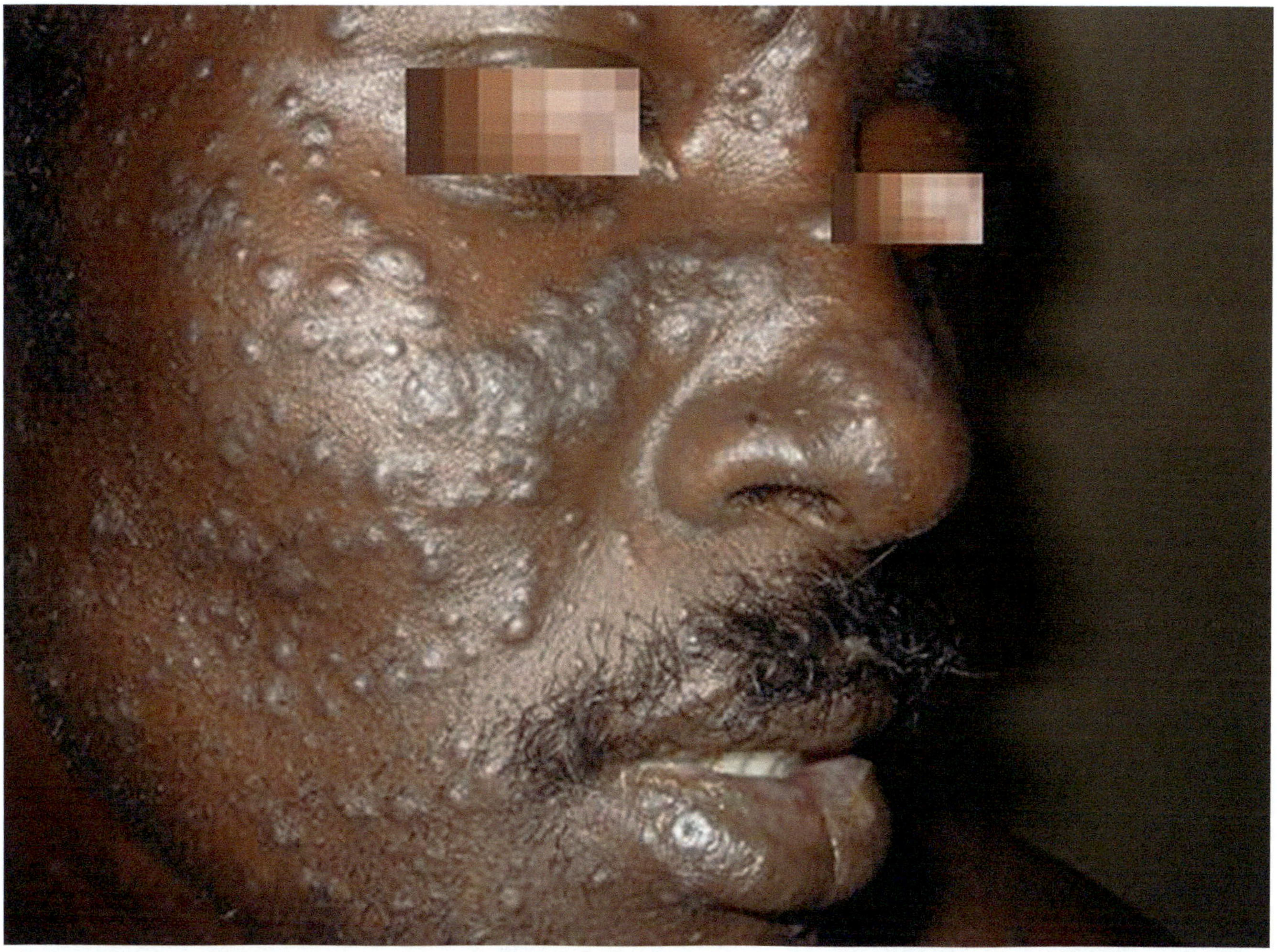

Fig. 6.11 *Cutaneous cryptococcosis* of the face in a HIV-positive male with 51/mm³ CD4+ T-cell count, before ART treatment. Cryptococcus meningitis was not diagnosed (Uganda)

histoplasmosis, its course and management, possibly due to under diagnosis.

Clinically, disseminated granulomatous nodules and plaques are presented with seropurulent fistules and crusting discharge from the openings (Fig. 6.14); differential diagnosis to other deep fungal infections is clinically difficult, and co-infections may occur (Fig. 6.15). The subcutaneous tissue and the bones may be affected; systemic dissemination involving the lungs, lymph nodes and other visceral organs is rarely described [26, 29]. Polymorphous ulcerative and budding skin lesions may occur. For treatment, it seems that itraconazole 400 mg/day offers favourable results. In patients with severe dissemination, 2–4 weeks of amphotericin B intravenously followed by maintenance management with oral itraconazole have been recommended. Posaconazole may serve as a rescue management [30].

6.6 Cutaneous Blastomycosis

Cutaneous blastomycosis occurs in the USA and the North American territory including Canada. Particularly in southern USA, states near to Ohio and Mississippi rivers endemic areas are known. In South America, only single infections have been reported. Further major foci are in Africa; in Congo, Uganda and Tanzania blastomycoses occur.

6.6.1 Pathogenesis

Causative agent is the dimorphic fungus *Blastomyces dermatitidis* which exists as a non-pathogenic form as a mould in nature and converts to pathogenic yeast at body temperature [31]. The infection is acquired via the air route after inhalation of spores causing primary pulmonary infection [32];

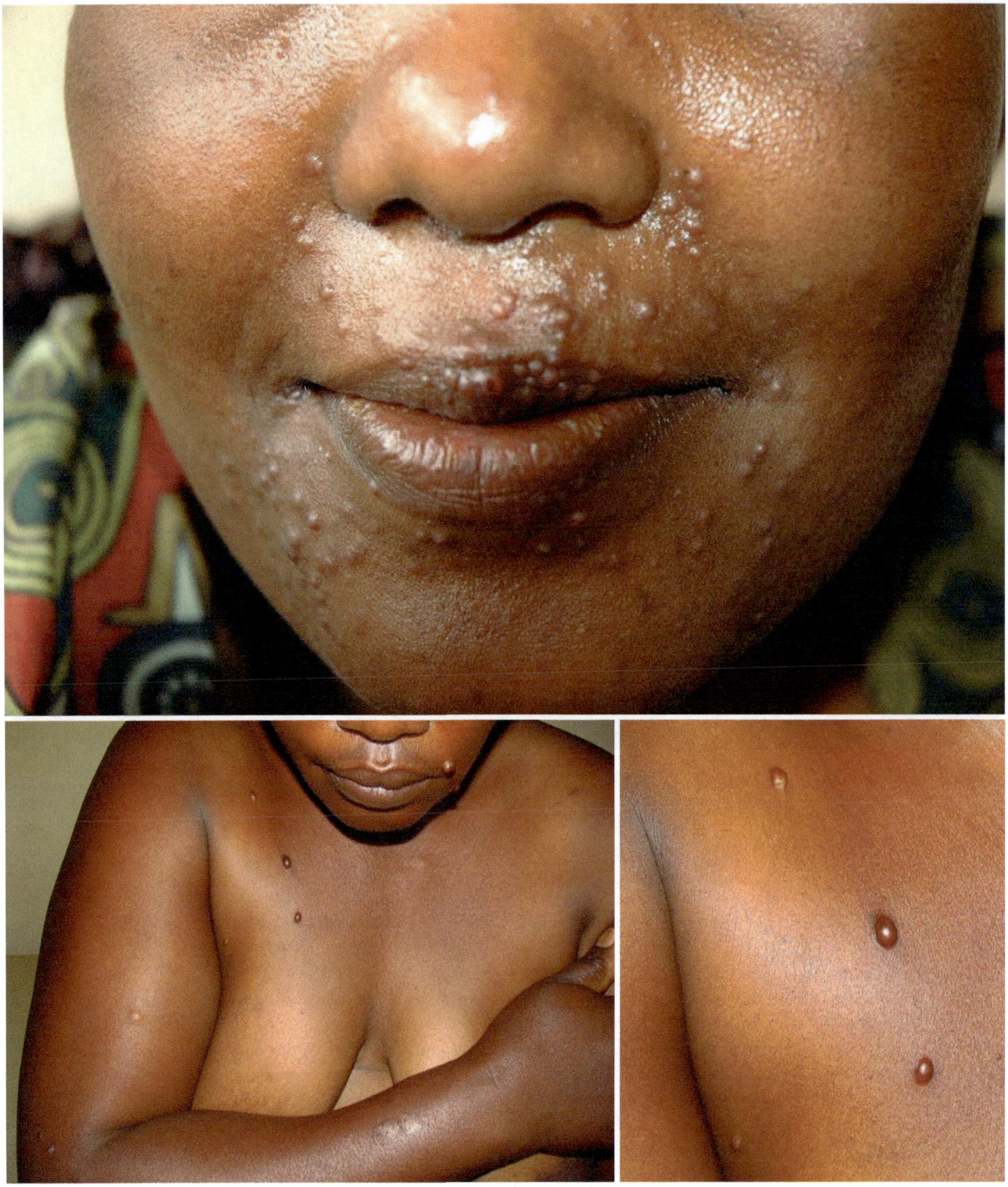

Fig. 6.12 *Disseminated cutaneous cryptococcosis* in HIV-positive females (Tanzania)

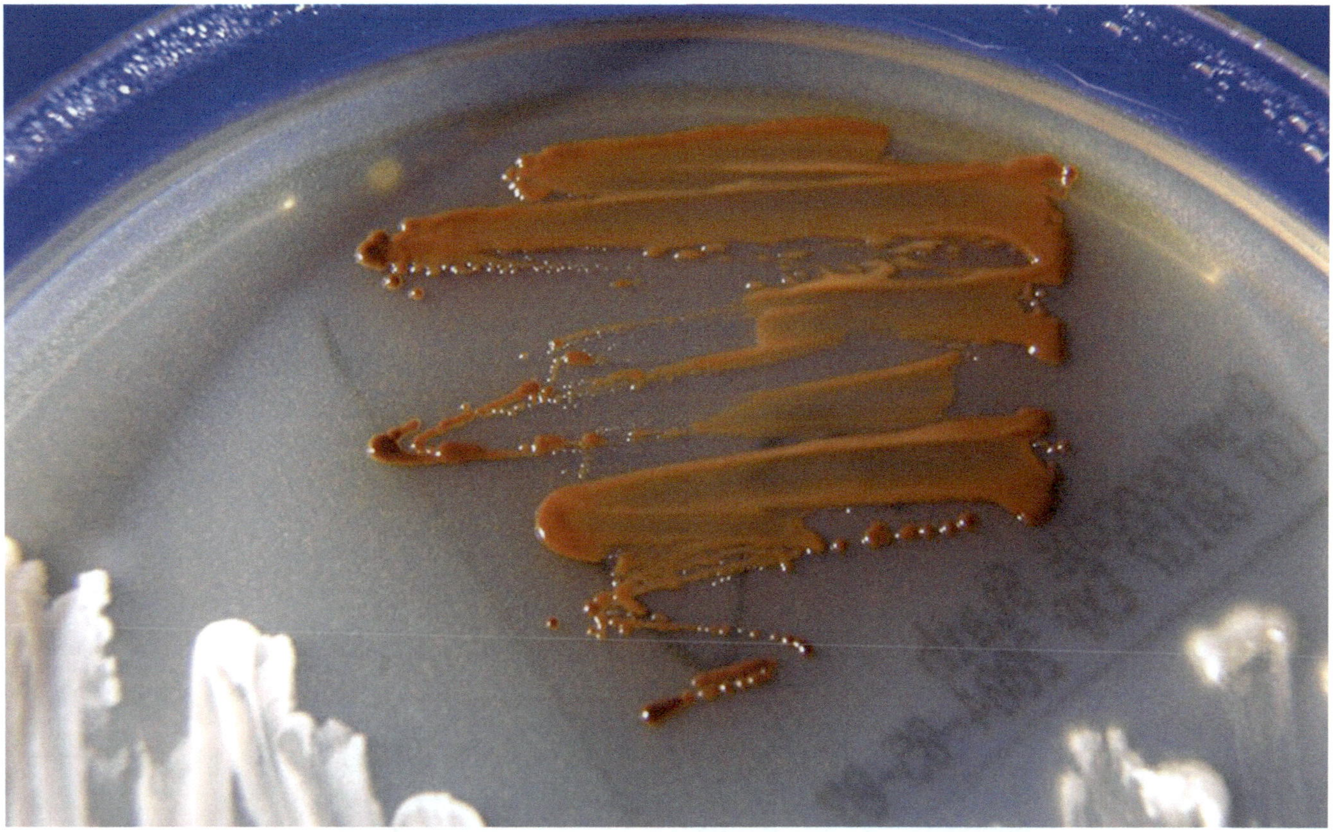

Fig. 6.13 *Cryptococcus neoformans* cultured on *Guizotia abyssinica* creatinine agar

systemic dissemination may follow. Primary cutaneous blastomycosis may rarely occur [31]. There is no indication for transmission person to person. Immunosuppressed patients are at risk to develop disseminated disease after haematogenous spread involving the skin and/or the bones. The infection also affects animals, e.g. dogs. *Blastomyces dermatitidis* has its natural habitat in the environment, particularly in soil and dust. In humid regions *Blastomyces* can be found in the soil with high organic content. In tissue, e.g. the lungs, the fungus grows in its yeast cell form with ellipsoid budding cells 8–15 µm in size. In cultural media the mycelial form develops under lower temperatures (20–28 °C); the fungus grows as mould.

6.6.2 Clinical Picture

Blastomycosis involves the skin following haematogenous spread from the lungs; the time of incubation is long, 45 days in average. Primary cutaneous blastomycosis following traumatic inoculation is rare. Skin infection initially presents papules which evolve to nodules. A verrucous variant has been described, and also ulcerations with livid red and elevated margin and erythematous indurations are seen. Panniculitis or erythema nodosum-like lesions may occur; lymphangitis and lymph node swelling like chancre are palpable.

In native KOH preparations from swabs unipolar sprouting budding cells are observed, whereas skin biopsies reveal epidermal microabscesses and necrosis together with inflammatory cell infiltrates in cutis and subcutis. In Grocott-Gomori and PAS stainings, 8–15 µm-sized unipolar budding cells can be seen in granulation tissue.

Differential diagnosis includes pyoderma, cutaneous leishmaniasis, skin tuberculosis and nontuberculous mycobacteria infection. Malignancies such as ulcerated basal cell or squamous cell carcinoma should be excluded.

6.6.3 Management

Management of choice for primary cutaneous blastomycosis is long-term administration of antifungals, itraconazole or fluconazole [33, 34]. Today, posaconazole is used in systemic blastomycosis for single patients. In complicated and severe courses, amphotericin B is given intravenously.

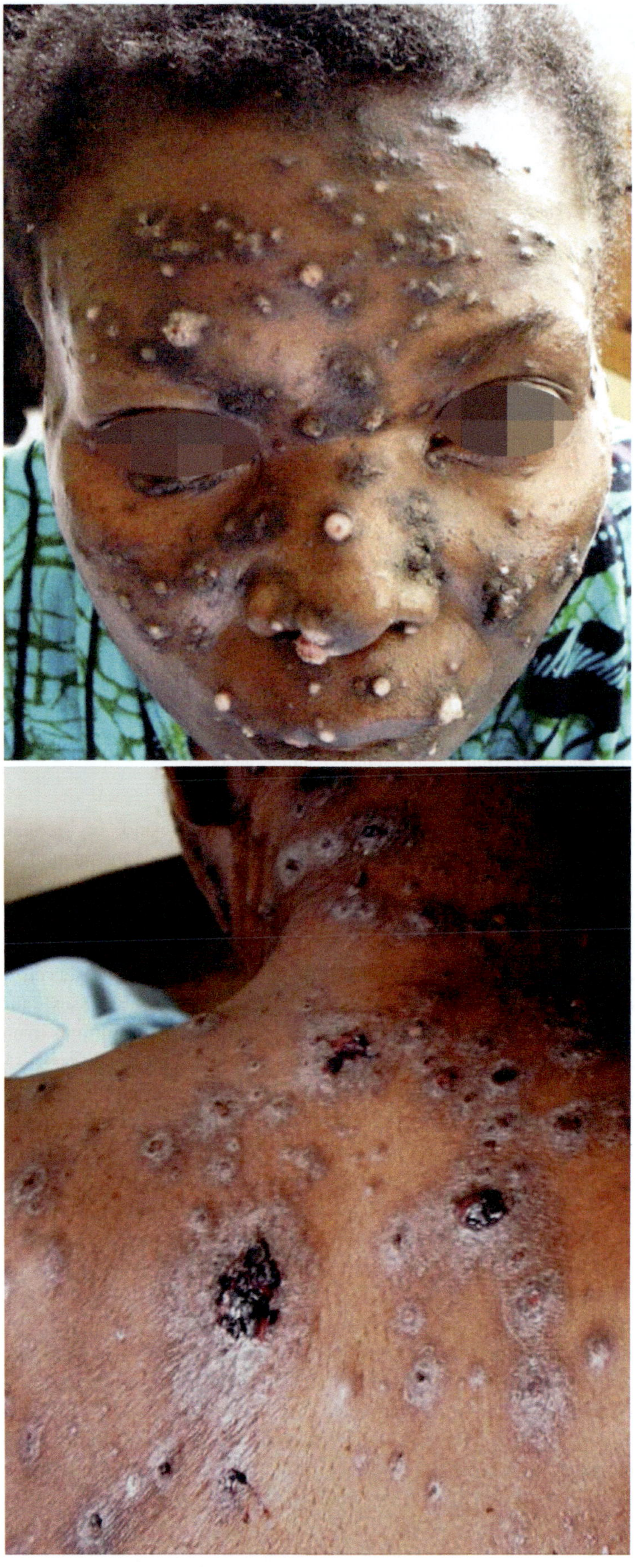

Fig. 6.14 *African histoplasmosis*: Cutaneous dissemination in a HIV-positive female, 2 weeks after initiation of treatment with itraconazole (400 mg/day). Courtesy Dr. M. Ketema, RDTC Moshi, Tanzania

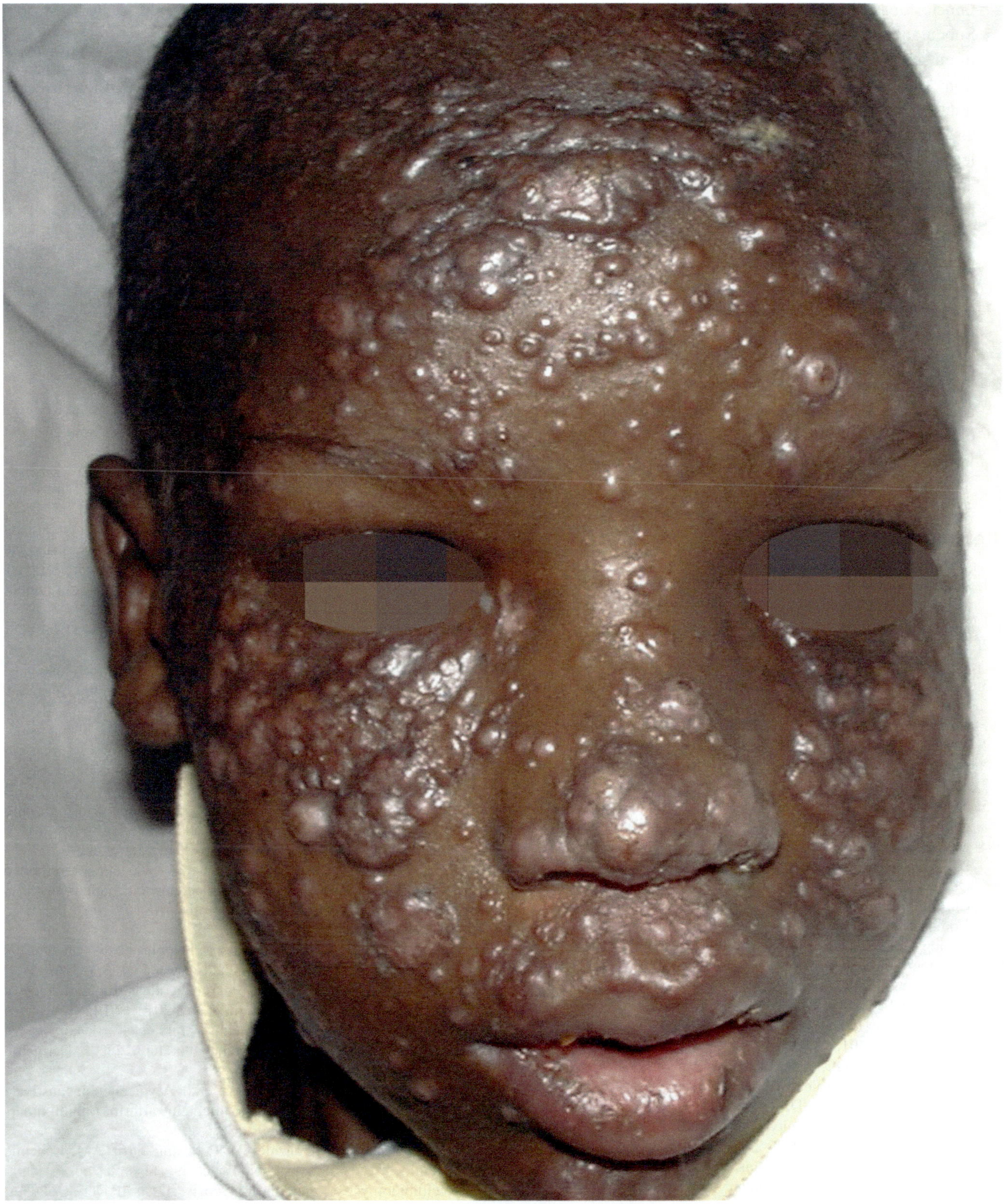

Fig. 6.15 *African histoplasmosis* DD: cryptococcosis. Co-infection? (RDTC Moshi, Tanzania; courtesy Dr. M. Ketema)

Conclusions

Subcutaneous and deep fungal infections of the skin are often seen in hot climate zones due to the climatic conditions, the low level of hygienic standards and the large numbers of HIV-infected immunocompromised individuals. They are considered as the diseases of the underprivileged and poor, may be seen in migrants and refugees and are difficult to treat. Saturated solution of potassium iodide remains as an antigranulomatous agent a first-line treatment choice, e.g. for uncomplicated cutaneous sporotrichosis. For any other subcutaneous/deep fungal infection of the skin, long-term administration of itraconazole, fluconazole or terbinafine is mainstay of treatment available in most countries; amphotericin B may be indicated in cases with systemic dissemination which often represent a therapeutic challenge. New potent antifungal azoles such as voriconazole and posaconazole were shown to be highly effective; however, they are expensive, still unattainable for most patients and countries with limited resources.

References

1. Mitjà O, Marks M, Bertran L, et al. Integrated control and management of neglected tropical skin diseases. PLoS Negl Trop Dis. 2017;11:e0005136.
2. Zijlstra EE, van de Sande WW, Fahal AH. Mycetoma: a long journey from neglect. PLoS Negl Trop Dis. 2016;10:e0004244.
3. Al-Hatmi AM, Bonifaz A, Tirado-Sánchez A, et al. *Fusarium* species causing eumycetoma: report of two cases and comprehensive review of the literature. Mycoses. 2017;60:204–12.
4. Tirado-Sánchez A, Calderón L, Saúl A, et al. Mycetoma: experience of 482 cases in a single center in Mexico. PLoS Negl Trop Dis. 2014;8:e3102.
5. Nenoff P, van de Sande WWJ, Fahal A, et al. Eumycetoma and actinomycetoma—an update on causative agents, epidemiology, pathogenesis, diagnostics and therapy. J Eur Acad Dermatol Venereol. 2015;29:1873–83.
6. Queiroz-Telles F, de Hoog S, Santos DW, et al. Chromoblastomycosis. Clin Microbiol Rev. 2017;30:233–76.
7. Gomes RR, Vicente VA, Azevedo CM, et al. Molecular epidemiology of agents of human chromoblastomycosis in Brazil with the description of two novel species. PLoS Negl Trop Dis. 2016;10:e0005102.
8. Radouane N, Hali F, Khadir K et al. [Generalized chromomycosis caused by Phialophora verrucosa]. Ann Dermatol Venereol. 2013;140:197–201.
9. Lima AM, Sacht GL, Paula LZ, et al. Response of chromoblastomycosis to voriconazole. An Bras Dermatol. 2016;91:679–81.
10. Milby AH, Pappas ND, O'Donnell J, et al. Sporotrichosis of the upper extremity. Orthopedics. 2010;33(4) doi: 10.3928/01477447-20100225-27.
11. Gremião ID, Miranda LH, Reis EG, et al. Zoonotic epidemic of sporotrichosis: cat to human transmission. PLoS Pathog. 2017;13:e1006077.
12. Chakrabarti A, Bonifaz A, Gutierrez-Galhardo MC, et al. Global epidemiology of sporotrichosis. Med Mycol. 2015;53:3–14.
13. McGuinness SL, Boyd R, Kidd S, et al. Epidemiological investigation of an outbreak of cutaneous sporotrichosis, Northern Territory, Australia. BMC Infect Dis. 2016;16:16.
14. Mahajan VK. Sporotrichosis: an overview and therapeutic options. Dermatol Res Pract. 2014;2014:272376.
15. Marques GF, Martins AL, Sousa JM, et al. Characterization of sporotrichosis cases treated in a dermatologic teaching unit in the state of São Paulo—Brazil, 2003–2013. An Bras Dermatol. 2015;90:273–5.
16. de Lima Barros MB, Schubach AO, de Vasconcellos Carvalhaes de Oliveira R, et al. Treatment of cutaneous sporotrichosis with itraconazole—study of 645 patients. Clin Infect Dis. 2011;52:e200–6.
17. Biancheri D, Kanitakis J, Bienvenu AL, et al. Cutaneous cryptococcosis in solid organ transplant recipients: epidemiological, clinical, diagnostic and therapeutic features. Eur J Dermatol. 2012;22:651–7.
18. Nenoff P, Reinel D, Krüger C, et al. Tropical and travel-related dermatomycoses: Part 2: cutaneous infections due to yeasts, moulds, and dimorphic fungi. Hautarzt. 2015;66:522–32.
19. Srivastava GN, Tilak R, Yadav J et al. Cutaneous *Cryptococcus*: marker for disseminated infection. BMJ Case Rep. 2015;2015. pii: bcr2015210898.
20. Wang J, Bartelt L, Yu D, et al. Primary cutaneous cryptococcosis treated with debridement and fluconazole monotherapy in an immunosuppressed patient: a case report and review of the literature. Case Rep Infect Dis. 2015;2015:131356.
21. Tsuji G, Matsuda T, Shigyo A, et al. Primary cutaneous cryptococcosis successfully managed by surgical debridement and liposomal amphotericin B/flucytosine therapy. Eur J Dermatol. 2017;27:96–7.
22. Lortholary O, Fernández-Ruiz M, Perfect JR. The current treatment landscape: other fungal diseases (cryptococcosis, fusariosis and mucormycosis). J Antimicrob Chemother. 2016;71(suppl 2):ii31–6.
23. Gugnani HC, Muotoe-Okafor F. African histoplasmosis: a review. Rev Iberoam Micol. 1997;14:155–9.
24. Gugnani HC. Histoplasmosis in Africa: a review. Indian J Chest Dis Allied Sci. 2000;42:271–7.
25. Ravindran S, Sobhanakumari K, Celine M, et al. African histoplasmosis: the first report of an indigenous case in India. Int J Dermatol. 2015;54:451–5.
26. Diadie S, Diatta B, Ndiaye M, et al. Multifocal histoplasmosis due to Histoplasma capsulatum var. duboisii in a 22 year-old Senegalese patient without proven immunodepression. J Mycol Med. 2016;26:265–70.
27. Zida A, Niamba P, Barro-Traoré F, et al. Disseminated histoplasmosis caused by Histoplasma capsulatum var. duboisii in a non-HIV patient in Burkina Faso. J Mycol Med. 2015;25:159–62.
28. Richaud C, Chandesris MO, Lanternier F, et al. Imported African histoplasmosis in an immunocompetent patient 40 years after staying in a disease-endemic area. Am J Trop Med Hyg. 2014;91:1011–4.
29. Raselli C, Reinhart WH, Fleisch F. Histoplasmosis—an unusual African souvenir. Dtsch Med Wochenschr. 2013;138:313–6.
30. Gonçalves D, Ferraz C, Vaz L. Posaconazole as rescue therapy in African histoplasmosis. Braz J Infect Dis. 2013;17:102–5.
31. Motswaledi HM, Monyemangene FM, Maloba BR. Blastomycosis: a case report and review of the literature. Int J Dermatol. 2012;51:1090–3.
32. Smith RJ, Boos MD, Burnham JM, et al. Atypical cutaneous blastomycosis in a child with juvenile idiopathic arthritis on infliximab. Pediatrics. 2015;136:e1386–9.
33. Bonifaz A, Vázquez-González D, Perusquía-Ortiz AM. Endemic systemic mycoses: coccidioidomycosis, histoplasmosis, paracoccidioidomycosis and blastomycosis. J Dtsch Dermatol Ges. 2011;9:705–14.
34. Bonifaz A, Morales D, Morales N, et al. Cutaneous blastomycosis. An imported case with good response to itraconazole. Rev Iberoam Micol. 2016;33:51–4.

7 Viral Infections

Sawko W. Wassilew

Viral infections involving the skin occur worldwide. Human papilloma (HPV), herpes simplex (HSV), and varizella/zoster (VZV) viruses are widely distributed all over the continents. In hot climate zones, the risk of acquiring viral infections is generally increased due to high population density, light clothing, and inadequate sanitary conditions for both ubiquitous and endemic agents. International travel of businessmen and holidaymakers facilitates the contacts with infected carriers or vectors which transmit viruses, and infections limited to tropical regions are occasionally imported by travelers to Europe, including dengue and chikungunya fever [1]. They often present exanthemas which can be subtle and may occur weeks after infection without any other distinctive clinical sign [2]. In addition, legal or illegal migrants with pigmented or dark skin and common viral skin diseases may enter countries in moderate climate zones.

A large number of viral infections present mucocutaneous manifestations; rashes with polymorphic maculopapular and vesiculobullous lesions often occur facing the physicians with unknown or unusual clinical pictures of diseases in dark skin [3], whereas malnourished or immunocompromised children and pregnant women carry the greatest risk of adverse outcome [4].

Agents such as human papilloma and pox viruses produce tumorlike papular skin lesions due to their replication in the epidermis; exanthemas can also appear as a secondary clinical manifestation of viral replication in other organs and cause fever, malaise, jaundice, arthralgia, and other constitutional symptoms. A significant amount of travelers to the developing world require medical care after their return to their home countries [5].

In well-known virus infections of the skin, the clinical picture is diagnostic; however, viral exanthemas are clinically not specific; history and course of the disease may be helpful to recognize uncommon infections.

S. W. Wassilew
Centre of Dermatology, Krefeld, Germany

7.1 Human Papilloma Virus Infections

Human papilloma viruses (HPV) are small DNA viruses that infect squamous epithelial cells generating various types of warty lesions. Subclinical and latent infections frequently occur; HPV-DNA was found at very low levels also in keratinocytes of normal epidermis and hair follicles [6]. Today, more than 100 different HPV types have been recognized, and their number is continuously increasing; among them are oncogenic types such as HPV 6, 11, 16, 18, 31, 33, and 45 and several others [6, 7]. They are usually transmitted by direct skin-to-skin contacts being easily inoculated into the skin with impaired barrier function, i.e., after maceration or in patients with atopic eczema.

Warts are most common in children and adults, and their management covers a large proportion of the daily practice in dermatological offices in the West. In developing countries their incidence is high, having as reservoir individuals with minor clinical or subclinical infections; sellers of meat or fish in markets and shops have often warts in their hands, and plantar warts occur frequently, most likely acquired in swimming areas, pools, or public shower rooms. Common warts may appear as flat (*verruca plana*), or hyperkeratotic lesions (*verruca vulgaris*), often localized in large numbers on the hands and feet. In children and young adults, also the face is a common localization; disseminated lesions occur occasionally depending on the immune status of the carrier, particularly in hot climate zones, found in large numbers and size as a marker of HIV-infected, immune-suppressed individuals (Figs. 7.1 and 7.2). In contrast to those at the hands, legs, and dorsal feet, plantar warts are often painful (Fig. 7.3).

Genital warts are sexually transmitted multiple lesions, localized in the perianal or genital region, caused by oncogenic strains (Fig. 7.4). They may increase to considerable tumorlike size and also lead to precanceroses and cervical cancer in females, depending on the properties of the causative viral strain (see Chap. 8). Spontaneous resolution may rarely occur.

C. E. Orfanos et al. (eds.), *Pigmented Ethnic Skin and Imported Dermatoses*, https://doi.org/10.1007/978-3-319-69422-1_7

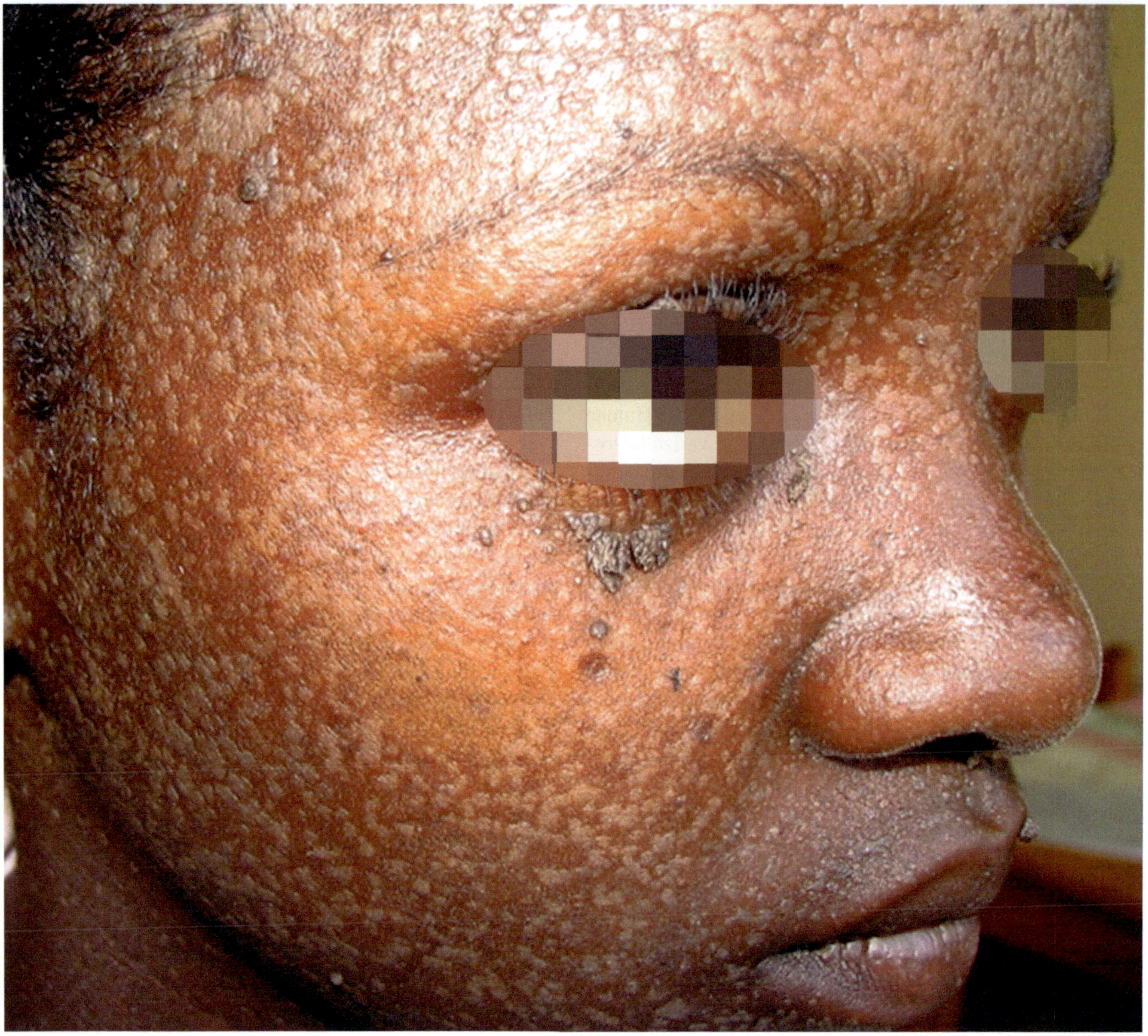

Fig. 7.1 Myriads of disseminated *plane warts* in a young African female. Hyperkeratotic, partly filiform *common warts* are also seen in the suborbital area; others occur in the hand and feet of the patient

Treatment: The management of warts depends on their number, size, and localization. Local application of chemicals (podophyllin, retinoic acid, imiquimod, etc.) or surgical intervention (electrocautery, cryosurgery, lasers) can be performed, particularly for treating painful lesions and those in the genital area (see Chap. 8). Restoration of the immune response of the carriers is an important goal for avoiding recurrences.

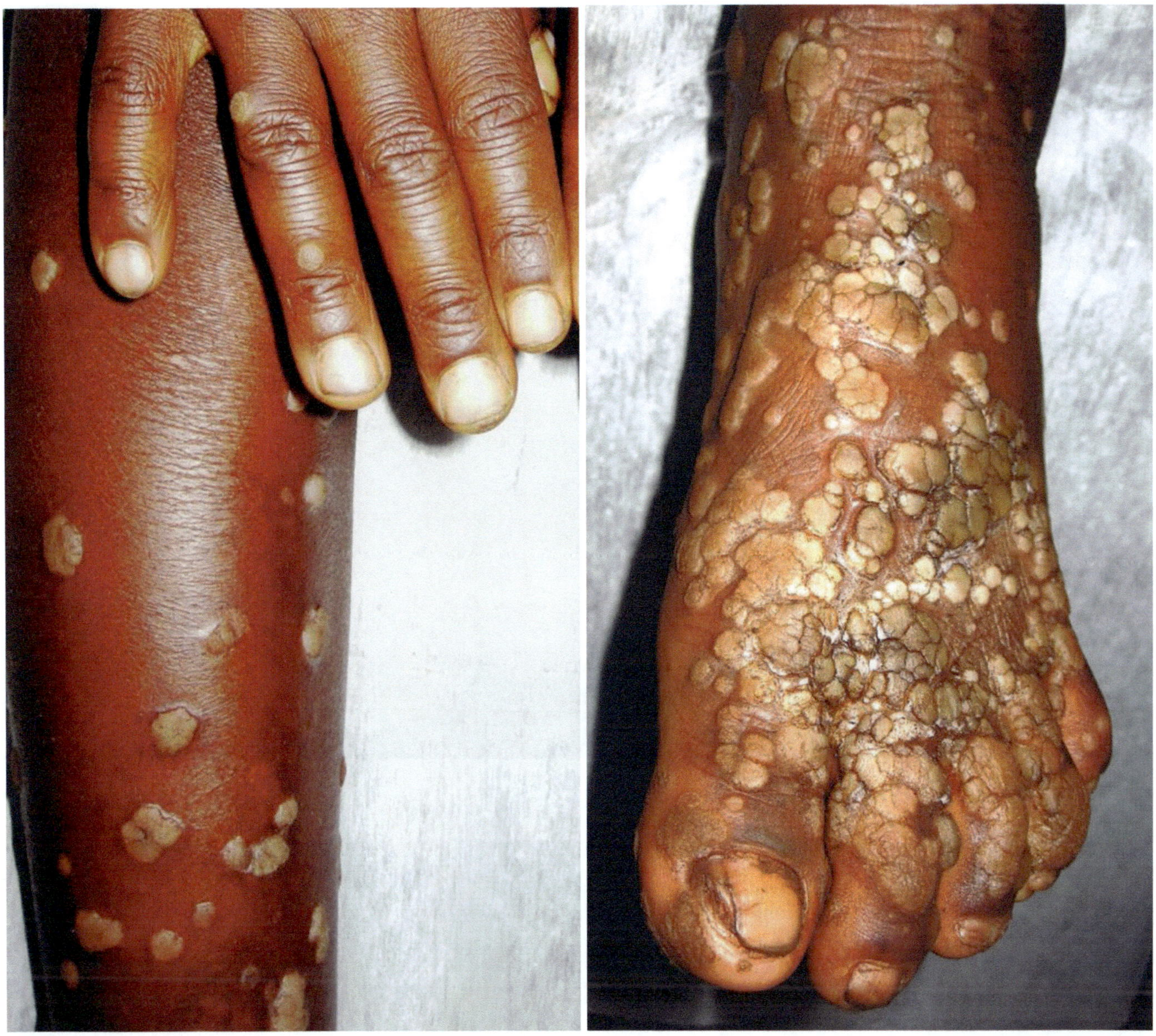

Fig. 7.2 Extensive dissemination of *common warts* on the extremities of an immune-compromised male patient, partly confluent

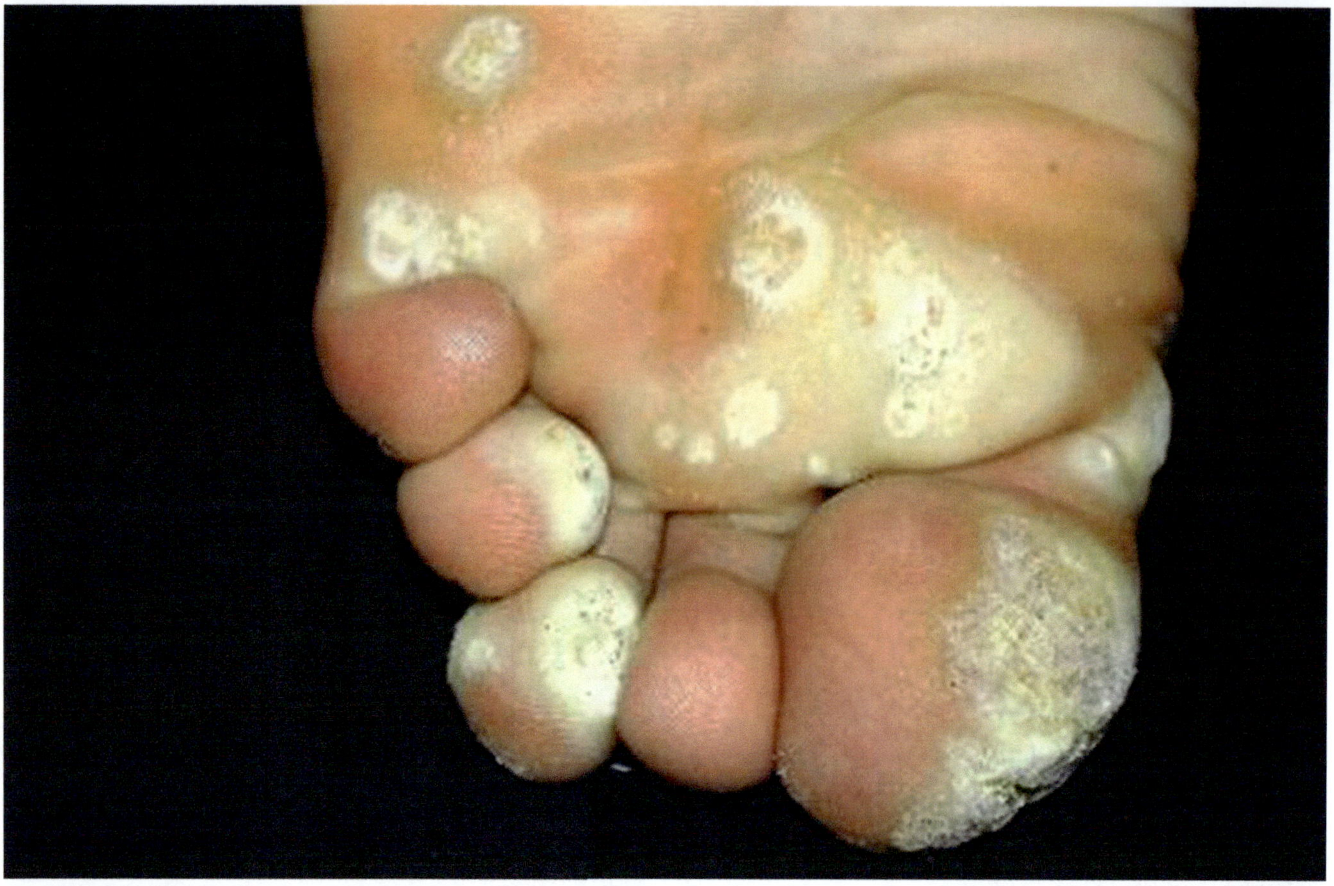

Fig. 7.3 Extensive plantar warts (under local treatment)

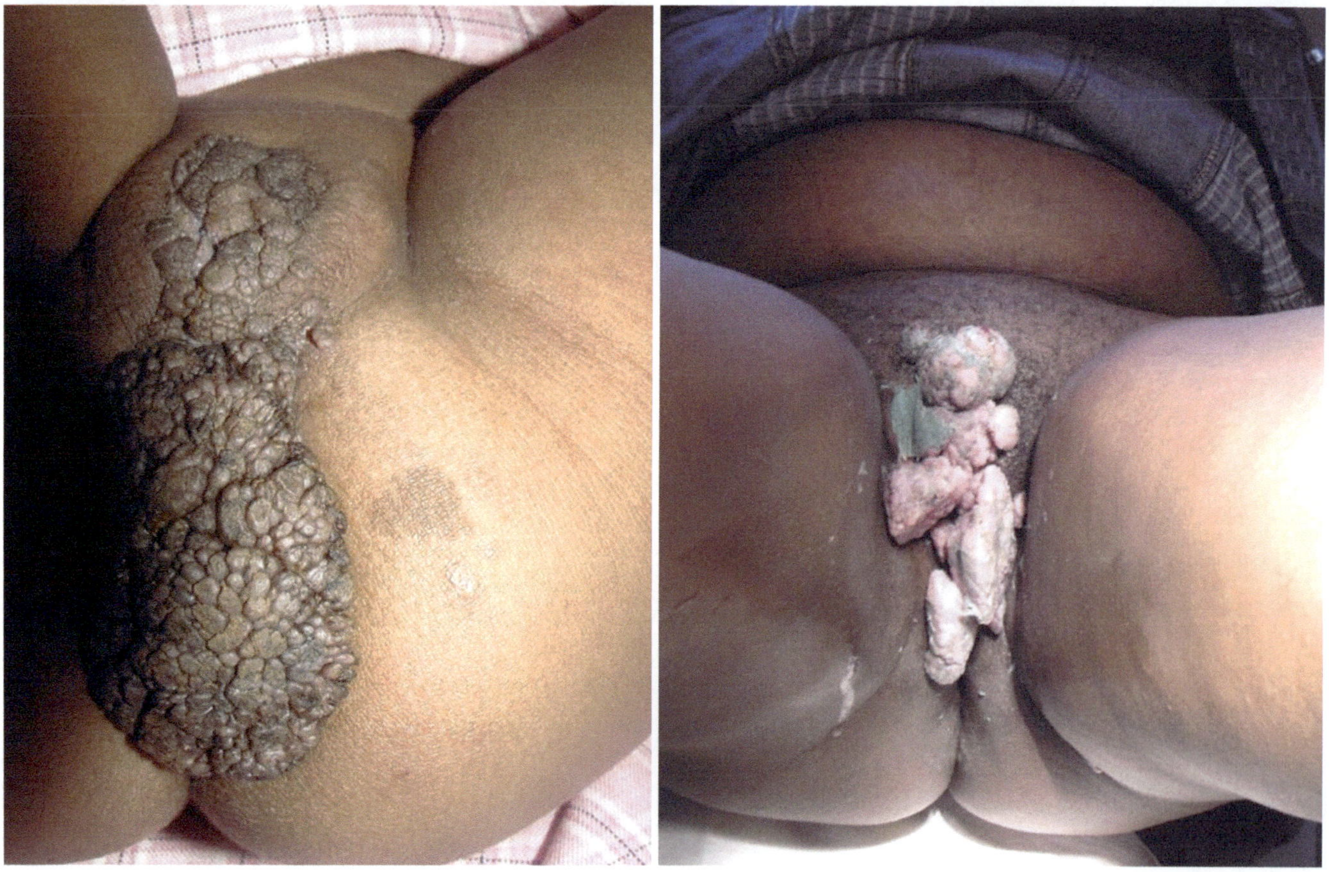

Fig. 7.4 Giant anogenital warts (*condylomata gigantea*) in two African females

7.2 Mollusca Contagiosa

The disease is caused by the *molluscipox virus* (MCV), a large double-stranded DNA virus visible even by light microscopy (MCV-I, MCV-II, MCV-III, and MCV-IV). MCV-I is the most prevalent infecting exclusively humans, mostly children; it replicates in the juvenile skin. Transmission occurs mainly by direct contact inoculation, with an incubation period of 2–7 weeks [8]. MCV-II is more commonly transmitted sexually. MCV-I infections are seen worldwide, with higher distribution in tropical areas where children are lightly dressed and in close contact to one another. Spread within the household is common. Peak incidence is reported in 1–4-year-old children in Fiji and the sub-Saharan Africa (Congo). In New Guinea, the annual attack rate for children under 10 years of age has been reported to be 6% of the total [8, 9]. The individual lesion is a skin-colored, dome-shaped umbilicated papule ranging from 2 to 6 mm in size, depending upon the stage of its development (Fig. 7.5); occasionally, mollusca papules may exceed 1 cm in size. The diagnosis is based on clinical examination; the course is usually benign and self-limited. However, mollusca easily disseminate in large numbers over the entire body and persist for 6–9 months, rarely for years, if untreated. They are more commonly found in patients with atopic dermatitis or eczema; use of swimming pools has been also correlated with childhood infections. Giant mollusca are seen in HIV-infected immune-suppressed patients.

Treatment: Management of mollusca contagiosa is not always required, their course is mostly benign and self-limited, and natural resolution is the rule in immunocompetent carriers. Active treatment may produce more complaints to affected children than the mollusca [10]. However, local treatment is often offered to prevent autoinoculation and transmission. Topical cantharidin 0.9% solution, 10% KOH solution, cryotherapy with liquid nitrogen, curettage, and manually expressing the central white core with or without cauterization with trichloroacetic acid or phenol solutions may be used. In HIV-infected and other immune-suppressed individuals, the lesions can affect adults, may become large and superinfected, and need surgical excision.

Parapoxvirus infections are self-limited zoonotic viral infections in individuals with close contact to infected animals, cattle, sheep, or goats. After a short incubation period of 4–7 days, erythematous macules or pustules develop usually on the hands of individuals with contact with the infected animal; the lesions are usually painless. Paravaccinia virus, also called pseudocowpox virus, causes *milker's nodule*, and a prototypic species of the genetically heterogeneous *Parapoxvirus* genus causes *orf disease* [9] with weeping pus-

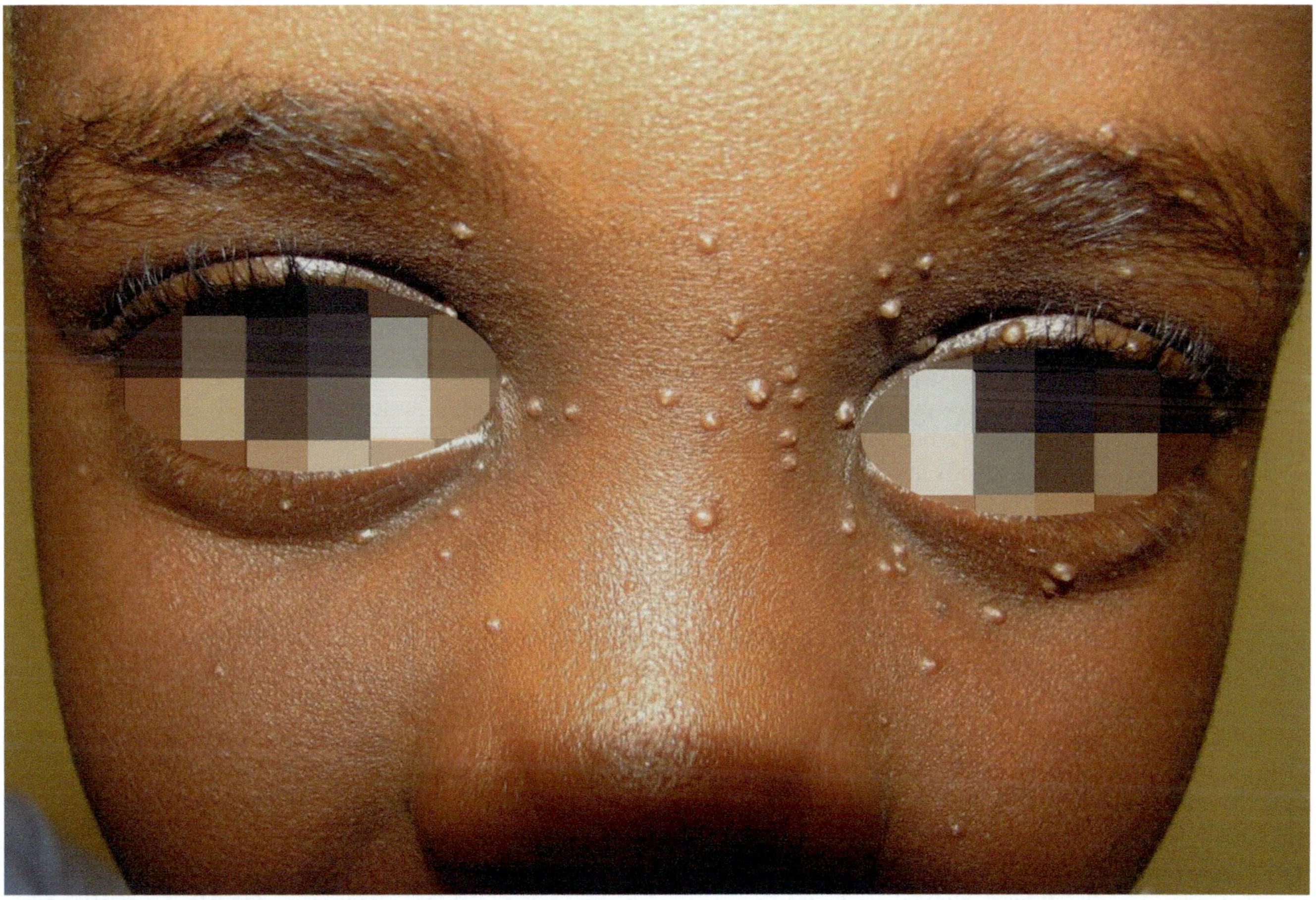

Fig. 7.5 *Mollusca contagiosa* in an African young boy

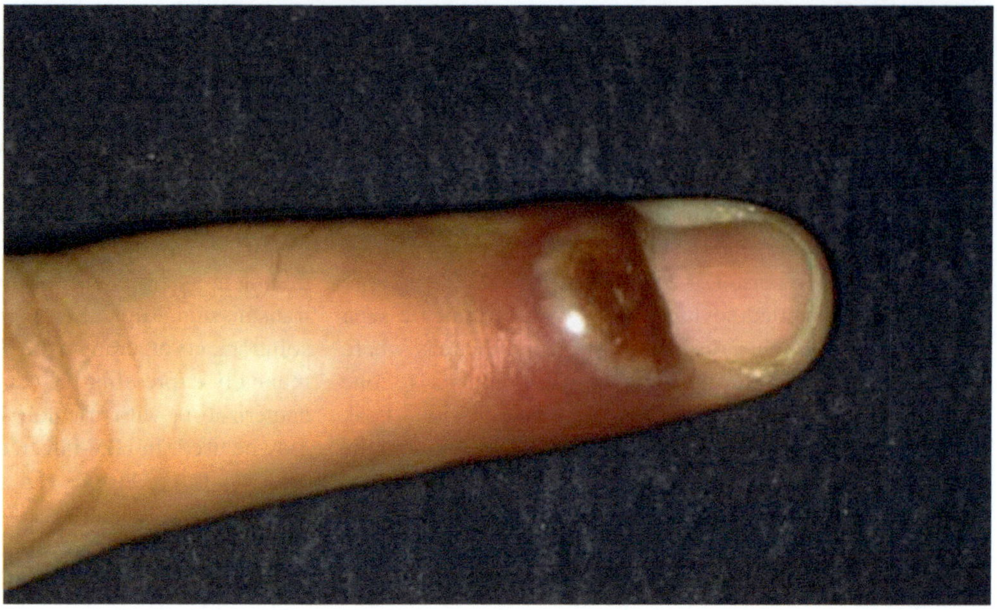

Fig. 7.6 *Parapoxvirus* infection (*orf disease*) presenting painless weeping pustule

tules developing within 2–3 weeks and regressing with papules and crusts without scarring (Fig. 7.6). Treatment is symptomatic, e.g., application of antiseptic compresses. For prevention use of gloves and good hand hygiene are recommended. Electron microscopy of blister fluid or crusts can identify the typical *Parapoxvirus*. For differential pyogenic granuloma, anthrax, unusual herpetic lesions, and keratoacanthoma are considered.

7.3 Herpes Simplex Virus Infection

Herpes simplex virus (HSV) infections are common worldwide with two separate antigenic types: HSV-1 associated with orofacial and HSV-2 with genitoanal infections (see Chap. 8), although there is considerable overlapping. The host's immune defense controls the viral replication but cannot fully eliminate the virus; thus, frequent recurrences occur following clinical recovery. Viruses persist throughout a person's life as a latent infection in the body, most likely in neural tissue, and can be easily reactivated after reexposure or under immune suppression [11].The molecular mechanisms responsible for reactivation are not clearly understood. Immune mechanisms are also responsible for the establishment of latent virus in ganglion cells. Viral transmission occurs via direct contact with infected skin or droplets from infected discharge during asymptomatic or symptomatic viral shedding.

Primary HSV-1 infections remain often subclinical but can also involve the oral mucosa as *gingivostomatitis herpetica* starting with mild fever and pain. The breath is foul and children often get difficulties in drinking or eating (Fig. 7.7). In elderly children or young adults, the infection can also appear with atypical clinical vesicular eruptions resembling herpetic eczema or shingles.

Recurrences arise in 30–50% of the cases. Possible triggers are fever, ultraviolet radiation, trauma, emotional stress, and others. Recurrent HSV-1 infections are often preceded by itching, burning, or mild painful sensation. Grouped vesicles develop on a slightly swollen skin area, most frequently around the mouth (*herpes labialis*), and tend to recur in the same area. Usually the lesions last for about 1 week. In immune-suppressed patients, the eruption may become larger and more severe and ulcerate or disseminate with longer duration (see Chap. 38).

Kaposi's varicelliform eruption (syn.: *eczema herpeticum*) is a rare complication resulting in patients with eczema, mostly atopic dermatitis, due to cutaneous dissemination and superinfection with HSV-1 or other herpes virus types (Fig. 7.8a, b). In severe cases hemorrhagic vesicopustules start often on the scalp and face and coalescence and further disseminate. The condition may remain misdiagnosed and be even fatal in children.

Treatment: Mild lesions of primary or recurrences of HSV-1 infection require symptomatic measures only or application of creams containing acyclovir. Topical antiseptic solutions may reduce the risk of secondary staphylococcal infection. If the lesions are severe or painful, early administration of oral acyclovir 5 × 800 mg/day over 5–7 days will be helpful and shorten the duration. Systemic acyclovir may be effective in reducing the duration of symptoms of recurrent HSV-1 infection, but the optimal timing and dose of treatment are uncertain [12]. In frequent (>6/year) painful recurrences, oral acyclovir 2 × 200–800 mg/day depending on the severity, valaciclovir 500–1000 mg/day, or famciclovir 2 × 250 mg/day is given as a prophylaxis over several months.

In cases with *varicelliform eruption* and in immunocompromised patients, full-dose antiviral treatment is indicated in most cases [13]. Acyclovir intravenously 3 × 5–10 mg/kg/day is given for at least 7–14 days; in the presence of severe

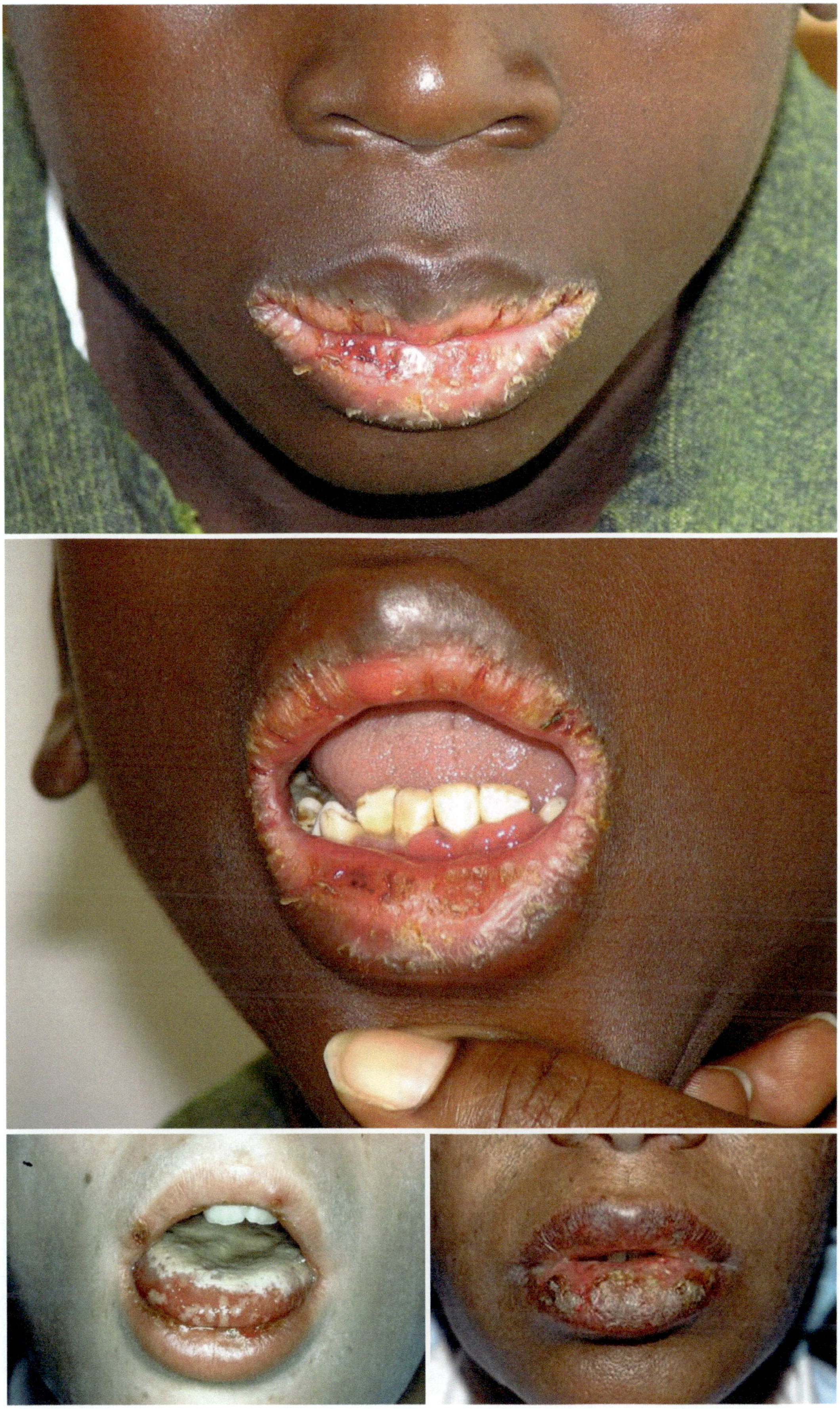

Fig. 7.7 *Gingivostomatitis herpetica* with accompanying glossitis and cheilitis

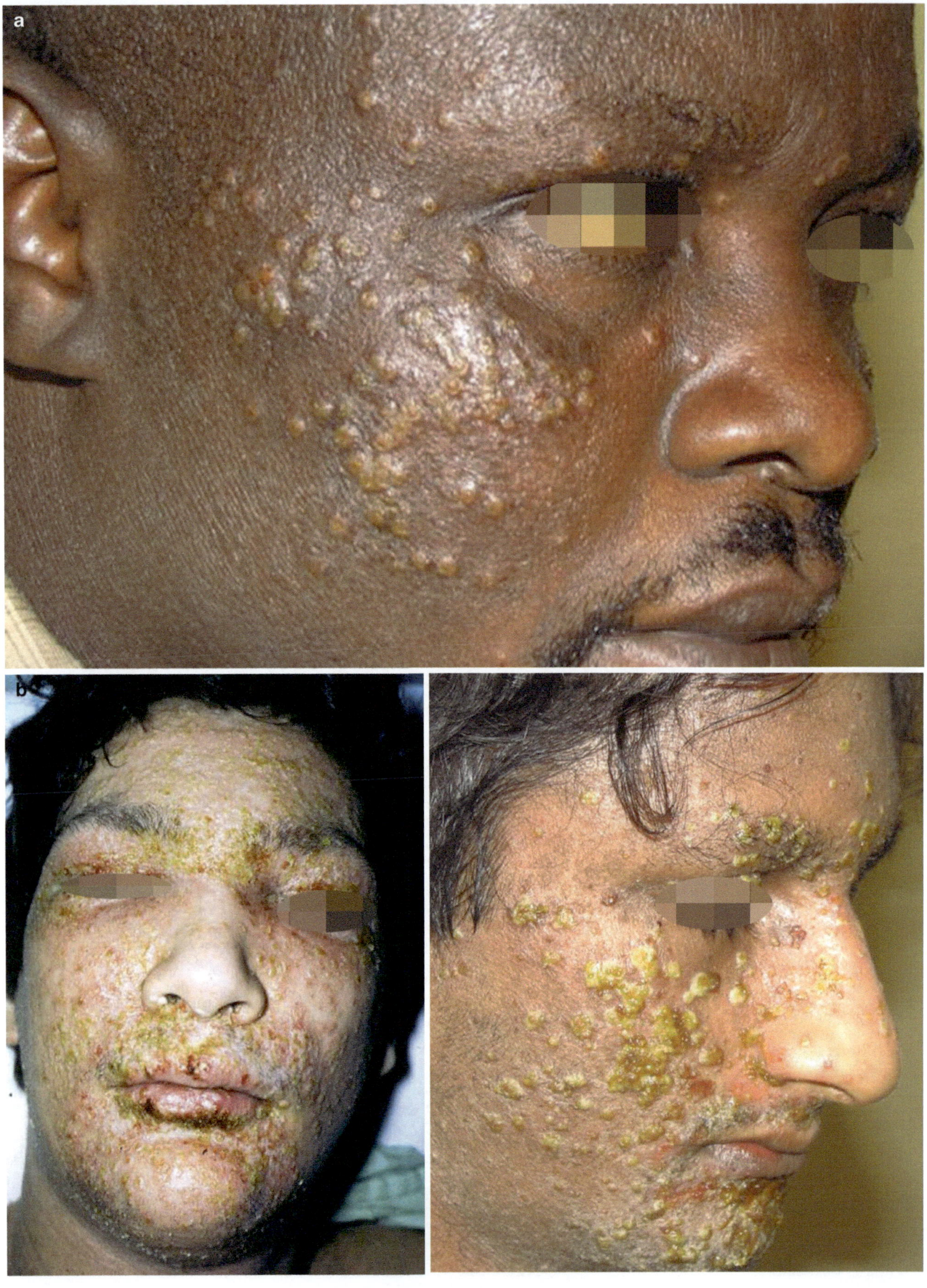

Fig. 7.8 (**a**) Early stage of *varicelliform eruption* (eczema herpeticum) in an African male (Tanzania). (**b**) Progressed stage of *varicelliform eruption* with heavy staphylococcal superinfection in two atopic patients (Indian origin) with constitutional symptoms

immune suppression, over 14–21 days is recommended. Alternatives are valaciclovir or fanciclovir orally 500–1000 mg 2×/day for 14–21 days.

7.4 Varicella

Varicella (chickenpox) is a common airborne-transmitted and highly contagious viral infection caused by the varicella zoster virus (VZV) especially among children. In hot climate regions, it occurs also in adults not easily recognizable in patients with heavily pigmented skin (Fig. 7.9) and may become clinically more extended and severe in malnourished children (Fig. 7.10). After an incubation period of 2–3 weeks and initial viral replication in the oropharynx (oral sore, *enanthema*) constitutional prodromi with fever and malaise appear, leading to VZV viremia and acute skin rash with macules, vesicles, and pustules accompanied by intense itching. The sterile pustules of the rash become umbilicated and develop crusts, leading to final clearing in 10–14 days; mild superficial scars may occur due to superinfections and scratching. In contrast to Caucasian skin, there are no macules found in pigmented skin; vesicles may develop into bullous lesions and become necrotic.

The polymorphism of the pruritic rash and its characteristic distribution initially involving the face, scalp, and the chest rapidly spreading all over the body are diagnostic for varicella. After the clinical recovery, the virus persists in neural tissue cells. The acute disease only rarely becomes a serious health problem in temperate zones, in contrast to the clinical picture that may arise in developing countries under tropical climatic conditions. In otherwise healthy children, possible complications such as pneumonia, hemorrhagic nephritis, purpura, and viral encephalitis rarely occur; they are more common in adults and immune-compromised patients. Reinfections may occur, but they remain subclinical.

In varicella infection during pregnancy, the virus may penetrate the placenta and infect the fetus. Early maternal infection during the first 28 gestational weeks may lead to severe fetal damage (*congenital varicella syndrome*) and late infection to premature delivery. *Neonatal varicella* often leads to severe complications of the newborn.

Treatment: In healthy children bed rest and topical application of calamine lotion or antiseptic creams to prevent superinfection are required; isolation of the affected individuals would prevent further viral spread. Sedating antihistamines are helpful to reduce the itch, and oral antibiotics may be necessary in a few cases with severe involvement to treat or prevent additional bacterial infection. In severely affected children, adults, or immune-suppressed patients, local measures are often combined with systemic antivirals, acyclovir 5 × 800 mg/day orally or 10 mg/kg/day intravenously for 10 days, and alternatives, oral valaciclovir 3 × 1000 mg/day or famciclovir 3 × 500 mg/day for 7–10 days. Vaccination is effective in preventing moderate varicella in children; it particularly prevents severe courses of the disease [14, 15].

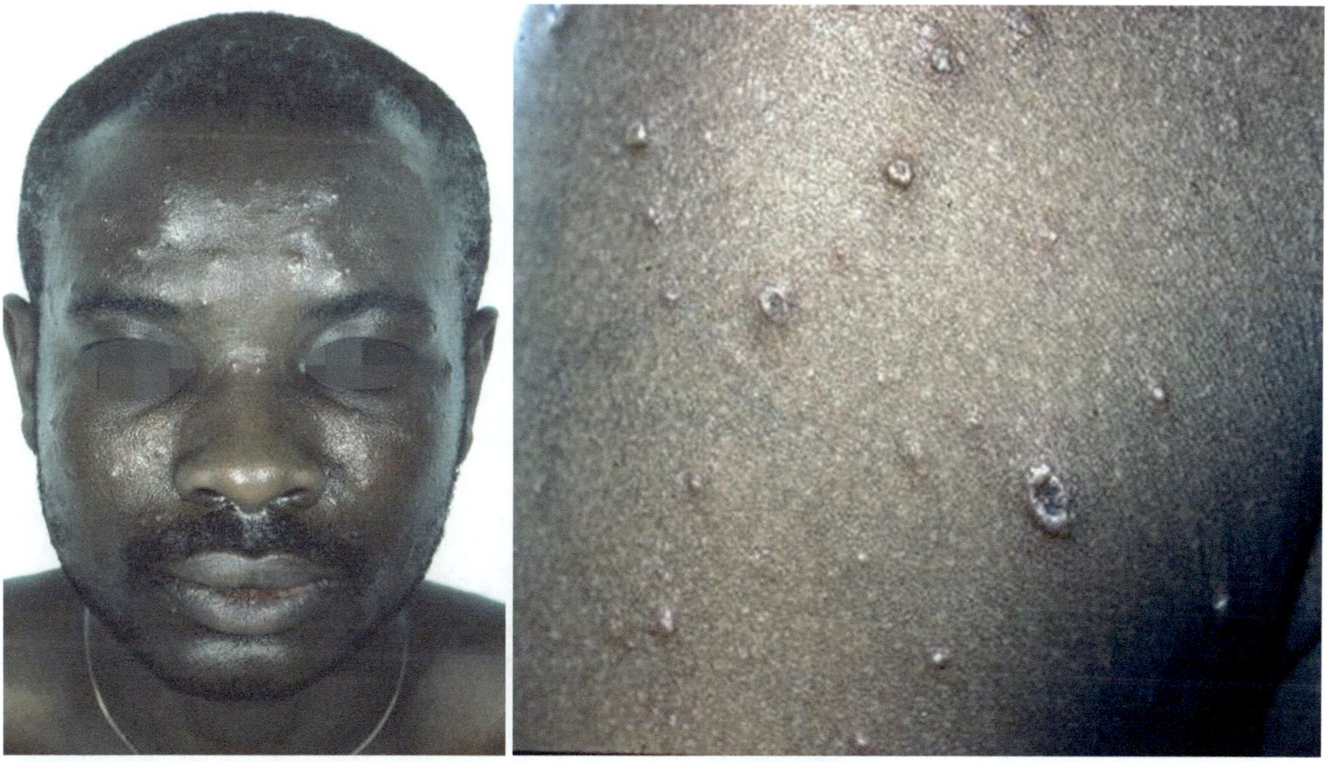

Fig. 7.9 *Varicella* infection in an African black-skinned adult

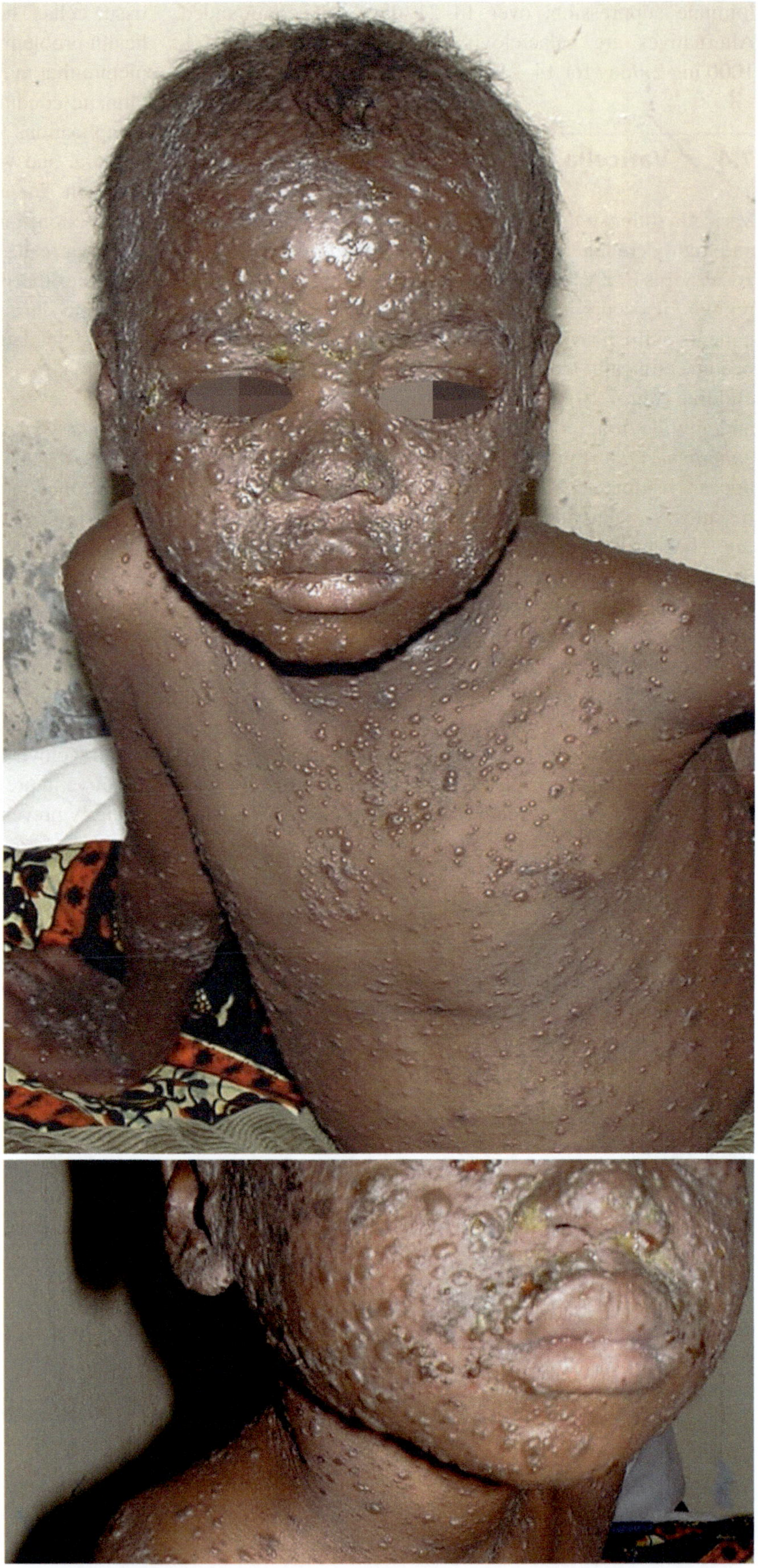

Fig. 7.10 *Severe varicella* in an African 5-year-old boy at first presentation and 3 days thereafter

7.5 Zoster

Zoster (shingles) is a clinical entity that results mainly in adults due to reactivation of VZV remaining in neural tissues after early chickenpox infection during childhood. The disease appears following triggering episodes, i.e., other infections, extensive UV exposure, stress, etc., particularly in individuals who are immune suppressed due to ongoing cancer disease, HIV infection, or other interfering conditions; 0.5–1% of the population may once present zoster during life [16, 17].

The first clinical sign of zoster is itching, burning, and painful sensation localized to areas of one or more dermatomes 3–5 days before the typical unilateral acute eruption with erythema and grouped blistering develops (*zoster segmentalis*); erythema is not recognizable and bullous lesions are more common in black skin (Fig. 7.11). Depending on the neural segment, mucous membranes can also be involved; the first branch of the trigeminal nerve and the eye (*zoster ophthalmicus*) or the ear with VZV reactivation in the ganglion geniculatum (*zoster oticus*, *Ramsay Hunt syndrome*) may be affected. Also muscle involvement occurs in about 5% of the cases and weakness usually follows the pain. The lesions of regular zoster usually clear in the majority of patients after 10–14 days without scarring. Severe multidermatomal involvement with necrotizing lesions may be registered in HIV-infected individuals (Fig. 7.12).

Treatment: Administration of systemic antivirals starting during the early stage of the eruption is the treatment of choice, preferably within the first 1–2 days after the eruption or as long as new blisters continue to develop [18]. Local treatment is symptomatic. Acyclovir is recommended orally 5 × 800 mg/day, or 3 × 10–15 mg/kg body weight intravenously for 7–10 days, which is more effective in respect to pain reduction, and alternatives oral valaciclovir 3 × 1000 mg/day for 7–10 days or famciclovir 3 × 250 or 500 mg/day for 7 days. Brivudin 125 mg once a day is as effective as famciclovir [19].

Postherpetic neuralgia is the commonest and most intractable complication of zoster, often seen in the elderly and multimorbid patients [20]. Painful sensations persist in the affected dermatome area long after the clinical recovery or arise 3 months after the onset of the initial eruption and may continue over several months or years. They represent a neuropathic pain consisting of continuous burning, spasmodic shooting, and allodynia, often triggered by nonspecific stimuli. Postherpetic neuralgia is difficult to control, frequently resistant to common analgesic drugs. If suspected, it seems

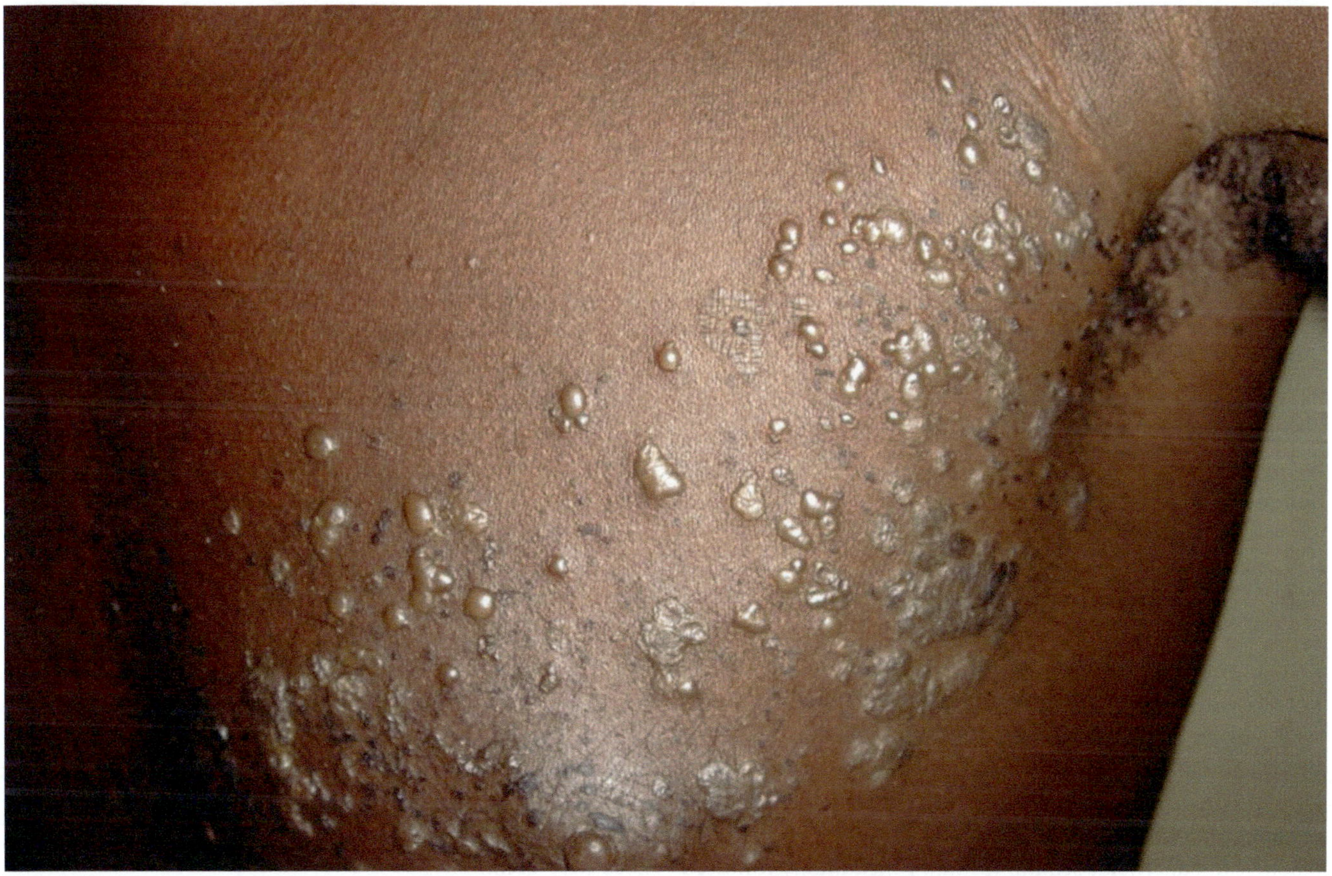

Fig. 7.11 *Zoster segmentalis* in an 18-year-old black-skinned male (no erythema is seen)

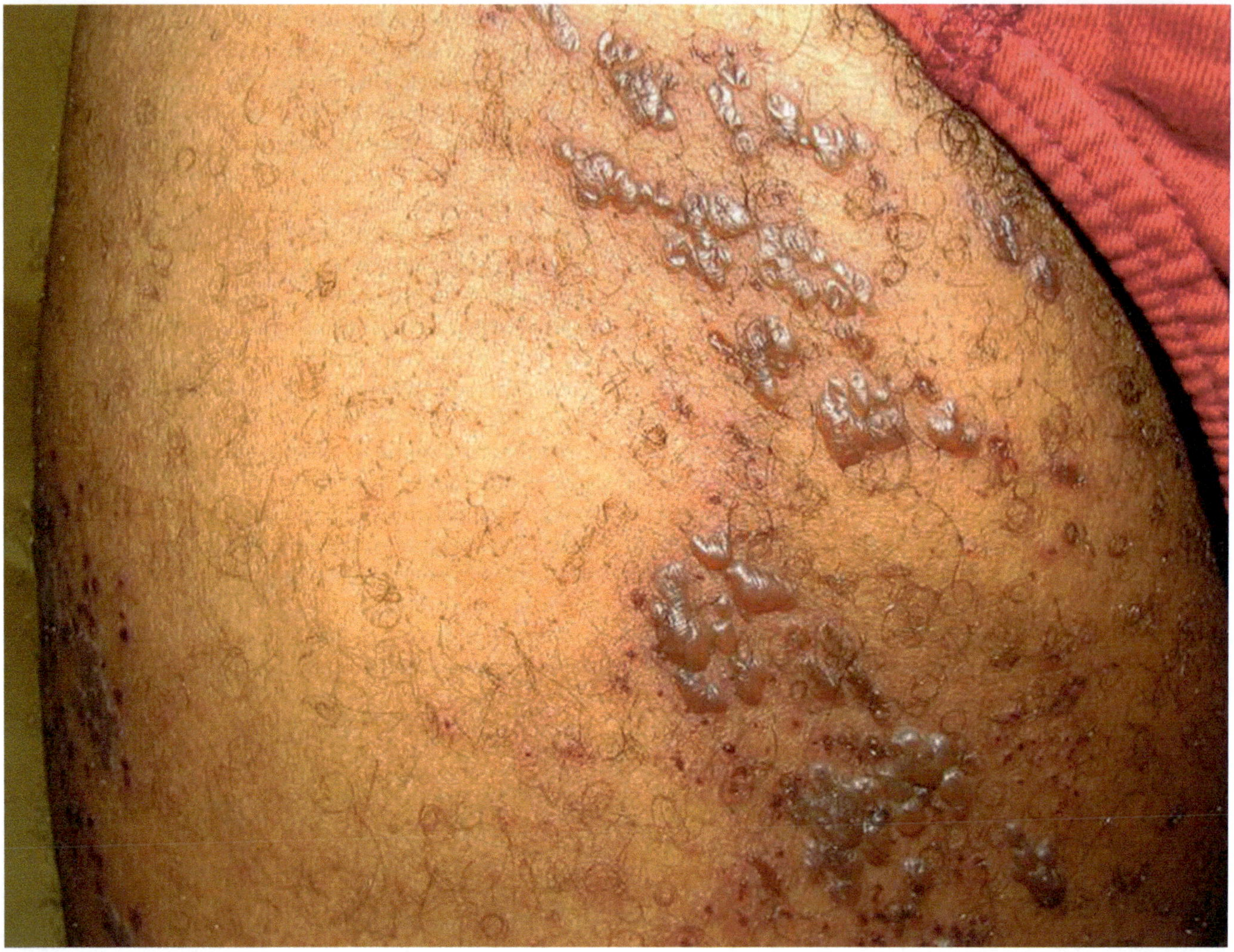

Fig. 7.12 *Multidermatomal zoster* in a HIV-infected, East African young male with Kaposi's sarcoma

beneficial to early administer valaciclovir 3 × 1000 mg/day or acyclovir 5 × 800 mg/day together with Carbamazepin 300 mg/day in increasing dose as a prophylactic measure. This combination is recommended particularly in patients who develop severe necrotizing zoster or the elderly who are at higher risk. For further interventions specialists on pain control may be contacted [18, 20].

7.6 Pityriasis Rosea

Pityriasis rosea is a common eruption which usually affects healthy children and adolescents, probably caused by reactivation of human herpes virus 6 (HHV-6), which is responsible for exanthema subitum (syn.: *roseola infantum*), and/or human herpes virus 7 (HHV-7), although the latter is still debatable [21]. The disease is first introduced by a herald-like patch with superficial scaling (*primary medallion*) followed by a generalized, often asymptomatic maculopapular eruption, mostly on the trunk and limbs. The scalp, palms, and soles are usually not involved. Spontaneous regression is to be expected in 2–6 weeks. A few patients complain of pruritus. Interestingly, pityriasis rosea in black children differs in several ways from classical descriptions [22]; atypical clinical pictures with facial and oral lesions have been described in dark-skinned patients [23, 24]. In contrast to Caucasians, cases with involvement of the face and neck have been reported in 29% of the patients in Nigeria [25] and in 30% of African American children [22], showing residual hypo- or hyperpigmentation. Mucosal involvement with partly erosive lesions, petechia, and temporary lymphadenopathy may also occur. Hypopigmented lesions of tinea versicolor should be considered as differential diagnosis [26].

For *management* topical application of calamine lotion and oral medication of antihistamines is recommended, if necessary at all.

7.7 Dengue Fever

Dengue is worldwide a rather common endemic virus infection in tropical America, sub-Saharan Africa, Southeast Asia, and also the Eastern Mediterranean Region. Travelers may spread the disease to non-endemic regions; today, dengue fever showing a subtle rash is more frequent than malaria in travelers returning to Europe from the tropics [2]. Numerous cases of vector-borne infections associated with traveling were reported in recent years, frequently by travelers returning from Southeast Asia, the Caribbean, and Oceania. The disease *is* caused by an arthropod-borne arbovirus with four distinct serotypes; 80 cases and all four genotypes were recently detected in Italy [27]. Vectors are mosquitoes, mainly *Aedes* species; person-to-person spread does not occur. After a short incubation period of about 1 week, patients present flu-like symptomatology with fever, myalgias, arthralgias, headaches, and typical retro-orbital pain. A severe hemorrhagic clinical form occurs, particularly when a second serotype reinfects an individual.

For *management* symptomatic measures, bed rest, supplementation of fluid, and fever and pain management are the main therapeutic modalities. Prognosis could be fatal; age is an important reliable in the outcome of secondary dengue infection. Death risk is nearly 15 times higher in children than in adults [28].

7.8 Chikungunya Fever

Outbreaks of chikungunya fever occur reportedly in tropical countries, mainly in Africa and South Asia, particularly in India, but recently also in the Americas (Colombia). In 2007 chikungunya fever was registered for the first time in Europe, presumably imported from an Indian traveler visiting relatives. In 2012 a total of 130 cases of dengue and chikungunya were reported in travelers returning to Italy; 40.4% of the imported cases with dengue had visited Asia within the incubation period, whereas 42.8% of the patients with chikungunya were imported from islands in the Indian Ocean, Mauritius, the Maldives, Bali, and Sri Lanka [29]. In a recent report, more than 41 cases have been confirmed by laboratory controls in Italy [27]. A few cases were also registered in France and Croatia. The disease is caused by an alphavirus of the family *Togaviridae* transmitted by mosquitoes (*Aedes aegypti*, *Aedes albopictus*).

Clinically, a rash with maculopapular lesions occurs, together with abrupt onset of fever, myalgias, fatigue, and joint pain. Arthralgias can persist for up to 1 year. The symptomatology is similar to that of dengue fever, sometimes overlooked or misdiagnosed, with a rather benign outcome; severe hemorrhagic courses rarely occur. Serological ELISA and PCR tests confirm the diagnosis.

Treatment is symptomatic to relieve malaise and pain.

7.9 Monkeypox Virus Infection

The disease is acquired from infected animals, e.g., monkeys, more often from rodents. It was recognized in 1970 described in tropical rainforest areas in Central and West Africa. Imported cases were reported after contact with cats or dogs which had contact with infected rodents [30]. The disease is caused by a zoonotic virus of the genus *Orthopoxvirus*. Patients in African countries, mainly children, develop a rash 1–3 days after the onset of fever with macules and papules and later umbilicated pustules. In Europe and the United States, affected individuals had only localized lesions.

There is no specific treatment. Symptomatic measures are indicated. Mortality ranges from 1 to 10%, mainly in children.

7.9.1 Prevention of Viral Infections

Individuals at risk to acquire viral infection, patients with atopic dermatitis, and other eczematous skin disease should be generally advised to avoid contact sports, shared towels, swimming pools, etc. for prevention.

Early vaccination is today recommended for prevention of genital warts since their vast majority and also genital cancer are associated with sexually transmitted HPV 16 and 18 and other oncogenic strains [31]. Commercial preparations such as *Gardasil®* or *Cervarix®* are given in developed countries to 4–14 years old females (0.5 mL day 1 and months 6) under yearly clinical monitoring, Pap smear examination, etc. Both vaccines induce detectable immunization and presence of circulating antibodies. A controlled vaccination program in Australia revealed marked declines in the proportions of diagnoses of genital warts in young indigenous women and men [32]. Overall, studies confirm that around >90% of genital warts and around 70% of cervical neoplasias can be prevented by early vaccination. It seems, however, that lack of affordability and also cultural barriers may be an intractable hindrance for implementing HPV vaccination programs in developing countries [33].

Vaccination is also the key for preventing a good number of other viral diseases including varicella. In several developed countries, routine immunization against VZV infection is recommended in early childhood and is regularly performed. Vaccination with two doses of a live attenuated VZV is the best prevention for varicella [34]; up to 90% of the vaccinated population becomes protected. Immunization is particularly effective for avoiding severe involvement and systemic complications of the disease.

A live attenuated VZV vaccine and a subunit vaccine are available in some countries to protect immune-competent adults from zoster and its complications or modify zoster pain [35].The subunit vaccine is more beneficial in the elderly reducing the risks of zoster and postherpetic neuralgia [36].

For vector-borne zoonotic infections like dengue and chikungunya fever, no vaccine exists. For prevention of monkeypox virus infection, it is recommended to avoid the proximity of vector-breeding sites and wear long sleeves and pants. Vector contact controls are necessary, e.g., with impregnated mosquito nets and clothes with repellents containing diethyltoluamide (DEET). For prevention CDC also recommends preexposure vaccination for health-care providers who are or may be in close contact with patients with monkeypox. The vaccination is also recommended for individuals directly exposed to the virus within 4 days after exposure.

Conclusions

Viruses are important pathogens in hot climate zones and tropical areas, more than any other infectious agent. They have a greater probability of mutation than bacteria and better possibilities to widespread; in addition, several viruses cross the skin barrier easily and infect both humans and animals in environments of great biodiversity. Tropical habitats also have been subject to major ecological changes in the last few decades. The collapse of eradication programs in many countries as well as population increases, and ecological qualifications have led to the spread of dengue fever and other tropical viral infections. Viruses previously strictly limited to certain geographic areas, e.g., chikungunya, are now entering new countries in the developed world. In most viral infections, mucocutaneous lesions occur; their knowledge should facilitate the diagnosis and help to prevent possible outbreaks.

References

1. Schwarz TF, Jäger G, Gilch S, et al. Travel-related vector borne virus infections in Germany. Arch Virol Suppl. 1996;11:57–65.
2. Fischer M, Schliemann S. Exanthems and fever in travelers returning from the tropics. Hautarzt. 2014;65:862–72.
3. Mays RM, Gordon RA, Javed S, et al. Viral diseases. In: Faber WR, Hay RJ, Naafs B, editors. Imported skin diseases. 2nd ed. Hoboken: Wiley-Blackwell; 2013. p. 123–47. Chapter 12.
4. Carneiro SC, Cestari T, Allen SH, et al. Viral exanthems in the tropics. Clin Dermatol. 2007;25:212–20.
5. Friedman DO, Weld LH, Kozarsky PE, et al. Spectrum of diseases and relation to place of exposure among ill returned travelers. N Engl J Med. 2006;354:119–30.
6. Androphy EJ, Kirnbauer R. Human papilloma virus infections. In: Goldsmith LA, Katz SI, Gilchrest BA, et al., editors. Fitzpatrick's dermatology in general medicine. 8th ed. New York: McGraw Hill; 2012. p. 2421–33. Chapter 196.
7. Bernard HU, Burk RD, Chen Z, et al. Classification of papilloma viruses (PVs) based on 189 PV types and proposal of taxonomic amendments. Virology. 2010;401:70–9.
8. Hanson D, Diven DG. Molluscum contagiosum. Dermatol Online J. 2003;9:2–8.
9. Piggott C, Friedlander SF, Tom W. Poxvirus infections. In: Goldsmith LA, Katz SI, Gilchrest BA, et al., editors. Fitzpatrick's dermatology in general medicine. 8th ed. New York: McGraw Hill; 2012. p. 2402–11. Chapter 195.
10. van der Wouden JC, van des Sande R, van Suijekom-Snit LW, et al. Intervention for cutaneous molluscum contagiosum. Cochrane Database Syst Rev 2009;(4):CD004767.
11. Fathazadeh W, Schwartz RA. Human herpes virus infections: epidemiology, pathogenesis, symptomatic, diagnosis and management. J Am Acad Dermatol. 2007;57:737–63.
12. Arduino PG, Porter SR. Oral and perioral herpes simplex virus type I infection: review of its management. Oral Dis. 2006;12:254–70.
13. Cernik C, Gallina K, Brodell RT. The treatment of herpes simplex infections. An evidence-based review. Arch Intern Med. 2008;168:1137–44.
14. Heininger U, Seward JF. Varicella. Lancet. 2006;368:1365–76.
15. Tognoti E. The eradication of smallpox, a success story for modern medicine and public health: what lessons for the future? J Infect Dev Ctries. 2010;4:264–6.
16. Cohen JI. Clinical practice: herpes zoster. N Engl J Med. 2013;369:255–63.
17. Bader MS. Herpes zoster: diagnostic, therapeutic, and preventive approaches. Postgrad Med. 2013;125:78–91.
18. Whitley RJ, Volpi A, McKendrick M, et al. Management of herpes zoster and postherpetic neuralgia now and in the future. J Clin Virol. 2010;48:20–8.
19. Gross G, Schoefer H, Wassilew S, et al. Herpes zoster guideline of the German Dermatology Society (DDG). J Clin Virol. 2003;26:277–89.
20. Johnson RW, Rice ASC. Postherpetic neuralgia. N Engl J Med. 2014;371:1526–36.
21. De Araujo T, Berman B, Weinstein A. Human herpes viruses 6 and 7. Dermatol Clin. 2002;20:301–6.
22. Amer A, Fischer H, Li X. The natural history of pityriasis rosea in black American children: how correct in the classic description? Arch Pediatr Adolesc Med. 2007;161:503–6.
23. Vano-Galvan S, Ma DL, Lopez-Neyra A, et al. Atypical pityriasis rosea in a black child: a case report. Cases J. 2009;2:6796.
24. Drago F, Ciccarese G, Thanasi H, et al. Facial involvement in pityriasis rosea: differences among Caucasian and dark-skinned patients. G Ital Dermatol Venereol. 2016;151:571–2.
25. Jacyk WK. Pityriasis rosea in Nigerians. Int J Dermatol. 1980;19:397–9.
26. Kallini JR, Riaz F, Khachemoune A. Tinea versicolor in dark-skinned individuals. Int J Dermatol. 2014;53:137–41.
27. Fortuna C, Remoli ME, Rizzo C, et al. Imported arboviral infections in Italy, July 2014-October 2015: a National Reference Laboratory report. BMC Infect Dis. 2017;17:216. https://doi.org/10.1186/s12879-017-2320-1.
28. Guzman MG, Kouri G, Bravo J, et al. Effect of age on outcome of secondary dengue 2 infections. Int J Infect Dis. 2002;6:118–24.
29. Napoli C, Salcuni P, Pompa MG, et al. Estimated imported infections of chikungunya and dengue in Italy, 2008 to 2011. J Travel Med. 2012;19:294–7.
30. McCallum AM, Damon IK. Human monkeypox. Clin Infect Dis. 2014;58:260–7.
31. zur Hausen H. Papilloma viruses and cancer: from basic studies to clinical application. Nat Rev Cancer. 2002;2:342–50.
32. Ali H, McManus H, O'Connor CC, et al. Human papillomavirus vaccination and genital warts in young indigenous Australians: national sentinel surveillance data. Med J Aust. 2017;206:204–9.
33. Venturas C, Umeh K. Health professional feedback on HPV vaccination roll-out in a developing country. Vaccine. 2017;35:1886–91. https://doi.org/10.1016/j.vaccine.2017.02.052. pii: S0264-410X(17)30265-7.
34. Marin M, Güris D, Chaves SS. Prevention of varicella: recommendations of the advisory committee on immunization practices (ACIP). MMWR Recomm Rep. 2007;56:1–50.
35. Oxman MN. Zoster vaccine: current status and future aspects. Clin Infect Dis. 2010;51:197–213.
36. Cunningham AL, Lal H, Kovac M, et al. Efficacy of the herpes zoster subunit vaccine in adults 70 years of age or older. N Engl J Med. 2016;375:1019–32.

8 Sexually Transmitted Infections in Dark Skin

Vishal Gupta, Adel Botros Zaghloul, and Somesh Gupta

The epidemiology of sexually transmitted infections (STIs) is ever-changing and reflects the prevalent sexual behaviors and the health-care services in the community. Knowledge of the various epidemiological factors is essential for designing effective control strategies. Developing nations account for the vast share of STIs, while the STI burden is quite low in the developed world. With the emergence of HIV infection, indiscriminate use of antibiotics, upgradation of health-care facilities at primary level, and success of a *syndromic approach* to STI treatment, we are currently witnessing a decline in bacterial STIs and a surge in viral infections. This change in the STI trends is common to both developing as well as developed countries. However, our understanding of the epidemiology of STIs in developing nations is limited by lack of good-quality community-based data: most of the data available are institution-based, with surveys in convenient populations like STI clinics or antenatal clinic attendees, which is not representative of the general population.

The WHO has published the 2012 global and regional estimates for the incidence and prevalence of four curable STIs: syphilis, gonorrhea, trichomoniasis, and *Chlamydia trachomatis* infections (Table 8.1).

The reported global incidence of these four STIs according to 2012 estimates is around 357 million. The highest burden of these STIs was found in the Western Pacific Region followed by the Americas and the African region. The low prevalence in Europe and Southeast Asia could be because of better socio-economic conditions, safer sexual behavior, or inadequate representation of the data from these regions. Because of the different methods used in the previous estimates, the 2012 data are not appropriate for trend analysis, and thus, one cannot comment whether the rates of infection have truly decreased over time (448 million in 2005, 498 million in 2008) [1].

This chapter aims to provide a brief review of the common STIs in dark-skinned populations. Syndromic approach to the management of these infections, which is commonly practiced in the developing world, is also discussed.

8.1 Syphilis

Syphilis is caused by *Treponema pallidum*, a spirochete. Syphilis was rare in the USA and Europe in the 1970s and 1980s. There was reemergence in the late 1990s, disproportionately affecting the African-Americans, men who have sex with men, drug abusers, and HIV patients [2]. In 1999, the WHO estimated around 12 million new cases of early syphilis, with over 2/3 cases in sub-Saharan Africa and Southeast Asia. The burden of syphilis has been gradually decreasing throughout the world, with around ten million and 5.6 million new cases in 2005–2008 and 2012, respectively. The highest prevalence is still in the Africa region, but other regions have shown a considerable reduction in the rates of infectious syphilis [1, 3]. It was estimated that between 0.75 and 1.5 million pregnancies were affected by syphilis in 2006. Congenital syphilis is now quite rare in industrialized nations but remains a significant problem in certain parts of the world (sub-Saharan Africa, East Europe). A slight resurgence was noted recently in the USA (2012–2014), mainly affecting individuals with black skin [4].

8.1.1 Clinical Manifestations

Untreated syphilis passes through the following stages: primary, secondary, latent, and tertiary syphilis. Approximately 1/3 patients develop primary chancre, around 3 weeks after

V. Gupta · S. Gupta (✉)
Department of Dermatology and Venereology, All India Institute of Medical Sciences, New Delhi, India

A. B. Zaghloul
Cairo Skin Clinik, VD Hospital, El Haud El Marsoud, Ministry of Health, Cairo, Egypt

C. E. Orfanos et al. (eds.), *Pigmented Ethnic Skin and Imported Dermatoses*, https://doi.org/10.1007/978-3-319-69422-1_8

Table 8.1 New cases in adults for the four major curable STIs in 2012 in selected regions worldwide[a]

STI	African region	Southeast Asia	Europe	The Americas	Western-Pacific	Global
Trichomoniasis	37.3	13.2	3.8	27.4	45.3	142.5
Chlamydia trachomatis infections	12.1	13.8	9.1	24.7	60.9	130.9
Gonorrhea	11.4	11.4	4.7	10.9	35.2	78.3
Syphilis	1.8	0.89	0.4	0.94	0.99	5.6
Total	62.5	39.3	18.1	63.9	142.4	357.3

[a]All numbers in millions

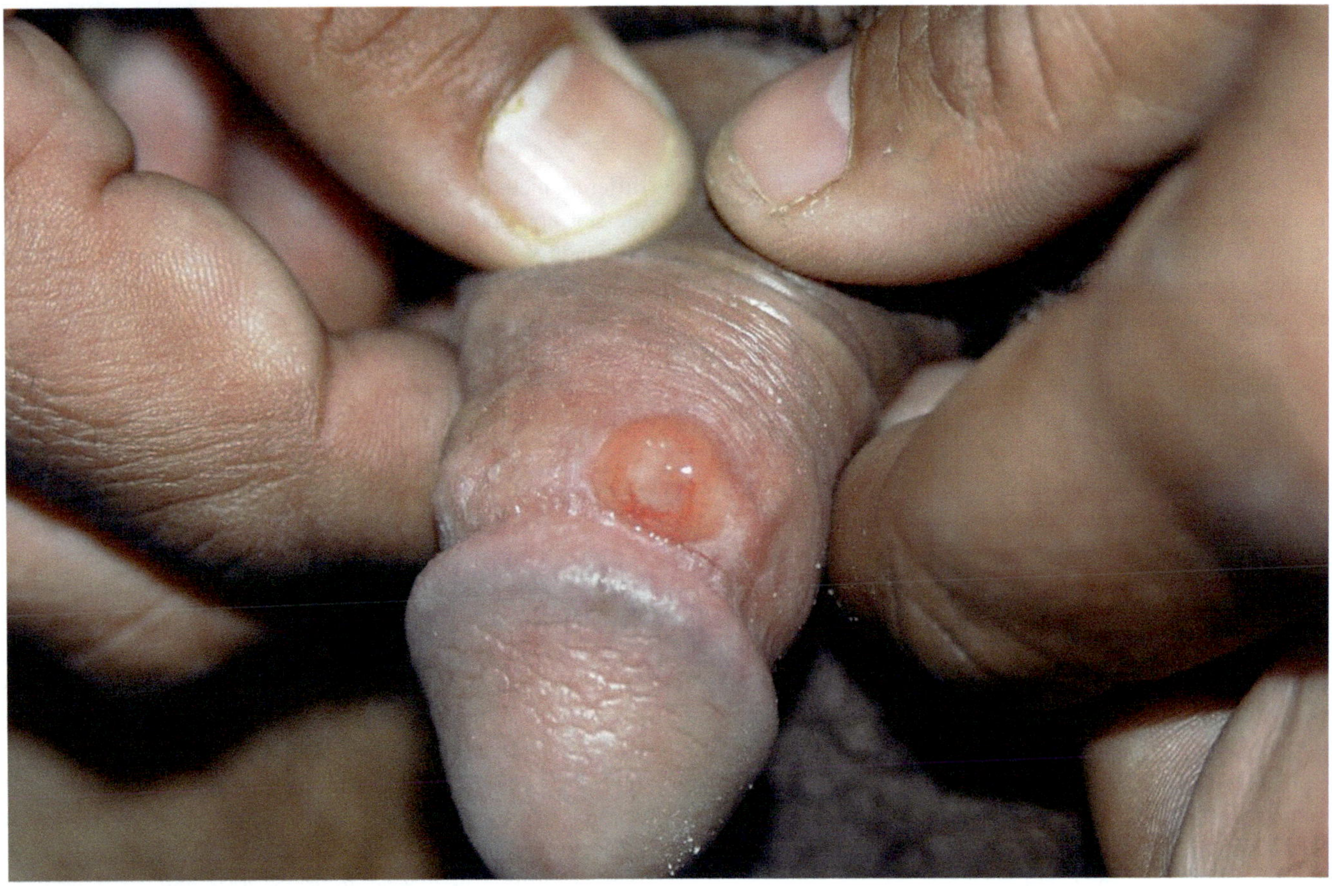

Fig. 8.1 Firm painless penile chancre in *primary syphilis*

contact. The primary stage may go unnoticed as the ulcer is painless and heals spontaneously in immune-competent patients in 3–8 weeks (Fig. 8.1). In immune compromised, the primary lesion may persist and enlarge in considerable size (Fig. 8.2).

The secondary stage is characterized by a self-limiting skin eruption: asymptomatic symmetric macules, papules, or papulosquamous lesions with generalized lymphadenopathy, often accompanied by fever and malaise. Moist syphilids, like *condylomata lata*, occur on intertriginous areas and are teeming with spirochetes (Fig. 8.3). Most characteristic is the appearance of brownish papulosquamous lesions on palms and soles (Figs. 8.4 and 8.5). Because of the wide spectrum of skin lesions seen in secondary syphilis, this stage of the infection is also called "the great imitator." After resolution of secondary syphilis, patents enter into a phase of latency, which is characterized by positive serology but no signs or clinical symptoms. Approximately 25% of the patients with latent syphilis can develop a relapse, mostly within the first year. If untreated, roughly one third of latent syphilis patients can progress to tertiary syphilis: gummatous, cardiovascular, or neurosyphilis. Neurosyphilis may also be seen during any stage of syphilis.

8.1.2 Diagnosis

Dark ground microscope for direct visualization of the treponemas from the genital ulcer, lymph node aspirates, or syphilids is not available widely. The diagnosis of syphilis rests on non-

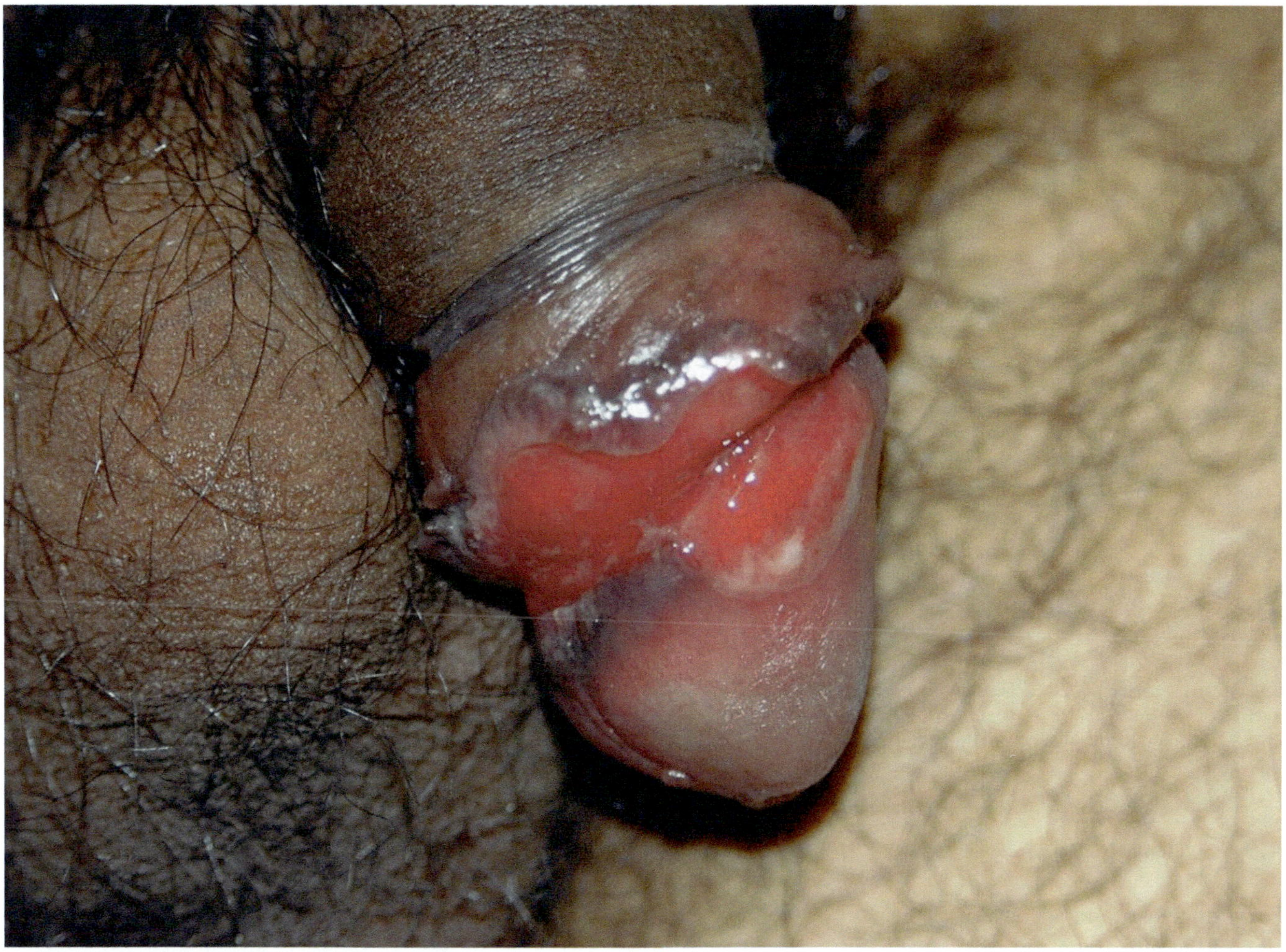

Fig. 8.2 Extended ulcerous *syphilitic chancre* in an immune compromised HIV-infected male

treponemal (VDRL, RPR) and treponemal serology tests (TPHA, FTA-Abs). Non-treponemal tests are commonly used for screening, followed by treponemal tests for confirming the diagnosis. As the titers of non-treponemal tests decrease with time and treatment, these can be used for monitoring the treatment response. However, the sensitivity of non-treponemal tests is low in late latent and tertiary syphilis. Cerebrospinal fluid examination is needed to diagnose neurosyphilis. Molecular tests like PCR and rapid point-of-care tests, available only in institutional settings, are not used routinely in clinical setting.

8.1.3 Treatment

Benzathine penicillin 2.4 mU given intramuscularly as a single dose for early syphilis (primary, secondary, early latent) and weekly for 3 weeks for late syphilis (late latent, tertiary syphilis except neurosyphilis) is the recommended treatment. For neurosyphilis, intravenous aqueous crystalline penicillin (3–4 mU every 4 h × 10–14 days) is given. Syphilis in pregnancy is treated according to the stage of the disease. For penicillin allergic patients, alternatives include doxycycline, erythromycin, and ceftriaxone. In pregnancy, de-sensitization followed by penicillin treatment is preferred as the efficacy of non-penicillin regimens is not completely known [5].

8.2 Chancroid

Haemophilus ducreyi, a facultative anaerobic gram-negative coccobacillus is the causative agent of chancroid. It has emerged as a cause of non-venereal chronic skin ulcers in children in the tropics [6].

In 1990s, the global prevalence of chancroid was approximately seven million, with high burden in Africa, Asia, Latin America, and the Caribbean. Once quite a common cause of sexually acquired genital ulcers, the incidence of chancroid has decreased drastically worldwide probably because of the success of syndromic approach. In the period from 2000 to 2014, studies across the globe reported low proportion of infections (<10%), except for Malawi (15%). No cases were reported from North America, Asia, and the Caribbean [6]. It is difficult

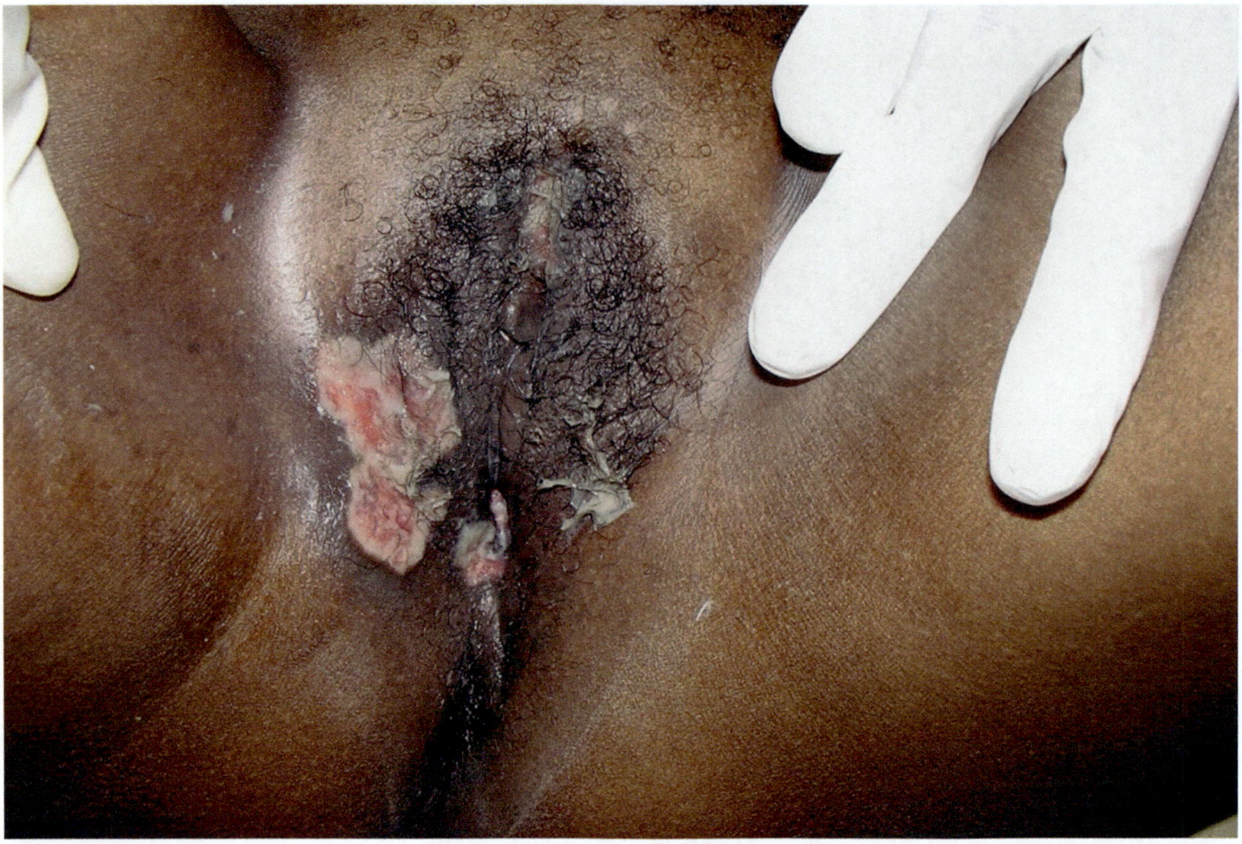

Fig. 8.3 Multiple *condylomata lata*, secondarily infected

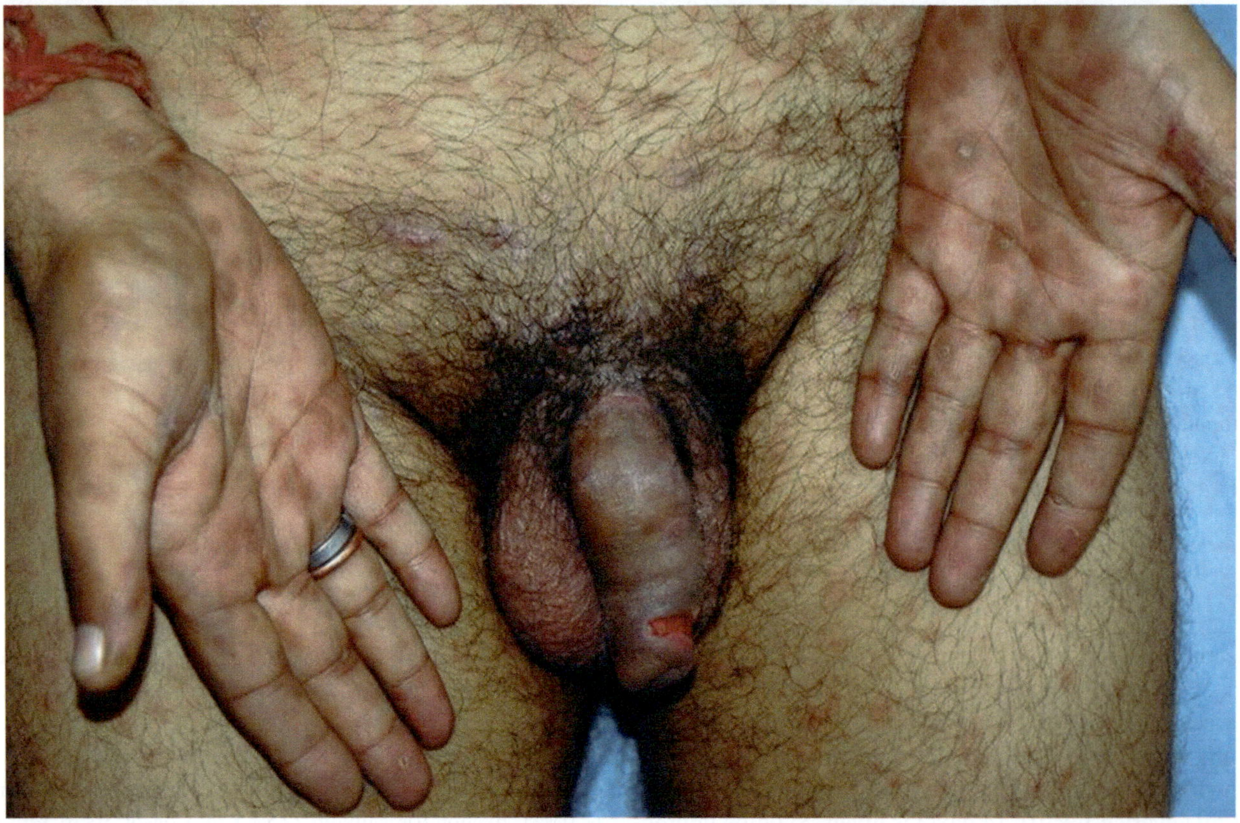

Fig. 8.4 Persisting *primary syphilitic chancre* and lesions on the palms indicating *secondary syphilis*

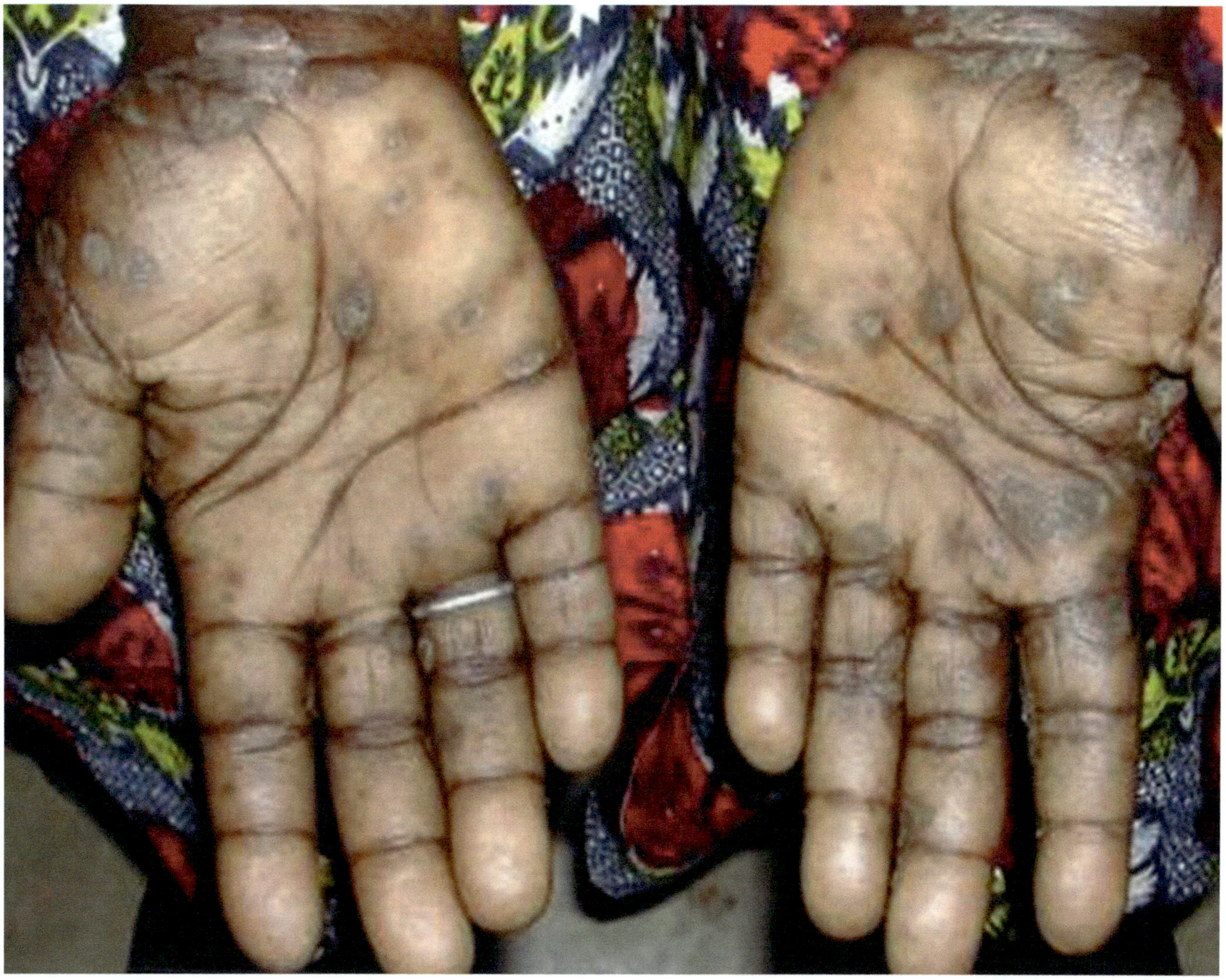

Fig. 8.5 Scaly lichenoid plaques on both palms in *secondary syphilis* (Courtesy Dr. Ketema, RDTC Moshi, Tanzania)

to estimate the true prevalence as a laboratory diagnosis is not always possible and clinical diagnosis is not reliable.

8.2.1 Clinical Manifestations

The initial lesion develops 1–14 days after contact, as an inflammatory papule or pustule which forms a painful ulcer with undermined edges and necrotic floor which bleeds easily on manipulation. About 50% patients have multiple ulcers. Unilateral painful inguinal lymphadenitis is seen in 30–60% of cases. The lymph nodes can suppurate (bubo) in about 25% cases, which can rupture to form a chancroidal ulcer or sinuses. Common sites in men include prepuce, coronal sulcus, urethral meatus, and penile shaft, while fourchette, labia, clitoris, vagina, and perianal area are the usual sites in females.

8.2.2 Diagnosis

Demonstration of gram-negative coccobacilli in the smear prepared from the ulcer floor has a low sensitivity. Culture, considered to be the gold standard, has a low sensitivity (0–80%) as *H. ducreyi* is a fastidious organism and the culture requires stringent conditions. Nucleic acid detection techniques like PCR are more sensitive than culture but are not commercially available. Clinical diagnosis is correct in not more than half of the cases but is usually relied upon for lack of cost-effective laboratory investigations with good sensitivity and specificity. The CDC proposes that a probable diagnosis of chancroid can be made based on the typical clinical features and negative tests for syphilis (dark ground microscopy, serology) and herpes [5].

8.2.3 Treatment

Azithromycin 1 g is the preferred treatment because it is given in a single oral dose. Intramuscular ceftriaxone 250 mg injection, ciprofloxacin (2 × 500 mg/day, 3 days), and erythromycin (3 × 500 mg/day, 7 days) are the other treatment options. Fluctuant buboes should be aspirated. Recent sexual partners should also be treated [5].

8.3 Gonorrhea

Gonorrhea is caused by *Neisseria gonorrhoeae*, an intracellular gram-negative diplococcus, which infects the columnar epithelium of the anogenital tract and conjunctiva. It is the second most common bacterial STI in the world. According to the 2012 WHO estimates, there were 78 million new cases worldwide. The highest prevalence was in Western Pacific Region (35 million), followed by Southeast Asia, African region, and the Americas (11 million in each). The prevalence in Europe was quite low (4.6 million) [1]. In the USA, the infection rates were the highest among African-Americans, followed by American Indians/Alaska Natives [7].

8.3.1 Clinical Manifestations

About 15% of men and roughly half of the women infected remain asymptomatic. Symptoms usually appear within 2–5 days of exposure. It presents as purulent or mucopurulent urethral discharge associated with dysuria, increased frequency and urgency in men. Women may develop features of cervicitis or urethritis. Gonococcal proctitis (more common in women and men who have sex with men) manifests as anal pruritus, altered bowel habits, tenesmus, rectal discharge, or bleeding per rectum. Pharyngeal infection may present as exudative pharyngitis or tonsillitis associated with cervical lymphadenopathy but is asymptomatic in over 90% of all cases. Coinfection with chlamydia is quite common, seen in about 25–30% of the cases. Untreated gonococcal infections can be complicated by periurethral abscesses (which can rupture leading to "water can perineum"), epididymitis, and prostatitis in men. Complications in women include pelvic inflammatory disease, infertility, ectopic pregnancy, and Bartholin's gland abscess. Disseminated gonococcal infection (seen in 0.5–3%, more common in women) is a rare complication, characterized by acral purpuric papulopustular skin lesions and polyarthritis. Neonatal gonococcal infections (*ophthalmia neonatorum*) are now rare in developed world but remain a serious concern in some developing countries.

8.3.2 Diagnosis

Demonstration of gram-negative diplococci within polymorphonuclear leukocytes in the smear prepared from genital swab has a high sensitivity (90–95%) in symptomatic men, but not in women and asymptomatic patients (50–70%) [8]. Culture on special media (like Thayer-Martin medium, New York City medium) allows not only confirming the diagnosis but also drug-sensitivity testing. Nucleic acid amplification tests like PCR are now available at many institutes. The availability of the rapid point-of-care tests which can detect gonococcal antigen from the urethral or genital swabs varies widely and are not used routinely.

8.3.3 Treatment

Since 2010, the CDC recommends dual management due to concerns regarding drug resistance: single intramuscular injection of ceftriaxone 250 mg for uncomplicated gonococcal infection plus single-dose azithromycin 1 g. Oral cefixime is no longer recommended as the first-line agent since 2012; however it is still prescribed in regions where ceftriaxone is not freely available. Another advantage of this dual regimen is covering for the concurrent chlamydial infection. All recent sexual partners (in the last 60 days) should also be treated empirically [5]. Resistance to oral cefixime was first reported from Japan in 1995. Since then, reports of documented resistance to cefixime have emerged across the globe, including Japan, several European countries, Canada, and South Africa [9].

8.4 Chlamydia Trachomatis Infections

Chlamydia trachomatis is an obligate intracellular bacterium, which infects the columnar epithelium of the urogenital tract. Approximately 105 million cases of *Chlamydia trachomatis* infection were reported worldwide in 2008 (a marginal increase of 4.1% from 2005 estimates), with the major burden being borne by Western Pacific Region (40 million new cases), followed by the Americas and the European region [3]. Chlamydial urethritis has now overtaken gonorrhea as the most common cause of urethritis worldwide. *Chlamydia trachomatis* serovars D–K are implicated in urethritis and cervicitis, while L1–L3 cause *lymphogranuloma venereum*.

8.4.1 Clinical Manifestations

It is estimated that about 85 and 40% of infected women and men, respectively, may be asymptomatic, thus serving as reservoir of infections. Women usually present with cervicitis (vaginal discharge, postcoital or intermenstrual bleeding, dyspareunia, friable cervical mucosa) and sometimes with symptoms suggestive of urethral infection (dysuria, increased urinary frequency). Infection can ascend to the endometrium and fallopian tubes and cause pelvic inflammatory disease (10–40%), ectopic pregnancy, infertility, and perihepatitis (*Fitz-Hugh-Curtis syndrome*). Chlamydial infection in pregnancy can lead to preterm delivery, premature rupture of membranes, low-birth weight, and neonatal conjunctivitis (*ophthalmia neonatorum*) and pneumonia. Symptomatic men develop dysuria, urethral discharge and per-urethral itching. Complications include epididymo-orchitis, prostatitis, and Reiter's disease. Rectal (rarely symptomatic) and conjunctival infections can occur in both the sexes.

Considering that majority of infections are asymptomatic, screening for genital chlamydial infections is recommended for at-risk population groups and pregnant women, but is not routinely carried out except in institutional settings where testing facilities are available.

8.4.2 Diagnosis

Presence of more than ten polymorphonuclear leukocytes (PMNs) per 1000× field in vaginal discharge and 30 PMNs/field in cervical discharge in the absence of detectable organisms on gram stain is indicative of chlamydial cervicitis. For urethritis, the corresponding figures are two PMNs/field in urethral swab or ten PMNs/field in urinary sediment. Nucleic acid amplification tests like PCR, the most sensitive and specific tests, are the mainstay of the diagnosis and are available at most of the research institutes. Direct fluorescent antibody test to detect chlamydial antigen and facilities for cell cultures are not widely available [10, 11].

8.4.3 Treatment

Doxycycline 2 × 100 mg/day for 7 days or azithromycin 1 g in a single oral dose is equally effective in treating uncomplicated anogenital chlamydial infection. All sexual partners in the last 60 days should be offered treatment [5].

8.5 Trichomoniasis

Trichomoniasis is caused by *Trichomonas vaginalis*, a protozoa of the order *Trichomonadida*. It is the most common curable sexually transmitted infection in the world. WHO estimated approximately 276 million new cases globally in 2008, an increase of 11.2% from 2005 (248 million) [12]. The majority of the cases were reported from WHO Western Pacific and African region [1].

8.5.1 Clinical Manifestations

Roughly half of the infected women are asymptomatic, but about 30% of these women become symptomatic when observed for 6 months. When symptomatic, it can present as vaginal discharge (copious, homogenous, malodorous, "frothy," yellow-green in color), vaginal itching, dysuria, pelvic pain, irregular bleeding, and/or dyspareunia. Punctate hemorrhages in the cervix, referred to as "strawberry cervix," are characteristic. Complications can include pelvic inflammatory disease, tubal infertility, adverse pregnancy outcomes (preterm birth, low-birth weight), and increased risk of cervical cancer [13]. It is also associated with an increased risk of HIV transmission: CDC estimates that up to 20% of HIV transmissions in African-Americans in the USA may be attributable to *Trichomonas vaginalis* infection [14]. Majority of the men are asymptomatic, and the infection can resolve spontaneously as well. It can cause urethral discharge or urethritis, prostatitis, epididymitis, and even potential infertility (decrease in sperm motility and viability) in men [13].

8.5.2 Diagnosis

Diagnosis based on clinical features is unreliable. Direct visualization of the motile protozoa by preparing a wet mount from the vaginal or urethral discharge is the most frequently used diagnostic test. However, it has a low sensitivity (50–65% sensitive, with higher sensitivity in women). Culture (on modified Diamond's medium) is the diagnostic gold standard, but facilities are available only at select tertiary care centers. Other diagnostic methods include molecular tests like nucleic acid amplification tests (most sensitive diagnostic test) and nucleic acid hybridization tests, which are not used routinely [15].

8.5.3 Treatment

Single oral dose of metronidazole or tinidazole 2 g is the recommended treatment, with a success rate of about 85%. Management of recent sexual partners is strongly recommended. Alternative treatment regimens include metronidazole (2 × 500 mg/day, 7 days) [5].

8.6 Genital Herpes

Genital herpes is the most common STI worldwide. The causative agent is herpes simplex virus (HSV), a double-stranded DNA virus. HSV-2 accounts for roughly 2/3 cases of genital herpes; however the incidence of genital HSV-1 infection is gradually increasing. The prevalence of HSV-2 infection varies greatly with different geographic regions, with generally higher estimates in developing countries. The prevalence was the highest in Africa (31.5%) followed by the Americas (14.4%) in 2012. Though the overall prevalence of HSV-2 infection was low in Southeast Asia and Western Pacific, these regions had a large burden of disease by virtue of their large population sizes. The risk of HSV infection increases with age and the number of sexual partners, while having protected sex and circumcision are protective. HSV infection is more common in women, men who have sex with men and HIV-positive individuals [16].

8.6.1 Clinical Manifestations

Many patients report developing prodromal symptoms (like tingling or burning sensation) prior to the onset of grouped vesicular lesions which rupture to form painful polycyclic erosions. The locoregional lymph nodes often become enlarged and tender. The first episode is more severe and longer lasting (2–3 weeks as compared to 5–7 days for recurrent episodes) and is usually accompanied by constitutional symptoms. The risk of viremia leading to systemic complications like aseptic meningitis, hepatitis, and pneumonitis is more with the first episode. The common sites in men include glans penis, prepuce, and penile shaft, while in women, labia, vagina, and cervix are usually affected. As HSV establishes a latent infection in the sensory ganglia, it can be reactivated by a trigger leading to a recurrence, which may be symptomatic or just asymptomatic viral shedding. Recurrences are more common and earlier in HSV-2 than in HSV-1 infections: 90% with HSV-2 infection and 60% with HSV-1 infection have at least one recurrence during the first year. The number of recurrences gradually decreases with time. Patients with HIV can develop extensive, necrotic, and non-healing ulcers with atypical morphologies like verrucous or vegetative plaques (Fig. 8.6).

8.6.2 Diagnosis

The diagnosis is usually made on clinical grounds in typical cases. However, its sensitivity is quite low as the characteristic lesions are seen only in a subset of patients. *Tzanck* smear (to look for multinucleated giant cells) is a simple bedside test, with a sensitivity and specificity of 80% and 93%, respectively. Direct fluorescent antibody testing can be used to detect HSV-1 or HSV-2 antigen on the genital specimen. Facilities for viral culture are available only in research settings. Amplification and detection of viral DNA by PCR is regarded as the test of choice as it is more sensitive than culture and requires less stringent transport conditions, however high cost limits its routine use in clinical settings. Serological testing is of limited value. Seroconversion or rising titers are more useful than a single reading [17].

8.6.3 Treatment

Acyclovir 3 × 400 mg/day for 7 days for the first episode and for 5 days for a recurrent episode is the recommended treatment. Acyclovir 2 × 400 mg/day can be given as suppressive management for patients who develop recurrent herpes frequently or those having a negative impact on their quality of

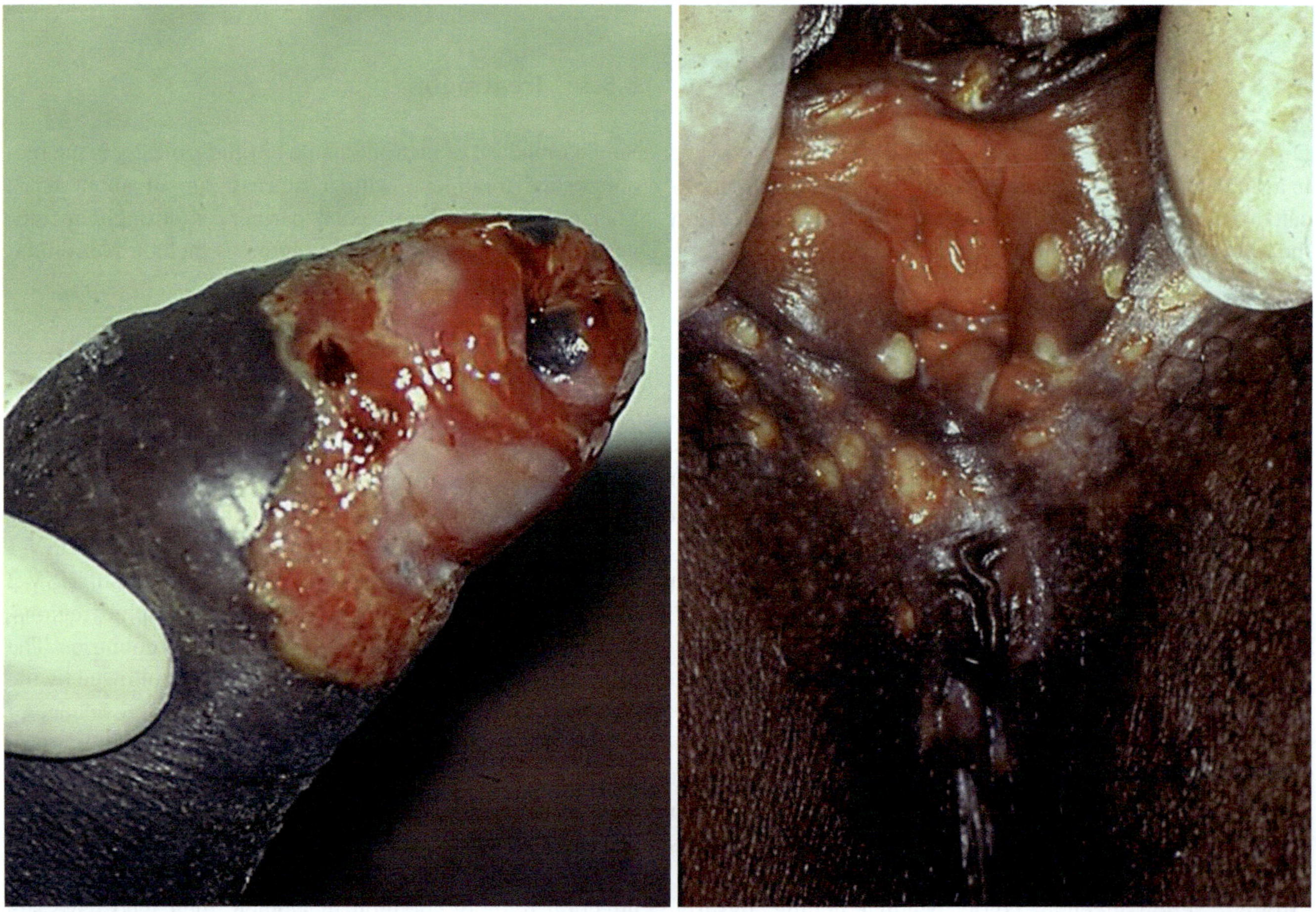

Fig. 8.6 *Genital herpes* (RDTC Moshi, Tanzania; courtesy Dr. M. Ketema)

life. Other options include valaciclovir and famciclovir with a similar efficacy and side effect profile. Sexual partners should be examined and offered treatment if symptomatic [5, 17].

8.7 Anogenital Warts

Anogenital warts are one of the most prevalent STIs worldwide. It is estimated that more than 50% of sexually active adults get infected with one or more HPV times in their lifetime. A systematic review on the epidemiology of the anogenital warts reported its prevalence ranging from 0.15 to 0.18% in the general population. Most of the studies included in the review were from the USA or European nations. Majority of the studies report a higher prevalence of HPV infections in men [18]. The worldwide prevalence of HPV infection in women with normal cervical cytology was estimated to be about 10% in a meta-analysis, with Eastern Africa having the highest regional prevalence (31.6%) and Southeast Asia with the lowest prevalence (6.2%) [19]. About 80% of all HPV-related cancers are seen in developing countries, with highest incidence rates in sub-Saharan Africa, Latin America, and the Caribbean and Asia. The risk of HPV infection increases with the number of sex partners that the woman or her partner has had over a lifetime. Circumcised men are less likely to have HPV infection, and even the risk of cervical cancer is reduced in women with circumcised male sex partners. HPV-16 seems to be the most frequently isolated HPV type in the world, with an estimated prevalence of 9% in Africa, 19% in Europe, and 21% in Asia [20].

8.7.1 Clinical Manifestations

Most of the genital HPV infection is asymptomatic and self-limited (70% infections self-resolved in 1 year and 90% in 2 years). The anogenital warts may be classified as *condylomata acuminata* (pink, fleshy, pedunculated, cauliflower-like growths on partially keratinized moist surfaces), papular warts, keratotic warts (*verruca vulgaris*), flat warts (*verruca plana*), and *bowenoid papulosis*, based on their clinical morphology. The common sites in men include prepuce, frenulum, glans, coronal sulcus, urethral meatus, scrotum, and penile shaft (Fig. 8.7), while posterior part of the introitus, labia, perineum, and perianal area are commonly affected in women (Fig. 8.8).

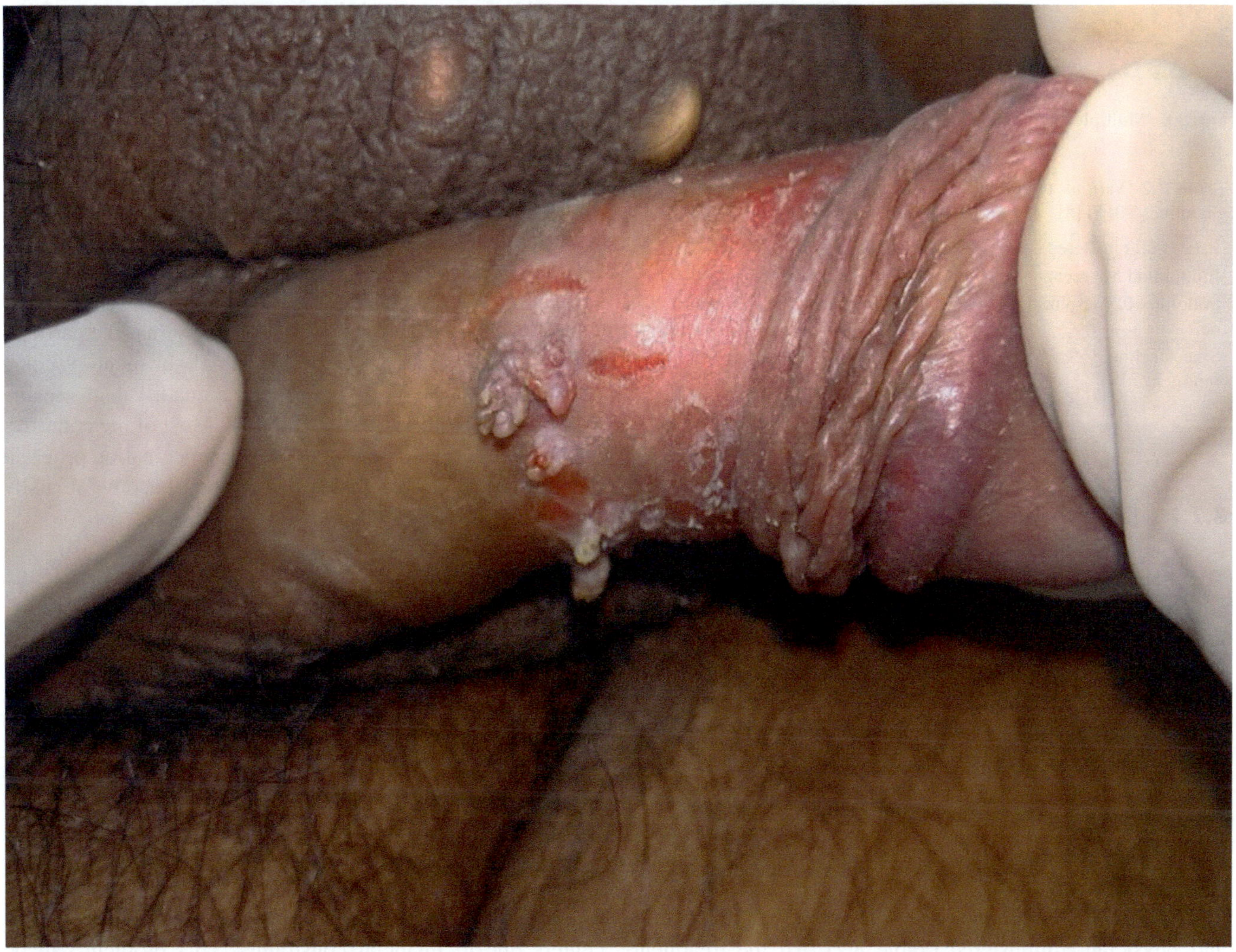

Fig. 8.7 *Genital warts* on penile shaft. The patient also has candidal balanoposthitis, as is evident by the linear fissures and erythema

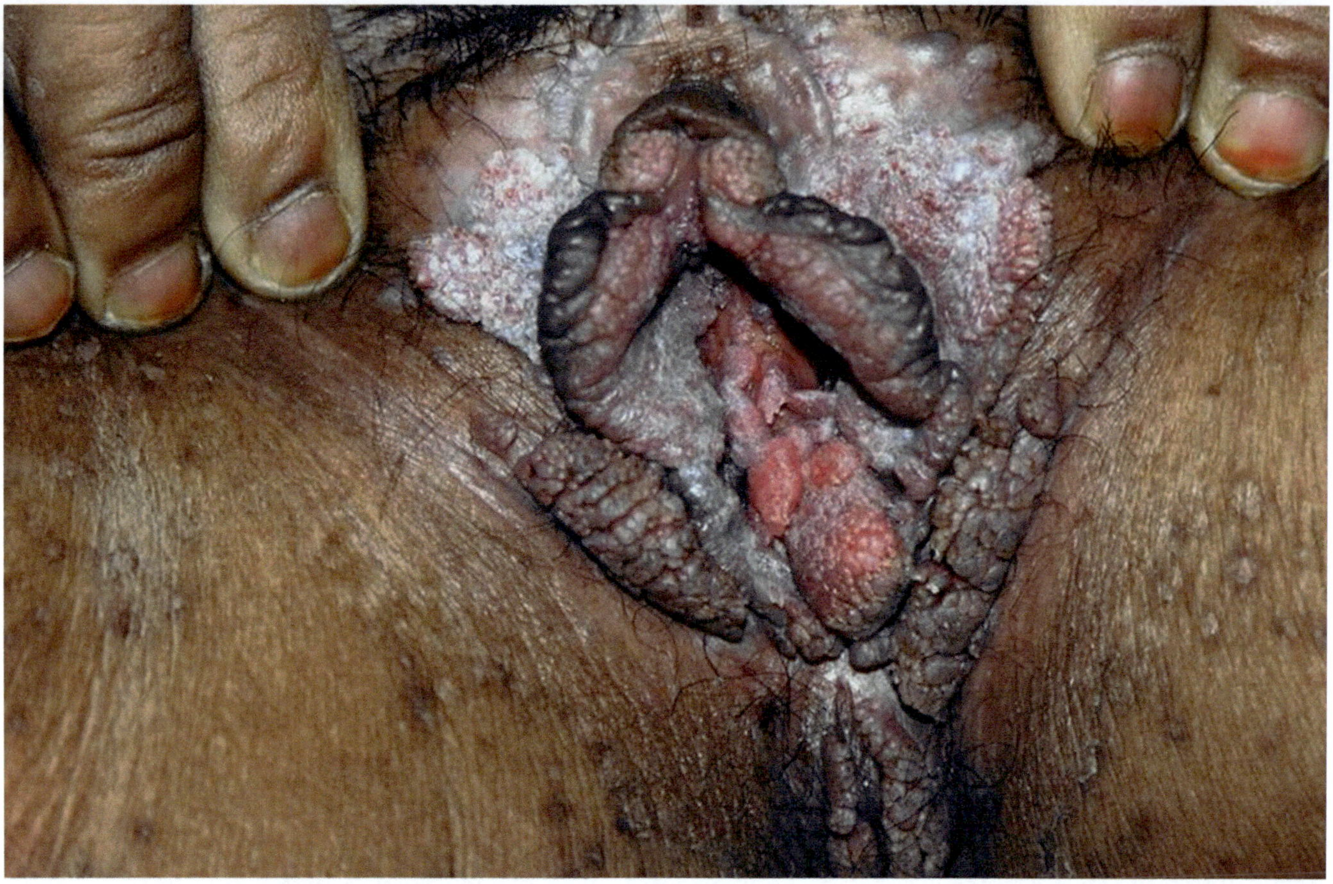

Fig. 8.8 Multiple anogenital *condylomata acuminata*

Table 8.2 Various treatment modalities for anogenital warts (CDC guidelines 2015) [5]

Patient-administered	Physician-administered
Imiquimod 5% cream	Bichloro- or trichloroacetic acid 80–90%
Podofilox 0.5% solution/gel	Podophyllin resin 15–25% in tincture benzoin
Sinecatechins 15% ointment	Cryosurgery with liquid nitrogen
	Electrosurgery
	Surgical excision

8.7.2 Diagnosis

The diagnosis is clinically straightforward when the lesions are present. A biopsy may be done to confirm the diagnosis, in case of doubt or to exclude premalignant changes. Detection of HPV DNA by PCR and HPV typing are primarily used as research tools. The Papanicolaou smear prepared from cervical tissue sample is a cytological test used for screening of cervical cancers and preneoplastic conditions.

8.7.3 Treatment

The available treatment options can be classified into patient- and physician-administered (Table 8.2). All the treatment modalities have a similar efficacy, with no evidence to suggest that one may be better than the other [5]. Immunotherapy with intralesional Mw vaccine (*Mycobacterium indicus pranii*) has been found to have similar efficacy and safety as imiquimod 5% cream [21].

HPV vaccines: Two prophylactic HPV virus-like particle-based vaccines are widely available: bivalent vaccine (*Cervarix*®) for HPV 16 and 18 and a quadrivalent vaccine (*Gardasil*®) for HPV 6, 11, 16, and 18. Most of the countries which have adopted the vaccine in their vaccination program are targeting young females before they become sexually active.

8.8 Syndromic Approach to the Management of Sexually Transmitted Infections

The treatment of any infection should ideally be directed toward the causative organism. This requires a laboratory equipped with trained personnel and facilities for performing microbiological tests that can identify the pathogen with good sensitivity and specificity, thus confirming the diagnosis. However, many of these laboratory tests are not widely available in developing countries, limited to only a few referral centers due to financial constraints. This problem can be

Table 8.3 STI-related syndromes and common causative organisms

STI syndrome	Common causative organisms
Genital ulcers	*Treponema pallidum, Haemophilus ducreyi, Herpes simplex virus, Klebsiella granulomatis, Chlamydia trachomatis (L1–L3)*
Urethral discharge	*Chlamydia trachomatis (D–K), Neisseria gonorrhoeae*
Cervical discharge	*Chlamydia trachomatis (D–K), Neisseria gonorrhoeae*
Vaginal discharge	*Chlamydia trachomatis (D–K), Neisseria gonorrhoeae, Trichomonas vaginalis, Candida albicans* anaerobic bacteria
Inguinal bubo	*Haemophilus ducreyi, Chlamydia trachomatis (L1–L3)*
Lower abdominal pain	*Pelvic inflammatory disease caused by Neisseria gonorrhoeae, Chlamydia trachomatis (D–K)*, and other bacteria
Acute scrotal swelling	*Chlamydia trachomatis (D–K), Neisseria gonorrhoeae*
Neonatal purulent conjunctivitis (*ophthalmia neonatorum*)	*Chlamydia trachomatis (D–K), Neisseria gonorrhoeae*

overcome, to a certain extent, by adopting a "syndromic approach" to the infections, which is based on the fact that a number of sexually transmissible pathogens produce a common pattern of easily recognizable signs and symptoms. Similar signs and symptoms forming a clinical pattern can be grouped together to form a syndrome. Though sexually transmitted infections are caused by a large number of different organisms, the resulting signs and symptoms can be clubbed into a limited number of syndromes. Though it is practical and cost-effective and ensures adequate management in case of lost to follow-up, this approach is applicable only in patients who are symptomatic [22]. For example, the usual causes of urethral discharge in men are *Chlamydia trachomatis* and *Neisseria gonorrhoeae*. So the syndromic approach would be to give treatment for both these organisms simultaneously. Though it has a high chance of success, this approach is of limited utility in case of the infection being caused by an uncommon organism, like *Mycoplasma* or *Trichomonas*. In case the patient does not respond adequately, referral to a higher center is warranted. The STI-related syndromes and their causes are summarized in Table 8.3.

The National AIDS Control Organization (NACO) provides free prepackaged color-coded kits at various health centers in India ("Suraksha clinics") as a part of its strategy to control and prevent sexually transmitted infections. The patients are offered HIV testing and counseled regarding safe sexual practices, including promotion of barrier contraceptives at these health centers. Sexual partners of the patients are also treated empirically. In Table 8.4 the various color-coded drug kits according to the STI syndrome are summarized [23].

Table 8.4 NACO color-coded kits for various STI syndromes

Kit	Color	STI syndrome	Drugs
1	*Gray*	Urethral discharge Cervical discharge Rectal discharge Painful scrotal swelling	Oral azithromycin 1 g stat + cefixime 400 mg stat
2	*Green*	Vaginal discharge	Oral secnidazole 2 g stat + fluconazole 150 mg stat
3	*White*	Genital ulcer–Non herpetic	Benzathine penicillin 2.4 mU im inj. Stat + oral azithromycin 1 g stat
4	*Blue*	Genital ulcer–Non herpetic, for penicillin allergic patients	Oral doxycycline 2 × 100 mg/day, 2 weeks + azithromycin 1 g stat
5	*Red*	Genital ulcer–Herpetic	Acyclovir 3 × 400 mg/day, 7 days
6	*Yellow*	Lower abdominal pain	Oral cefixime 400 mg stat + metronidazole 2 × 400 mg/day, 2 weeks + doxycycline 2 × 100 mg/day, 2 weeks
7	*Black*	Inguinal bubo	Doxycycline 2 × 100 mg/day, 3 weeks + azithromycin 1 g stat

For genital ulcers, kits 3 and 4 provide treatment for syphilis and chancroid. Genital herpes is treated by kit 5. The genital ulcer in *lymphogranuloma venereum* is transient and thus is not included in the kits 3 or 4 (treated by kit 7 for inguinal bubo), while donovanosis has become extremely rare and its treatment is not included in the syndromic management.

There is no kit provided by NACO for neonatal purulent conjunctivitis (*ophthalmia neonatorum*). The treatment should cover both *Neisseria gonorrhoeae* (single dose intramuscular injection of ceftriaxone 50 mg/kg, maximum 125 mg) and *Chlamydia trachomatis* (oral erythromycin syrup 50 mg/kg/day, 14 days).

Conclusions

Sexually transmitted infections pose an enormous burden on health-care services in the developing world, especially among women and children who have to bear their sequelae. The disparities seen in the distribution of various STIs are confounded by the socioeconomic status and the prevalent sexual behavior in the populations. Though the number of new STI cases has declined globally, certain geographic areas continue to have a high prevalence. Syndromic management has been successful in bringing the infection rates down in resource-poor countries. Overall, the proportion of viral STIs has increased considerably; they now account for the majority of the cases seen in STI clinics. As viral STIs cannot be completely cured with the currently available treatment, greater emphasis should be laid on education and promotion of safe sexual behavior as part of control programs to further decrease the STI burden.

References

1. Newman L, Rowley J, Vander Hoorn S, et al. Global estimates of the prevalence and incidence of four curable sexually transmitted infections in 2012 based on systematic review and global reporting. PLoS One. 2015;10:e0143304.
2. Savage EJ, Hughes G, Ison C, et al. Syphilis and gonorrhoea in men who have sex with men: a European overview. Euro Surveill Bull Eur Sur Mal Transm Eur Commun Dis Bull. 2009;14(47).
3. http://apps.who.int/iris/handle/10665/75181
4. https://www.cdc.gov/mmwr/preview/mmwrhtml/mm6444a3.htm
5. Workowski KA, Bolan GA. Sexually transmitted diseases treatment guidelines, 2015. MMWR Recomm Rep. 2015;64:1.
6. González-Beiras C, Marks M, Chen CY, et al. Epidemiology of Haemophilus ducreyi infections. Emerg Infect Dis. 2016;22:1–8.
7. Sexually transmitted disease surveillance. 2014. http://www.cdc.gov/std/stats
8. Hook EW, Handsfield HH. Gonococcal infections in adults. In: Holmes KK, Sparling PF, Stamm WE, Piot P, Wasserheit JN, Corey L, Cohen MS, Watts DH, editors. Sexually transmitted diseases. 4th ed. New York: McGraw-Hill; 2007.
9. Unemo M, del Rio C, Shafer WM. Antimicrobial resistance expressed by Neisseria gonorrhoeae: a major global public health problem in the 21st century. Microbiol Spectr. 2016;4(3).
10. Malhotra M, Sood S, Mukherje A, et al. Genital chlamydia trachomatis: an update. Indian J Med Res. 2013;138(3):303–16.
11. Workowski KA, Berman S, Centers for Disease Control and Prevention (CDC). Sexually transmitted diseases treatment guidelines, 2010. MMWR Recomm Rep. 2010;59(RR-12):1–110.
12. Abu-Raddad LJ, Schiffer JT, Ashley R, et al. HSV-2 serology can be predictive of HIV epidemic potential and hidden sexual risk behavior in the Middle East and North Africa. Epidemics. 2010;2:173–82.
13. Swygard H, Seña AC, Hobbs MM, et al. Trichomoniasis: clinical manifestations, diagnosis and management. Sex Transm Infect. 2004;80:91–5.
14. Sorvillo F, Smith L, Kerndt P, et al. Trichomonas vaginalis, HIV, and African-Americans. Emerg Infect Dis. 2001;7:927–32.
15. Nye MB, Schwebke JR, Body BA. Comparison of APTIMA trichomonas vaginalis transcription-mediated amplification to wet mount microscopy, culture, and polymerase chain reaction for diagnosis of trichomoniasis in men and women. Am J Obstet Gynecol. 2009;200:188.e1–7.
16. Looker KJ, Magaret AS, Turner KME, Vickerman P, Gottlieb SL, Newman LM. Global estimates of prevalent and incident herpes simplex virus type 2 infections in 2012. PLoS One. 2015; 10:e114989.
17. Gupta V, Bhari N, Gupta S. Genital herpes. http://www.aaus.info/mediawiki/index.php/Genital_herpes
18. Patel H, Wagner M, Singhal P, et al. Systematic review of the incidence and prevalence of genital warts. BMC Infect Dis. 2013;13:39.
19. de Sanjosé S, Diaz M, Castellsagué X, et al. Worldwide prevalence and genotype distribution of cervical human papillomavirus DNA in women with normal cytology: a meta-analysis. Lancet Infect Dis. 2007;7:453–9.
20. Clifford GM, Rana RK, Franceschi S, et al. Human papillomavirus genotype distribution in low-grade cervical lesions: comparison by geographic region and with cervical cancer. Cancer Epidemiol Biomark Prev. 2005;14:1157–64.
21. Kumar P, Dar L, Saldiwal S, et al. Intralesional injection of mycobacterium w vaccine vs imiquimod, 5%, cream in patients with anogenital warts: a randomized clinical trial. JAMA Dermatol. 2014;150:1072–8.
22. Latif AS. The syndromic approach for the management of STIs: an overview. In: Gupta S, Kumar B, editors. Sexually transmitted infections. 2nd ed. New York: Elsevier; 2012.
23. Amin AR. Enhanced syndromic case management of reproductive tract infection/sexually transmitted infection cases as per National AIDS Control Organization guidelines. Indian J Sex Transm Dis. 2010;31:61–2.

9 Cutaneous Leishmaniasis

Mansour Nassiri Kashani, Ali Khamesipour,
and Alireza Firooz

Leishmaniasis is a vector-borne disease, caused by more than 20 different species of the protozoan parasite *Leishmania*, transmitted to humans by 30 species of various sand flies. Leishmania infection depends upon the causative species and the host genetic profile which governs the immune responses. The disease may be clinically presented as *cutaneous* (CL), *mucocutaneous* (MCL), and *visceral leishmaniasis* (VL) with *post-kala-azar dermal leishmaniasis* (PKDL) as a particular entity of the latter (Fig. 9.1).

Currently leishmaniasis is endemic in 98 mostly developing countries, the WHO estimated that a tenth of the world's population are at risk of contracting a form of the disease. Poverty, lack of sanitary facilities, deforestation, and urbanization are major factors facilitating the widespread of the vector and the risk of infection. The loss in disability-adjusted life years is around 2.4 million. Cutaneous leishmaniasis is worldwide the most common clinical form, consisting 75% of all cases with approximately 1.5 million new infections reported from 88 countries each year. Around 90% of these occur in Afghanistan, Algeria, Brazil, Iran, Peru, Saudi Arabia, and Syria (Fig. 9.2).

Cutaneous leishmaniasis is either zoonotic or anthroponotic; recently several cases in non-endemic areas have been reported in war refugees and soldiers [1–3].

9.1 Etiology

Leishmania is an intracellular parasite showing two forms of life cycle: the flagellate form (promastigote) is seen in sand flies and culture media, and the nonflagellate (amastigote) is found in vertebrate hosts. After the bite of an infected female sand fly, the promastigotes are inoculated into the skin, attach and enter tissue macrophages, and transform into the amastigote form.

The most common causative agents of CL in Old World include *L. major*, *L. tropica*, *L. aethiopica*, and rarely *L. infantum*, transmitted by various species of *Phlebotomus* sand fly. In the New World, *L. braziliensis*, *L. mexicana*, and *L. amazonensis* are the most common organisms transmitted by *Lutzomyia* species [4–6].

9.2 Clinical Entities

The clinical presentation of cutaneous leishmaniasis is protean, depending on the species of *Leishmania* and the cell-mediated immune response of the host. Lesions are more common on exposed areas of the body, the face, and the upper and lower extremities. In endemic areas they are mostly seen in children; in new foci or in travelers, lesions can be seen at any age [7, 8].

9.2.1 Leishmaniasis in the Old World

Acute zoonotic CL: Wet or rural CL is usually caused by *L. major*. A few weeks to 2 months later, an erythematous papule appears at the site of the bite of the infected sand fly affected which gradually develops to a plaque or nodular lesion and may ulcerate (Fig. 9.3a). Its base is indurated by palpation, offering a helpful diagnostic sign. The number of lesions depends on the number of bites; they may even be tens to hundreds (Fig. 9.3b). All lesions heal spontaneously in a time period less than 1 year, leaving mild pale scars (Fig. 9.4).

Acute anthroponotic CL: Dry or urban cutaneous leishmaniasis is caused by *L. tropica*. The incubation period is longer, and the number of lesions is less than in zoonotic CL. They are usually not painful, present the characteristic

M. N. Kashani (✉) • A. Khamesipour • A. Firooz
Center for Research and Training in Skin Diseases and Leprosy, Tehran University of Medical Sciences, Tehran, Iran

C. E. Orfanos et al. (eds.), *Pigmented Ethnic Skin and Imported Dermatoses*, https://doi.org/10.1007/978-3-319-69422-1_9

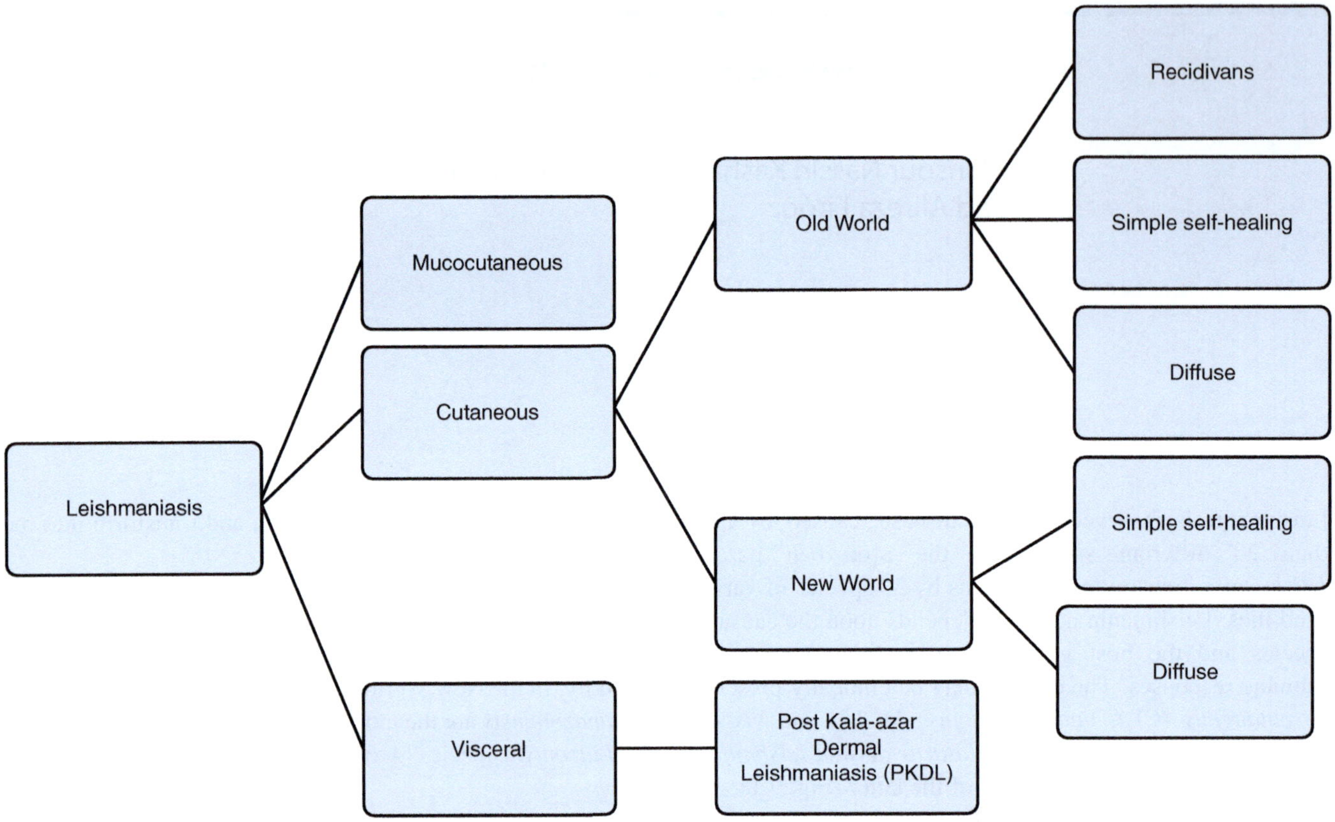

Fig. 9.1 Classification of leishmaniasis

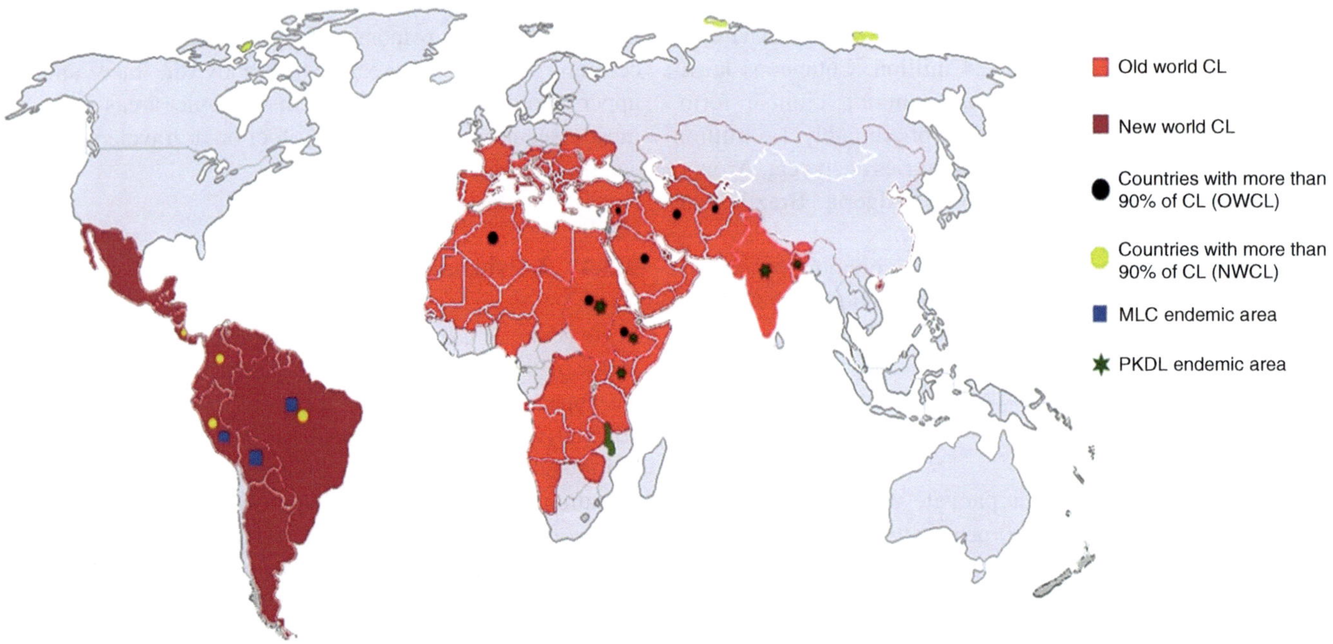

Fig. 9.2 World map of different forms of cutaneous leishmaniasis

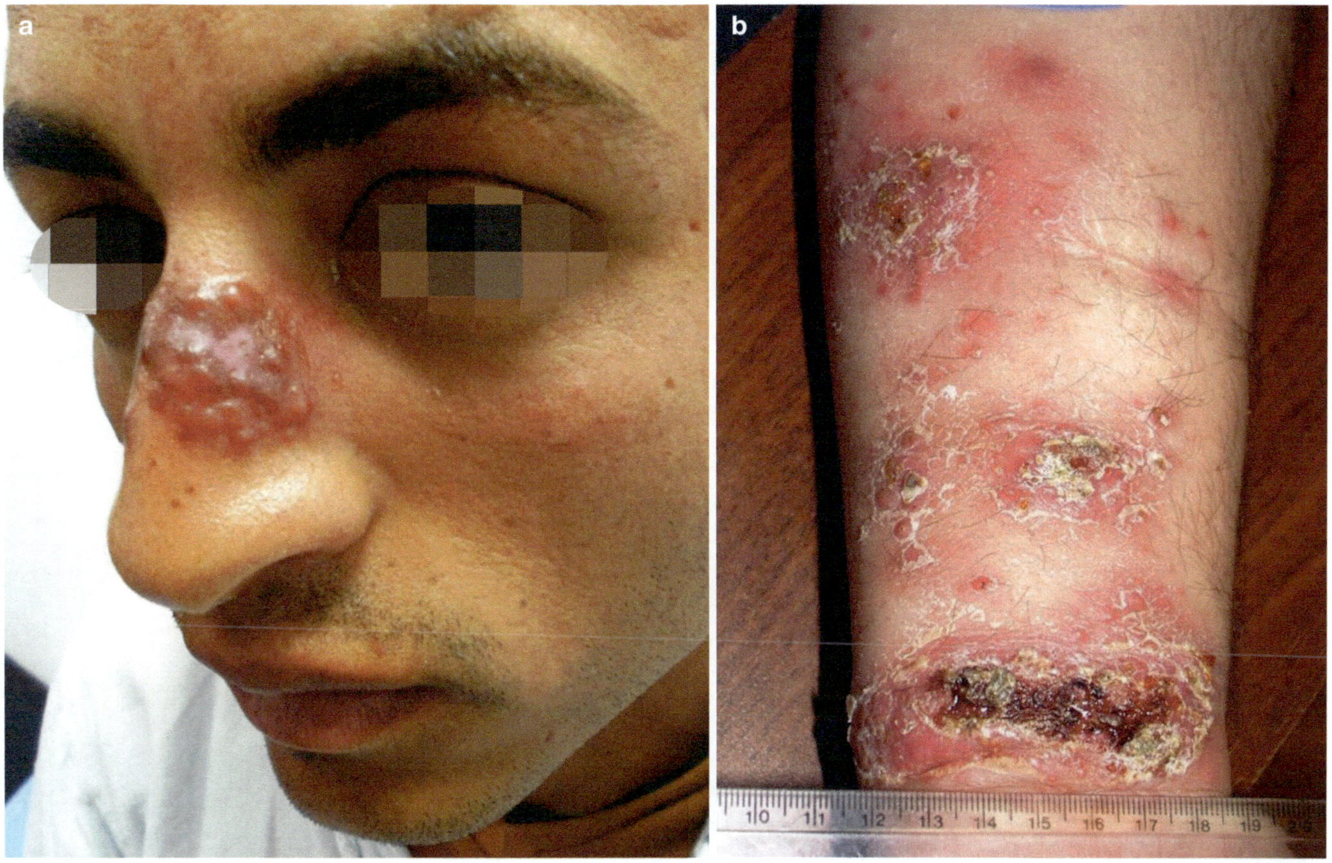

Fig. 9.3 (**a**) *Nodular cutaneous leishmaniasis* in an Egyptian soldier after servicing in areas near Sudan (courtesy Maadi Military Hospital, Cairo; Photo: CEO). (**b**) Ulcerated lesions of *acute zoonotic leishmaniasis*, *partly superinfected*

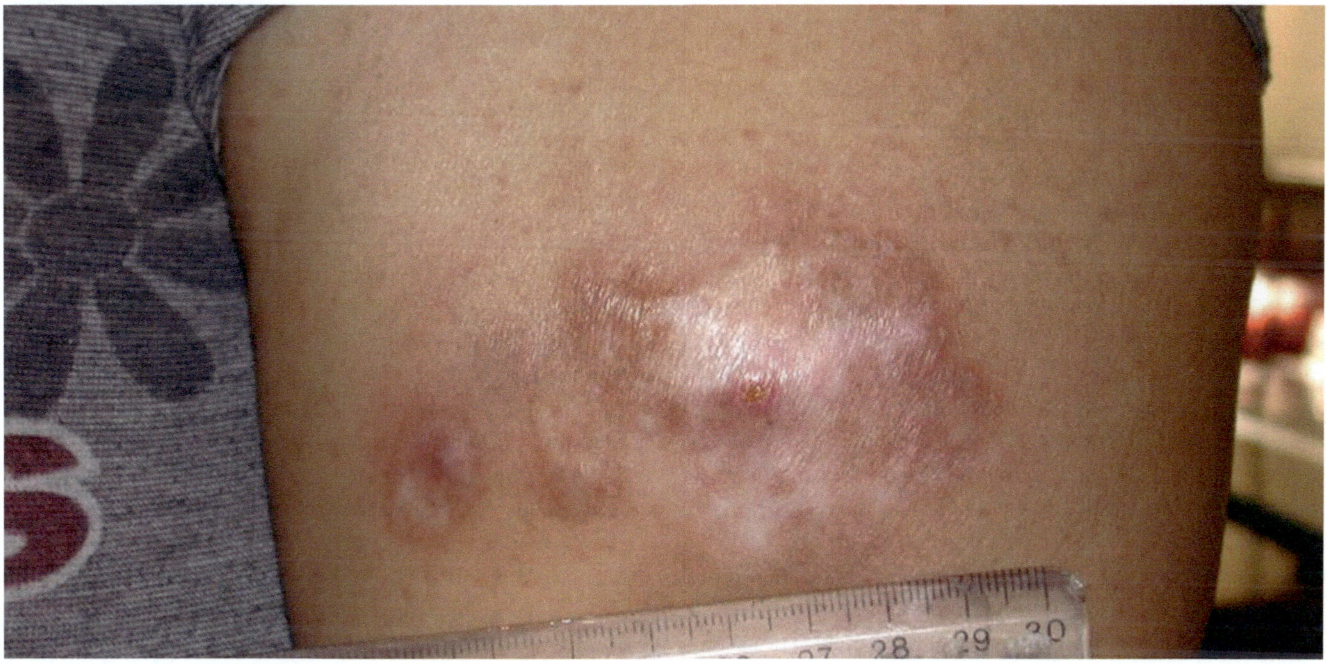

Fig. 9.4 Scarring lesion of cutaneous leishmaniasis after topical treatment. Papules may indicate relapse

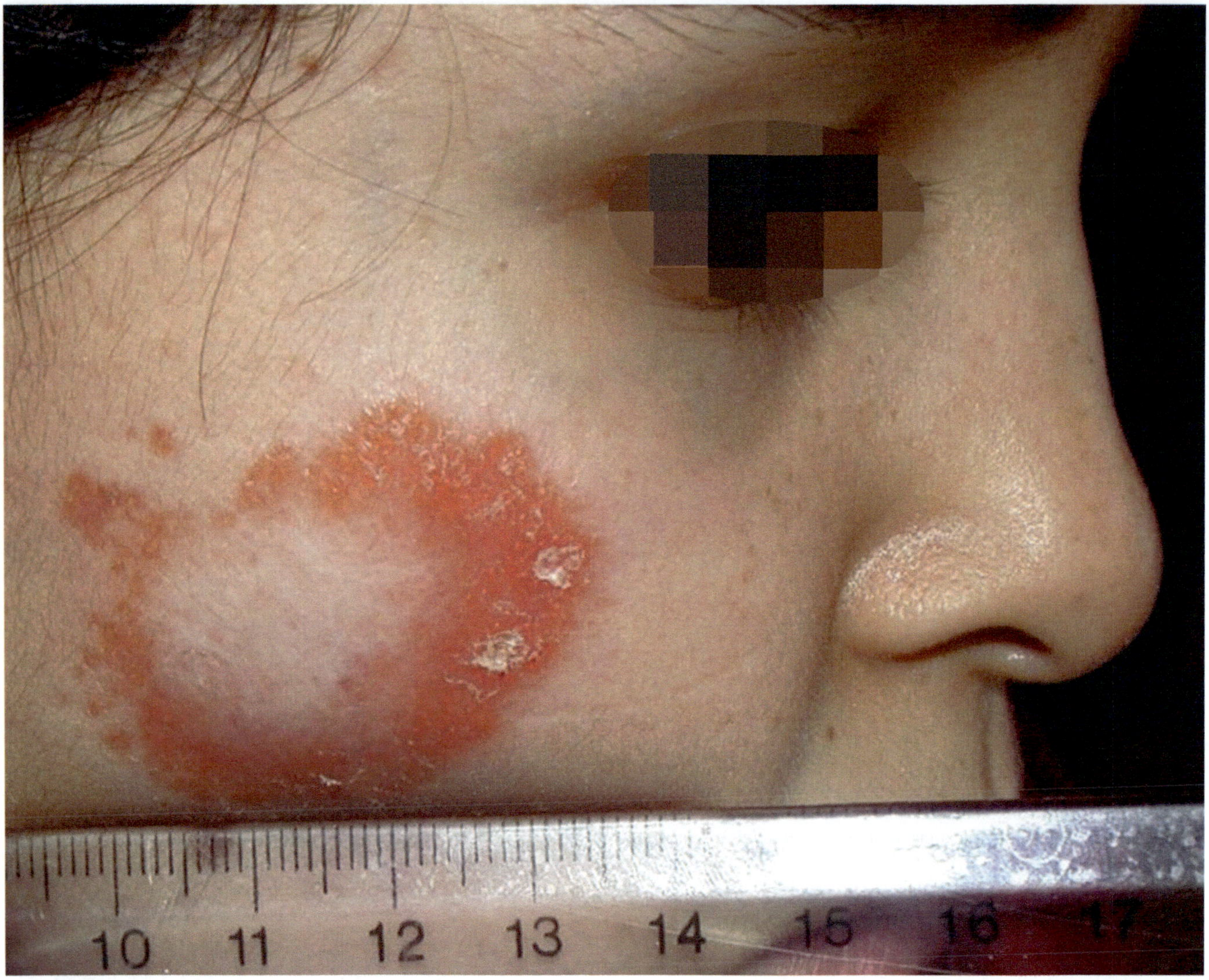

Fig. 9.5 Translucent papules and plaques of *leishmaniasis recidivans* at the periphery of a leishmaniasis scar

induration, rarely ulcerate, and are occasionally crusted or hyperkeratotic. The course of the disease is longer; the lesions usually heal in 1–2 years, even without treatment. This CL variant may clinically mimic several other dermatoses; atypical forms such as erysipeloid, sporotrichoid, verrucous, and eczematoid may occur.

Chronic or non-healing CL: Although the majority of cases of CL heal spontaneously in 1–2 years, a few cases do not heal during the expected time period and also do not respond to treatment, probably due to a defect of the cell-mediated immunity.

Lupoid CL or leishmaniasis recidivans: This uncommon form of CL is usually caused by *L. tropica*, presenting small, translucent, yellow, or reddish-brown papules. They often develop at the periphery of an old scar of CL, usually on the face, after several years. The lesion occasionally mimics apple-jelly lesions of skin tuberculosis (lupus vulgaris) and gradually coalesces into a plaque (Fig. 9.5). There is a strong hypersensitivity reaction marked by a positive leishmanin skin test; usually the parasites cannot be detected in the lesions [9].

Diffuse CL: This unusual form of CL consists of several generalized non-ulcerated papules and nodules without any systemic involvement. It is often caused by hematogenous spread of *L. aethiopica*, in anergic patients, similar to lepromatous leprosy. In endemic areas crusted nodular and mucocutaneous lesions may occur (Figs. 9.6 and 9.7).

In the *post-kala-azar* dermal leishmaniasis, skin lesions develop months to years after treatment and recovery from visceral leishmaniasis. They present hypopigmented macules and patches on trunk and extremities, erythematous patches on the face similar to malar rash, or soft, non-ulcerated and asymptomatic nodules on face and trunk.

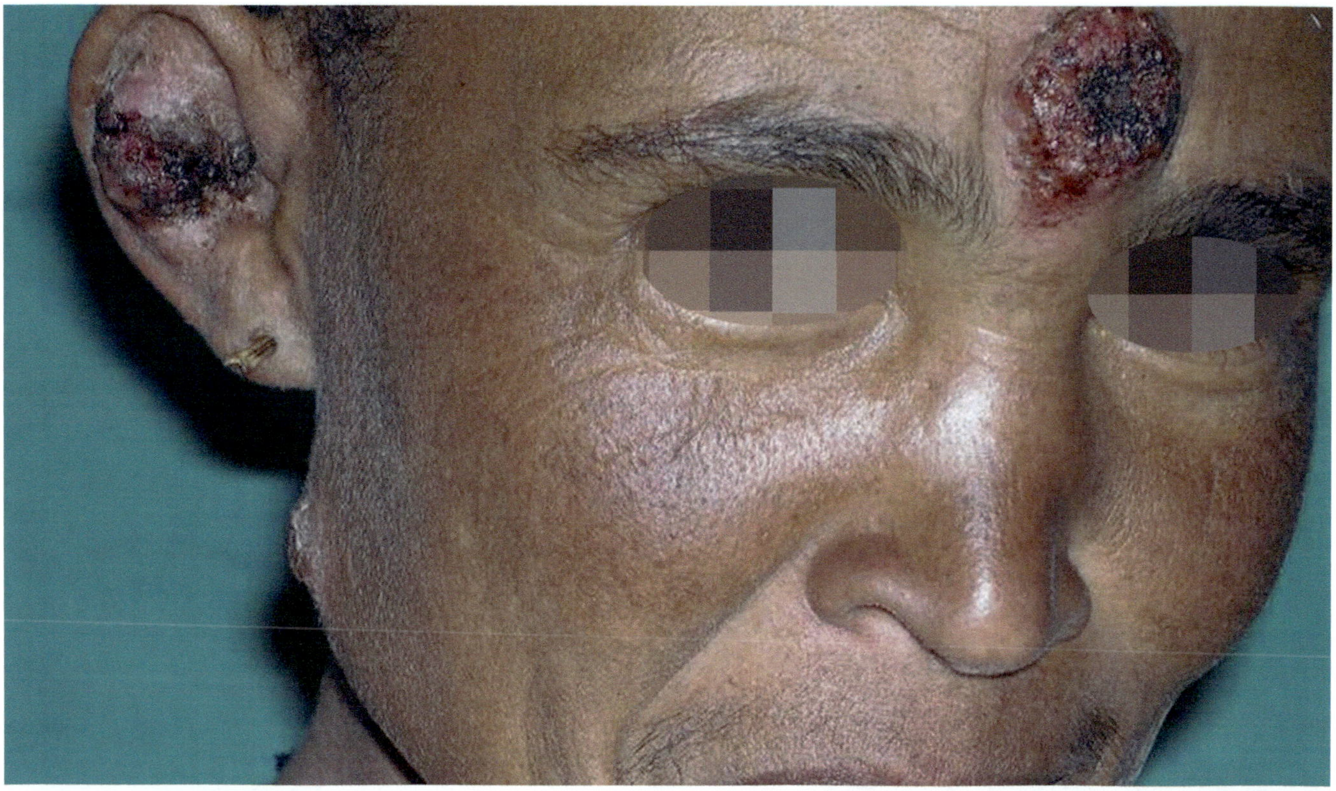

Fig. 9.6 Crusted papulonodular lesions of cutaneous leishmaniasis of the face in an Ethiopian female (spp. *L. aethiopica* confirmed by PCR; courtesy V. Padovese)

9.2.2 Leishmaniasis in the New World

Typical lesions of cutaneous leishmaniasis in the New World are similar to the lesions of zoonotic or azoonotic leishmaniasis in the Old World. *L. braziliensis* causes *mucocutaneous leishmaniasis*, involving the mucous membranes of the nose, lips, and the oral cavity. The mucocutaneous lesions heal spontaneously in a few months leaving scars; however, months or years after their development become destructive.

Diffuse cutaneous leishmaniasis is also caused by *L. amazonensis* due to a defect of the cell-mediated immunity of the host.

9.3 Diagnosis

The country of residence of a patient or history of traveling to an endemic area weeks or months before the development of skin lesions in an exposed body area, the indurated basis of the presented lesions by palpation, and their painlessness will help the clinician to consider leishmaniasis. If clinically suspected the detection of the agent in smears and biopsies will confirm the diagnosis. In all forms of the disease, the parasite can be detected under the microscope [10, 11]. In endemic areas smears are done by skin scraping from the margin of an active lesion, smeared on a glass slide, fixed with methanol, and stained with Giemsa to be checked for 2–4 μm inclusions in tissue macrophages, the *Leishmania amastigotes* (Leishman-Donovan bodies). Occasionally, culture in NNN medium and histological examination of a skin biopsy sample will also be helpful to confirm the diagnosis. Sensitive identification of *Leishmania* species DNA is possible with PCR.

9.4 Treatment

A large number of different chemical, physical, and immunological modalities have been used to treat cutaneous leishmaniasis; only a few of them delivered satisfactory results [12, 13]. Since the skin lesions in CL are self-healing, especially in the Old World, only well-designed randomized controlled trials can define the efficacy of a candidate modality. Pentavalent antimonials have been used for treatment of different forms of CL for more than half a century as intralesional, intramuscular, or intravenous injections; they are still considered today as the most effective antileishmanial modality. Nonetheless, a series of side

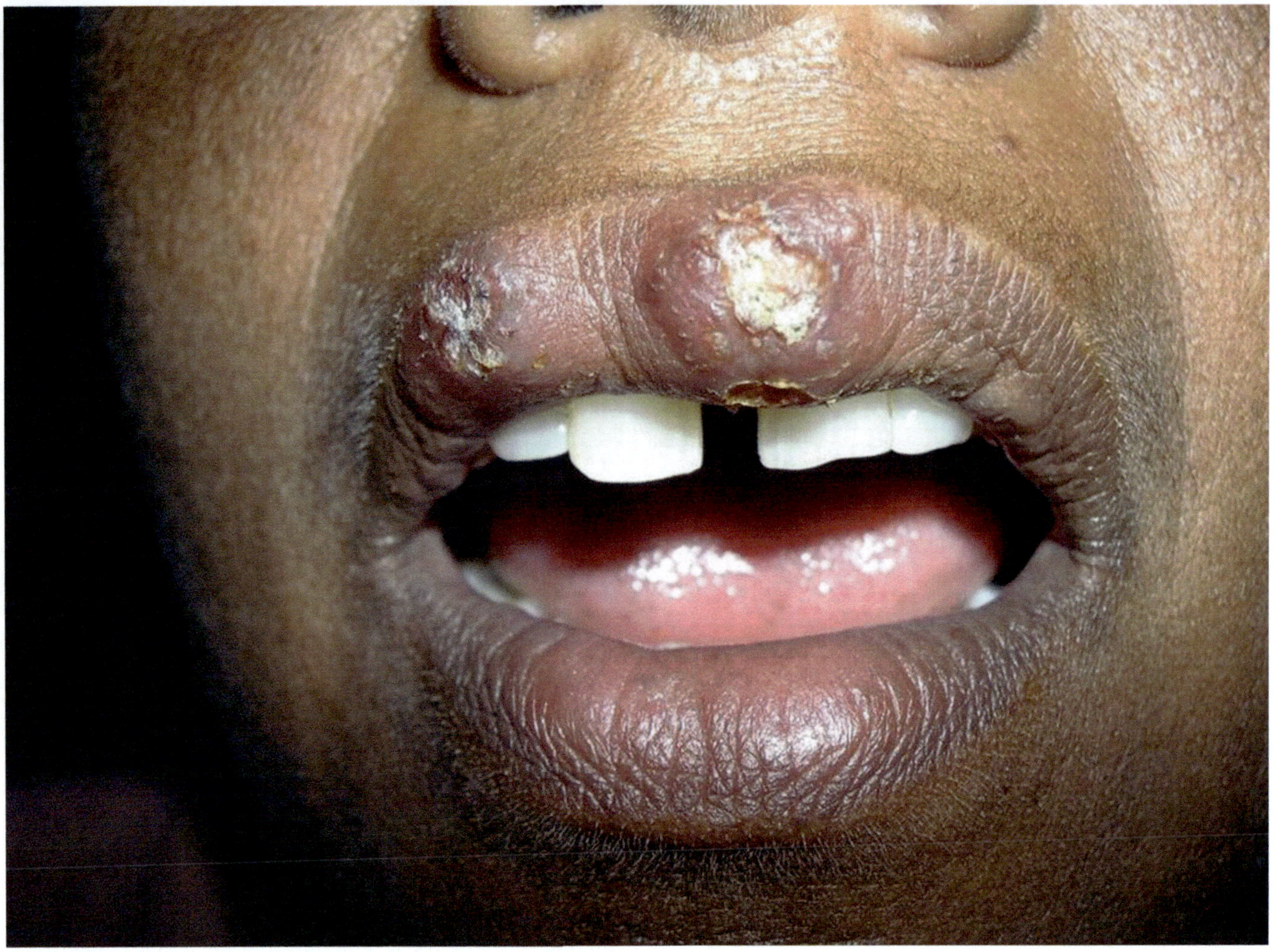

Fig. 9.7 *Mucocutaneous leishmaniasis* in an Ethiopian female with multiple nodular lesions on the upper lip (spp. *L. aethiopica*; courtesy V. Padovese)

effects of these drugs (heart, liver, kidney, pancreas, etc.) have been reported; administration of antimonials is painful, their medication is expensive, and the rate of drug resistance is increasing.

There is strong evidence to recommend *local therapies* for small and limited numbers of CL lesions [14–18]: (a) Intralesional antimonial injections one to two times per week, (b) cryotherapy with liquid nitrogen for 10–30 s every 1–2 weeks (alone or combined with intralesional antimonial injections), (c) thermotherapy by local 50 °C heat application using radiofrequency devices for 30 s in a single application or with repeated applications for up to 4 weeks, and (d) topical 15% paromomycin ointment 2×/day for over 4 weeks in lesions caused by *L. major.*

Systemic treatment is recommended in patients with multiple or large lesions, lesions on sensitive areas amenable for local treatment (such as eyelid, nose, ear, and joints), lesions with sporotrichoid features, those caused by *L. braziliensis* and all others resistant to topical applications. Systemic administration of pentavalent antimonials 20 mg/kg/day over 2–4 weeks is considered as the gold standard of treatment for different forms of CL.

Pentamidine, amphotericin B, azole-based antifungal drugs, and miltefosine can be used in selected cases.

9.5 Prevention

The wide variations in the epidemiologic features, the species of the agent involved, the vectors, and their reservoirs together with the unpredictable individual susceptibility of the affected populations have made all efforts to control the disease in endemic areas unsuccessful on a long term. Control measures for vectors and reservoirs, insecticide impregnated bed nets and clothes, and different Leishmania vaccines have provided short term results [19, 20]. Vicinity of wild rodents' burrows to cities and villages plays an important role in transmission of zoonotic CL to humans [21]. Indoor residual spraying, application of chemicals in rodent burrows, impregnation of bed nets and curtains with insecticides, the use of insect repellents, impregnation of dog collars, etc. are important measures [22]. Education of the population living in endemic areas on the factors controlling the transmission is mandatory for personal protection, together with health strategies to prevent expansion.

Conclusions

Leishmaniasis is a global health problem, a vector-borne parasitic disease caused by more than 20 different species of an intracellular protozoon, *Leishmania donovani*, transmitted by the bite of an infected female sand fly. It affects millions of people around the world; the WHO estimated that a tenth of the world's population is at risk to contract one form of the disease, mostly in developing countries. Poverty, lack of facilities, and urbanization are important contributory factors. The clinical presentation of CL is protean and depends on the species of *Leishmania* and the host cell-mediated immune response. Residence in or travelers to endemic areas have a risk to acquire the infection. Development of lesions in exposed skin areas of tourists, migrants, and refugees weeks or months after traveling, together with the palpable induration and the painlessness of the lesion(s), may facilitate the clinical diagnosis, to be confirmed by the detection of the amastigote in smears and biopsies or by PCR. Pentavalent antimonials and other drugs used for treatment of leishmaniasis are effective but toxic and cause high costs; new low-cost drugs with antileishmanial activity are needed.

References

1. Alvar J, Vélez ID, Bern C, et al. Leishmaniasis worldwide and global estimates of its incidence. PLoS One. 2012;7:e35671.
2. WHO: leishmaniasis. 2012. http://www.who.int/leishmaniasis/en/2. Accessed 4 Jan 2017.
3. Du R, Hotez PJ, Al-Salem WS, et al. Old world cutaneous leishmaniasis and refugee crises in the Middle East and North Africa. PLoS Negl Trop Dis. 2016;10:e0004545. https://doi.org/10.1371/journal.pntd.0004545. eCollection
4. Postigo JA. Leishmaniasis in the World Health Organization eastern Mediterranean region. Int J Antimicrob Agents. 2010; 36:S62–5.
5. Reithinger R, Dujardin JC, Louzir H, et al. Cutaneous leishmaniasis. Lancet Infect Dis. 2007;7:581.
6. Gontijo B, de Carvalho ML. American cutaneous leishmaniasis. Rev Soc Bras Med Trop. 2003;36:71–80.
7. Momeni AZ, Aminjavaheri M. Clinical picture of cutaneous leishmaniasis in Isfahan, Iran. Int J Dermatol. 1994;33:260–5.
8. Dowlati Y. Cutaneous leishmaniasis: clinical aspects. Clin Dermatol. 1996;14:425–31.
9. Sharifi I, Fekri AR, Aflatoonian MR, et al. Leishmaniasis recidivans among school children in Bam, South-East Iran, 1994–2006. Int J Dermatol. 2010;49:557–61.
10. Markle WH, Makhoul K. Cutaneous leishmaniasis: recognition and treatment. Am Fam Physician. 2004;69:1455–6.
11. Goto H, Lindoso JAL. Current diagnosis and treatment of cutaneous and mucocutaneous leishmaniasis. Expert Rev Anti-Infect Ther. 2010;8:419–33.
12. Khatami A, Firooz A, Gorouhi F, et al. Treatment of acute Old World cutaneous leishmaniasis: a systematic review of randomised controlled trials. J Am Acad Dermatol. 2007;57:335.e1–e29.
13. González U, Pinart M, Reveiz L, et al. Interventions for Old World cutaneous leishmaniasis. Cochrane Database Syst 2008;Rev 8:CD005067.
14. Khatami A, Firooz A, Gorouhi F, et al. Systematic review of New World cutaneous leishmaniasis: several points. Int J Dermatol. 2009;48:201–2.
15. Khatami A, Firooz A, Zartab H, et al. Cutaneous leishmaniasis. In: Maibach H, Gorouhi F, editors. Evidence based dermatology. 2nd ed. Shelton: PMPH-USA; 2011.
16. Cardona-Arias JA, Vélez ID, López-Carvajal L. Efficacy of thermotherapy to treat cutaneous leishmaniasis: a meta-analysis of controlled clinical trials. PLoSOne. 2015;10:e0122569.
17. López-Carvajal L, Cardona-Arias JA, Zapata-Cardona MI. Efficacy of cryotherapy for the treatment of cutaneous leishmaniasis: meta-analyses of clinical trials. BMC Infect Dis. 2016;16:360.
18. López-Carvajal L, Hoyos M, et al. Systematization of clinical studies on the efficacy of treatments for cutaneous leishmaniasis 1980-2015. Arch Med. 2016;12(3):8. https://doi.org/10.3823/1307.
19. Noazin S, Khamesipour A, Moulton LH, et al. Efficacy of killed whole-parasite vaccines in the prevention of leishmaniasis: a meta-analysis. Vaccine. 2009;27:4747–53.
20. González U, Pinart M, Sinclair D, et al. Vector and reservoir control for preventing leishmaniasis. Cochrane Database Syst Rev. 2015;(8):CD008736.
21. Sofizadeh A, Vatandoorst H, Rassi Y, et al. Spatial analysis of the relation between rodent's active burrows and incidence of zoonotic cutaneous leishmaniasis in Golestan province, northeastern of Iran. J Arthropod Borne Dis. 2016;10:569–76.
22. Yaghoobi-Ershadi MR. Control of phlebotomine sand flies in Iran: a review article. J Arthropod Borne Dis. 2016;10:429–44.

Mycobacterioses in Pigmented Ethnic Skin

10

Federica Dassoni and Bernard Naafs

Mycobacterial organisms have reemerged as an important cause of infectious disease worldwide. Both tuberculosis and nontuberculous mycobacterial infections remain endemic in many parts of the globe, especially in low- and middle-income countries, becoming more common in patients with iatrogenic immunosuppression and HIV infection. Mycobacteria responsible for most cutaneous diseases are *M. tuberculosis*, *M. marinum*, *M. ulcerans*, *M. fortuitum*, *M. chelonae*, and *M. avium-intracellulare*. More rare are skin infections caused by *M. scrofulaceum*, *M. szulgai*, *M. kansasii*, or *M. haemophilum*.

Infections caused by *M. leprae* and *M. ulcerans* (Buruli ulcer) will be discussed separately.

10.1 Cutaneous Tuberculosis

Tuberculosis (TB) is one of the world's deadliest diseases. In 2014 more than nine million people worldwide contracted the infection caused by *M. tuberculosis*, and 1.5 million deaths were registered [1]. It frequently affects the lungs, but in about 14% of cases (in children up to 20%) it affects other body sites extrapulmonary tuberculosis (EPTB). Out of these cases, about 2% are cutaneous tuberculosis (CTB), which is especially seen in developing countries and impoverished populations. Most of the affected individuals (82%) live in 22 high burden countries. The advent of the HIV epidemic and an increase in immunosuppressive therapies has led to an increase of all forms of TB, as has the emergence of resistant strains. TB is the leading cause of mortality in people living with HIV.

One third of the world's population is infected with TB bacilli. Out of these, only 5–10% of those who are immune competent will clinically develop tuberculosis [2–5].

F. Dassoni, M.D. (✉)
Ospedale Alessandro Manzoni, Lecco, Italy

B. Naafs, M.D., Ph.D.
Stichting Global Dermatology, Munnekeburen, Netherlands
e-mail: benaafs@dds.nl

Cutaneous tuberculosis has become a rare disease in the western hemisphere. The majority of CTB cases will be diagnosed in immigrants coming from high TB burden low-income settings (Africa, Asia, South America, and Middle East). In developing countries of hot climate zones, the clinical picture may be particularly severe and long lasting, due to the late access to hospitals from remote areas, costs of transport, use of traditional or domestic remedies first, missed diagnosis, poor living conditions, immunosuppression, and sometimes insecurity of the roads. Although no age is exempt, CTB is frequent in the first three decades of life and is more common in men.

10.1.1 Pathogenesis

M. tuberculosis is the predominant etiologic agent causing granulomas in cutaneous TB. Occasionally *M. bovis*, *bacille Calmette-Guérin* (the attenuated strain of *M. bovis*), and NTB may affect the skin and cause similar lesions. The agent disseminates by inhalation, ingestion, or inoculation. As mycobacteria are intracellular microorganisms, the immunological response of the host is cell mediated, resulting in a granulomatous tissue reaction. Once the bacteria have invaded, the interaction of T lymphocytes with mycobacterial antigens displayed on the surface of antigen presenting cells induces the liberation of lymphokines, interleukins (IL-1, IL-6, IL-12, later IL-17 and IL-23), and interferon (IFN-γ). They promote the activation and expression of MHC class II antigens and IL-2R on T lymphocytes, macrophages accumulate, and tissue granuloma is formed [6]. The sensitization status of the host, e.g., previously infected vs. never exposed, the degree of cell-mediated immunity, the route of infection, and the pathogenicity of the infective strain together with the size and frequency of the inoculum, determine the type of the resulting clinical picture. In HIV-infected individuals, cell-mediated immunity is impaired, and there may be reactivation of quiescent disease.

C. E. Orfanos et al. (eds.), *Pigmented Ethnic Skin and Imported Dermatoses*, https://doi.org/10.1007/978-3-319-69422-1_10

10.1.2 Diagnosis and Classification

The various clinical forms of cutaneous tuberculosis can be classified into four categories, based on the inoculation mechanism in each case, and the sensitization of the host with tuberculous mycobacteria:

1. Primary infection (in tuberculin-negative persons, first exposure)
2. Secondary or postprimary infection (in tuberculin-positive individuals, previously exposed patients):
   (a) Exogenous inoculation.
   (b) Endogenous inoculation by contiguous spread.
   (c) Endogenous inoculation by hematogenous route
3. Bacille Calmette-Guérin (BCG) and *M. bovis* infection
4. Immunological reactions of the host to the infectious agent (tuberculids)

The clinical diagnosis can be confirmed by smear, biopsy, culture, and/or PCR. Because biopsies, cultures, and PCR techniques are often not available, diagnosis is particularly difficult in developing countries. The differential diagnosis should consider cutaneous leishmaniasis, Buruli ulcer, actinomycosis, malignancies, etc. Even when mycobacteria are found on skin smears or in biopsies, they cannot be differentiated from nontuberculous mycobacteria (NTM), which sometimes cause a similar clinical picture.

The clinical manifestations of the infection results from the interactions between the environment, the resistance of the agent, and the defense resources of the host also depending on age, immune status, malnutrition, and any coexisting intercurrent disease. Inflammatory papules, verrucous plaques, suppurative nodules, chronic ulcers, etc. may occur, presenting a wide spectrum of skin lesions. There are several classifications of CTB variants; the most widely used is based on the *inoculation mechanism.* Lesions can be caused by direct inoculation of *M. tuberculosis* from an exogenous source such as in tuberculous chancre, in warty tuberculosis, and, occasionally, in lupus vulgaris. Others are due to endogenous spread and appear as contiguous (scrofuloderma, orificial tuberculosis), lymphatic (lupus vulgaris), or hematogenous spread (miliary tuberculosis, tuberculous gumma, lupus vulgaris).

Other clinical classifications are often based on the *bacterial load*, in a continuous spectrum as it is used in leprosy [7, 8]. *Multibacillary* forms such as tuberculous chancre, scrofuloderma, orificial tuberculosis, miliary tuberculosis, and tuberculous gumma, in which bacilli are easily detected in skin tissue or isolated in exudates, are usually associated with low cellular immunity and high humoral host response. Paucibacillary forms, such as tuberculosis verrucosa cutis, lupus vulgaris and the tuberculids, in which visualization or isolation of the organisms is difficult, are seen in immune competent patients.

10.1.3 Clinical Pictures

10.1.3.1 Cutaneous Primary Complex

Primary tuberculosis, also called tuberculous chancre, accounts for 2% of all cases of cutaneous tuberculosis; it is rare and develops as a result of exogenous inoculation into the skin of an individual not previously sensitized or without natural immunity to the tuberculous bacilli. Children in endemic areas with low vaccination coverage are affected. Local trauma, often unnoticed by the patient, is necessary as the bacilli cannot penetrate the intact skin barrier. Two to four weeks after inoculation, a firm papule or nodule appears slowly enlarging into a plaque which later ulcerates (Fig. 10.1a, b). Face and limbs are frequently involved. The ulcer has undermined edges and is painless. After 3–8 weeks, the bacilli spread to regional lymph nodes, resulting in a lymphocutaneous complex analogous to the Ghon complex seen in pulmonary infections. The evolution is variable; healing may occur spontaneously with atrophic scarring in 3–12 months; when untreated, it may cause lupus vulgaris, tuberculosis verrucosa cutis, or miliary TB. The regional lymph nodes may suppurate, producing scrofuloderma, or the ulcer can persist. Mycobacteria are usually easily detected with a skin smear. Other causes of ulceration such as Buruli ulcer, subcutaneous mycoses, cutaneous leishmaniasis, sporotrichosis, and cat scratch disease should be considered [9].

10.1.3.2 Tuberculosis Verrucosa Cutis

Warty tuberculosis is a common form of CTB in the East, particularly in India. It is the result of exogenous inoculation of the bacilli through injured skin in previously sensitized individuals with moderate to high immunity against *M. tuberculosis*. Due to a rapid cell-mediated response, the infection often remains localized; regional lymphadenopathy is not prominent. In endemic hot climate zones, this form is seen in children walking or sitting on contaminated soil. The lesions are usually solitary, painless, and develop from a reddish-brown papule into verrucous plaques of varying shape and size. The plaque increases by peripheral extension and is usually firm, although areas of softening and atrophic scarring may be present within the same lesion (Fig. 10.2a, b). The verrucous fissures may become superinfected or heal spontaneously in the course of months to years. An identical lesion may be seen among cattle workers. Here the species involved is most commonly *M. bovis*. In developing countries, the lower

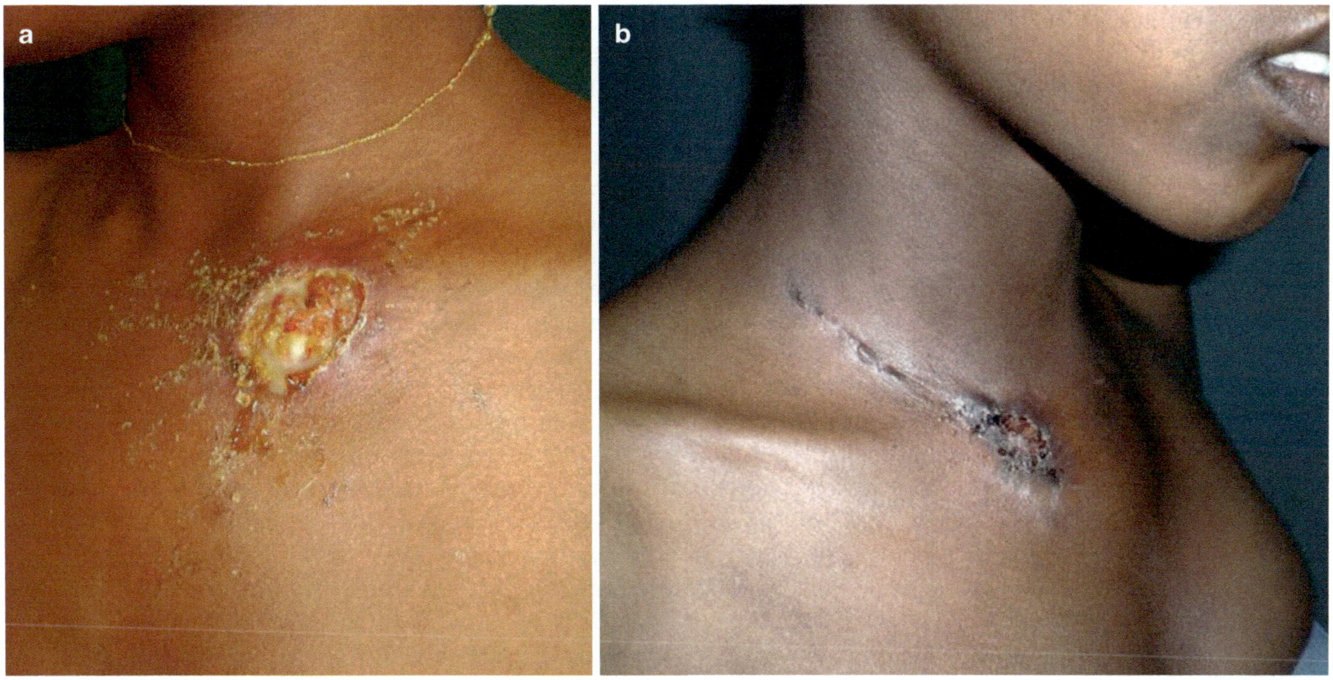

Fig. 10.1 *Cutaneous primary complex* (**a**) ulcer and (**b**) cutaneous primary complex with partial spontaneous scarring (courtesy INMP Institute, Rome; photo FD)

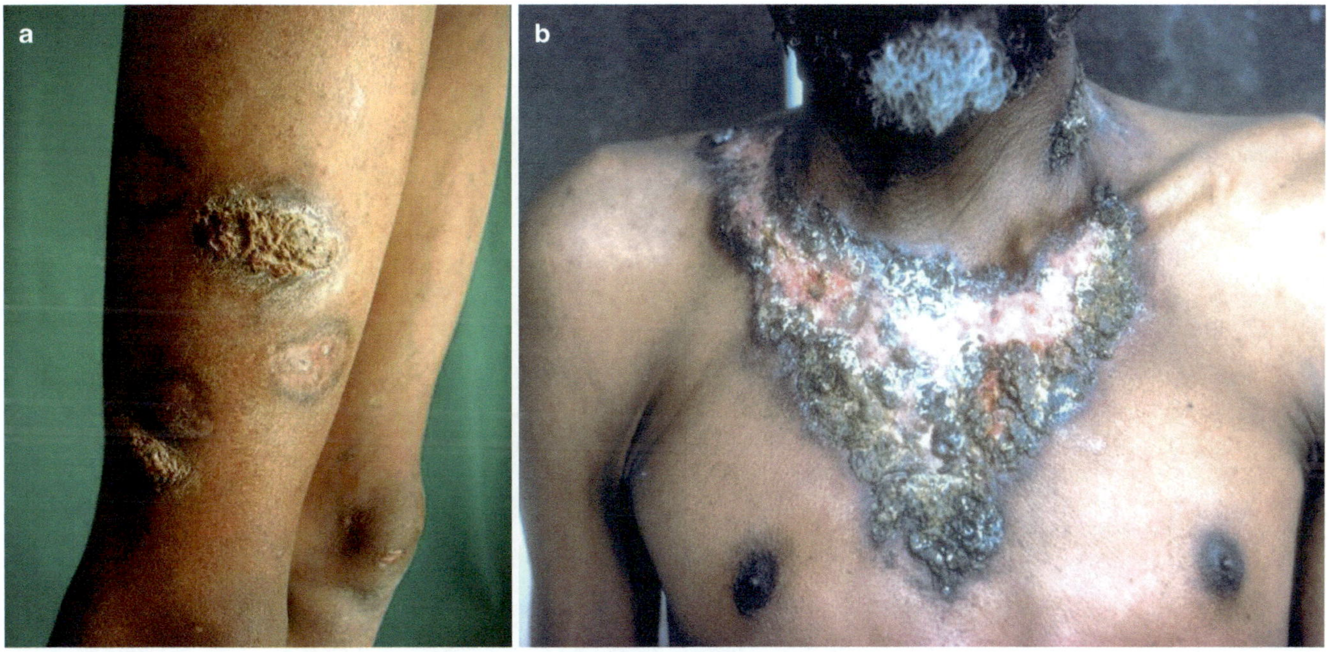

Fig. 10.2 *Verrucous TB*. (**a**) Multiple lesions of *verrucous TB* on the lower limbs in a young boy (courtesy INMP Institute, Rome; photo FD); (**b**) Warty lesions on the chest. Features of lupus vulgaris are also present (central scarring, enlarging plaque) (courtesy ALERT Addis Ababa Ethiopia; photo BN)

extremities are affected frequently, especially in children. Hypertrophic lichen planus, verrucous lesions caused by NTM or deep mycoses, some forms of leishmaniasis, verrucous tertiary syphilis, and squamous cell carcinoma should be considered [8, 9].

10.1.3.3 Tuberculosis Cutis Colliquativa

This clinical type, also called *scrofuloderma*, is the most common form of CTB in developing countries [10, 11]. Children, teenagers, and elderly are frequently affected because of the higher risk of immunologic failure. The clinical picture of scrofuloderma is the result of a contiguous spread from an underlying mycobacterial infection, commonly in lymph nodes or the bone, joints, and also the epididymis. Due to suppuration asymptomatic fluctuating abscesses develop which may ulcerate and form sinuses, ulcers have undermined edges and granulating floors (Fig. 10.3a, b). Watery, purulent, or caseous discharge may drain from the sinuses. In the course of time, cord-like scars develop. Cervical lymph nodes are often involved, although in widespread disease, parasternal, axillary, supraclavicular, epitrochlear, and the inguinal lymph nodes can be affected (Fig. 10.4a, b). Coexistence with pulmonary tuberculosis is possible, and mixed type lesions may exist in the skin and heal over years leaving retractions, atrophic and keloid scars, particularly in immunosuppressed patients. Recurrences of drainage are common (Figs. 10.5a, b and 10.6a–c).

Other mycobacteria known to cause scrofuloderma are the MAIS group (*M. avium-intracellulare* complex, *M. scrofulaceum*) and *M. haemophilum*. For differential diagnosis, deep mycoses such as sporotrichosis, actinomycosis, hidradenitis suppurativa in axillary lesions, granuloma inguinale and lymphogranuloma venereum in inguinal lesions, and chronic bacterial osteomyelitis should be considered when localized over the bone.

10.1.3.4 Lupus Vulgaris

This classical form of CTB has become rare in the West, but it still occurs in developing countries, especially in India. It is chronic and progressive, due to reactivation by contiguity, autoinoculation or lymphoematogenous spread of a mycobacterial infection in sensitized individuals with moderate to high degree of cellular-mediated immunity. Lupus vulgaris may rarely follow primary inoculation, BCG vaccination, or be localized around warty tuberculosis [12]. Classic lesions start as brown-red soft papules extending to plaques with active, irregular borders and central healing with atrophic, depigmented scarring. The surface may be smooth or sometimes covered with scales resembling psoriasis. In tropical countries, lesions on the legs and buttocks are common. The translucency of the flat papules and soft plaques can be rarely seen in dark skin, and the "apple jelly" aspect found by diascopy in light skin is not visible in dark-skinned individuals (Fig. 10.7a, b). In the lesions only a few bacilli are found. If untreated, the lesions persist for years, gradually growing in size, leading to scarring. Flat, hypertrophic, ulcerative, and vegetating forms have been described. Lesions on the ear lobe are usually hypertrophic and resemble a tumor. In rare cases, squamous cell carcinoma may develop. The buccal, nasal, or conjunctival mucosa may rarely become affected either primarily or by extension of

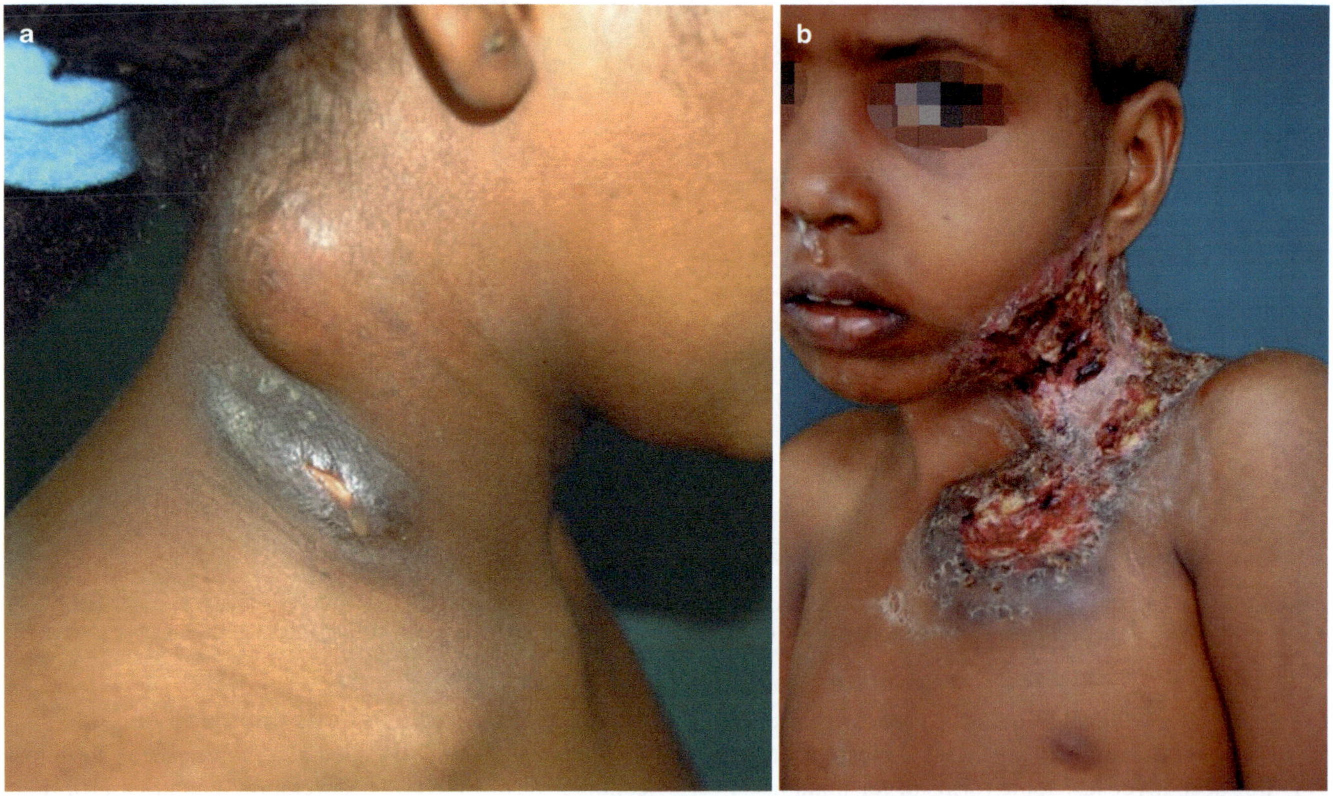

Fig. 10.3 *Scrofuloderma.* (**a**) Different stages of lymph nodes involvement; (**b**) severe ulcerations and crusts after 1 year duration and rupture of the cervical lymph nodes (courtesy INMP Institute, Rome; photo FD)

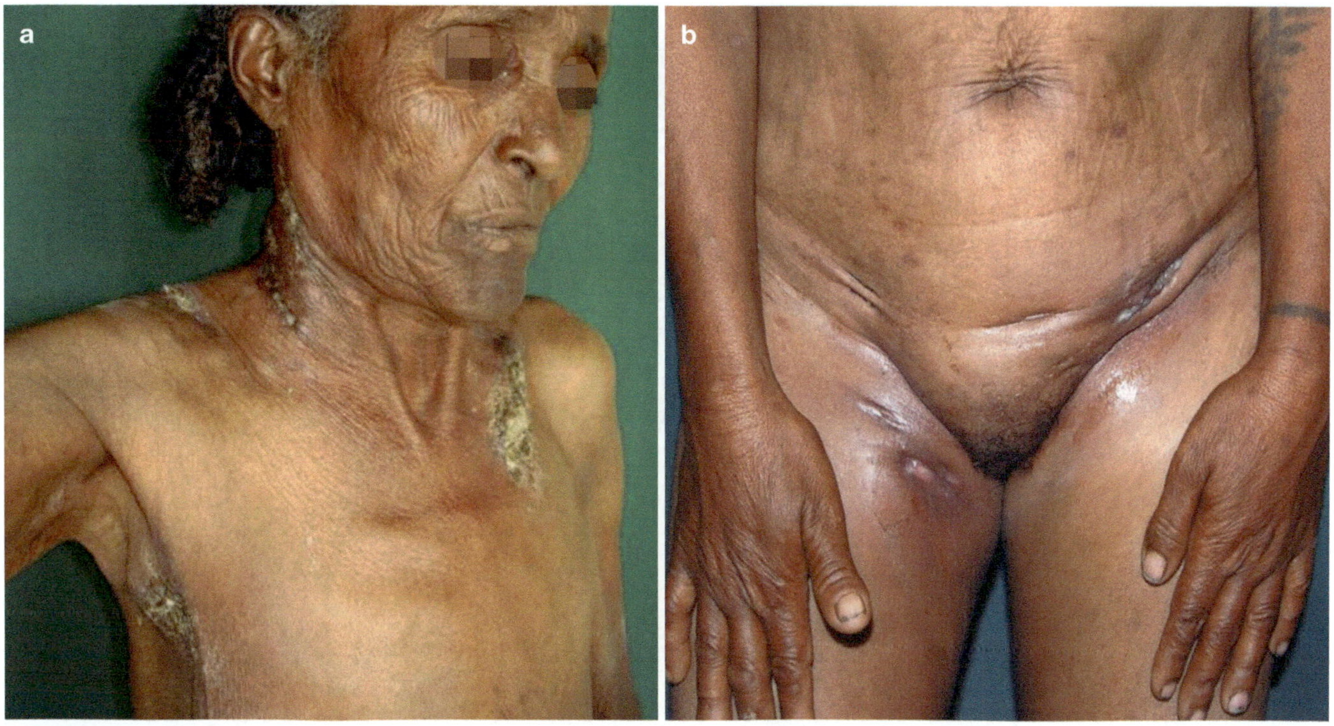

Fig. 10.4 *Scrofuloderma*. (**a**) Multiple lymph node involvement in a woman with crusted lesions; (**b**) bilateral involvement of the inguinal lymph nodes (courtesy INMP Institute, Rome; photo FD)

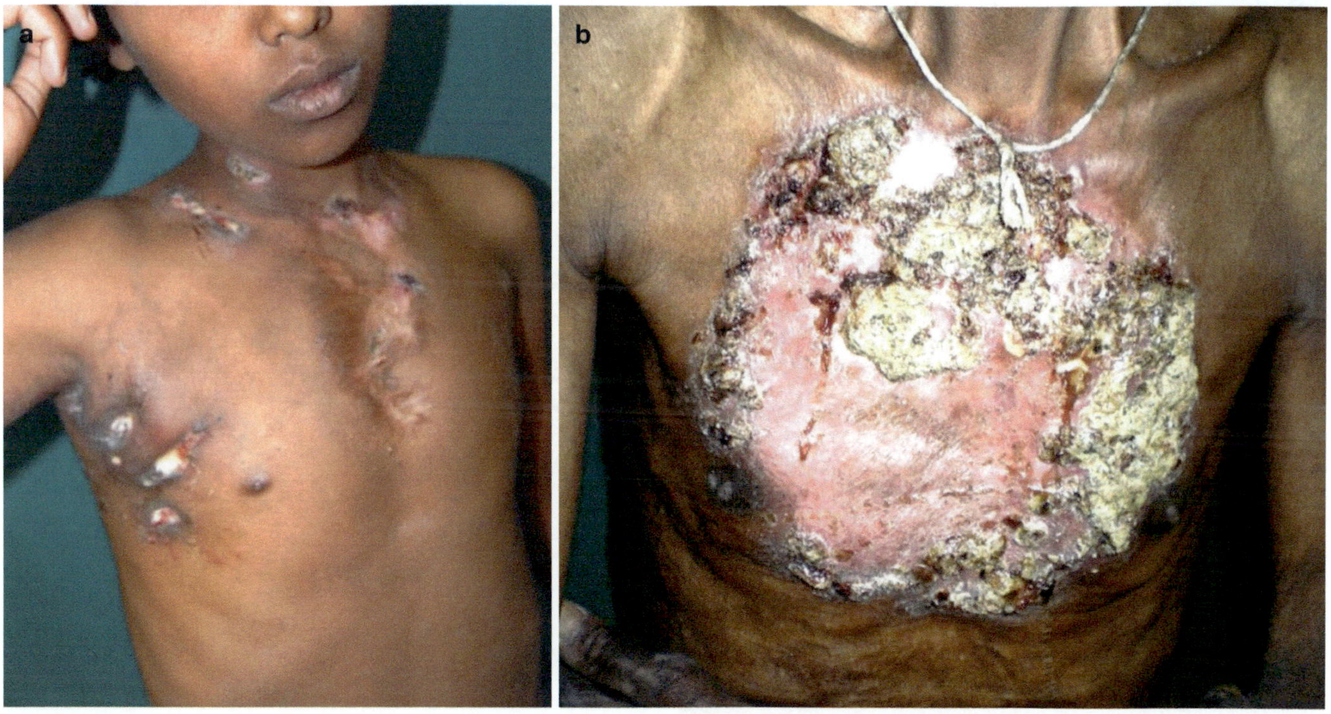

Fig. 10.5 *Scrofuloderma*. (**a**) Multiple active and scarring lesions; (**b**) features of scrofuloderma (discharging sinuses, crusts) are present in this lesion in the presternal area. Features of lupus vulgaris are also present (enlarging plaque, central scarring) (courtesy INMP Institute, Rome; photo FD)

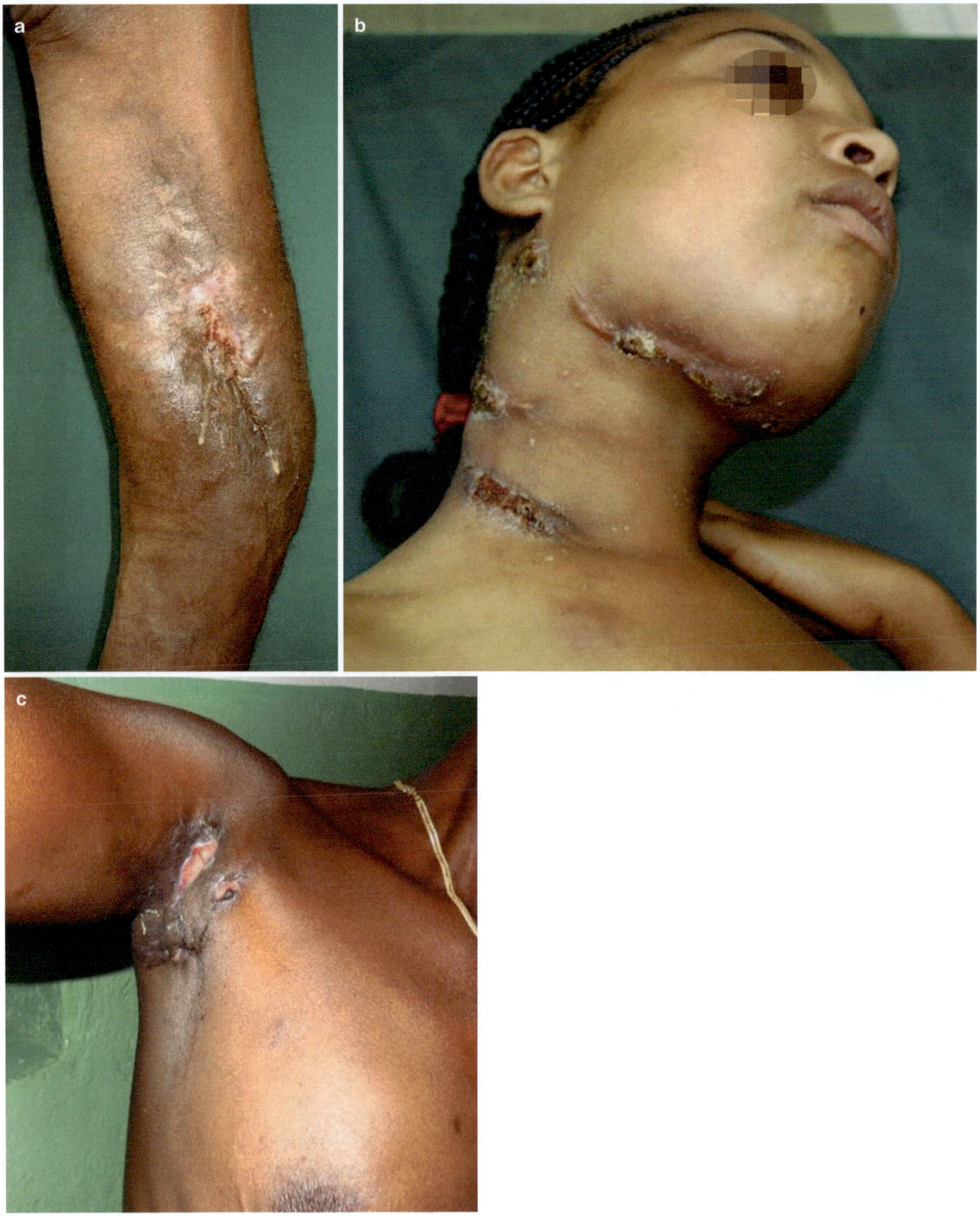

Fig. 10.6 (**a**) Tuberculous osteomyelitis of the femoral bone, with secondary cutaneous involvement. Differential: bacterial osteomyelitis; (**b**) typical cord-like scars on the neck (courtesy INMP Institute, Rome; photo FD). (**c**) *Scrofuloderma* in an immunosuppressed patient: Ulceration of axillary lymph nodes simulating hidradenitis suppurativa (courtesy Nzara hospital; South Soudan; photo FD)

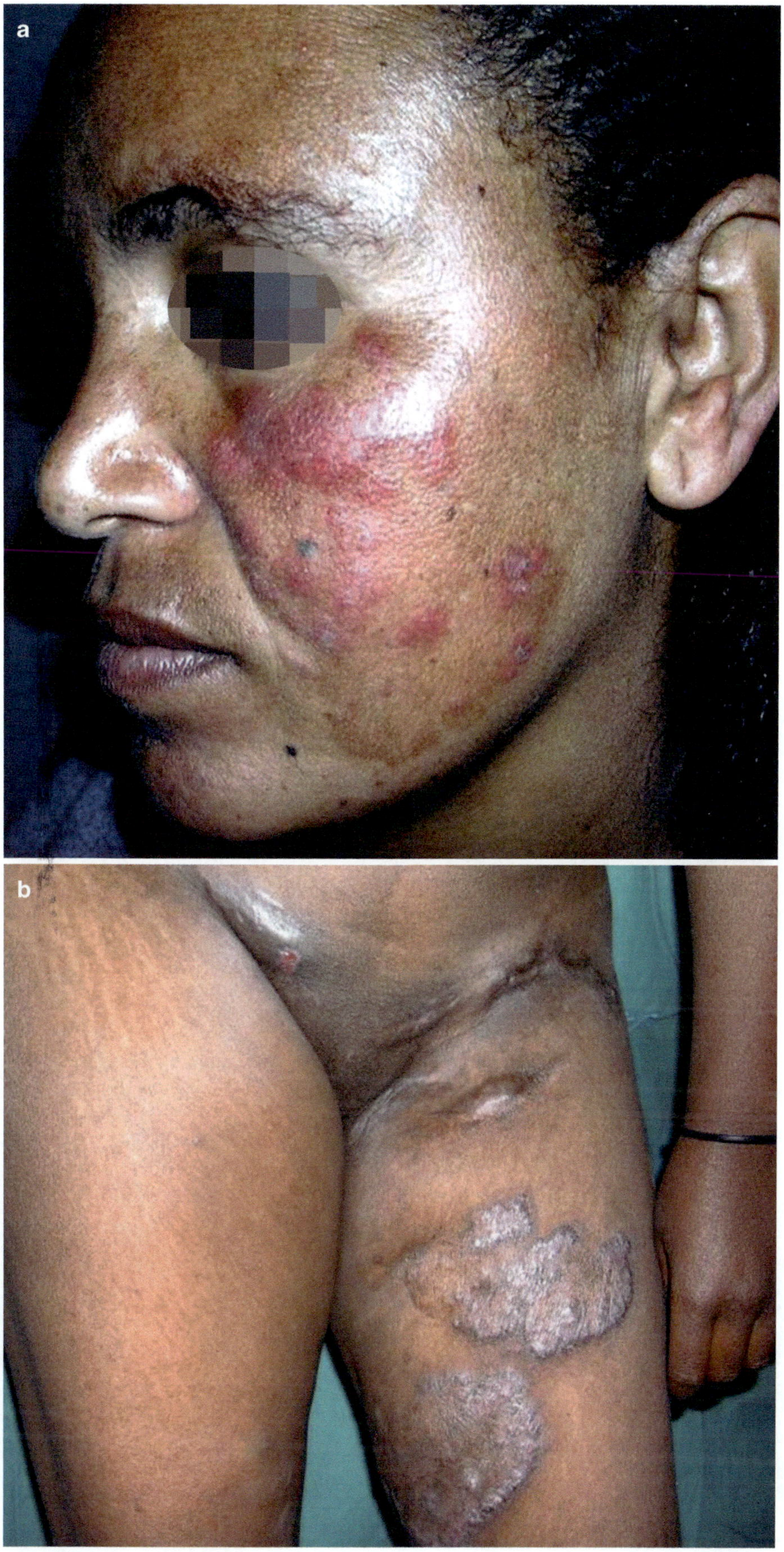

Fig. 10.7 (**a**) *Lupus vulgaris.* Classical lesions on the face in an Ethiopian female. Courtesy INMP Institute, Rome (F.D.). (**b**) *Lupus vulgaris.* Plaques on the upper leg associated with tuberculous lymphadenitis (courtesy INMP Institute, Rome; photo FD)

skin lesions. Often is the nose affected, leading to destruction of the cartilage. Direct or lymphatic spread may involve the palate, larynx, and pharynx [13].

10.1.3.5 Orificial Tuberculosis

This rare form starts with single or multiple papules and nodules close to the orifice which spread, become fluctuant, and lead to painful mucosal ulcers due to autoinoculation, often in elderly or immunocompromised individuals (Fig. 10.8). Pain is a cardinal feature. The affected individual is usually in poor health with long-standing advanced tuberculosis involving internal organs. The prognosis is poor.

10.1.3.6 Tuberculous Abscesses (Gumma)

Abscesses and gummas may develop in skin due to hematogenous dissemination of the infection from an underlying primary focus, during periods of decreased cellular immunity of the patient (Fig. 10.9). Malnourished children and immunocompromised adults are affected. A subcutaneous fluctuant nodule results in an undermined ulcer with sinus formation, also known as metastatic tuberculous abscess or ulcer, resembling scrofuloderma (Fig. 10.10a, b). There are usually a few lesions affecting the trunk and extremities, often without regional lymphadenopathy. As a rule, prognosis is poor.

10.1.3.7 Miliary Tuberculosis

This rare and severe form of tuberculosis may develop due to hematogenous dissemination of the bacilli in immunocompromised individuals and in anergic children, also showing fever, anorexia, asthenia, and weight loss. The initial focus of infection is either pulmonary or meningeal. Multiple disseminated lesions may occur on the trunk, thighs, buttocks, and genitalia. They begin as red to brown papules upon which bursting vesicles appear forming crusts overlying umbilication. They tend to regress in 1–4 weeks, leaving depressed scars. Macules, pustules, ulceration, purpuric lesions, and subcutaneous nodules may also be present. The disease is usually fatal.

10.1.3.8 Tuberculids

Tuberculids are considered as a reaction to dissemination of *M. tuberculosis* or its antigenic particles in immune competent patients. The lesions are usually widespread and symmetrical, with absence of mycobacteria, low positivity in PCR, positive PPD, and good therapeutic outcome. They

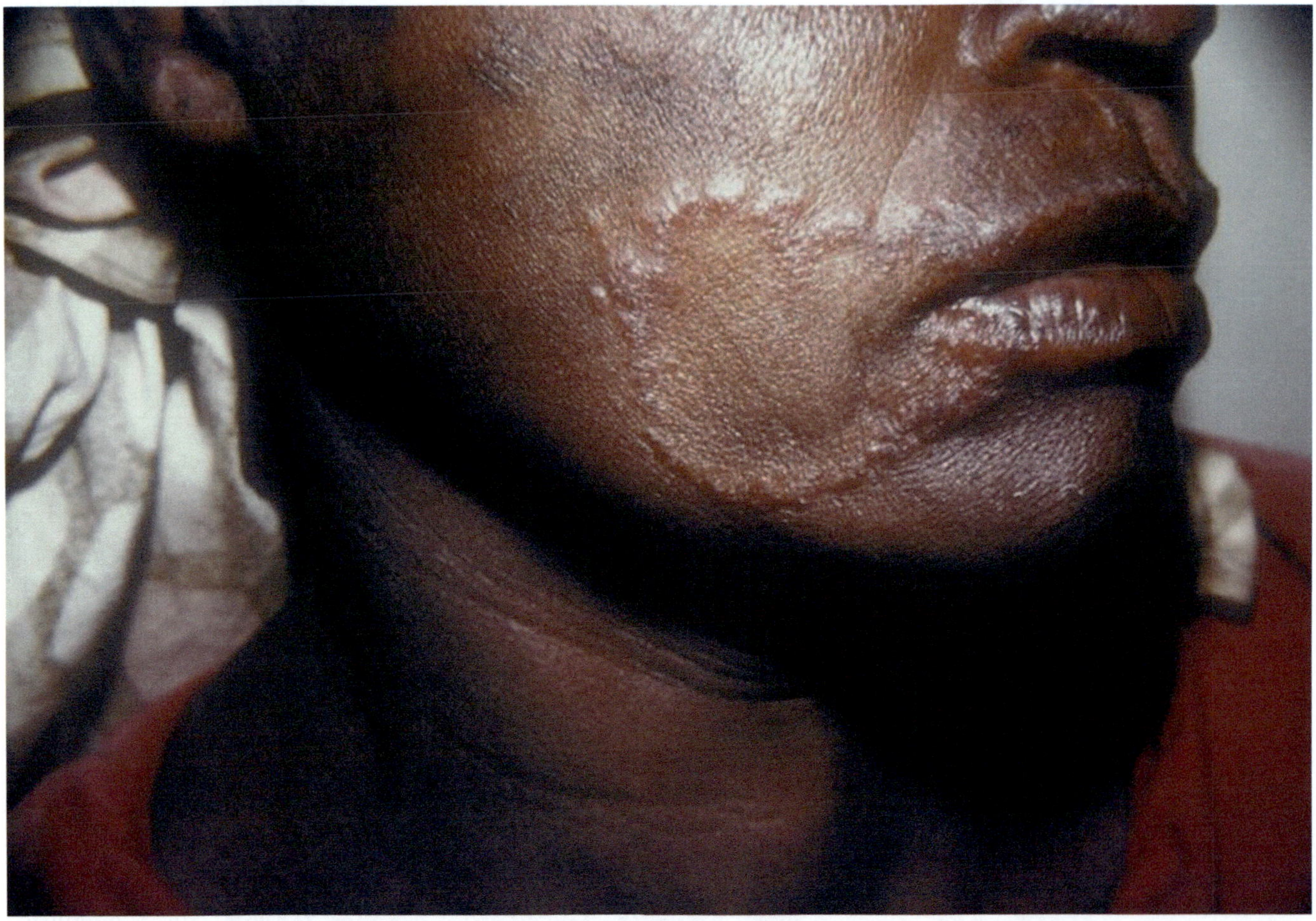

Fig. 10.8 *Orificial tuberculosis* (courtesy RDTC Moshi, Tanzania; photo BN)

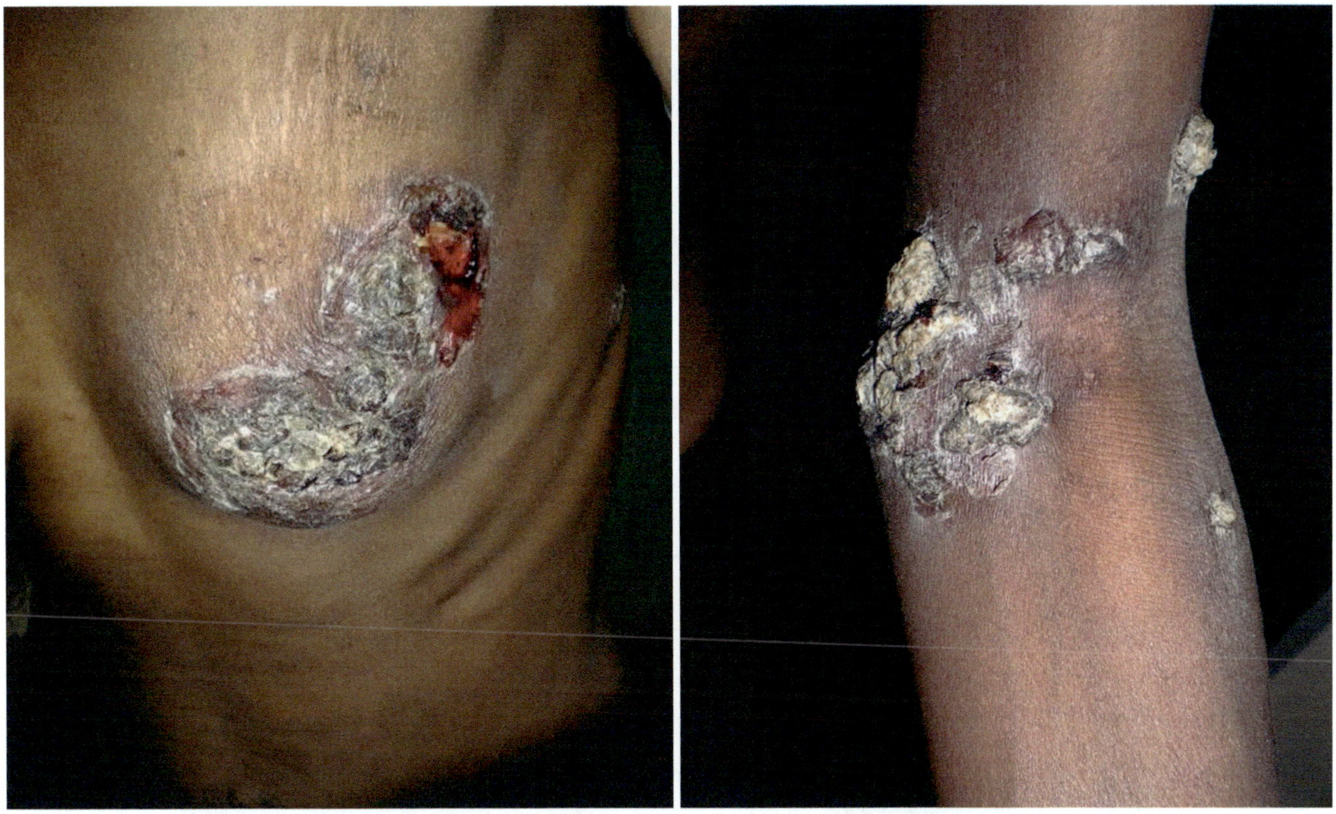

Fig. 10.9 *Metastatic tuberculous abscesses* (gumma) in a immunosuppressed female (courtesy INMP Institute, Rome; photo FD)

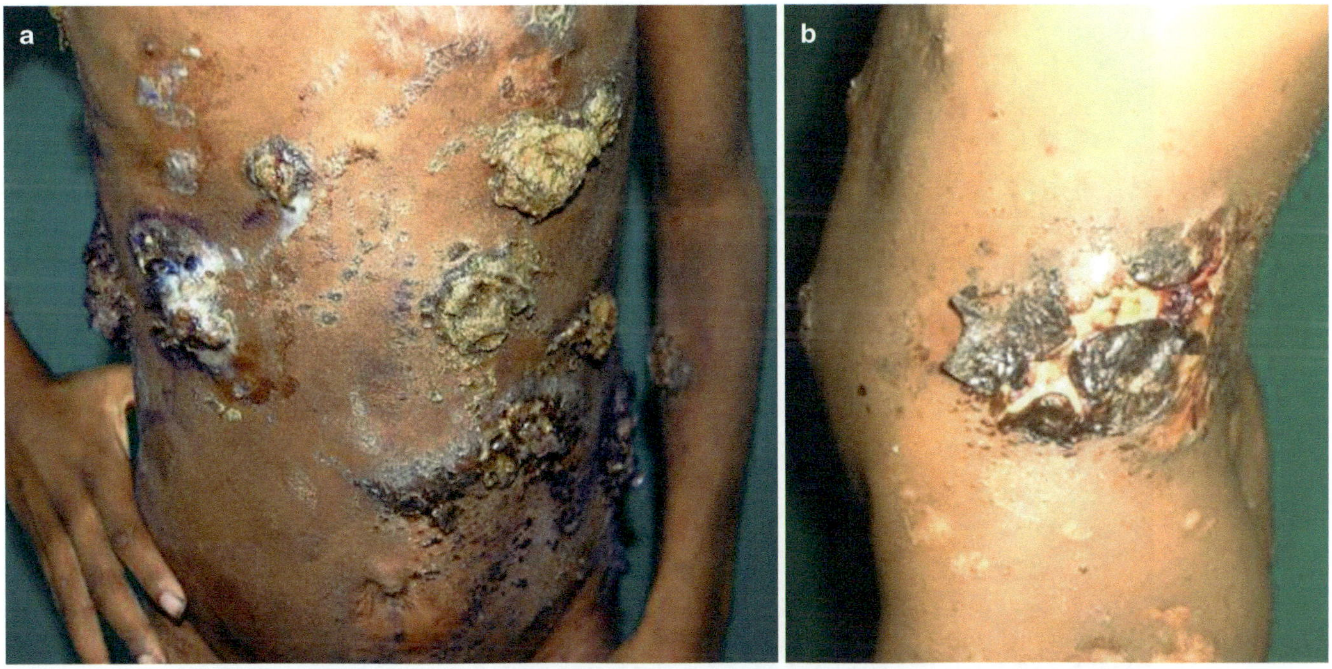

Fig. 10.10 (**a**, **b**) *Metastatic tuberculous abscesses* (gumma) in a malnourished child (first episode and relapse) (courtesy INMP Institute, Rome; photo FD)

often develop in the presence of NTM infection or even after BCG vaccination, being more common among children and young adults.

(a) *Papulonecrotic tuberculid* shows symmetrical crops of small, inflammatory papulonodular lesions, mostly on the acral and dorsal surfaces. Lesions may undergo central ulceration and heal spontaneously within weeks, leaving depressed varioliform scars. PCR positivity and response to specific treatment are observed.
(b) *Lichen scrofulosorum*, also known as tuberculosis cutis lichenoides or lichenoid tuberculid, is mostly observed in children and adolescents. It is characterized by round-shaped lesions consisting of closely grouped, asymptomatic, skin-colored to brown follicular, or perifollicular papules commonly located on the trunk or the proximal limbs. The eruption is usually associated with a strongly positive tuberculin reaction. Studies with PCR have shown the presence of *M. tuberculosis* DNA in lesions. Proper treatment leads to complete resolution of the lesions in weeks, and spontaneous regression in months or years is possible.
(c) *Erythema induratum Bazin* is induced by numerous mycobacterial triggers including CTB. It presents as recurrent subcutaneous poorly defined erythematous plaques and tender violaceous nodules, sometimes ulcerating, on the lower legs of otherwise healthy young and middle-aged females (Fig. 10.11). Histopathology reveals nodular vasculitis. In lesional biopsies, *M. tuberculosis* DNA has been demonstrated. Lesions may regress even without treatment after weeks to months, leaving depressed hyperpigmented scars; recurrences frequently occur.

10.1.4 Management

Cutaneous tuberculosis is curable in virtually 100% of the cases sensitive to antituberculous drugs. HIV testing is recommended before treatment, after having the consent of the patient. If together with the involvement of the skin pulmonary, bone, lymph node, or renal tuberculosis is found, an approach together with the responsible physician is essential. Treatment should be administered according to local regional or national guidelines. Pulmonary TB is treated using a

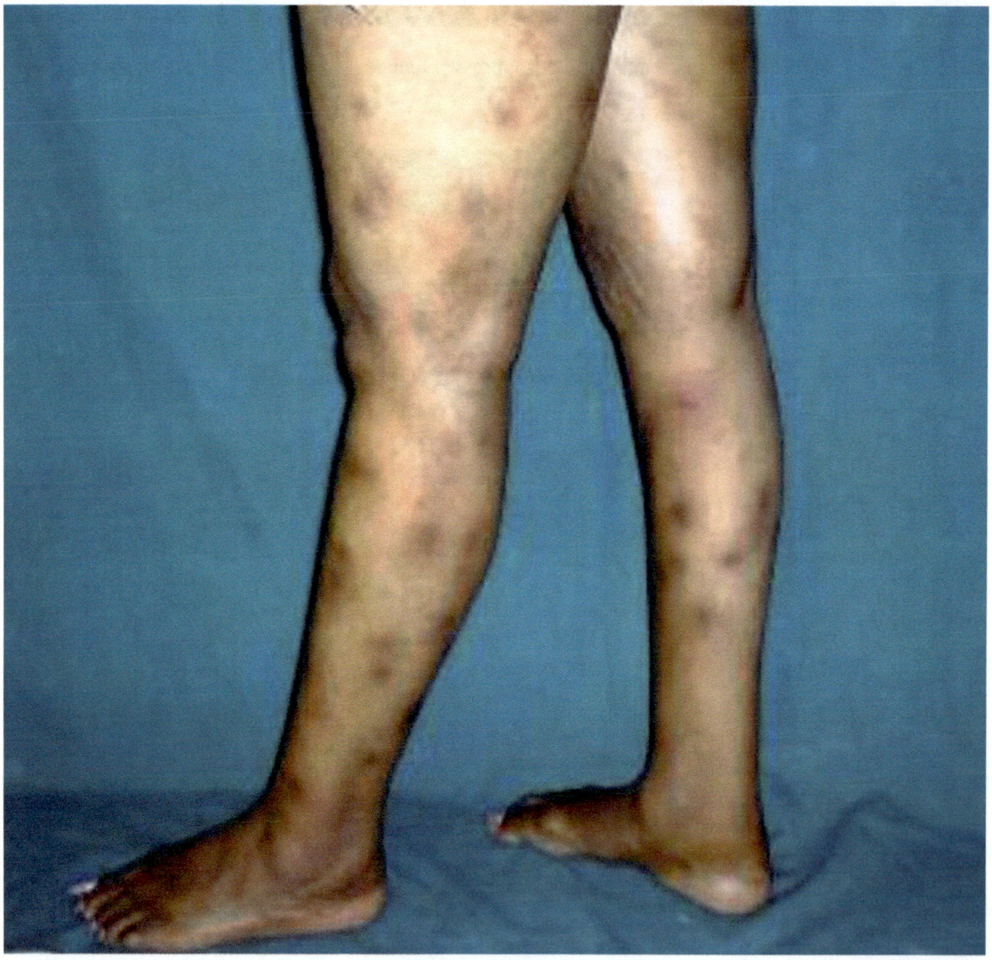

Fig. 10.11 *Erythema induratum Bazin*. Multiple lesions on the legs in an Ethiopian female (courtesy INMP Institute, Rome; photo FD)

6-month course with a combination of antibiotics in order to avoid drug resistance. The usual course for adults is the combination of isoniazid 300 mg/day and rifampicin 150 mg/day for 6 months and of two additional drugs, ethambutol 275 mg/day and pyrazinamide 400 mg/day for the first 2 months (HREZ schedule). For children <10 years old, the recommendation is HRZ, without ethambutol, in doses depending on body weight. Cutaneous and other extrapulmonary forms can be treated using the same schedule, although the duration may be longer. The US recommendation is 2HREZ/7HR. However, there is good evidence from randomized controlled trials that a 6-month regimen is equivalent to the 9-month 2HREZ/4HR regimen [14].

Streptomycin is added in cases with relapses or reinfections in some countries for the first 2 months, and the duration of treatment is longer. In countries with high resources, the necessary medication should be started until cultures and susceptibility tests are made. Special attention should be given to the treatment of groups considered at high risk for toxicity, e.g., the elderly, individuals in poor general health, alcohol addicts, HIV-infected, those under anticonvulsant treatment, and with hepatic disease. For pregnant women, the HREZ scheme can be administered as above; however, the additional administration of pyridoxine (50 mg/day) during pregnancy is recommended because of the risk of neurological toxicity to the newborn due to isoniazid. There is no contraindication to breastfeeding if the mother does not have tuberculous mastitis.

Unfortunately, multidrug-resistant infections with mycobacteria are becoming a major global problem. About 3.7% of all new TB patients have multidrug-resistant strains (MDR-TB), defined as resistance to rifampicin and isoniazid, with or without resistance to the other antituberculous drugs. Current estimates are that about 450,000 new cases of MDR-TB occur worldwide each year, and their number may be even higher since not all resource-poor countries perform testing for drug resistance.

XDR (extensively drug-resistant) tuberculosis, a denomination for MDR strains with resistance to at least three of the main six classes of second line antituberculous drugs, had been officially reported in 84 countries in 2013. On average, an estimated 9.6% of the patients with MDT strains cases may have XDR tuberculosis [15]. Treatment of these patients is complex, most difficult in many developing countries as they lack adequate primary care facilities and the necessary investigational tools. Furthermore, the cost of third-line drugs is not sustainable.

10.1.5 Course and Monitoring

Treatment of all patients should be supervised by physicians, as patient non-compliance is currently one of the most important factors limiting successful treatment, especially in developing countries [15]. Directly observed therapy (DOT), where the ingestion of every drug dose is witnessed, has shown improved cure rates in a number of countries. The WHO advocates universal DOT as part of their overall strategy. Fixed-dose combination tablets should be used to improve adherence in countries in hot climate zones [16].

Apart from antituberculous chemotherapy, local dressings and surgery play a role during the course of treatment of tuberculosis. Excision, surgical drainage, and debridement are useful adjuvants to oral medication. Corrective plastic surgery may be necessary in mutilated and deformed cases, especially when scarring and contractures in the face, neck, and joints cause functional impairment. This may be difficult to perform in developing countries.

10.2 Skin Infections with Nontuberculous Mycobacteria

Nontuberculous mycobacteria (NTM) are species other than *M. tuberculosis* and *M. leprae*, also causing cutaneous infections. Denominations such as atypical mycobacteria (ATM), mycobacteria other than TB (MOTT), environmental mycobacteria, opportunistic mycobacteria, etc. are in broad use [17–20].

NTM are environmental organisms residing in soil and water. More than 140 species are known, and 25 of those have been associated with skin diseases. They are usually transmitted from environmental sources by ingestion, inhalation, or inoculation. These sources may include aerosols, water, soil, dust, food products, and contaminated medical equipment. Culture is the golden standard for the diagnosis of these entities. HIV-related immunosuppression, TNF-alpha inhibitors, and other immunosuppressive drugs have caused an increase in the number of mycobacterial skin infections, in particular of infections with *Mycobacterium avium complex* in the West. Patients with intrinsic innate immunity against mycobacteria are protected.

In settings with a high burden of tuberculosis, little data for the epidemiology and the appearance of NTM disease are available, and several cases remain unspecified (Fig. 10.12), since the ability to confirm mycobacterial disease is limited and NTM-specific treatment options are not widely available. A diagnostic and therapeutic problem is therefore evident in low-resource settings. The global epidemiology of NTM varies. Attempts to understand the burden of NTM infections are hampered by inadequate reporting. Most of the cases seen are diagnosed as tuberculosis or management-resistant tuberculosis.

In children, NTM infection causes lymphadenitis, skin and soft tissue lesions, and occasionally also lung or disseminated disease. These manifestations can be indistinguishable from true tuberculosis on the basis of clinical and radiological findings and tuberculin skin testing. In

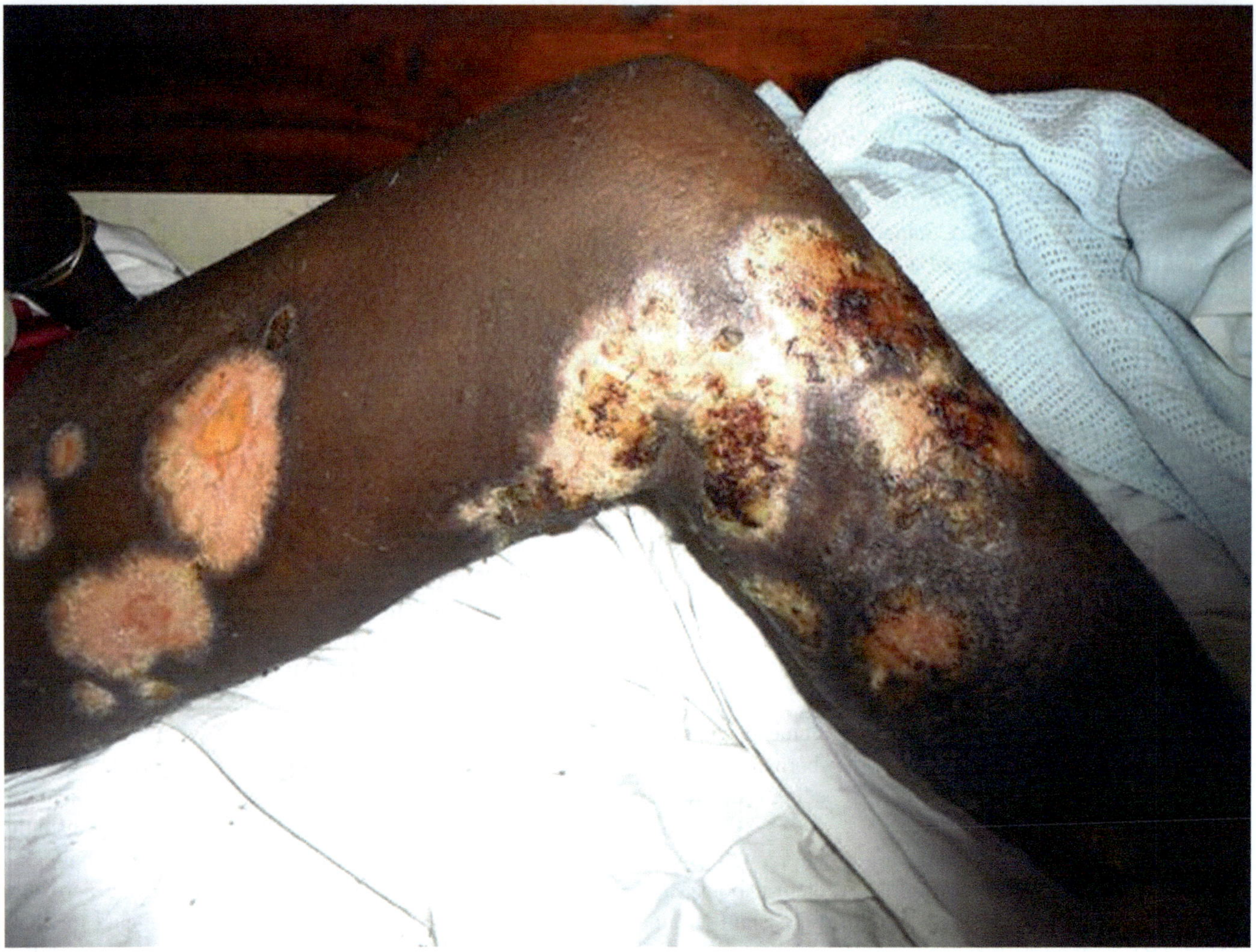

Fig. 10.12 *Atypical mycobacteriosis* (unspecified) in an African patient. The patient improved with management for NTM, but not with anti-TB treatment (courtesy RDTC Moshi, Tanzania; photo BN)

immune competent patients, cutaneous infection is usually a consequence of trauma, and skin lesions tend to be localized. Immunocompromised hosts show a tendency to develop widespread or disseminated lesions.

The group of NTM can be divided into *slow-growing* and *fast-growing*, based on the interval to colony formation by subculture on solid media. For treatment of cutaneous NTM infections, it is preferable to select the drugs based on the antimicrobial susceptibility profile of the responsible agent. However, testing is useful only for fast-growing not for slow-growing NTM, since the in vitro results in this group do not correlate with the in vivo response. Empiric management with clarithromycin is preferred or acceptable in case the identification of the responsible agent by culture or PCR is not indicative or not possible. The overall duration of treatment of NTB infection is generally based on clinical judgment, 6–9 months in most cases. AIDS patients being on treatment with HIV protease inhibitors should not receive rifampicin because the drug significantly increases the breakdown of the antiretrovirals. Rifabutin is a suitable alternative.

10.2.1 Infections with *Mycobacterium marinum*

M. marinum causes disease in fish and occasionally in humans, known as swimming pool or fish tank granuloma. It is found in aquariums, pools, natural water supplies, and in salt water. It is the most common NTM known to cause opportunistic infection in humans. The infection is preceded by trauma due to fish-related activities or swimming in open water. After an average incubation period of 2–6 weeks, the initial inflammatory papule appears, gradually enlarging into violaceous-brown nodules or plaques which may ulcerate or remain verrucous. The lesions are painless, often multiple, mainly localized on hands or feet. They may heal spontaneously in the course of months to years. In approximately

20% of cases, sporotrichoid nodules extend along the lymphatic vessels, whereas the regional lymph glands may be enlarged. The clinical diagnosis should be confirmed by histopathology, culture, or PCR.

Monotherapy with minocycline, clarithromycin, doxycycline, and trimethoprim-sulfamethoxazole can be effective; however, a combination management of two or three drugs is preferable and recommended. Clarithromycin has been considered the drug of choice, particularly in combination with ethambutol. The agent is resistant to isoniazid and pyrazinamide. Azithromycin is considered as an alternative to clarithromycin, and also ciprofloxacin has shown considerable effectiveness. In cases of severe infection, including those with sporotrichoid pattern, a combination of rifampicin and ethambutol is the recommended regimen. Response to treatment is slow. The medication is continued until 4 weeks after clinical cure, often over 4–9 months. Cryotherapy, X-ray management, electrodessication, photodynamic management, and local hyperthermic management have been reported as effective alternatives.

10.2.2 Infections with *Mycobacterium kansasii*

M. kansasii is primarily a pulmonary pathogen, and cutaneous infection is rare and often associated with AIDS. It has been isolated from cattle and swine, water is most likely its true habitat, and affects patients of all ages. Inoculation into the skin occurs through a small wound. Cutaneous lesions are diverse, composed of papules and pustules, often forming verrucous or granulomatous plaques and nodules, which may ulcerate. They can resemble pyogenic abscesses, cellulitis, or sporotrichosis. Cervical lymphadenitis is reported in children. Management usually consists of combinations of isoniazid, rifampicin, ethambutol, or rifampicin and macrolides. Monotherapy is not recommended.

10.2.3 Infections with *Mycobacterium scrofulaceum*

This agent is included in the so-called MAIS group together with *M. avium* and *M. intracellulare.* It causes pulmonary infections and may lead to cervical lymphadenitis in children. Cutaneous lesions are rare, usually part of disseminated infection; multiple subcutaneous abscesses and sporotrichoid infections have been described. For cervical lymphadenitis in childhood induced by *M. scrofulaceum,* surgery without chemotherapy is the recommended treatment. For oral medication, isoniazid, rifampin, and streptomycin are given. Good results have been described with a combination of isoniazid, ethambutol, rifampin, and ofloxacin.

10.2.4 Infections with *Mycobacterium avium*-Intracellulare Complex

The infection is caused by two closely related and difficult to distinguish agents, *M. avium* and *M. intracellulare,* with several other related species (MAC). They are all slow-growing organisms and ubiquitous saprophytes found in water, soil, animals, and dust. It is the most common group of NTM infections associated with AIDS in the West causing opportunistic infections in immunosuppressed individuals. MAC may be isolated in more than 30% of fecal samples. *M. intracellulare* primarily tends to affect the lung; *M. avium* causes lung disease and lymphadenitis in children and disseminated disease in the immunocompromised. Fever, night sweats, weight loss, and diarrhea occur in disseminated infection. Skin involvement is uncommon, often secondary to disseminated disease, rarely by inoculation. Depending on the degree of immunosuppression, widespread skin involvement may present as papules, nodules, plaques with possible abscess formation, and ulcers. Lymph node involvement can occur, showing sinus formation indistinguishable from tuberculous scrofuloderma. For treatment, two or three antimicrobials for at least 18–24 months are given. First-line drugs include clarithromycin or azithromycin, ethambutol, and rifampicin. In HIV-associated MAC disease, a macrolide in combination with ethambutol is the minimum recommended schedule. Surgical excision is considered for lymph nodes and localized cutaneous lesions.

10.2.5 Infections with *Mycobacterium haemophilum*

Such infections have been reported in a broad geographical range. The natural habitat and route are unknown. *M. haemophilum* causes skin, joint, bone, and pulmonary infections in immunocompromised persons and submandibular lymphadenitis in children. Most infections are seen in patients with AIDS, transplant recipients, patients with hematologic malignancies, and those receiving immunosuppressive treatment including biologics. Skin lesions are papules and nodules which enlarge to become painful abscesses or ulcers. In vitro, *M. haemophilum* appears to be susceptible to ciprofloxacin, clarithromycin, rifabutin, and clofazimine but is resistant to isoniazid and ethambutol.

10.2.6 Infections with *Mycobacterium fortuitum*

M. fortuitum is a common, fast-growing mycobacterium isolated from water, soil, and dust. Primary cutaneous disease is seen at all ages. The agent has been implicated in numerous outbreaks of hospital infections. Clinical manifestations are localized cellulitis, frequently with draining abscesses and nodules. History of a penetrating injury with possible soil or water contamination is reported; postoperative infections are possible. The agent responds to treatment with ciprofloxacin, amikacin, and cefoxitin. Alternative drugs are doxycycline, imipenem, ethambutol, and co-trimoxazole. A combined regimen, preferably with three drugs, should be used for 2–4 weeks, followed by ciprofloxacin and a companion drug (e.g., clarithromycin) for 3 months.

10.2.7 Infections with *Mycobacterium chelonae* and *M. abscessus*

The two closely related species are responsible for approximately 95% of cutaneous infections caused by rapidly growing mycobacteria. The clinical picture may present localized or disseminated lesions with cellulitis and multiple, often draining subcutaneous nodules in immunocompromised patients. Localized infections often occur after traumas or surgical incisions. Monotherapy is not recommended, tobramycin and clarithromycin are drugs of choice for *M. chelonae*, and cefoxitin and amikacin are active against both subspecies of *M. abscessus*.

Conclusions

Tuberculosis (12 patients per 10,000 inhabitants worldwide) is according to the WHO criteria still a common disease; however, involvement of the skin is rather rare (0.24 patients per 10,000 inhabitants). This fact together with the prevalence of the disease in developing countries and impoverished populations makes it difficult for non-specialized physicians in the western hemisphere to recognize tuberculous skin lesions. Immigration from high tuberculosis burden, low-income settings requires physicians' awareness in order to diagnose and manage the several variants of cutaneous tuberculosis.

References

1. WHO. Global tuberculosis report; 2015.
2. Portaels F. Epidemiology of mycobacterial diseases. Clin Dermatol. 1995;13:207–22.
3. Hautmann G, Katsambas A, Lotti T. Non-tuberculous mycobacterial skin infections. J Eur Acad Dermatol Venereol. 1997;9:1–35.
4. Naafs B, Van Hees CLM, Van Ingen J. Mycobacterial skin infections. In: Olafsson JH, Hay RJ, editors. Antibiotic and antifungal therapies in dermatology. New York: Springer; 2016. p. 81–139.
5. Faber WR. Mycobacterial infections. In: Faber WR, Hay JR, Naafs B, editors. Imported skin diseases. 2nd ed. New York: Wiley; 2013. p. 64–78.
6. Belo dos Santos J, et al. Cutaneous tuberculosis: epidemiologic, etiopatogenetic and clinical aspects. Part I. An Bras Dermatol. 2014;89:219–28.
7. Sehgal VN, Wagh SA. Cutaneous tuberculosis. Current concepts. Int J Dermatol. 1990;29:237–52.
8. Sehgal VN, Bhattacharya SN, Jain S, et al. Cutaneous tuberculosis: the evolving scenario. Int J Dermatol. 1994;33:97–104.
9. Bolognia JL, Jorizzo JL, Rapini RP. Dermatology. 2nd ed. St. Louis: Mosby; 2003. Chapter 75
10. Bilcha KD, Norton SA. African dermatology handbook. Gondar: University of Gondar; 2014. Chapter II
11. Terranova M, Padovese V, Fornari U, et al. Clinical and epidemiological study of cutaneous tuberculosis in Northern Ethiopia. Dermatology. 2008;217:89–93.
12. Motta A, Feliciani C, Toto P, et al. Lupus vulgaris developing at the site of misdiagnosed scrofuloderma. J Eur Acad Dermatol Venereol. 2003;17:313–5.
13. Reis Gavazzoni Dias MF, Quaresma MV, da Costa Nery JA, et al. Update on cutaneous tuberculosis. An Bras Dermatol. 2014;89:925–38.
14. Yates VM, Walker SL. Mycobacterial infections. In: Griffiths C, Barker J, Bleiker T, Chalmers R, Creamer D, editors. Rook's textbook of dermatology. 9th ed. New York: Wiley; 2015. Chapter 27.
15. European Centre for Disease Prevention and Control/WHO Regional Office for Europe. Tuberculosis surveillance and monitoring in Europe. Stockholm: European Centre for Disease Prevention and Control; 2012.
16. Varshney A, Goyal T. Incidence of various clinico-morphological variants of cutaneous tuberculosis and HIV concurrence: a study from the Indian subcontinent. Ann Saudi Med. 2011;31:134–9.
17. Lopez-Varela E, et al. Non-tuberculous mycobacteria in children: muddying the waters of tuberculosis diagnosis. Lancet Respir Med. 2015;3:244–56.
18. Alcaide F, Esteban J. Cutaneous and soft skin infections due to nontuberculous mycobacteria. Enferm Infecc Microbiol Clin. 2010;28(Suppl 1):46–50.
19. Elston D. Nontuberculous mycobacterial skin infections: recognition and management. Am J Clin Dermatol. 2009;10:281–5.
20. Dodiuk-Gad R, Dyachenko P, Ziv M, et al. Nontuberculous mycobacterial infections of the skin: a retrospective study of 25 cases. J Am Acad Dermatol. 2007;57:413–20.

Leprosy

11

Alireza Firooz, Mansour Nassiri Kashani,
Lila Izadi Firouzabadi, and Mohammad Shizarpoor

11.1 Epidemiology

Leprosy (*Hansen's disease*) is a chronic infection caused by *Mycobacterium leprae*. It predominantly involves the skin and the peripheral nervous system. Although in multibacillary forms of the disease the agents can be detected in a majority of body organs, (except the central nervous system, the gastrointestinal system, and the lungs), their dissemination causes no clinical symptoms [1].

A recent WHO report has shown that the global prevalence of leprosy is 0.32 per 10,000, i.e., a total of 180,618 cases at the beginning of 2014. The exact incidence is unknown because of the number of subclinical infections present in endemic areas, the long incubation period, and the possibility of self-cure, particularly in children. The number of new detected cases in 2013 was 215,656 (3.81 per 100,000), with the highest prevalence in tropical parts of Southeast Asia (India, Nepal, Bangladesh, Myanmar, and Indonesia), South America (Brazil), and Africa (Ethiopia, Tanzania, Congo, and Madagascar), mostly in overpopulated countries with high rates of poverty. More than 80% of all new cases of leprosy are registered in India, Brazil, and Indonesia [2]. In 1991, the World Health Organization introduced the target of eliminating, not eradicating, leprosy reducing its prevalence rate to <1 case per 10,000 persons, achieved in 2013 [3].

The incubation period of leprosy is long, with an average of 2–5 years in paucibacillary and 8–12 years in multibacillary clinical forms. The disease affects preferably men in most parts of the world; paucibacillary forms of the disease are more common, with two peak ages at 10–15 and 30–60 years [4].

11.2 Etiology

In 1873, the Norwegian scientist, Armauer Hansen, discovered the infectious agent of leprosy, *Mycobacterium leprae*. This acid-fast bacillus has several exclusive features. Its reservoir is only in humans and probably armadillos in some parts of the world. It is an obligatory intracellular organism, and cell-mediated immunity is the only mechanism of defense against it. The division time of the bacilli is long (12–14 days), thus expanding the incubation period of the disease to several years. The best temperature for its growth is 30–33 °C; therefore, the agents grow in the cooler regions of the body such as the skin and the peripheral nerves. In vitro culture is not available to date, and mouse foot pads or armadillos are used for replication in vivo. This has led to difficulties in the laboratory diagnosis, evaluation of sensitivity and resistance to antibiotics, and discovery of new anti-leprosy drugs. Unlike the *Mycobacterium tuberculosis*, its genetic mutational rate is low and the DNA genome rather stable, as completely sequenced in 2001 [5].

The main reservoir in humans is the upper respiratory tract of untreated patients with multibacillary leprosy; the disease is transmitted to the healthy via close and lengthy contact through nasal secretions. After inhalation, *Mycobacterium leprae* replicates in the upper respiratory tract of the new host, has a short phase in blood, and finally binds to the Schwann cells of the peripheral nerves and skin macrophages. Undamaged skin is resistant to transmission, but rare cases of leprosy have been reported after traumatic inoculation such as vaccination, penetrating trauma, tattoo, and surgery. In the USA, some rare cases of leprosy have been described in patients who had no history of travel to or contact in endemic areas but had contact with armadillo.

A. Firooz, M.D. (✉) · M. Nassiri Kashani, M.D.
L. Izadi Firouzabadi, M.D. · M. Shizarpoor, M.D.
Center for Research and Training in Skin Diseases and Leprosy,
Tehran University of Medical Sciences, Tehran, Iran
e-mail: firozali@tums.ac.ir

C. E. Orfanos et al. (eds.), *Pigmented Ethnic Skin and Imported Dermatoses*, https://doi.org/10.1007/978-3-319-69422-1_11

Overall, the significance of armadillo for a transmission of leprosy is not clearly elucidated [6].

About 90% of humans are genetically resistant to leprosy. Others may acquire the disease only if they have close, prolonged, and continuous household contact with multibacillary patients for months or years.

11.3 Classification

There are several systems for classifying the clinical forms of leprosy, the two most commonly used are the WHO and Ridley-Jopling classifications. The classification of WHO [7] is more practical, especially for healthcare providers in endemic areas. It is primarily based on skin smear results, dividing patients into two groups: *Paucibacillary* (PB) forms with negative smear and *multibacillary* (MB) with positive smear. Due to the absence of facilities for preparing and evaluating skin smears in many medica in poor endemic areas, WHO later recommended a new scheme of classification based on the number of skin lesions. Patients who have five or fewer skin lesions are considered as *paucibacillary*, and those with >5 lesions are considered *multibacillary*. The main obstacle for such classification is that some MB patients might have less than five skin lesions, be classified as PB group, and receive insufficient treatment. As a result, if there is any doubt regarding MB or PB, the patient should be considered as MB for treatment.

A system based on clinical and histopathological findings has been proposed by Ridley and Jopling [8], taking into account the cell-mediated immune reaction against the agent. The patients are divided into six groups: *Indeterminate* (I), *tuberculoid* (TT), *borderline tuberculoid* (BT), *mid-borderline* (BB), *borderline lepromatous* (BL), and *lepromatous leprosy* (LL). The first three groups almost match with paucibacillary, whereas the last three are compatible with multibacillary patients. The skin smear is usually negative in the first three groups and positive in the rest. After a strong immune response, the patient develops tuberculoid leprosy (TT), a moderate response results in borderline, and minimal or lacking response to lepromatous leprosy [9, 10]. Patients in the tuberculoid pole of leprosy have few asymmetric cutaneous and nervous lesions. Toward the lepromatous pole of the disease, there is an increase in the number of lesions with more diversity and symmetry in the morphology of the lesions. Although an involvement of the peripheral nerves is more obvious in the first group, such symptoms can also be seen in advanced stages of the second group.

11.4 Clinical Features

A wide spectrum of clinical signs and symptoms can be seen in patients with leprosy, depending on the immune response of the patient [11, 12].

Indeterminate (I) leprosy: This is the early phase of the infection, usually seen in children. It usually presents with a single hypopigmented patch, particularly in dark-skinned patients, with an ill-defined margin. In fair-skinned patients, there is a fade erythema within this patch. The lesion often develops on the face, upper arm, upper leg, and buttock. It does not involve the scalp, axilla, and inguinal areas as these areas are warmer. The patient may complain from paresthesia, but there is no sensory impairment. Indeterminate leprosy generally improves spontaneously; a few cases develop into progressive disease.

TT leprosy: This type involves the skin and peripheral nerves only. There is usually a single elevated annular plaque or a few asymmetric macules or flat patches, sometimes showing a prominent border. The center may be erythematous in light skin or hypopigmented in dark-skinned individuals (Fig. 11.1). The scalp, axillae, and inguinal areas are usually spared. On physical examination, the TT lesions are hypo- or anesthetic. Temperature sensation is the first to get lost, followed by loss of sensation of light touch, pain, and deep touch. As a rule, a peripheral nerve close to the skin lesion is enlarged and palpable. Involvement of the autonomic innervations can lead to lack of perspiration and decrease in hair growth.

BT leprosy: Likewise in TT type, the lesions have a well-demarcated border and hypopigmented center. There is a possibility for erythematous appearance in fair skin. The number of lesions in BT leprosy is higher than in TT patients but usually less than five. Small satellite lesions may be seen at their periphery, revealing a symmetric pattern of distribution. Peripheral nerve involvement is common, and large nerve trunks are asymmetrically involved. Impairment of the sensory function is a significant feature.

BB leprosy: This form is usually unstable, and the patient often upgrades or downgrades to other types of leprosy. The

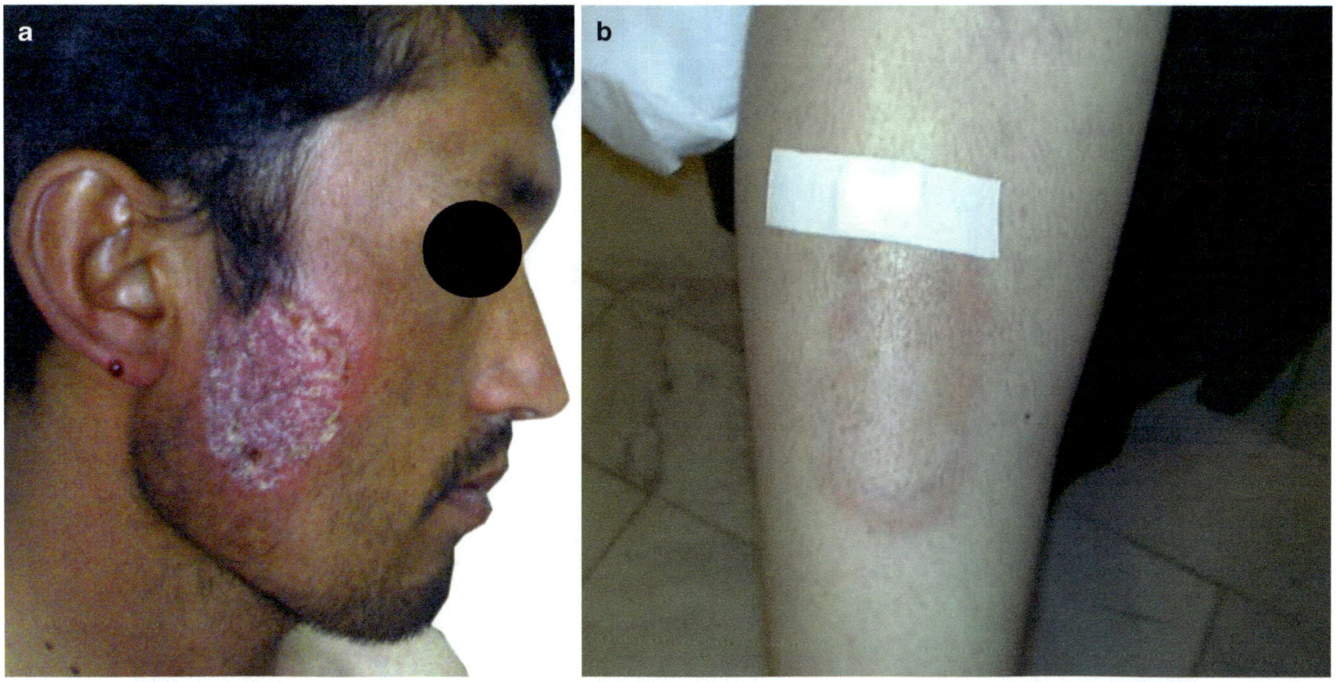

Fig. 11.1 Patients with *TT leprosy*. (**a**) Single erythematous plaque, (**b**) asymmetric dissemination of hypopigmented, hypoanesthetic macules on the trunk

number of lesions is high, but not as much as in LL leprosy. Their distribution tends to be more symmetric than BT, presenting macules, papules, and plaques. A rare but typical feature is a punch out erythematous plaque with well-demarcated inner border and a fade, nonspecific outer border. Nerve enlargement and symmetrical peripheral neuropathy is often found.

BL leprosy: Involvement of the skin is in this type diffuse, multiple, and almost symmetric. Fade macules are followed by papules, plaques, and nodules (Fig. 11.2), often with ill-defined borders and asymptomatic symmetric enlargement of large peripheral nerves. Patients also show distal sensory loss in a stock-and-glove pattern, reduced sweating, and in late stages muscle atrophy and contractures (Fig. 11.3). In early stages, there are no signs and symptoms of oral and nasal involvement such as epistaxis, septal perforation, saddle nose, and madarosis (thinning or loss of eyebrows and lashes). The incidence of immunological reactions, both types 1 and 2, is high in BL leprosy.

LL leprosy: High and unrestrained replication of *Mycobacterium leprae* in the skin, nerve tissue, and several other organs is the cause for the clinical features of lepromatous leprosy. Widespread and symmetric papules, nodules, and plaques are seen, but still the scalp, axillae, and groins are spared. Diffuse infiltration of bacillus in the skin leads to multiple lesions and in some cases to the typical and characteristic feature of leonine facies (Figs. 11.4, 11.5 and 11.6). Saddle nose deformity, destruction of nasal bridge, and epistaxis may occur due to heavy infiltration of the agent. Madarosis, lagophthalmos due to facial nerve paralysis, and ichthyosis-like xerosis are also features in late-stage LL. The auricle may be infiltrated, enlarged, and swollen. Neuropathy in the form of glove-and-stocking anesthesia is seen in the late and progressive stages of lepromatous leprosy. The nerve damage permits blisters, cuts, burns, and infections of the extremities due to repetitive or unsuitable traumas. Later secondary infections, cellulitis, osteomyelitis, loss of tissue, and permanent deformities and disabilities may occur.

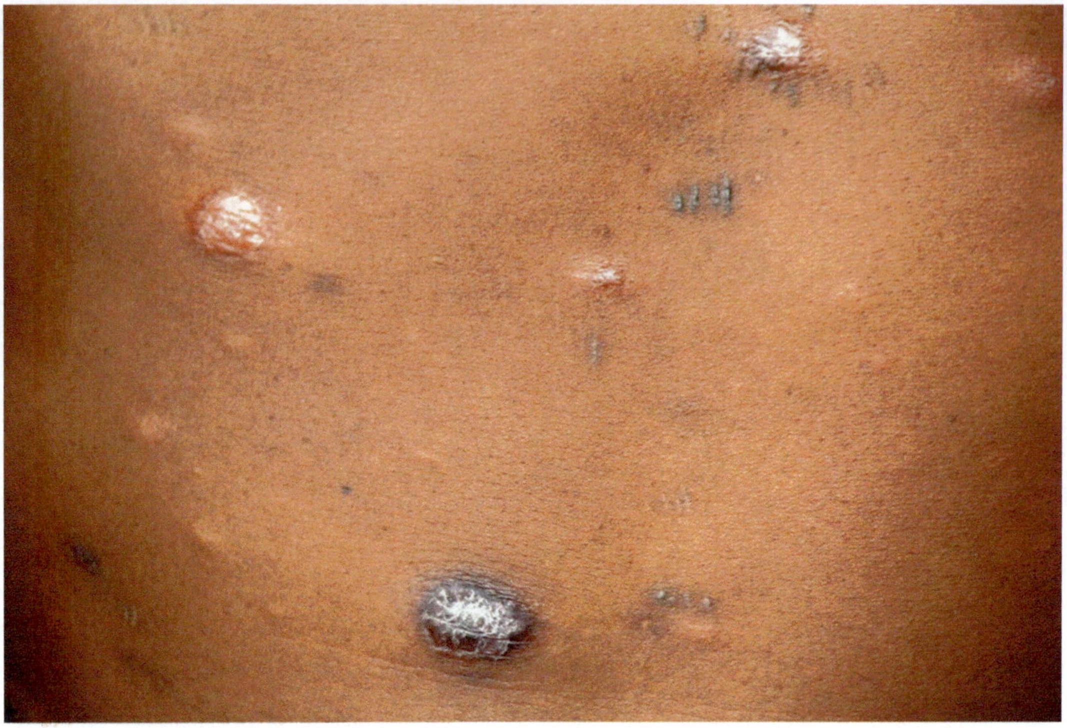

Fig. 11.2 *BL leprosy* showing macules plaques and nodules

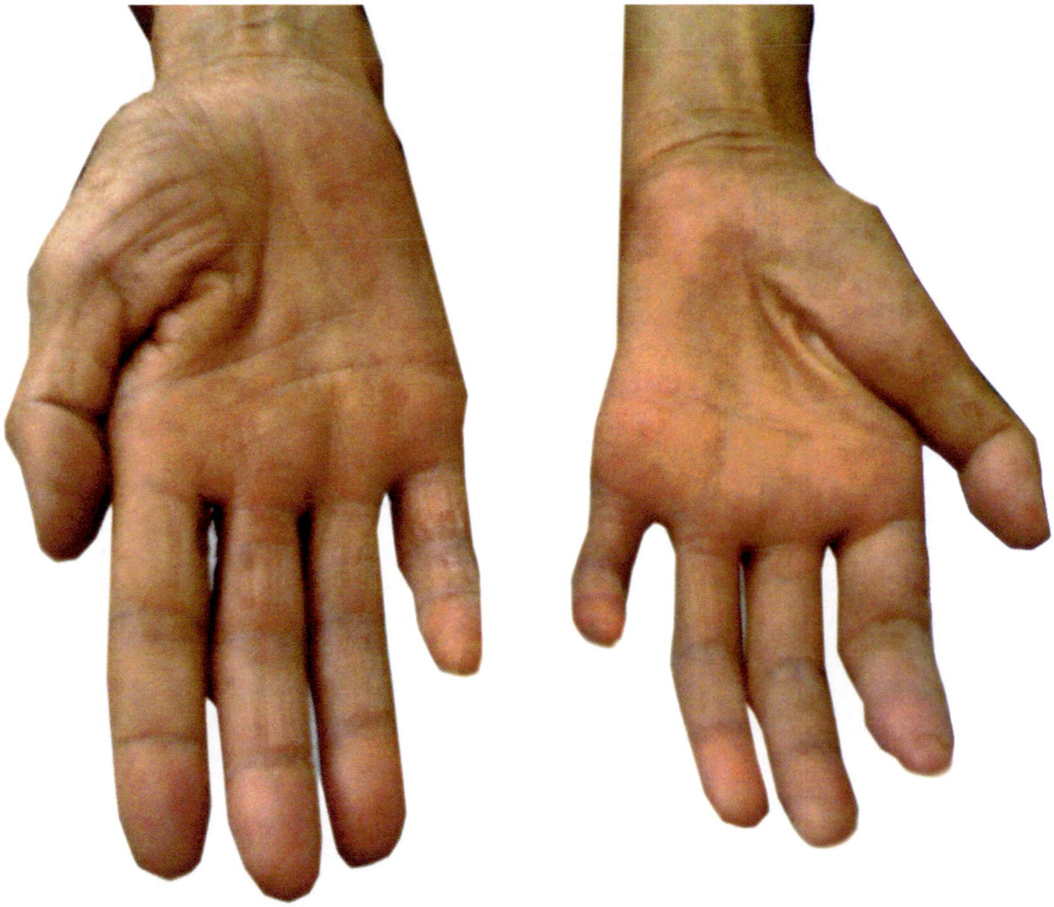

Fig. 11.3 Muscle atrophy and contractures in *BL leprosy*

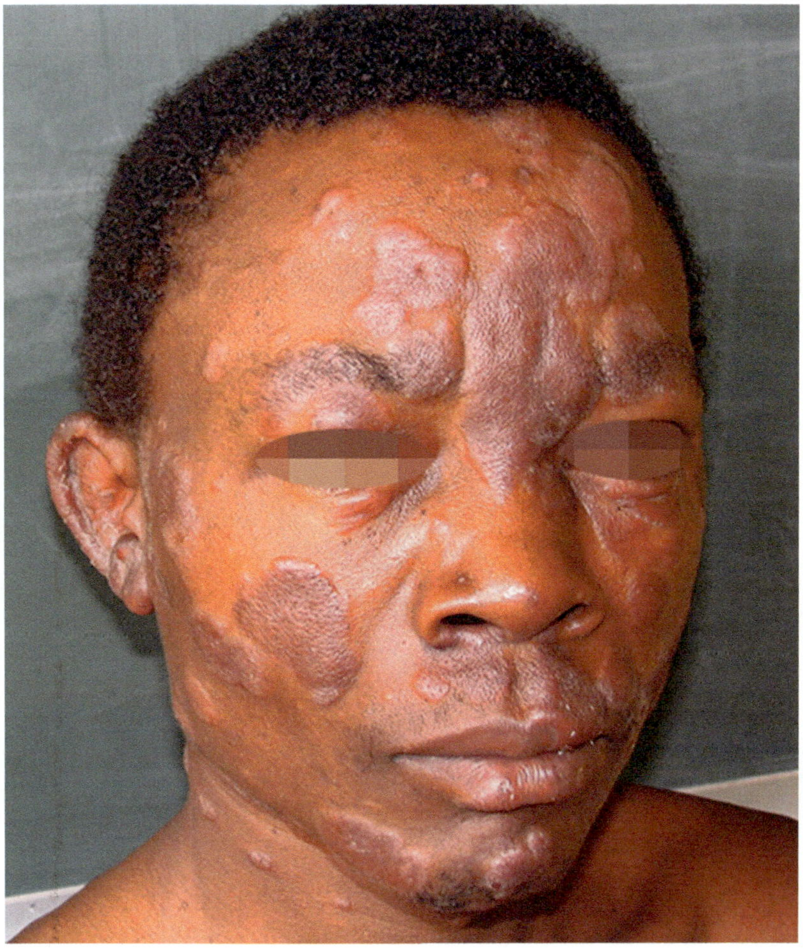

Fig. 11.4 Elevated plaques and leonine aspect of the face in *lepromatous leprosy* (Courtesy RDTC in Moshi, Tanzania (Photo: CEO))

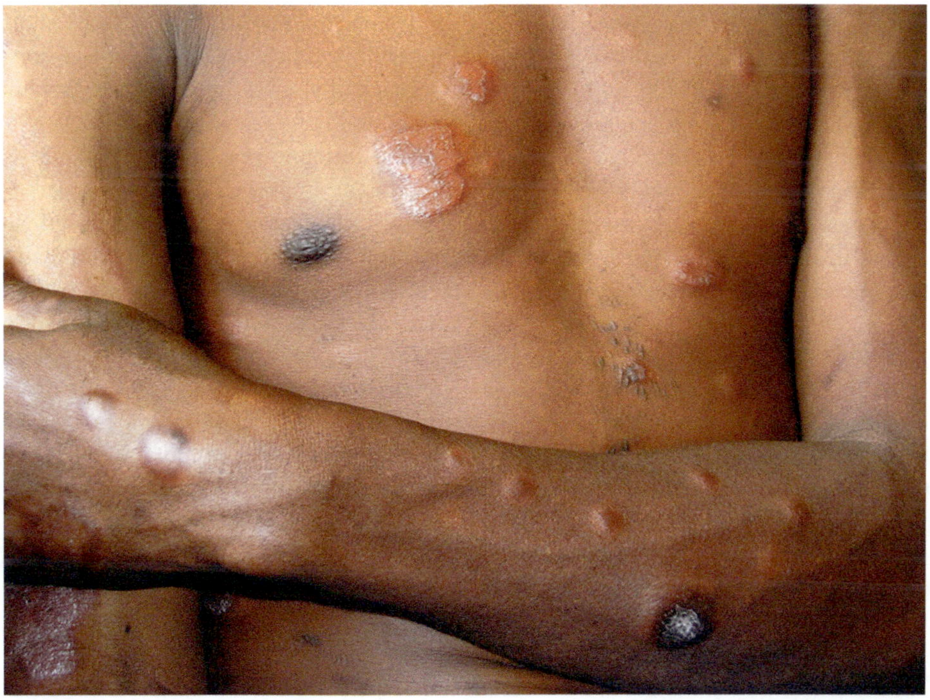

Fig. 11.5 *LL leprosy*. Characteristic lesions on the trunk and extremities (Courtesy RDTC Moshi, Tanzania (Photo: CEO))

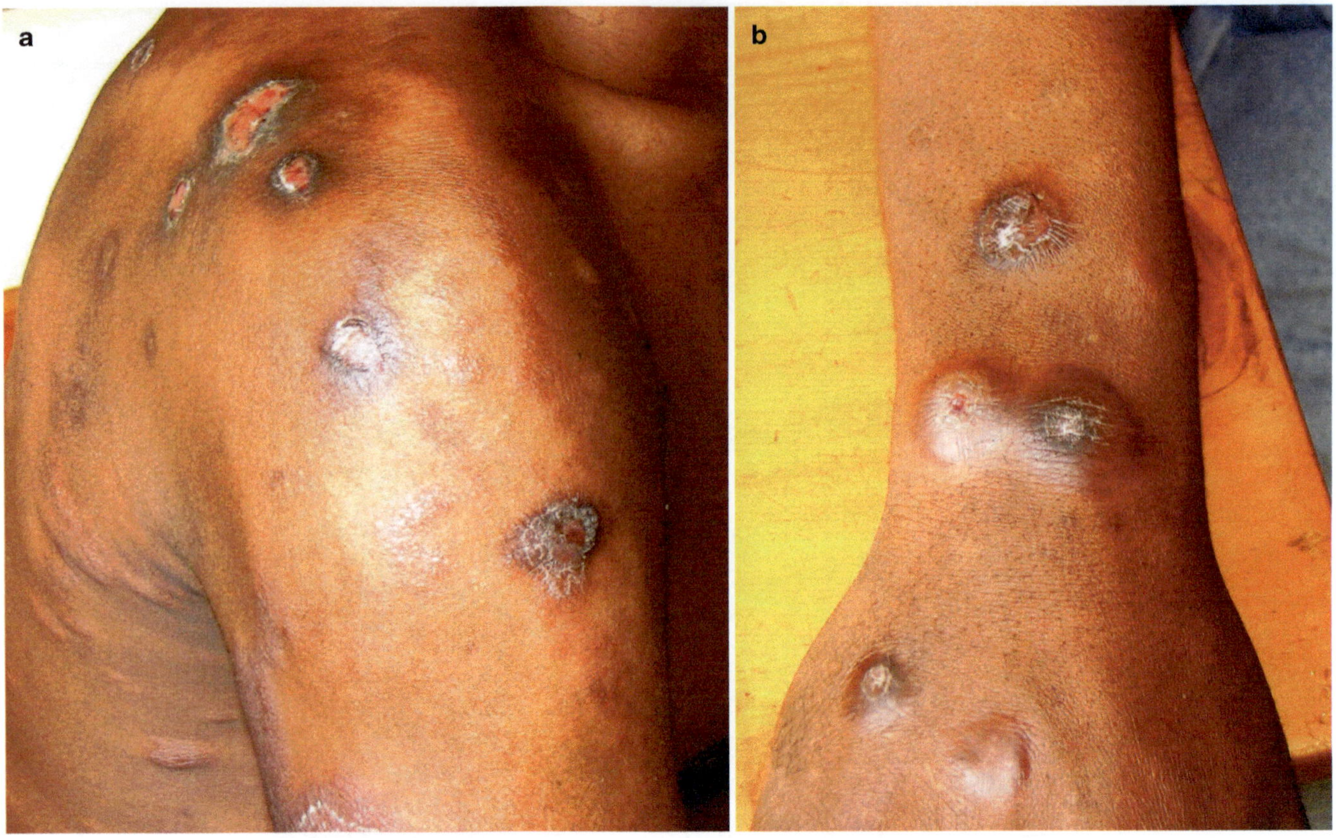

Fig. 11.6 (**a**, **b**) Tumor-like lesions in late *lepromatous leprosy*

11.5 Immunologic Reactions

Type 1 reactions can occur in borderline leprosy patients before, during, or even after treatment due to changes of the cell-mediated immune response, considered as a type IV hypersensitivity reaction. Patients develop acute symptoms of inflammation in the skin and peripheral nerves. On examination, pain, swelling, and erythema in cutaneous lesions and/or in nerve fibers occur. New skin lesions can appear abruptly with inflammation and erythema (Fig. 11.7a). This phenomenon is a destructive process and can damage nerves permanently.

Type 2 leprosy reactions are due to the formation and deposition of antigen-antibody complexes (type III hypersensitivity) and occur in around 50% of the patients with BL and LL types of the disease, particularly after the onset of oral medication. It is a multi-systemic process representing leukocytoclastic vasculitis. Uveitis, orchitis, arthritis, lymphadenopathy, and hepatosplenomegaly may be diagnosed. *Erythema nodosum leprosum* (ENL) is a cutaneous manifestation of type 2 reaction, consisting of multiple, painful subcutaneous nodules (Fig. 11.7b). Unlike ordinary erythema nodosum, the nodules in ENL last shorter and involve the upper limbs, face, and trunk, in addition to the lower limbs. Occasionally, ENL may be the first manifestation of the infection.

The immune reactions in patients with leprosy are of significant importance and considered as an emergency condition to be instantly diagnosed and treated. If they remain untreated, persistent complications and disabilities may follow. Both physicians and patients should be aware that reactions arising during treatment are not side effects of the drugs or signs of failure of the medication and that treatment must continue. It may be difficult to differentiate mild type 2 reaction from a relapse after termination of treatment; however, immune reactions are always acute and show rapid response to corticosteroids. In contrast, relapses are much less frequent and usually arise years after the treatment is stopped; they do not respond to corticosteroids and slowly progress.

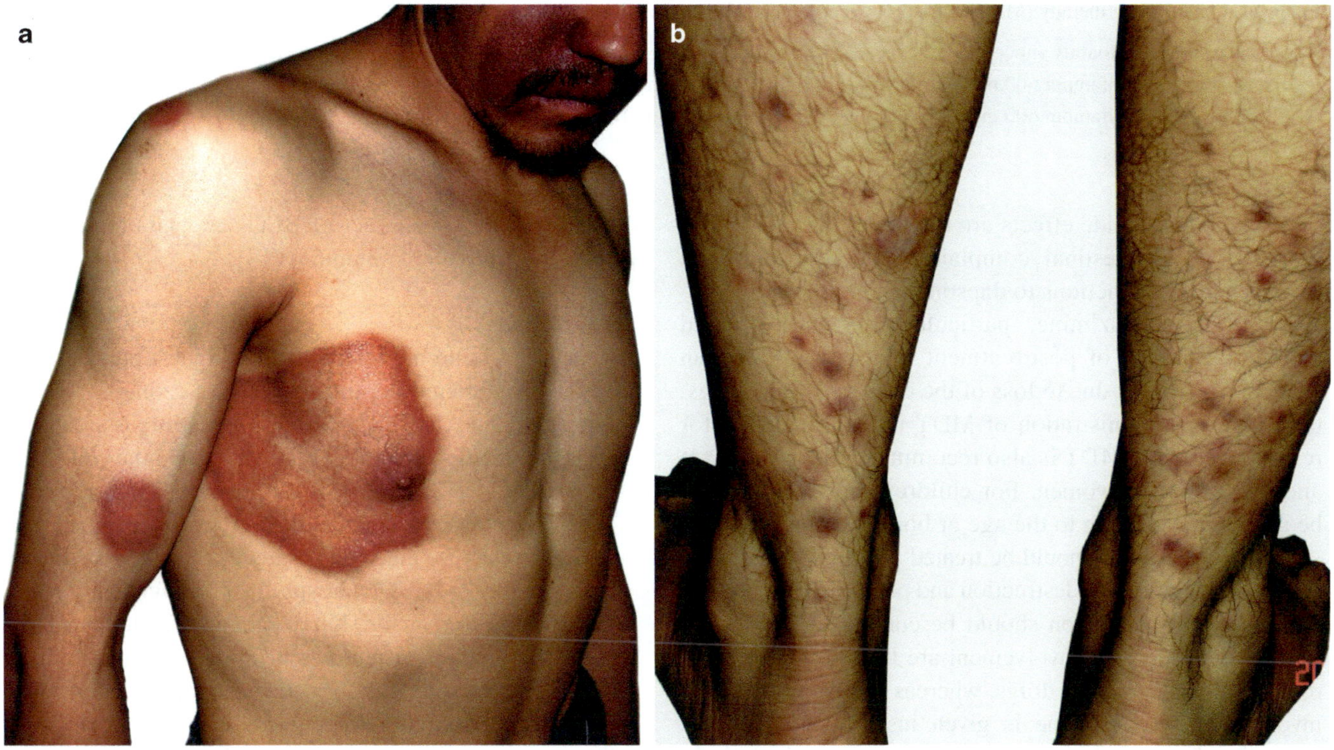

Fig. 11.7 (**a**) Elevated plaques representing type 1 reaction and (**b**) erythema nodosum leprosum (ENL) as a type 2 reaction in leprosy

11.6 Diagnosis

The diagnosis of leprosy is usually clinical, based on the history and accurate examination of the patient. When leprosy is suspected, a complete and thorough physical examination of the entire skin is necessary. None of the existing laboratory methods are sensitive enough or available in endemic areas.

The main diagnostic criteria are (*a*) presence of cutaneous lesions compatible with leprosy, (*b*) sensory impairment on skin lesions in tuberculoid pole or extremities in lepromatous pole, and (*c*) palpable thickening of peripheral nerves. Due to the diverse features in its different clinical types, almost any skin lesions can be related to leprosy. The peripheral nerves should be then palpated for thickening and tenderness. Following that, the sensory function should be thoroughly examined and carried out by test tubes containing warm and cold water for thermal sensation, a cotton wool or feather for light touch, pinprick for pain, and pinch test for deep sensation. Examinations should be performed on the cutaneous lesions of paucibacillary leprosy; for excluding multibacillary forms, all limbs should be examined, together with evaluation of strength of the distal muscles and the presence of atrophy or muscle contractures. Hypohidrosis or loss of hair can be a sign of impairment of autonomic nerves. Examination of the eyes is mandatory in all patients suspected for leprosy.

Hypopigmented lepromatous lesions must be differentiated from pityriasis alba, vitiligo, post-inflammatory hypopigmentation, and achromic or anemic nevi. The well-demarcated erythematous lesions of paucibacillary forms can imitate dermatophytosis, granuloma annulare, cutaneous tuberculosis, mycosis fungoides, or allergic contact dermatitis; erythematous lesions in multibacillary forms may resemble psoriasis, pityriasis rosea, secondary syphilis, cutaneous lymphoma, and sarcoidosis. The leonine facies is most characteristic for LL, but not pathognomonic; it can be also seen in leishmaniasis, lymphoma, and pseudolymphoma.

Although the WHO does not recommend any laboratory evaluation for confirming the diagnosis, slit skin smears, histopathology of the skin and/or the peripheral nerves with special stains, and PCR investigations will be helpful.

11.7 Management

A multidrug regimen (MDT) has been introduced by the WHO for treatment of leprosy [7, 13], and monthly packages of the necessary drugs are distributed free of charge. The combination of drugs recommended is highly effective

Table 11.1 Multidrug therapy (MDT) for leprosy recommended by the WHO

Type of leprosy	Monthly supervised	Daily oral intake	Duration
Paucibacillary	Rifampin 600 mg + clofazimine 300 mg	Dapsone 100 mg + clofazimine 50 mg	6 months (over 6–9 months)
Multibacillary	Rifampin 600 mg + clofazimine 300 mg	Dapsone 100 mg + clofazimine 50 mg	12 months (over 12–18 months)

(Table 11.1). The side effects are tolerable; the most common are gastrointestinal complaints due to rifampicin, hypersensitivity reactions to dapsone, and hyperpigmentation due to clofazimine, particularly in dark-skinned patients. The rate of posttreatment relapses is less than 1:1000, mostly not due to loss of the efficacy of the drugs; therefore, re-administration of MDT is recommended for relapsed patients. MDT is also recommended for pregnant and breastfeeding women. For children, the dosage must be adjusted according to the age or body weight.

Leprosy reactions should be treated promptly since there is a possibility of rapid destruction and permanent damage of nerves; MDT medication should be continued. Mild reactions without nervous involvement are treated with nonsteroidal anti-inflammatory drugs, whereas in cases with nerve involvement, prednisolone is given instantly (40–60 mg/day). The dose should be gradually tapered, particularly in type 1 reactions, and be withdrawn when the reaction is controlled. Thalidomide (100–200 mg/day) is a drug of choice for type 2 reactions including ENL, with or without prednisolone. Its use in childbearing women is limited due to high risk of teratogenicity. High-dose clofazimine (300 mg/day) might be effective in some ENL patients. When it is difficult to differentiate between immune reactions and relapse, it is advised to administer corticosteroids in order to avoid possible nerve injury [12].

11.8 Prevention

Early diagnosis, prompt treatment, and patient education are the main strategies of WHO for prevention of leprosy and its complications. Household contact persons of leprosy, particularly in multibacillary cases, should be followed for the development of signs and symptoms of the infection. Regular monitoring of the sensory and motor functions of the hands, feet, and eyes is mandatory to early diagnose nerve damage. Patients should be instructed to apply ointments on the skin to prevent xerosis, wear appropriate shoes, massage the muscles and do physiotherapy to prevent contractures, and clean all abrasions. In cases with lagophthalmos, frequent use of artificial tears and occlusion of the eyes with an ointment at night are recommended [13]. Efforts to develop a vaccine for leprosy were unsuccessful before the introduction of MDT. The protective effect of BCG vaccination was quite variable in different communities [14].

Conclusions

Leprosy is a chronic infection with highest prevalence in developing countries in hot climate zones of Asia, America, and Africa. *Mycobacterium leprae* is an obligatory pathogenic intracellular organism, and the cell-mediated immunity is the only mechanism of defense. About 90% of humans are genetically resistant to the agent; their immune response inactivates and destroys the bacilli after entering the body. A wide spectrum of signs and symptoms can be seen on the skin of patients affected, resulting into various clinical pictures depending on the immune response of the host. Early diagnosis and prompt introduction of treatment sustainable over several months are the main strategies for prevention. The multidrug regimen (MDT) introduced and supported by the WHO for the management of leprosy is highly effective; however, profound education of patients and all health workers involved is an essential precondition for eradicating the disease in developing countries under the circumstances of poverty.

Immunological reactions in patients under antilepromatous treatment must be diagnosed instantly and treated appropriately as emergencies, in order to prevent persistent complications and disabilities.

References

1. James WD, Berger TG, Elston DM, editors. Andrews' diseases of the skin: clinical Dermatology. Toronto: Elsevier; 2006. p. 343–52.
2. WHO. Weekly epidemiological record, 2014;36(89):389–400. 2016. www.who.int/wer/2014/wer8936.pdf?ua=1
3. Leprosy Elimination Group.World Health Organization; 2003.
4. Sugita Y. Leprosy. Clin Dermatol. 1995;13:235–43.
5. Monot M, Honore N, Garnier T. Comparative genomic and phylogeographic analysis of Mycobacterium leprae. Nat Genet. 2009;41:1282–9.
6. Balamayooran G, Pena M, Sharma R, et al. The armadillo as an animal model and reservoir host for Mycobacterium leprae. Clin Dermatol. 2015;33:108–15.
7. World Health Organization. Chemotherapy of leprosy for control programmes: technical report series 675, Geneva; 1982.
8. Ridley DS, Jopling WH. Classification of leprosy according to immunity. Int J Lepr. 1966;34:255–73.

9. Yamamura M, Uyemura K, Deans RJ, et al. Defining protective responses to pathogens: cytokine profiles in leprosy lesions. Science. 1991;254:277–9.
10. Sampaio EP, Moraes MO, Pessolani MCV, et al. Role of Th1 cytokines in host defense against Mycobacterium leprae. In: Kotb M, Calandra T, editors. Cytokines and chemokines in infectious diseases handbook. Totowa: Humana Press; 2003. p. 163–86.
11. Prasad PVS. All about leprosy. New Delhi: Jaypee Brothers Medical Publishers; 2005.
12. Firooz A, Dowlati Y, Ayatollahi A. Leprosy. In: McDowell MA, Rafati S, editors. Neglected tropical diseases-Middle East and North Africa. Wien: Springer; 2014. p. 172–92.
13. Firooz A. Multidrug therapy regimen for leprosy. J Am Acad Dermatol. 2006;55:1115.
14. Lockwood DNJ. Leprosy. BMJ Clin Evid. 2007;2007:pii: 0915.

12 Endemic Treponematoses

Valeska Padovese

Endemic treponemal diseases are non-venereal infections closely related to syphilis. They consist of *yaws*, *bejel* (endemic syphilis), and *pinta*. They are endemic in tropical rural areas and very rare in Europe. Increasing worldwide migration from endemic areas requires recognition of these diseases by physicians in developed countries.

12.1 Epidemiology

The endemic treponemal diseases, consisting of yaws, bejel (endemic syphilis), and pinta, are non-venereal infections closely related to syphilis and are recognized by the World Health Organization as neglected tropical diseases. They are endemic in tropical rural areas among poor communities living in overcrowded conditions. Few cases of imported yaws and endemic syphilis have been described in Europe. However, the escalating military presence in many world areas and the increasing worldwide travel and migration of people from endemic areas to developed countries may present clinicians with diagnostic dilemmas [1].

Yaws is the most prevalent non-venereal treponematosis. Data available from a number of endemic countries demonstrate that yaws is endemic mainly in warm, humid equatorial regions of Africa, Southeast Asia, and Western Pacific [2]. Elimination of yaws has been reported in Ecuador; additional data on yaws in the Americas are limited. West Africa is an important reservoir for yaws, particularly in Ghana (18,702 cases in 2013) and Cote d'Ivoire (2256 cases in 2013). There is also a growing number of cases in the Pacific region, including Papua New Guinea (19,710 cases in 2013), the Solomon Islands (14,909 cases in 2013), and Indonesia (2043 cases in 2013). Reporting of yaws is not mandatory; these figures likely reflect underreporting. India reported elimination of yaws in 2006, and the World Health Organization officially declared India free of yaws in May 2016 [3].

Bejel occurs mainly in the arid areas of the Sahel (southern border of the Sahara desert), including Senegal, Burkina Faso, Mali, and Niger. In these areas, high rates of seropositivity (10–20% of children <15 years) have been reported. Bejel has also been described among the nomadic people of the Arabic Peninsula, Iraq, and Syria. There was a report of three cases of bejel in Turkey in 1995 (where the disease was considered to be eliminated), as well as a case report from Iran in 2012 [4].

Data on the prevalence of *pinta* are limited; there is the perception that the disease has sustained a marked decline over the past century. Pinta might remain endemic in remote regions of Mexico and Central and South America (among Indian tribes in the Amazon region of Brazil, Colombia, Venezuela, and Peru) [5].Yaws and bejel usually occur in children; 65–75% of new cases arise in individuals <15 years, and children are the primary reservoir of infection. The age range for pinta is 15–50 years (median 30–34 years) [6].

12.2 Clinical Picture

Yaws and bejel affect the skin and bones (Figs. 12.1, 12.2 and 12.3); pinta affects the skin only. Data on the incubation period of endemic treponematoses are limited; the range is 9–90 days (mean 21 days). Infected individuals may develop immunity to reinfection, which may be strain specific.

12.2.1 Yaws (Frambesia)

Yaws consists of primary, secondary, and tertiary phases. The infection may become latent at any time, with only serologic evidence of the infection. Relapses may occur for up to 5–10 years. The primary lesion ("mother yaw")

V. Padovese
Genito-Urinary Clinic, Mater Dei Hospital, Ministry of Health, Msida, Malta

C. E. Orfanos et al. (eds.), *Pigmented Ethnic Skin and Imported Dermatoses*, https://doi.org/10.1007/978-3-319-69422-1_12

appears at the inoculation site, most commonly on the legs and ankles (65–85% of cases), but can also occur on the buttocks, arms, hands, or face. It is usually a localized papule that may develop into a large nodule (2–5 cm in diameter) that ulcerates. Ulcers characteristically have a red, moist base reminiscent of a raspberry, hence the name "frambesia." Yellow-brown crusts often overlie areas of ulceration. It usually heals after 3–6 months, regressing into a depigmented pitted scar with dark margins. In 9–15% of patients, the primary lesion persists at the onset of the secondary stage. Secondary lesions are the result of lymphatic and hematogenous spread of organisms; they appear a few weeks to 2 years after the primary lesion. Arthralgia is probably the most common symptom of secondary yaws. Secondary skin lesions consist of multiple smaller excrescences, sometimes resembling the primary lesion ("daughter yaws"), that may ulcerate. Multiple scaly patches or plaques with discoid or irregular shapes also may develop. Other manifestations of secondary yaws include regional lymphadenopathy, palmar and plantar hyperkeratotic plaques, and nocturnal bone pain due to osteoperiostitis of the proximal phalanges of the fingers (dactylitis) or long bones (forearm, tibia, or fibula). Yaws is a polyostotic disorder; the mean number of affected bones is three. Involvement of the hands and feet is common. Tertiary yaws is not common nowadays and occurs in approximately 10% of untreated patients; it consists of late lesions that develop after 5 or more years of infection. This stage is characterized by gummatous lesions of the skin, bones, and overlying tissues. Massive necrotic tissue destruction can occur, followed by debilitating scarring. Manifestations include juxta-articular subcutaneous nodules, extensive osteoperiostitis of long bones, hyperostosis of the nasal processes of the maxillae, and ulceration of the palate and nasopharynx

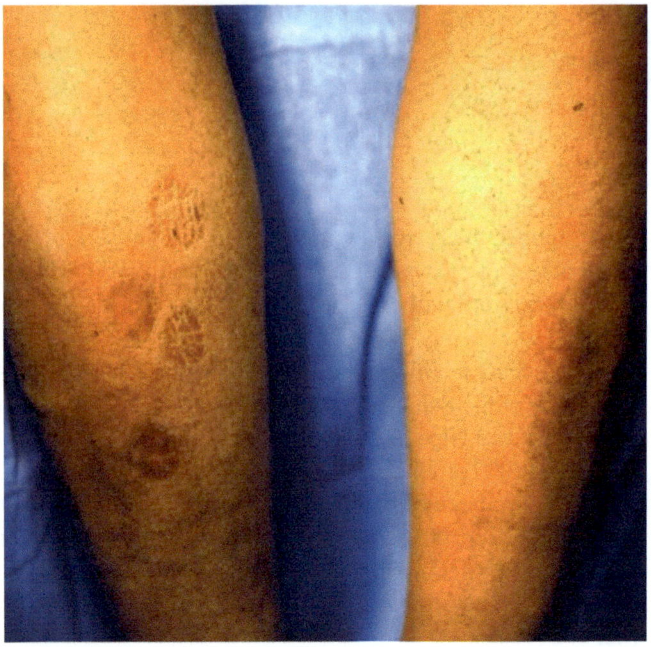

Fig. 12.1 Scars of *yaws* on the legs of a patient (Courtesy Prof. J. L. Pace)

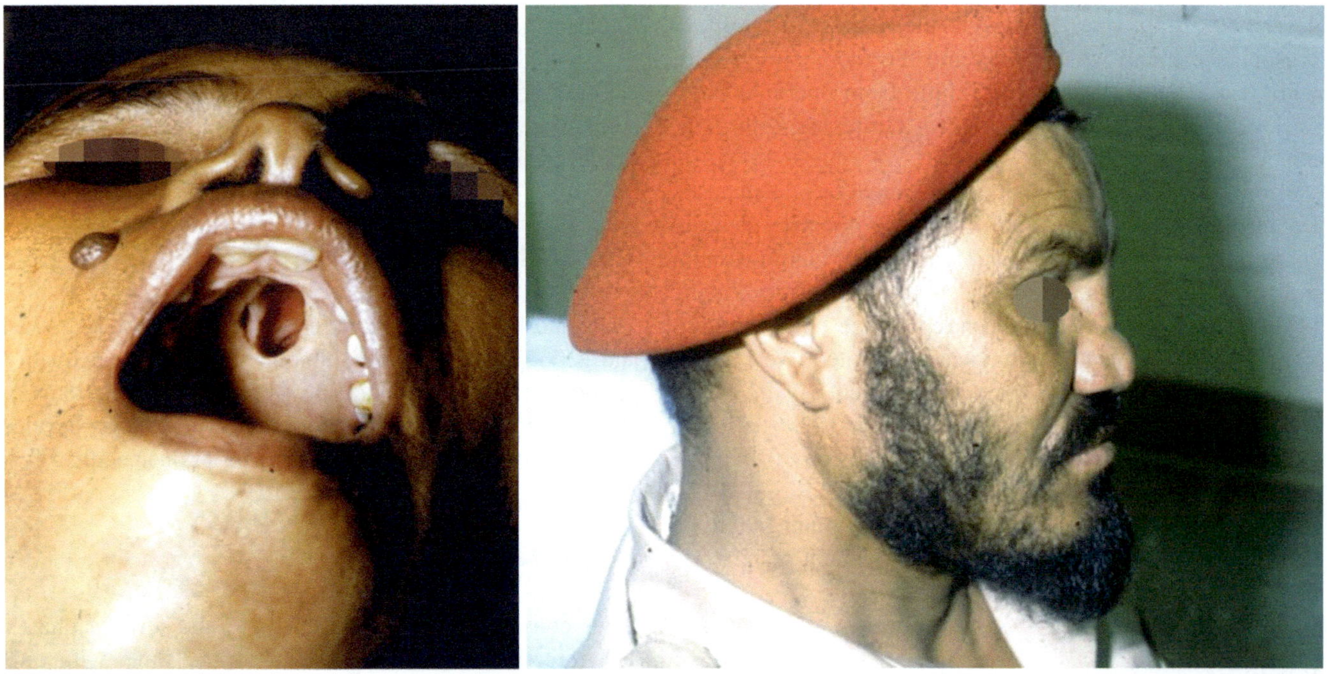

Fig. 12.2 *Bejel*. Late destruction changes, such as soft palate ulcer (left) and destructive lesions of the nasal septum (right) (Courtesy Prof. J. L. Pace)

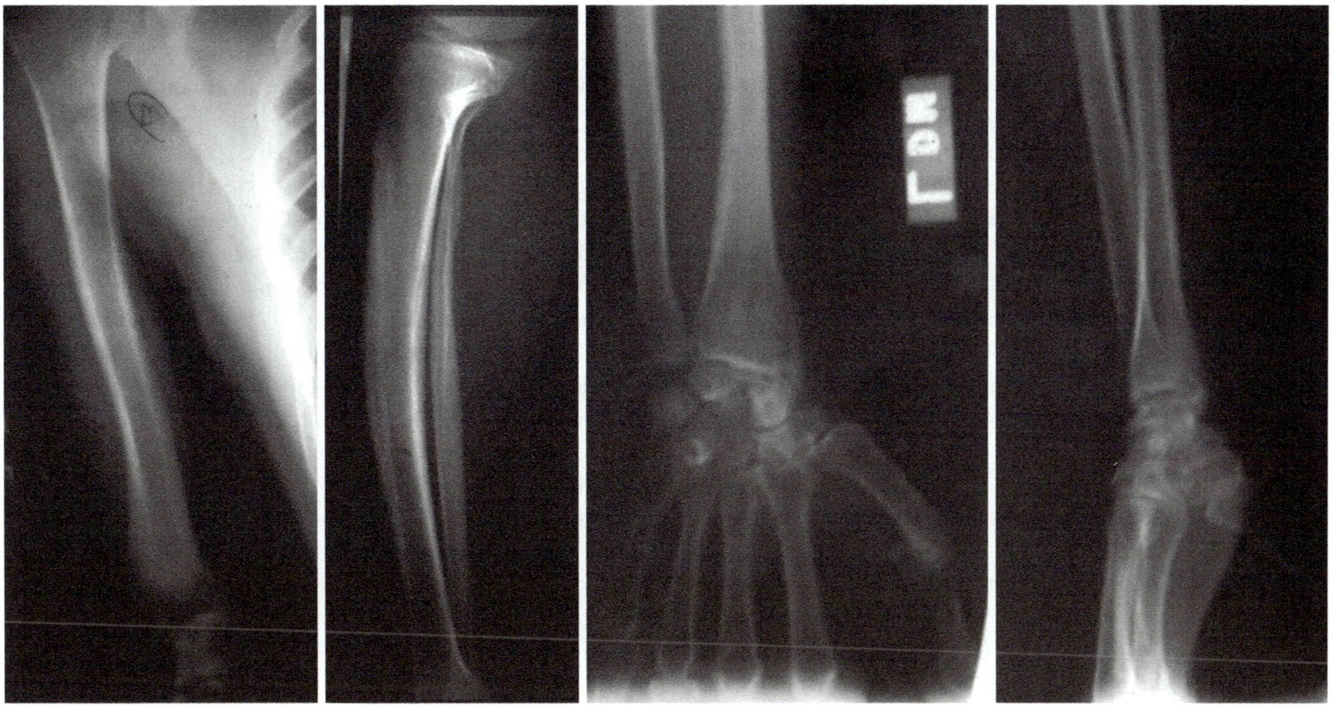

Fig. 12.3 *Bejel*. Changes in the long bones (Courtesy Prof. J. L. Pace)

(rhinopharyngitis mutilans or gangosa) with secondary infection resulting in foul-smelling discharge [7].

12.2.2 Bejel

The primary lesions of bejel are usually painless mucinous ulcers within the oral and oropharyngeal mucosa. Secondary stage manifestations include mucous patches (i.e., shallow, painless ulcers in the oropharynx and on the lips) and bone pain due to periostitis (particularly of the long bones of the leg). Other common manifestations include hoarseness related to laryngitis and cutaneous involvement that favors warm and moist areas of the body and manifests as split papules or angular stomatitis at the labial commissures or condylomata lata in intertriginous areas. Later, the patient may enter the latent phase, which may be prolonged; after this, some patients develop juxta-articular nodules and late destructive lesions, especially of the nose, nasal septum, nasopharynx, and soft palate, which are similar to those seen in yaws [8].

12.2.3 Pinta

Pinta is confined to the skin and is the mildest of the treponematoses. The primary lesion is an itchy, red, scaly papule or a plaque that expands to >10 cm but does not ulcerate. Like primary yaws, this sentinel lesion is most commonly found on the exposed lower extremities and is teeming with treponemes. Satellite lesions and regional lymphadenopathy are common. The secondary stage develops several months later in other areas with the appearance of pintids, which are similar to the initial lesions and are also pruritic. They undergo a variety of color changes from red to copper colored, gray, and bluish-black. The secondary lesions remain active and infectious for many years, leading to extensive depigmentation resembling vitiligo. The late lesions are characterized by varying degrees of hypochromia, discoloration, atrophy, and achromia. No severe mutilations occur.

12.3 Pathogenesis

The etiological agents of endemic treponematoses are Gram-negative bacteria that belong to the order of the *Spirochaetales*, family *Spirochaetaceae*, and genus *Treponema*. The causative organisms of yaws and bejel were originally classified as separate species but are now considered to be subspecies of *T. pallidum* and are, respectively, *T. pallidum* subsp. *pertenue* and *T. pallidum* subsp. *endemicum*. The lack of availability of an isolate of the agent of pinta has precluded genetic analyses of this organism, and it retains its separate name, *T. carateum*.

Our overall understanding of the pathogenesis of human treponematoses is limited by the inability to grow these spirochetes in vitro, requiring expensive and difficult continual propagation in laboratory animals, by their remarkably fragile cellular ultrastructure, permitting only limited mechanical manipulation of the pathogen to preserve its integrity and viability, and by the bacterium limited viability outside a host. The rabbit is widely used for propagation of isolates of the *T. pallidum* subspecies.

Endemic treponematoses are transmitted by direct skin-to-skin, nonsexual contact with infectious lesions. Transmission may be facilitated by a breach in the skin of the recipient, such as a scratch or insect bite. These diseases may be clustered in households, but transmission also occurs between children in the community, schools, and other public places [9].

12.4 Course and Further Monitoring

The diagnosis of all endemic treponematoses must be confirmed by serology or via direct visualization of the organism in a clinical specimen. The serological tests are the same as those used to diagnose syphilis and involve a nonspecific non-treponemal antibody test followed by a more specific treponemal test for diagnostic confirmation. Existing serologic tests cannot differentiate between endemic treponematoses and syphilis; until more specific laboratory tools are available, diagnosis requires use of serologic tests correlated with clinical manifestations and epidemiologic and demographic characteristics.

Non-treponemal agglutination tests (RPR or VDRL) are positive in untreated patients and can also be used as a test of cure since the quantitative titers fall following treatment. The non-treponemal tests may give rise to false positives in patients with other conditions, including syphilis, malaria, leprosy, and rheumatological diseases. They are often performed on serial dilutions of serum to give a quantitative titer, defined as the highest dilution that yields a positive result.

Non-treponemal tests become positive within 2–4 weeks after appearance of the primary lesion. There is a negative correlation between the duration of yaws infection and the titer, and nontreponemal tests may be nonreactive in end-stage disease. Treponemal tests (TPHA, TPPA) are more specific than non-treponemal tests. These assays cannot distinguish between active (untreated) and previously treated infection and remain positive even after successful treatment.

Rapid point-of-care tests that can be used in the field are widely available. However, most of them are treponemal-based and cannot distinguish between past and current infection. Recently dual treponemal and non-treponemal rapid tests have become available, thus simplifying diagnosis in the field. These tests are able to detect both present and past infections to guide treatment of people with active infection [10].

Patients should be examined 4 weeks following administration of antibiotic treatment. The lesions of yaws and bejel become noninfectious within 24 of treatment, and, in most cases, complete healing of the primary and secondary lesions is observed within 2–4 weeks following treatment. Skin lesions of pinta heal more slowly after treatment (within 6–12 months). Administration of antibiotic treatment during early pinta infection results in cure in nearly all patients; antibiotic treatment administered in the setting of advanced pinta infection cannot reverse skin changes. Patients should undergo follow-up non-treponemal testing at 6 and 12 months after treatment. The RPR or VDRL titers usually decline within 6–12 months; in most cases, they become negative within less than 2 years. The RPR reversal rates depend on the pretreatment titer and stage of disease; patients with first infection and low titers are more likely to revert. In some patients, the RPR or VDRL may remain positive at low titer (below 1:8); this is called a serofast reaction. The treponemal tests (TPHA, TPPA) remain positive for life [11].

12.5 Treatment

Treponemes are highly sensitive to azithromycin and penicillin, which are the drugs of choice. Penicillin G benzathine is administered at a single intramuscular dose of 1.2 million units for adults and 600,000 units for children. Cure rates for patients with early active yaws lesions are >95%. A single oral dose of azithromycin (30 mg/kg bw, maximum 2 g) was shown to be non-inferior to intramuscular penicillin G benzathine for treatment of yaws in a randomized trial including 250 children in Papua New Guinea [12]. Efficacy of azithromycin was 91% for patients with primary-stage lesions and 100% for patients with secondary-stage disease, including polyarthralgia or bone pain and swelling. Azithromycin may also be used for treatment of bejel and pinta. A single high-dose azithromycin is generally well tolerated; the most commonly observed adverse events in 10–15% of cases are related to the gastrointestinal tract, and these are all transient and short-lived.

In 2012, the World Health Organization officially set a goal for yaws eradication by 2020. Treatment with azithromycin avoids the need for injection and could enable yaws elimination through mass treatment programs. Contacts of any confirmed case of yaws (household residents, friends, schoolmates, playmates, etc.) should be treated with the same regimen as the index case [13].

Surveillance for treatment failure and resistance will be essential if azithromycin is used widely for treatment and eradication of yaws. Macrolide resistance in *T. pallidum* is associated with alteration of the target site due to a single-step mutation of the 23S ribosomal RNA gene. A real-time PCR assay for detection of the above-mentioned mutations has been developed that would enable molecular surveillance for rapid identification of macrolide resistance in *T. pallidum pertenue*, though this may be challenging in resource-limited settings [12]. Alternative agents are only appropriate if first-line drugs cannot be used; they include doxycycline (100 mg p.o. 2×/day for 15 days) or tetracycline (500 mg p.o. 4×/day for 15 days). Erythromycin (8–10 mg/kg bw p.o. 4×/day for 15 days) has been used for penicillin-allergic children <12 years. These regimens are based on clinical efficacy observed in small case series. Adverse effects and frequent dosing for these second-line antibiotics can result in poor compliance and, therefore, higher rates of treatment failure [14].

An early-stage yaws or bejel lesion that has not healed within 4 weeks is considered a treatment failure. Patients with clinical treatment failure should be switched to an alternative regimen.

Serological treatment failure is defined as ≥4-fold increase in the RPR titer, titer persistently ≥1:64, or ≤4-fold decrease in titer over 12 months. Patients who do not have an appropriate decline in serological titer should be managed with another course of treatment. Most serologically defined treatment failures are considered to be caused by either reinfection following treatment or slow decline in non-treponemal test titers rather than by relapse or true antibiotic resistance. In addition, it is important to ensure that all household and community contacts are treated to decrease the risk of reinfections.

References

1. Engelkens HJ, Oranje AP, Stolz E. Early yaws, imported in The Netherlands. Genitourin Med. 1989;65:316.
2. Marks M, Lebari D, Solomon AW, et al. Yaws. Int J STD AIDS. 2015;26:696–703.
3. Narain JP, Jain SK, Bora D, et al. Eradicating successfully yaws from India: the strategy and global lessons. Indian J Med Res. 2015;141:608–13.
4. Abdolrasouli A, Croucher A, Hemmati Y, et al. A case of endemic syphilis, Iran. Emerg Infect Dis. 2013;19:162.
5. Koff AB, Rosen T. Nonvenereal treponematoses: yaws, endemic syphilis, and pinta. J Am Acad Dermatol. 1993;29:519.
6. Farnsworth N, Rosen T. Endemic treponematosis: review and update. Clin Dermatol. 2006;24:181–90.
7. Giacani L, Lukehart SA. The endemic treponematoses. Clin Microbiol Rev. 2014;27:89–115.
8. Marks M, Solomon AW, Mabey DC. Endemic treponemal diseases. Trans R Soc Trop Med Hyg. 2014;108:601–7.
9. Fanella S, Kadkhoda K, Shuel M, et al. Local transmission of imported endemic syphilis, Canada, 2011. Emerg Infect Dis. 2012;18:1002.
10. Mitjà O, Šmajs D, Bassat Q. Advances in the diagnosis of endemic treponematoses: yaws, bejel, and pinta. PLoS Negl Trop Dis. 2013;24:e2283.
11. Mitjà O, Houinei W, Moses P, et al. Mass treatment with single-dose azithromycin for yaws. N Engl J Med. 2015;372:703–10.
12. Mitjà O, Hays R, Ipai A, et al. Single-dose azithromycin versus benzathine benzylpenicillin for treatment of yaws in children in Papua New Guinea: an open-label, non-inferiority, randomised trial. Lancet. 2012;379:342–427.
13. Backhouse JL, Hudson BJ, Hamilton PA, et al. Failure of penicillin treatment of yaws on Karkar Island, Papua New Guinea. Am J Trop Med Hyg. 1998;59:388.
14. Lukehart SA, Godornes C, Molini BJ, et al. Macrolide resistance in Treponema pallidum in the United States and Ireland. N Engl J Med. 2004;351:154.

13 Onchocerciasis and Lymphatic Filariasis

Achim Hoerauf and Anna Albers

Infections with parasitic worms are widespread in tropical and sub-tropical areas of the world. In particular, infections with filarial nematodes occur in hot climate zones including *lymphatic filariasis*, *onchocerciasis* and *loiasis*; *Mansonella* species which occur in parts of Central Africa and Central and South America usually cause mild clinical symptoms. All filarial infections are transmitted by flying insects; humans are the only reservoir. Throughout the hot climate zones in Africa, approximately 130–150 million people are affected; the prevalence has clear association with poverty. Despite ongoing control programmes, lymphatic filariasis and onchocerciasis have been included in the list of *neglected tropical diseases (NTD)* by the WHO.

Today, filarial infections are occasionally seen in Europe in immigrants from the sub-Saharan countries [1]. Particularly, onchocerciasis may occur as an imported disease in the developed world; physicians should consider this tropical infection when caring for refugees, migrants and travellers with pruritus, skin lesions and eosinophilia [2]. Filariasis was one of the most frequent causes for eosinophilia and hyper-IgE among 362 immigrant children studied in Spain coming from sub-Saharan Africa [3]. Especially in patients with clinical pictures and findings suggestive of atopic dermatitis, onchocerciasis should be considered and excluded [4].

13.1 Onchocerciasis

Onchocerciasis is caused by the filarial nematode *Onchocerca (O.) volvulus* transmitted by *Simulium* black flies. According to recent estimates by the *African Programme for Onchocerciasis Control* (APOC), 21 million people are still infected, with main foci in Central Africa [5]. The adult worms may grow to a length up to 70 cm situated in subcutaneous nodules, whereas, the offspring *microfilariae* (MF) remain in the upper dermis and in the anterior chamber of the eye causing local damage. Accordingly, the main symptoms of onchocerciasis are related to skin lesions and eye inflammation.

13.1.1 Epidemiology

Transmission of *O. volvulus* occurs in tropical Africa, Latin and Central America and Yemen. More than 99% of the estimated 21–25 million infected individuals live in Africa, with 187 million people located in areas with potential risk for transmission [6]. Recent estimates calculate the overall burden of the disease by 1.1 million *disability-adjusted life years* (DALYs) in 2015. Exposure begins after birth; in adulthood, it is associated with physical work such as farming, where it is difficult to eliminate the vector despite the fact that the black flies need several minutes to sit on the victims before they start biting. *Simulium* is active during the day, does not enter houses, and mosquito nets are ineffective for prevention. Large-scale insecticide spraying programmes have been successful in West Africa, but vector control is difficult to implement in forested areas in the central part of the continent. *Mass drug administration* (MDA) with ivermectin has been the first successful drug donation programme for *neglected tropical diseases* (NTDs); it brought down the number of infected people by >50% and averted millions of DALYs and blindness.

13.1.2 Pathogenesis

Infection is caused by third-stage larvae (L3) transmitted by *Simulium* black flies during biting. They mature within 12 days from microfilariae (L1) taken up in a previous blood meal from an infected human host. The larvae moult

A. Hoerauf (✉) · A. Albers
Institut für Med. Mikrobiologie, Immunologie und Parasitologie, Deutsches Zentrum für Infektionsforschung, Universitätsklinikum Bonn, Bonn, Germany
e-mail: achim.hoerauf@ukb.uni-bonn.de

C. E. Orfanos et al. (eds.), *Pigmented Ethnic Skin and Imported Dermatoses*, https://doi.org/10.1007/978-3-319-69422-1_13

twice during a few months, migrate through the body and settle in subcutaneous nodules (*onchocercomata*) which may contain several dozen adult female worms, thus increasing the size of the nodules to several cm. A fertile female releases up to several thousand MF up to 300 μm in length, which migrate into the papillary dermis; a load of several hundred MF per mg skin may result. Nevertheless, the skin often appears clinically not noticeably inflamed, due to active immunosuppression by adult female worms and also by the MF themselves. Immunosuppression is mediated by regulatory T cells leading to downregulation by macrophages, deactivation of eosinophils and neutrophils by TGF-β or IL10 and production of the immune regulatory subclass IgG4 [7]. A minority of infected people mount strong Th2-dependent immune responses with high eosinophilia, low or absent MF in their skin but strong dermal reaction.

Besides the skin, the eye is affected: MF in the anterior chamber induce chronic inflammation leading to sclerosing keratitis and blindness if untreated, giving the disease its popular name *river blindness*. Iridocyclitis with elliptical shape papillae, vasculitis and other damages of the retina and the optical nerve may occur.

13.1.3 Clinical Picture

The clinical picture of onchocerciasis is characterised by skin changes showing scattered pruritic papules, plaques and excoriations as a leading symptom, together with variable lymphadenopathy and inflammation of the eye, which is often absent in forest foci. In different geographic regions, varying types of onchodermatitis are seen, each type being graded for its severity, activity and distribution [8]. It is a cutaneous inflammatory response of the host to dying MF. The following types may occur, also depending on the stage of the infection:

(a) *Acute papular onchodermatitis,* highly pruritic, consisting of small papules mostly at the extremities, shoulder and trunk (Fig. 13.1). Progression of the lesions to hyalinised scar tissue is often seen, particularly after microfilaricidal treatment with ivermectin.
(b) *Chronic papular onchodermatitis*, mostly seen in hyperendemic areas, with flat hyperpigmented papules symmetrically located mainly on the buttocks, waist and shoulders, while the intensity of the pruritus decreases.
(c) *Lichenified onchodermatitis* with strongly pruritic papules and plaques (Fig. 13.2). In skin biopsies, MF can be detected in the upper dermis.
(d) *Skin atrophy* with loss of cutaneous elasticity due to chronic inflammation and release of elastase by eosinophils. Atrophic skin folds are seen, also called "hanging groins", containing groups of enlarged lymph nodes (Fig. 13.3).
(e) *Spotted depigmentation* called "leopard skin", particularly involving the interfollicular epidermis with the openings of the follicles still pigmented, mainly seen on the lower legs; the forearm and dorsum of the hand and the trunk may also be involved (Fig. 13.4).

Severe grade onchodermatitis may also occur localised, usually in one leg, often associated with considerable swelling of the regional lymph nodes [9], called *sowda* in Yemen (*sowda* = Arabic for black).

Most characteristic are *onchocercomata*, i.e. indolent cutaneous nodules, isolated or multiple, usually 0.5–3 cm in diameter, palpable in the subcutaneous tissue representing a marker for onchocerciasis. Preferred localisations are the iliac crest, the trochanter of the femoral bone, os sacrum, thorax, head and the median side of the knees (Figs. 13.5 and 13.6). Up to 50% of the nodules are less palpable, deeply located along the bones. Involvement of the eye initially shows punctate keratitis starting from the lower half of the cornea, progressing to sclerosing keratitis and leading to blindness. Inflammation of the posterior chamber includes changes of the retinal pigment with chorioretinitis, chorioretinal atrophy and atrophy of the optical nerve.

High eosinophilia (20–30%) is always present in patients with onchocerciasis, and eosinophilic cardiomyopathy is a cause of death if untreated.

13.1.4 Diagnosis

Serology shows cross reactivity to other filarial nematodes including *strongyloides*; it can only be applied in travellers who have not stayed long in endemic areas. Gold standard for diagnosis is to take from the suspected areas thin *skin snips* using a corneoscleral biopsy instrument (*Holth* punch), incubate the skin material taken in isotonic saline at room temperature for a minimum of 12 h, best done in a microtiter plate, and then examine the fluid at 40×. If present, motile MF can be seen and counted. If blood vessels were also opened, MF from other filarial infections such as *W. bancrofti*, *M. perstans* or *L. loa* can be present and misdiagnosed. The preferred site for the skin snips is the high end iliac crest. MF of *O. volvulus* should be differentiated from the smaller MF of *M. streptocerca* which have no sheath. If a patient has been recently infected, MF detection can be negative during prepatency for up to 2 years. If the procedure cannot be carried out in a local laboratory, it is also possible to preserve the biopsy for PCR.

During and up to 6 months after oral intake of ivermectin, there are no MF detectable in the tissue, but the patient is still

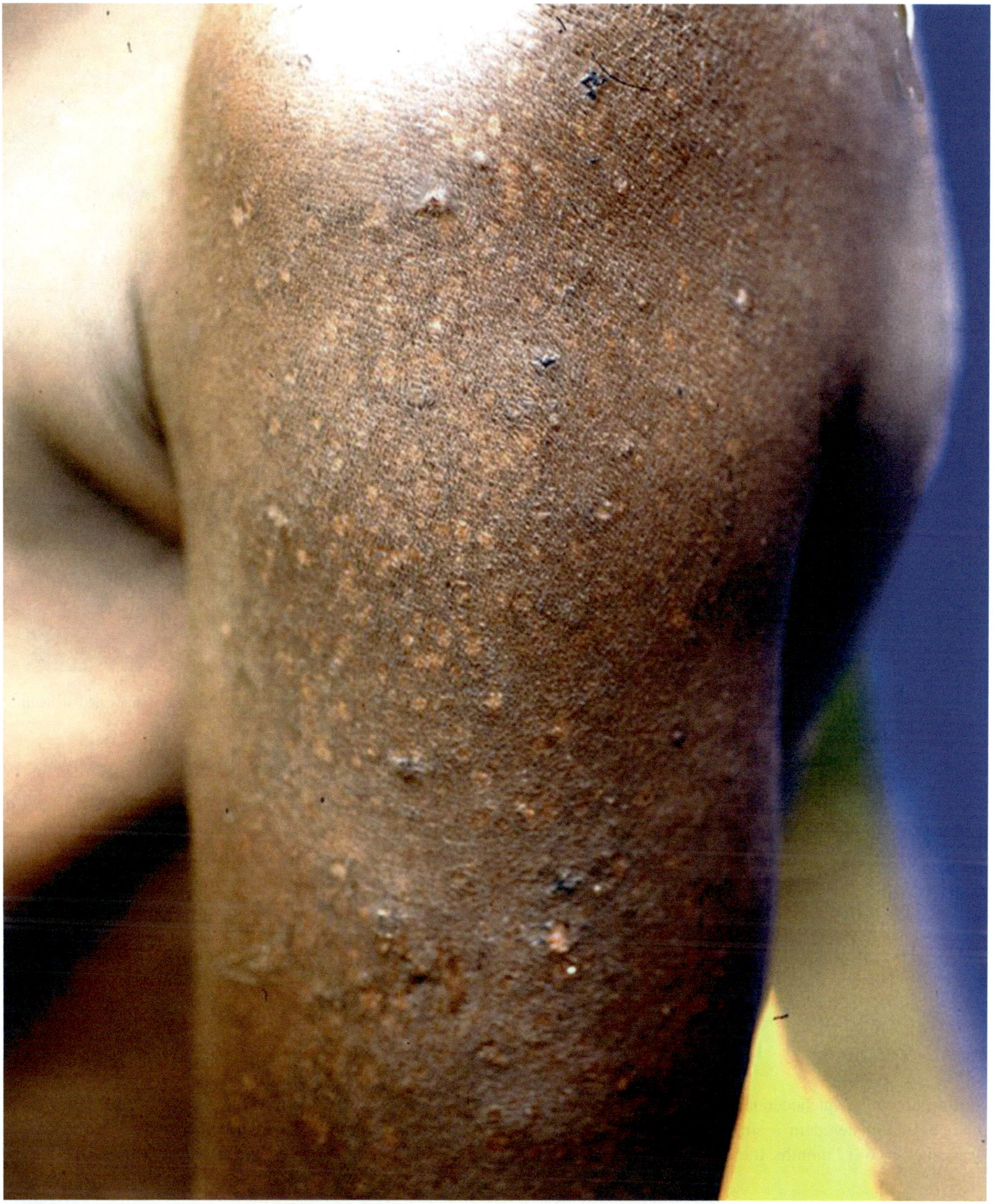

Fig. 13.1 Characteristic clinical presentation of *onchodermatitis* (acute type), associated with intense pruritus and scratching

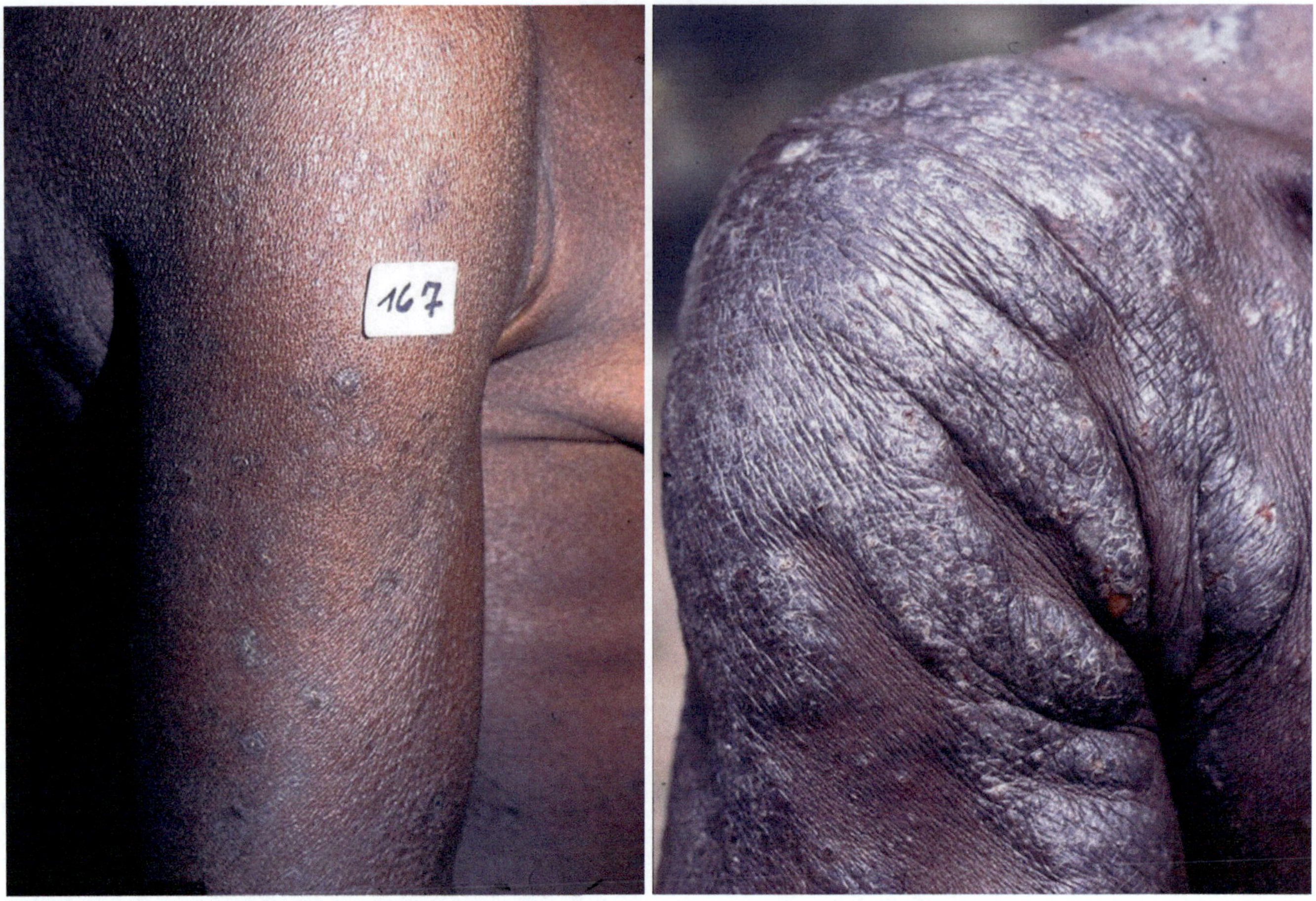

Fig. 13.2 *Chronic onchodermatitis*, with hyperpigmented pruritic papules (left); *Chronic onchodermatitis* with well-demarcated lichenified plaques, highly pruritic with excoriations (right)

infected. Since no markers to diagnose MF-negative onchocerciasis exist, one may pick up movements of the adult worms by using sonography of an onchocercoma. The *Mazzotti* patch test (topical application of diethylcarbamazine) is rarely used today, because the test is only positive if MF are present and also because the test cannot differentiate between *O. volvulus* and *M. streptocerca* infection, which clinically presents similar skin changes (Fig. 13.7).

13.1.5 Treatment

For treatment of onchocerciasis, *ivermectin* is the drug of choice, administered in a single dose of 150 μg/kg body weight every 6–12 months. It inactivates the glutamate sensitive chloride channels present only in nematodes and leads to >90% reduction of MF within 3 months. However, since the drug does not sterilise or kill the female adult worms, MF and skin lesions reappear after 6 months. Adverse events of treatment due to MF killing are prominent in patients with heavy infestation (>20 mg/kg skin) including dermatitis, cutaneous oedema as well as orthostatic low blood pressure; the latter may require that the patient lay down the days during drug intake. Adverse reactions can be mitigated by premedication of cortisone. The drug is not administered to children below the age of 5, respectively, 15 kg body weight, as well as to pregnant and breast-feeding women. The beneficial effect of albendazole has been discussed; however, recent controlled trials were not supportive [10]. The comfortable administration 1–2x per year makes ivermectin the

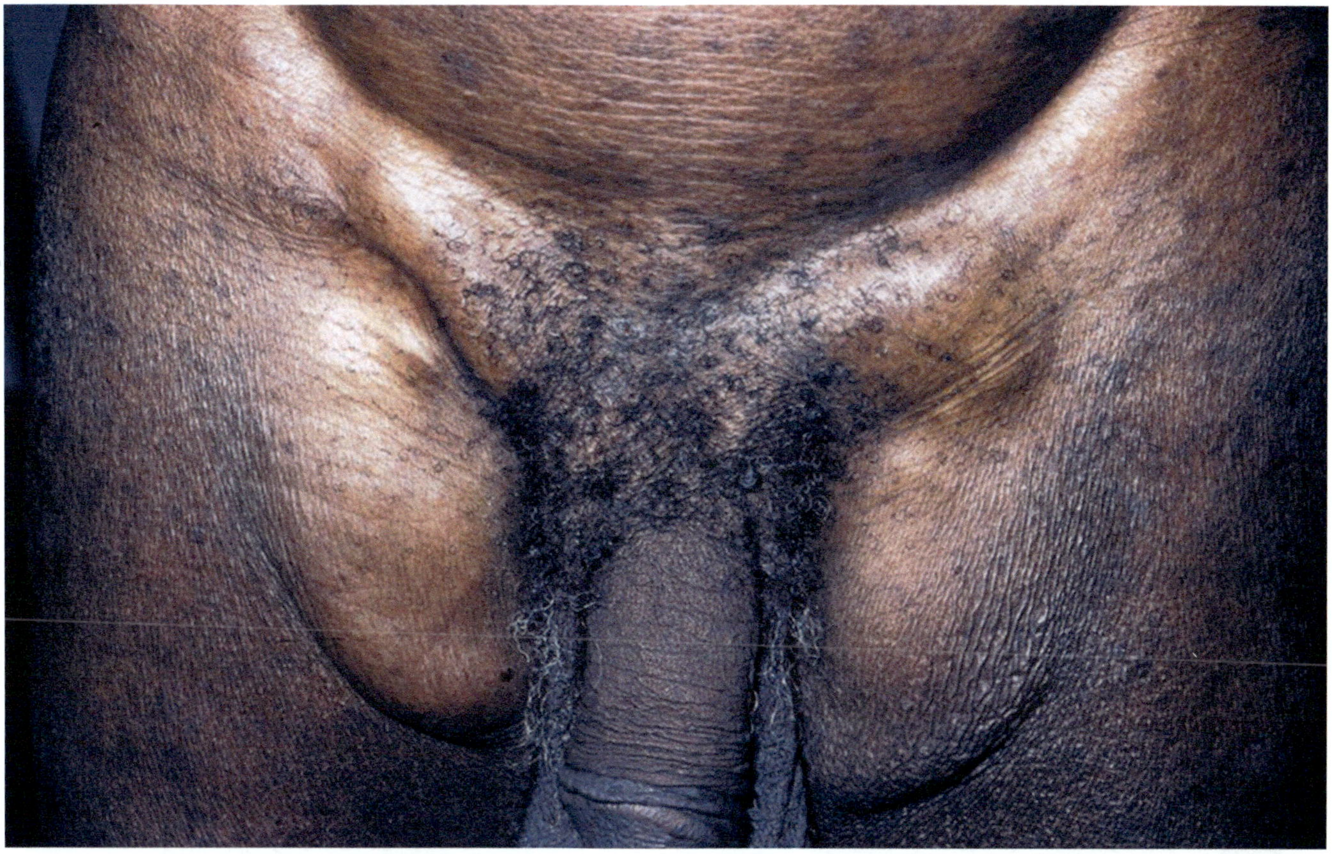

Fig. 13.3 *Hanging groins* in atrophic skin folds containing enlarged lymph nodes in onchocerciasis

drug of choice particularly for patients living in endemic areas under the risk of reinfection. MDA covering 80% of the eligible population living in endemic areas is the basis of WHO control programmes. Since ivermectin does not kill adult worms, MDA has to be repeated over many, in some areas >20 years until adult worms will have been eliminated in a given population.

Doxycycline was recently shown in randomised controlled trials to be a safe macrofilaricidal drug for onchocerciasis [11]; it targets *Wolbachia* endosymbiotic bacteria, necessary for reproduction and survival of the adult worms. The drug leads by depletion to worm sterility and death, administered at 100 mg/day for 5 weeks or 200 mg/day for 4 weeks. While doxycycline is indicated for all those who are not living in endemic areas and cures the individual patient, the long time required for treatment precludes its broad administration in MDA programmes. Contraindications for doxycycline are pregnancy or breast-feeding, and it is not administered to children below 9 years of age.

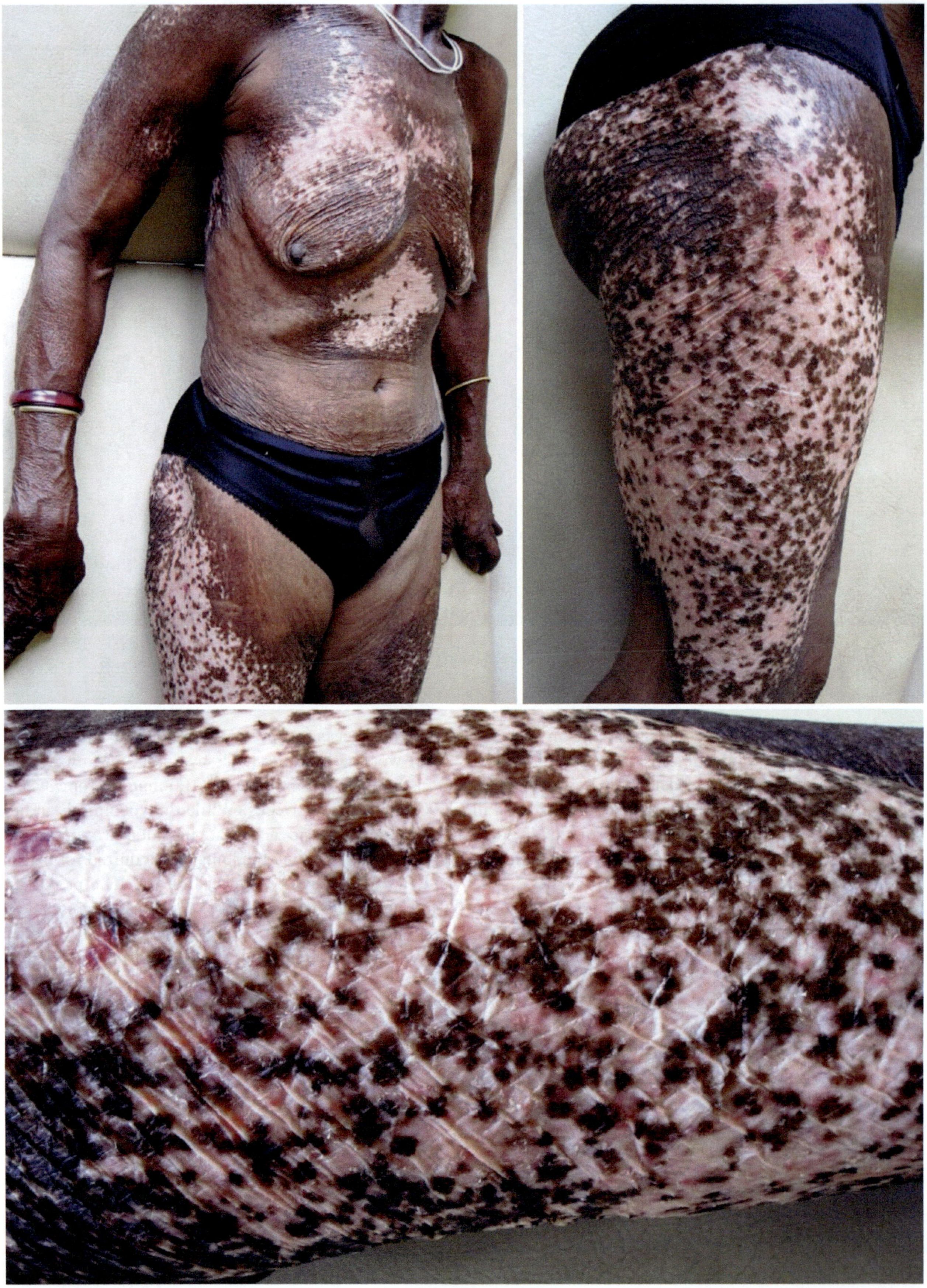

Fig. 13.4 Chronic onchocerciasis in an aged Maasai female with characteristic dyspigmentations, so-called *leopard skin*. Enlarged lymph nodes are seen in the inguinal area (left)

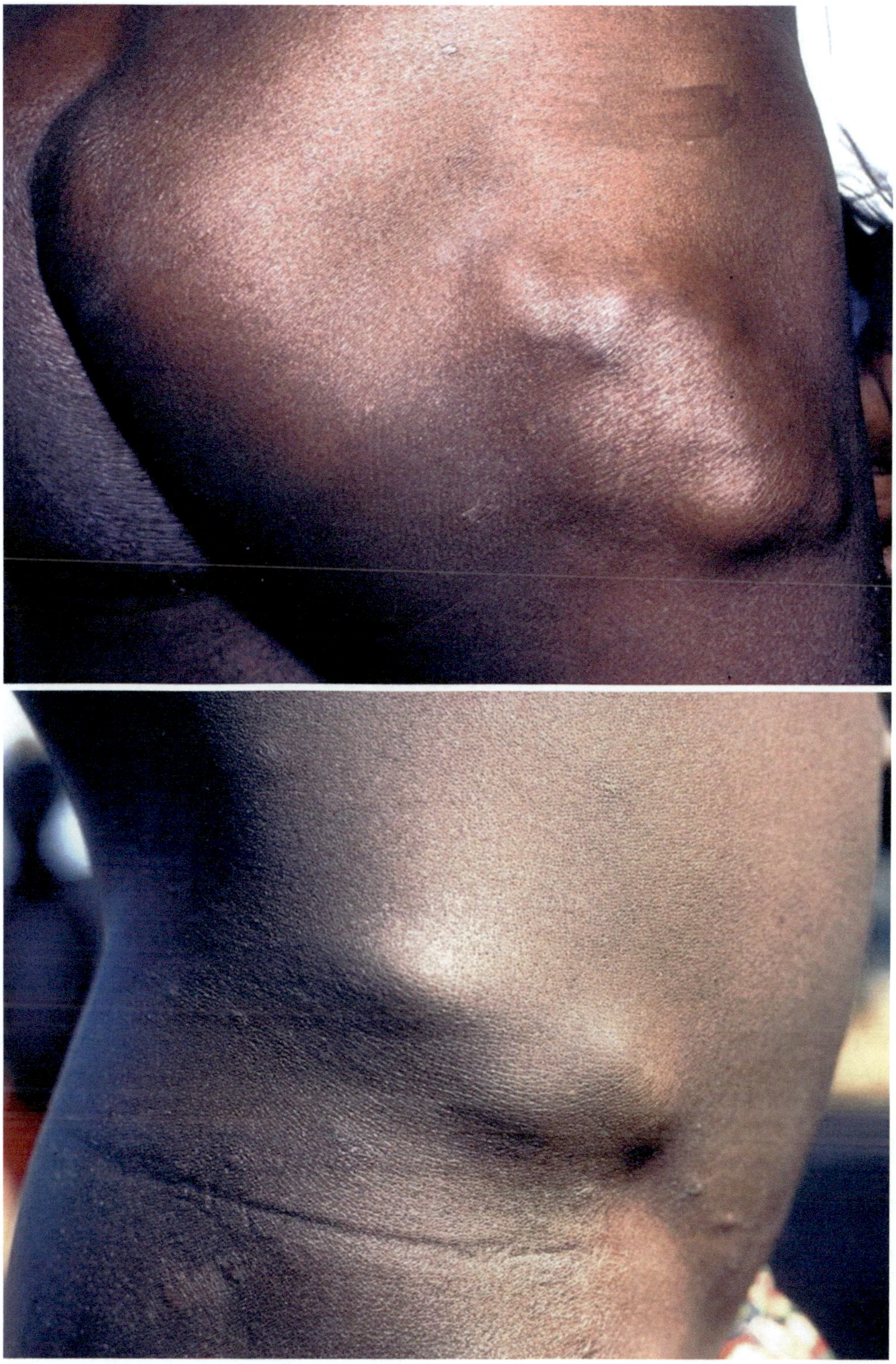

Fig. 13.5 *Onchocercomata* in typical localisation

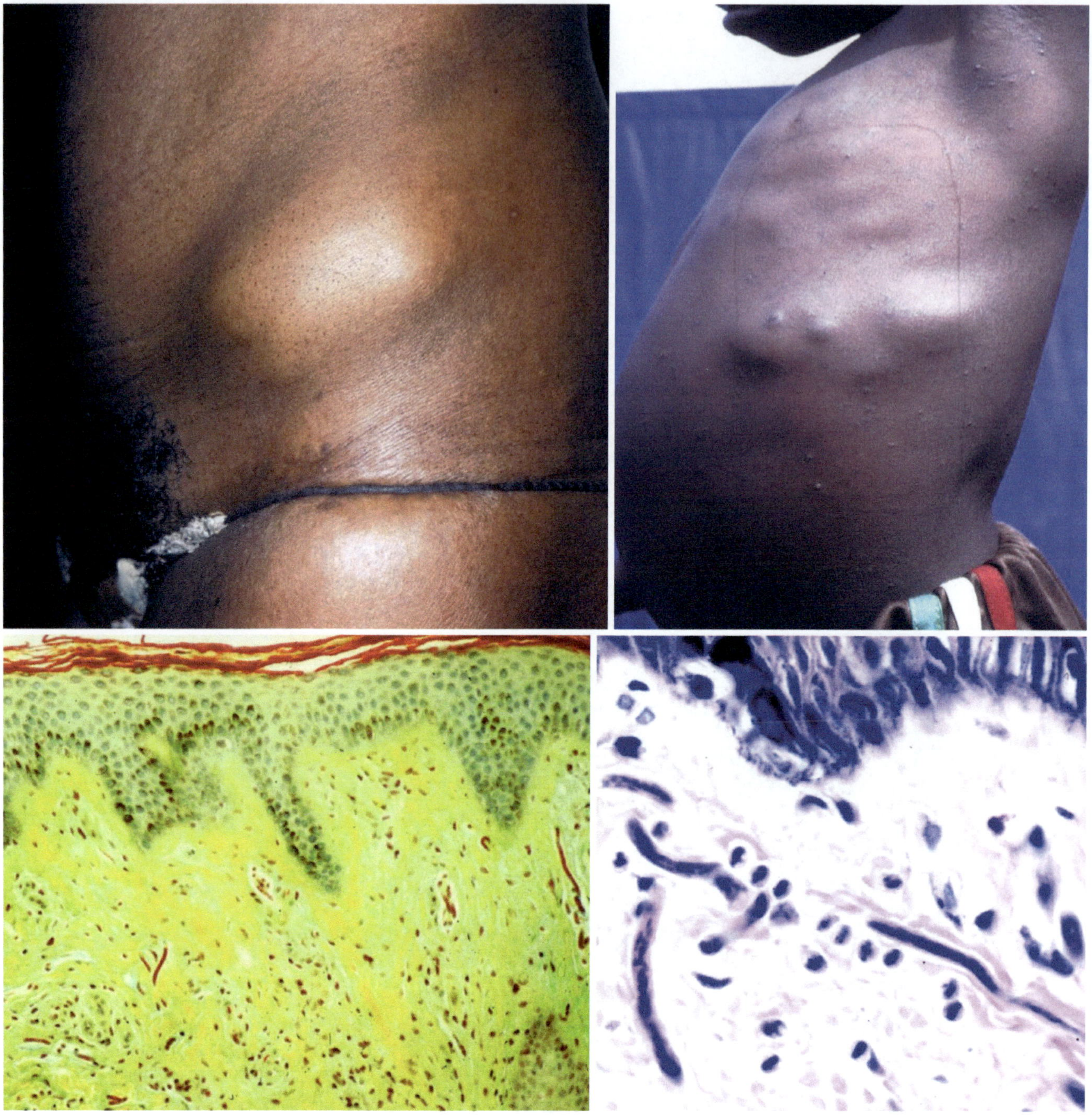

Fig. 13.6 Large conglomerates of *onchocercomata*. In skin biopsies, numerous MF of *O. volvulus* are seen in the upper papillary dermis

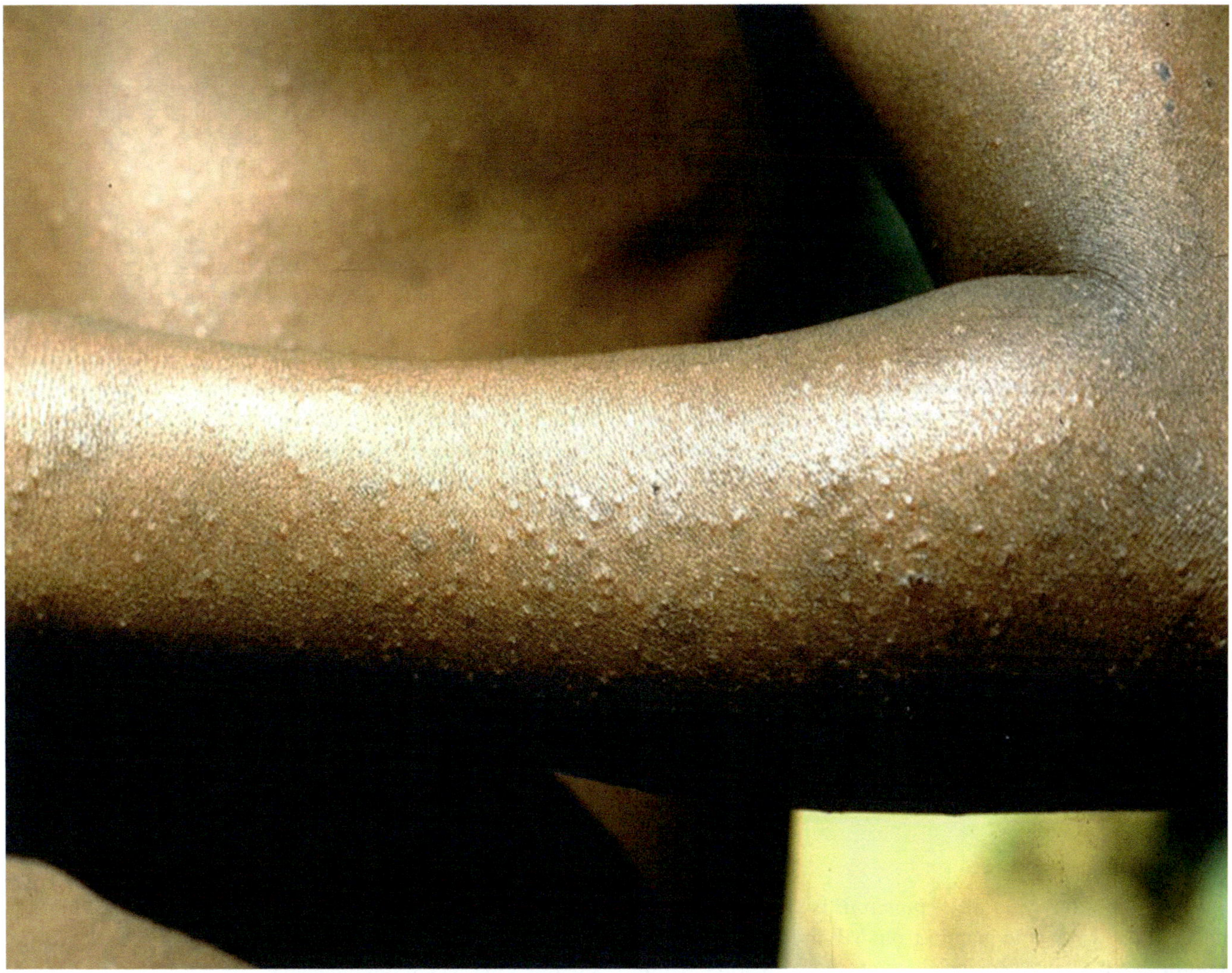

Fig. 13.7 Pruritic dermatitis due to infection with *Mansonella streptocerca*, seen in West and Central Africa, to be considered in differential diagnosis. Lymph nodes may be enlarged

13.2 Lymphatic Filariasis

Lymphatic filariasis (LF) is prevalent in all tropical regions except in Australia. The disease is commonly caused by *Wuchereria (W.) bancrofti*; the species *Brugia malayi* and *Brugia timori* are only found in Southeast Asia and will not be further considered here. *W. bancrofti* infective third-stage (L3) larvae are transmitted by bites of several infected mosquito species, including *Anopheles* in Africa, *Culex* mainly in Asia and *Aedes* in the Pacific islands. The adult worms live in the human lymphatic system, vessels and lymph nodes, grow to a length of 10–20 cm and cause inflammatory and mechanical aberrations to the vessels leading to lymphoedema (*lymphatic elephantiasis*) and hydrocele. Their offspring MF can be detected in the peripheral blood. Therapeutic modalities should not only prevent the transmission of MF but also be directed against the adult worms to prevent clinical damage.

13.2.1 Epidemiology

Updated figures on LF prevalence are yearly presented in epidemiological WHO reports. Successful implementation of MDA in endemic areas has greatly reduced the prevalence of LF from formerly 120 million down to 68 million cases and an estimated 36 million MF carriers. Not all infected individuals suffer from disease symptoms; around 66% of the infected individuals remain clinically symptomless. There are 19 million with lymphoedema and another 16 with hydrocele; however, the relative proportion of disabled people increases as infection is controlled, since the clinical damage is largely irreversible.

The prevalence of LF varies considerably in endemic areas with 30% in a given village and <1% in another, without noticeable differences in the mosquito environment; only in Papua New Guinea >70% can be observed. This is an obstacle for control programmes and measurements of prevalence. In addition, only 50% of the individuals affected present MF in their peripheral blood, the rest merely shows positivity for circulating filarial antigen measured by an antigen detection card test applicable in the field. The measurements correlate well with the detection of moving adult worms by ultrasound in the scrotal area of adult men.

LF has been assigned as one of NTDs amenable to preventive chemotherapy and control by the WHO. A Global Alliance for Elimination of Lymphatic Filariasis (GAELF) unites WHO and private NGOs as well as governments with the goal to eliminate LF in many areas of the world by 2020, and from all countries by 2025. This ambitious goal is aimed by implementing MDA with *diethylcarbamazine* (DEC; "mass deworming") at 6 mg/kg combined with a single dose of *albendazole* 400 mg outside Africa and of *ivermectin* 200 μg/kg plus albendazole 400 mg in Africa. DEC is not distributed in African countries because of the eye damage it causes in patients suffering from concomitant onchocerciasis.

13.2.2 Pathogenesis

The transmission cycle of *W. bancrofti* is similar to that of *O. volvulus*: L3 larvae mature from MF in the insect vector within 12–14 days and develop into adult worms within lymphatic tissue in a few months. Adult worms live in lymphatic tissue, in lymph vessels and lymph nodes. They are most stable in the scrotal tissue of men after puberty and can be detected by ultrasound over time periods of years. Chronic filarial inflammation induced by the worms leads to *elephantiasis* via lymph vessel dilation and lymph angiogenesis, visualised in its initial stages by sonography or lymphoscintigraphy. However, MDA against LF does not roll back the progression of lymphoedema once it is established, it may continue after eliminating filarial infection clustered in families with genetic predisposition. Individuals with lymphoedema have a much stronger immune reaction of Th1 and Th17 cell types, as opposed to patients with high worm load and microfilaremia who often present no clinical symptoms showing strong immunosuppression mediated by regulatory T-cell responses and high IL10 [12].

Hydrocele is a second most important feature seen in *W. bancrofti* infections due to inflammatory changes of the lymph vessels by draining the fluid secreted between the two layers of the *tunica vaginalis*. As secretion continues, lymph efflux is impaired and fluid accumulates. Lymphoedema and/or chyluria in the genital area in men and women are all consequences of the impaired lymph efflux.

13.2.3 Clinical Picture

The clinical manifestations of LF comprise lymphangitis and lymphadenitis, lymphedema/elephantiasis and hydrocele. Acute manifestations of the disease impose as *acute filarial lymphangitis* (AFL) or *acute filarial dermatolymphangioadenitis* (ADLA). Lymph vessel dilation impairs lymph transport, leading to extravasation of fluid particularly in the lower limbs and feet. Fissures and open wounds may then result and bacterial super infection perpetuate the inflammatory process. Genital manifestations in women, e.g. oedema of the labia majora, are much less frequent than those in men. Chyluria and tropical pulmonary eosinophilia are relatively rare.

AFL is a skin reaction of the carrier against dying worms in lymph vessels or lymph nodes (natural or drug-induced) which can ulcerate releasing a serous fluid and heals with scarring. It is frequently seen in femoral lymph nodes in endemic areas. The process tends to heal without chronic lymph vessel dilation, but after several episodes of chronic lymphangiectasia with subcutaneous oedema may occur, leading to the development of interdigital fissures and bacterial super infection even in the absence of filarial worms. In ADLA, different to AFL, there is always cutaneous oedema with a few enlarged and painful lymph nodes. ADLA episodes heal and the skin peels off after 1 week. Such episodes occur repeatedly, thus enlarging the size of lymphedema.

In the lower extremities, chronic lymphoedema with thickening of the skin and the underlying tissues occurs, usually starting at the ankles, but can also involve the arms, breasts, scrotum, vulva and penis. Based on the staging by *Dreyer* early stages are more easily reversible, whereas late stages usually progress towards elephantiasis (Figs. 13.8 and 13.9). The extensive chronic lymphoedema often present additional findings, such as other bacterial co-infections and ulcers; lymphoedema due to Kaposi's sarcoma or podoconiosis may complicate and/or mimic lymphatic filariasis (Figs. 13.10 and 13.11).

Hydrocele is most frequently found in men (after puberty) and silently progresses accompanied by attacks of funiculitis and epididymitis. In the majority of cases, the tunica vaginalis thickens and the efflux obliterates (Fig. 13.12). Hydroceles due to LF can reach the size of a basketball due to continuous secretion of fluid. Small hydroceles can disappear spontaneously, occasionally triggered by worm-killing drugs such as DEC.

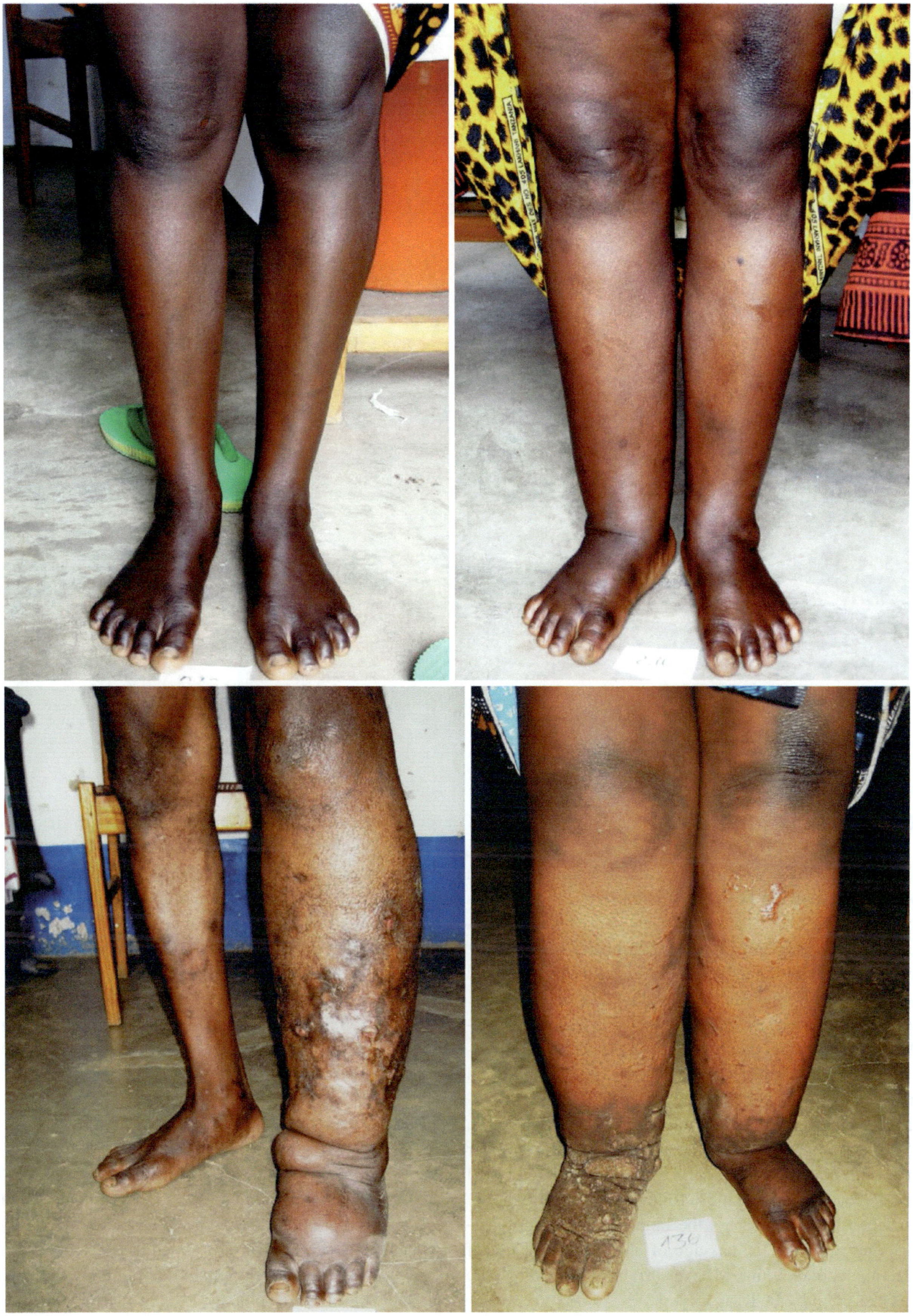

Fig. 13.8 *Lymphatic filariasis* presenting elephantiasis in different stages: *Dreyer* stages 1 and 2 (up); stages 4 and 6–7 (down)

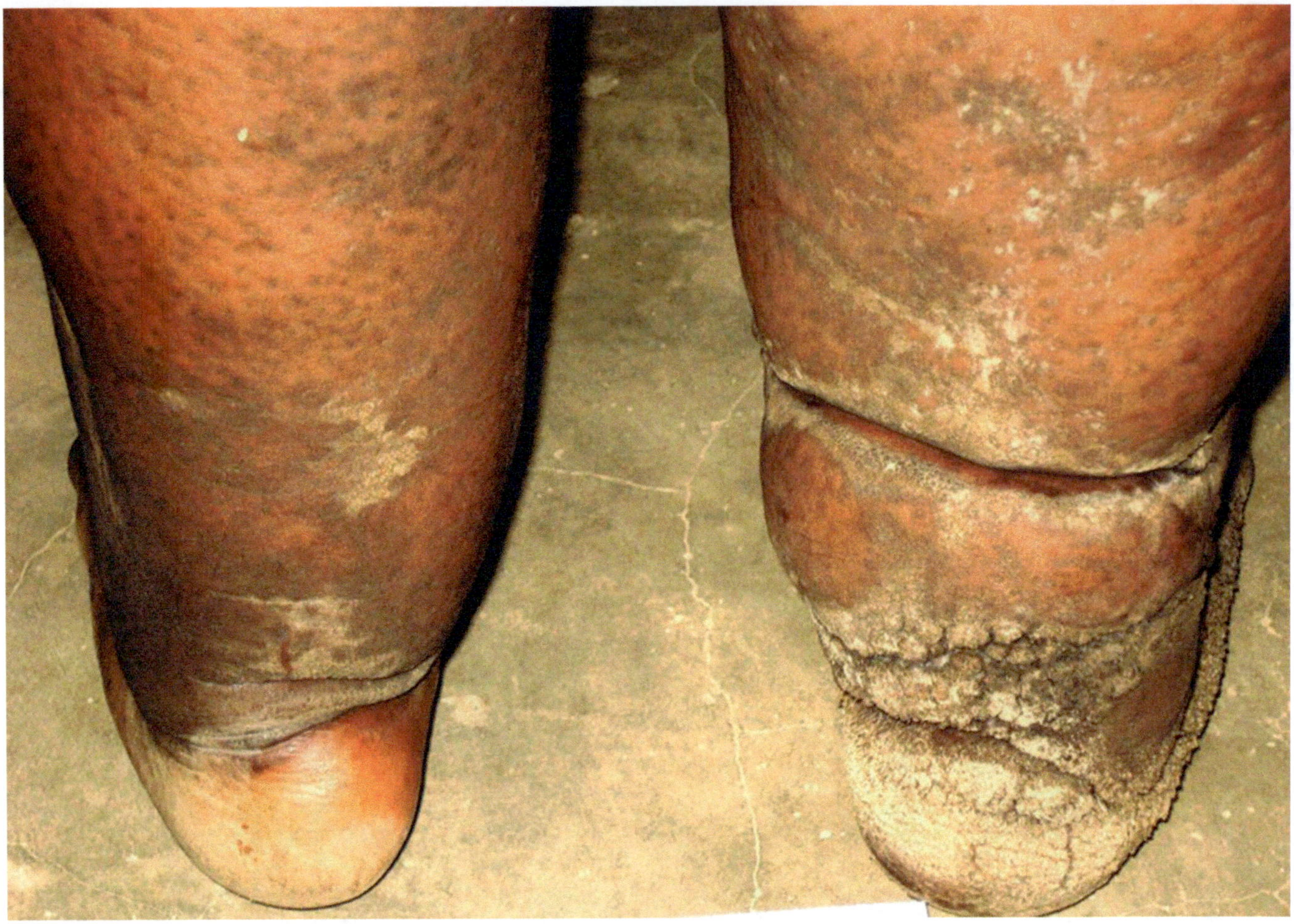

Fig. 13.9 Lymphatic elephantiasis *Dreyer* stage 7

13.2.4 Diagnosis

The diagnosis of LF is confirmed by the detection of MF in the peripheral blood, to be differentiated from other species of nematodes such as *L. loa* and *M. perstans* by their size, presence of a sheath and characteristic nuclei in their tail. Depending on the biting habits of the vectors, MF are found in the peripheral blood either at night (*Anopheles, Culex, Mansonia*) or during the day (*Aedes*). EDTA blood (10–20 μL) will allow detecting higher numbers of MF, approximately 500 MF/mL; since MF are 20–50× larger in size than erythrocytes, low magnifications are sufficient for microscopic examination with a light microscope. In patients with low MF load, the blood has to be enriched in a thick smear (such as with malaria) or lysis of 3 mL anticoagulated blood with 6 mL formalin solution 2% followed by centrifugation. Another possibility is to pass the blood through a polycarbonate filter allowing the passage of blood cells but not of the MF (nucleopore 3 μm). MF can also be amplified and the species classified by PCR.

A more recent diagnostic technique is to determine the circulating filarial antigen (CFA) by a rapid immunochromatographic card test that can be used in the field. Positivity does not vary between day and night so that examination can be made at all times. By using the *CFA test* in endemic areas, twice as many individuals were found positive than the number of those showing presence of MF in their blood, indicating an equal number of occult infections. There is also the possibility to detect moving filariae in scrotal areas of men or, less easily, in lymph node areas in men and women [13].

13.2.5 Treatment

Mass drug administration programmes for treatment of LF are organised in endemic areas by governmental health services in collaboration with the WHO and NGOs. In areas where onchocerciasis is not endemic or present, a single-dose albendazole 400 mg plus DEC 6 mg/kg was given and albendazole 400 mg plus 200 μg/kg ivermectin in African

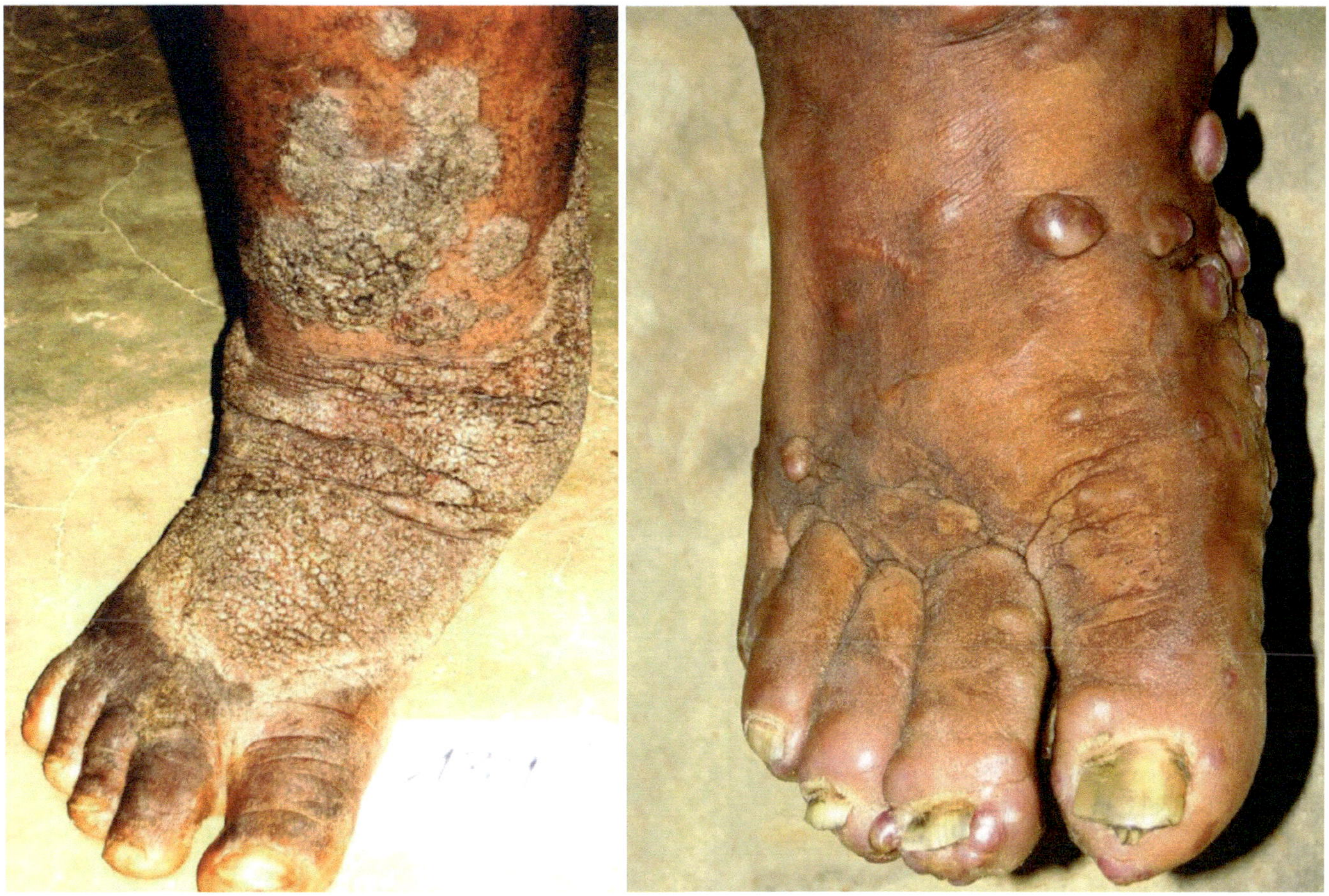

Fig. 13.10 *Podoconiosis* (left) and possible co-infection with *bacillary angiomatosis* (right)

countries with coexistence of onchocerciasis. These drug combinations deplete MF in infected patients over a period of >6 months, also having an additional but epidemiologically not relevant macrofilaricidal activity. A biannual MAD with albendazole on LF diagnosed with the CFA test in Congo has been recently reported successful [15].

Treatment with doxycycline 200 mg for 4–6 weeks has been shown effective against adult worms [14, 16], in recent studies also in a lower dose, 100 mg for 4–5 weeks; efficacy up to 90% has been observed after 12–18 months (Klarmann-Schulz et al.; in preparation). The mode of action is the same as in onchocerciasis targeting *Wolbachia* endobacteria. Doxycycline also reverts early stages of lymphoedema (Dreyer 1–3), recommended to be administered in 6-week courses every 1–2 years [16, 17].

Triple combinations of single doses of DEC, ivermectin and albendazole showed strong macrofilaricidal activity in pilot studies [18]; if confirmed, this may introduce a change in the recommendations for individual therapies, as well for MDA. As an alternative to doxycycline, rifampicin has been recently reported to be effective and safe in preclinical models [19].

Since lymphoedema progresses even without the initial trigger, management of LF is not limited to antifilarial treatment. The effect of doxycycline may be due to impairment of lymph angiogenesis rather than to infection control [17]. In addition, it is essential to instruct the patients that hygiene is a key to impede the entry of opportunistic bacteria through skin lesions with proper footwear and daily washings with local antiseptics. WHO issues a series of instructions (http://www.who.int/lymphatic_filariasis/resources/training/en/) for patients and physicians. Surgical intervention is necessary in large hydroceles in order to prevent relapses.

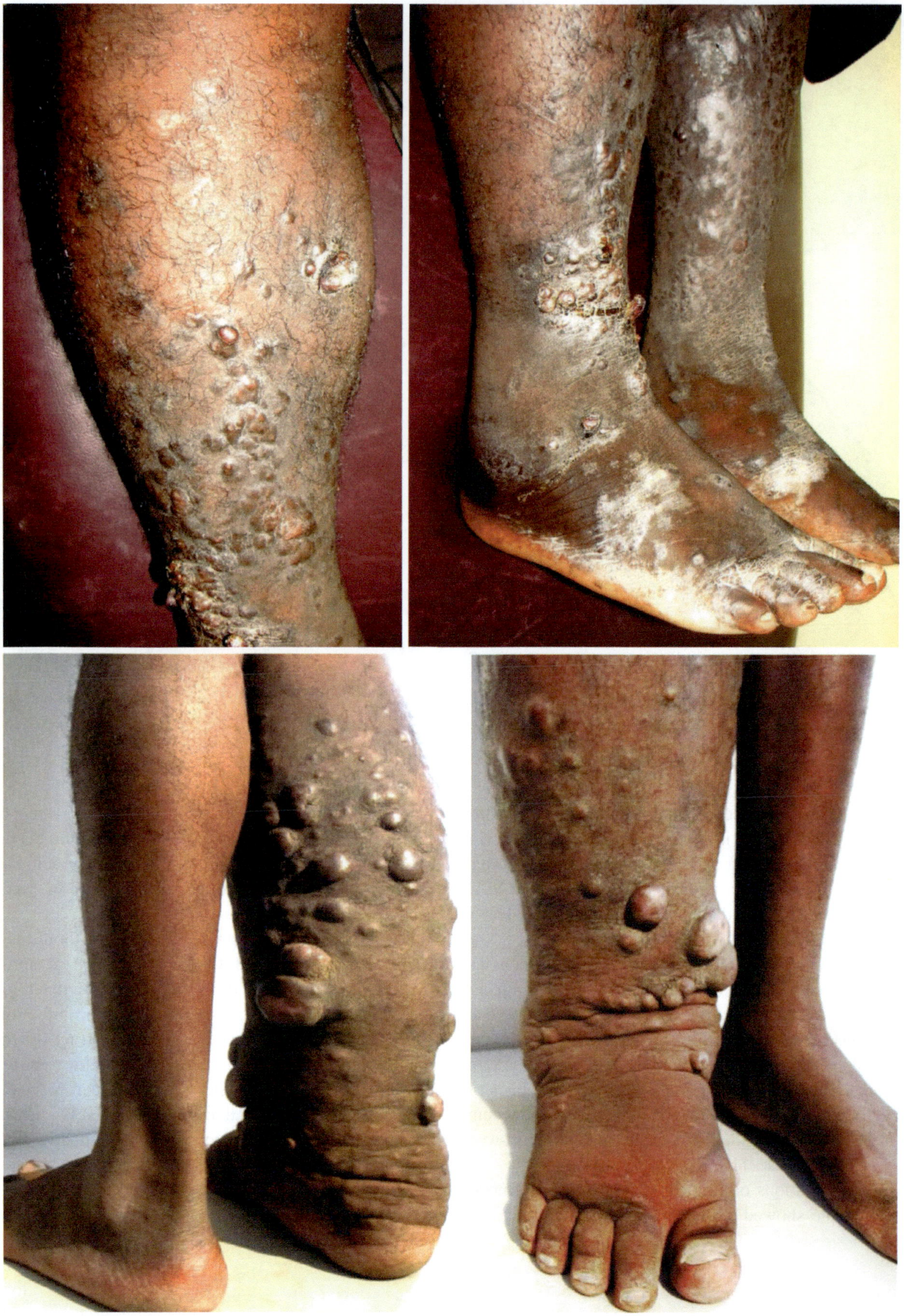

Fig. 13.11 Comorbidities: Bacterial super infections (up) and nodular type of *African Kaposi's sarcoma* (down)

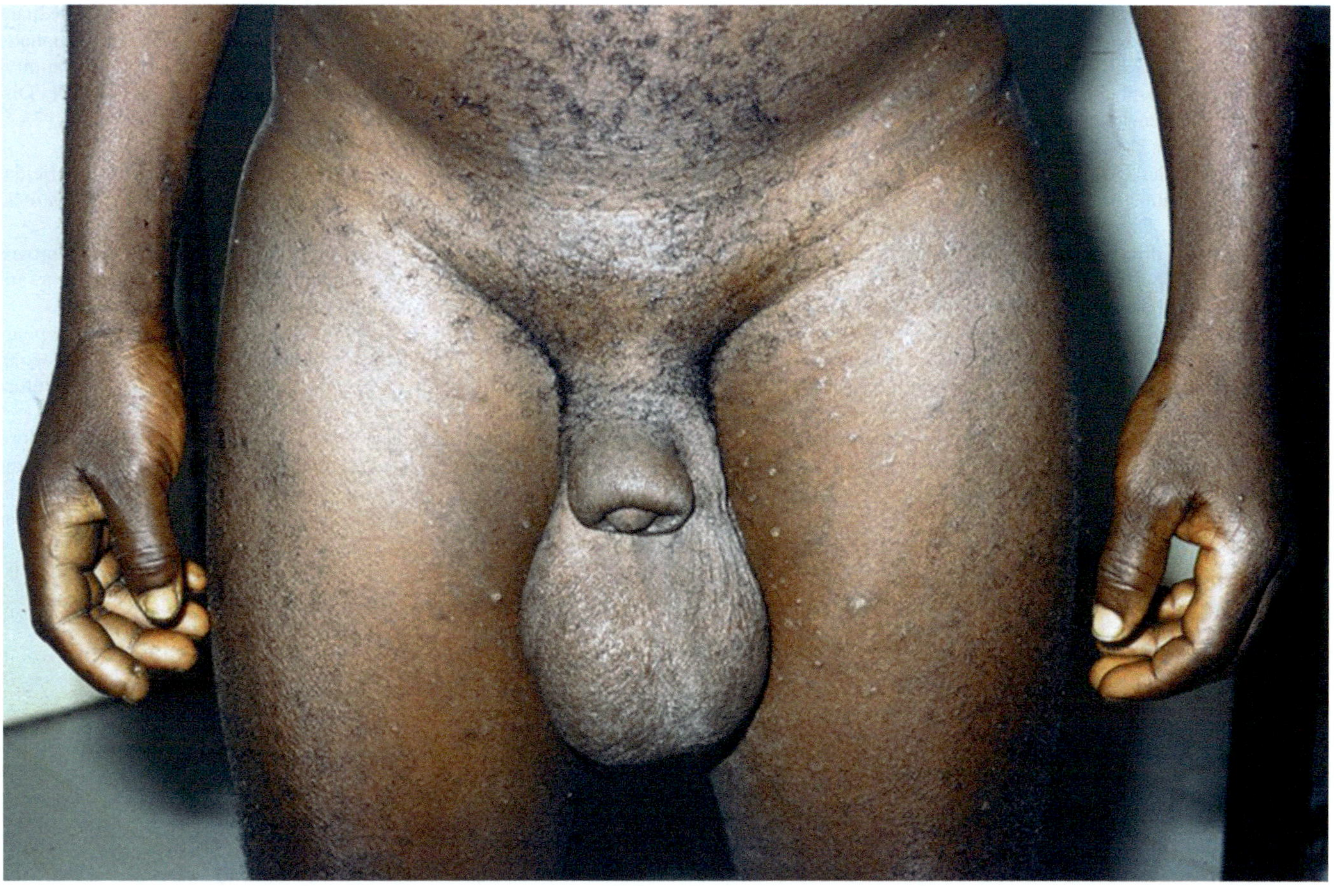

Fig. 13.12 Scrotal *hydrocele* due to lymphatic filariasis

Conclusions

Onchocerciasis and lymphatic filariasis are major infections with widespread parasitic worms transmitted by insect bites in hot climate zones. They are associated with local environmental conditions and poverty and represent a major public health issue of the populations in endemic areas. Several mass drug administration programmes have been introduced by governmental agencies and the WHO which reduced the prevalence of these infestations; however, filariases are still a challenge. In recent years, cases were imported to developed countries by immigrants and refugees or by international travellers not following hygienic rules and prevention. Recognition of these tropical infestations and treatment with antifilarial drugs such as ivermectin, diethylcarbamazine and albendazole are required. Physicians should be aware of their clinical picture, diagnosis and management, since these entities are not included in medical curricula and routine medical education in the Western world.

References

1. Develoux M, Hennequin C, Le Loup G, et al. Imported filariasis in Europe: a series of 31 cases from Metropolitan France. Eur J Intern Med. 2017;37:e37–9. https://doi.org/10.1016/j.ejim.2016.09.021.
2. Antinori S, Parravicini C, Galimberti L, et al. Is imported onchocerciasis a truly rare entity? Case report and review of the literature. Travel Med Infect Dis. 2017;16:11–7. https://doi.org/10.1016/j.tmaid.2017.02.006. pii: S1477-8939(17)30012-1.
3. Belhassen-García M, Pardo-Lledías J, Pérez del Villar L, et al. Relevance of eosinophilia and hyper-IgE in immigrant children. Medicine (Baltimore). 2014;93:e43. https://doi.org/10.1097/MD.0000000000000043.
4. Baum S, Greenberger S, Pavlotsky F, et al. Late-onset onchocercal skin disease among Ethiopian immigrants. Br J Dermatol. 2014;171:1078–83.
5. Coffeng LE, Stolk WA, Zouré HG, et al. African programme for onchocerciasis control 1995-2015: updated health impact estimates based on new disability weights. PLoS Negl Trop Dis. 2014;8:e2759. https://doi.org/10.1371/journal.pntd.0002759.
6. WHO weekly epidemiological record. 2016;91:501–16.
7. Adjobimey T, Hoerauf A. Induction of immunoglobulin G4 in human filariasis: an indicator of immunoregulation. Ann Trop Med Parasitol. 2010;104:455–64.

8. Murdoch ME, Hay RJ, Mackenzie CD, et al. A clinical classification and grading system of the cutaneous changes in onchocerciasis. Br J Dermatol. 1993;129:260–9.
9. Korten S, Wildenburg G, Darge K, et al. Mast cells in onchocercomas from patients with hyperreactive onchocerciasis (sowda). Acta Trop. 1998;70:217–31.
10. Klarmann-Schulz U, Batsa-Debrah L, Osei-Mensah J, Dubben B, Fischer K, Mubarik Y, Ricchiuto A, Fimmers R, Weil GJ, Kazura JW, King CL, Debrah AY, Hoerauf A. The addition of albendazole to ivermectin does not reduce female worm fertility in onchocerciasis. Am J Trop Med Hygiene. 2017;97:166.
11. Debrah AY, Specht S, Klarmann-Schulz U, et al. Doxycycline leads to sterility and enhanced killing of female *Onchocerca volvulus* worms in an area with persistent microfilaridermia after repeated ivermectin treatment: a randomized, placebo-controlled, double-blind trial. Clin Infect Dis. 2015;61:517–26.
12. Arndts K, Deininger S, Specht S, et al. Elevated adaptive immune responses are associated with latent infections of *Wuchereria bancrofti*. PLoS Negl Trop Dis. 2012;6:e1611. https://doi.org/10.1371/journal.pntd.0001611.
13. Mand S, Marfo-Debrekyei Y, Dittrich M, et al. Animated documentation of the filaria dance sign (FDS) in bancroftian filariasis. Filaria J. 2003;2:3.
14. Debrah AY, Mand S, Specht S, et al. Doxycycline reduces plasma VEGF-C/sVEGFR-3 and improves pathology in lymphatic filariasis. PLoS Pathog. 2006;2:e92.
15. Pion SD, Chesnais CB, Weil GJ, et al. Effect of 3 years of biannual mass drug administration with albendazole on lymphatic filariasis and soil-transmitted helminth infections: a community-based study in Republic of the Congo. Lancet Infect Dis. 2017;17:763–9. https://doi.org/10.1016/S1473-3099(17)30175-5. pii: S1473-3099(17)30175-5.
16. Debrah AY, Mand S, Marfo-Debrekyei Y, et al. Macrofilaricidal effect of 4 weeks of treatment with doxycycline on *Wuchereria bancrofti*. Trop Med Int Health. 2007;12:1433–41.
17. Mand S, Debrah AY, Klarmann U, et al. Doxycycline improves filarial lymphedema independent of active filarial infection: a randomized controlled trial. Clin Infect Dis. 2012;55:621–30.
18. Thomsen EK, Sanuku N, Baea M, et al. Efficacy, safety, and pharmacokinetics of coadministered diethylcarbamazine, albendazole, and ivermectin for treatment of bancroftian filariasis. Clin Infect Dis. 2016;62:334–41.
19. Aljayyoussi G, Tyrer HE, Ford L, et al. Short-course, high-dose rifampicin achieves wolbachia depletion predictive of curative outcomes in preclinical models of lymphatic filariasis and onchocerciasis. Sci Rep. 2017;7:210. https://doi.org/10.1038/s41598-017-00322-5.

14 Cutaneous Manifestations of Schistosomiasis

Joachim Richter

Human schistosomiasis remains a public health problem in many parts of the world, mostly affecting poor rural communities. Two hundred forty to 400 million people are infected in large parts of Africa, the Arabic Peninsula, South America and East and Southeast Asia [1]. In Africa live millions of people who require chemotherapy for schistosomiasis in order to prevent complications such as hepatic fibrosis, portal hypertension, urinary tract obstruction, hydronephrosis and bladder cancer, as well as sequelae involving the reproductive tract [1, 2]. Of the 78 countries considered endemic for schistosomiasis, 52 countries have populations requiring preventive chemotherapy. The total number of people in need of preventive chemotherapy for 2012 was estimated 249 million, of which 114.3 million were school age children, vulnerable through contacts to contaminated waters. Severe morbidity starts to occur in adolescents or even in childhood [3]. In women urogenital schistosomiasis may be also a risk factor for HIV infection. Recently, autochthonous schistosomiasis has reappeared in southern Europe [4]. The disease with its various, often serious, complications disables rather than kills.

14.1 Epidemiology

Human schistosomiasis is caused by the species *Schistosoma (S.) haematobium*, *S. mansoni*, *S. intercalatum*, *S. guineensis*, *S. japonicum*, or *S. mekongi*. Cutaneous manifestations after freshwater exposure to schistosomal larvae can be caused not only by species pathogenic to humans but also by zoonotic species, such as avian species including *Trichobilharzia* sp. and bovine *Schistosoma bovis* which are endemic also in temperate regions of the world or by hybrids between zoonotic and human species [4, 5]. In some regions, zoonotic *Schistosoma* species have been described which may cause *cercarial dermatitis* after exposure in marine waters or rivers and lakes [3, 4].

14.2 Clinical Picture

Cercarial dermatitis appears 30–60 min after exposure to contaminated fresh water following the penetration of schistosomal larvae into the skin ("swimmer's itch"). The cutaneous lesions are urticarial, occasionally eczematous in part, located mostly on the trunk, with persisting pruritus (Fig. 14.1). Children who grow up in endemic areas are protected during their first months of life by antischistosomal antibodies of the mother and later experience an immunomodulation. In these endemic areas, swimmer's itch is usually not observed. Cercarial dermatitis may be otherwise observed in immune-naive individuals, males and females, who are newly exposed to schistosomiasis. On the dark skin, the erythematous lesions are difficult to recognize; however, one feels the roughness of the skin by touching the itchy lesions with the back of the hand. Differential diagnosis includes other non-specific or allergic contact dermatitis [1, 2].

Acute schistosomiasis occurs 3–5 weeks after the infection, usually with fever, accompanied by a flare of urticarial lesions [6]. The skin lesions may change their localization over time. Differential diagnosis includes other urticarial rashes or immune reactions to helminthic antigens which may occur, e.g., in acute fascioliasis, paragonimiasis, ascariasis, toxocariasis, strongyloidiasis, hookworm infections, filariasis, or echinococcosis. In some patients vasculitis-like petechiae may be observed [6]. Blood eosinophilia is high as it is in most helminthic infections.

Chronic schistosomiasis: In endemic areas, although generally rarely observed, skin lesions, single or multiple, nodular

J. Richter
Institut für Tropenmedizin und Internationale Gesundheit, Charité—Universitätsmedizin Berlin, Berlin, Germany
e-mail: joachim.richter@charite.de

C. E. Orfanos et al. (eds.), *Pigmented Ethnic Skin and Imported Dermatoses*, https://doi.org/10.1007/978-3-319-69422-1_14

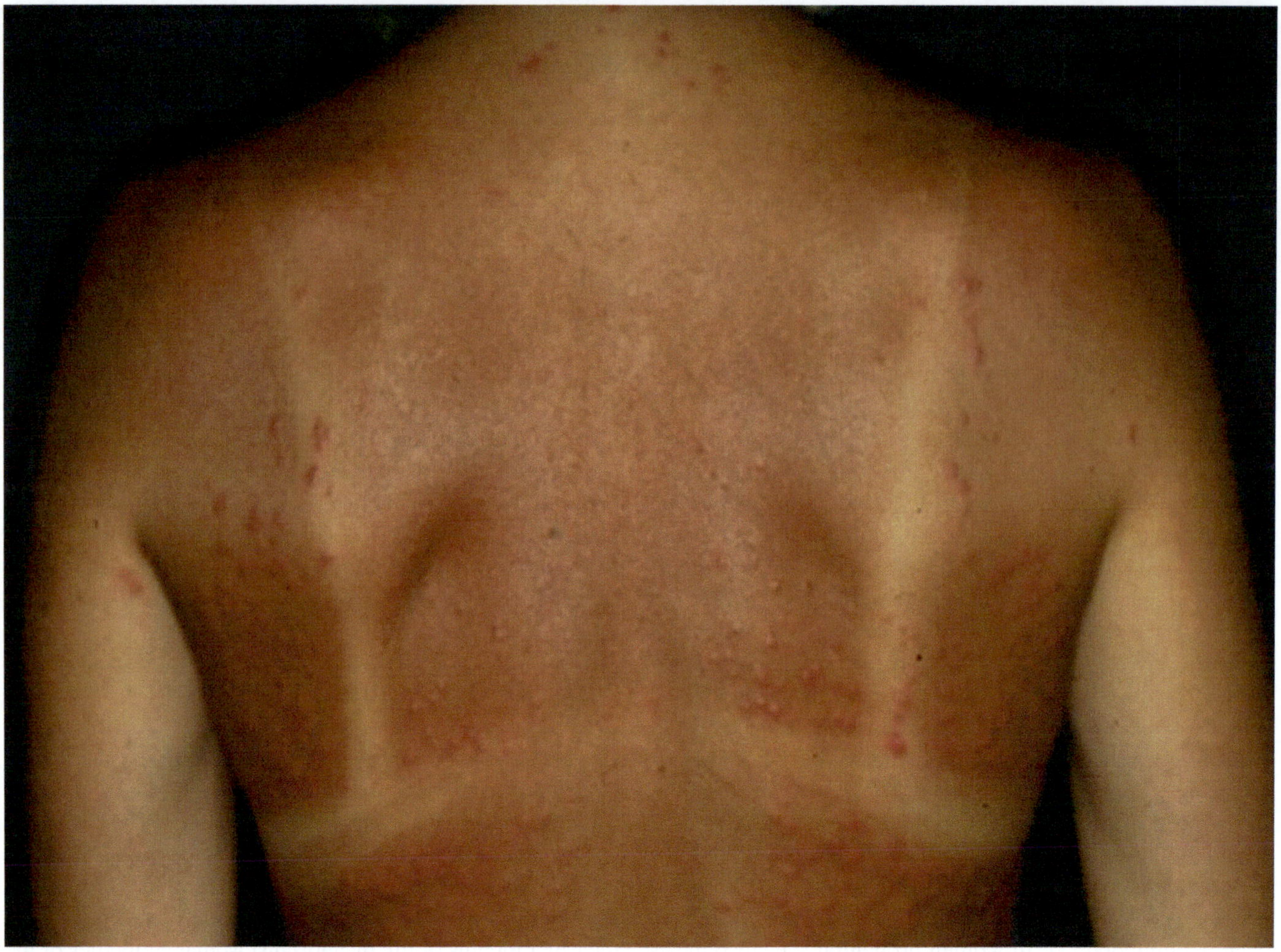

Fig. 14.1 *Cercarial dermatitis* (swimmer's itch) in a young female (courtesy Dept. of Dermatology Krefeld, Germany)

or papillomatous, may occur in patients with long-lasting infection, often localized on the external genital or perineal skin (Fig. 14.2). Occasionally, lesions are localized on the trunk or other sites [7]. In women nodules and ulcers in the vulva with vaginal bleeding may occur. Differential diagnosis includes infection by human papilloma virus, syphilis, and other sexually transmitted diseases. Occasionally, ova of schistosomes and HPV genome may be co-localized in the same lesion. In adolescents and young males, cutaneous schistosomiasis may also present as phimosis or paraphimosis.

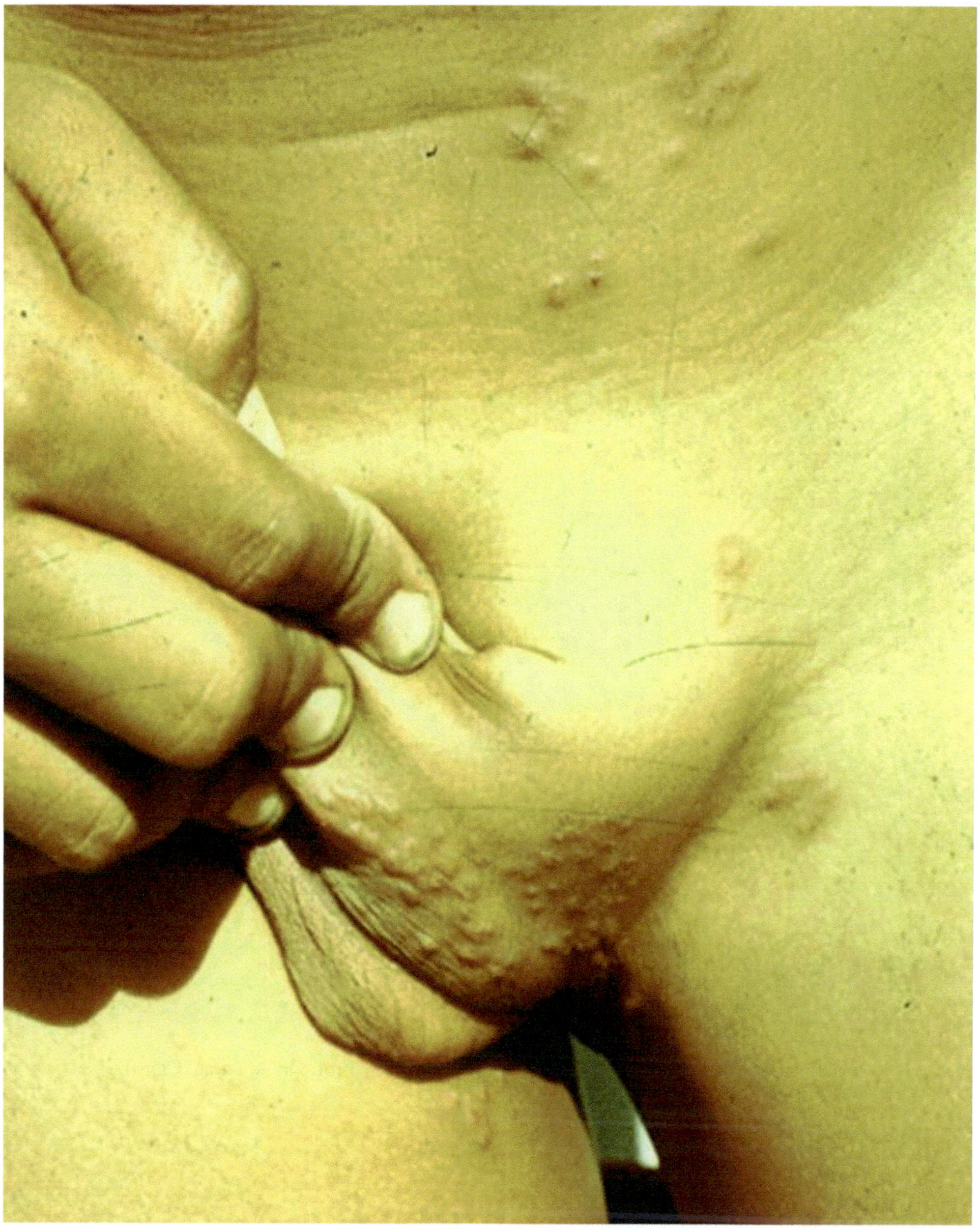

Fig. 14.2 *Cutaneous schistosomiasis* showing perigenital and abdominal nodular lesions in a young Egyptian male (courtesy Prof. Dr. A. Farag, Cairo)

14.3 Etiology and Diagnosis

Cercarial dermatitis is an allergic response to antigens of the cercariae which enter the intact skin. In acute and chronic schistosomiasis, the lesions are typically urticarial showing cutaneous lesions consisting of granulomatous nodules containing deposited ova. The diagnosis of schistosomiasis is confirmed by the detection of typical worm ova in faeces or urine. Sensitivity is increased by enrichment laboratory methods and microscopy of urine passed through microfilters. Antibody testing is particularly useful in previously immune-naïve patients such as travellers from nonendemic areas. In patients who have grown up in endemic areas, serology does not allow differential diagnosis of a passed versus an active schistosomal infection. Cutaneous perineal or genital lesions may also mimic cutaneous amoebiasis and sexually transmitted diseases. The proof of the schistosomal aetiology of a suspicious cutaneous lesion is provided by bioptical detection of schistosomal ova in the granulomatous lesion (Figs. 14.3 and 14.4). Microscopy of a wet biopsy crushed between two cover slides and stained by malachite green is easily performed also in areas with limited resources. Tissue sections are best stained with Ziehl-Neelsen to better reveal the worm ova.

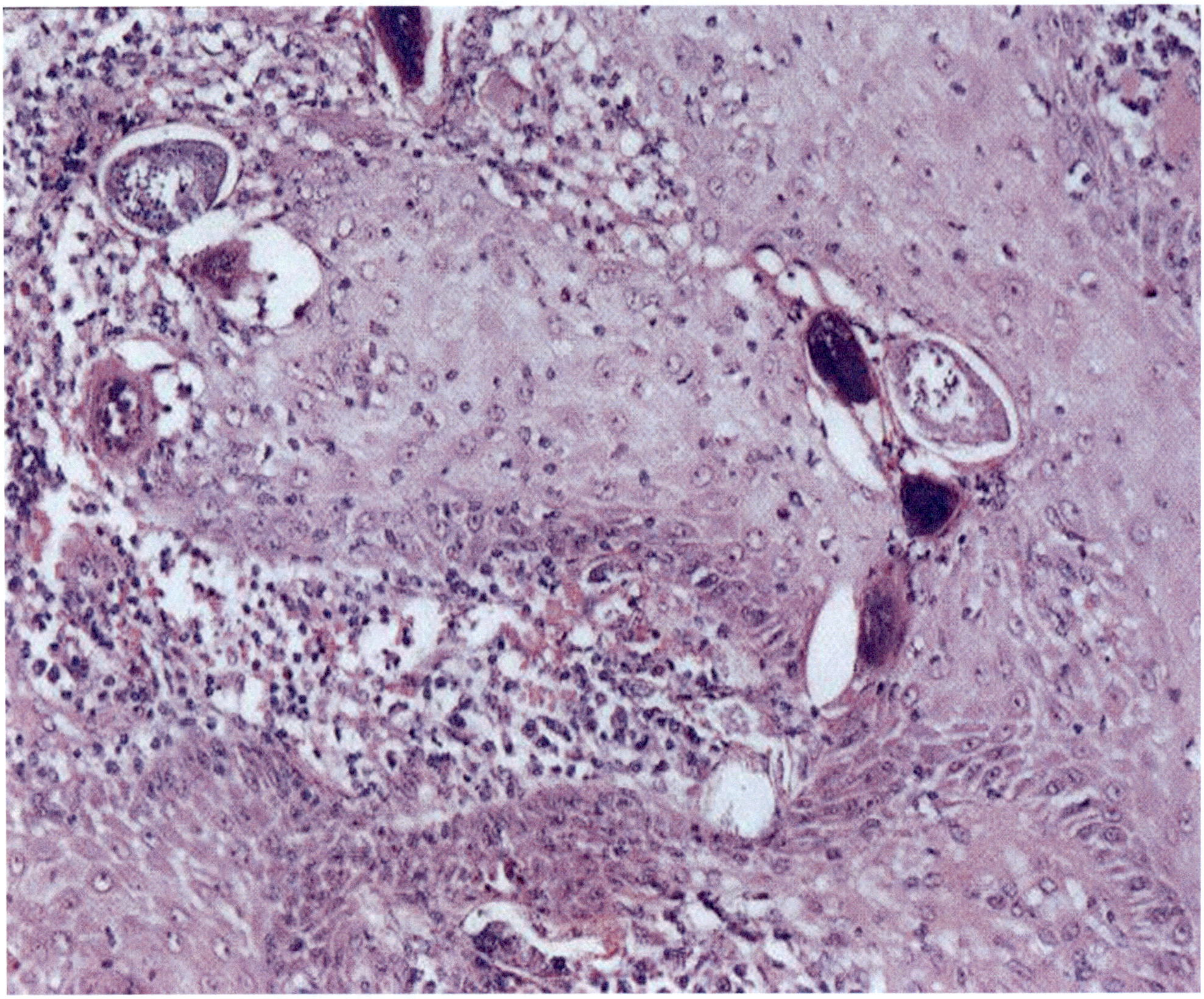

Fig. 14.3 Histology of a schistosomal perigenital nodule (courtesy Prof. Dr. A. Farag, Cairo)

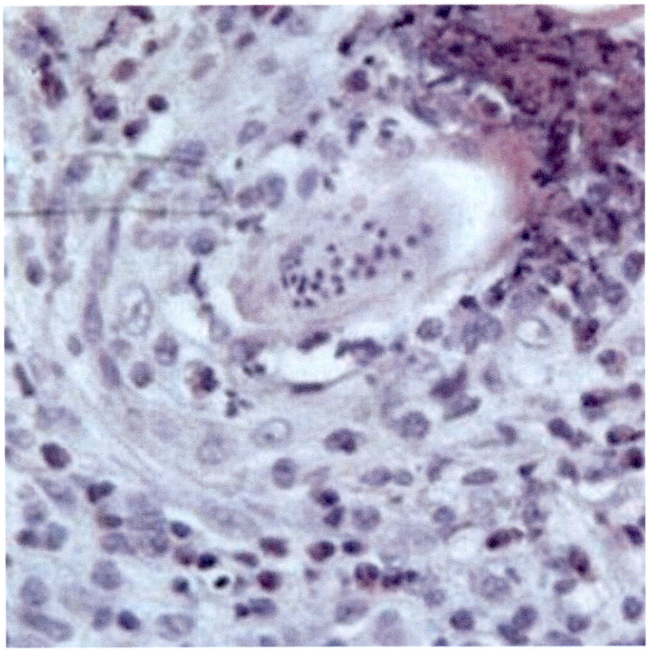

Fig. 14.4 Granulomatous tissue reaction surrounding a schistosomal egg

Antibodies against schistosome are frequently not yet detectable; parasitological examination of faeces or nuclepore filtration is positive 35 days after exposure, since ova are not yet produced by the immature worms. In specialized laboratories, schistosomal DNA can be detected in blood by PCR. Most frequently, suspicion relies on clinical grounds: skin exposure to contaminated fresh water 3–6 weeks earlier suggests a schistosomal aetiology to be confirmed by serological and/or parasitological tests 2–5 weeks later.

14.4 Management

Cercarial dermatitis can be treated with topical antihistaminics and/or corticosteroids. In this stage antiparasitic management is not warranted because the larvae are too immature to be susceptible to antihelminthics. The patients should be advised, however, to present again after 6 weeks or when symptoms indicating acute schistosomiasis ("Katayama fever") occur.

In *acute schistosomiasis*, antiallergic treatment with topic or systemic antihistaminics and/or corticosteroids may be warranted. Antihelminthic treatment should be deferred if allergic phenomena are important. Otherwise, antihelminthic management with praziquantel may be started. Treatment has to be repeated after 3 months when all larvae have matured to adult worms. Antiparasitic management is then most effective and has less pseudo-allergic side-effects.

In patients with long-lasting and repeated schistosomal infections, praziquantel is the drug of choice, active against the adult worms but not against the juvenile worms or ova. Depending on the species, praziquantel is given at doses of 40 mg/kg in South American and African schistosomiasis and at 60 mg/kg in *S. japonicum* and *S. mekongi* infections. The drug can be given either as a single dose or especially if allergic reactions are feared in two doses divided by 6 h. Thereby, a cure rate of around 80% is achieved. An approximately 100% cure rate is achieved by repetition of a single-dose treatment for 2 days, best after 6 and 12 weeks. Patients with lesions of the external genital tract must be counselled regarding the non-sexual transmission of the infection to avoid stigmatization. Furthermore, genital schistosomiasis may facilitate the transmission of STD including HIV and HBV and cause infertility as well as ectopic pregnancy due to occlusion of the fallopian tube.

Management is warranted also in pregnant women at least from the third trimester on, since praziquantel is safe, whereas the infection causes maternal anaemia and impairs intrauterine foetal growth and preterm birth [8].

The further course is uneventful. Parasitologic stool and urine control examinations are performed not earlier than 6 weeks after management because worm ova are still excreted also after the adult worms are eliminated. Superficial lesions usually regress within 6 months, but calcified ova may sometimes persist for longer. Control of eosinophilia in blood and antibody titre after 6 and/or 12 months may be used to confirm complete cure.

References

1. Bustinduy AL, King CH. Schistosomiasis. In: Farrar J, et al., editors. Manson's tropical diseases. 23rd ed. Edinburgh: Elsevier; 2014. p. 698–725. Chapter 49.
2. Hotez PJ, Fenwick A. Schistosomiasis in Africa: an emerging tragedy in our new global health decade. PLoS Negl Trop Dis. 2009;3:e485.
3. Brant SV, Andrew N, Cohen AN, et al. Cercarial dermatitis transmitted by exotic marine snail. Emerg Infect Dis. 2010;16:1357–65.
4. Moné H, Holtfreter MC, Allienne JF, et al. Introgressive hybridizations of *Schistosoma haematobium* by *Schistosoma bovis* at the origin of the first case report of schistosomiasis in Corsica (France, Europe). Parasitol Res. 2015;114:4127–33.
5. Horak P, Kolarova L. Bird schistosomes: do they die in mammalian skin? Trends Parasitol. 2001;17:66–9.
6. Lambertucci JR. Acute schistosomiasis mansoni: revisited and reconsidered. Mem Inst Oswaldo Cruz. 2010;105:422–35.
7. Grossetete G, Diabate I, Pichard E, et al. Manifestations cutanées des bilharzioses à propos de 24 observations au Mali. Cutaneous schistosomiasis among 24 cases in Mali. Bull Soc Pathol Exot. 1989;82:225–32.
8. Friedman JF, Mital P, Kanzaria HK, et al. Schistosomiasis and pregnancy. Trends Parasitol. 2007;23:159–64.

15 Insect Bites, Tick Bites, and Stings

Valeska Padovese, Federica Dassoni, and Christos C. Zouboulis

Bites and stings typically result from an insect or tick trying to obtain a blood meal from a host. Clinically, they appear as erythematous papules that can be distributed singly, grouped, or generalized, depending on the amount of accessible skin and the number and type of the biting; a robust host response can produce bullae. Pruritus often results either as a direct result of the bite or as a host response to proteins injected into the skin by the insect. Stings involve the injection of venom into the victim and may cause reactions ranging from local irritation to life-threatening anaphylaxis. Although worldwide distributed, insects are numerous in humid hot climate zones, and, therefore, insect bite and sting-induced diseases commonly occur in dark skin populations. They are also common complains of visitors and returning travelers.

15.1 Insect Bites

Insect bite and sting reactions are common in hot climate zones. In India, children <14 years of age show prevalence of 5.3–10.6%, depending on the residential area, with seasonal variations (rainy season 16.7%, summer 6.7%, winter 5.8%) [1]. The most commonly occurring insect bites are inflicted by mosquitoes of the family Culicidae (order Diptera); the genera *Anopheles*, *Culex*, and *Aedes* are usually responsible. Mosquitoes are often found around standing waters, since they need an aquatic environment to complete their life cycle. The bites of insects may be a minor nuisance or may lead to serious medical problems, including transmission of insect-borne illnesses and severe allergic reactions. Skin reactions are mostly due to allergens contained in the saliva of the insect which contains pharmacologically active compounds inhibiting body's innate immune response, causing anticoagulation, impaired platelet formation, vasodilation, and anti-inflammatory activities [1].

V. Padovese
Genito-Urinary Clinic, Mater Dei Hospital, Ministry of Health, Msida, Malta

F. Dassoni, M.D.
Ospedale Alessandro Manzoni, Lecco, Italy

C. C. Zouboulis (✉)
Departments of Dermatology, Venereology, Allergology and Immunology, Dessau Medical Center, Brandenburg Medical School Theodor Fontane, Dessau, Germany
e-mail: christos.zouboulis@klinikum-dessau.de

15.1.1 Clinical Picture

Local erythema and painful pruritus are clinically typical for mosquito bites or stings. In dark skin, erythema is not visible, but indurated pruritic papules appear resolving after a few days or weeks [1], and hyperpigmentation often occurs as a response to the inflammatory reaction (Fig. 15.1). Secondary bacterial infection may lead to flat ulcerations (Fig. 15.2). In white Caucasians with sensitive skin, uncommon local reactions to insect bites and stings in hot climate zones include ecchymosis, vesiculation, or blistering resembling hemorrhagic vasculitis (Fig. 15.3). In young children, edema may surround the site of the bite accompanied by fever and can be mistaken as streptococcal infection. Lesions of various origin due to bites and stings of mosquitoes, fleas, and/or bedbugs may lead to recurrent and itchy *papular urticaria* on exposed areas, involving the arms, lower legs, upper back, and scalp, reported predominantly in young infants 2–10 years of age (Fig. 15.4). The genital, perianal, and axillary areas are usually spared. The 0.5–1 cm lesions may be urticarial at the start of the episode and become persistent, papular, and/or nodular with time. The diagnosis of papular urticaria is made clinically, although there may be a delay between the inciting bite(s) and the onset of lesions, or insect bites may not have been noticed at all. New pruritic lesions appear sporadically leading to reactivation of older lesions, a chronic cycling disorder lasting a few months to years. Symptoms of acute anaphylaxis such as generalized urticaria,

C. E. Orfanos et al. (eds.), *Pigmented Ethnic Skin and Imported Dermatoses*, https://doi.org/10.1007/978-3-319-69422-1_15

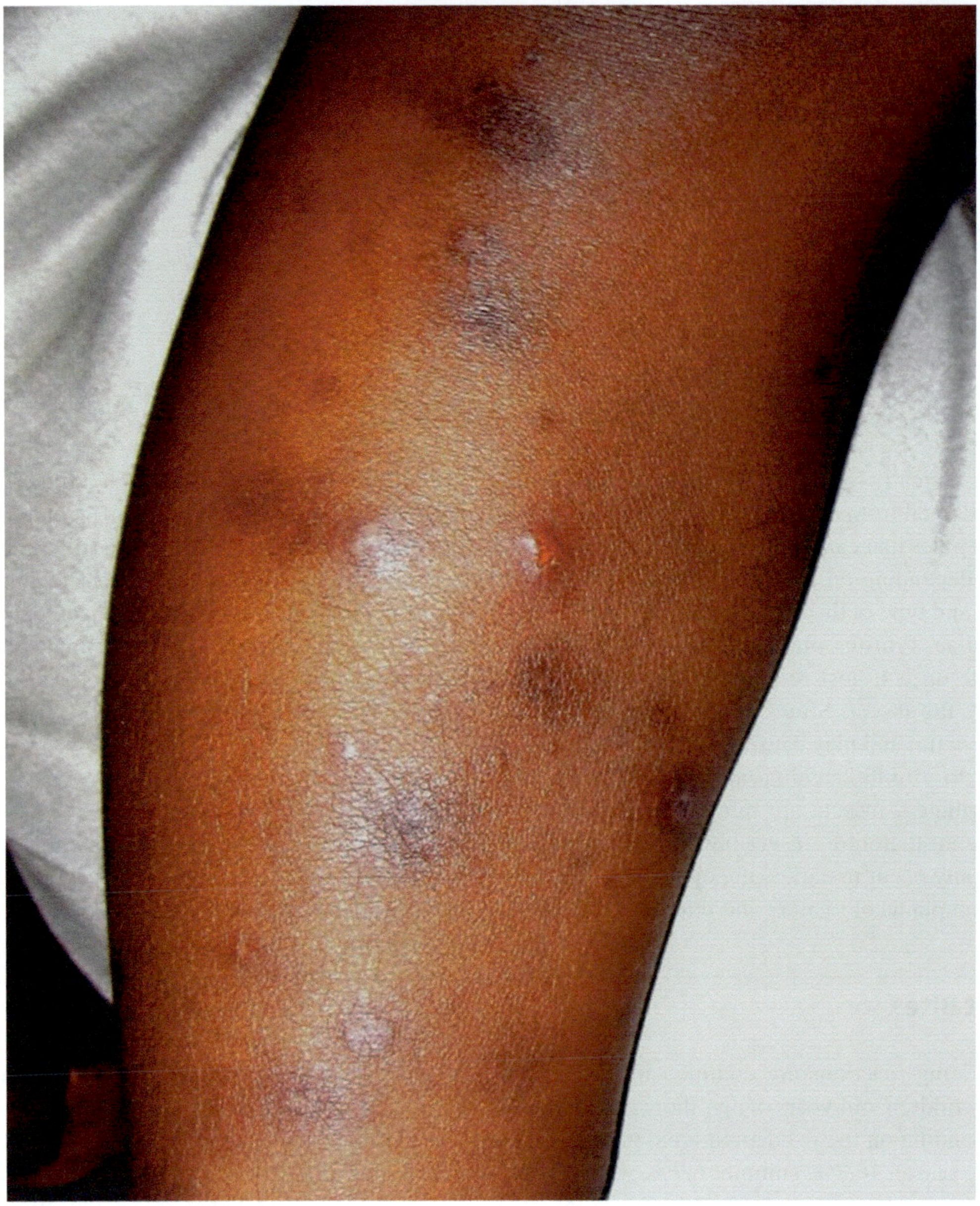

Fig. 15.1 Indurated papules on the leg of a child in East Africa due to insect bites. Hyperpigmented macules indicate previous episodes (photo: CEO)

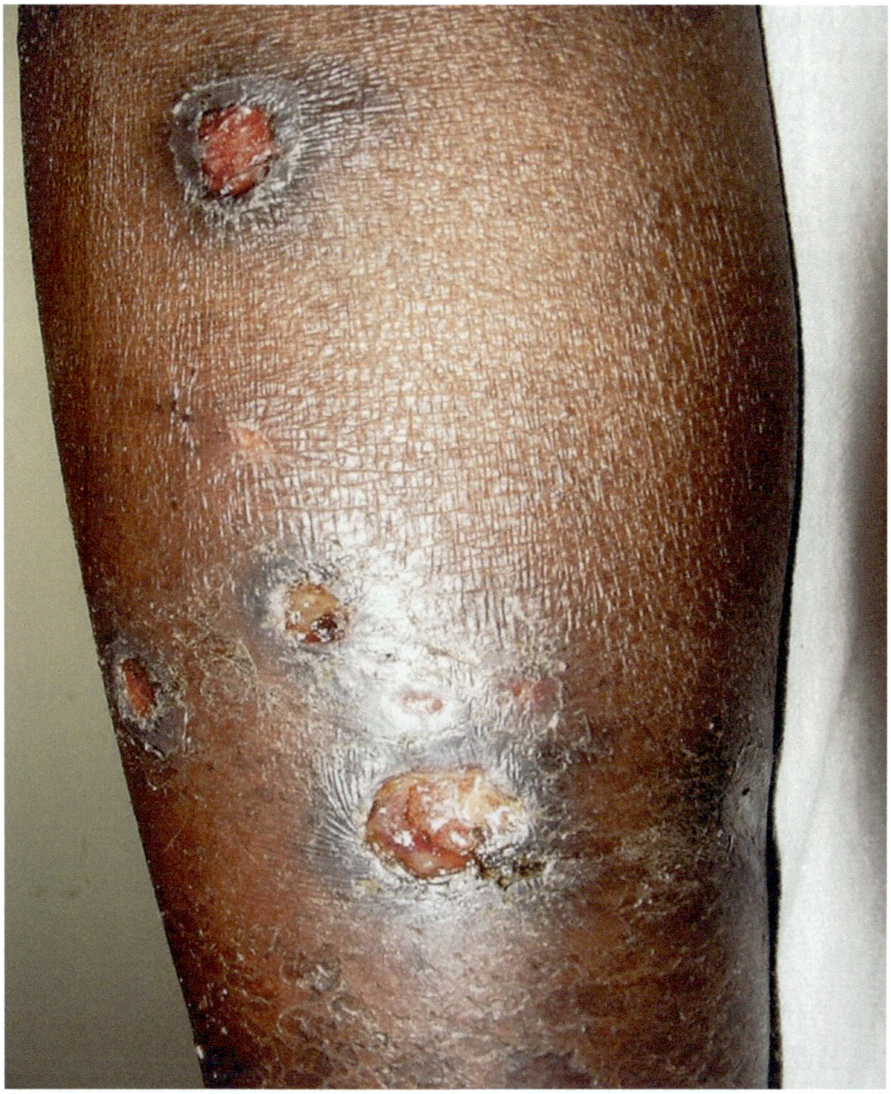

Fig. 15.2 Flat ulcerations on the legs of an African adult due to secondary bacterial super infection of insect bites (photo: CEO)

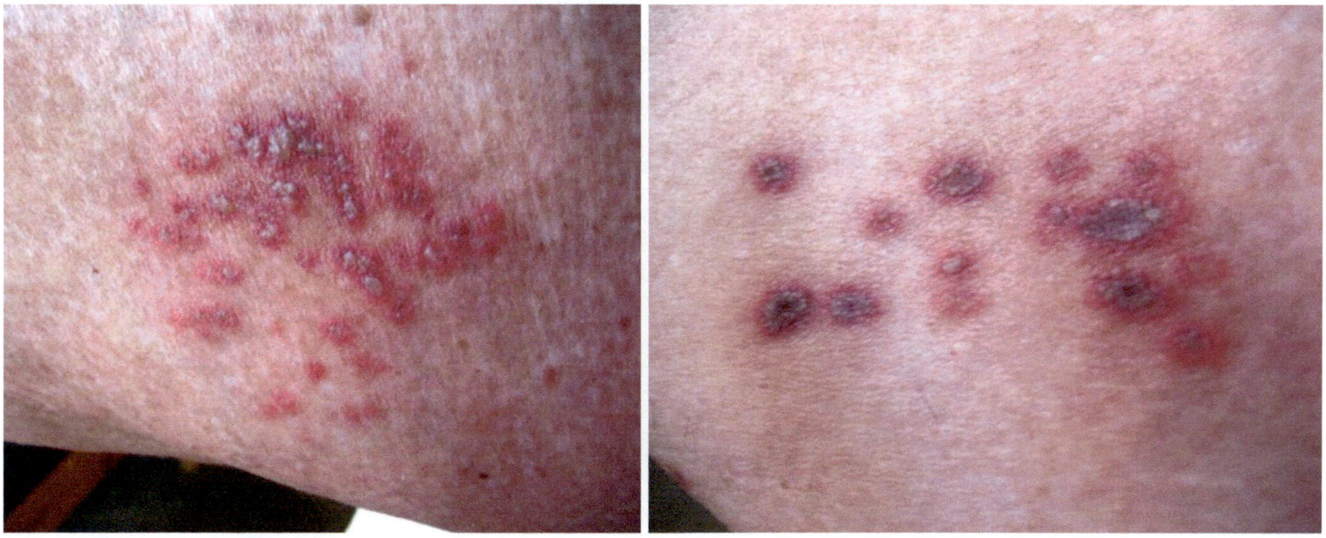

Fig. 15.3 Insect bites or stings in a European female after visiting Kenya showing hemorrhagic blistering in acute stage (left) and a week later (right)

angioedema, wheezing, vomiting, hypotension, and loss of consciousness may occur.

15.1.2 Treatment

Non-sedating oral antihistamines such as cetirizine or loratadine (10 mg 1×/day) may be helpful for controlling pruritus. A combination of topical antibiotics and mid-potency corticosteroids applied to the individual lesions is used to decrease the inflammatory reaction and prevent secondary bacterial infections. Dramatic local swelling can be reduced with a brief course of oral glucocorticosteroids; however, systemic medication should be reserved for severe cases only. Anaphylaxis associated with insect bites needs to be treated promptly with epinephrine.

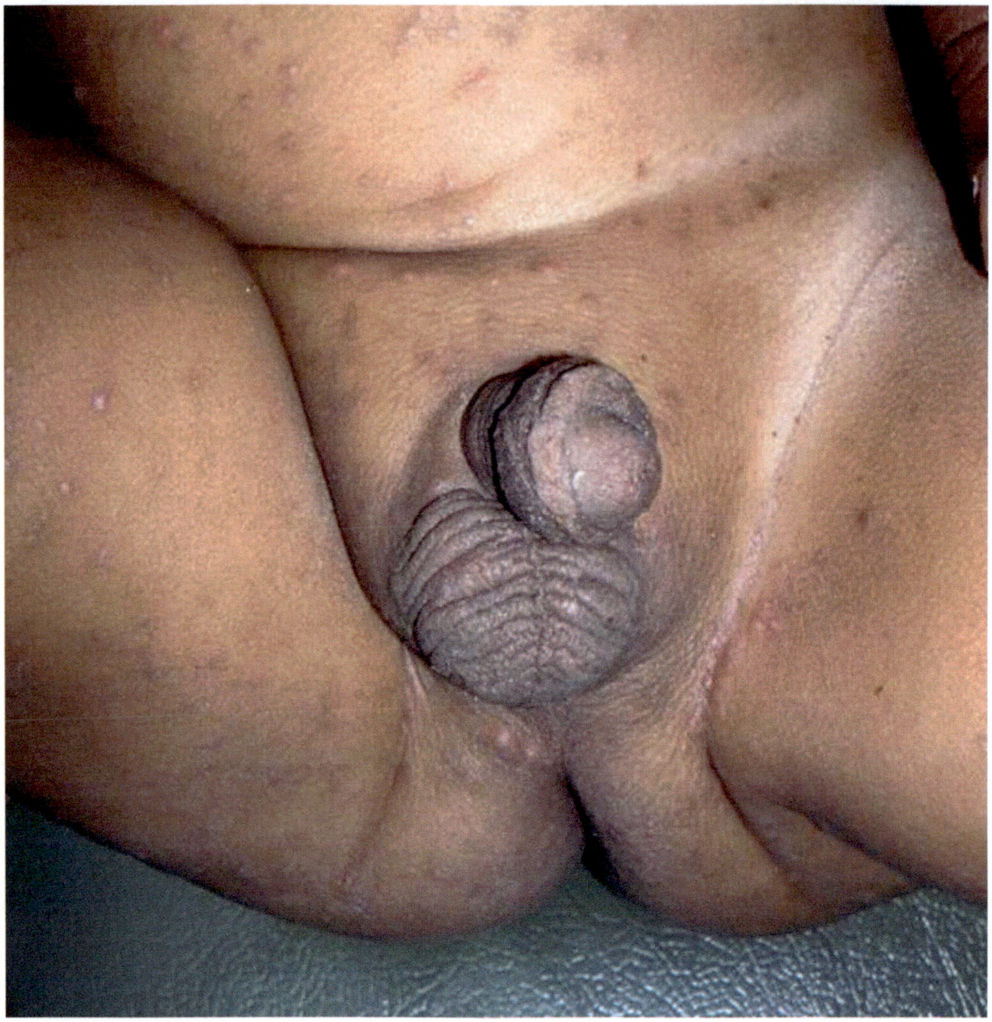

Fig. 15.4 Insect bites and stings in a child clinically presenting as *papular urticaria*

15.2 Insect Bites and Vector-Borne Diseases

15.2.1 Malaria

According to the WHO, there were around 212 million cases of malaria in 2015 and 429,000 deaths worldwide registered, with sub-Saharan Africa continuing to carry a disproportionately high share of the global malaria burden. It was home up to 90% of malaria cases and 92% of malaria deaths in 2015. Some 13 sub-Saharan countries account for 76% of all malaria cases and 75% deaths globally. Malaria is a life-threatening disease caused by *Plasmodium* spp. transmitted to humans through the bites of an infected female mosquito of the genus *Anopheles*. In 2015 nearly half of the world population was at risk of malaria. Infants, children <5 years, pregnant women, and patients with HIV/AIDS, as well as nonimmune migrants, mobile populations, and travelers, are at considerably higher risk of getting ill with malaria and developing severe disease than others [2].

Clinical symptoms usually occur 10–30 days after infection. Patients coming from endemic areas may not have any clinical signs. The most common is sudden development of fever, often with arthralgias, headache, malaise, cough, chills, jaundice, sweating, vomiting, tachycardia, and hypotonus. Hepatomegaly as well as splenomegaly with abdominal pain and anemia may be detected. The diagnosis is based on the clinical criteria, especially the sudden occurrence of fever. Giemsa blood smears allow the detection of detection of the agent in the erythrocytes.

Treatment depends on the type and severity of the case. Simple or uncomplicated malaria may be treated with oral artemisinin in combination with other antimalarials: amodiaquine, lumefantrine, mefloquine, or sulfadoxine/pyrimethamine and artemisinin-combination therapy (ACT). Another recommended combination is dihydroartemisinin and piperaquine. ACT is about 90% effective in uncomplicated malaria [3]. During pregnancy, the WHO recommends the use of quinine plus clindamycin early in the first trimester and ACT in later stages (second and third trimesters) [4]. In the 2000s, malaria with partial resistance to artemisinins emerged in Southeast Asia. Infections with *P. vivax*, *P. ovale*, or *P. malariae* usually do not require hospitalization. Treatment of *P. vivax* requires both treatment of blood stages with chloroquine or ACT and clearance of liver forms with primaquine. Treatment with tafenoquine prevents relapses after confirmed *P. vivax* malaria [5].

15.2.2 Dengue Fever

Dengue is a vector-borne disease transmitted by the bite of infected mosquitoes of the *Aedes* family (*A. aegypti* and *A. albopictus*) [6]. The ship and air travel have led to both mosquito species now being present throughout the world, though *A. aegypti* primarily resides in hot climate zones. The mosquitoes can live in forested, rural, and urban areas. There are four serotypes of the RNA flavivirus that causes dengue (DEN-1, DEN-2, DEN-3, DEN-4). Dengue outbreaks have largely been confined to the tropics, though cases have been reported in the United States. It is estimated that there are over 50–100 million cases of dengue worldwide each year and 3 billion people living in dengue endemic countries [7]. *A. aegypti* and other species are highly adaptive and their combined distribution can spread dengue higher up north across Europe or North America during summer. Travelers and migrants already infected with the virus also spread the disease when they get bitten by the local *Aedes* mosquito population.

After inoculation the incubation period for the virus averages 4–7 days. Symptoms are non-specific including fever, headache, severe myalgias, arthralgias, and gastrointestinal symptoms. Cutaneous manifestations occur in about half of the patients and consist of diffuse erythema or a morbilliform rash with islands of sparing. Petechiae may also be noted on the skin [8]. Diagnosis is confirmed by RT-PCR or by immunoassays to detect antibodies against the virus.

Treatment is aimed at symptom control, as the disease is usually self-limited and fever resolves within 2–7 days, though fatigue can persist following infection. Complications may occur with reinfection in form of dengue hemorrhagic fever or dengue shock syndrome. In experienced centers, the mortality rates are <1% [7].

15.2.3 Yellow Fever

The *yellow fever* virus is a single-stranded positive sense RNA virus of the *Flaviviridae* family, like the *Zika* virus, and is transferred by the vector mosquito *Aedes aegypti* [9]. Yellow fever occurs only in tropical areas of Africa and the United States. It is currently a rare illness because most countries have regulations and requirements for yellow fever vaccination [10]. Until 1946, the use of yellow fever vaccine led to a notable reduction of the disease in endemic countries. Every year about 200,000 cases still occur with 30,000 deaths in 33 countries, with 90% occurring in Africa. A recent analysis of African data sources estimates that 84,000–170,000 severe cases and up to 29,000–60,000 deaths occurred due to yellow fever in Africa during 2013

[10]. Over the past decade, the prevalence has increased [11]. In 2005, 2 cases were imported to Europe from Africa [12], and 11 imported cases were reported in 2016 from China [9]. The infection may clinically present in a mild acute and a severe toxic phase. The acute symptoms include fever, headache, nausea, and dizziness; severe yellow fever virus infection usually presents with viremia, fever, and renal and myocardial injury with hemorrhages resulting in 20–50% lethality [9]. The infection is difficult to diagnose. Several studies have shown that most infections with flaviviruses exhibit antibodies cross-reacting with the *yellow fever* virus, so the differentiation between *dengue* and *yellow fever* virus infection may remain clinical. The treatment is symptomatic in both entities.

15.2.4 Chikungunya Fever

Chikungunya virus is an *RNA toga virus* transmitted by the *Aedes* mosquito species as dengue. Outbreaks are generally confined to the tropics, though cases have been reported in temperate climates such as Northern Italy and the Midwestern United States. Similar to dengue, the *Chikungunya* virus incubates for 3–7 days. Symptoms include high fever, symmetric polyarthritis, and gastrointestinal symptoms. Pruritic light pink papules that can progress to bullae occur in 40–50% of the patients 2–5 days after the fever occurrence. The arthritis can be chronic, with more than half of patients reporting joint pain for longer than 18 months. Diagnosis is made by RT-PCR or serology for IgM or IgG against the virus. The *treatment* is primarily supportive; nonsteroidal anti-inflammatory drugs and oral corticosteroids are used for the joint pain associated with the virus [13].

15.2.5 Zika Virus Infection

Zika virus was first discovered in macaque monkeys in 1947 in the Zika Forest region of Uganda. It is a member of the *Flaviviridae* family related to West Nile, yellow fever, Dengue, St. Louis, and the equine encephalitis viruses. Since its discovery in 2015 at the coast of South America, it has rapidly spread to the South Pacific and western hemisphere; Zika cases have been found in 35 countries in the entire American continent. Zika has the potential to spread to new areas where the responsible mosquito vector is present (*A. aegypti*, *A. africanus*, and *A. albopictus*); therefore, it could be a risk for Southern Europe. Zika infection remains clinically asymptomatic in most cases. Patients who are symptomatic experience mild fever, arthralgias in the small joints of their hands, headaches, a nonsuppurative conjunctivitis, and morbilliform rash [14]. The diagnosis is confirmed by RT-PCR in serum, urine, or amniotic fluid in pregnancy. Complications of *Zika* virus infection include *Guillain-Barré* syndrome and microcephaly of fetus in pregnant women infected during the first trimester.

Treatment is primarily supportive; management includes preventive measures, such as insect repellant and protective clothing, paramount in anyone traveling to areas where they might be exposed to *Zika* virus [14].

15.3 Myiasis

Myiasis is commonly seen in patients from sub-Saharan Africa, Latin America, and the Caribbean, and less commonly from northeast Asia, and represents 1–5% of the diseases seen in travelers returning from these regions. However, cases of myiasis have been also reported across North America and Southern Europe [6]. Cutaneous myiasis is a skin infestation by the larvae of certain fly species. Myiasis involves the larvae (maggots) of two-winged (dipterous) flies. Three clinical types of cutaneous infestation exist, depending on the species involved, namely, follicular/furuncular, wound, and migratory myiasis. Other organs are rarely involved, e.g., nasopharynx, gastrointestinal, and genitourinary tract.

15.3.1 Follicular/Furuncular Myiasis

Bot flies, such as *Dermatobia hominis*, native to South and Central America, are a common cause in travelers arriving from these geographic areas. Other species include *Cordylobia anthropophaga* (*tumbu fly* in sub-Saharan Africa), various *Cuterebra* spp. (rabbit or rodent bot flies; in North America), and *Wohlfahrtia vigil* and *opaca* (in North America, Europe, and Pakistan). Many of the flies do not lay their eggs on humans but on other insects, mosquitoes, or objects that may come in contact with the skin, e.g., on lying laundry. Eggs on the skin hatch into larvae, which quickly burrow into the skin, where they mature and feed on the host blood for 5–10 weeks and develop through successive stages (instars) into mature larvae, 1–2 cm long, depending on the species. If the infestation is untreated, larvae eventually emerge from the skin and drop to the ground continuing their life cycle. Typical symptoms of infestation include itching, sensation of movement, and sometimes lancinating pain. The initial lesion may resemble one or more erythematous papules or nodules, ranging in size from 0.2 to 2 cm with a central pore or *punctum*, which is the caudal spiracle of the larva through which it breathes and expels waste. It resembles an arthropod bite or bacterial furuncle but may be distinguished by the presence of the central pore with serosanguineous drainage (larva waste); sometimes a small portion of the end of the larva is visible. *Dermatobia hominis* lesions are more common on the face, scalp, and extremities, whereas *Cordylobia anthropophaga* lesions tend to occur in areas that are covered by clothing and appear on the head, neck, and back (Fig. 15.2). Symptoms may also include fever, chills, and local lymphadenopathy.

15.3.2 Wound Myiasis

Open wounds and mucous membranes, often in the homeless, alcoholics, and other people in poor social circumstances, may be infested by fly larvae, most often from *Cochliomyia hominivorax*, *Chrysomya bezziana*, and *Wohlfahrtia magnifica* (green or black blowflies). Unlike larvae of common houseflies, most agents of wound myiasis invade healthy as well as necrotic tissue. The female fly lays eggs around the edges of wounds or on mucous membranes, particularly the nose and orbit. Eggs hatch in 1–2 days, and larvae feed on tissue for approximately 1 week, which can increase the size of the wound. The spines on the body of the larvae serve as an anchor to the wound base, which can make removal of the larvae difficult. Infestation of the wound produces a characteristic odor that attracts more flies to lay eggs. After maturing, the larvae fall to the ground to complete maturation to an adult fly. The entire life cycle is approximately 24 days.

15.3.3 Migratory Myiasis

The most common flies are *Gasterophilus intestinalis* and *Hypoderma bovis* and *lineatum*. The female fly lays eggs on the leg hairs of the distal extremities of horse or cattle. The eggs remain dormant until the animal bites or lick the areas where the eggs are laid. The larvae subsequently hatch and burrow into the oral mucosa; from there, they are ultimately swallowed and remain in the gut for 8–11 months until they pass through the feces to the ground where they pupate. Humans are an accidental host in migratory myiasis and acquire the eggs by contact with the horse coat or by accidental deposition of eggs by the fly onto human skin. On hatching, the larvae burrow into the epidermis and migrate 1–30 cm per day, causing pruritic, advancing lesions, which may be mistaken for cutaneous larva migrans. However, fly larvae are much larger than nematodes, and the lesions created by fly larvae last longer. At last, they ultimately die as they are unable to pupate.

15.3.4 Diagnosis and Treatment

Diagnosis is primarily clinical and often strengthened by the travel history. If the furuncle is closely observed, movement can often be appreciated around the *punctum*, and the spiracle can be appreciated on dermoscopy. If the nodules are submerged in water and the organism is alive, air bubbles may appear at the punctum. Differential diagnosis includes an inflamed cyst, abscess, folliculitis, or other arthropod bite.

In follicular/furuncular and migratory myiasis, occlusion of the location of the burrowed larva with petrolatum over 24 h will cause the larva to come closer to the surface, facilitating its removal with a needle or a forceps (Fig. 15.5). Dead larvae are difficult to remove and often trigger intense inflammatory reactions; they should be extracted through eccentrically placed cruciform incision (Fig. 15.3). Single dose of oral ivermectin 200 μm/kg bw will kill the larvae or induce migration. In wound myiasis, the usual treatment is irrigation and manual debridement.

15.4 Fleas and Skin Infections/Infestations

Fleas belonging to the order Siphonaptera inflict bites that usually present small papules arranged in a non-follicular pattern, with a punctate hemorrhage at the site of the bite. Despite any negligible skin reaction, flea bites play a role as a component of epidemiologic cascades for the transmission of other infectious diseases involving animals and humans. Examples include *plague*, *bartonellosis*, *endemic typhus*, and *tungiasis*.

Clinically, papular urticaria is a most common skin manifestation of flea bites (Fig. 15.6), with varying severity depending on the site, the age of the patient, and the status of previous sensitization. First episodes in newborn infants are usually prominent, showing urticarial lesions at the exposed areas of the face and the extremities. In highly sensitized individuals, wheals and even bullous lesions may occur. After the first attack, the reaction may later be minimal and pass without notice in adults who have been often exposed to repeated flea bites.

For *treatment*, mild emollients, topical corticosteroids, and oral antihistamines are helpful. Eradication of the fleas from clothes and domestic animals is performed by spraying chemicals such as DDT 5%.

15.4.1 Tungiasis

Tungiasis is a cutaneous parasitosis caused by the female sand flea *Tunga penetrans* (chigger flea, jigger flea, chigoe), which is endemic in equatorial and subtropical regions including sub-Saharan Africa. Both the male and the non-fertilized female flea feed on warm-blooded hosts, but only the impregnated female flea anchors invades the skin by using biting mouthparts and burrows with most of her body into the epidermis. Tungiasis is widely distributed in tropical and subtropical regions [15]; in South America, tungiasis has been reported from Columbia to Argentina and is documented in Trinidad, Tobago, and Haiti in the Caribbean, where the prevalence is up to 15–50%. Also historical records indicate that tungiasis occurred in almost all countries in Central America. Tourism in endemic regions and globalization may import

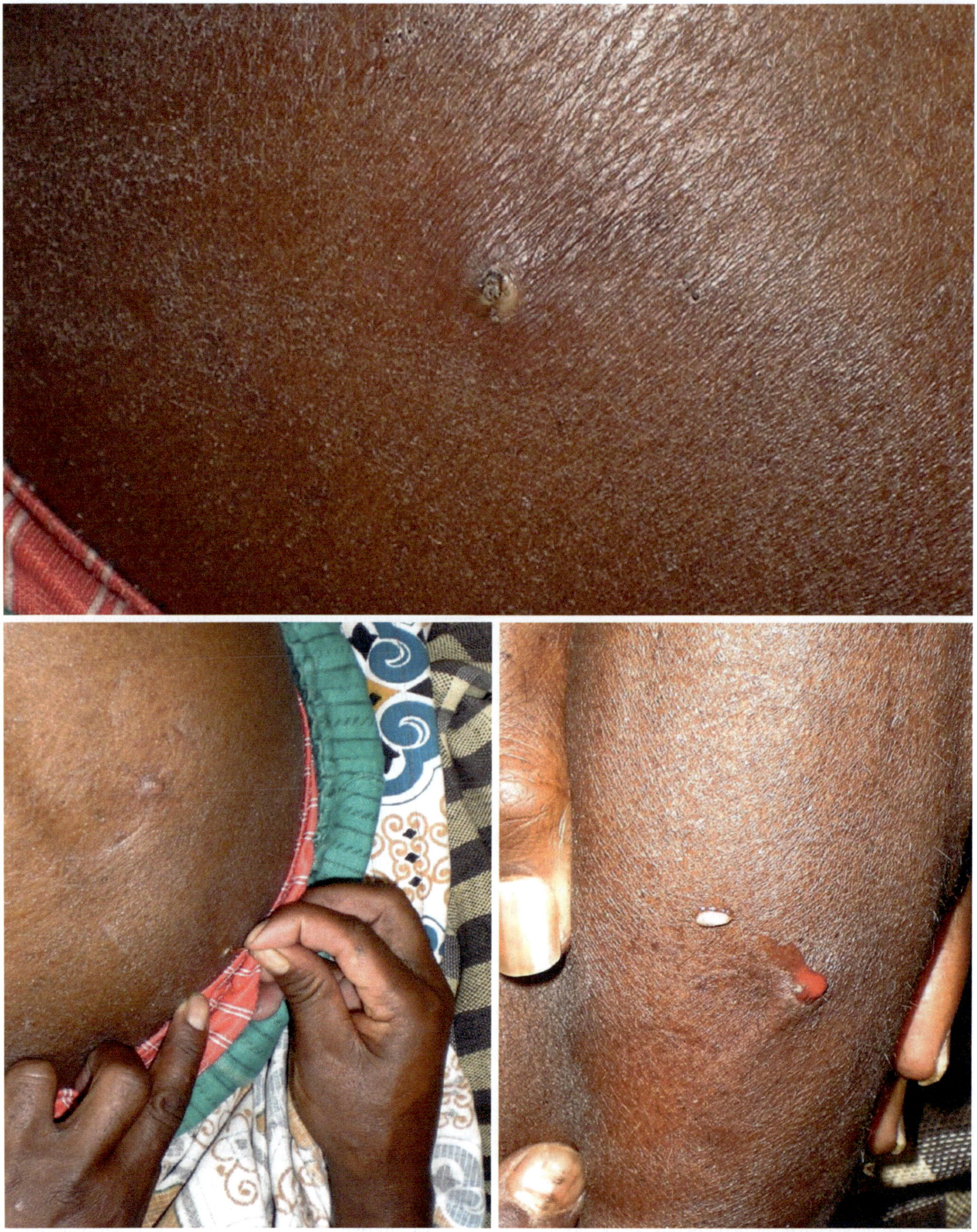

Fig. 15.5 *Myiasis* presenting a suppurating nodule (up) and extraction of the larva with a needle (down, left, and right)

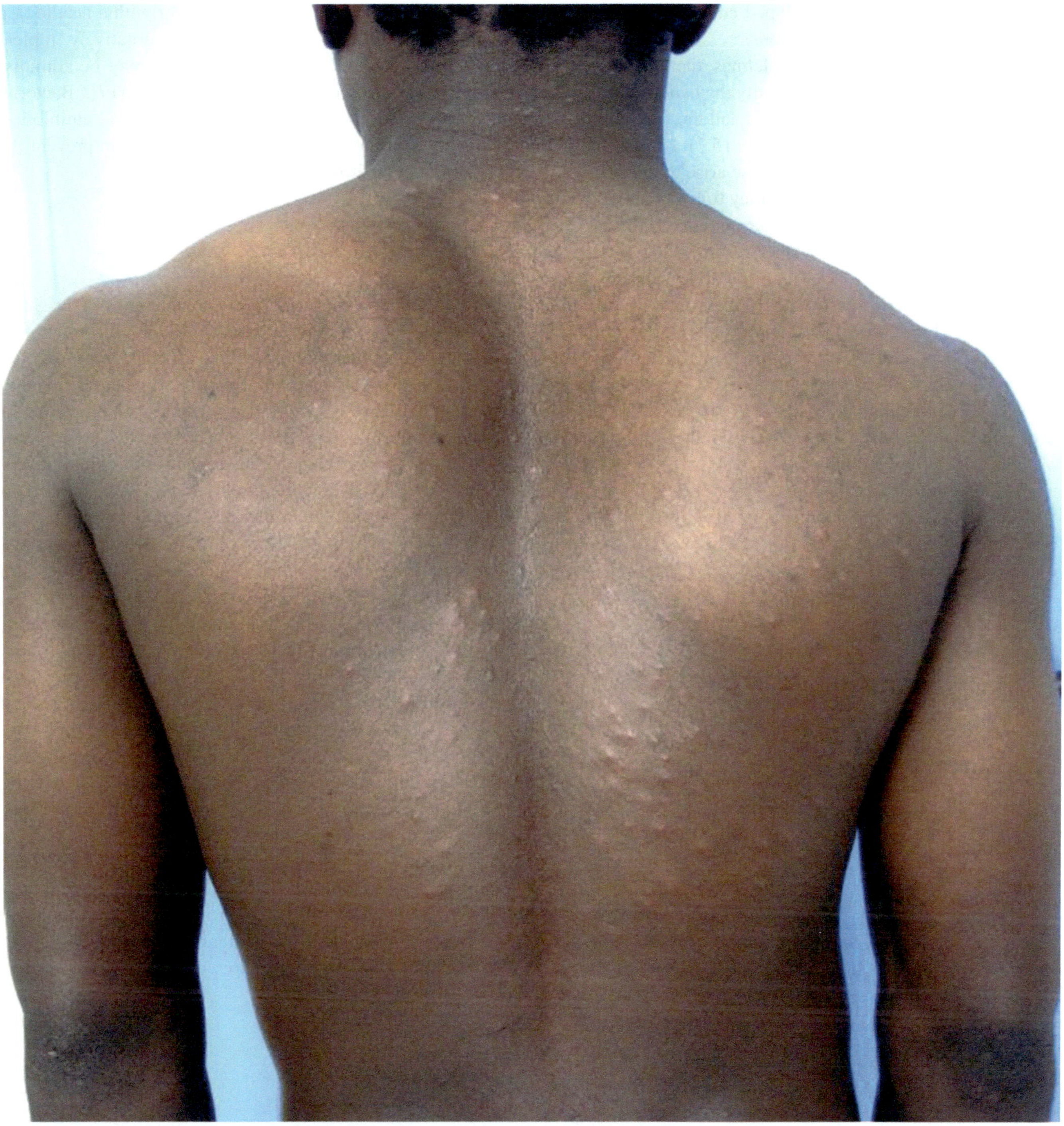

Fig. 15.6 Multiple non-follicular papules due to *flea bites* on the back of an African migrant

new cases of tungiasis in developed countries and in previously unaffected geographic regions.

The Fortaleza classification defines the five stages of tungiasis [16] (Table 15.1). Clinically the hands, particularly the interdigital and subungual areas, and the feet (toes, sole, and heals) are predilection sites (Fig. 15.7). Hard itchy nodules with local inflammatory response arise at the site where the female fleas suck blood, while they fully develop increasing their body volume by 2000× within 2 weeks [17]. Multiple lesions coalesce together forming boggy nodular-pustular eruptions (Fig. 15.8); suppurating pustules occur whereby the posterior part of the female fleas is seen as a dark plug (Fig. 15.9). Bacterial super infection with abscesses, bacteremia, lymphangitis, gangrene, and septicemia can develop and rarely be fatal [15]. Multiple lesions and intense local inflammation restrict mobility. In endemic areas, the burden of the disease is particularly high in individuals afflicted by multiple organisms.

Treatment: Petrolatum applied over 12–24 h or gauze soaked with chloroform or ether applied a few minutes to the area will be enough to kill the flea. The pustule should be opened and the flea removed manually or with a needle or a dissecting forceps [18] (Fig. 15.10). Alternatively, topical ivermectin, metrifonate, or thiabendazole may be administered in patients with widespread disease [17]. Bacterial infections should be treated with topical or oral antibiotics. The patients are to protect the exposed skin and prevent the infestation by wearing socks and shoes.

Table 15.1 Fortaleza classification of tungiasis [16]

Stage	Definition	Time (days)
I	Penetration (beginning of penetration of the epidermis by the female chigoe flea with its proboscis)	1
II	Beginning hypertrophy (complete penetration of the flea with most of its body borrowed into the skin)	1–2
III	White halo [maximum hypertrophy of flea's midsection (IIIa) and release of eggs and fecal coils into the skin (IIIb)]	3–6 (IIIa) 7–21 (IIIb)
IV	Involution [loss of flea's vitality (IVa) and death of flea and elimination of the parasite through skin repair mechanisms (IVb)]	22–26 (IVa) 26–42
V	Residues in the host's skin (expulsion of flea carcass)	43–50

15.4.2 Endemic Typhus

Rat fleas transmit murine typhus or endemic typhus [19], while epidemic typhus is caused by *Rickettsia prowazekii*, which is transmitted by lice. The clinical signs of both endemic and epidemic typhus are similar, whereas the ones of endemic disease are milder. Prodromal symptoms appear after an incubation period of about 1 week. They include fever, chills, aches, and generalized pain. The skin manifestations are a pinkish macular eruption, which appears 5 days after the infection on the trunk, transforming later in hemorrhagic lesions affecting mainly the fingers, toes, nose, and the ear lobes. The face palms and soles are usually spared. There is conjunctival injection with photophobia. At last, general manifestations psychic disturbances, such as delirium and hallucination, which is characteristic of the disease, myocardial damage, which leads to pulse irregularities and hypotension that may lead to coma can occur. The patient becomes week and debilitated. Leukopenia and anemia are detected. The complement fixation test OX-19 test demonstrates the antibodies in infected persons.

Treatment should be performed with broad-spectrum antibiotics and is curative. Tetracyclines are the drugs of choice; treatment with oral tetracycline 500 mg 4×/day should be started as soon as the clinical diagnosis is made. Also doxycycline (200 mg po single dose) is effective in epidemic typhus and scrub typhus [20]. Chloramphenicol is also effective. General supportive measures are necessary in severe cases.

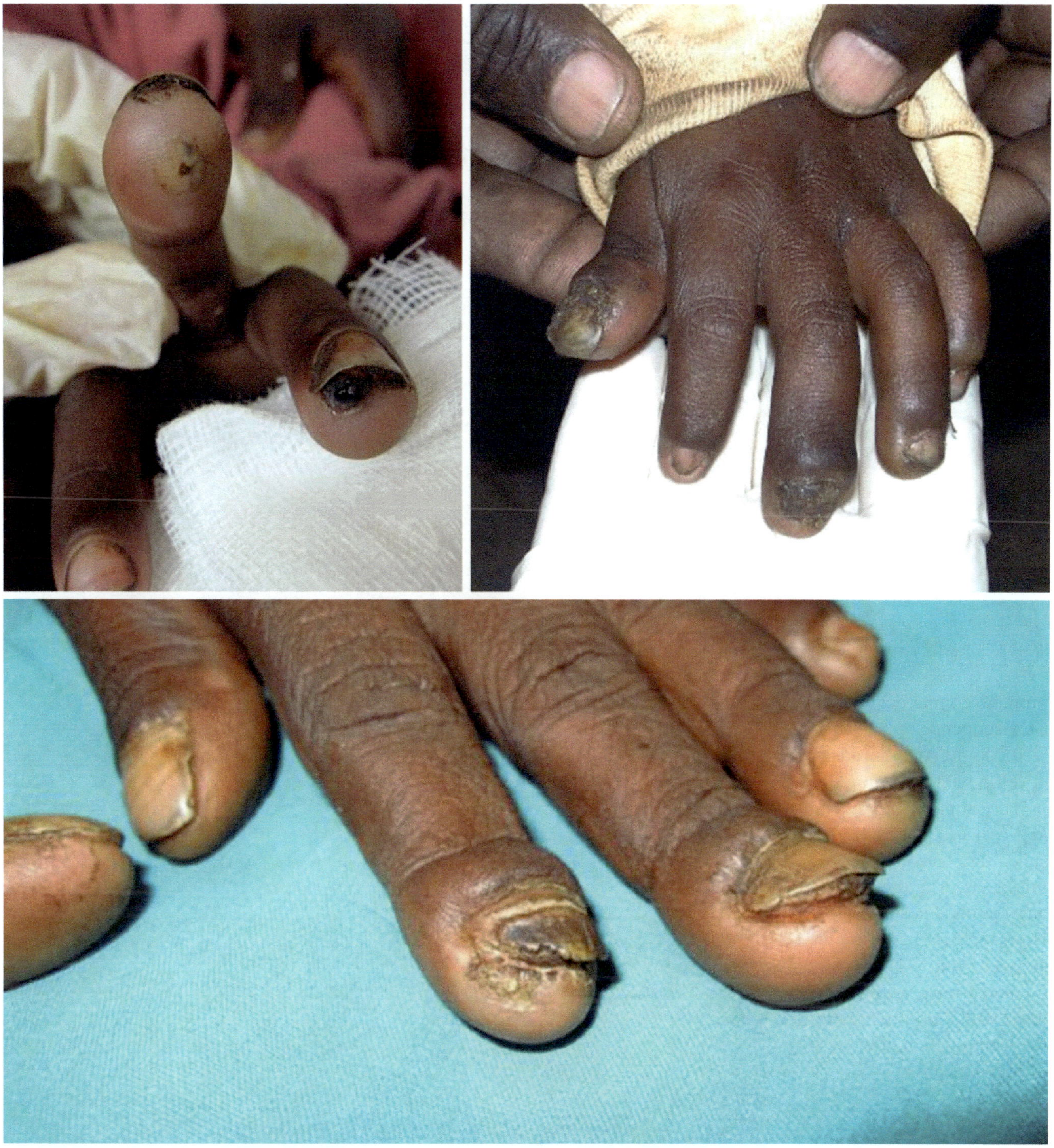

Fig. 15.7 *Tungiasis*: Involvement of the nails in a child (up) and chronic deformities with nail dystrophy in an adult (down)

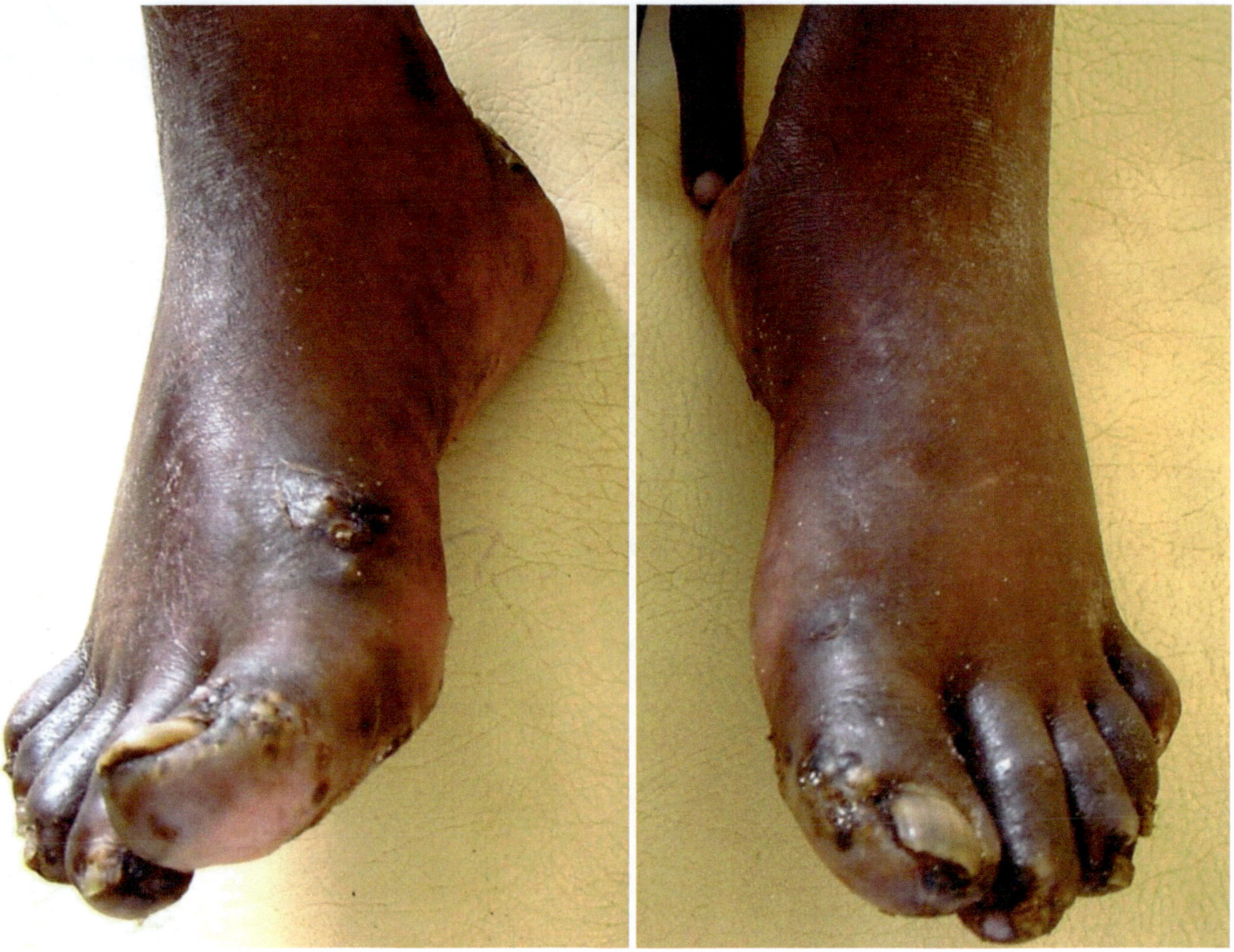

Fig. 15.8 Severe *tungiasis* of the feet due to chronic infestation with multiple fleas

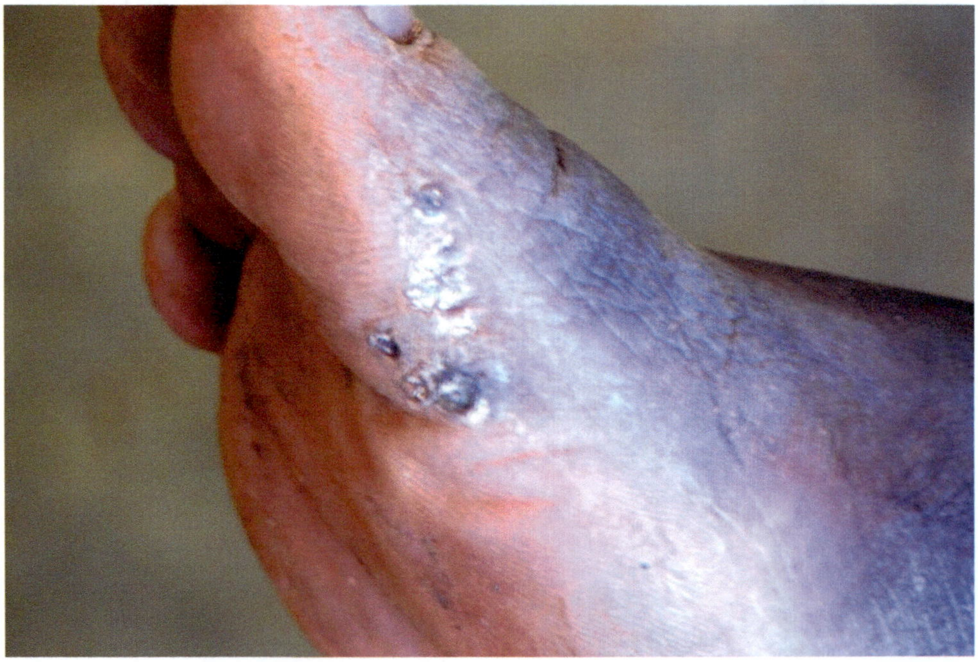

Fig. 15.9 *Stage IV* of tungiasis with dead *Tunga penetrans* at the rim of the right toe

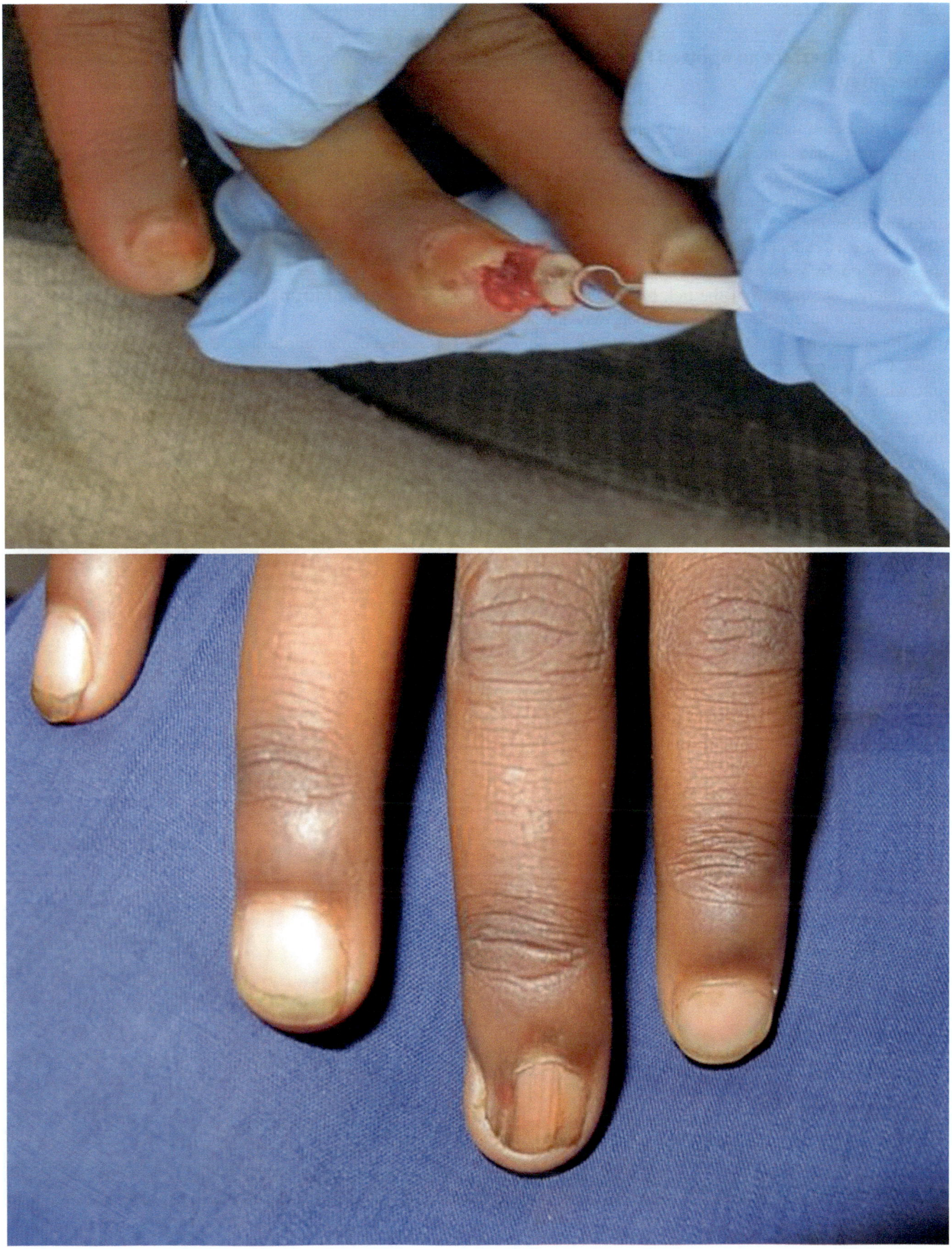

Fig. 15.10 *Tungiasis*. Excision of the flea with deep ulceration (up), swelling of the fingers and sequelae (down)

15.5 Tick Bites

15.5.1 Mediterranean Spotted Fever (fievre boutonneuse)

Bites of ticks are usually a harmless episode causing transient erythema and some itching (Fig. 15.11); however, ticks may transmit other infections that may be life-threatening. Mediterranean spotted fever is caused by *Rickettsia conorii* transmitted by the dog tick *Rhipicephalus sanguineus* [21]. The disease is endemic in countries of the Mediterranean area, in northern parts of Africa and in India, mainly affecting children. At the site of the tick bite, erythema and an indurated papule appear (*bouton*), which may ulcerate; a maculopapular eruption later occurs on the trunk, palms, and soles. Characteristic black eschar develops at the site of the bite with febrile exanthema. The course, manifestation, and treatment of the disease are roughly the same as that of epidemic typhus. Management includes protection from tick bites and effective delousing, which is necessary to control spread of infection. Treatment with oral tetracyclines 500 mg 4×/day over 5–7 days is curative, started as soon as early as the clinical diagnosis is made [20]. Also a single dose of oral doxycycline 200 mg is reported effective. General supportive measures may be necessary in severe cases.

Another spotless variant of tick bite fever seen in travelers returning from South Africa is a disease caused by *R. africae* transmitted by *Amblyomma ticks*, characterized by multiple taches noire, lymphadenopathy, lymphangitis, and edema, but no or only a discrete rash [22].

15.5.2 Rocky Mountain Spotted Fever

This is an endemic febrile disease caused by *Rickettsia rickettsii* transmitted by ticks from various types of animals such as rabbits, rodents, and ticks living in shrubs and grasses [19]. It is the most virulent type of the rickettsia infections. If the tick is infected, it remains so throughout its life where the virulence of the organisms increases after the tick takes a blood

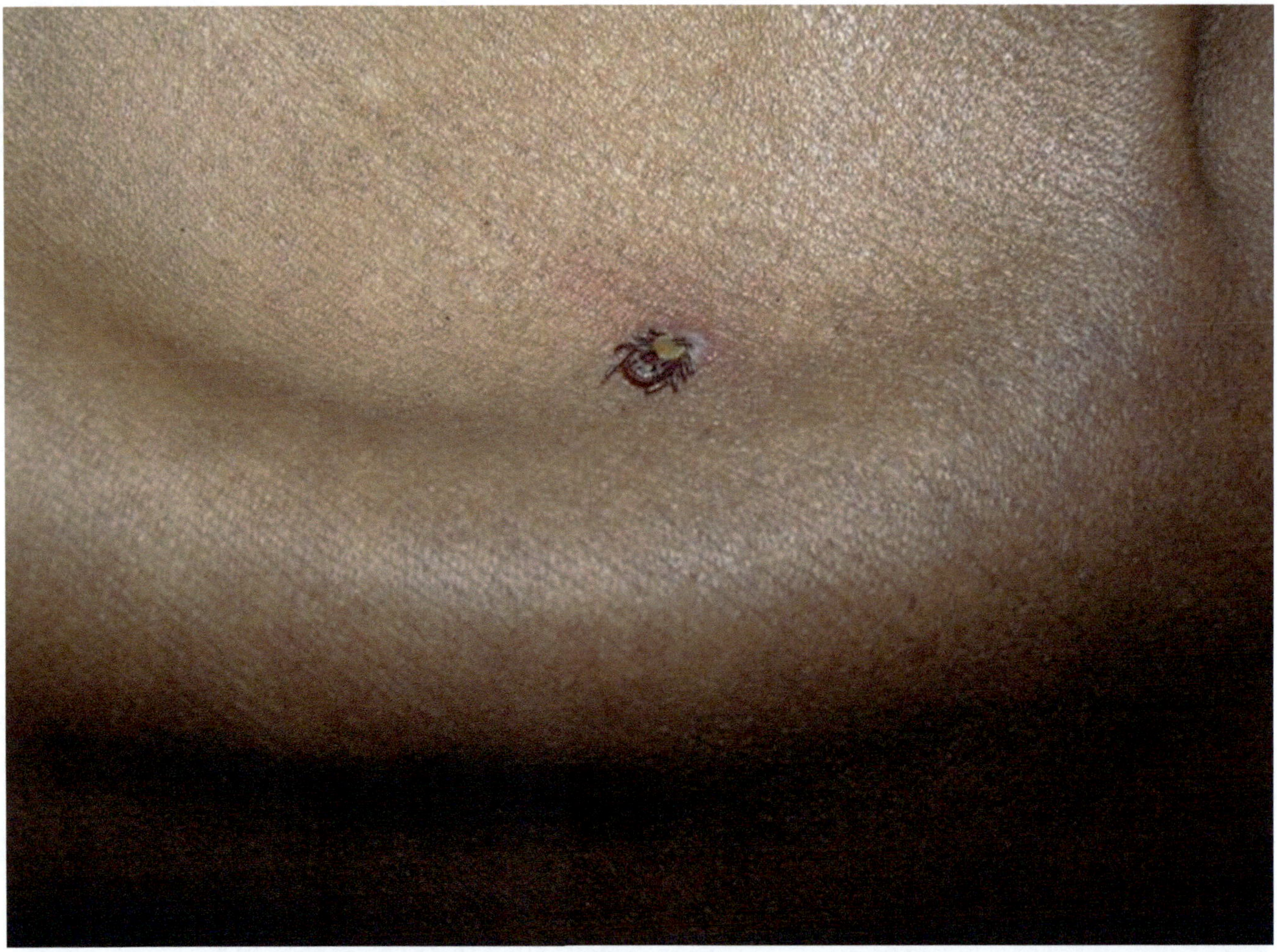

Fig. 15.11 Tick having a meal on dark skin

meal. The incubation period is about 1 week. The onset of the disease begins with prodromal high fever lasting for 2–3 weeks, chills, generalized pain, and prostration. A skin eruption appears on the first week, begins on the wrists and ankles, and then becomes generalized with purpuric eruptions. Systemic manifestation is due to involvement of other systems, such as meningeal irritation, which leads to convulsions and disorientation and gastrointestinal disturbances. Flushing of the face and epistaxis is a common manifestation.

For *treatment* tetracyclines are the drugs of choice and treatment with tetracycline (500 po mg 4×/day) should be started as soon as the clinical diagnosis is made. Doxycycline 200 mg po single dose) is also effective. Chloramphenicol has been recommended in pregnant women and children <8 years old. General supportive measures are necessary in severe cases [20].

15.5.3 Bedbugs

The most common bedbugs affecting humans are *Cimex lectularius* in temperate climates and *Cimex hemipterus* mainly in tropical climates. They hide in cracks and crevices of bed frames, mattresses, cushions, and walls of mud houses and thatched roofs in developing countries. The parasite punctures human skin with its *proboscis* where it injects vasodilators and irritating substances into the human skin. Bedbugs bite exposed skin, usually at night. A feeding is completed in 5–10 min. With the introduction of DDT 60 years ago, the bedbug population significantly decreased. Since DDT's prohibition, coupled with increased travel and heightened resistance to over-the-counter insecticides, the bedbug population has reemerged exponentially [23]. Infestations have been reported worldwide. In Australia, infestations have risen 4500% in the last 10–15 years. In the United States, the incidence of bedbug infestation is rising. New York City experienced a 2000% increase in bedbug complaints between 2004 and 2009.

Bedbugs can be transmitted either through active migration of colonies from one area to another adjacent living area through wall spaces or ventilation or through passive transportation in luggage, clothing, furniture, used mattresses, book bags, and other personal items [24]. Although infestation affects people of all socioeconomic classes and backgrounds, the likelihood increases in people, who frequently travel and people, who live in lower income neighborhoods with tightly packed apartments. Bedbug infestations are also common in refugee camps: 98% of the rooms in a refugee camp in Sierra Leone had bedbugs, and almost 90% of the residents had signs of bites [25]. Unlike scabies, direct person-to-person transfer is rare.

Clinically, the bites of bedbugs may result in punctate erosions, purpuric macules, erythematous macules, papules, or wheals, often pruritic, each with a central hemorrhagic punctum [26]. The lesions may form linear patterns or may be seen in groups. Older adults develop symptoms less often than do younger people. Lesions usually resolve after about 1 week but can last longer. Secondary infection can develop. Diagnosis based on lesion appearance may be difficult; however, bedbug bites are usually larger and more edematous than flea bites. Identification of bedbugs can help confirm the diagnosis. Bedbugs have flat, oval, reddish-brown bodies. After a blood meal, the body is less flat and more reddish. Adult *C. lectularius* are about 5–7 mm in length, and *C. hemipterus* are slightly longer. Bedbug feces or blood may be evident on bed linens or behind wallpaper.

The *treatment* is symptomatic. Bedbugs should be eradicated using physical and/or chemical means [26]. Physical means include vacuuming affected areas and laundering suspect articles, then drying on the dryer's hottest setting. When possible, infested rooms should be treated professionally with overheat up to temperatures ≥50 °C and/or with multiple insecticides. Chemical means include malathion 0.5% and pyrithium or trichlorfon spray to dust small holes in the furniture, walls, and floors. Moreover, methyl bromide fumigation for infested houses may be enough to eradicate the bugs. Fumigation using sulfur is also effective.

15.6 Stings

15.6.1 Stings by Bees, Yellow Jackets, and Ants

These are Hymenoptera belonging to the Apidae family (honey bees and bumble bees), the Vespidae family (yellow jackets, yellow hornets, white-faced hornets, and paper wasps), and the Formicidae family (fire ants, harvester ants, bulldog ants, and jack jumper ants). They generally sting humans in self-defense, to protect their nests or hives. Their stings are acutely painful and patients become aware that a sting has occurred, although they may not have visualized the insect. Identification of the responsible winged Hymenoptera after the sting can be difficult since the resultant lesions are similar in appearance. Bees and occasionally yellow jackets have a barbed stinging apparatus that becomes lodged in the skin and rips away, along with the venom sac, from the insect body following a sting event.

Clinically, reactions to stings may be graded as local, urticaria without systemic symptoms, or generalized. Large local reactions do not predispose patients to generalized reactions. Local reactions may be life-threatening, if local swelling at the sting site compromises the airway, and they can cause peripheral nerve block. Most people develop only minor local reactions, but patients with venom allergy are at risk for systemic allergic reactions (i.e., anaphylaxis) [6]. Local reactions to a Hymenoptera sting is redness and an area of painful swelling (1–5 cm) at the site of the sting that develops within minutes and resolves within a few hours. Some people develop exaggerated redness and swelling at the site of the sting that gradually enlarges over 1–2 days, to resolve over 5–10 days. The area of swelling typically measures about 10 cm in diameter. The stinging apparatus may have been seen in the wound and removed prior to presentation. Urticaria may occur with or without the symptoms noted in local reaction. Imported fire ant stings typically cause pustule-like lesions at the site of the sting within about 24 h. These pseudopustules are sterile, and patients should be advised not to open them, as this can lead to infection. In the absence of this advice, patients tend to unroof the lesions.

Management: If the insect or stinger can be flicked off of the skin immediately, it may help limit the amount of venom injected. However, if the patient presents minutes later, immediate stinger removal is not critical, because the venom will have already been fully expelled. Remaining stingers should eventually be removed since they occasionally cause foreign body reactions. Imported fire ants grasp the skin firmly with their mandibles and inflict multiple stings per insect, so these should be promptly removed as well.

Treatment of a local reaction involves cleansing, removal of the stinging apparatus if present, and application of ice packs. The limb should be elevated if the sting is on an extremity. In case of severe reactions, oral prednisone 40–60 mg given as a single dose or rapidly tapered over 2–5 days may help reduce significant swelling [6]. Pruritus can be treated with oral cetirizine 10 mg p.o. 1×/day and high-potency topical corticosteroids (e.g., clobetasol 0.05% ointment 4–6×/day) until the itching subsides. A tetanus booster is not necessary following a sting unless there was a concomitant soil-contaminated injury. A self-administered injectable form of epinephrine should be available for individuals at risk for anaphylactic reactions. Secondary bacterial infections may occur; systemic antibiotic treatment (e.g., oral amoxicillin 500 mg 4×/day for 7 days) is suggested.

15.6.2 Stings by Centipedes

Centipedes are found in moist and usually warm climates worldwide, and human envenomations are typically reported from Asia, Indonesia, India, Hawaii, South America, and Australia [27]. The *Scolopendra* represents the best-known genus of centipede. Centipedes are largely nocturnal, and most human stings occur during the night; they inject their venom through forcipules, pincer-like appendages extending from the insect head that are used to immobilize prey. Stings of centipedes often affect the extremities, and two small puncture marks may be visible; they are usually painful, and erythema and edema are common. Most centipede stings resolve without complications, although various sequelae are reported, including local infection and necrosis, myocardial infarction, rhabdomyolysis with renal failure, and anaphylaxis. Laboratory examinations may show leukocytosis and an increase in erythrocyte sedimentation rate. Complete remission can be achieved within 2 weeks by means of paracetamol and oral prednisolone [28].

References

1. Singh S, Mann BK. Insect bite reactions. Indian J Dermatol Venereol Leprol. 2013;79:151–64.
2. World Health Organization. 2016a. http://www.who.int/mediacentre/factsheets/fs094/en/.
3. Howitt P, Darzi A, Yang GZ, et al. Technologies for global health. Lancet. 2012;380:507–35.
4. Manyando C, Kayentao K, D'Alessandro U, et al. A systematic review of the safety and efficacy of artemether-lumefantrine against uncomplicated Plasmodium falciparum malaria during pregnancy. Malar J. 2011;11:141.
5. Rajapakse S, Rodrigo C, Fernando SD. Tafenoquine for preventing relapse in people with Plasmodium vivax malaria. Cochrane Database System Rev 2015;(4):CD010458.
6. Vasievich MP, Villarreal JD, Tomecki KJ. Got the travel bug? A review of common infections, infestations, bites, and stings among returning travelers. Am J Clin Dermatol. 2016;17:451–62.
7. World Health Organization. 2016b. http://www.who.int/denguecontrol/epidemiology/en/.
8. Chen LH, Wilson ME. Dengue and chikungunya infections in travelers. Curr Opin Infect Dis. 2010;23:438–44.
9. Wang L, Zhou P. Yellow fever virus: increasing imported cases in China. J Infect. 2016;73:377–80.
10. World Health Organization. 2016c. http://www.cdc.gov/ncidod/dvbid/yellowfever/index.htm.
11. Chan M. Yellow fever: the resurgence of a forgotten disease. Lancet. 2016;387:2165–6.
12. Bae HG, Drosten C, Emmerich P, et al. Analysis of two imported cases of yellow fever infection from Ivory Coast and The Gambia to Germany and Belgium. J Clin Virol. 2005;33:274–80.
13. Bautista-Reyes E, Núñez-Avellaneda D, Alonso-Palomares LA, et al. Chikungunya: Molecular aspects, clinical outcomes and pathogenesis. Rev Invest Clin. 2017;69:299–307.
14. Saiz JC, Vazquez-Calvo A, Blazquez AB, et al. Zika virus: the latest newcomer. Front Microbiol. 2016;7:496.
15. Feldmeier H, Heukelbach J, Ugbomoiko US, et al. Tungiasis—a neglected disease with many challenges for global public health. PLoS Negl Trop Dis. 2014;8:e3133.
16. Eisele M, Heukelbach J, Van Marck E, et al. Investigations on the biology, epidemiology, pathology and control of Tunga penetrans in Brazil: I. Natural history of tungiasis in man. Parasitol Res. 2003;90:87–99.
17. Karagiannidis I, Kanaki T, Brunner B, et al. Multiple, schwärzliche Papeln an beiden Fußsohlen einer 20-jährigen Patientin. Hautarzt. 2016;67:586–8.
18. Cestari TF, Pessato S, Ramos-e-Silva M. Tungiasis and myiasis. Clin Dermatol. 2007;25:158–64.

19. Graves SR, Stenos J. Tick-borne infectious diseases in Australia. Med J Aust. 2017;206:320–4.
20. Song JH, Lee C, Chang WH, et al. Short-course doxycycline treatment versus conventional tetracycline therapy for scrub typhus: a multicenter randomized trial. Clin Infect Dis. 1995;21:506–10.
21. Parola P: Rickettsioses in sub-Saharan Africa Ann NY Acad Sci 2006;1078:42–47.
22. Brouqui P, Harle JR, Delmont J, et al. African tick-bite fever. An imported spotless rickettsiosis. Arch Intern Med. 1997;157:119–24.
23. Davies TG, Field LM, Williamson MS. The re-emergence of the bed bug as a nuisance pest: implications of resistance to the pyrethroid insecticides. Med Vet Entomol. 2012;26:241–54.
24. Ibrahim O, Syed UM, Tomecki KJ. Bedbugs: helping your patient through an infestation. Cleve Clin J Med. 2017;84:207–11.
25. Gbakima AA, Terry BC, Kanja F, et al. High prevalence of bedbugs *Cimex hemipterus* and *Cimex lectularis* in camps for internally displaced persons in Freetown, Sierra Leone: a pilot humanitarian investigation. West Afr J Med. 2002;21:268–71.
26. McMenaman KS, Gausche-Hill M. Cimex lectularius ("bed bugs"): recognition, management, and eradication. Pediatr Emerg Care. 2016;32:801–6.
27. Haddad V Jr, Amorim PC, Haddad WT, et al. Venomous and poisonous arthropods: identification, clinical manifestations of envenomation, and treatments used in human injuries. Rev Soc Bras Med Trop. 2015;48:650–7.
28. Veraldi S, Cuka E, Gaiani F. Scolopendra bites: a report of two cases and review of the literature. Int J Dermatol. 2014;53:869–72.

Infestations and Parasitoses

16

Christos C. Zouboulis and Federica Dassoni

Parasitism is a form of symbiosis in which an organism (parasite) lives in or on another organism and benefits at the expense of the host. This host-parasite association may eventuate to the injury of the hosting organism. Parasites may be grouped in *endo-* and *ectoparasites*. Infections with endoparasites can cause systemic diseases with possible dermatological signs, whereas infestations with ectoparasites only cause cutaneous lesions. The burden of parasitoses often rests on communities in countries of hot climate zones, but parasitic infections and infestations are also on the rise in clinical practices in developed countries due to the increase of traveling individuals and migrating populations. The debilitating impact which a persistent itch of certain parasitosis may have must be taken into account when assessing these conditions. Ectoparasites can also be vectors of pathogens, as discussed in other chapters; in humans they are comprised of two major animal groups, parasitic *arachnids* and parasitic *insects* [1], whereby parasitic arachnids include ticks and mites. As for the ectoparasitic insects, they are exemplified by mosquitoes, tsetse flies, fleas, and lice (Table 16.1).

Table 16.1 Cutaneous parasitic infestations

	Parasites	Cutaneous infestations
Ectoparasites	*Sarcoptes scabiei* var. *hominis*	Scabies
	Pediculus humanus (capitis, corporis)	Pediculosis (capitis, corporis)
	Pthirus pubis	Pediculosis pubis
Helminths	*Ancylostoma* spp.	Cutaneous larva migrans
	Strongyloides spp.	Larva currens
	Schistosoma spp.	Cutaneous schistosomiasis
	Enterobius vermicularis	Cutaneous enterobiasis
	Taenia solium	Cutaneous cysticercosis
	Wuchereria bancrofti, *Brugia malayi*, *Brugia timori*	Acute dermatolymphangioadenitis (lymphatic filariasis)
Protozoa	*Entamoeba histolytica*	Cutaneous amoebiasis

16.1 Scabies

Scabies is one of the most common parasitic conditions, accounting for a substantial proportion of dermatological care in developing countries. Globally, scabies affects more than 130 million people at any time. It is an important communicable endemic disease in resource-poor countries and has been added in 2013 to the list of neglected tropical diseases by the World Health Organization [2, 3]. Rates of scabies occurrence vary in the recent literature from 0.2% in several countries to 71% on the islands of the Pacific Ocean (Oceania) [4]. In countries with Arabic populations, the approximate prevalence of scabies is up to 2.2%, in African countries up to 9.2%. In 2010, it was estimated that the direct effects of scabies infestation on the skin alone led to more than 1.5 million years lived with disability, and the indirect effects of complications on renal and cardiovascular function are far greater. In resource-poor tropical settings, the sheer burden of scabies infestation, as well as their complications, imposes a major cost on health-care systems.

The disease is caused by the human scabies mite *Sarcoptes scabiei* acquired by personal direct skin contact. The mite lays eggs in a previously burrowed tunnel of up to 4 mm into the superficial layer of the epidermis.

C. C. Zouboulis (✉)
Departments of Dermatology, Venereology, Allergology and Immunology, Brandenburg Medical School Theodor Fontane, Dessau Medical Center, Dessau, Germany
e-mail: christos.zouboulis@klinikum-dessau.de

F. Dassoni
Ospedale Alessandro Manzoni, Lecco, Italy

C. E. Orfanos et al. (eds.), *Pigmented Ethnic Skin and Imported Dermatoses*, https://doi.org/10.1007/978-3-319-69422-1_16

16.1.1 Clinical Pictures

Highly pruritic papules with or without excoriations and S-shaped burrows are the classical skin lesions leading to the clinical diagnosis of scabies. At first infestation, symptoms usually do not appear for up to 2–6 weeks; during that time, however, affected persons can spread the mites even without showing visible clinical features. At reinfestation, lesions appear much sooner, 1–4 days after exposure.

Itching and rash may be limited to common predilection sites, such as the finger web spaces, the flexor surfaces of the wrists and elbows, armpits, genital organs, nipples, along the belt line, lower buttocks, and shoulder, or affect much of the body surface (Fig. 16.1). The posterior auricular folds, head, face, neck, palms, and soles often are involved in infants and young children. In chronic scabies, the lesions may become eczematous and hyperkeratotic, thus masking the disease (Fig. 16.2). In dark skin, scabies may also manifest as granulomatous small nodules [5]. The most common and characteristic symptom of scabies infestation is severe pruritus, especially at night, followed by a non-characteristic papular rash caused by sensitization of the host to the proteins and feces of the parasite. Generalized involvement may remain unrecognized and be treated with topical corticosteroid creams and ointments (Figs. 16.3 and 16.4).

Crusted (Norwegian) scabies is a severe form that often affects the elderly, patients with conditions that prevent from itching or scratching (spinal cord injury, paralysis, loss of sensation, mental debility), and also immunocompromised individuals. Vesicles and thick crusts occur that usually contain large numbers of mites (Figs. 16.5 and 16.6). Notably, itching may be absent due to the reduced general condition of the patient. Patients with crusted scabies are highly contagious.

The intense itching of all types of scabies often leads to super infections with *S. aureus* or β-hemolytic streptococci, with the risk of post-streptococcal glomerulonephritis, particularly in children (Fig. 16.7).

Diagnosis of scabies is suspected when pruritus is out of proportion to the physical findings [6] and is confirmed by finding the mite, ova, or fecal pellets on microscopic examination. Scrapings should be obtained after placing glycerol, mineral oil, or immersion oil over a burrow or papule to prevent dispersion of mites while unroofing the papule with the edge of a scalpel. The obtained material is placed on a slide and covered with a cover slip for examination under a light microscope.

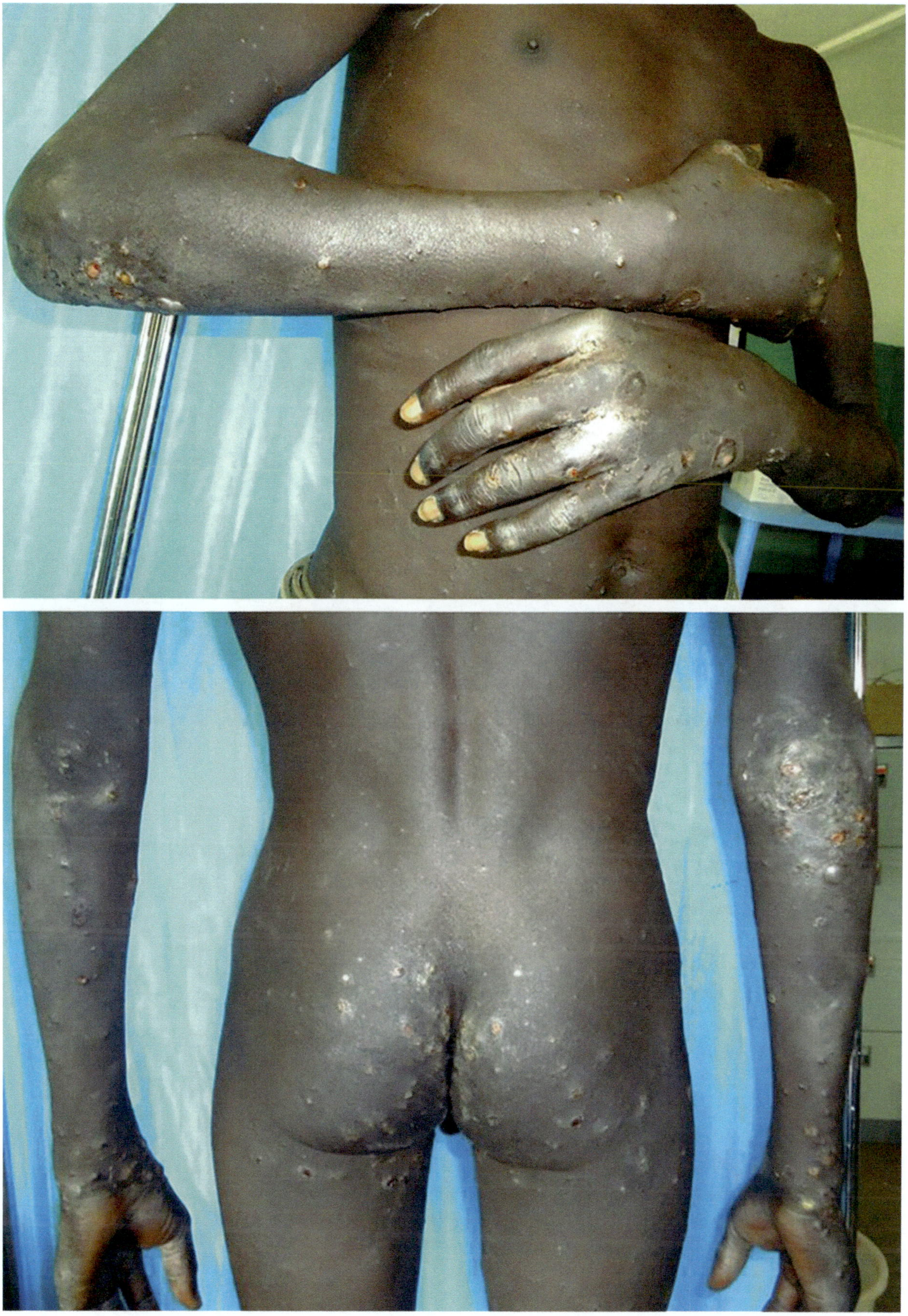

Fig. 16.1 *Scabies.* Disseminated lesions in an immunocompetent adult localized at predilection areas between the fingers, the elbows, and flexor surfaces of the wrists and the buttocks, partly super infected

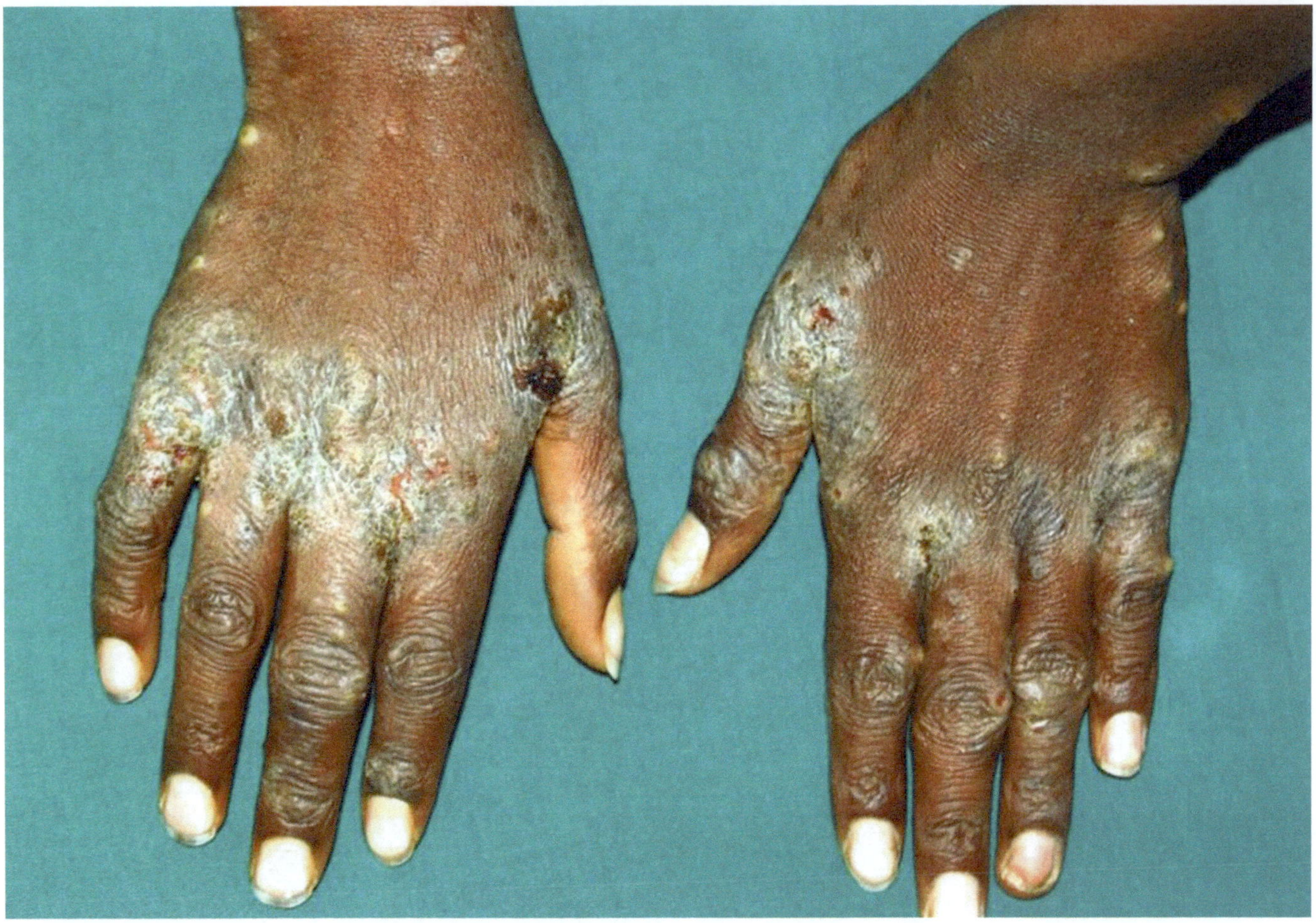

Fig. 16.2 Eczematization of chronic *scabies* with crusts on both hands

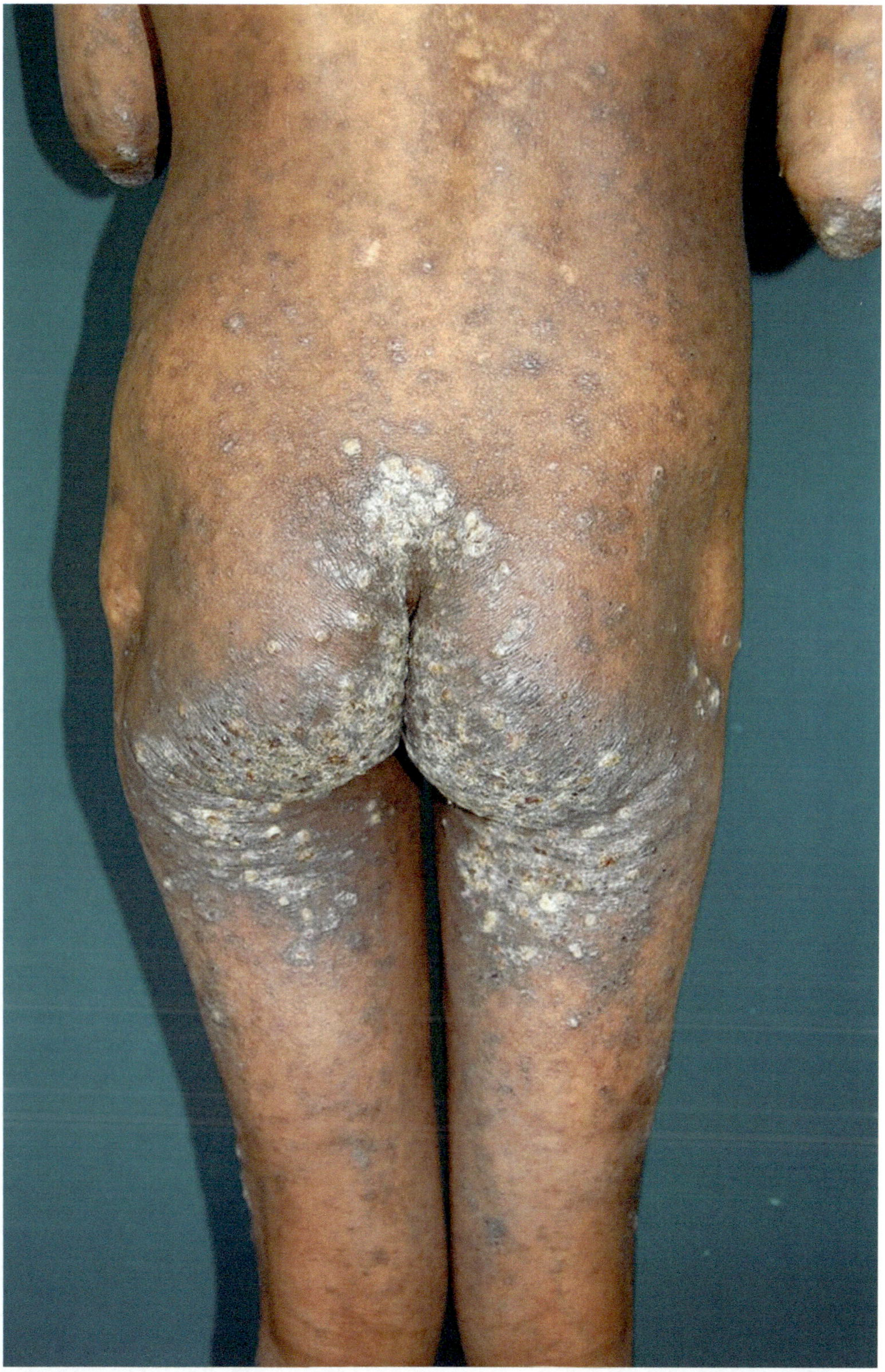

Fig. 16.3 Severe *generalized scabies* in an Ethiopian female immunosuppressed patient, partly eczematized and scaly. Scabies in immunosuppressed individuals is clinically more severe

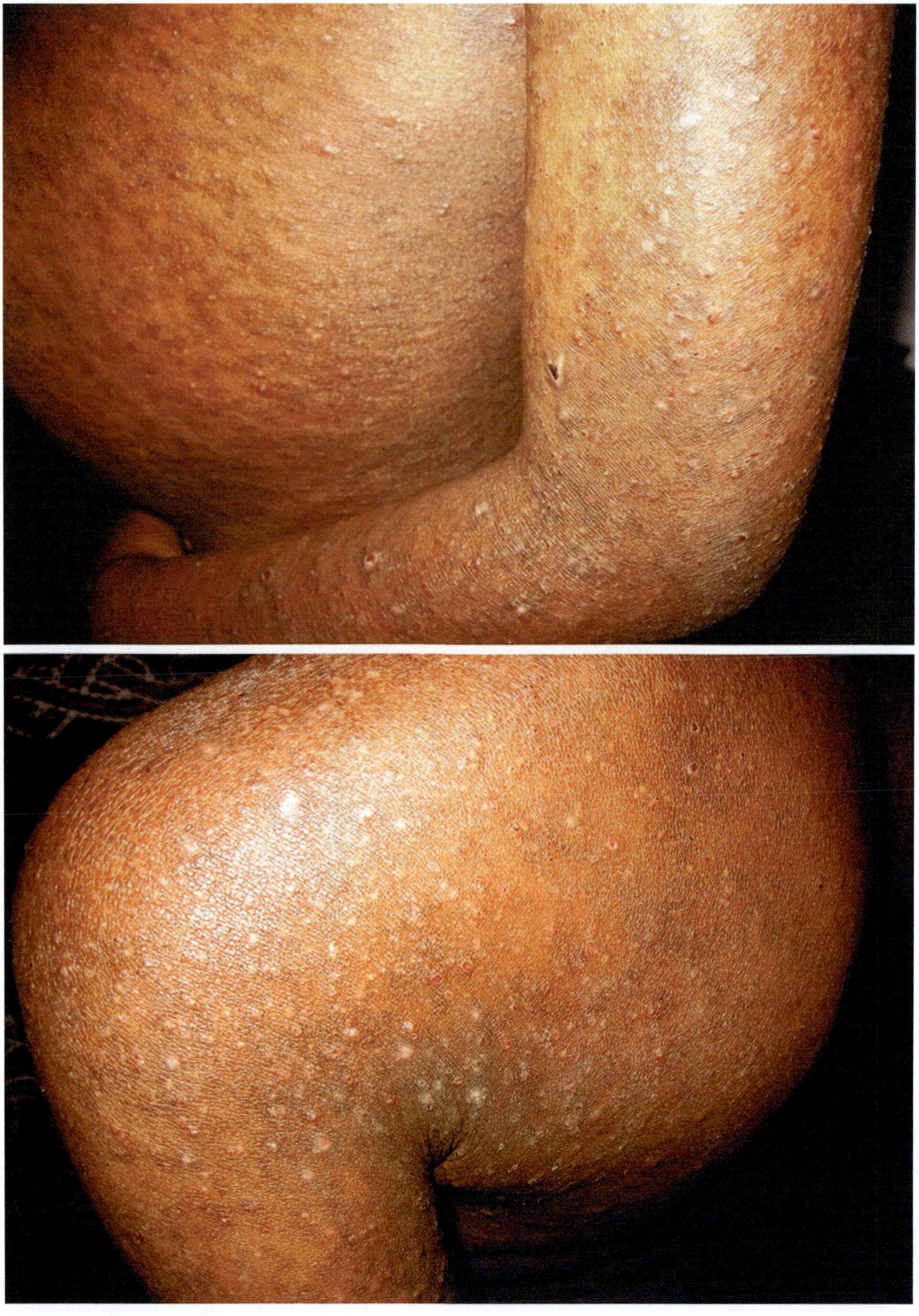

Fig. 16.4 *Generalized scabies*, treated with topical corticosteroids in an East-African young male (Photos: CEO)

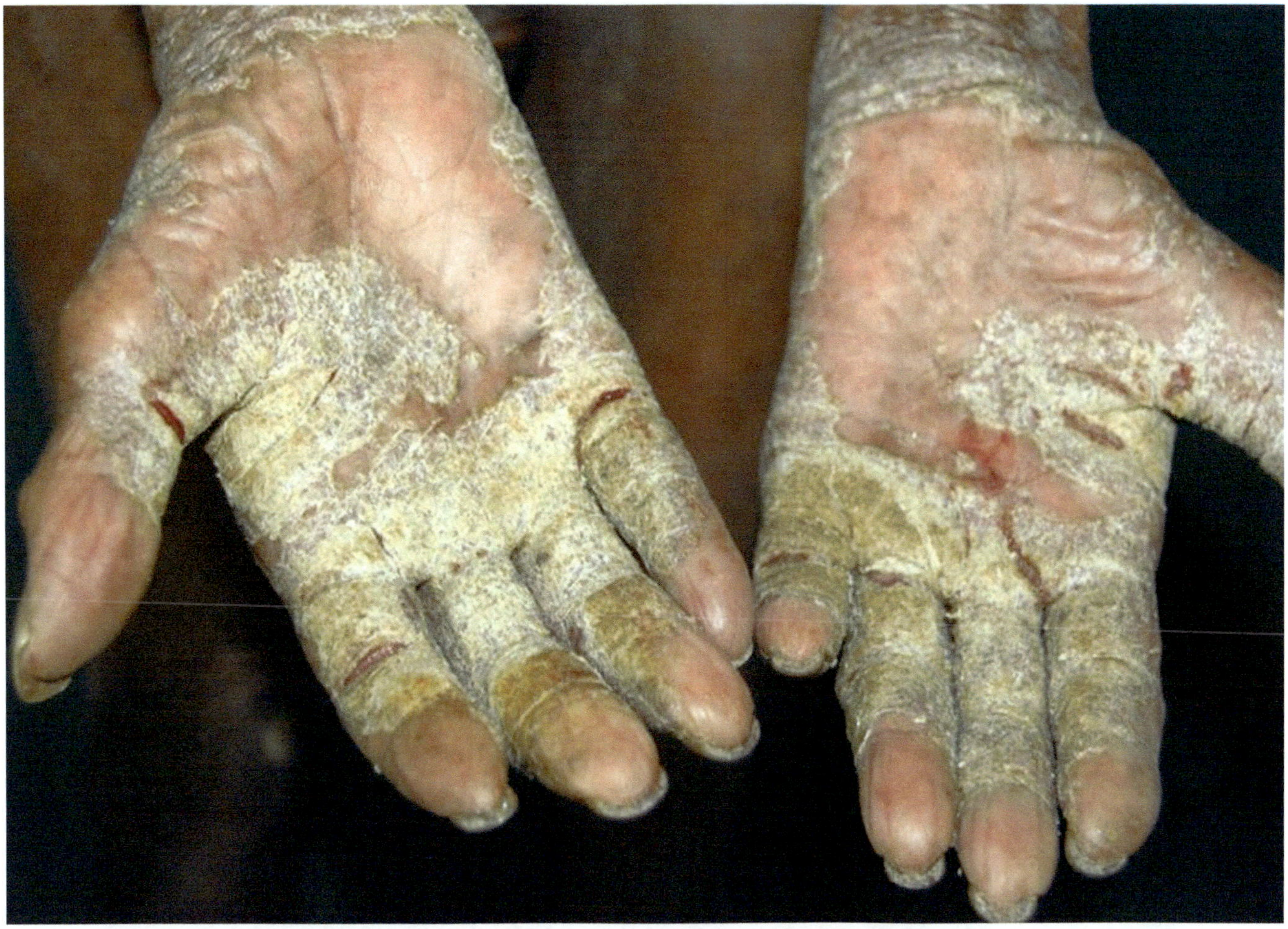

Fig. 16.5 *Norwegian scabies* presenting hyperkeratotic plaques in both hands of an elder immunocompetent patient

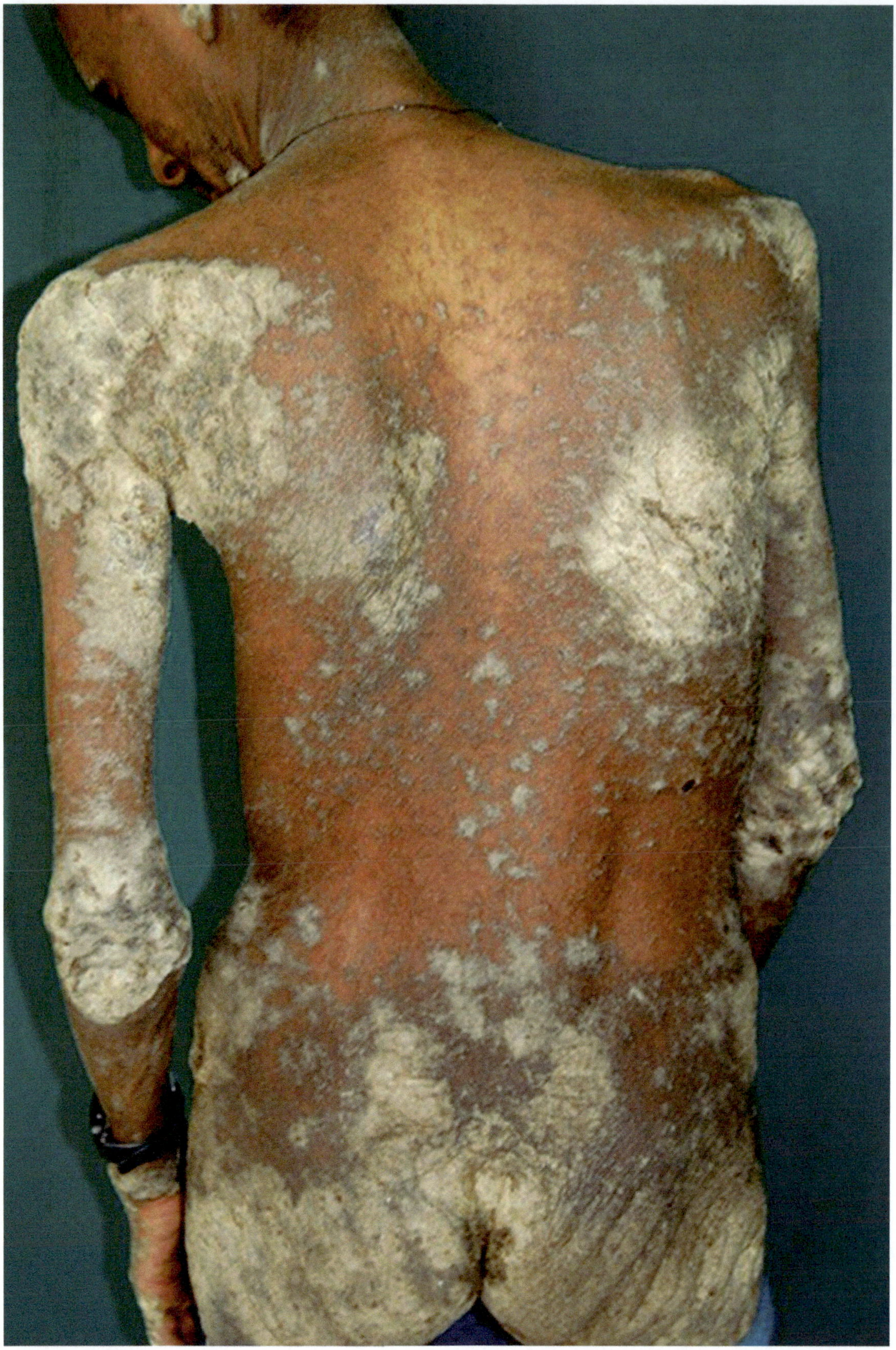

Fig. 16.6 Severe generalized *scabies of the Norwegian type* in an immunocompromised patient

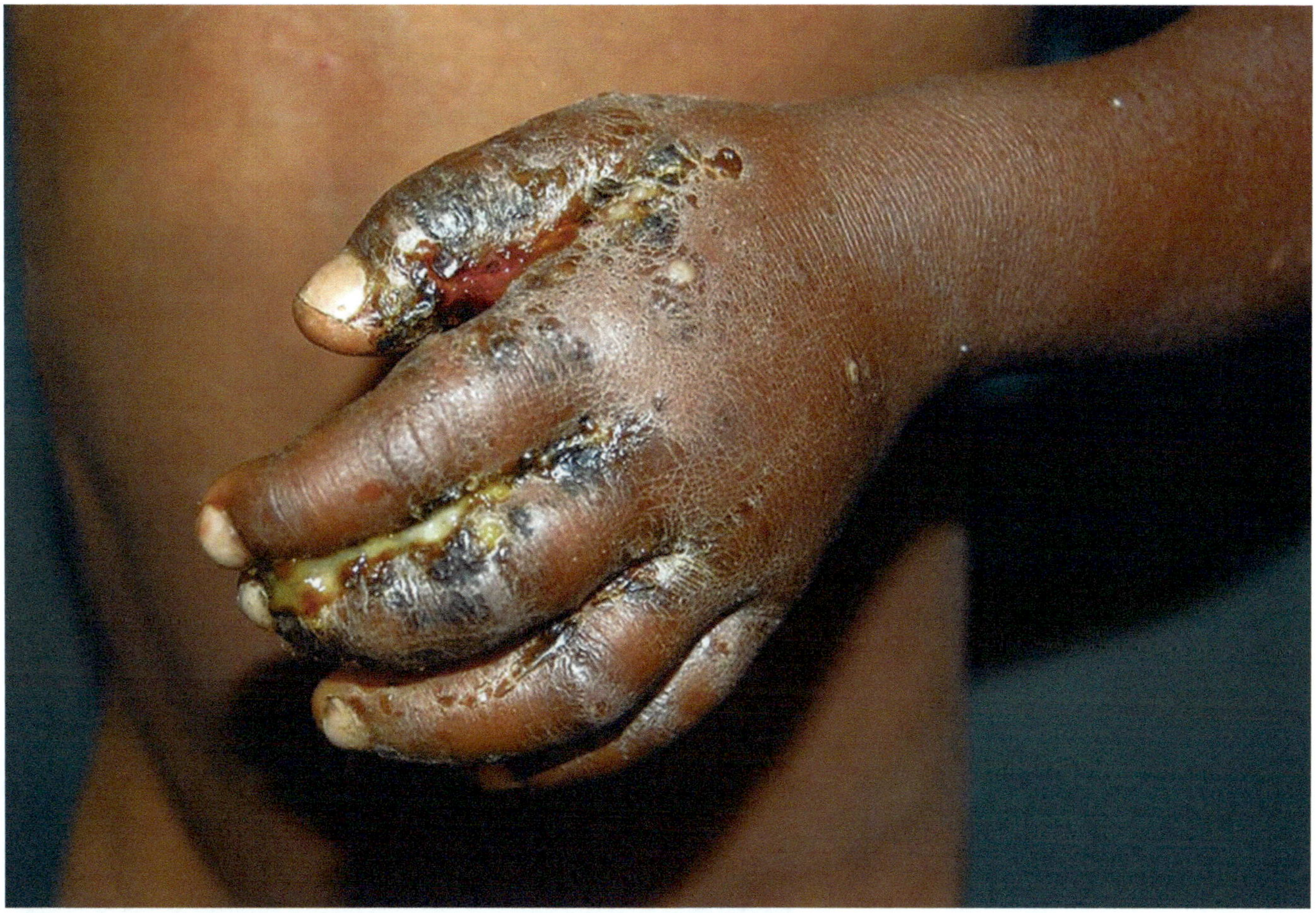

Fig. 16.7 *Scabies*. Severe super infection of the hand in a child. The intense itch often leads to super infections with S. aureus or β-hemolytic streptococci, with the risk of post-streptococcal glomerulonephritis, particularly in children

16.1.2 Treatment

Primary treatment is the administration of topical or oral scabicides [7]. Permethrin, a synthetic pyrethroid, is the first-line topical drug; older children and adults should apply 5% cream (60 g) to the entire body from the neck down, wash it off after 8–14 h, and repeat the procedure after 7 days. Periorbital and perioral regions should be avoided; special attention should be given to intertriginous areas and the umbilical area, fingers, and toes. Alternative medications are emulsions of 10–25% benzyl benzoate or crotamiton (5% gel, 10% lotion, cream, or ointment) to be applied on 3–5 consecutive days. Topical application of precipitated sulfur 6–10% in petrolatum over 24 h for 3 consecutive days is safe and effective for infants <2 months of age.

Ivermectin in a single oral dose 200 μg/kg bw (to be repeated after 7–10 days) is indicated for patients who do not respond or are unable to adhere to topical regimens and in those with widespread crusted scabies. The drug has been successfully used in epidemics in nursing homes, etc. Close contacts should be treated and personal items such as towels, clothing, bedding, etc. should be washed in hot water and dried in a hot drier or isolated in a closed plastic bag for at least 3 days.

Pruritus can be managed with topical corticosteroids and/or oral antihistamines (e.g., hydroxyzine up to 25 mg orally 4×/day). Caution is required when given to elderly patients with hepatic, renal, or cardiac disorders, not recommended for pregnant or lactating women and children <5 years old or with <15 kg body weight.

Secondary infection should be considered in patients with weeping, yellow-crusted lesions and treated with systemic or topical antibiotics against *Staphylococcus aureus* and *Streptococcus pyogenes*. Symptoms and lesions take up to 3 weeks to resolve despite killing of the mites; treatment failures due to resistance, poor penetration, reinfection, or nodular scabies are difficult to recognize. Skin scrapings can be done periodically to check for persistent mites.

16.2 Pediculosis

Pediculosis is worldwide a most common ectoparasitic infestation affecting hundreds of millions of people [8], mainly school children. In the USA, 6–12 million children are afflicted annually [9]. Independent of the country and culture, girls are usually more frequently infested than boys [10]. Although there is no clear association between head lice and poor hygiene or low socioeconomic status [11], crowded urban slums, migrants, refugees, and similar communities are preferred. In a study in Israel, 65% of all Ethiopian migrants were infested with head lice [12]. During the civil wars in Burundi, Rwanda, and Zaire in the 1990s, the prevalence of lice infestations reached 90–100% [13]. The prevalence of pediculosis capitis ranges from 1 to 20% in European countries, occurring in small epidemics mostly in play groups, kindergartens, and schools [10]. To some degree, there has been an increase in the incidence of pediculosis during the last decades, also due to treatment-resistant lice and treatment failures. Pediculosis often results in substantial personal embarrassment and social distress.

The scalp, body, pubis, and eyelashes are infested by three species, the head louse (*Pediculus humanus capitis*), the body louse (*Pediculus humanus corporis*), and pubic louse (*Pthirus pubis*) [10], all of them causing inflammation, itching, and skin discoloration. Head and body lice are transmitted by close contacts mostly under cramped, crowded conditions and pubic lice via sexual contact. The three species differ substantially in morphology and clinical features. Head and pubic lice live directly on the host while body lice in garments. The body louse may also be vector of infectious agents and cause relapsing fever and typhus [14]. Pediculosis corporis differs from scabies by the absence of skin burrows, and the hands and feet are not involved.

16.2.1 Clinical Picture

Louse infestation typically affects the hair of the scalp although it may involve any other hair-bearing areas, causing severe discomfort and pruritus (Fig. 16.8). Physical examination often reveals mild excoriations. Secondary bacterial infection

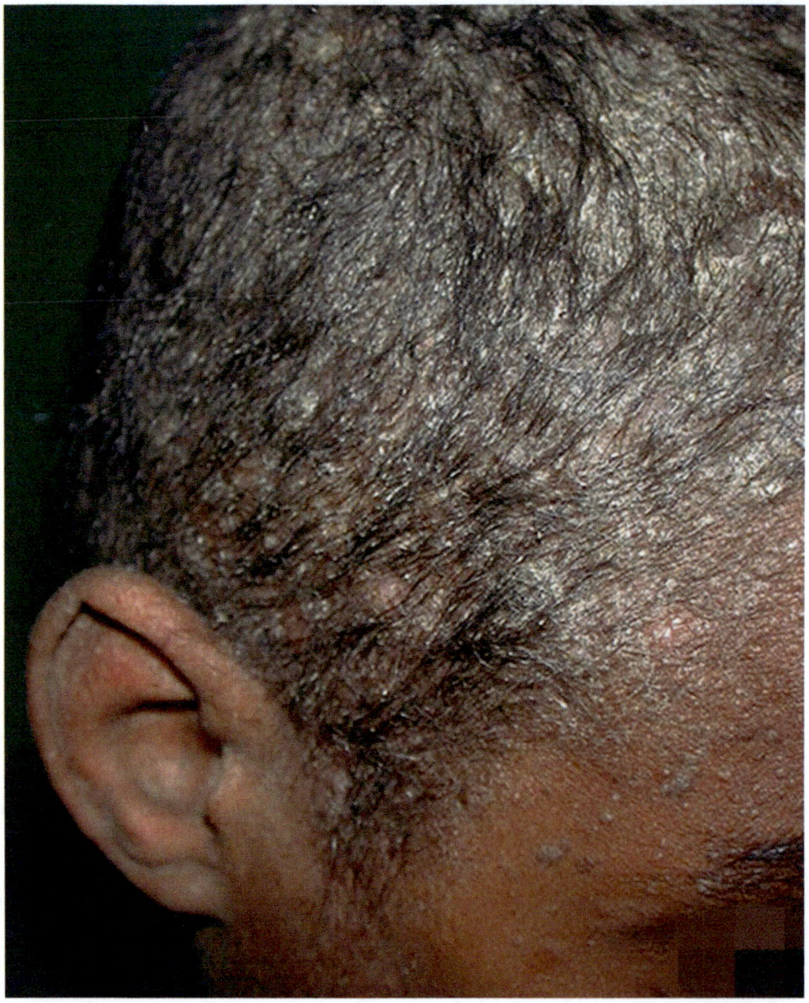

Fig. 16.8 *Pediculosis capitis* with scaly excoriations in an immunocompromised child

may cause folliculitis and regional lymphadenopathy; impetigo and furunculosis are occasionally detected and constitutional symptoms may occur, especially in infants and young children. Infestation of the eyelashes manifests as eye itching, burning, and local irritation. Lice are found usually at the back of the head or behind the ears by combing the wet scalp hair with a fine-tooth comb; in a case, usually ≤20 lice are present; nits are commonly fixed on the basis of the hair shafts. Each adult female louse lays three to five eggs/day; nits typically vastly outnumber the lice. Diagnosis of body lice is by demonstration of lice and nits in clothing, especially at the seams.

16.2.2 Treatment

Secondary bacterial infections should be treated first before eliminating the lice. Wet-crusted lesions are treated by wet compresses with potassium permanganate 1:9000 2×/day, followed by topical mupirocin or other antibacterial preparation.

Management of pediculosis often requires rotation of pediculicides to avoid resistance. Gamma-benzene hexachloride is rubbed to the scalp at night and then shampooed next night, with permethrin 1% creams/ointments or malathion 0.5% solution as alternatives, following their particular instructions. A second course may be required after 7–14 days, if lice are still seen. After applying the topical treatment, nits have to be removed by using a fine-tooth comb on wet hair, in order to prevent reinfestation; shaving of the area may facilitate the efficacy. Most pediculicides also kill nits. Dead nits remain after successful treatment; however, they do not signify active infestation and do not have to be removed; they grow away from the scalp with time. Absence of nits less than 7 mm from the scalp rules out current active infection. An alternate schedule on days 0, 7, and 14 has been proposed for nonovicidal pediculicides. New topical compounds such as benzyl alcohol 5% (nonovicidal) and spinosad 0.9% (ovicidal) were recently introduced and were found effective in cases with resistant lice [15].

A single oral dose of ivermectin 200 μg/kg, repeated in 10 days, has been shown to be effective against head pediculosis; however, ivermectin should not be used for young children with <15 kg body weight. The drug is also available as 0.5–1% topical preparations.

Hot air has been shown to kill >88% of the nits but is variably effective in killing hatched lice. Thirty minutes of hot air, slightly cooler than a blow drier, may be an effective adjunctive measure to treat head lice.

Controversy surrounds the need to clean the personal items of the afflicted persons and the need to exclude children with head lice or nits from school; there are no conclusive data supporting either approach. However, some experts recommend replacement of personal items or thorough cleaning, followed by drying at 55 °C for 30 min. Items that cannot be washed may be placed in airtight plastic bags for 2 weeks to kill the lice, which live only about 10 days. Primary treatment of body lice is thorough cleaning (e.g., cleaning, followed by drying at 65 °C) or replacement of clothing and bedding. Oral antihistamines may be required to alleviate itching.

16.3 Cutaneous Larva Migrans

Cutaneous larva migrans, often called *creeping eruption*, is one of the most common diseases transmitted to travelers, accounting for about 10% of all skin diseases seen when returning from hot climate zones [16]. The disease occurs worldwide, most often in tropical environments. It is usually acquired on sandy soils in Asia, Africa, South or Central America, and the Caribbean [17], caused by the animal hookworm *Ancylostoma* spp.; however, other species such as *Gnathostoma* spp. or even non-hookworm species such as *Dirofilaria conjunctivae*, *Capillaria*, and *Strongyloides* may also be the causative agent [5]. The eggs of the worms in dog or cat feces develop into infective larvae when left in warm moist ground or sand and penetrate into the unprotected skin, when it directly contacts contaminated soil or sand. As a rule, the feet, legs, buttocks, or the back are affected, while the larvae remain confined to the upper dermis.

16.3.1 Clinical Picture

Cutaneous larva migrans causes intense pruritus; classical signs are papules at the site of entry, followed by a growing linear or serpiginous, subcutaneous trail of inflammation that can reach 15–20 cm in length, justifying the designation of a creeping eruption. Most common localization is the dorsal side of the feet (Fig. 16.9), followed by the hands, arms, buttocks, and genitalia (Figs. 16.10 and 16.11). Patients may also develop papules and vesicles resembling folliculitis ("hookworm folliculitis"). The lesions are found occasionally in various other sites such as the scalp, oral mucosa, and the trunk [5]. As a rare complication, patchy pulmonary infiltrates with peripheral blood eosinophilia occur (self-limiting *Löffler syndrome*).

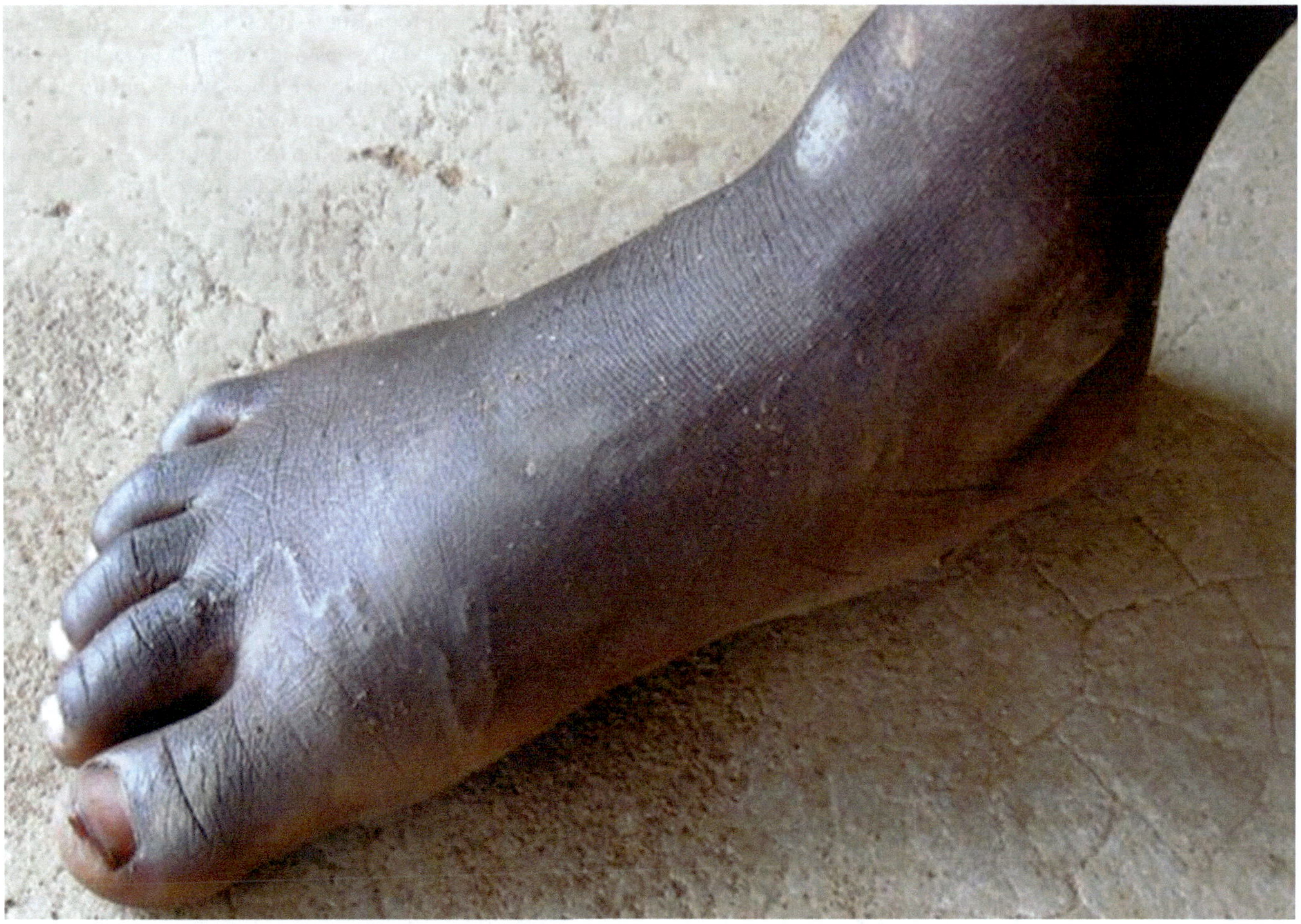

Fig. 16.9 *Cutaneous larva migrans*. Classical serpiginous, subcutaneous trail at the dorsal side of the foot

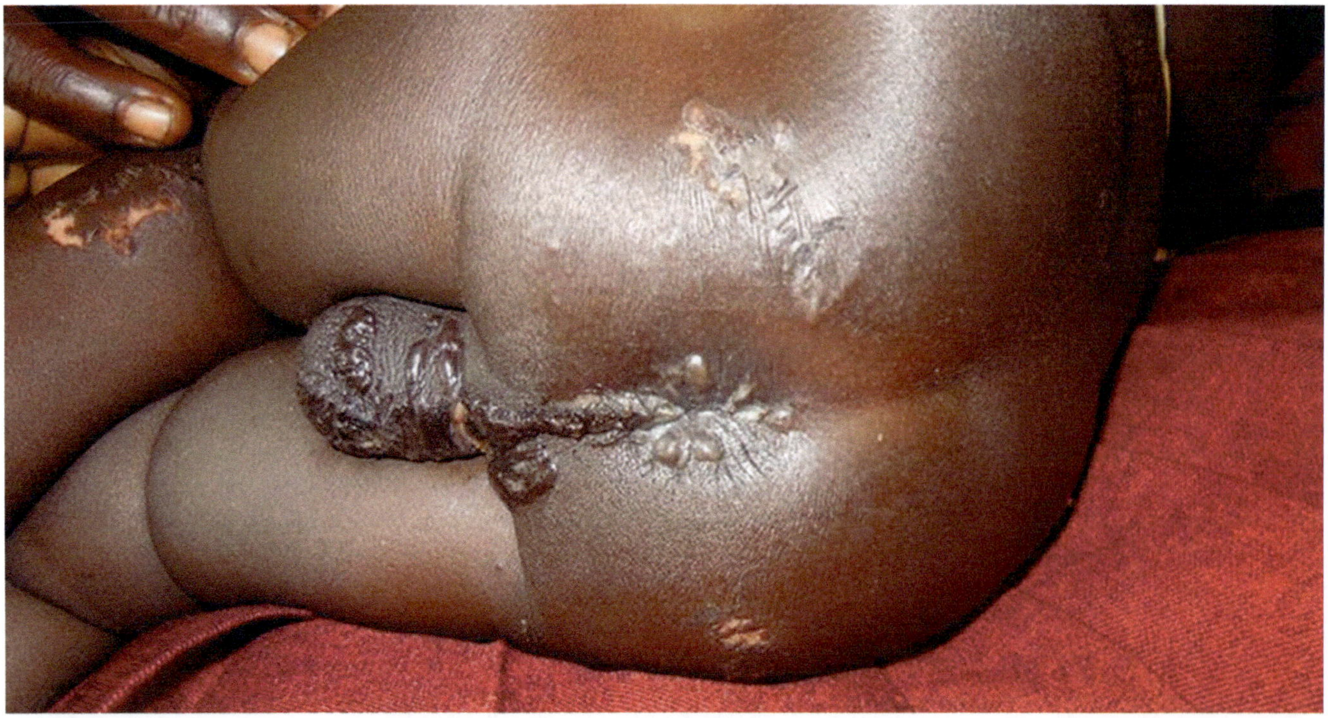

Fig. 16.10 *Cutaneous larva migrans*. Creeping eruption at the buttocks and the genitalia of a child

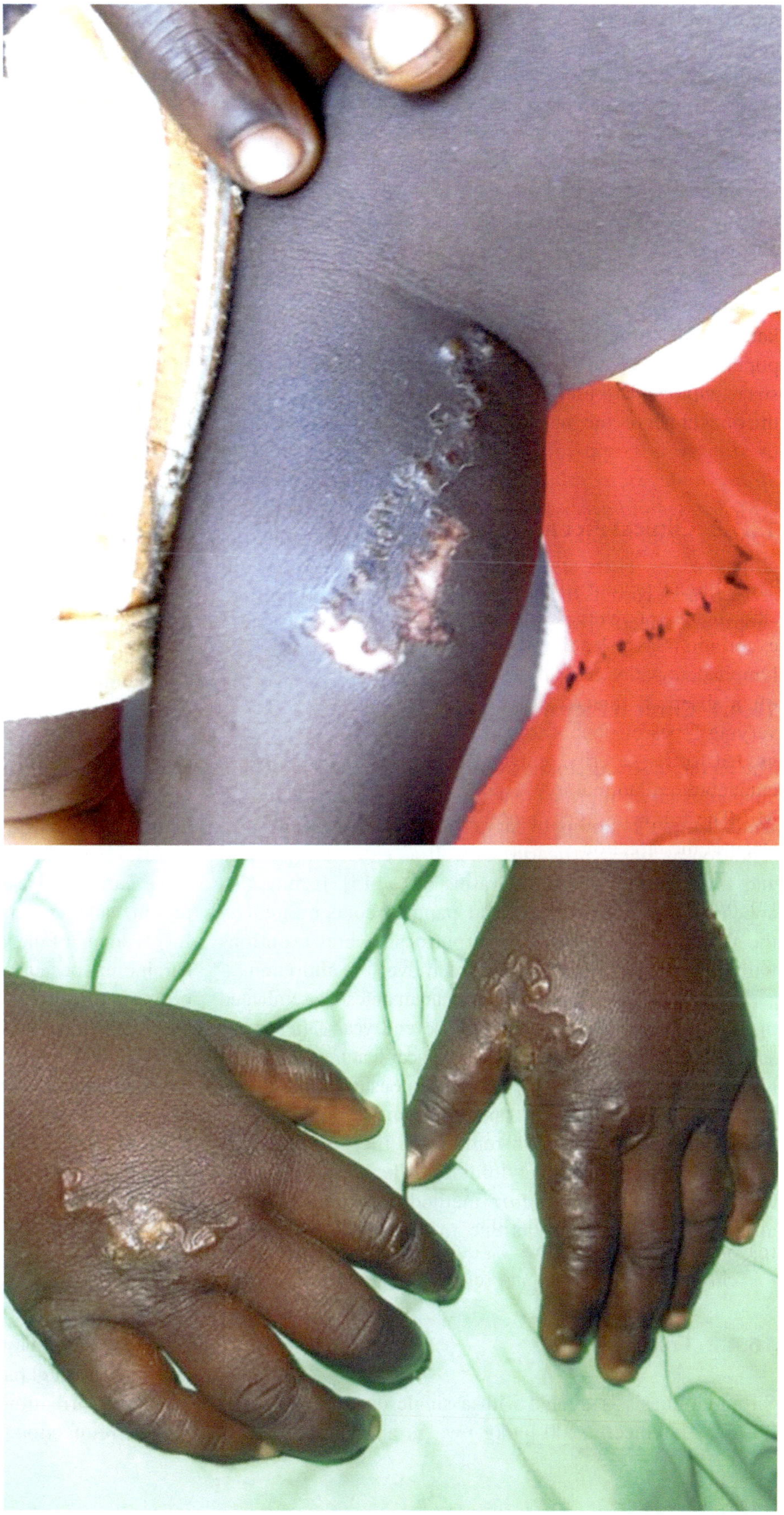

Fig. 16.11 *Cutaneous larva migrans*. Chronified, partly bullous multiple lesions in children

16.3.2 Treatment

Although the infestation resolves spontaneously after a few weeks, discomfort and the risk of secondary bacterial infection require treatment. Topical thiabendazole 15% liquid or cream (compounded) 2–3×/day for 5 days is effective. Oral thiabendazole is rarely used since it is not well tolerated. Oral albendazole (400 mg 1×/day for 3–7 days) and ivermectin 200 μg/kg bw 1×/day for 1–2 days are well tolerated and cure the infestation.

16.4 Larva Currens

Larva currens is a recurrent serpiginous maculopapular or urticarial rash on the buttocks, perineum, and thighs caused by *Strongyloides* spp. [5]. The condition is most often due to *Strongyloides stercoralis*, rarely to *Strongyloides fulleborni* [18]. *Strongyloidiasis* is known to occur in all continents but is most common in the tropics, subtropical regions, and hot climate zones. There are limited epidemiological data available on larva currens, but it is estimated that 30–100 million people are affected by strongyloidiasis worldwide [19].

16.4.1 Clinical Picture

The larvae in strongyloidiasis migrate more rapidly than in cutaneous larva migrans, reaching up to 10 cm/h. Unusual clinical manifestations of larva currens may include presentation as linear urticaria, as well as extensive purpura and skin invasion due to migrating larvae [5]. It may also appear as generalized petechial papules concentrated on the trunk or as progressive purpuric petechial eruptions with reticulated pattern concentrated over the abdomen.

The infestation may remain latent and manifest disseminated in immunocompromised individuals several years after exposure. The diagnosis is based on the clinical features and travel history. Filariform larvae may also be demonstrated in biopsies taken from the site of the rash and/or in dermal granulomas.

Serial stool examination remains as the gold standard for the diagnosis of strongyloidiasis. The *Baermann* concentration and *Harada-Mori* methods are also used as alternative diagnostic tools due to the low sensitivity of other techniques.

16.4.2 Treatment

Strongyloidiasis is treated with a single dose or two daily doses of ivermectin 200 μg/kg bw. As an alternative, oral albendazole may also be given 400 mg 2×/day for 7 days. If not treated, larva currens has been reported to persist for as long as 65 years due to autoinfection [5].

16.5 Cutaneous Enterobiasis (Oxyuriasis)

Cutaneous enterobiasis is common among children and institutionalized persons. It is estimated that more than 200 million people are infected worldwide [5].The disease is caused by *Enterobius vermicularis* transmitted through ingestion or inhalation of embryonated eggs and autoinfection through hand-to-mouth spread. The primary cutaneous manifestation of enterobiasis is nocturnal anal and perianal pruritus that begins 4–6 weeks after infection and may last for months. This is caused by the migration of female worms depositing eggs in the perianal area.

16.5.1 Clinical Picture

Scratching may cause skin irritation, and in more serious cases eczematous dermatitis, hemorrhage, or secondary bacterial infections occur. *Enterobius vermicularis*, if found in ectopic locations, can elicit severe granulomatous inflammation. Ectopic migration often results in infestation of the genital tract in women. This may cause granuloma of the uterus, ovary, fallopian tubes, and pelvic peritoneum [5]. In some cases, this may result in a polypoid mass in the anal region and pruritus vulvae with vaginal discharge. Involvement of the vulva in enterobiasis may be mistaken for carcinoma because of the presence of differentiated cell proliferation.

The disease is diagnosed using a Scotch test from the perianal area or cellulose-tape slide test, performed in the morning before defecation [19]; the presence of *Enterobius* can also be diagnosed by demonstrating eggs of the helminths in the feces (Fig. 16.12), perianal scrapings, or swabs from under the fingernails or by clinically detecting adult worms around the anus, usually at night.

16.5.2 Treatment

Albendazole is the treatment of choice, although mebendazole and pyrantel pamoate are also effective. Considering its familial distribution, the entire family should be treated to prevent reinfection [5].

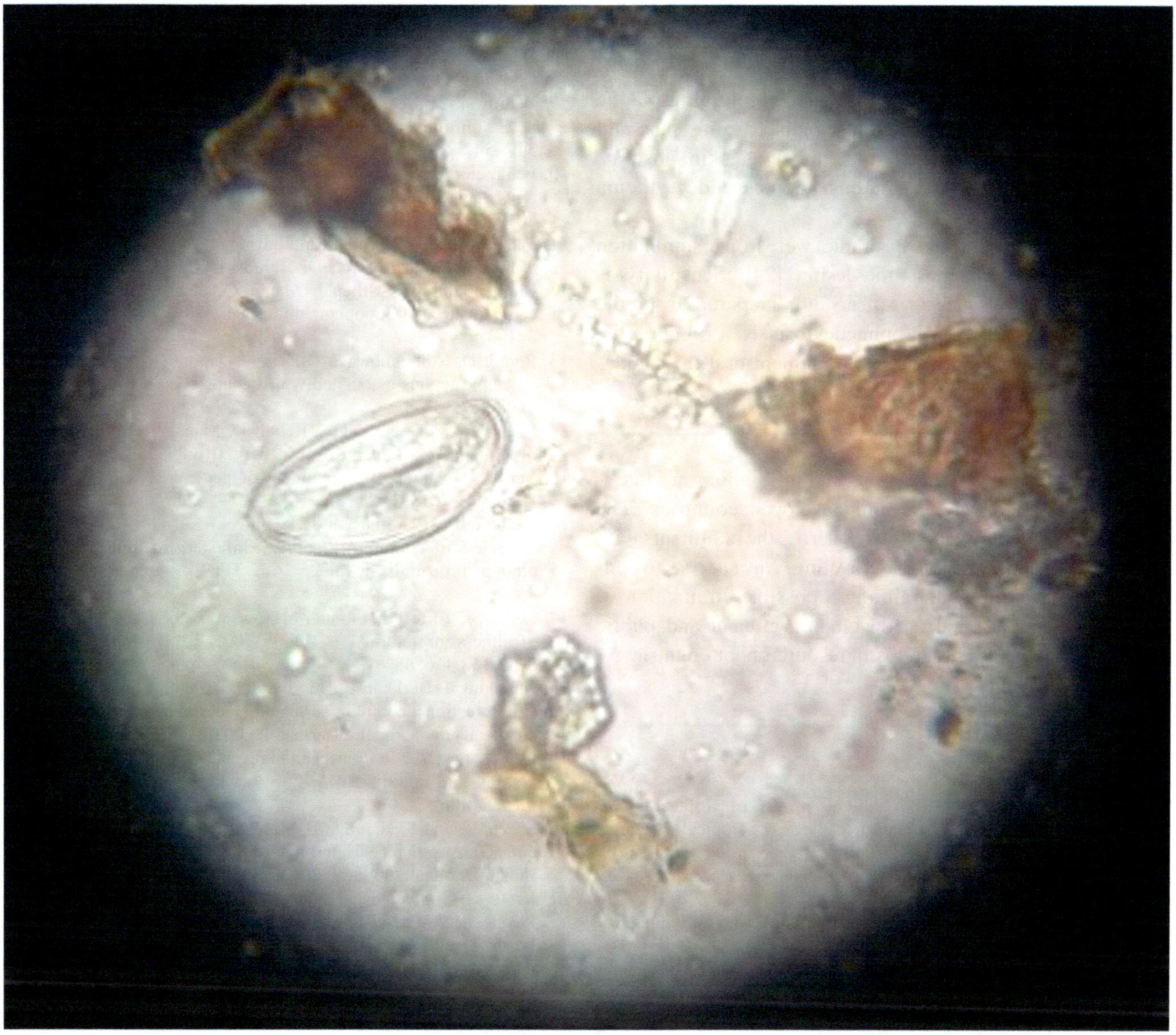

Fig. 16.12 *Enterobiasis*. Microscopical detection of *Enterobius vermicularis* eggs in the feces of a patient

16.6 Cutaneous Cysticercosis

Cases with cutaneous involvement have been reported in India, Africa, Mexico, and South America [20]. Cysticercosis, caused by the larvae of *Taenia solium*, occurs when a person ingests the parasite's eggs. The larvae lodge in the tissues, including the muscle and brain, and form spherical milky white cysts or cysticerci [19]. Approximately half of all cases present cutaneous manifestations, detectable as well-defined anechoic or hypoechoic lesions with or without calcification. The number of lesions may vary and may be too many to count. Cysticercosis also has the uncommon etiology of subcutaneous swellings in children [21]. Although less common, cutaneous cysticercosis may also result in neurocysticercosis. Diagnosis of the disease requires imaging and serological examinations. The history of travel and food intake should be also considered.

Treatment of cutaneous cysticercosis includes the use of anthelminthics such as albendazole or praziquantel together with surgery. There is, however, no generally accepted treatment regimen for the condition [21].

16.7 Cutaneous Amoebiasis

Cutaneous amoebiasis is caused by infection of wounds with *Entamoeba histolytica* trophozoites, a protozoan parasite found worldwide. It is transmitted via direct or indirect fecal-oral route [22]. Cutaneous amoebiasis is a rare skin manifestation of the infestation; amoebiasis can destroy various human tissues, such as the intestinal mucosa, the liver, and to a lesser extent the brain and skin.

The disease initially presents as a deep-seated, well-defined, indurated, painful, progressively enlarging plaque with overlying ulcers and sinuses discharging pus and blood. Amoebiasis may also manifest as skin abscess, which may start as erythematous nodules and erythema nodosum [23].

Clinical suspicion and a simple wet drop examination may be used to diagnose the lesion [24]. Sensitivity is increased when tissues or smears are prepared from the edges of the ulcer. Erythrophagocytosis is a sign of the pathogenicity of the disease. For treatment oral metronidazole is the drug of choice [19].

Conclusions

A series of parasitic infections and infestations are in rising, both in developing and developed countries. The causative agents are transferred across the continents with increased globalization and traveling. Any success to control these entities, first aiming a possible elimination of scabies, will depend on developing clinical and public large-scale health programs in resource-poor countries.

References

1. Goldsmith JM, Leggat PA, editors. primer of tropical medicine. Brisbane: The Australasian College of Tropical Medicine Publications; 2005. p. 10.2.1–10.2.18.
2. Currie BJ. Scabies and global control of neglected tropical diseases. N Engl J Med. 2015;373:2371–2.
3. World Health Organization. 2017. http://www.who.int/lymphatic_filariasis/epidemiology/scabies/en/.
4. Romani L, Steer AC, Whitfeld MJ, et al. Prevalence of scabies and impetigo worldwide: a systematic review. Lancet Infect Dis. 2015;15:960–7.
5. Belizario V Jr, Delos Trinos JP, et al. Cutaneous manifestations of selected parasitic infections in western pacific and southeast asian regions. Curr Infect Dis Rep. 2016;18:30.
6. Johnston G, Sladden M. Scabies: diagnosis and treatment. BMJ. 2005;331:619–22.
7. Sunderkötter C, Feldmeier H, Fölster-Holst R, et al. S1 guidelines on the diagnosis and treatment of scabies—short version. J Dtsch Dermatol Ges. 2016;14:1155–67.
8. Chosidow O. Scabies and pediculosis. Lancet. 2000;355:819–26.
9. Wadowski L, Balasuriya L, Price HN, et al. Lice update: new solutions to an old problem. Clin Dermatol. 2015;33:347–54.
10. Feldmeier H. Pediculosis capitis: new insights into epidemiology, diagnosis and treatment. Eur J Clin Microbiol Infect Dis. 2012;31:2105–10.
11. Falagas M, Matthaiou D, Rafailidis P, et al. Worldwide prevalence of head lice. Emerg Infect Dis. 2008;14:1493–4.
12. Mumcuoglu KY, Miller J, Manor O, et al. The prevalence of ectoparasites in Ethiopian immigrants. Isr J Med Sci. 1993;29:371–3.
13. Raoult D, Ndihokubwayo JB, Tissot-Dupont H, et al. Outbreak of epidemic typhus associated with trench fever in Burundi. Lancet. 1998;352:353–8.
14. Sangaré AK, Doumbo OK, Raoult D. Management and treatment of human lice. Biomed Res Int. 2016;2016:8962685.
15. Verma P, Namdeo C. Treatment of pediculosis capitis. Indian J Dermatol. 2015;60:238–47.
16. Vasievich MP, Villarreal JD, Tomecki KJ. Got the travel bug? A review of common infections, infestations, bites, and stings among returning travelers. Am J Clin Dermatol. 2016;17:451–62.
17. Leder K, Torresi J, Libman MD, et al. GeoSentinel surveillance of illness in returned travelers, 2007–2011. Ann Intern Med. 2013;158:456–68.
18. Meinking T, Burkhart C, Burkhart C. Changing paradigms in parasitic infections: common dermatological helminthic infections and cutaneous myiasis. Clin Dermatol. 2003;21:407–16.
19. Centers for Disease Control and Prevention. Parasites–scabies: prevention and control. 2015. http://www.cdc.gov/parasites/scabies/prevent.html.
20. Sacchidanand S, Namitha P, Mallikarjuna M, et al. Disseminated cutaneous cysticercosis and neurocysticercosis: a rare occurrence. Indian Dermatol Online J. 2012;3:135–7.
21. Kraft R. Cysticercosis: an emerging parasitic disease. Am Fam Physician. 2007;76:91–6.
22. World Health Organization. Amoebiasis. 2015. http://www.who.int/ith/diseases/amoebiasis/en/.
23. Verma G, Sharma N, Shanker V, et al. Amoebiasis cutis: clinical suspicion is the key to early diagnosis. Australas J Dermatol. 2010;51:52–5.
24. Fernández-Díez J, Magaña M, Magaña M. Cutaneous amoebiasis: 50 years of experience. Cutis. 2012;90:310–4.

17 Ulcers in Hot Climate Zones

Federica Dassoni

Skin ulcers are a common problem in the Western world, where most ulcers localized on the legs are due to venous insufficiency, arterial disease, neuropathies (usually diabetic), malignancies, or combinations of those. In addition, physicians may be consulted for imported skin ulcers because of the increasing travels to exotic locations. The prevalence of leg ulcers in hot climate zones is largely unknown; there have been no studies on large series. The most common causes for ulcers in a global perspective are thought to be infections, including pyoderma, mycobacterial infections, tropical ulcer, diphtheria, anthrax, and others. In some parts of the world, cutaneous leishmaniasis is one of the most prevalent causes; this is also one of the ten most frequent causes of skin diseases in travelers returning from tropical countries.

Infection with *Mycobacterium (M) ulcerans*, *M. marinum*, *M. leprae*, and *M. tuberculosis* may cause ulcers. Cutaneous tuberculosis is rare in travelers but may be well encountered in immigrants from developing countries. Neuropathy secondary to leprosy often leads to ulcer formation. Buruli ulcer, caused by *M. ulcerans*, is endemic in foci in Africa and has been reported as an imported disease in the West. Cutaneous diphtheria and anthrax (caused by *Bacillus anthracis*) are still endemic in many tropical countries. Sporotrichosis, chromo(blasto)mycosis, and mycetoma are the most common mycoses that may be accompanied by ulceration; these infections are restricted to certain regions and result from direct penetration of the agent into the skin by minor trauma. Some forms of *filariasis* (e.g., *Wuchereria bancrofti*) and podoconiosis (mossy foot) may also lead to ulceration, secondary to lymphedema and/or scratching. Myiasis and tungiasis are also possible causes of skin ulcers. Other ulcers in the tropics are of mixed vascular etiology, secondary to hemopathies, malignancies, endemic Kaposi's sarcoma, and herpes simplex infections in immunosuppressed patients, and of traumatic origin (e.g., burns), neuropathic secondary to diabetes or paraplegia and idiopathic or secondary to lymphedema and osteomyelitis. Ulcers in hot climate zones are occasionally non-specific and cannot be attributed to a clear etiology. In developing countries diagnosis is often made on clinical grounds because of lacking health facilities and diagnostic techniques.

17.1 Tropical Ulcer

Tropical ulcers are common in hot humid tropical or subtropical areas; their exact prevalence is unknown. There are reports from Western, Central, and Eastern Africa, India, New Guinea, East Asia, and Fiji islands, also on travelers and after sport injuries [1–3]. Ulcers are more commonly seen in children and young adults, often following minor trauma and contact with mud and contaminated water. The more commonly involved sites are lower leg and foot, rarely arms and upper leg. Malnutrition and poor health do not seem to be risk factors for the development of a tropical ulcer [6]. Both sexes are affected; some authors reported a male and some others female predominance. Tropical ulcer is more frequent during the hot rainy seasons, attributed to sweating, maceration of the skin, and scratching, thus introducing the agents.

The rising numbers of travelers visiting tropical rural areas, especially ecotourists, workers or foreign aid workers, and military personnel returning from tropical regions, as well as in immigrants from endemic geographic regions, have led to increasing numbers of imported tropical ulcers in Western countries [4].

17.1.1 Etiology

Tropical ulcers are thought to be a combined infection with anaerobic and aerobic bacteria. Anaerobes are always present, together with aerobes or facultative anaerobes, particularly in the early phase of the ulcers, suggesting that their combination is important for the pathogenesis. The anaerobic *Fusobacterium ulcerans* has

F. Dassoni, M.D.
Ospedale Alessandro Manzoni di Lecco,
Centro Medico Santagostino, Milano, Italy

C. E. Orfanos et al. (eds.), *Pigmented Ethnic Skin and Imported Dermatoses*, https://doi.org/10.1007/978-3-319-69422-1_17

been isolated in about 60% of the cases, as well as *Bacteroides* spp., *E. coli*, enterobacteria, staphylococci, and streptococci [5, 6]. Spirochetes have been also identified; their pathogenetic role is unclear. Anaerobic bacteria showing similar morphology to the ones causing ulcers have been isolated in soil and water in endemic regions. A hot and humid climate is necessary for the survival of the causative organisms, and small skin abrasions allow penetration from the contaminated mud or stagnant water into the skin. The release of toxins is thought to cause tissue necrosis.

17.1.2 Clinical Picture

Tropical ulcers are ulcerative necrotic lesions which result from mixed bacterial infection. They are most frequently seen on the lower legs but may occasionally occur on thighs and arms, showing ragged, rolled, and undermined edges surrounded by edema in early stages (Figs. 17.1 and 17.2). The ulcer initially occurs at the site of minimal trauma; the maximum size is reached after 6 weeks. It starts acutely as a small pustule which enlarges gradually to involve the dermis and subcutaneous tissue. When it ruptures foul-smelling blood-stained pus exudes. A gray crusting may cover the ulcer in the early stages, and considerable tissue necrosis develops. With time, granulation tissue is formed. If untreated, the ulcer usually runs a chronic course [7].

In the acute phase, the wound will be painful; regional lymphadenopathy is absent. If the wound becomes chronic, the pain abates and the ulcer becomes asymptomatic. Long-standing lesions may be very difficult to differentiate from other types of ulceration. Complications of these lesions may be bacterial superinfections (including tetanus), necrosis/gangrene, and septicemia. If untreated, the ulcer may involve the underlying periosteum (about 10% of the cases) with the risk of developing osteomyelitis. Squamous cell carcinoma may develop from the ulcer or scar after several years [8]. In endemic areas, patients usually present with large and complicated ulcers of long-standing duration. The diagnosis in rural areas of developing countries is difficult as cultures are rarely available. Histopathology is non-specific.

Differential diagnosis includes vascular ulcers, ulcerative pyoderma (which have a more rapid evolution), cutaneous diphtheria, Buruli ulcers (only in endemic areas), pyoderma gangrenosum, neuropathic ulcers secondary to leprosy, ulcerative cutaneous leishmaniasis, traumatic ulcers, and neoplasms (Figs. 17.3, 17.4, 17.5, 17.6, 17.7, 17.8 and 17.9).

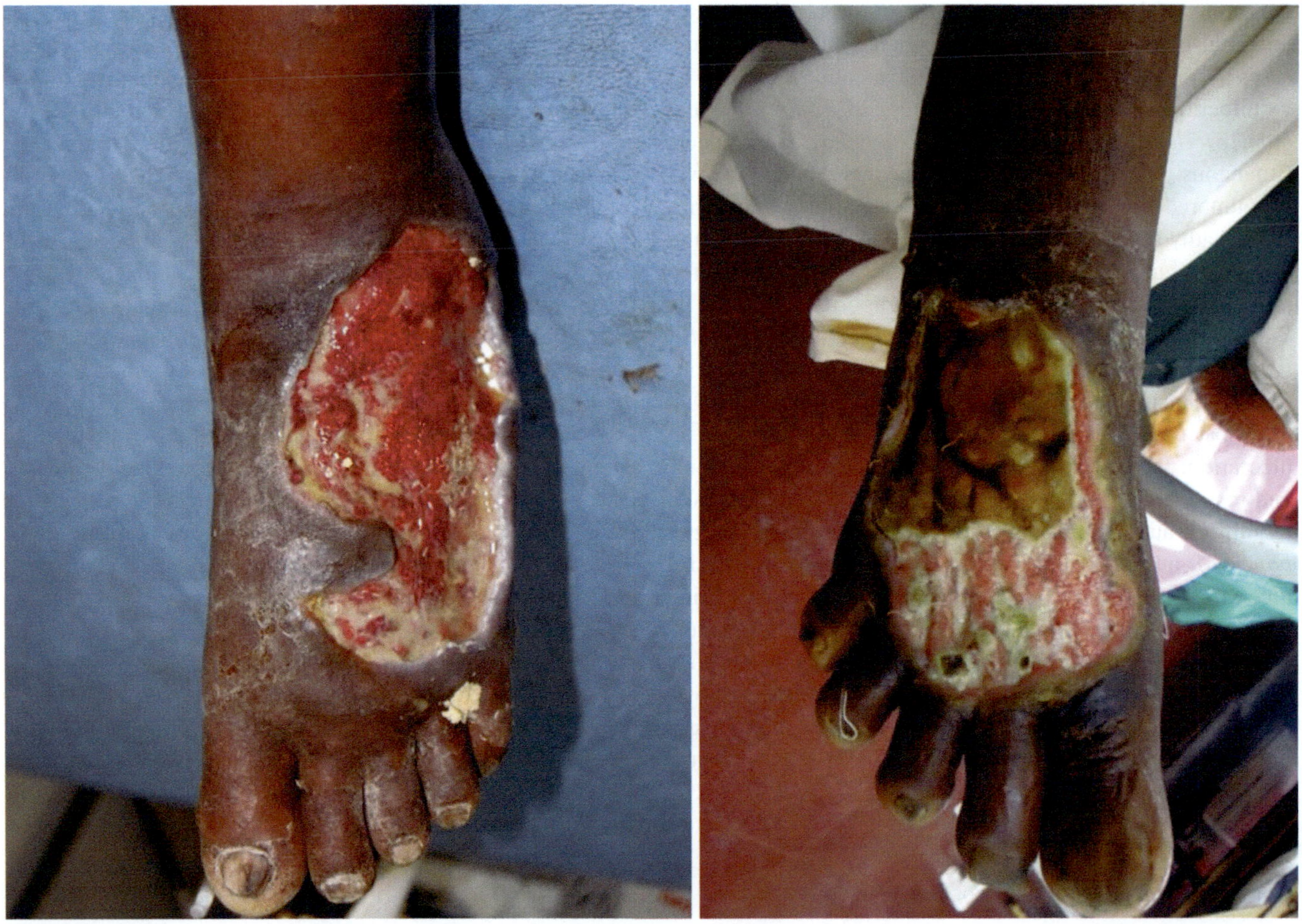

Fig. 17.1 *Left*: tropical ulcer on the foot of a young boy (Ethiopia) (courtesy INMP Institute, Rome; photo FD). *Right*: tropical ulcer partly covered by necrotic tissue (courtesy Chaaria Mission Hospital, Kenya)

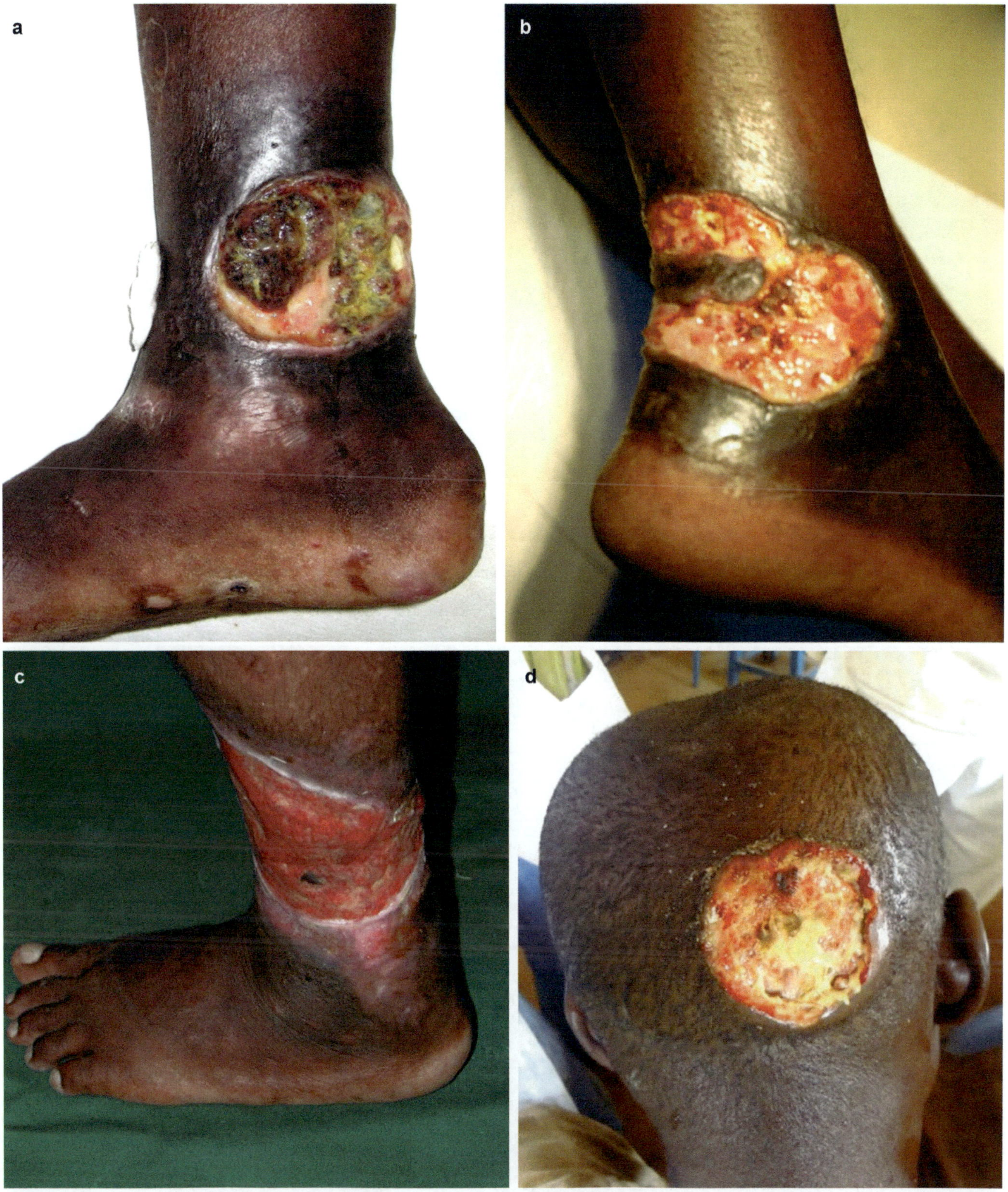

Fig. 17.2 *Tropical ulcers*. (**a**) Acute deeply progressive, Ziehl-Neelsen smear negative. DD: Buruli ulcus (RDTC Moshi, Tanzania; courtesy CEO), (**b**) recurrent and chronified (RDTC, Moshi Tanzania; courtesy CEO), (**c**) in healing phase, and (**d**) unsually sited on the scalp (courtesy Nzara Mission Hospital, South Sudan)

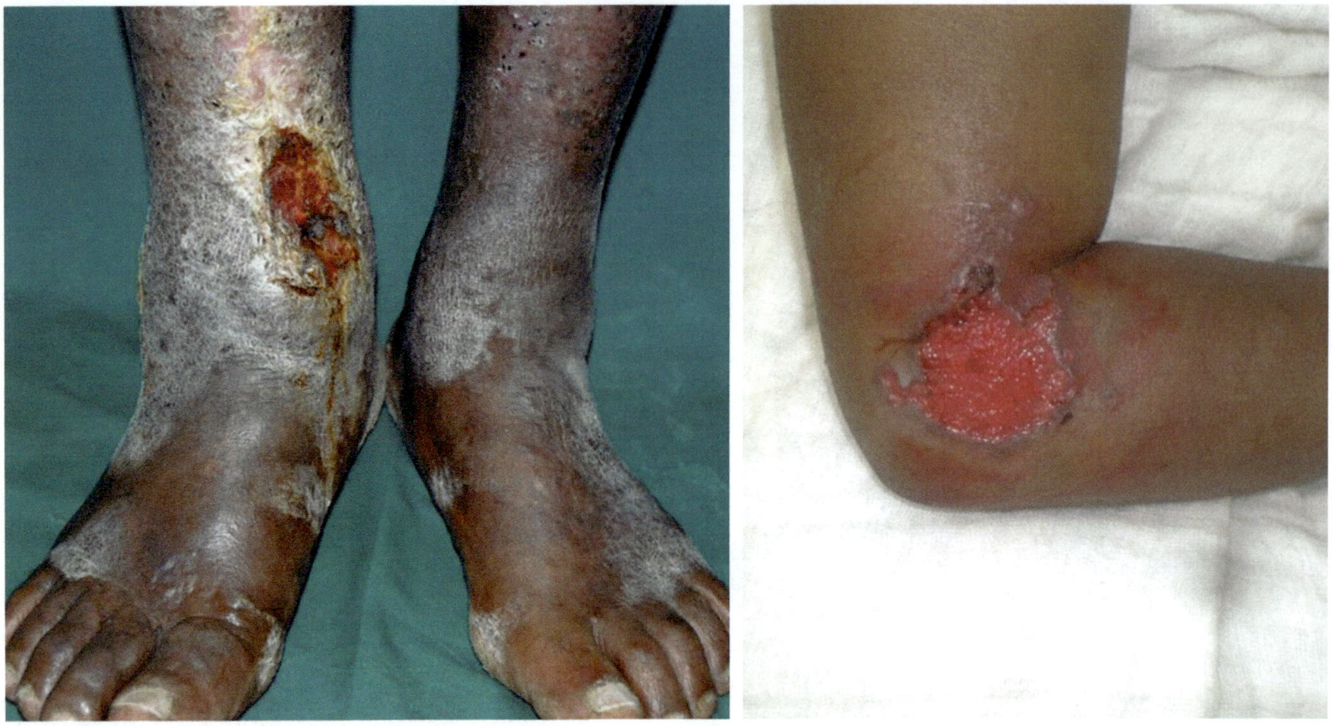

Fig. 17.3 Differential diagnoses *Left*, *venous ulcer* in a farmer. DD: tropical or Buruli ulcer; *right*, ulcerative *leishmaniasis* in a child (Ethiopia). DD: tropical ulcer (Ethiopia) (courtesy INMP Institute FD)

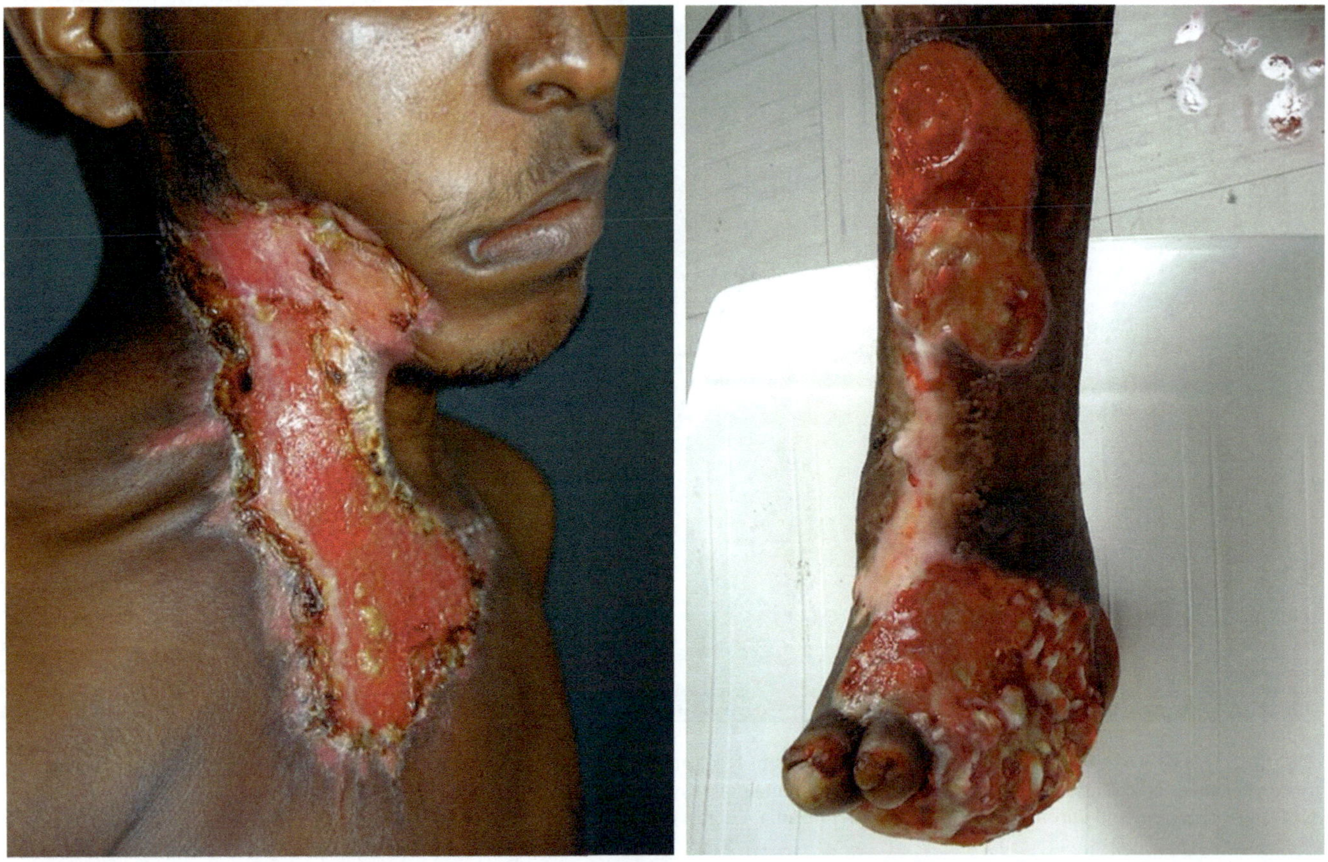

Fig. 17.4 Differential diagnoses *Left*, ulcerous *cutaneous tuberculosis* (scrofuloderma), 4–5 years duration. DD: tropical ulcer, Buruli ulcer. Skin smear confirmed the presence of mycobacteria; *right*, *neuropathic ulcer* secondary to leprosy. DD: neuropathic diabetic ulcer, other neuropathies (Ethiopia) (courtesy INMP Institute, Rome; photo FD)

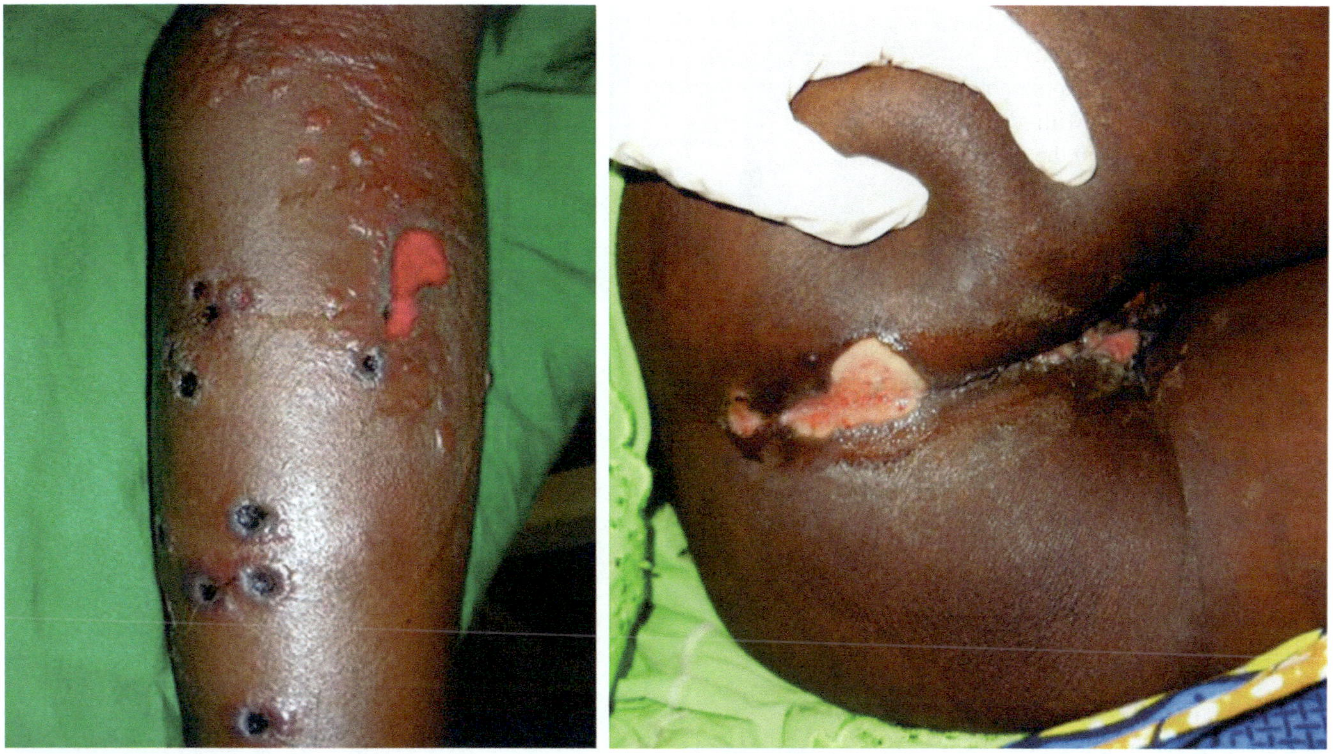

Fig. 17.5 Differential diagnoses *Left*, multiple ulcers in *anthrax*, showing necrotic areas and surrounding blisters (courtesy Chaaria Mission Hospital, Kenya); *right*, multilesional *genital herpes* simplex in an immunosuppressed HIV-positive patient (courtesy Nzara Mission Hospital, South Sudan)

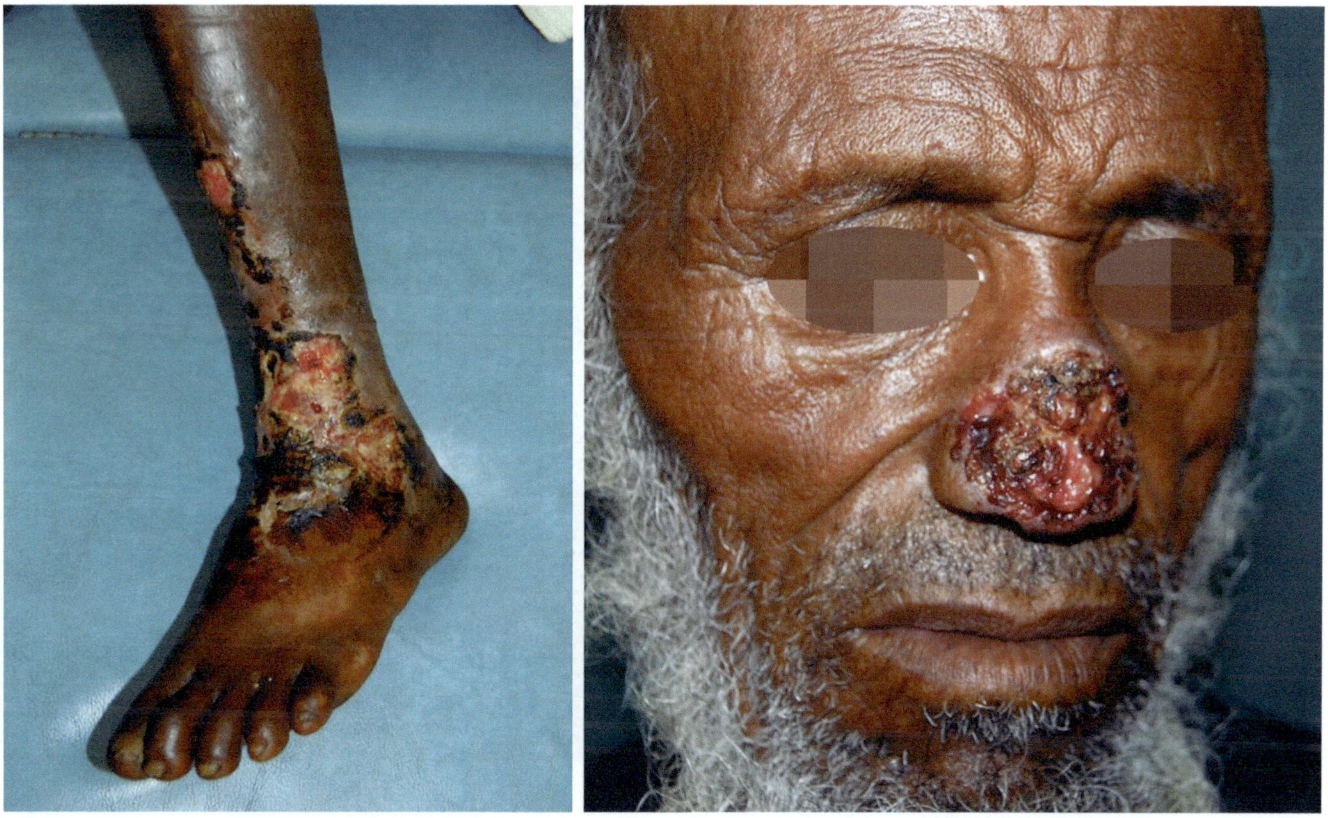

Fig. 17.6 Differential diagnoses *Left*: Ulcers in *segmental scleroderma*; *right*: Ulcerated *basal cell carcinoma* (ulcus rodens) (Ethiopia) (courtesy INMP Institute, Rome; photo FD)

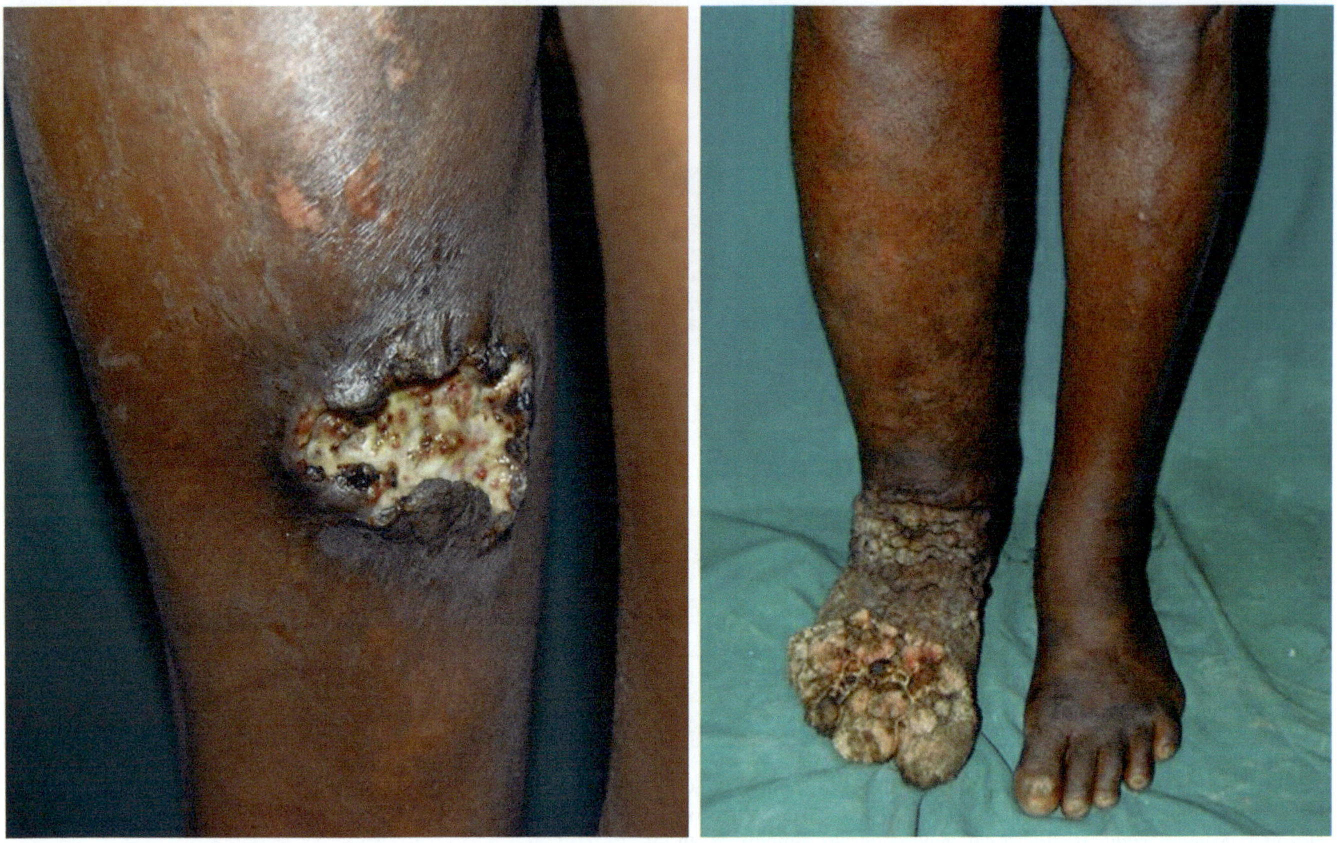

Fig. 17.7 Differential diagnoses *Left*, ulcerated *squamous cell carcinoma* increasing in size with indurated margins, histologically confirmed; *right*, ulcerated *podoconiosis* in chronic lymphedema. DD: ulcers in secondary to venous insufficiency, Kaposi's sarcoma. (Ethiopia) (courtesy INMP Institute, Rome; photo FD)

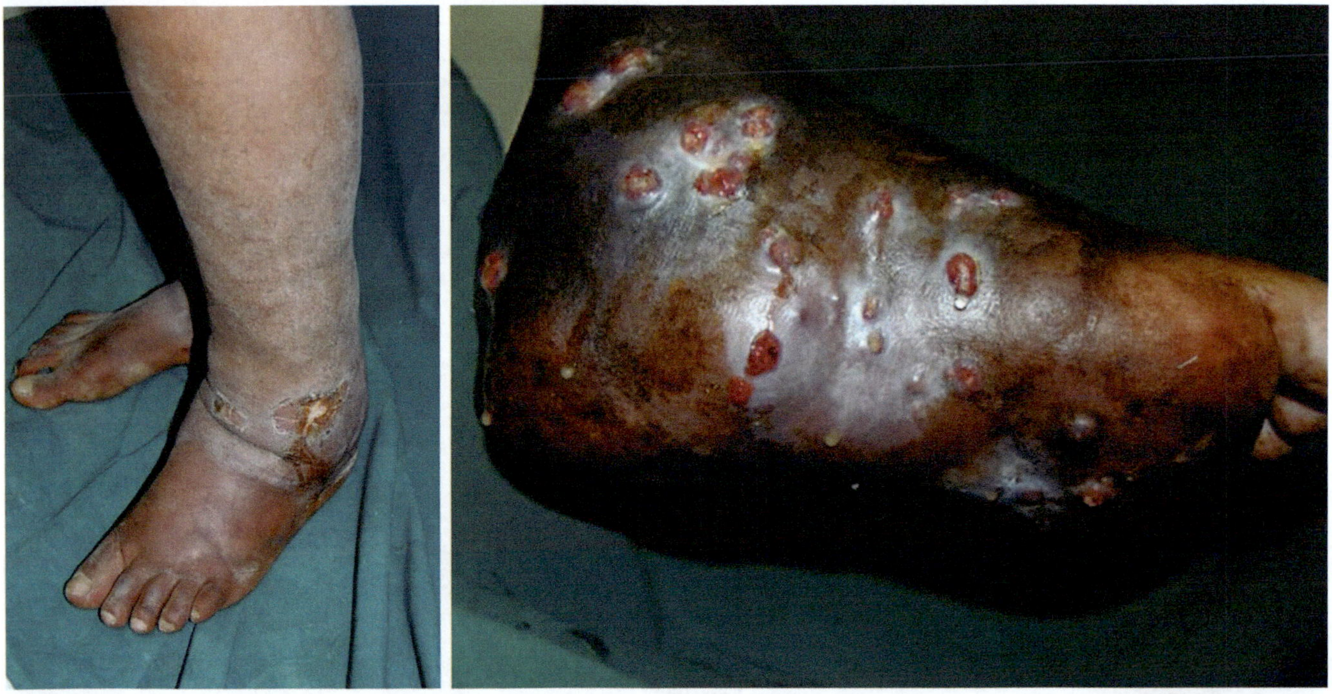

Fig. 17.8 Differential diagnoses Left, leg ulcers in *congenital lymphedema*; right, progressed *eumycetoma* with multiple sinuses, vegetations, pus, and granules with multiple ulcerations. (Ethiopia) (courtesy INMP Institute, Rome; photo FD)

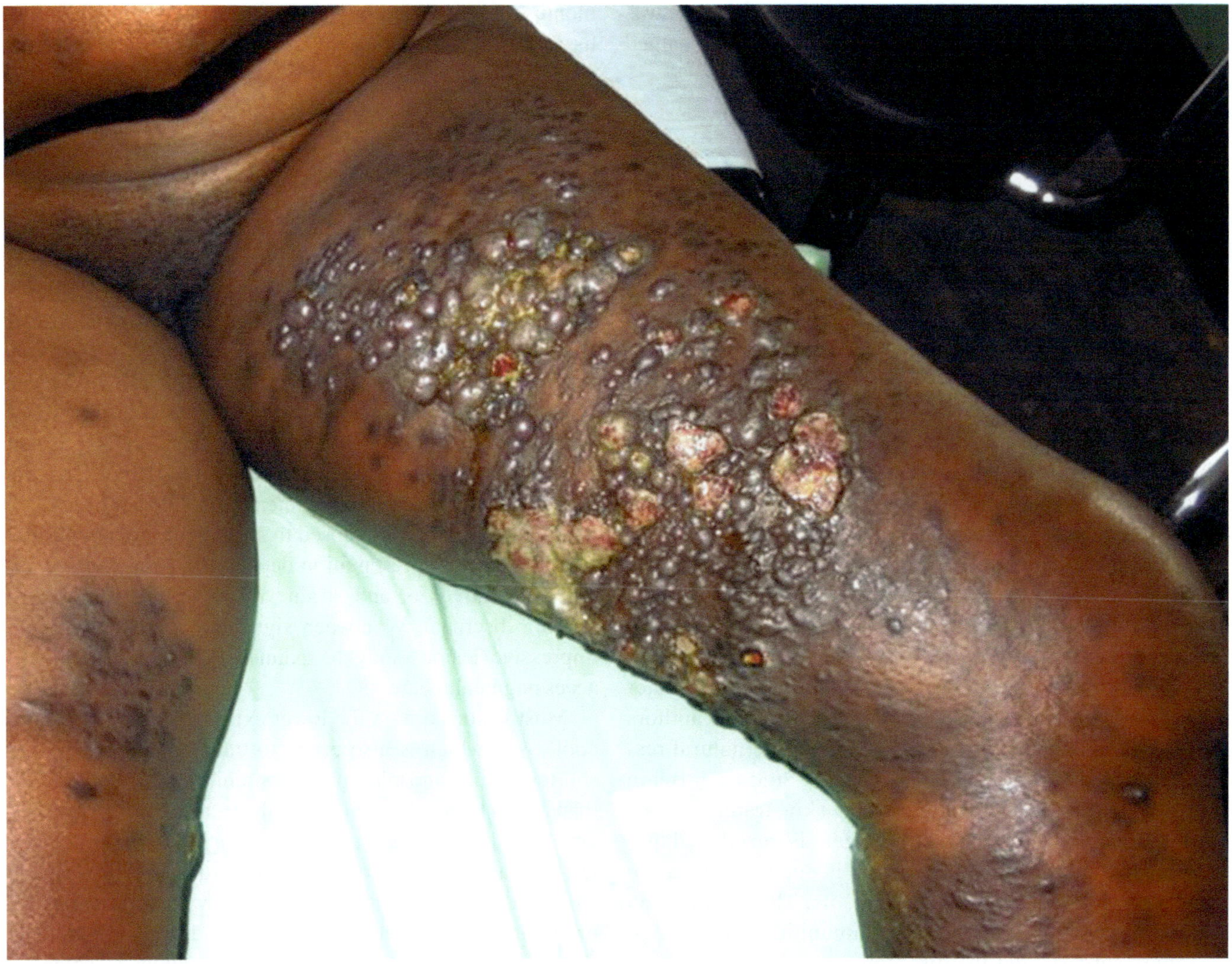

Fig. 17.9 Ulcerative lesions in *Kaposi's sarcoma* (courtesy Nzara Mission Hospital, South Sudan)

17.1.3 Management and Prevention

First-line treatment is a combination of penicillin (500 mg every 6 h over 1 week) and metronidazole (250 mg every 8 h over 10 days). For patients allergic to penicillin, tetracyclines (minocycline 100 mg 2×/day or doxycycline 100 mg 2×/day) can be given instead. Antibiotic treatment should be combined with careful wound care and nutritional support. Effective wound care includes cleansing with clean boiled water or saline, treatment with a topical antibacterial agent such as gentian violet paint and/or tetracycline ointment, regular dressing changes every other day with clean vaseline gauzes and bandages if available, or otherwise steam-sterilized banana leafs. Large ulcers (>5 cm) may require surgical debridement and/or skin grafting, if possible.

It is thought that most tropical ulcers start with a small traumatic lesion, e.g., an insect bite or a puncture wound; therefore, wearing shoes, cleaning small wounds and dressings, and cleaning mud off the legs should prevent the development of an ulcer by protecting from and removing bacteria which could penetrate the skin.

17.2 Buruli Ulcer

Buruli ulcer (BU) is an indolent necrotizing disease of the skin, the subcutaneous tissue, and the bone caused by *Mycobacterium ulcerans*. BU is the third most common mycobacterial disease of humans, after tuberculosis and leprosy, and the least understood of the three. It is considered a public health problem in endemic countries. The disease was named 1961 after the first large epidemic in an area named "Buruli" near Lake Kyoga in Uganda [9].

17.2.1 Epidemiology

BU is endemic in tropical countries in West Africa, mostly in Benin, Ghana, and Cote d'Ivoire, but occurs also in other countries such as in Kenya, Tanzania, and Uganda. Less commonly is BU seen in America (French Guiana, Surinam, Mexico, Peru), Asia (Malaysia, China, Japan), and Australia. Seasonal variations have been reported. Little is known on the epidemiology because of underreporting, spontaneous healing, socioeconomic factors, and the use of traditional medicine in endemic areas. BU is strongly associated with rural wetlands, especially those with slow flowing or stagnant water. An inverse relationship between the prevalence of BU and distance from a river has been observed. Aquatic insects have been suspected to be potential vectors of *M. ulcerans* by carrying the mycobacteria in their salivary glands, thus spreading the infection to some distance from the source of water [10]. This hypothesis has been contested by other authors [11]. The exact mode of transmission and the natural reservoir of *M. ulcerans* are still not known. Studies in Benin indicate that minor often unnoticed skin trauma is the most frequent means by which the agent is introduced into the body. Contamination of the skin is due to exposure to stagnant water, insect bites, or aerosols. The predilection of the disease for poor rural communities, the cost of complex surgery, and the disabling sequelae after recovery make BU a major socioeconomic burden in areas of prevalence.

17.2.2 Etiology

M. ulcerans is a slow-growing, environmental mycobacterium that infects the skin and subcutaneous tissue through minor breaks in the skin. It grows optimally at 30–32 °C. There is a latent period of 2–4 months or more before an infection becomes clinically evident. After inoculation *M. ulcerans* proliferates and produces the polyketone toxin mycolactone, causing tissue destruction and suppressing host immune responses. The development of lesions takes place preferentially in cooler body sites, especially the skin and subcutaneous tissues. In early stages, a toxin-induced necrosis of dermal and subcutaneous tissue develops with secondary leukocytoclastic vasculitis and septal panniculitis. Necrosis of the dermis extends laterally, leading to the characteristic undermining of the ulcer edge. The muscle is usually spared, possibly because of its higher temperature. Healing starts after some months, accompanied by lymphocytic and/or granulomatous tissue reaction. Fibrosis and scarring complete the sequence.

17.2.3 Clinical Picture

Contact with environmental mycobacteria may result in colonization or primary infection. The development of clinical symptoms depends largely on the defense of the host. More than 70% of all patients are children <15 years old. Adults of >60 years of age or older are also at increased risk to develop BU. Thus, exposure of the traumatized skin to *M. ulcerans* may lead to several outcomes: infection occurs and clears spontaneously without any symptom; clinical disease manifests 2–3 months after inoculation as primary BU; or subclinical/asymptomatic infection (latent BU) develops that may later reactivate and be clinically manifested. It is likely that many individuals exposed to *M. ulcerans* do not develop BU. The clinical presentation depends on host immune status, inoculum size, and strain virulence. There may be a striking discrepancy between signs and symptoms as even impressive lesions may be painless, leading to delays in accessing health care.

Most lesions are on the lower extremities, on a relatively cooler site which is also prone to trauma. Because of their shorter stature and play practices, children are more likely than adults to develop lesions on the trunk, upper arms, neck, and head [12]. Three stages are recognized: non-ulcerated lesions, ulcerated lesions, and a third stage of scarring. However, there may be mixed forms, with different stages presenting in the same site or at a different body site. Disseminated forms also occur, continuously enlarging through contiguous spread of *M. ulcerans* or more generalized by lymphohematogenous spread. Approximately 10% of all patients with BU develop osteomyelitis by contiguity or by lymphohematogenous spread (Fig. 17.10). HIV-associated immunosuppression may cause severe BU with large and edematous lesions [13]. Clinical criteria suggesting the diagnosis of BU include:

- ≥1 painless ulcers lasting several weeks with undermined edges.
- Nodules, plaques, or wheals.
- Swelling over a painful joint suggesting bone involvement.
- No fever or regional lymphadenopathy (if no bacterial superinfection).
- Patient <15 years of age.
- Patient lives in or has traveled to a BU endemic region, particularly in West Africa.

For differential, many conditions resemble BU, including tropical ulcers, leishmaniasis, anthrax, necrotizing fasciitis,

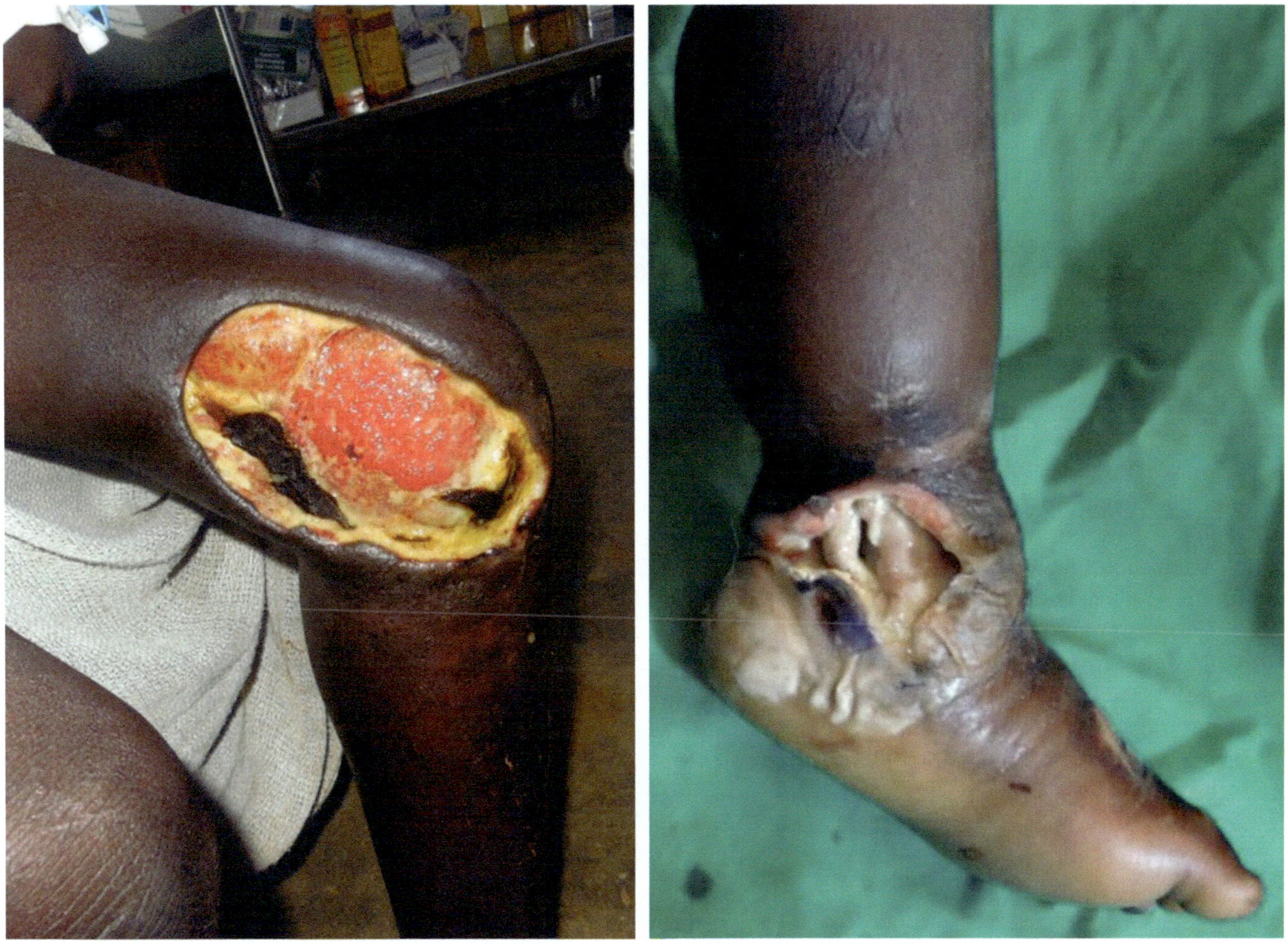

Fig. 17.10 *Left*, *Buruli ulcer* in a young boy with undermined edges; *right*, *Buruli ulcer* in a child, extending to deep tissues with bone involvement. Smear showed mycobacteria on Ziehl-Neelsen stain. (courtesy Nzara Mission Hospital, South Sudan)

and others ([14]; Figs. 17.3, 17.4, 17.5, 17.6, 17.7, 17.8 and 17.9). Most of these conditions are painful, unlike BU, and tropical ulcers usually present with a foul smell. However, painful ulcers may indicate secondary infection of a BU. The most often available technique for diagnosis in endemic areas is smear examination from the ulcer stained with Ziehl-Neelsen or auramine to detect acid-fast bacilli. Cultures, histopathology, and PCR are not widely available in regions where BU is endemic. Microbiologic confirmation of BU is essential for determination of the true prevalence and incidence in a given area. WHO recommends at least two different laboratory tests to be positive among direct smear, culture, histopathology, and PCR, to consider a patient as confirmed BU.

17.2.4 Management

In 2004, WHO advocated an evidence-based antibiotic regimen, composed of oral rifampicin with intramuscular streptomycin and surgery as needed. Its routine implementation has dramatically improved healing and reduced relapses of BU [15]. The current regimen comprises oral rifampicin (10 mg/kg/day) plus intramuscular streptomycin (15 mg/kg/day), both administered over 8 weeks under supervision. Amikacin (15 mg/kg/day) can be used to substitute streptomycin administered intramuscularly or intravenously. A pilot study from Benin using oral chemotherapy with rifampicin plus clarithromycin showed promising results [16]. Patients with lesions less than 5 cm in diameter should receive antibiotics alone and wound care [17, 18]. The current WHO recommendations for treatment are:

- Combination of specific antibiotics over 8 weeks as first-line treatment for all forms of active disease
- Wound care.
- Prevention of disability.
- Surgery to remove necrotic tissue, cover large skin defects, and correct deformities.

In general, recurrence rates in lesions of less than 15 cm in longer diameter after completing a rifampicin + streptomycin-based regimen are low (1–2%). Surgery should be considered in addition after 4 weeks of antibiotic management for lesions 5–15 cm in diameter and after 1 week for lesions more than 15 cm in diameter, for multifocal lesions; lesions at critical sites such as the eye, breast, and genitalia; or bone involvement; the antibiotics are then continued for a total of 8 weeks after surgery.

17.2.5 Prevention

In endemic rural areas where scantily dressed people work and play, avoiding contact with the contaminated environment is almost impossible. Wearing protective clothing and cleansing of any skin injury with clean water may reduce rates of infection; however, these measures are difficult to achieve in low-income settings with inadequate water supplies. The use of protected sources of water for domestic use (drilling wells, providing pumps) can reduce the exposure to *M. ulcerans* and consequently the BU prevalence rate by reducing the exposure to contaminated water sources. Reducing risk factors for agricultural workers, fishermen, and other workers at risk remains a serious task.

Educational programs for behavioral changes to the community, although not easy to be implemented, should be included in BU control strategies. *M. ulcerans*, as an intracellular organism, triggers cell-mediated immunity. A protective effect of BCG vaccination is controversial: in some studies, it has been reported to reduce the rate of osteomyelitis in BU patients; in others no evidence of a protective role of BCG vaccination against BU was found. BURULIVAC, a collaborative project funded by the European Union under the Seventh Framework Programme, supports efforts to identify vaccine candidates based on DNA engineering and virulence factors, including mycolactone.

17.3 Ulcers in Sickle Cell Disease

Sickle cell disease (SCD) is an inherited disorder of hemoglobin (Hb) characterized by rigid, sickle-shaped red blood cells, hemolytic anemia, and endothelial dysfunction with occlusion of the blood vessels, pain, organ injury, and early mortality [19, 20]. SCD is caused by homozygosis for the β-globin S gene mutation. The clinical manifestations of SCD are diverse, and disabling leg ulcers are relatively common.

17.3.1 Epidemiology

Inherited hemoglobin disorders (sickle cell disorders and thalassemias) were originally characteristic of the tropics and subtropics but are now common worldwide due to migration. Sickle cell disease has a significant prevalence worldwide, occurring not only in Africa but also throughout the Mediterranean basin, the Middle East, and India. SCD is one of the most common inherited genetic disorders affecting African and Caribbean populations. Approximately 8% of the African American and Caribbean American populations are heterozygous carriers of the sickle cell gene. SCD is common throughout sub-Saharan Africa, affecting up to 3% of births in some parts of the continent. Around 85% of sickle cell disorders and over 70% of all affected births occur in Africa [21]. The distribution of the mutated allele displays a close association with the endemic distribution of *Plasmodium falciparum*. SCD carriers do not experience the clinical problems associated with the homozygous disorder. In high-income countries that provide neonatal diagnosis and adequate health care for patients, most SCD patients survive well into adult life. Most affected children born in low-income countries continue to die undiagnosed. In Africa, sickle cell disease (SCD) is reported to be associated with high rate of childhood mortality [20], 50–90%, yet there is limited up-to-date information from the continent.

Leg ulcers are the most common cutaneous manifestation of SCD resulting in significant morbidity. The prevalence rate varies, being low before 10 years of age and increasing with age. Leg ulcers are reported to be more common in males in some studies. The geographical distribution of ulcers is variable, affecting 75% of homozygous SCD patients in Jamaica but only 8–10% of the patients in North America. Data from Africa are scarce.

17.3.2 Etiology

The pathogenesis of chronic ulcerations in SCD is complex. Microvascular obstruction by dense sickled erythrocytes and ischemia, bacterial infections, abnormal autonomic control with excessive vasoconstriction, in situ thrombosis, anemia with decrease in oxygen-carrying capacity, minor trauma (scratching, insect bites), and decreased nitric oxide bioavailability lead to altered endothelial function. They have been proposed as potential contributing factors. Venous insufficiency is not considered as a primary cause although it worsens prognosis if present. Arteriovenous shunting has been postulated as a factor promoting ulcer formation as it deprives the skin from oxygen. Combinations of all these factors contribute to ulcerations in the lower extremities of patients with SCD. Superinfection with common pathogens such as staphylococci, *Pseudomonas* spp., *Streptococcus* spp., and others is the most commonly described.

17.3.3 Clinical Picture

Leg ulcers are a disabling complication of SCD as they are painful, relapsing, and often intractable and heal slowly over months to years. The pain may be severe, sharp, and stinging

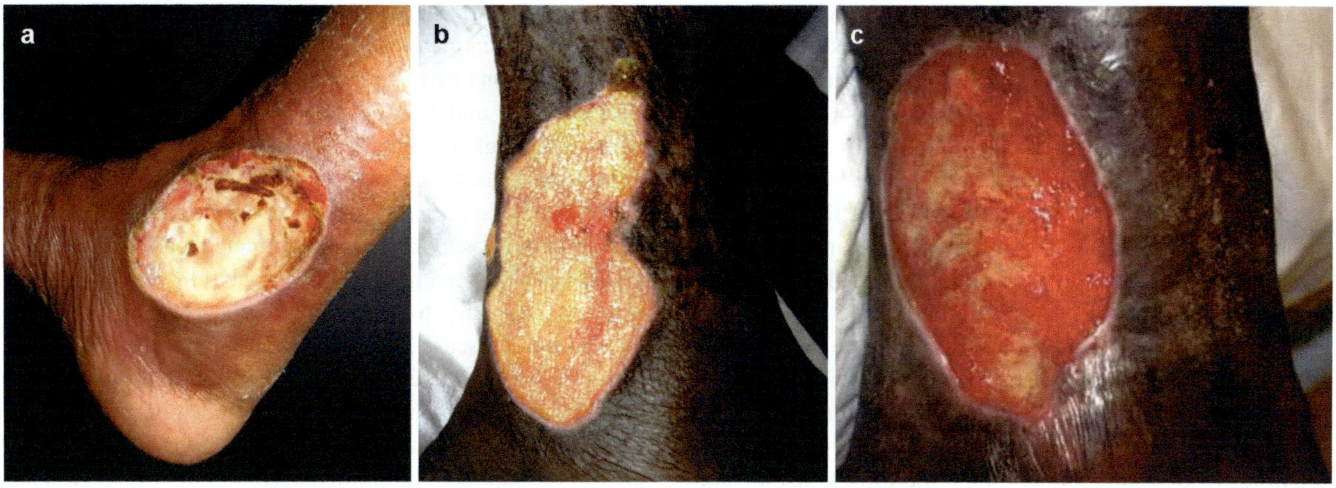

Fig. 17.11 (**a**), Recurrent, chronified *ulcus in sickle cell disease* in typical localization; (**b**, **c**), *ulcer in sickle cell disease* under intensive wound cleansing and care. (**a** and **b**), RDTC, Moshi, Tanzania (courtesy CEO). (**c**), Nzara Mission Hospital, South Sudan (courtesy Dr. C. Tassi)

in nature. The leg ulcers are often associated with a more severe clinical course including hemolysis, pulmonary hypertension, stroke, priapism, and low Hb levels [22]. Cutaneous leg ulcers should be viewed by the attending physicians as an indicator for severe SCD. They occur in areas with less subcutaneous fat, thin skin, and decreased blood flow. The commonest sites are the medial and lateral malleoli (Fig. 17.11). The medial malleolus is more commonly involved than the lateral; the ulcers often become circumferential if not controlled early. Less common sites are the anterior tibial area, dorsum of the foot, and Achilles tendon. Many severity indices for leg ulcers are based on its size, depth, and duration. Staging of leg ulcers in SCD based on depth is as follows:

Stage 1: Erythema of intact skin heralds skin ulceration. In individuals with darker skin, only discoloration of the skin may be observed. In any skin type, warmth, edema, induration, or hardness may be indicators of impending ulceration.

Stage 2: Partial-thickness skin loss involving epidermis, dermis, or both. The lesion is superficial and presents clinically as a flat erosive ulcer or blister.

Stage 3: Full-thickness skin loss involving damage to or necrosis of subcutaneous tissue that may extend down to the underlying fascia. The ulcer presents clinically as a deeper crater with or without undermining of the adjacent tissue.

Stage 4: Full-thickness skin loss with extensive destruction, tissue necrosis, or damage to the muscle, bone, or tendon. Undermining and sinus tracts may also be present.

Leg ulcers may be classified as acute or chronic according to their duration; however, there is no consensus as to a specific length of time to define chronicity. An acute ulcer should usually heal in less than a month; a chronic ulcer may last up to 6 months. In some cases, recurrent ulcers can last many years, often closing and reopening repeatedly.

Table 17.1 Recommendations for cutaneous ulcers in SCD

Prevention	Hygiene	General and local hygiene Avoid synthetic fabric
	Venous stasis reduction	Avoid longtime standing
	Trauma prevention	Wear comfortable shoes Prevent insect bites
Local treatment	Washing	Delicate washing Soft curettage
	Venous stasis control	Elastic bandages if needed Bed rest with elevation of leg
	Improving cutaneous trophism	Zinc oxide bandages Topical antibiotics/honey Skin graft
Systemic treatment		Oral zinc sulfate Oral antibiotics

17.3.4 Treatment

Controlled clinical trials regarding SCD ulcers are scarce. Some therapeutic methods used are based on their efficacy on other ulcers (diabetic, venous, etc.). Management schedules may target the local wound environment including debridement, infection control, education of the patient, and protection. Local treatment is based on wound care using wet-to-dry dressings; those persisting >6 months may require additional measures such as skin grafting, hyperbaric oxygen, etc. Hydroxyurea or transfusion management is used as disease-modifying agents together with compression stockings and topical therapies [23]. Standard procedures are summarized in Table 17.1.

Recent advances in the management of leg ulcers in general include systemic and topical applications of analgesics, including opioids, topical application of a platelet-derived growth factor prepared either autologously or by recombinant technology, and the use of skin grafts. A study proposed a topical synthetic extracellular matrix as a temporary substitute for the damaged natural extracellular matrix [24]; topical application of GM-CSF as growth factor for tissue trophism has also been described as effective. The effect of hydroxyurea as the most commonly used chemotherapy for the disease on the SCD leg ulcers remains controversial. It is advisable to rule out osteomyelitis. There is no systematic or controlled data showing efficacy of blood transfusions on SCD ulcers. Zinc deficiency is known to be common in individuals with sickle cell diseases. Studies showed that administration of zinc sulfate 220 mg 2×/day resulted in more rapid healing. In tropical rural settings, the topical use of natural honey is well known and often used [25]. Recurrences are frequent; nevertheless, the general outcome of therapeutic efforts is satisfactory once the disease is recognized and treated [26].

17.3.5 Prevention

Clinical observations and epidemiological studies document the important role of local trauma in the onset of SCD leg ulcers. A number of simple interventions can be taught to SCD patients to potentially reduce the ulcers such as the regular use of protective bandages. Although not all studies support the importance of venous stasis in the development of leg ulcers, control of venous stasis may be essential for successful interventions. Bed rest and limiting the amount of standing time seem to have an impact on wound healing as well.

17.4 Noma (Cancrum Oris)

Noma is an acute necrotizing phagedenic ulcerative gingivitis that primarily affects the mouth and face. The exact cause of noma is unknown but is likely due to bacteria. The term "noma" originates from the Greek word *nemo* which means "consume, destroy." The disease is common among severely malnourished children 2–5 years of age, with approximately 140,000 new cases each year [27], mostly in sub-Saharan Africa. South America (Argentina, Colombia, Uruguay, Paraguay, Suriname) and Asia (India, Pakistan, Cambodia, Thailand) are also involved [27]. Most cases are reported from the so-called noma belt that stretches from Mauritania to Ethiopia. The true incidence and prevalence of the disease are not known because of the high associated mortality rate and its occurrence in underdeveloped countries with migrant populations and poor general health services limiting registration, treatment, and follow-up. It is believed that only <15% of patients with acute disease seek medical care [28]. Social stigma associated with noma further complicates identification of cases [29].

In conditions of poverty, where many children are malnourished or undernourished, the prevalence of noma is likely to be higher. Noma has been described less frequently in neonates, adults, and chronically ill elderly. Recently, isolated cases have been reported from developed countries [30] and in immunosuppressed HIV-infected patients [29, 31]. Noma has also been reported in association with cyclic neutropenia, herpetic stomatitis, leukemia, Down's syndrome, and Burkitt's disease [32]. However, the most important risk factor for noma is severe or moderate malnutrition. Other risk factors depend on poverty and include poor hygiene and inadequate sanitation, unsafe drinking water, intrauterine growth retardation, and limited access to high-quality health care. Hypotheses about predisposing conditions to the disease include febrile communicable illnesses such as measles, varicella, malaria, tuberculosis, and HIV infection. The role of malnutrition and HIV seropositivity as co-predisposing factors needs further investigation [33].

17.4.1 Etiology

The etiology of noma is not known, but it is believed to be multifactorial. It is suggested that factors such as poverty and consequent malnutrition, weakened immune functions, and viral infections, all associated with poor oral hygiene, could lead to the development of oral ulcers. These ulcers can be entry sites for microorganisms responsible for the disease [35]. The role of specific microorganisms in the pathogenesis of noma has not been explained; the polymicrobial environment of the oropharynx and the rapid development of the disease in remote geographic areas make an early microbiological analysis difficult [35]. Lastly, preexisting poor oral hygiene makes superinfections common and bacteriological studies potentially misleading. It is accepted that several bacterial species operate in concert, releasing biological mediators that disrupt the local vasculature and degrade extracellular proteins.

Recent advancements in microbial identification techniques have helped to better characterize the microorganisms present in noma ulcers. A number of potential pathogens have been found in abundance from the oral flora in patients with noma ulcers, including *Prevotella melaninogenica*, *Corynebacterium pyogenes*, *Fusobacterium nucleatum*, *Bacteroides fragilis*, *Bacillus cereus*, *Prevotella intermedia*, and *Fusobacterium necrophorum* [27]. Recent studies showed that bacteria from healthy and affected individuals (either by noma or necrotizing gingivitis) are similar and differ in the prevalence of a limited group of phylotypes, namely, *Prevotella intermedia* and *Peptostreptococcus* genus; no evidence was found for a specific infection-

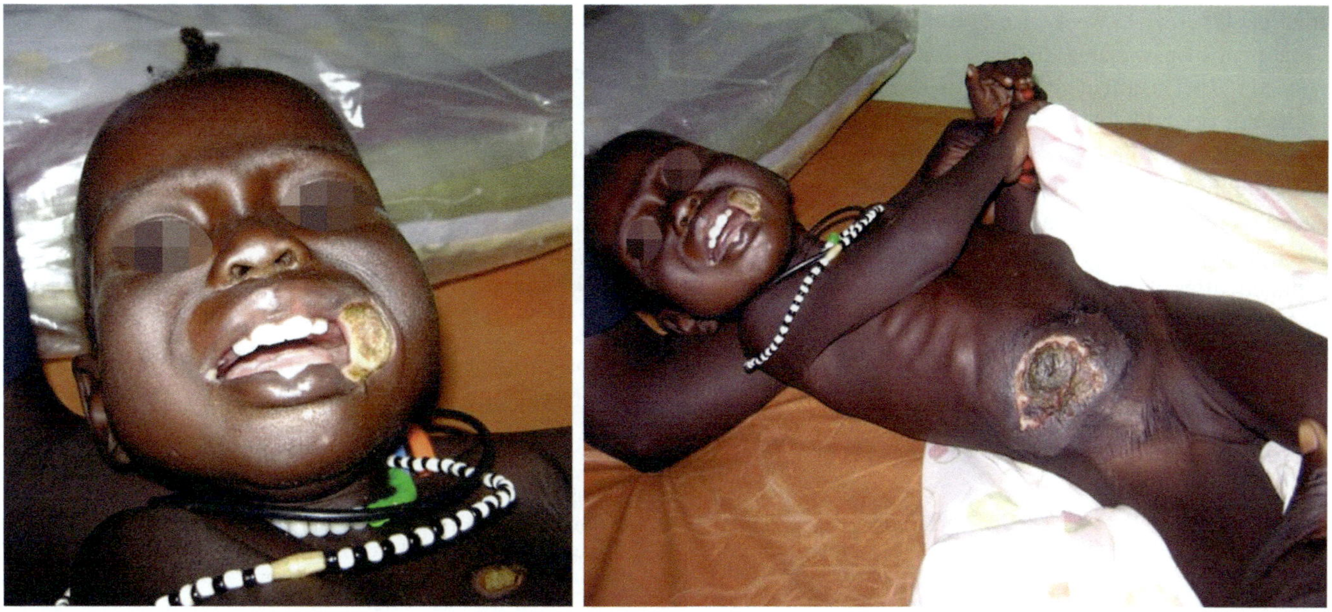

Fig. 17.12 *Noma* in a severely malnourished child. Early stage ulceration (Nzara Mission Hospital, South Sudan; Dr. M. Martinelli)

triggering agent [34, 35]. The disease, though considered of infectious origin, is believed to be opportunistic rather than communicable.

17.4.2 Clinical Picture

Noma is a multistage, opportunistic, rapidly progressive, and painless disease characterized by destructive necrosis of oral tissues and underlying bone. The course is rapid and death can occur in days [33]. It is believed that noma is an extension of necrotizing ulcerative gingivitis (NUG) characterized by gingival edema, necrosis, bleeding, and pain in the early stage [27]. NUG may progress to necrotizing periodontitis and later to necrotizing stomatitis. The first recognized sign of noma is edema of the cheek, gingiva, or both (Fig. 17.12). A grayish black area appears on the external surface of the cheek opposite to the intraoral lesion within the next few days, which later becomes a well-defined black painless necrotic zone. This necrotic zone rapidly sloughs away [27]. Intraoral manifestations include sequestration of the exposed bone and teeth, halitosis, pseudomembranes, excessive salivation, spontaneous gingival bleeding, and loss of the tips of interdental gingival papilla. Sometimes the necrosis is so severe that the maxilla and mandible are destroyed; it extends up to the nose or involves the upper lip, premaxilla, and the infraorbital margin [33], leading to facial deformity and oral incontinence. The patient is sick, anemic, apathetic, and dehydrated. Systemic manifestations include malodorous breath, fever, tachycardia, lymphadenopathy, anorexia, general edema, and ascites as symptoms of acute illness. Medical history usually reveals a parasitic or viral infection (measles, malaria) in the recent past, recurrent fever and diarrhea. Blood examinations show low hemoglobin and white blood cell count.

Differential diagnosis includes leprosy, leishmaniasis, clostridial or streptococcal gangrene, midfacial lymphoma, and several other conditions (Fig. 17.4). Noma can be distinguished from cellulitis caused by pyogenic cocci by the foul odor, the thin uncolored exudates rather than pus, and the relatively rapid and widespread tissue destruction. Bacterial fermentation with gas formation is not a feature of noma, differentiating it from gangrenous necrosis induced by *Clostridium perfringens*. Necrosis of muscle tissues in the infected field occurs within 1–3 days as the infection spreads due to the massive proteolytic action of released bacterial enzymes.

17.4.3 Management

Noma is devastating clinically and socially. Untreated, only 10–20% of children with acute disease will survive. Early treatment with antibiotics and nutrition increases survival in childhood to greater than 90%. Even with medical treatment, oral disfigurement and oral incontinence as a consequence of the rapidly progressive gangrene often requires reconstruction to achieve functionality and acceptable cosmesis. Treatment is aimed at arresting the acute infection and correcting the underlying deficits in nutrition and hydration. Fluid hydration (via nasogastric tube or intravenously), correction of electrolyte imbalance, nutritional support, and broad-spectrum antibiotics (ampicillin-cloxacillin and metronidazole) for 1 week are the first-line management. Treatment of associated diseases like malaria or anemia is needed [27]. The affected area has to be cleaned with diluted hydrogen peroxide/chlorhexidine gluconate if available, or saline, and any remaining tissue slough and sequestrate be removed by surgical debridement. The patient has to be screened for HIV infection or other immune deficiencies and referred appropriately. Surgical correction/reconstruction is initiated after a period of disease quiescence of at least 6–18 months. The aim of the surgical procedure is to restore speech, oral competence, and acceptable aesthetics.

References

1. Gupta SK, Shukla VK. Leg ulcers in the tropics. Int J Low Extrem Wounds. 2002;1:58–61.
2. Ziegelaar JE, Faber WR. Imported tropical infectious ulcers in travelers. Am J Clin Dermatol. 2008;9:219–32.
3. Webb J, Murdoch DA. Tropical ulcers after sports injuries. Lancet. 1992;339(8785):129–30.
4. Veraldi S, Caputo R. Dermatologia di importazione. 2nd ed. Milan: Poletto Editore; 2000. p. 108–10.
5. Adriaans B, Drasar BS. The isolation of fusobacteria from tropical ulcers. Epidemiol Infect. 1987;99:361–72.
6. Adriaans B. Tropical ulcer—a reappraisal based on recent work. Trans R Soc Trop Med Hyg. 1988;82:185.
7. Robinson DC, Adriaans B, Hay RJ, et al. The clinical and epidemiologic features of tropical ulcer (tropical phagedenic ulcer). Int J Dermatol. 1988;27:49–53.
8. Spencer H, et al. Tropical pathology. Berlin: Springer; 1973. p. 706.
9. Walsh DS, Meyers WM, Portaels F. Buruli ulcer. In: Faber WR, Hay JR, Naafs B, editors. Imported skin diseases. 2nd ed. New York: Wiley-Blackwell; 2013. p. 94–106.
10. Marsollier L, Robert R, Aubry J, et al. Aquatic insects as a vector for *Mycobacterium ulcerans*. Appl Environ Microbiol. 68:4623–8. https://doi.org/10.1128/AEM.68.9.4623-4628.2002.
11. Benbow ME, Williamson H, Kimbirauskas R, et al. Aquatic invertebrates as unlikely vectors of Buruli ulcer disease. Emerg Infect Dis. 2008;14:1247–54.
12. Phanzu DM, Mahema RL, Suykerbuyk P, et al. Mycobacterium ulcerans infection (Buruli ulcer) on the face: a comparative analysis of 13 clinically suspected cases from the Democratic Republic of Congo. Am J Trop Med Hyg. 2011;85:1100–5.
13. Vincent QB, Ardant MF, Marsollier L, et al. HIV infection and Buruli ulcer in Africa. Lancet Infect Dis. 2014;14:796–7.
14. Toutous Trellu L, Nkemenang P, Comte E, et al. Differential diagnosis of skin ulcers in a mycobacterium ulcerans endemic area: data from a prospective study in Cameroon. PLoS Negl Trop Dis. 2016;10:e0004385.
15. WHO. Provisional guidance on the role of specific antibiotics in the management of Mycobacterium ulcerans disease (Buruli ulcer). Geneva: WHO; 2004.
16. Etuaful S, Carbonnelle B, Grosset J, et al. Efficacy of the combination rifampin-streptomycin in preventing growth of mycobacterium ulcerans in early lesions of Buruli ulcer in humans. Antimicrob Agents Chemother. 2005;49:3182–6.
17. Nienhuis WA, Stienstra Y, Thompson WA, et al. Antimicrobial treatment for early, limited mycobacterium ulcerans infection: a randomised controlled trial. Lancet. 2010;375:664–72.
18. Chauty A, Ardant MF, Marsollier L, et al. Oral treatment for mycobacterium ulcerans infection : results from a pilot study in Benin. Clin Inf Dis. 2011;52:94–6.
19. Weatherall DJ, Clegg JB. Inherited haemoglobin disorders: an increasing global health problem. Bull World Health Organ. 2001;79:704–12.
20. Grosse SD, Odame I, Atrash HK, et al. Sickle cell disease in Africa. A neglected cause of early childhood mortality. Am J Prev Med. 2011;41:S398–405.
21. Modell B, Darlison M. Global epidemiology of haemoglobin disorders and derived service indicators. Bull World Health Organ. 2008;86:417–96.
22. Minniti CP, Eckman J, Sebastiani P, et al. Leg ulcers in sickle cell disease. Am J Hematol. 2010;85:831–3.
23. Delaney KM, Axelrod KC, Buscetta A, et al. Leg ulcers in sickle cell disease: current patterns and practices. Hemoglobin. 2013;37:325–32.
24. Wethers DL, Ramirez GM, Koshy M, et al. Accelerated healing of chronic sickle-cell ulcers treated with RGD peptide matrix. RGD Study Group. Blood. 1994;84:1775–9.
25. Okany CC, Atimomo CE, Akinyanju OO. Efficacy of natural honey in the healing of leg ulcers in sickle cell anaemia. Niger Postgrad Med J. 2004;11:179–81.
26. Ndiaye M, Niang SO, Diop A, et al. Leg ulcers in sickle cell disease: a retrospective study of 40 cases. Ann Dermatol Venerol. 2016;143:103–7.
27. Enwonwu CO, Falkler WA, Phillips RS. Noma (cancrum oris). Lancet. 2006;368(9530):147–56.
28. Tonna JE, Lewin MR, Mensh B. A case and review of noma. PLoS Negl Trop Dis. 2010;4:e869.
29. Baratti-Mayer D, Gayet-Ageron A, Hugonnet S, et al. Risk factors for noma disease: a 6-year, prospective, matched case-control study in Niger. Lancet Glob Health. 2013;1:e87–96.
30. Chiandussi S, Luzzati R, Tirelli G, et al. Cancrum oris in developed countries. Aging Clin Exp Res. 2009;21:475–7.
31. Marck KW. Noma: a neglected enigma. Lancet Glob Health. 2013;1:e58–9.
32. Ashok N, Tarakji B, Darwish S, et al. A review on noma: a recent update. Glob J Health Sci. 2015;8:53–9.
33. Masipa JN, Baloyi AM, Khammissa RA, et al. Noma (cancrum oris): a report of a case in a young AIDS patient with review of pathogenesis. Head Neck Pathol. 2013;7:188–92.
34. Bolivar I, Whiteson K, Stadelmann B, et al. Bacterial diversity in oral samples of children in Niger with acute noma, acute necrotizing gingivitis, and healthy controls. PLoS Negl Trop Dis. 2012;6:e1556.
35. Huyghe A, Francois P, Mombelli A, et al. Microarray analysis of microbiota of gingival lesions in noma patients. PLoS Negl Trop Dis. 2013;7:e2453.

Acne in Dark Skin

18

Christos C. Zouboulis, Emeka Okoro, and Raj Kubba

Acne vulgaris is a chronic, inflammatory disease of the sebaceous follicle characterized by increased sebum secretion and formation of follicle-associated closed and open comedones, papules, pustules and nodules; pseudocysts and several types of scars are sequelae of the primary lesions [1]. Acne is a most common skin disease seen worldwide. However, its incidence and clinical presentation differ in various geographic areas and ethnicities. The disease is less commonly seen in populations with dark skin living in developing countries in Africa. In contrast, acne is on the top list of dermatoses seen in African Americans in the USA [2, 3], indicating that environmental factors may play a prominent role in the pathogenesis of the disease. Acne vulgaris in dark skin is frequently either mild comedonal or nodular, in contrast to the classical presentation of acne papulopustulosa in fair skin (Table 18.1). In addition, facial acneiform dermatoses are frequently seen in patients with dark skin in Africa and India, more often than acne vulgaris itself. On the other hand, it seems that metabolic abnormalities associated with acne are overrepresented in India. Overall, the disease has a significant impact on the quality of life of young individuals worldwide and requires medical assistance and continuing support.

C. C. Zouboulis (✉)
Departments of Dermatology, Venereology, Allergology and Immunology, Dessau Medical Center, Brandenburg Medical School Theodor Fontane, Dessau, Germany
e-mail: christos.zouboulis@klinikum-dessau.de

E. Okoro
Dermatology Unit, Department of Medicine, Federal Medical Centre, Keffi, Nasarawa State, Nigeria

R. Kubba
Delhi Dermatology Group, Kubba Clinic, New Delhi, Delhi, India

18.1 Epidemiology

18.1.1 Acne Is Common in Dark Skin

Acne vulgaris is the most common reason for dermatology consultation among adults (≥18 years) in Africa [5]. Its prevalence has been reported to vary between 35.5 and 90.7% in African adolescents [6–8]. The low prevalence of 2.8–17.5% among hospitalized African patients indicates the ambulatory character of the disease [5, 9, 10]. The prevalence of acne in Africa is higher among girls in early adolescence age (10–13 years) but reverses to become higher in males in late adolescence (14–16 years) [8].

Table 18.1 Simplified classification of acne [4]

Classification	Definition
After the clinical picture	• Comedonal acne • Papulopustular acne • Papulopustular/nodular acne • Conglobate acne • Acne fulminans
After the age of occurrence	• Neonate acne • Infantile acne • Acne praecox • Acne vulgaris • Acne tarda
After the disease severity	• Mild acne (comedonal and papulopustular acne without scars) • Moderate acne (papulopustular acne with initial scarring) • Severe acne (nodular acne with scarring)

C. E. Orfanos et al. (eds.), *Pigmented Ethnic Skin and Imported Dermatoses*, https://doi.org/10.1007/978-3-319-69422-1_18

18.1.2 Acne Is Less Common in Developing Countries

Acne prevalence rates in South Asia, North Africa and the Middle East, sub-Saharan Africa, Latin America and the Caribbean, geographical areas where people with dark skin predominate, are lower than those in Europe, North America, Southeast Asia and East Asia [11, 12]. Furthermore, a slower increase of the prevalence rates during the last decades has been assessed in Africa as compared to North America, Southeast Asia and East Asia [12]. In contrast, acne is more prevalent in African American (37%) and Hispanic women (32%) than in Continental Indian, Caucasian and Asian women (23%, 24%, 30%, respectively) [13] and is on the top list of dermatoses seen in African Americans in the USA [2, 3]. These observations corroborate earlier pronouncements that acne is a disease of civilization [14] and is linked to socioeconomic prosperity and affluence through changing dietary and lifestyle patterns.

18.2 Pathogenesis

Acne is a multifactorial disease of the sebaceous follicle, which represents an anatomic form of the pilosebaceous unit with distribution over the face, the central torso line and the shoulders. Some of the key features underlying acne development include disturbed sebaceous gland activity associated with excessive sebum production and alterations in sebum fatty acid composition, dysregulation of the hormone microenvironment, interaction with neuropeptides, follicular hyperkeratinization, induction of inflammation and dysfunction of the innate and adaptive immunity. These processes impair functioning of the pilosebaceous unit, which leads to the transition of a normal pore to microcomedone and further to comedone and inflammatory lesion. Bacterial antigens can potentiate the inflammatory process [1, 15–18]. Genetic studies of heterozygous and homozygous twins, family and population studies have produced evidence for the role of hereditary factors, especially the influence of the mother, in the development risk of acne lesions [19, 20]. Acne can also be triggered or worsened by ultraviolet radiation and other environmental factors, dietary factors, smoking, stress and lifestyle [17, 18].

Whether hyperkeratinization of the follicular duct precedes the onset of inflammation in acne or vice versa is under debate [21]. IL-1 activity is increased around still uninvolved follicles leading to the initiation of disturbed differentiation of follicular keratinocytes. The sebaceous gland expresses functional receptors for several neuropeptides, whose activation in human sebocytes modulates the production of cytokines and sebaceous lipogenesis [22, 23].

Sebum is secreted by the sebaceous gland and comprises an oily mixture of triglycerides, wax esters, squalene, free fatty acids and small amounts of cholesterol, cholesterol esters and diglycerides. Sebum production is regulated by several factors that activate pathways involved in cell proliferation and differentiation, lipogenesis, hormone metabolism, and cytokine and chemokine release [1, 15, 16]. Excessive sebum is thought to be a key contributor to acne development. However, not all patients with acne experience hyperseborrhea. Acne is further associated with alterations in the free fatty acid composition of sebum. Pro-inflammatory lipid fractions (unsaturated fatty acids and lipoperoxides) in sebum have been associated with the development of acne lesions, and the skin surface lipid oxidant to antioxidant ratio is another acne stimulus [1, 16]. Different ethnic groups have different lipid profiles; for example, specific wax ester lipid fractions differ in quantity between fair skin and skin of African Americans [24].

Systemic and local hormonal imbalance may cause acne; however, whether the primary abnormality causing acne is in the level of circulating hormones or in the processing of hormones in the peripheral tissue is debated [1, 15, 18]. Typically, acne begins during puberty when the hormone balance begins to change dramatically. In addition to systemic changes in hormone levels, local overproduction of steroids, in particular androgens, is associated with the disease. Other hormonal factors might influence the sebaceous gland [25, 26], with peroxisome proliferator-activated receptors (PPAR) and their natural ligands, circulating lipids, being the primary candidates.

Adult women and men with acne can have increased serum levels of insulin-like growth factor 1 (IGF1), which is detected in maturing sebocytes and suprabasal sebaceous duct cells. In women, serum IGF1 levels are correlated with the number of acne lesions, facial sebum excretion rate in postadolescents and serum levels of 5α-dihydrotestosterone and dehydroepiandrosterone sulphate [27, 28]. A high-glycemic Western diet correlates with activation of IGF1 signalling and the PPARγ-stimulated lipid uptake and differentiation of sebocytes, suggesting that circulating IGF1 and local androgen production will have a pivotal role in sebum synthesis and acne [25].

Cutaneous microbiota might also be involved in acne pathogenesis. Although the amount of *Propionibacterium*

(P.) acnes on the skin is similar between patients with acne and healthy controls, the strain populations are different between the two groups [18]. Through their direct antimicrobial characteristics and by inducing the expression of antimicrobial peptides, sebum free fatty acids are involved in the disinfecting activity of the human skin and the enhancement of its innate immune defence [16].

At last, the modern lifestyle, which includes diet, stress, urban noise, socioeconomic pressure, light stimuli and variations in sleep patterns, is a potential risk factor for acne [18]. Among Africans, environmental factors appear to play a major role in the pathogenesis of acne. The careless use of steroid creams in the process of skin whitening leads to the appearance of steroid-induced acne. The use of thick hair oils, petrolatum and other oils on the face stimulates comedogenesis. Other factors that may contribute to the increased occurrence of acne among Africans are the westernization of their diet and enhanced stress.

18.3 Clinical Picture and Course

18.3.1 Acne Vulgaris

It is widely believed that acne is a common accomplice of puberty and adolescent age; therefore, it does not require active treatment except in severe cases. However, acne is a chronic disease [15], which if untreated usually progresses [29]. Acne can occur since adrenarche or further through the puberty (≥10 years). Late onset acne flairs or starts with ≥25 years.

The disease usually starts as a gradual onset of follicular hyperkeratotic (comedones, initially closed and later open) and follicular inflammatory lesions (papules, pustules and nodules), localized at the sebaceous follicle-rich areas, mainly on the face but sometimes also on the chest, upper back and shoulders. The closed comedones are approximately 1 mm large skin-coloured follicular papules (Fig. 18.1), while the open comedones are similar in size with dilated follicles filled with keratinous material (Fig. 18.2). In deeply pigmented skin, closed comedones are difficult to appreciate unlike the open ones. The papules are 1–5 mm skin-coloured elevated solid follicular lesions, occasionally with perilesional inflammation, and the pustules are similar in size with infiltrated follicular lesions filled with pus (Fig. 18.3). The nodules are larger in size three-dimensional follicular infiltrates (Fig. 18.4). Cysts, occurring from liquefied nodules, are secondary lesions of acne. Various combinations of these lesions are found in patients with acne vulgaris. These lesions later give rise to postinflammatory hyperpigmentation, hypopigmentation and scars (Fig. 18.5).

Acne in dark skin is morphologically different than acne in fair skin [29–32]. All ethnic groups display equal prevalence of comedonal and inflammatory types of acne with the exception of Asians, for whom inflammatory acne is more prevalent than comedonal acne (20% vs. 10%), and in Caucasians, for whom comedonal acne is more prevalent than inflammatory acne (14% vs. 10%). Postinflammatory hyperpigmentation is the commonest complication of acne among patients with dark skin, whereas it is more prevalent in African American and Hispanic women (65%, 48%, respectively) than in Asian, Continental Indian and Caucasian ones (18%, 10%, 25%, respectively) [13].

Adolescent acne mainly comprises comedones, while adult acne mainly occurs with clinically inflammatory lesions. In female patients, premenstrual exacerbation of acne lesions may occur. In addition, patient should be examined for additional features of hyperandrogenism, such as hirsutism (Fig. 18.6a). In general, acne is persisting longer in females, and the prevalence of acne tarda is rising worldwide [33]. In India, acne tarda makes up nearly 50% of all acne cases in both sexes (Fig. 18.6b). Acne vulgaris is associated with significant psychological problems, especially in the presence of complications, such as hyperpigmentation and scars.

18.3.2 Acneiform Dermatoses

The differential diagnosis of acne vulgaris includes a large group of acneiform dermatoses induced by Pityrosporum, Demodex, *Staphylococcus* spp. and Gram-negative bacteria [17].

Among acneiform dermatoses, Pityrosporum folliculitis commonly occurs in tropical and subtropical areas of the world. In the Philippines, 56% of acne-considered patients were reported to have Pityrosporum folliculitis [34], and the infection is also common in Korea [35] and India [31]. The following distinctive constellation of morphologic features characterize the disease: upper face distribution with predilection for skin along the hairline, mild severity typically as a few small papules and/or small superficial pustules, with little or no physical discomfort appearing on first impression to be consistent with superficial folliculitis. However, these patients also have superficial comedones on the forehead and

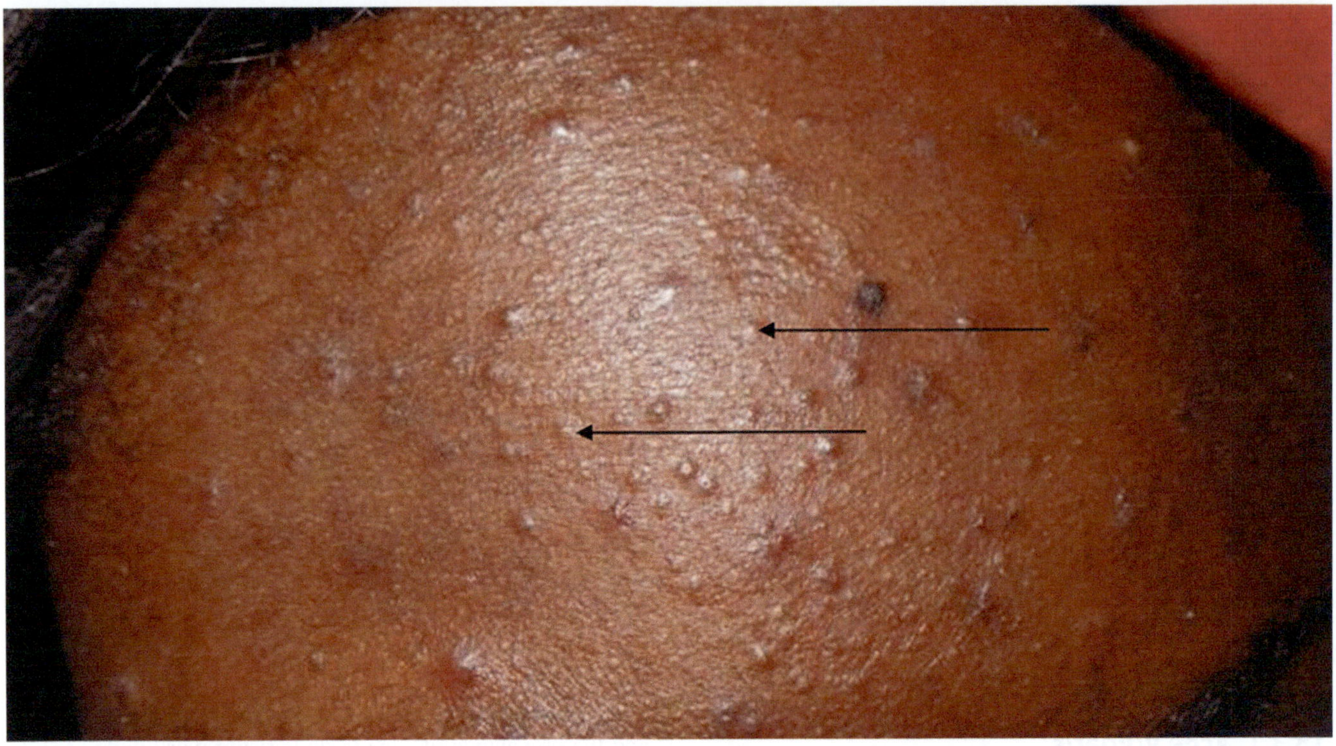

Fig. 18.1 Closed comedones on the forehead. They are skin-coloured lesions of about 1 mm in size (arrows)

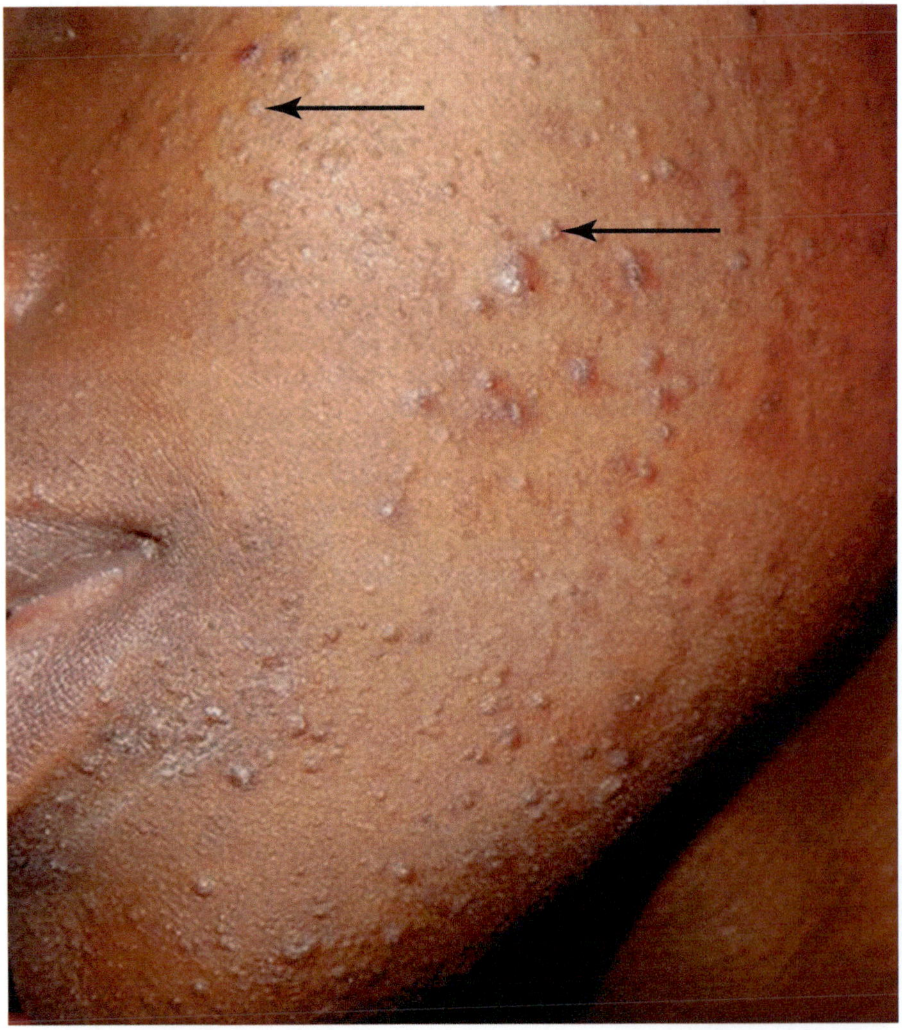

Fig. 18.2 Open comedones on the cheek (arrows). These are small lesions with dilated ducts filled with keratinous material

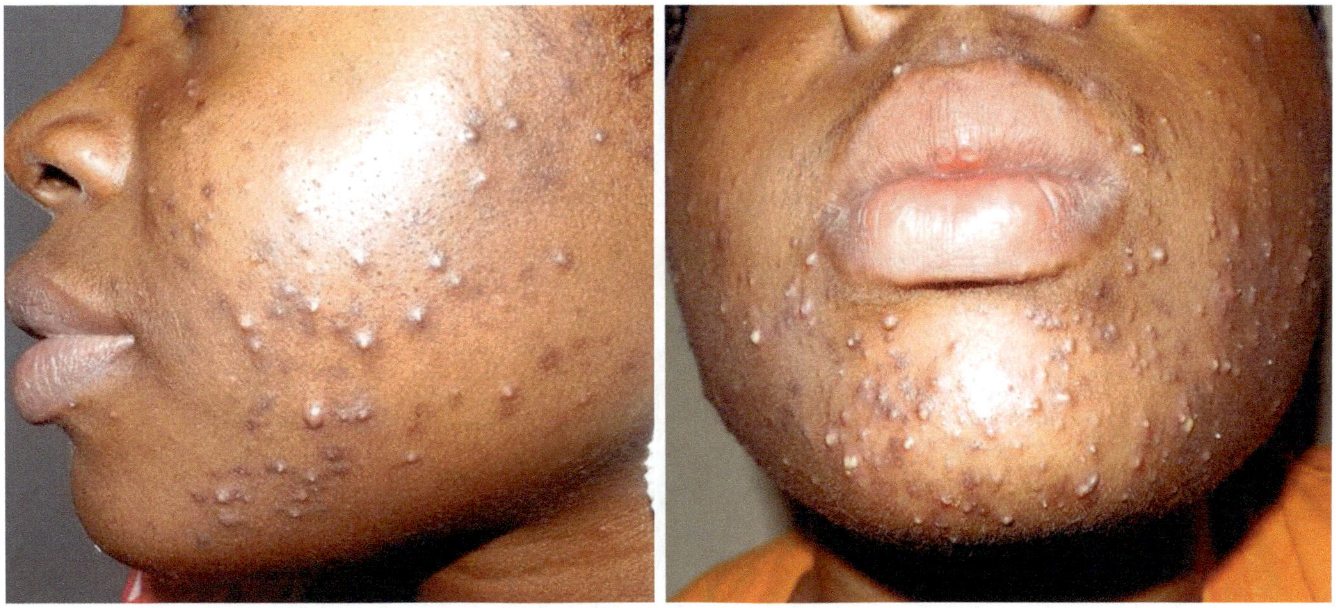

Fig. 18.3 Papules and pustules in acne patients. A few comedones are also present

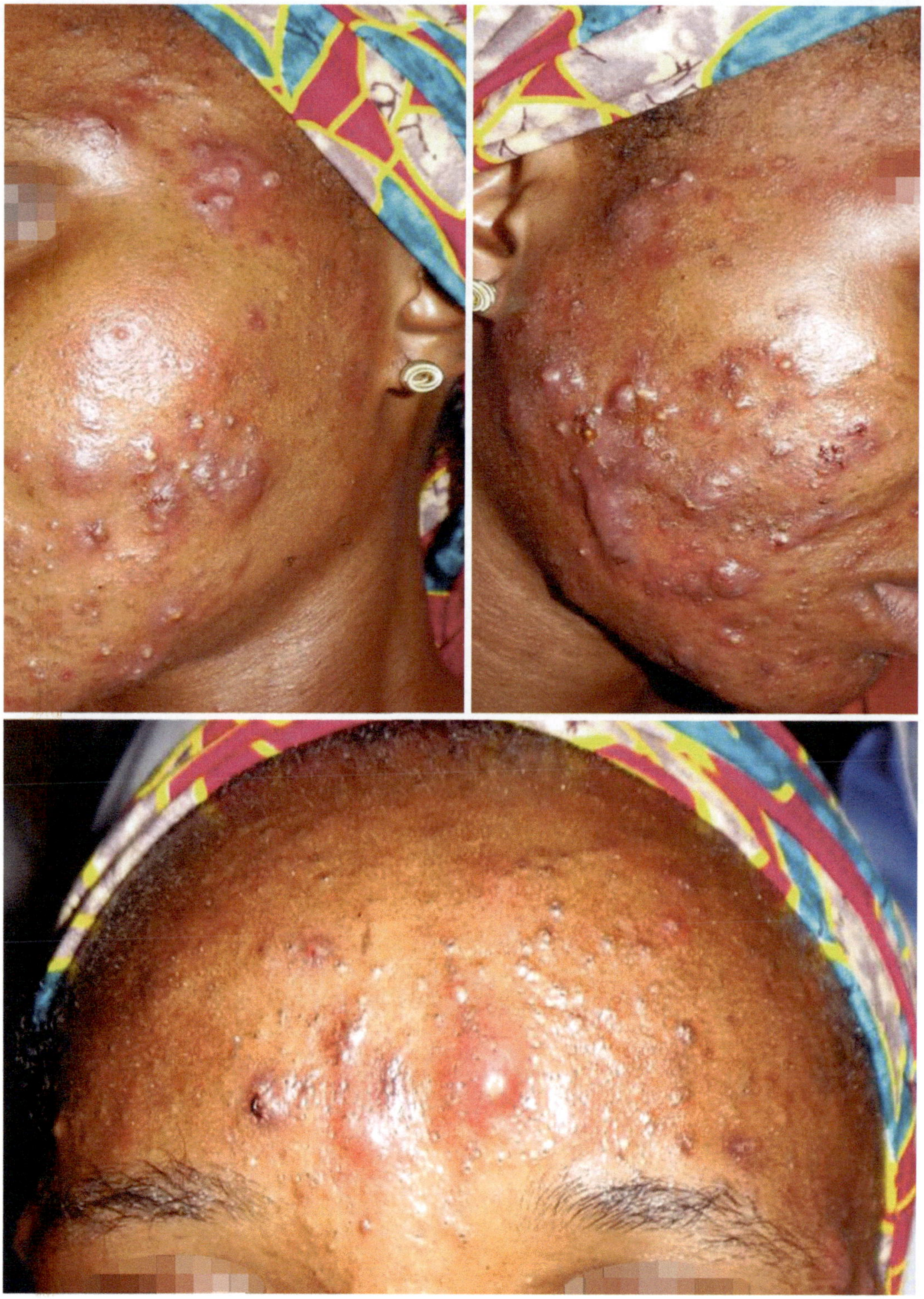

Fig. 18.4 Severe acne with multiple nodules as well as secondary acne lesions, such as cysts and sinus-forming scars

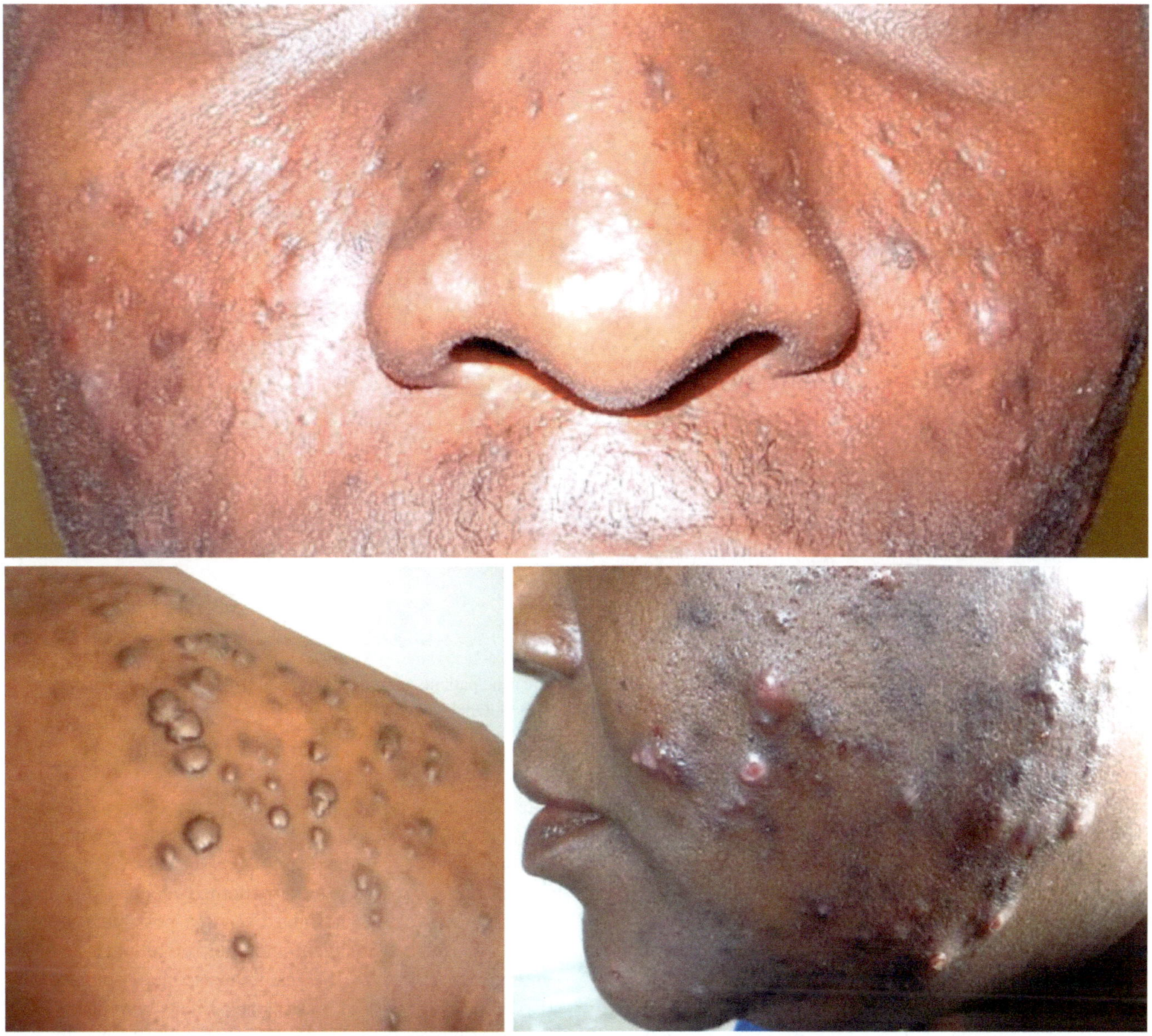

Fig. 18.5 Atrophic acne scars on the cheeks (up), hypertrophic acne scars and keloids on the back (down left), inflammatory acne lesions with postinflammatory hyperpigmentation and development of initial keloids over the jaw angles (down right)

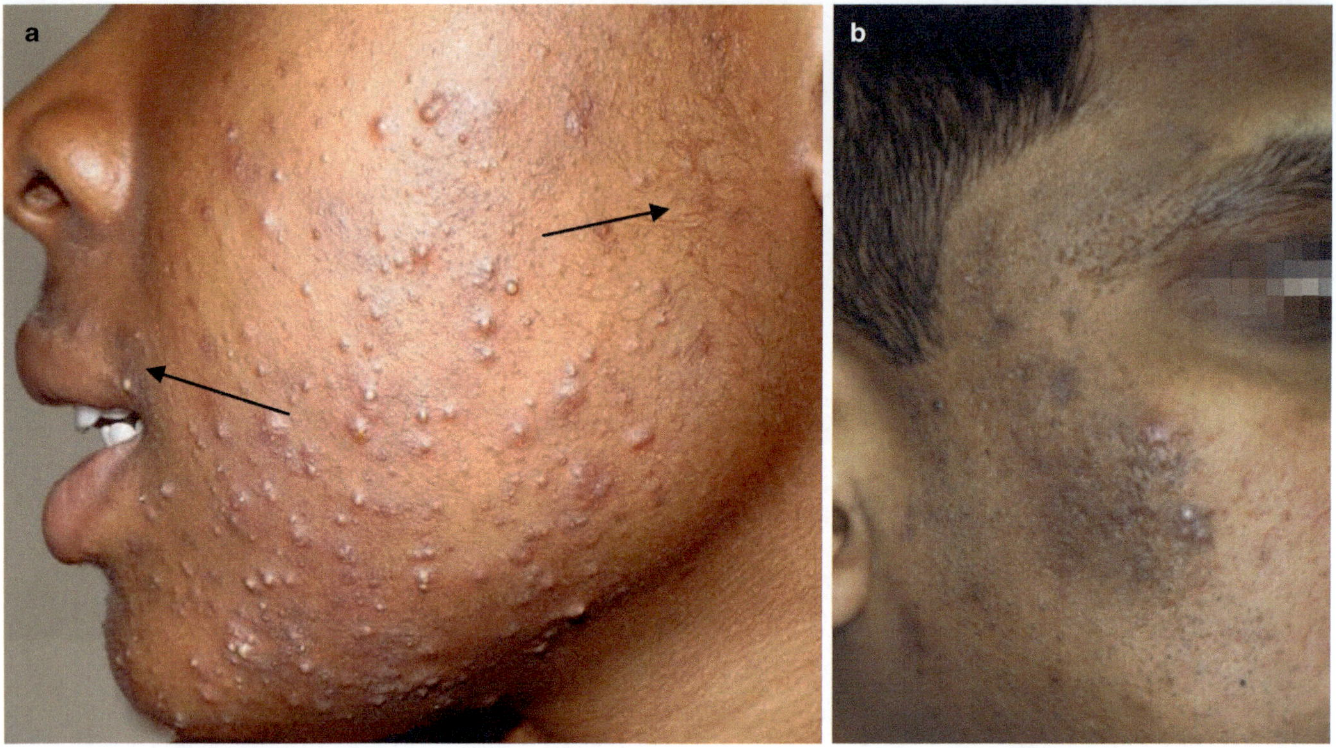

Fig. 18.6 (**a**) Minor hirsutism (arrows), a sign of hyperandrogenism in female acne patients with dark skin, and (**b**) acne tarda with dermal elastosis, comedones, ice-pick scars, hyperinsulinemia and acanthosis nigricans in a male adult patient from India

temples (Fig. 18.7) and mini scars mostly on the temples. The disease may imitate preadolescent acne [35] (Fig. 18.8); however, typical Pityrosporum folliculitis is characterized by recurrent, superficial, fine pustules arising in nasal folds, on the upper lip, glabella and sometimes on the eyelids. Such pustules are relatively asymptomatic and transient and resolve without sequelae.

Nodular elastosis with cysts and comedones (Favre-Racouchot syndrome) in dark skin is the emerging pattern of relatively mild upper face acne of young adults in the background of dystrophic pigmentation/dermal elastosis in a photo-distribution pattern (overlying zygomas and temples). There are sparse and subtle open and closed comedones in the dystrophic area (Fig. 18.9), accompanied by superficial comedones (at the periphery) and mini scars. There is bilateral asymmetry. The clinical morphology in such cases suggests exogenous/environmental factors, particularly air pollution and ultraviolet radiation, which are often possible to validate through diligent history [36].

18.3.3 Acne and Endocrine/Metabolic Diseases

Acne patients with marked seborrhea, obesity, insulin resistance, prolactinemia, polycystic ovary syndrome (PCOS) and male equivalent of PCOS are commonly observed in India [32] and only occasionally in Africa. The hyperandrogenism-insulin resistance-acanthosis nigricans (HAIR-AN) syndrome also features acne [37]. Acne-patterned alopecia-acanthosis nigricans (APAAN) syndrome [32] is a possible variant of the seborrhea-acne-hirsutism-androgenetic alopecia (SAHA) syndrome [38] (Fig. 18.10). Insulin resistance associated acne (IRAA) refers to dark-skinned acne patients with a characteristic clinical pattern (Table 18.2, Fig. 18.11). IRAA is the prototype for Indian acne. It represents approximately 75% of the acne patients from urban areas in India, independent of gender and age. IRAA onsets early, sometimes as adrenarche/preadolescent acne, peaks in adolescence and tends to persist as post-adolescent acne/acne tarda. It is comparatively mild, more comedonal, strongly associated with postinflammatory hyperpigmentation and less scarring and generally less responsive to standard acne treatments. Biochemical signs of metabolic syndrome appear at late stage. IRAA patients are more likely to have PCOS and male equivalent of PCOS [39]. Indian, African and Hispanic patients with dark skin seem to have predilection for insulin resistance [40] and, therefore, for acne. In women, IRAA may be confused with HAIR-AN syndrome. The latter is a relatively uncommon hereditary disorder wherein severe insulin resistance results from a genetic mutation in the tyrosine kinase domain on the insulin receptor [41]. It is often compounded by lifestyle maladjustments resulting in a clinical syndrome, in which hyperandrogenism as hirsut-

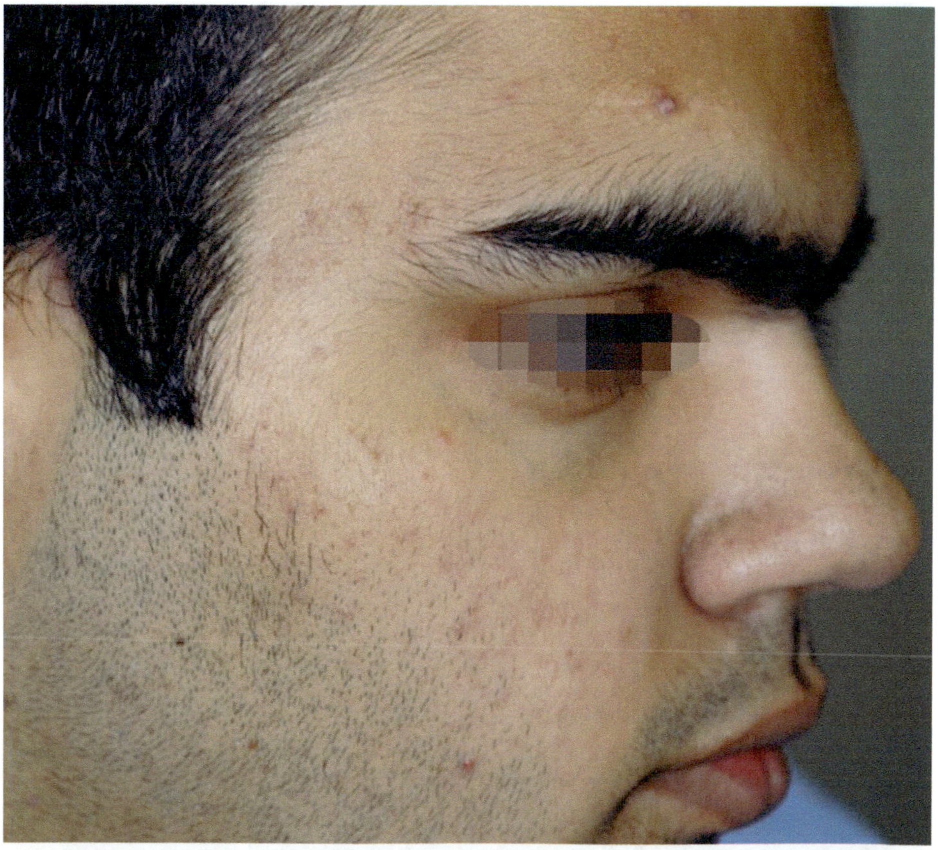

Fig. 18.7 Pityrosporum folliculitis acneiform dermatosis. Mild adult acne showing characteristic distribution and morphology, mini scars on the temple and subtle malar seborrheic dermatitis

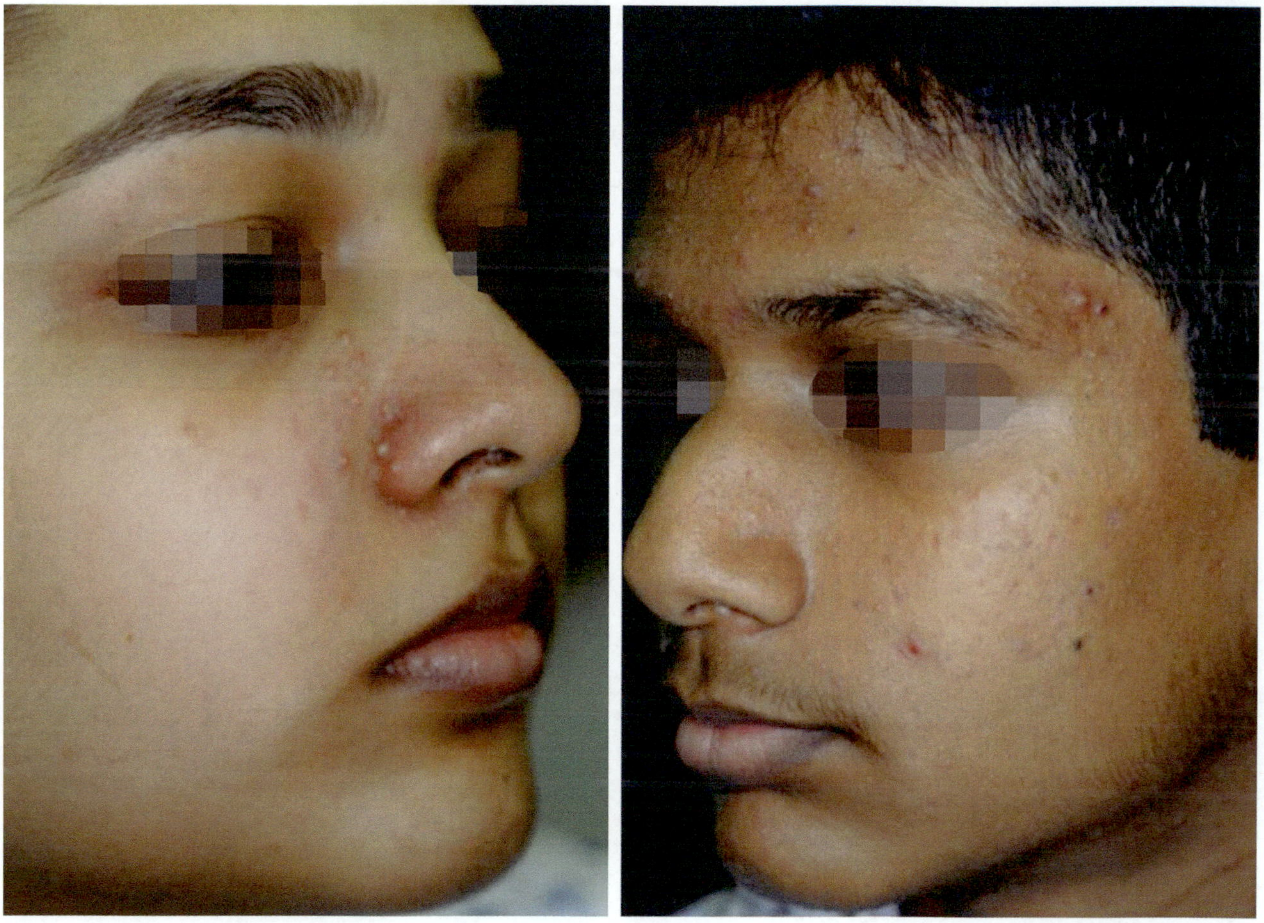

Fig. 18.8 Pityrosporum folliculitis imitating preadolescent acne (acne praecox)

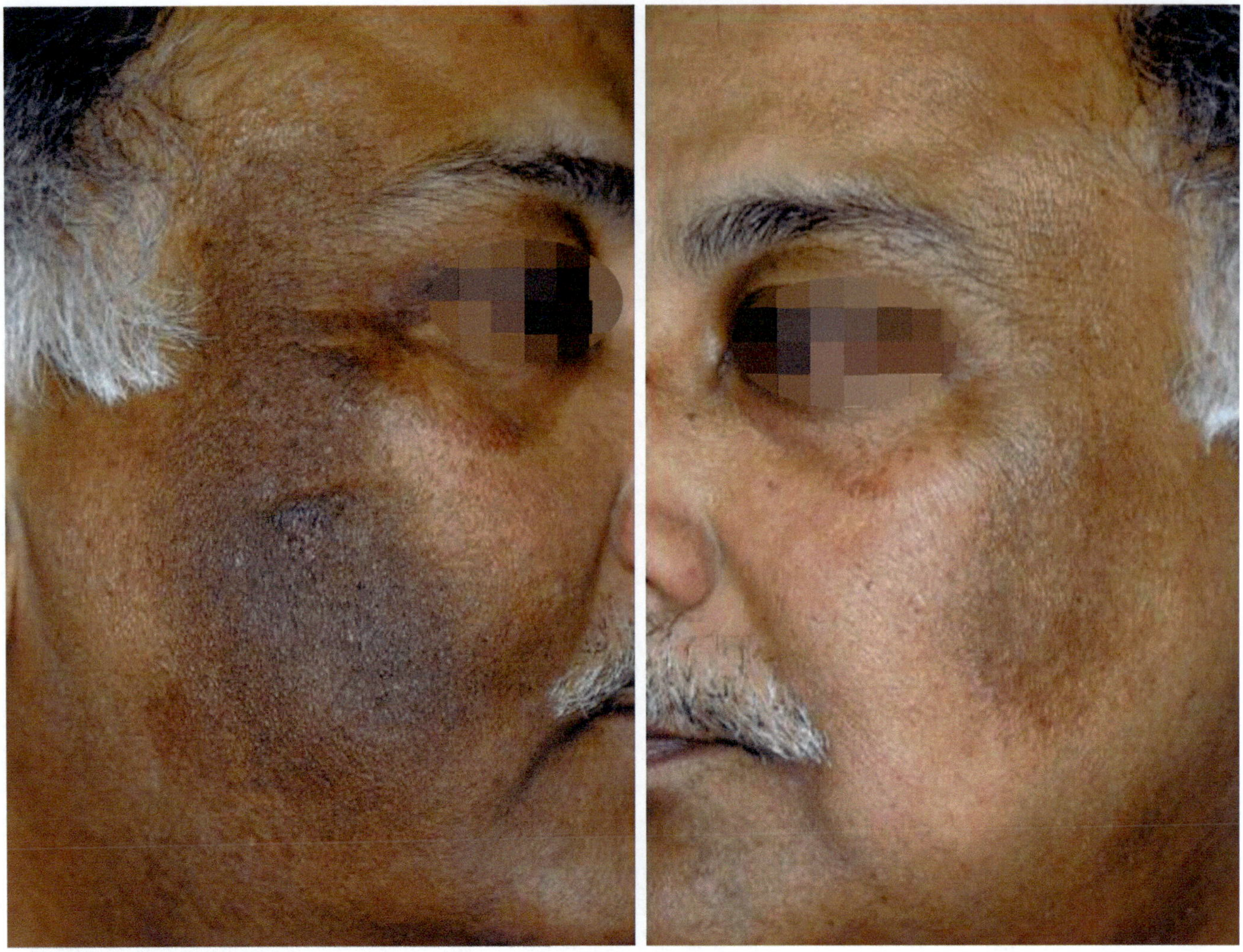

Fig. 18.9 Asymmetrical dystrophic acneiform dermatosis (Favre-Racouchot syndrome) showing dermal elastosis and subclinical acne as subtle secondary comedones

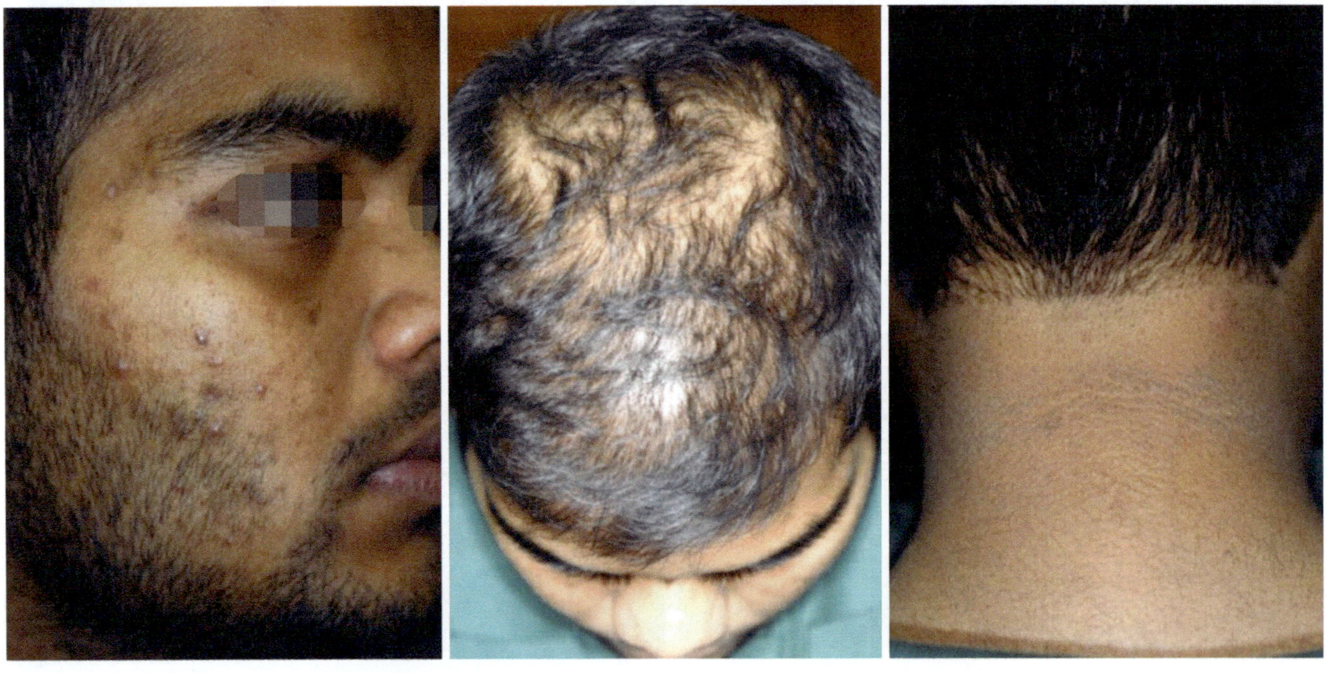

Fig. 18.10 Acne-patterned alopecia-acanthosis nigricans (APAAN) syndrome in a male patient

Table 18.2 Clinical characteristics of acne with metabolic disorders in dark skin

Facial acanthosis nigricans signs	• Periocular dark circles • Shaded chin and forehead with accentuated skin markings
Darkening of skin colour	• "Persistent tan"
Acrochordons	• Frictional areas (neck, axillae) • Periocular location
Benign hyperplasias	• Syringomata • Melanocytic nevi • Actinic lentigines • Seborrheic keratosis • Xanthelasma • Angiomas
Patterned hypertrichosis	• Jaw angles • Zygomas • Forehead • Ear rims • Confluent hypertrichosis on the nape of the neck extending to adjacent back in women • Generalized hypertrichosis in men
Patterned hair loss	• Androgenetic alopecia of male or female pattern • Diffuse hair loss • Hair thinning in both women and men
Pigment irregularities	• Melasma-like pigmentation • Lentigines
Signs of Pityrosporum overcolonization	• Recalcitrant dandruff • Malar seborrheic dermatitis
Recurrent scalp folliculitis	
Recurrent deep folliculitis	• Furuncles in the bathing trunk area
Chronic folliculitis	• Associated with waxing in women

ism is the important presenting feature rather than acne, acanthosis nigricans is pronounced, PCOS is frequent and, more importantly, the insulin response to administered glucose is attenuated [42]. In IRAA, hyperinsulinemia is initially acute (elevated postprandial insulin), and with time it becomes chronic (elevated fasting insulin), and the proposed mechanism is IGF1 gene polymorphism [43]. Acne in HAIR-AN syndrome has no known specificity, and a possible explanation for this may be that this is not a diagnosis dermatologists often make.

Non-classic congenital adrenal hyperplasia (NCAH) is the most common, autosomal recessive disorder with prevalence rate of 1:1000 and Indians, Arabs, Ashkenazi Jews and Mediterranean residents more commonly afflicted [44] (Table 18.3). The genetic defect is mutation in gene CYP21A2 expressing as variable deficiency of enzyme 21-carboxylase impacting on steroidal biosynthesis pathway.

18.3.4 Steroid Acne

Corticosteroids, both topical and systemic, can cause de novo acne as well as aggravate pre-existing acne [45]. In contrast to developed countries, steroid creams are available over the counter and are being used widely as "fairness creams" or as "after-shave creams" in the developing countries with dark skin populations, and, therefore, steroid acne is common [46]. Facial acne with 38–58% is the most common reported clinical sign in such individuals. Topical steroid acne is observed mainly on the face, while systemic steroid-induced acne generally spares the face, occurring instead on other seborrheic areas

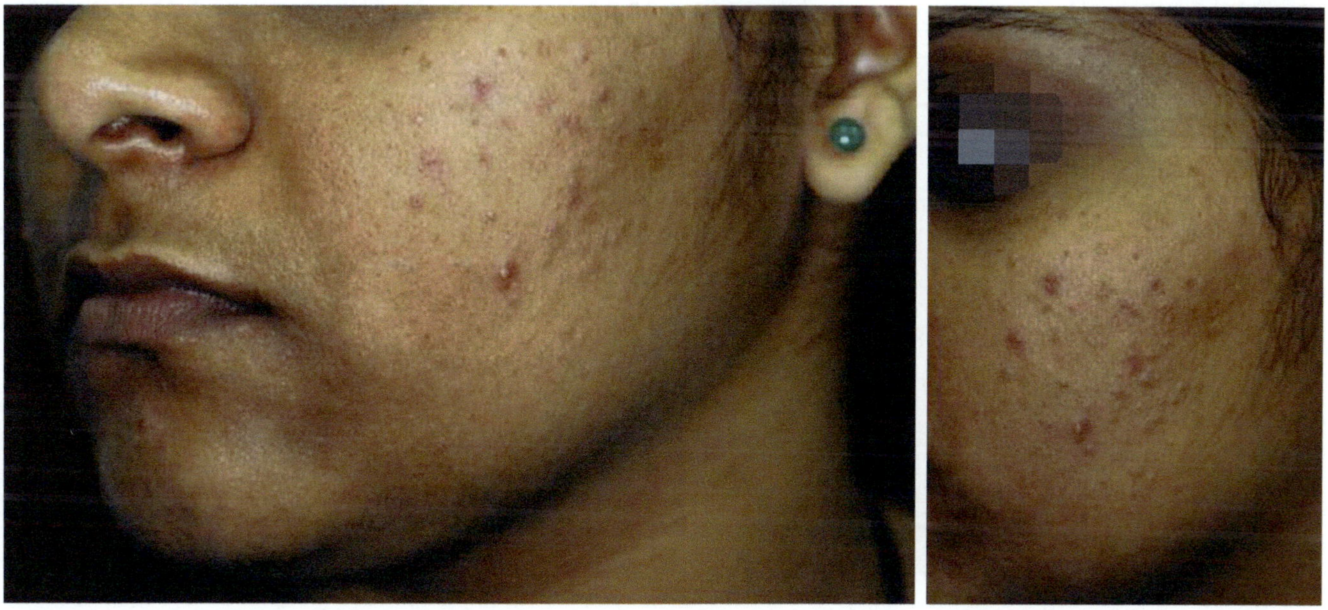

Fig. 18.11 Facial acanthosis nigricans shaded chin (left) and dark periorbital circles (right) in a patient with HAIR-AN

(Fig. 18.12). Systemic steroid-induced acne is monomorphic, devoid of comedones, erupts abruptly and the component lesions evolve and resolve in unison; topical steroid acne, on the other hand, is dominated by secondary features such as atrophy, telangiectasia, flushing, dyspigmentation and hypertrichosis with comedones and papules being few and far between. Unlike acne vulgaris, the comedone formation in topical steroid acne is a secondary phenomenon.

Table 18.3 Diagnostic features of acne in non-classic congenital adrenal hyperplasia

• Family history of persistent acne (particularly from the maternal side)
• Early onset of acne (often as acne praecox)
• Variable degree of androgen excess
• Therapeutic unresponsiveness
• Elevated 17-hydroxyprogesterone with variable hyperandrogenemia (elevated dehydroepiandrosterone sulphate, androstenedione, 5α-dihydrotestosterone)

18.3.5 Acne Sequelae

Postinflammatory hyperpigmentation and scarring are important sequelae of acne and both express differently in dark skin. Postinflammatory hyperpigmentation is more pronounced in dark skin and is associated with a greater impact on quality of life. Evaluating postinflammatory hyperpigmentation in acne is not easy [47]. It can be mistaken for erythema and vice versa in darker skin types especially during the active phase. Postinflammatory hyperpigmentation can also easily be confused with pigmentary companion morphologies, such as ephelides and lentigines in HAIR-AN and solar elastosis in environmental acne. Vague dyschromias on the upper back are common in Pityrosporum folliculitis. Dark-skinned patients are considered to suffer less from atrophic acne scars, and this, at least in some part, is on account of comparatively less severe acne. Mini scars, thus, may be the commonest type of acne scars in dark skin. Furthermore, mini scars are often encountered in mild forms of acne [48]. Hypertrophic

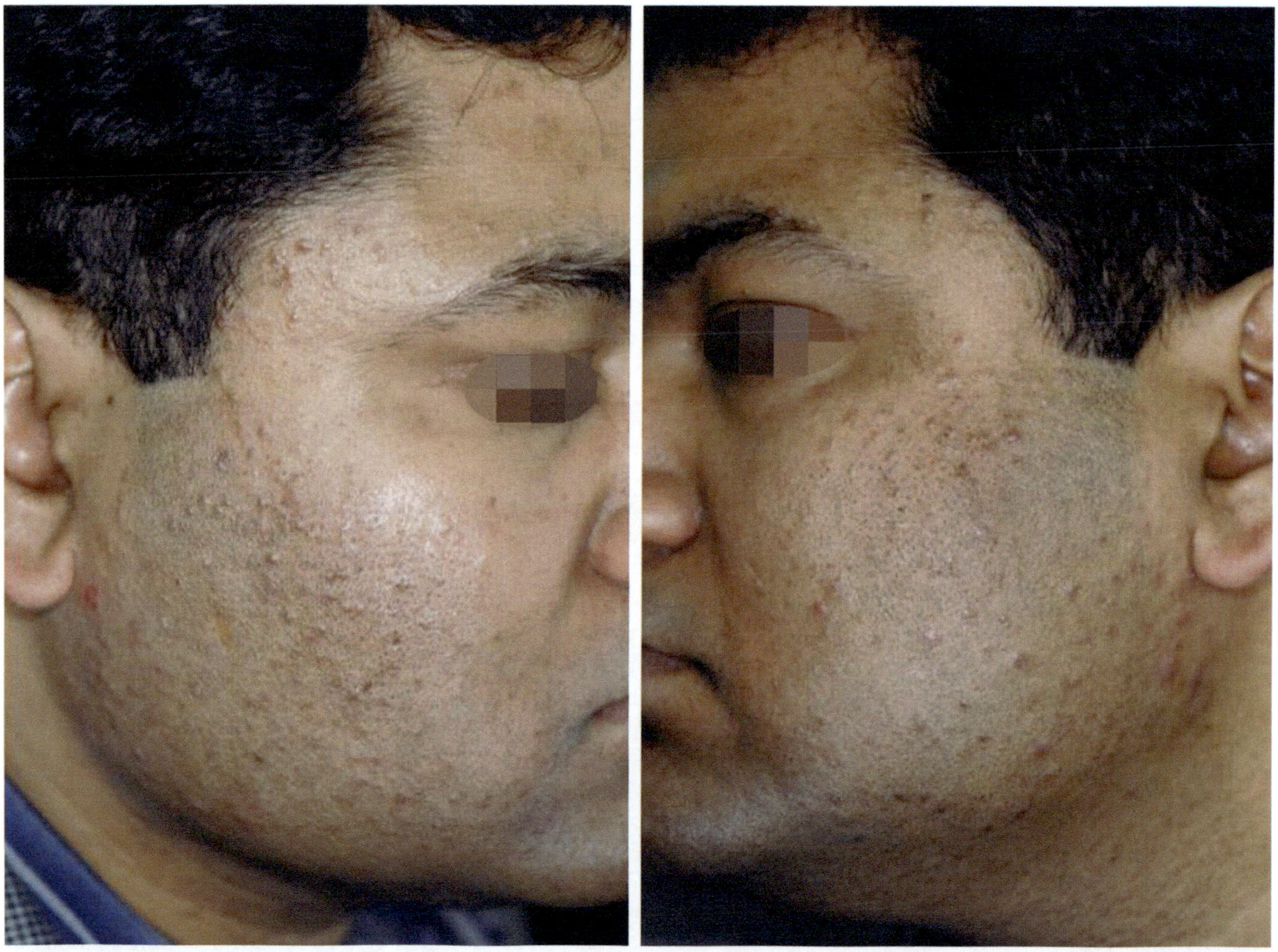

Fig. 18.12 Topical steroid-induced acne from clobetasol gel prescribed for lichen planopilaris in the scalp

scars and keloids are recognized to be more common in dark skin, especially in Africans and Afro-Americans. Hypertrophic scars ordinarily do not occur on the face; however, occasionally they develop over the jaw angles in dark skin (Fig. 18.5).

Diagnosis of acne vulgaris is related with the detection of characteristic follicular lesions, especially comedones, at the specific localizations, namely the sebaceous follicle-rich areas of the body. There are several classification models for acne with a most simplified one shown in Table 18.1.

18.4 Treatment

Acne in dark-skinned individuals is managed differently in different countries, where such people reside reflecting local ground realities, institutional/governmental regulation or lack of it and socioeconomic factors. Acne guidelines that recognize such differences have been created, but physicians/patients do generally not adhere to them [27]. Adequate treatment of acne requires the assessment of the severity of the disease including the psychological status of the patient. A simple way to do this is to classify the disease according to its severity as shown in Table 18.1.

18.4.1 Mild Comedonal Acne

Topical retinoids, such as tretinoin (0.025–0.5%), adapalene (0.1%) or tazarotene, are the treatment of choice [49]. Tretinoin 0.05% cream is readily available in most African countries unlike other topical retinoids. Dark-skinned patients certainly experience more irritation in the initial phase of treatment with topical retinoids and are recommended to adopt escalating regimens [50]. This has been not only shown in Afro-Americans, but also in Indians, Chinese and Malays. Topical retinoids are helpful in both preventing and treating acne-associated postinflammatory hyperpigmentation [28].

18.4.2 Mild Papulopustular Acne

Combinations of topical retinoids, antibiotics (clindamycin 1%) or antimicrobials (benzoyl peroxide 2.5%, 5%) are required. These can be used separately or in fixed-dose combinations. Topical antibiotics are losing favour and are currently available in combination with benzoyl peroxide and topical retinoids. Topical nadifloxacin and azelaic acid are available in some countries.

18.4.3 Moderate Acne

A combination of systemic and topical drugs is essential. Systemic antiacne drugs include oral antibiotics, such as tetracyclines (tetracycline 2 × 250–500 mg/day, doxycycline 2 × 50–100 mg/day, minocycline 2 × 25–50 mg/day and lymecycline 2 × 150–300 mg/day) and macrolides (erythromycin 2 × 250–500 mg/day and azithromycin 1–2 × 250 mg/day), hormonal anti-androgens (only for females) and isotretinoin. The oral antibiotics also possess an anti-inflammatory effect and can only be used for 8–12 weeks to avoid the development of resistant bacteria. The expected side effects are minimal. Despite the global consensus on restricting the use of antibiotics in acne to short periods and to avoid monotherapy and the use of dissimilar oral and topical antibiotics concomitantly, such recommendations are commonly flouted. Antibiotic resistance is thus rampant. In India, *P. acnes* has been reported to be resistant to azithromycin (100%), erythromycin (98%), clindamycin (90%), doxycycline (44%) and tetracycline (31%), whereas low resistance was observed to minocycline (2%) and levofloxacin (10%) in a recent study [51]. Similar (but less bleak) reports have emanated from Japan, Korea, Hong Kong, Singapore, Australia, Iran, Egypt, Mexico, Costa Rica, Columbia and Chile [48].

In *female acne patients*, who do not respond to antibiotics, hormonal anti-androgens can be introduced, especially if the patients have features of hyperandrogenism. Combinations of estrogen (20 or 30 μg) and progesterone (drospirenone 3 mg) or anti-androgens, such as cyproterone acetate (2 mg/day), chlormadinone acetate or dienogest are effective after 6–12 months of treatment [52]. Spironolactone (50–100 mg/day) or flutamide (62.5–250 mg/day) can also be administered, if no contraceptive effect is required.

18.4.4 Severe Acne

In severe acne or no response to antibiotics and hormonal anti-androgens (females), isotretinoin at 0.2–0.5 mg/kg/day at best in two doses can be used for a period of 6 months (cave: teratogeneity) [53]. Low-dose isotretinoin has mainly its appeal in reducing mucocutaneous toxicity [54] but also in being more economical. On review of published studies, the efficacy of low-dose isotretinoin in dark-skinned patients varies from 69 to 99.8% with the relapse rate of 0–39% [55]. Oral isotretinoin has additional beneficial effects in acne patients with dark skin. It is helpful in reversing acanthosis nigricans when used in combination with metformin [56]. It also reverses darkening of skin colour encountered in HAIR-AN. Oral isotretinoin is also the most effective medication to prevent and repair acne sequelae including acne scars and postinflammatory hyperpigmentation.

Additional measures that will help to improve the acne lesions are:

(a) The use of a short course of systemic steroids (prednisolone 10–30 mg/day) in addition to isotretinoin for 2 weeks in cases of severe acne.
(b) Intralesional triamcinolone injection (0.1 mL of 2.5 mg) in abscesses/cysts (after aspiration) and in nodular lesions.
(c) Metformin 500 mg 2×/day is increasingly being used by dermatologists as additional treatment (not as monotherapy) in treating acne of patients with metabolic syndrome [57]. Metformin reduces serum insulin and inhibits the expression of gene coding for multiple inflammatory cytokines.
(d) The definitive treatment of NCAH-related acne is low-dose suppressive oral prednisolone (5 mg/day) administered at bedtime. The therapeutic response is prompt with acne remitting, whereas the amelioration of androgen excess occurs more slowly.
(e) Extraction of comedones using comedone extractors.
(f) Salicylic acid 20% peels every 4–6 weeks.

Maintenance management using topical retinoids (0.05% tretinoin, adapalene), fixed combinations of retinoids with benzoyl peroxide or azelaic acid (15%, 20%) is important to prevent reoccurrence of the lesions. Salicylic acid (2%) facial washes may help to temporarily open the closed comedones and reduce skin oiliness in patients with seborrhea. Dermatologists in developed countries must be aware for the varieties of acne and acneiform dermatoses, which occur in dark skin, and take into consideration that several environmental factors may be responsible for the patient's disease in order to exclude them and be able to treat the patient properly.

References

1. Zouboulis CC. Acne as a chronic systemic disease. Clin Dermatol. 2014;32:389–96.
2. Alexis AF. Acne vulgaris in skin of color: understanding nuances and optimizing treatment outcomes. J Drugs Dermatol. 2014;13:s61–5.
3. Davis SA, Narahari S, Feldman SR, et al. Top dermatologic conditions in patients of color: an analysis of nationally representative data. J Drugs Dermatol. 2012;11:466–73.
4. Zouboulis CC. Acne vulgaris. Hautarzt. 2014;65:733–50.
5. Okoro OE, Sani H. Pattern of skin diseases at the dermatology clinic of Jos University Teaching Hospital, Jos Plateau state Nigeria. Jos J Med. 2014;8:15–21.
6. Ogunbiyi AO, Omigbodun Y, Owoaje E. Prevalence of skin disorders in school children in South-West Nigeria. Int J Adolesc Med Health. 2009;21:235–41.
7. Yahaya H. Acne vulgaris in Nigerian adolescents—prevalence, severity, beliefs, perceptions, and practices. Int J Dermatol. 2009;48:489–505.
8. Okoro OE, Ogunbiyi AO, George AO. Prevalence and pattern of acne vulgaris among adolescents in Ibadan, south-west Nigeria. J Egypt Women Dermatol Soc. 2016;13:7–12.
9. Hartshorne ST. Dermatological disorders in Johannesburg, South Africa. Clin Exp Dermatol. 2003;148:193–4.
10. Ogunbiyi AO, Daramola OOM, Alese OO. Prevalence of skin diseases in Ibadan Nigeria. Int J Dermatol. 2004;43:31–6.
11. Henshaw EB, Olasode OA, Ogedegbe EE, et al. Dermatologic conditions in teenage adolescents in Nigeria. Adolesc Health Med Ther. 2014;5:79–87.
12. Lynn DD, Umari T, Dunnick CA, et al. The epidemiology of acne vulgaris in late adolescence. Adolesc Health Med Ther. 2016;7:13–25.
13. Perkins A, Cheng C, Hillebrand G, et al. Comparison of the epidemiology of acne vulgaris among Caucasian, Asian, Continental Indians and African American women. J Eur Acad Dermatol Venereol. 2011;25:1054–60.
14. Cordain L, Lindeberg S, Hurtado M, et al. Acne vulgaris: a disease of western civilization. Arch Dermatol. 2002;138:1584–90.
15. Zouboulis CC. Acne and sebaceous gland function. Clin Dermatol. 2004;22:360–6.
16. Zouboulis CC, Jourdan E, Picardo M. Acne is an inflammatory disease and alterations of sebum composition initiate acne lesions. J Eur Acad Dermatol Venereol. 2014;28:527–32.
17. Gollnick H, Zouboulis CC. Not all acne is acne vulgaris. Dtsch Arztbl Int. 2014;111:301–12.
18. Moradi-Tuchayi S, Makrantonaki E, Ganceviciene R, et al. Acne vulgaris. Nature Rev Dis Primers. 2015;1:15029.
19. Herane MI, Ando I. Acne in infancy and acne genetics. Dermatology. 2003;206:24–8.
20. Ghodsi SZ, Orawa H, Zouboulis CC. Prevalence, severity, and severity risk factors of acne in high school pupils: a community-based study. J Invest Dermatol. 2009;129:2136–41.
21. Zouboulis CC. Is acne vulgaris a genuine inflammatory disease? Dermatology. 2001;203:277–9.
22. Zouboulis CC, Seltmann H, Hiroi N, et al. Corticotropin releasing hormone: an autocrine hormone that promotes lipogenesis in human sebocytes. Proc Natl Acad Sci U S A. 2002;99:7148–53.
23. Ganceviciene R, Graziene V, Fimmel S, et al. Involvement of the corticotropin-releasing hormone system in the pathogenesis of acne vulgaris. Br J Dermatol. 2009;160:345–52.
24. Pappas A, Fantasia J, Chen T. Age and ethnic variations in sebaceous lipids. Dermatoendocrinology. 2013;5:319–24.
25. Zouboulis CC, Eady A, Philpott M, et al. What is the pathogenesis of acne? Exp Dermatol. 2005;14:143–52.
26. Zouboulis CC, Schagen S, Alestas T. The sebocyte culture: a model to study the pathophysiology of the sebaceous gland in sebostasis, seborrhoea and acne. Arch Dermatol Res. 2008;300:397–413.
27. Cappel M, Mauger D, Thibutot D. Correlation between serum levels of insulin-like growth factor 1, dehydroepiandrosterone sulfate, and dihydrotestosterone and acne lesion counts in adult women. Arch Dermatol. 2005;141:333–8.
28. Vora S, Ovhal A, Jerajani H, et al. Correlation of facial sebum to serum insulin-like growth factor-1 in patients with acne. Br J Dermatol. 2008;159:990–1.
29. Kubba R, Bajaj AK, Thappa DM, et al. Acne in India: guidelines for management—IAA consensus document. Ind J Dermatol Venereol Leprol. 2009;75:S1–62.
30. Silverberg JI, Silverberg NB. Epidemiology and extracutaneous comorbidities of severe acne in adolescence: an U.S. population-based study. Br J Dermatol. 2014;170:1136–42.
31. Davis EC, Callender VD. A review of acne in ethnic skin: pathogenesis, clinical manifestations, and management strategies. J Clin Aesthet Dermatol. 2010;3:24–38.
32. Kubba R. Acne in dark skin people. In: Schwartz RA, Micali G, editors. Acne. Gurgaon: Macmillan; 2013. p. 39–50.

33. Kubba R, Chatrath V. Acne expression and management in Indians. World Clin Dermatol. 2013;1:105–27.
34. Jacinto-Jamora S, Tamesis J, Katigbak MI. Pityrosporum folliculitis in the Philippines: diagnosis, prevalence and management. J Am Acad Dermatol. 1991;24:693–6.
35. Youn NH, Cha SH, Park S. Malassezia yeasts in acne vulgaris. Korean J Dermatol. 2002;40:1453–60.
36. Ju Q, Yiang K, Zouboulis CC, et al. Chloracne: from clinic to research. Dermatol Sin. 2012;30:2–6.
37. Adler YD, Zouboulis CC, Geilen CC, et al. Eine seltene Variante des SAHA syndroms. Z Hautkr. 2001;76:327–8.
38. Orfanos CE, Adler YD, Zouboulis CC. The SAHA syndrome. Horm Res. 2000;54:251–8.
39. Sanke S, Chander R, Jain A, et al. A comparison of the hormone profile of the early androgenetic alopecia in men with the phenotypic equivalent of polycystic ovarian syndrome in women. JAMA Dermatol. 2016;152:986–91.
40. Svetlana T, Maclaren N. Insulin resistance syndrome in children. J Clin Endocrinol Metab. 2004;89:2526–34.
41. Globerman H, Carnieli E. Analysis of the insulin receptor gene tyrosine kinase domain in obese patients with hyperandrogenism, insulin resistance and acanthosis nigricans. Int J Obes Relat Metab Disord. 1998;22:349–53.
42. Dunaif A, Finegood DT. Beta-cell dysfunction independent of obesity and glucose intolerance in the polycystic ovary syndrome. J Clin Endocrinol Metab. 1996;81:942–7.
43. Rahman MA, De D, Handa S, et al. Association of insulin-like growth factor (IGF-1) gene polymorphisms with plasma levels of IGF-1 and acne severity. J Am Acad Dermatol. 2016;75:768–73.
44. Honour JW. 17-Hydroxyprogesterone in children, adolescents and adults. Ann Clin Biochem. 2014;51:424–40.
45. Plewig G, Kligman AM. Induction of acne by topical steroids. Arch Dermatol Forsch. 1973;247:29–52.
46. Saraswat A, Lahiri K, Chatterjee M, et al. Topical corticosteroid abuse on the face: a prospective, multicentre study of dermatology outpatients. Ind J Dermatol Venereol Leprol. 2011;77:160–6.
47. Goh CL, Abad-Casinthan F, Chow SK, et al. Evaluating acne-related post-inflammatory hyperpigmentation is a challenge even amongst experts. J Dermatol. 2014;41:1106–8.
48. Hayashi N, Miyachi Y, Kawashima M. Prevalence of scars and "mini-scars", and their impact on quality of life in Japanese patients with acne. J Dermatol. 2015;42:690–6.
49. Nast A, Dréno B, Bettoli V, et al. European evidence-based (S3) guidelines for the treatment of acne. J Eur Acad Dermatol Venereol. 2012;26(suppl 1):1–29.
50. Taylor SC, Cook-Bolden F, Rahman Z, et al. Acne vulgaris in skin of color. J Am Acad Dermatol. 2002;46:S98–106.
51. Sardana K, Gupta T, Kumar B, et al. Cross-sectional pilot study of antibiotic resistance in Propionibacterium acnes strains in Indian acne patients using 16S-RNA polymerase chain reaction: a comparison among treatment modalities including antibiotics, benzoyl peroxide, and isotretinoin. Ind J Dermatol. 2016;61:45–52.
52. Zouboulis CC, Rabe T. Hormonelle Antiandrogene in der Aknetherapie. J Dtsch Dermatol Ges. 2010;8(suppl 1):S60–74.
53. Ganceviciene R, Zouboulis C. Isotretinoin for acne vulgaris: state-of-the-art treatment for acne vulgaris. J Dtsch Dermatol Ges. 2010;8(suppl 1):S47–59.
54. Borghi A, Mantovani L, Minghetti S, et al. Low-cumulative dose isotretinoin treatment in mild-to-moderate acne: efficacy in achieving stable remission. J Eur Acad Dermatol Venereol. 2011;25:1094–8.
55. Dhaked DR, Meena RS, Maheshwari A, et al. A randomized comparative trial of two low-dose isotretinoin regimens in moderate to severe acne vulgaris. Ind Dermatol Online J. 2016;7:378–85.
56. Walling HW, Messingham M, Myers LM, et al. Improvement of acanthosis nigricans on isotretinoin and metformin. J Drugs Dermatol. 2003;6:677–81.
57. Fabbrocini G, Izzo R, Faggiano A, et al. Low glycaemic diet and metformin therapy: a new approach in male subjects with acne resistant to common treatments. Clin Exp Dermatol. 2016;41:38–42.

Hidradenitis Suppurativa

19

Christos C. Zouboulis and Mankul Goyal

Hidradenitis suppurativa (HS) or *acne inversa* is a chronic, inflammatory, recurrent, debilitating skin disease of the hair follicles that usually presents after puberty with painful, deep-seated, inflamed lesions in the apocrine gland-bearing areas of the body, most commonly the axillae, inguinal, and anogenital regions [1]. The disease affects mainly young adults with a female predominance (female to male ratio 2.4–3.3:1). Among the various populations and skin types, prevalence and incidence often differ, but there are no differences in major clinical characteristics. Spontaneous resolution of the disease is rare. Medical treatment targets the inflammatory response, and surgical intervention reduces the burden of the disease offering an overall better outcome. In addition, lifestyle modifications like weight loss and smoking cessation play an important role in improving the prognosis of HS. In recent studies, patients with blistering diseases, leg ulcers, psoriasis, and eczemas had the highest risk for reduction of health-related quality of life among all other non-tumor dermatological conditions [2].

19.1 Epidemiology

HS has a global distribution; its prevalence in Europe is 1%, as estimated in studies on representative samples of French and Danish populations [3, 4]. Among immigrants in Alicante, Spain, the frequency of HS was lower than in a cross section of the autochthonous patient population (0.2% vs. 0.9%) [5]. In the USA, a markedly lower prevalence of 0.053–0.1% has been reported [6, 7], with a mean incidence rate of 6.0/100,000 person-years. Notably, a 2.5-fold increase has been registered between the years 1968 and 2008 [8]; the average annual incidence over the last 10 years was 8.6/100,000 involving disproportionally women, young adults, and African Americans [9]. The prevalence of HS in the African American population is 2.0– to 3.1– fold higher than in the group with fair skin, and the incidence among African Americans was found to be 30.6/100,000, i.e., 2.6 fold higher [9, 10]. Studies on the prevalence and incidence of HS in Asian and African populations are lacking. While Asians seem to be less affected, Indians may exhibit a higher prevalence; they constitute 80% of the HS patients in Malaysia although they only represent 8% of its population.

19.2 Pathogenesis

The occlusion of the infrainfudibulum is considered as the primary event in HS, caused by hyperplasia of the follicular epithelium and infundibular hyperkeratosis; accumulation of cellular debris then leads to cyst formation [11]. Eventually the hair follicle ruptures, followed by secondary inflammatory response and granulomatous tissue reaction.

Genetic factors have been considered to play a role in this process. In case series approximately one-third of all patients with HS had a family history of the condition, and an autosomal dominant inheritance pattern with incomplete penetrance has been suggested [12]. Genetic research has demonstrated loss of function mutations in three out of four subunits of γ-secretase (presenilin-1, presenilin enhancer-2, and nicastrin) [13]. In mouse models, γ-secretase deficiency results in conversion of hair follicles into epidermal cysts and absence of sebaceous glands, the latter observation in keeping with a reduction of sebaceous gland number and volume in uninvolved hair follicles. Potential target proteins

C. C. Zouboulis (✉)
Departments of Dermatology, Venereology, Allergology and Immunology, Dessau Medical Center, Brandenburg Medical School Theodor Fontane, Dessau, Germany
e-mail: christos.zouboulis@klinikum-dessau.de

M. Goyal
Delhi Dermatology Group, Kubba Clinic, New Delhi, Delhi, India

C. E. Orfanos et al. (eds.), *Pigmented Ethnic Skin and Imported Dermatoses*, https://doi.org/10.1007/978-3-319-69422-1_19

of γ-secretase are type I integral membrane proteins like Notch, E-cadherin, or CD44. Notch plays a significant role in normal hair follicle development and T cell-mediated immune response. After initial link of γ-secretase gene to HS in Han Chinese families, mutations have also been reported in other populations, including an African American family in the USA [14]. In genotype-phenotype correlation, patients with γ-secretase mutations tend to have more severe disease with involvement of non-flexural sites and increased risk for development of squamous cell carcinoma; however, γ-secretase mutations only underpin a minority of cases of HS, even in those individuals with positive family history.

Environmental factors such as obesity, smoking and mechanical stress may represent important precipitating factors in HS. Nicotine activates acetylcholine and aryl hydrocarbon receptors in keratinocytes, leading to infundibular epithelial hyperplasia with increased cornification [15]; it contributes to inhibition of Notch signaling, hence fueling the follicular occlusion. Tobacco smoke also induces proinflammatory cytokines, like TNF-α, IL-1α, IL-1β, and IL-8, leading to neutrophil chemotaxis and Th17 cell induction. Obesity may aggravate HS by worsening insulin resistance as well as by increasing local friction in skin folds. Regarding mechanical stress, it has been postulated that constant mechanical forces, such as friction in the axillae and groins, contribute to intrafollicular hyperkeratinization, dilatation, and eventually rupture of the follicle wall with ensuing abscesses. In tropical climate, increased sweating and secondary maceration are additional aggravating factors.

The onset of HS after puberty, premenstrual flares of the disease, and female predominance further suggest that *hormones* may play a pathogenetic role. High concentration of total testosterone, increased free androgen index, and good response to antiandrogen therapies support the role of androgens [16], although normal androgen profiles have mostly been documented in HS patients. In addition, an association between metabolic syndrome and HS has been detected, which is further validated by the therapeutic efficacy of metformin. Insulin resistance, hyperprolactinemia, and hyperandrogenemia are likely to represent key pathogenetic factors.

Although many studies have attempted to identify the role of *bacteria* in HS, missing colonization in mild disease and bacterial diversity in moderate and severe stages do not support a bacterial etiology. Gram-positive cocci and rods, including coagulase-negative staphylococci, have been frequently cultured from HS lesions [17].

Last but not least, drugs known to induce HS include lithium, sirolimus, cyclosporine, and vemurafenib.

19.3 Clinical Picture

HS presents a variable clinical picture and course with recurrent inflammatory lesions in skinfolds, although other areas may also be affected [1, 18]. Inguinal, axillary, perineal and perianal, as well as the submammary and/or intermammary folds in females, buttocks, mons pubis, scalp, retroauricular area, and eyelids are often involved. Initial single or multiple transient superficial follicular papules and pustules are not diagnostic. Transient or persisting nodules and abscesses are part of the diagnostic definition; they can gradually coalesce to form plaques. Recurrences occur in a period of 6 months at inverse regions of the body and lead to formation of tunnels (fistulae, sinuses) as well as of other secondary lesions such as pseudo-comedones, cysts, and/or scars. 23–30% of HS patients are also affected by a pilonidal disease.

There are no studies evaluating differences in clinical features of HS between fair and pigmented ethnic skin; the clinical presentation is similar in different skin types (Figs. 19.1, 19.2, 19.3, 19.4, 19.5, and 19.6). However, patients with HS living in hot climate zones face more frequent secondary infections. Rare cases of associated tubercular and non-tubercular mycobacterial infections have been reported in India [19, 20]. Due to the chronic inflammatory process, secondary scrotal or vulvar lymphedema and fistula formation in the vagina, urethra, peritoneum or bladder can develop. Lymphangioma circumscriptum of the vulva is possible. Squamous cell carcinoma developing on HS is a rare life-threatening complication reported with early metastatic spread and a devastating mortality rate of 50% [21]. Patients with coexisting HS and human immunodeficiency virus infection tend to have more severe disease and involvement of ectopic sites. Diagnostic criteria both for the primary care setting and for dermatologists are presented in Table 19.1. Despite the simplification of diagnosis, the average duration between first manifestation of the disease and diagnosis is 7.2 years [23].

Inflammatory cases of HS are classified as *mild*, *moderate*, and *severe* based on the International Hidradenitis Suppurativa Severity Score System (IHS4) (Table 19.2), whereas, noninflammatory cases are classified in *stages I*, *II*, *and II* according to the Hurley score (Table 19.3). Several other classification score systems exist.

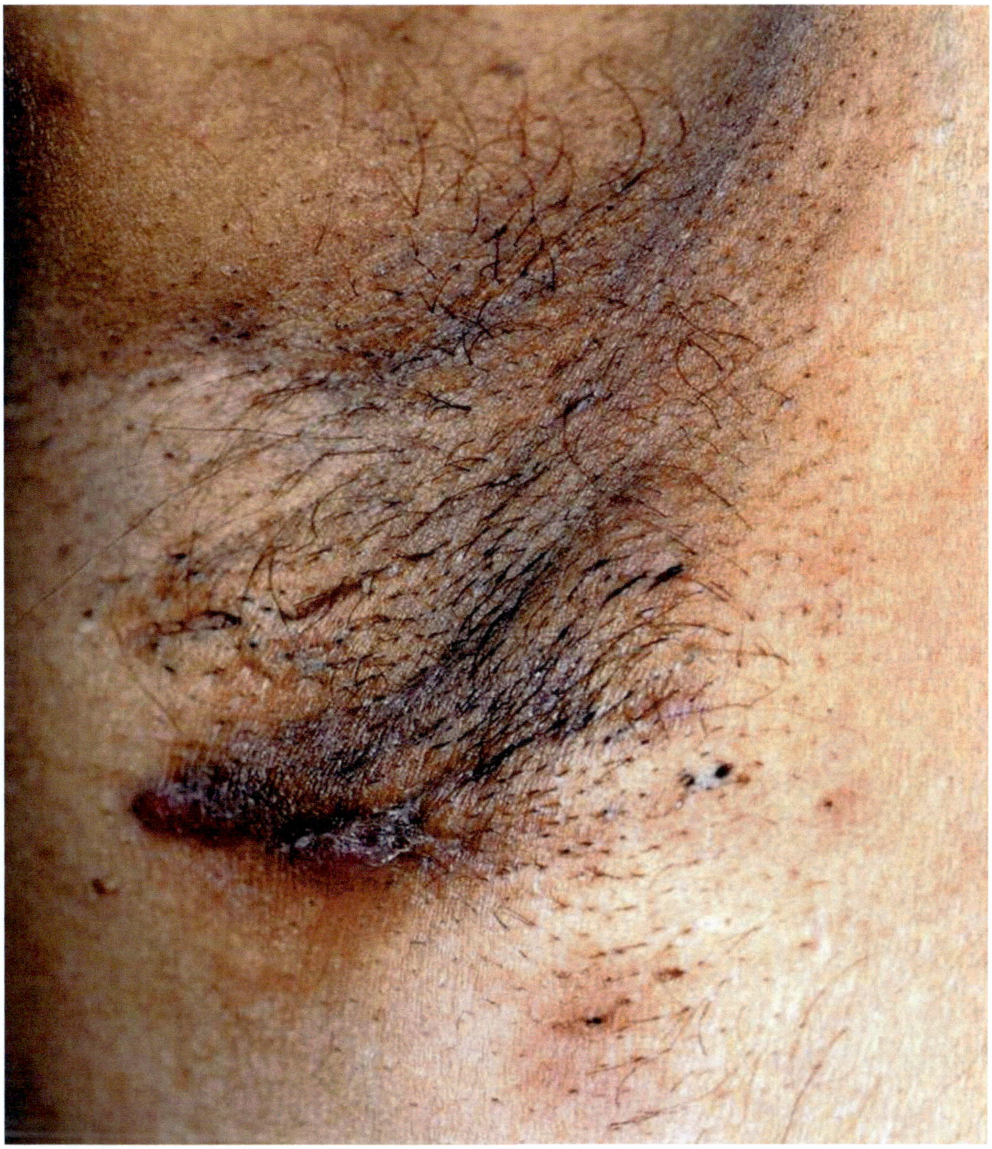

Fig. 19.1 Abscesses and double pseudo-comedones at the axillary area of an Indian patient with early *hidradenitis suppurativa*; Hurley I, moderate IHS4

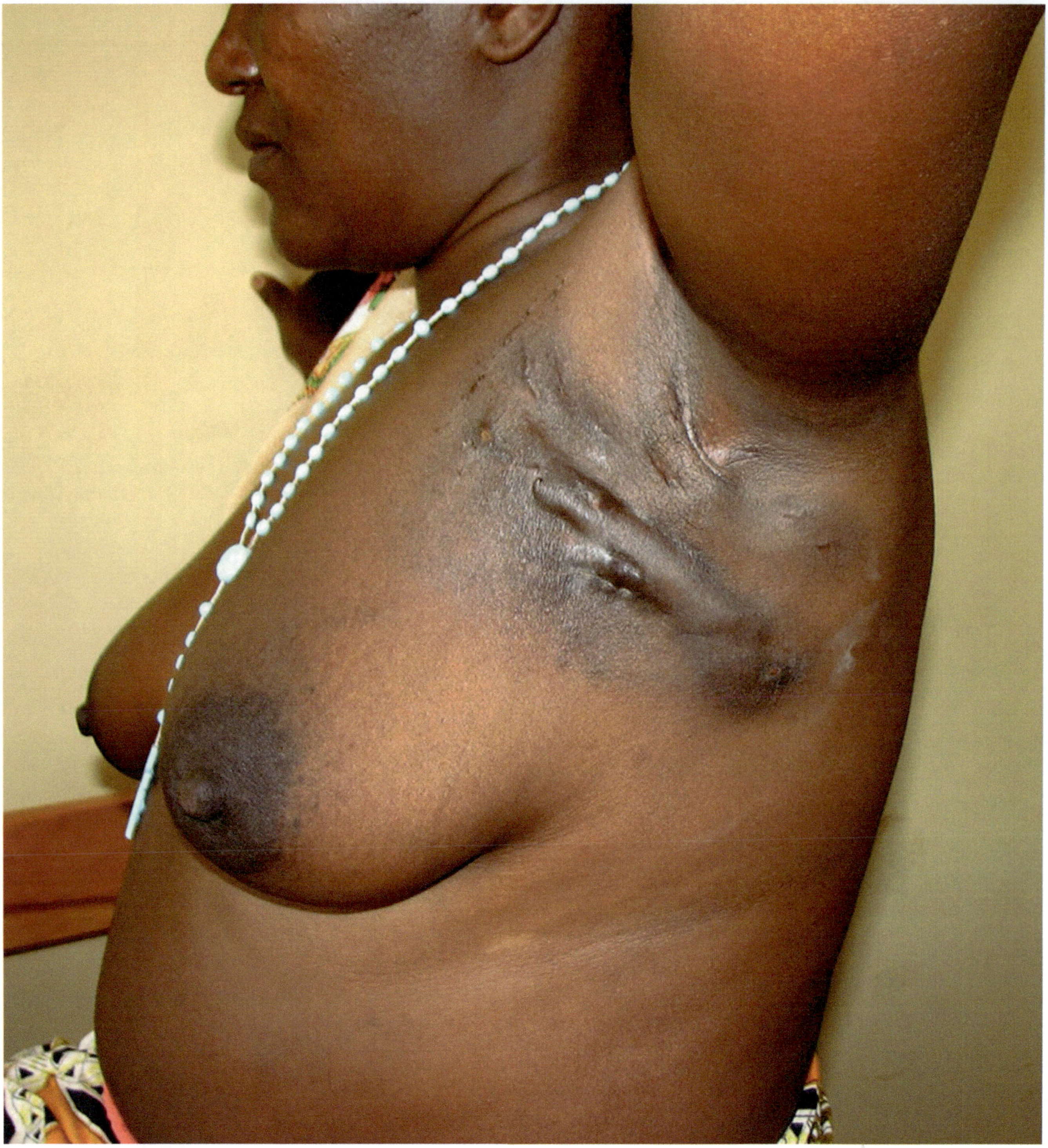

Fig. 19.2 Tunnels of *hidradenitis suppurativa* in an African female; Hurley III, severe IHS4 (RDTC Tanzania, photo: CEO)

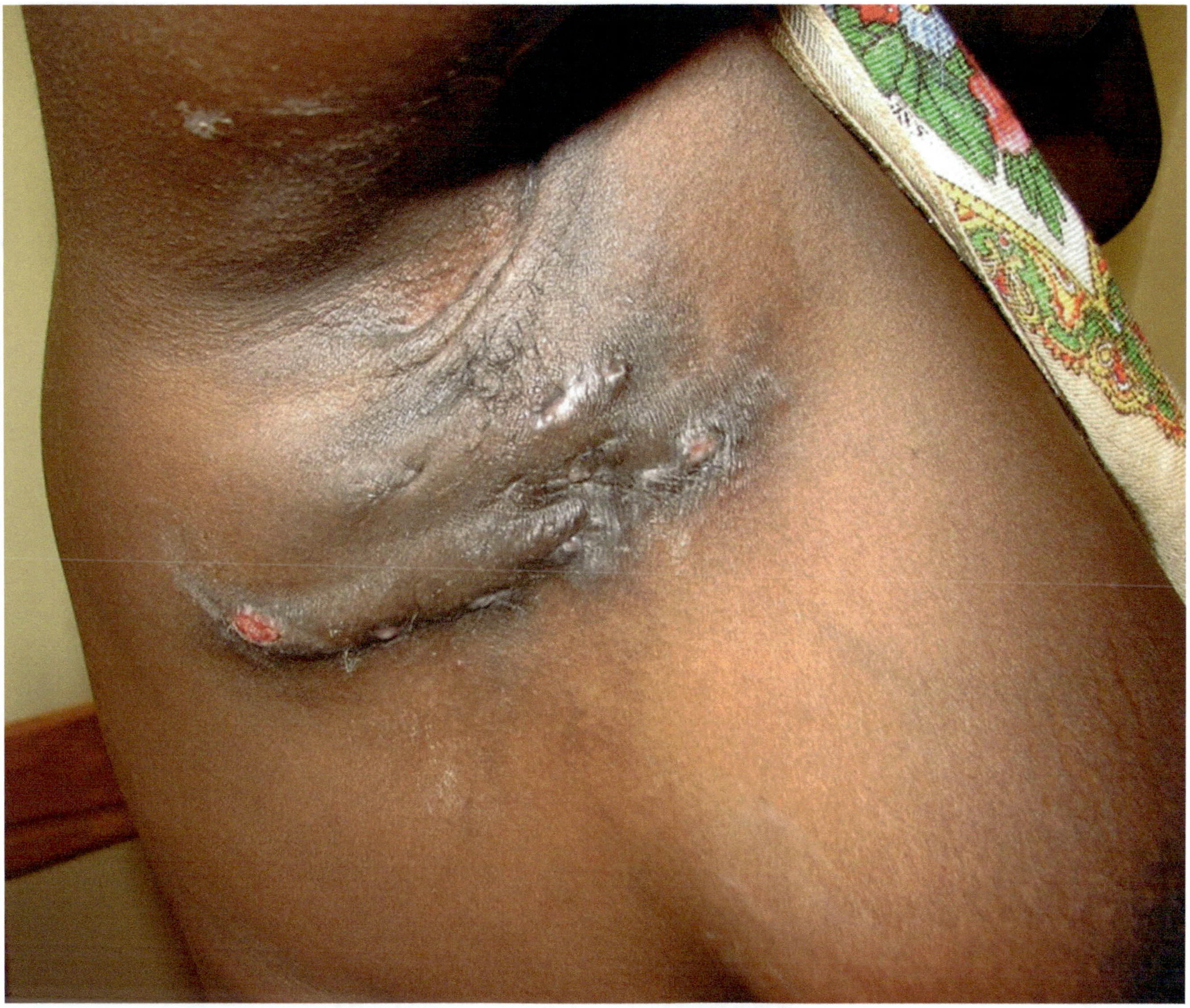

Fig. 19.3 *Hidradenitis suppurativa* in an African female a few weeks after treatment with tetracyclines; Hurley III, moderate IHS4 (RDTC Tanzania, photo: CEO)

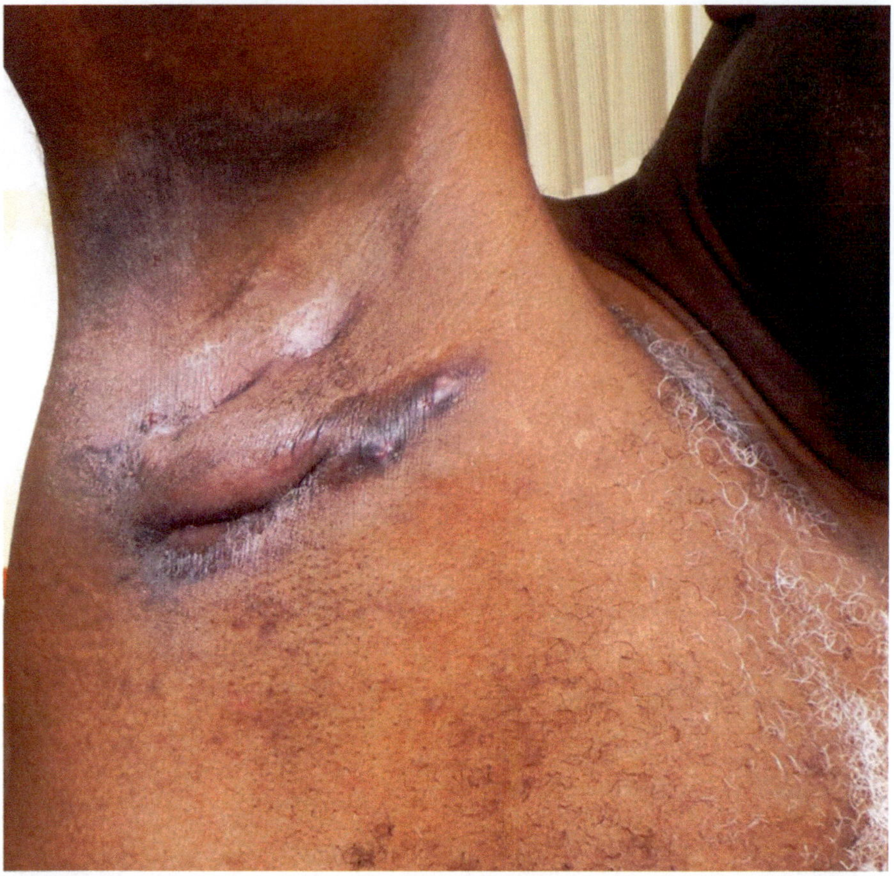

Fig. 19.4 *Hidradenitis suppurativa* at the axillary area of an African male (Hurley II, moderate IHS4) (courtesy: Dr. E.O. Okoro, Nigeria)

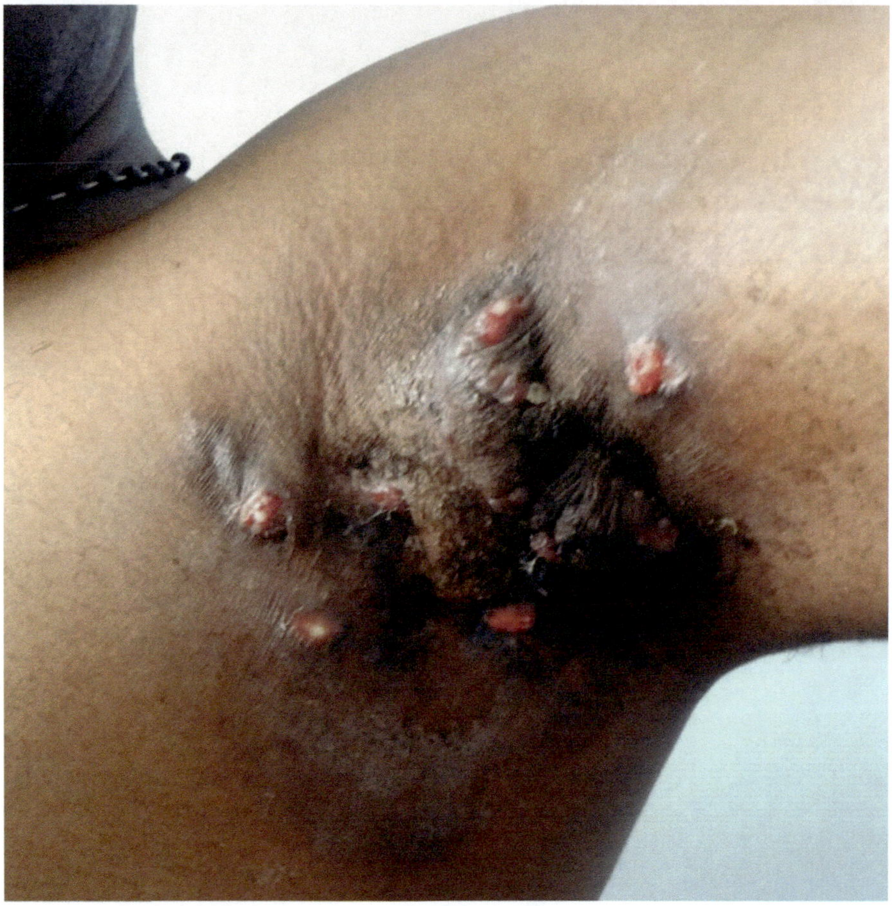

Fig. 19.5 Prominent network of draining abscesses and tunnels in *hidradenitis suppurativa*; Hurley III, severe IHS4 (courtesy: Dr. E.O. Okoro, Nigeria)

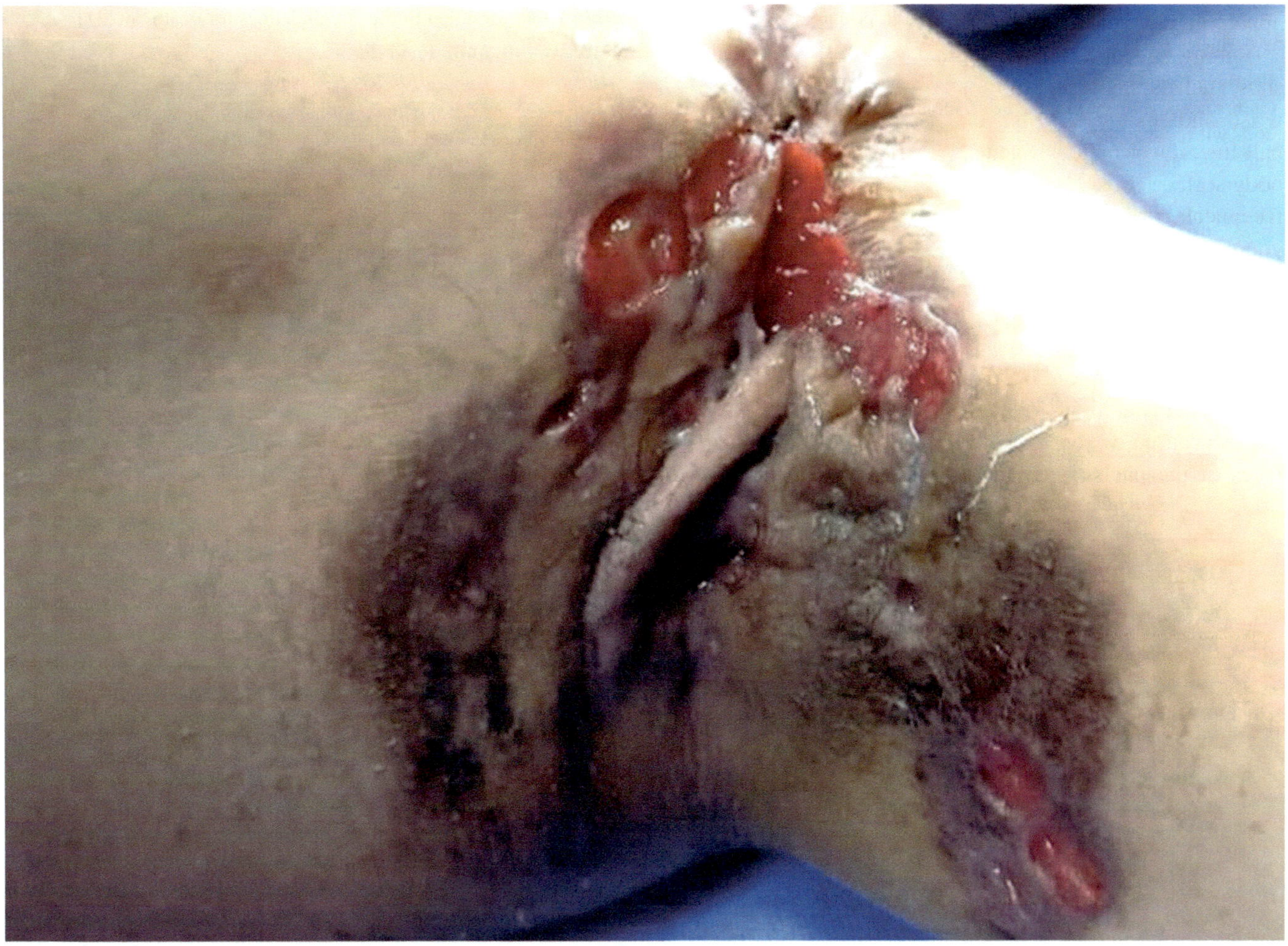

Fig. 19.6 Large network of draining tunnels at the axillary area of an Indian patient with long-standing *hidradenitis suppurativa*; Hurley III, severe IHS4

Table 19.1 Diagnostic criteria to be used in primary care setting and by dermatologists [22]

Primary care setting Outbreaks of boils during the last 6 months with a minimum of two boils with five different location options [axilla, groin, genitals, under the breasts, and other locations, e.g., perianal, neck, and abdomen]
Dermatology clinic setting (a) Obligatory criteria • History: Recurrent painful or purulent lesions more than 2×/6 months • Location: Groin, armpit, perineum, buttock area, and submammary/intramammary fold (women) • Clinical signs: – *Primary lesions* Follicular papules/pustules (folliculitis), **nodules** (**inflammatory** or noninflammatory), **abscesses** , **tunnels** (**fistula/sinus**; **draining** or non-draining) – *Secondary lesions* Cysts, double pseudo-comedones, scars (atrophic, netlike, erythematous, hypertrophic, linear, or bridged) (b) Additional criteria (not obligatory) • History: HS-positive family history • Microbiology: No evidence of pathogens or presence of normal skin microflora at the predominant primary type of lesions
Diagnosis of HS if: • All three obligatory criteria are present • One or more obligatory locations are involved • One or more types of diagnostic lesions are present (**primary lesions in bold letters are diagnostic lesions**)

Table 19.2 International Hidradenitis Suppurativa Severity Score System (IHS4) [24]

IHS4 (*points*) = • Number of inflammatory nodules multiplied by 1 + • Number of abscesses multiplied by 2 + • Number of draining tunnels (fistulae/sinuses) multiplied by 4	
Mild HS	1–3 points
Moderate HS	4–10
Severe HS	11 or more points

Table 19.3 Hurley's clinical classification of HS [25]

Stage	Definition
I	Individual primary lesions and/or cysts without fistulae or scarring
II	Individual primary lesions and/or cysts with presence of fistulae and scarring
III	Confluent primary and secondary lesions at involved surface(s) with fistulae and scars

Table 19.4 Modified European guidelines for treatment [31]

I. Active (inflammatory) disease		
Mild	***Moderate–severe***	
Topical: Clindamycin 1%	Conventional systemic management: Clindamycin + rifampicin/tetracyclines/acitretin	
	Treatment with biologics: Adalimumab (registered)/infliximab (off label)	
II. Inactive (noninflammatory) disease		
Hurley I	***Hurley II***	***Hurley III***
No surgery	Deroofing, lasers, local excision	Radical surgical excision (with secondary wound healing)
Adjuvant: Weight loss and tobacco abstinence (essential), pain management, treatment of superinfection		

19.3.1 Comorbid Disorders

Obesity, diabetes, hypertension, metabolic syndrome, dyslipidemia, depression, and substance dependence are often associated with HS [26], together with increased risk for cardiovascular diseases [27]. HS is also often associated with acne conglobata, dissecting cellulitis, and pilonidal sinus forming together a so-called follicular occlusion tetrad [1]. Further associations are those with inflammatory bowel conditions (Crohn's disease, ulcerative colitis), seronegative arthritis, and spondyloarthritis [28]. Co-occurrence of HS with Crohn's disease has been estimated in 0.6–38% and with ulcerative colitis in 14% of the cases. In contrast, only 0.8% HS patients also present Crohn's disease and 1.3% ulcerative colitis [29]. HS can also co-occur with pyoderma gangrenosum. Manifestations of HS with other genetic or acquired syndromes such as the *SAPHO syndrome*, *KID syndrome*, the *Dowling-Degos disease*, *steatocystoma multiplex*, *Sjogren syndrome*, and other rare entities have been reported [30].

19.4 Management

The treatment of HS is challenging for any physician since it requires a long-term strategy with consecutive measures together with careful monitoring. General therapeutic recommendations have been recently standardized in Europe including *topical*, *systemic*, and *surgical* measures, depending on the stage of the disease and the patient characteristics (Table 19.4). In mild cases topical agents such as 1% clindamycin, benzoyl peroxide, and 15% resorcinol peel may be successful to prevent or delay progression. Intralesional triamcinolone injections (2.5–10 mg/ml) in combination with oral and topical management act as an effective anti-inflammatory intervention in isolated HS nodules.

In more progressed cases, *systemic antibiotics* are the treatment of choice. Tetracycline 4 × 500 mg/day or doxycycline 2 × 50 to 2 × 100 mg/day is preferred because of good safety profile and low cost. In addition, zinc supplementation (90 mg/day) has been reported to be useful in mild to moderate HS. Clindamycin 2 × 300 mg/day and rifampicin 2 × 300 mg/day for up to 12 weeks are the most well-studied drug combination recommended for HS [1]. In countries with high tuberculosis, prevalent use of rifampicin has been discouraged since it is first-line medication for tuberculosis. For severe or management-resistant cases, the combination of rifampicin, moxifloxacin, and metronidazole has been suggested as an alternative therapeutic option.

Hormonal therapies may be an effective approach in management of HS in women with menstrual abnormalities. The 5α-reductase inhibitors finasteride and dutasteride, spironolactone, or oral hormonal contraceptive pills may be administered; nevertheless, strong clinical evidence is still missing.

Metformin 0.5–1.0 g/day, increased to 2–2.5 g/day bw depending on the degree of insulin resistance, has been found to be effective as add-on management in HS patients who have failed antibiotic and hormonal therapies. It acts as an insulin sensitizer and also has antiandrogenic properties. Currently, it is being used as a second-line add-on management for HS at most centers due to its good safety profile, efficacy, and low cost; metformin may be considered as first-line or add-on treatment in documented cases of HS with insulin resistance in the future.

Retinoids may be considered; acitretin 0.5 mg/day kg bw has been more promising in treating HS as compared to isotretinoin which primarily acts on the sebaceous gland. Recently, also alitretinoin (30 mg/day) has been introduced in the treatment of HS. Due to the markedly shorter half-life, it makes a better treatment option for female patients.

Among other immunomodulating drugs, *dapsone* (50–200 mg/day) may represent an option due to its low cost, but current evidence is weak.

Biologic compounds such as adalimumab and infliximab are beneficial for patients with severe HS, with adalimumab being the only registered drug in several countries. Clinical experiences with ustekinumab and anakinra is very limited. Phase II and III studies with other compounds are still ongoing. Since the use of biologics is associated with the risk of reactivation of latent infections, there is some concern that this risk could be higher in patients living in or have migrated from tropical countries [32].

Surgical interventions aim to remove and clear all primary lesions, including nodules, abscesses, and preexisting tunnels together with the resulting scar tissue, preferably through excision of the whole involved skin area en bloc. Surgical deroofing through electrosurgery or with a CO_2 laser is recommended for patients in Hurley stage I/II. For Hurley stage II/III, wide excision is regarded as the preferred surgical method. The "skin-tissue-saving excision with electrosurgical peeling" (STEEP) procedure may be a promising alternative to wide excision since it conserves healthy tissue to a maximum and achieves complete removal of lesional tissue. Simple sutures can be used in small defects surrounded by loose skin. Split-thickness skin grafts are used for large wounds after skin granulation. Especially in genital and inguinal areas, flaps can be used successfully. However, flap reconstruction may not be appropriate in HS since there is significant risk of progression [33]. IPL and lasers such as Nd:YAG, alexandrite, and diode laser may be used selectively in Hurley stage I–II to reduce the number of hair follicles and sebaceous glands involved, whereas, CO_2 laser ablatively debulks the diseased tissue and established sinus tracts and is hence more useful in stages II/III.

19.4.1 Lifestyle Adjuvant Measures

Obesity and smoking are two key factors in the pathogenesis of HS, and emphasis on losing weight and quitting smoking should be laid. Improvement or resolution of the disease can occur after weight loss either through dietary measures alone or with the help of bariatric surgery [34]. Smoking cessation has failed to show instant improvement in HS, but in a study where patients were asked 22 years after the diagnosis was made if they still suffered from HS, nonsmokers and ex-smokers were more often disease-free than active smokers [35]. Hence, educating patients about long-term benefits is important. Other lifestyle modifications which may benefit include maintaining good local hygiene and use of antiperspiring agents, especially in tropical climates.

In the diet, avoiding dairy products and whey protein and consuming low-glycemic food could improve HS by reducing excess IGF-1 and insulin production, respectively. Both IGF-1 and insulin are known to repress androgen receptor expression and also aggravate metabolic syndrome. However, conducting a formal clinical trial on such a complex problem is still a challenge [36].

References

1. Zouboulis CC, Desai N, Emtestam L, et al. European S1 guideline for the treatment of hidradenitis suppurativa/acne inversa. J Eur Acad Dermatol Venereol. 2015;29:619–44.

2. Balieva F, Kupfer J, Lien L, et al. The burden of common skin diseases assessed with the EQ5D™: a European multicentre study in 13 countries. Br J Dermatol. 2017;176:1170–8.
3. Jemec GB, Heidenheim M, Nielsen NH. The prevalence of hidradenitis suppurativa and its potential precursor lesions. J Am Acad Dermatol. 1996;35:191–4.
4. Revuz JE, Canoui-Poitrine F, Wolkenstein P, et al. Prevalence and factors associated with hidradenitis suppurativa: results from two case-control studies. J Am Acad Dermatol. 2008;59:596–601.
5. Albares MP, Belinchón I, Ramos JM, et al. Estudio epidemiológico de la patología cutánea en la población inmigrante de Alicante. Actas Dermosifiliogr. 2012;103:214–22.
6. Cosmatos I, Matcho A, Weinstein R, et al. Analysis of patient claims data to determine the prevalence of hidradenitis suppurativa in the United States. J Am Acad Dermatol. 2013;68:412–9.
7. Garg A, Kirby JS, Lavian J et al. Sex- and age-adjusted population analysis of prevalence estimates for hidradenitis Suppurativa in the United States. JAMA Dermatol. 2017;153:760–4.
8. Vazquez BG, Alikhan A, Weaver AL, et al. Incidence of hidradenitis suppurativa and associated factors: a population-based study of Olmsted County, Minnesota. J Invest Dermatol. 2013;133:97–103.
9. Garg A, Lavian J, Lin G, et al. Incidence of hidradenitis suppurativa in the United States: a sex- and age-adjusted population analysis. J Am Acad Dermatol. 2017;77:118–22.
10. Vlassova N, Kuhn D, Okoye GA. Hidradenitis suppurativa disproportionately affects African Americans: a single-center retrospective analysis. Acta Derm Venereol. 2015;95:990–1.
11. von Laffert M, Stadie V, Wohlrab J, et al. Hidradenitis suppurativa/acne inversa: bilocated epithelial hyperplasia with very different sequelae. Br J Dermatol. 2011;164:367–71.
12. Ingram JR. The genetics of hidradenitis suppurativa. Dermatol Clin. 2016;34:23–8.
13. Prens E, Deckers I. Pathophysiology of hidradenitis suppurativa: an update. J Am Acad Dermatol. 2015;73(suppl 1):S8–S11.
14. Chen S, Mattei P, You J, et al. γ-Secretase mutation in an African American family with hidradenitis suppurativa. JAMA Dermatol. 2015;151:668–70.
15. Kurzen H, Kurokawa I, Jemec GB, et al. What causes hidradenitis suppurativa? Exp Dermatol. 2008;17:455–72.
16. Karagiannidis I, Nikolakis G, Zouboulis CC. Endocrinologic aspects of hidradenitis suppurativa. Dermatol Clin. 2016;34: 45–9.
17. Nikolakis G, Join-Lambert O, Karagiannidis I, et al. Bacteriology of hidradenitis suppurativa/acne inversa: a review. J Am Acad Dermatol. 2015;73(suppl 1):S12–8.
18. Jemec GB. Clinical practice. Hidradenitis suppurativa. N Engl J Med. 2012;366:158–64.
19. Peters NJ, Kapoor R. Gluteal and perianal hidradenitis suppurativa associated with tuberculosis. Indian J Surg. 2012;74:194–5.
20. Patnaik S, Mohanty I, Panda P, et al. Disseminated mycobacterium chelonae infection: complicating a case of hidradenitis suppurativa. Ind Dermatol Online J. 2013;4:336–9.
21. Fabbrocini G, Ruocco E, De Vita V, et al. Squamous cell carcinoma arising in long-standing hidradenitis suppurativa: an overlooked facet of the immunocompromised district. Clin Dermatol. 2017;35:225–7.
22. Zouboulis CC, del Marmol V, Mrowietz U, et al. Hidradenitis suppurativa/acne inversa: criteria for diagnosis, severity assessment, classification and disease evaluation. Dermatology. 2015;231: 184–90.
23. Saunte DM, Boer J, Stratigos A, et al. Diagnostic delay in hidradenitis suppurativa is a global problem. Br J Dermatol. 2015;173:1546–9.
24. Zouboulis CC, Tzellos T, Kyrgidis A et al. Development and validation of IHS4, a novel dynamic scoring system to assess hidradenitis suppurativa/acne inversa severity. Br J Dermatol. 2017; 177:1401–9.
25. Hurley HJ. Axillary hyperhidrosis, apocrine bromhidrosis, hidradenitis suppurativa and familial benign pemphigus. Surgical approach. In: Roenigk RK, Roenigk Jr HH, editors. Dermatologic surgery. Principles and practice. 2nd ed. New York: Marcel Dekker; 1996. p. 623–45.
26. Shalom G, Freud T, Harman-Boehm I, et al. Hidradenitis suppurativa and metabolic syndrome: a comparative cross-sectional study of 3207 patients. Br J Dermatol. 2015;173:464–70.
27. Tzellos T, Zouboulis CC, Gulliver W, et al. Cardiovascular disease risk factors in patients with hidradenitis suppurativa: a systematic review and meta-analysis of observational studies. Br J Dermatol. 2015;173:1142–55.
28. Fimmel S, Zouboulis CC. Comorbidities of hidradenitis suppurativa (acne inversa). Dermatoendocrinology. 2010;2:9–16.
29. Egeberg A, Jemec GBE, Kimball AB, et al. Prevalence and risk of inflammatory bowel disease in patients with hidradenitis suppurativa. J Invest Dermatol. 2017;137:1060–4.
30. Cugno M, Borghi A, Marzano AV. PAPA, PASH and PAPASH syndromes: pathophysiology, presentation and treatment. Am J Clin Dermatol. 2017;18:555–62.
31. Zouboulis CC, Desai N, Emtestam L, et al. Partial actualization of the European S1 guideline for the treatment of hidradenitis suppurativa/acne inversa. Exp Dermatol. 2016;25(suppl 2):13.
32. Bartalesi F, Bartoloni A, Bisoffi Z, et al. The emerging problem of biological treatment in migrant and travelling populations: it is time to extend guidelines for the screening of infectious diseases. Ann Rheum Dis. 2014;73:794–6.
33. Janse I, Bieniek A, Horváth B, et al. Surgical procedures in hidradenitis suppurativa. Dermatol Clin. 2016;34:97–109.
34. Kromann CB, Ibler KS, Kristiansen VB, et al. The influence of body weight on the prevalence and severity of hidradenitis suppurativa. Acta Derm Venereol. 2014;94:553–7.
35. Kromann CB, Deckers IE, Esmann S, et al. Risk factors, clinical course and long-term prognosis in hidradenitis suppurativa: a cross-sectional study. Br J Dermatol. 2014;171:819–24.
36. Danby FW. Diet in the prevention of hidradenitis suppurativa (acne inversa). J Am Acad Dermatol. 2015;73(suppl 1): S52–4.

20 Rosacea in Dark Skin

Uwe Wollina, Adebola Ogunbiyi, Shyam B. Verma, and Karalikkattil T. Ashique

20.1 Epidemiology

Rosacea is a common chronic inflammatory facial dermatosis, which mainly affects adults of Caucasian origin and among them mostly individuals with fair skin, as expressed by the term "blessing of the Celts" [1]. The ethnic background influences the prevalence and the frequency of the clinical subtypes of rosacea, possibly also any subjective symptoms and comorbidities. There is an impact of geographical and social factors as well. In contrast to Western countries, rosacea research in populations with dark skin is rudimental. However, despite all differences, the response of the disease to treatment is not dependent on patients's skin type.

There is an increasing prevalence of rosacea from South to North Europe with highest prevalence reported in Sweden (10%) and in Estonia (22%). The disease usually starts earlier among females, while rhinophyma is almost exclusively seen among adult males. Ocular involvement is the most common extracutaneous manifestation and affects 6–50% of all Caucasian patients with rosacea. A few rare cases have been observed during childhood and adolescence. The prevalence of rosacea in dark skin is very low; in a US study using the database of the National Ambulatory Medical Care Survey of 1993–2010 for ethnic distribution of patients with rosacea, only 2.0% were patients with dark skin, 2.3% were Asians or Pacific Islanders, and 3.9% were Hispanics or Latinos [2]. The prevalence of the disease in Colombia was currently estimated 2.9% [3]. In contrast, rosacea is a common diagnosis in China, Taiwan, Japan, and Korea [4].

In the African continent, rosacea is an uncommon observation. In a study of 2254 consecutive new patients seen at the dermatology clinic of Komfo Anokye Teaching Hospital in Kumasi, Ghana, not a single case of rosacea has been recorded [5]; rhinophyma in black-skinned Africans is rare [6]. In Egypt, the Maghreb states, and the Middle East, rosacea can occasionally be diagnosed [7]. In a study from Tunisia with 244 hospitalized patients, the prevalence of rosacea was 0.2% with a male-to-female ratio of 0.4 [8], while in India steroid-induced rosacea is seen more frequent than the classical type [9].

20.2 Pathogenesis

The pathophysiology of rosacea is complex, not fully elucidated. It involves various cell types and molecules in the skin and has various subtypes [10]. The clinical observation of a tight association of rosacea with sensitive fair skin generated the concept of a disturbed epidermal barrier function leading to activation of certain epidermal pro-inflammatory proteins. Serine proteases of the stratum corneum may represent a link between impaired barrier function and inflammation [11]. In addition, the trypsin-like serine protease kallikrein 5 was found increased in lesional rosacea, responsible for the cleavage and activation of cathelicidin LL37 [12] which possesses antimicrobial, pro-inflammatory, and angiogenic properties [13]. Also LL-37 levels were found remarkably increased [14], leading to activation of the toll-like receptor 2, a pattern recognition receptor tightly bound to innate immunity.

U. Wollina (✉)
Department of Dermatology and Allergology, Hospital Dresden-Friedrichstadt, Teaching Hospital of the Technical University of Dresden, Dresden, Germany
e-mail: wollina-uw@khdf.de

A. Ogunbiyi
Department of Medicine, University of Ibadan, Ibadan, Oyo, Nigeria

S. B. Verma, MBBS, DVD, FRCP, FAAD
Nirvana Skin Clinic, Vadodara, Gujarat, India

K. T. Ashique
Kims Alshifa Hospital, Malappuram, Kerala, India

C. E. Orfanos et al. (eds.), *Pigmented Ethnic Skin and Imported Dermatoses*, https://doi.org/10.1007/978-3-319-69422-1_20

Prolonged flush with persistent erythema is a hallmark of disturbed facial blood flow in rosacea. The vascular endothelial growth factor is expressed by cells infiltrating the epidermis, contributing to the vascular changes present in rosacea. Moreover, the vasoactive intestinal peptide receptor is also increased in cutaneous blood vessels of phymatous rosacea and in patients' serum [15]. Due to dysregulation of markers specific for lymphatic vessels in sebaceous gland-rich skin, rosacea has also been considered as an actinic lymphatic vasculopathy [16, 17].

The skin of rosacea patients has a significantly lower heat pain threshold than normal skin. Since transient receptor potential ion channels of the vanilloid type 1 and ankyrin 1 function as cellular sensors for phenomena such as cold and heat and have a prominent role in inflammation and pain sensation, they are possibly involved in rosacea. The activation of such receptors may increase the release of substance P. The different vanilloid receptors have an impact on local immune function, vascular regulation, nociception, and epidermal integrity [18].

The prevalence of demodex mites in rosacea has been estimated to be as high as 60% in in vivo tests and 80% in skin biopsies with *Demodex folliculorum* being the dominant infestation agent. The odds ratio was 8.1 for Chinese patients suffering from rosacea [19, 20]. In a study from Egypt, *Helicobacter pylori* infection was found in 49 rosacea patients (72%) and 25 controls (46.3%). Analysis of genotypes revealed that *vacAs1m1* was dominant in papulopustular subtypes (54.8%), compared with 22.2% in erythematotelangiectatic rosacea and 16% in controls; after administration of the eradication regimen, significant improvement was observed in 55.6% of papulopustular rosacea but only in 17.6% of the patients with the erythematotelangiectatic subtype, indicating that *Helicobacter pylori* may play a significant role in pathogenesis, especially in patients who had dyspeptic symptoms [21, 22]. Overall, increased density of demodex in rosacea has been accepted as an aggravating factor in rosacea but not as a causative one [23].

20.3 Clinical Picture and Course

According to its clinical picture, rosacea has been classified into four subtypes (Table 20.1). Primary clinical features of the disease include transient and persistent erythema in the centrofacial region, inflammatory papulopustules, and telangiectasias. Secondary clinical features are dry and sensitive facial skin, fine scaling, persistent nasal and perinasal edema, plaque formation, phymatous growth, and ocular and extrafacial manifestations [1]. This classification is also used for patients with dark skin showing similar features of rosacea, as seen in African countries (Figs. 20.1, 20.2 and 20.3) and also in India (Figs. 20.4 and 20.5).

Table 20.1 Classification of rosacea according to the USA National Rosacea Society Expert Committee [24]

Subtype	Descriptive term	Clinical signs
1	*Erythematotelangiectatic*	Flushing and centrofacial erythema with telangiectasias. Additional features: Edema, stinging and burning sensations, roughness, and/or scaling
2	*Papulopustular*	Persistent centrofacial erythema and transient papules or pustules (inflammatory subtype)
3	*Phymatous*	Thickened skin, irregular surface nodularities, and enlargement of the affected areas (chin, forehead, cheeks, ears, and nose)
4	*Ocular*	Conjunctivitis, keratitis, and blepharitis

Rosacea has a negative impact on the quality of life, generating stigmatizing feelings and anxiety. Rosacea patients also have an increased risk for cardiovascular disease, namely, dyslipidemia (odds ratio 1.41), coronary artery disease (odds ratio 1.35), and hypertension (odds ratio 1.17) [20]. Coronary artery disease remained independently associated with rosacea after adjustment for hypertension, diabetes mellitus, and dyslipidemia. Male patients with rosacea had higher risks for all comorbidities than female patients. Other known comorbidities include dementia, Alzheimer, and Parkinson disease [25, 26].

Erythema in rosacea varies and can be subdivided into (a) sole erythema, (b) erythema with telangiectasias, (c) erythema with edema, and (d) erythema with inflammatory papules and nodules. It is of great therapeutic importance to differentiate the perilesional erythema of inflammatory lesions from the diffuse facial erythema [27]. In patients of skin phototypes IV–VI, erythema is often missing for the naked eye inflicting the clinical diagnosis. Dermoscopy may be a valuable tool to assess erythema in dark skin types.

In Tunisia the major triggering factors of rosacea were sun exposure (64%) and thermal stimuli (25%), whereas, the frequency of subtypes differed from that in Northern Europe. The leading clinical subtype among 244 patients was papulopustular rosacea (69%), followed by the erythematotelangiectatic type (12%) and rhinophyma (3.7%) [8]. Ocular rosacea was frequent [28]. In Saudi women extrafacial lesions affecting the chest, back, and ears were identified in 14%. Severe erythematotelangiectatic rosacea is seen more often in skin type IV compared with its frequency in skin types V and VI. The severe papulopustular subtype of rosacea was noted in 20% with skin type IV and 14% with

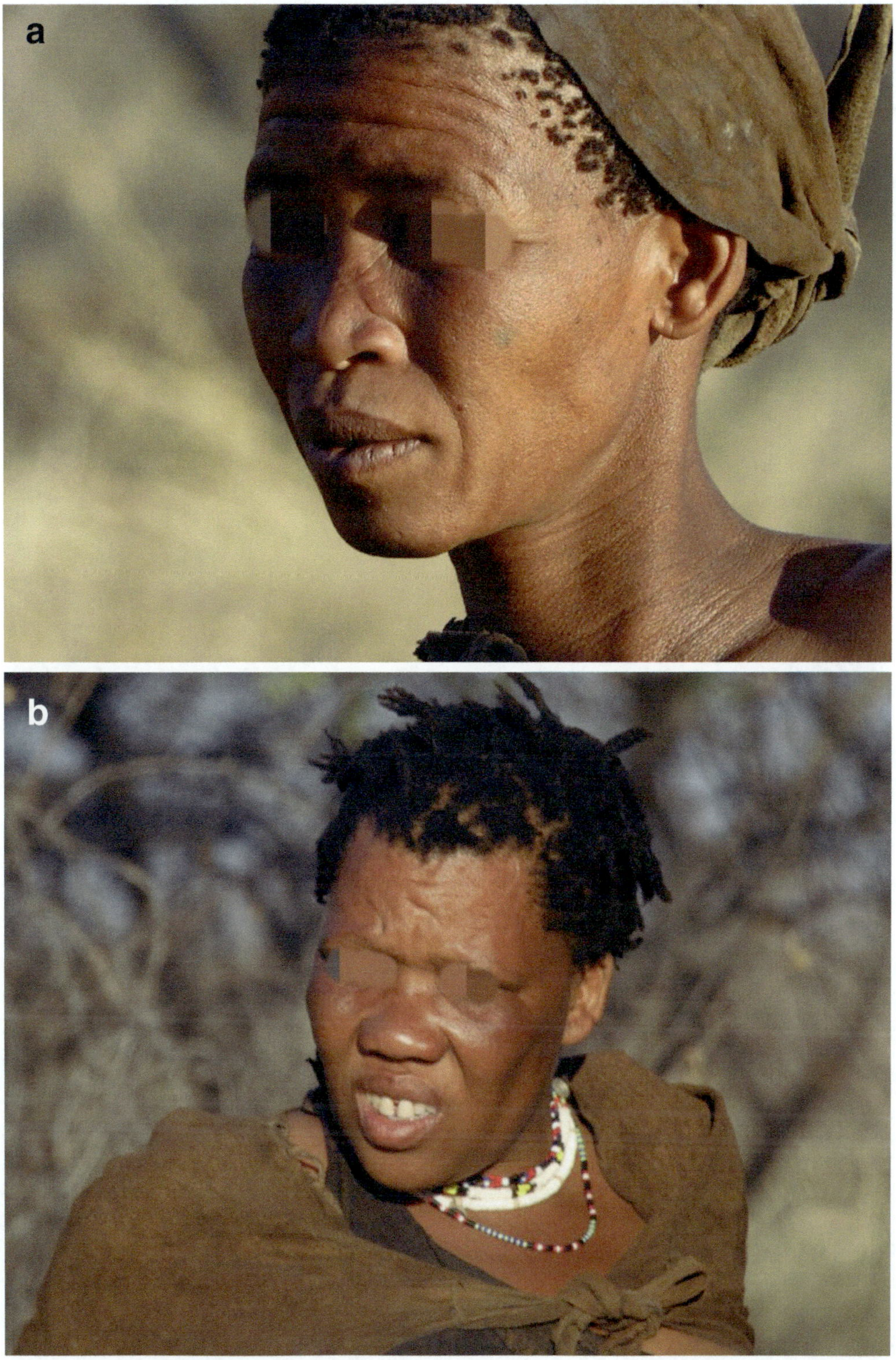

Fig. 20.1 Rosacea manifestations in Botswana: (**a**) younger San female with nasal edema; (**b**) another San female with metophyma

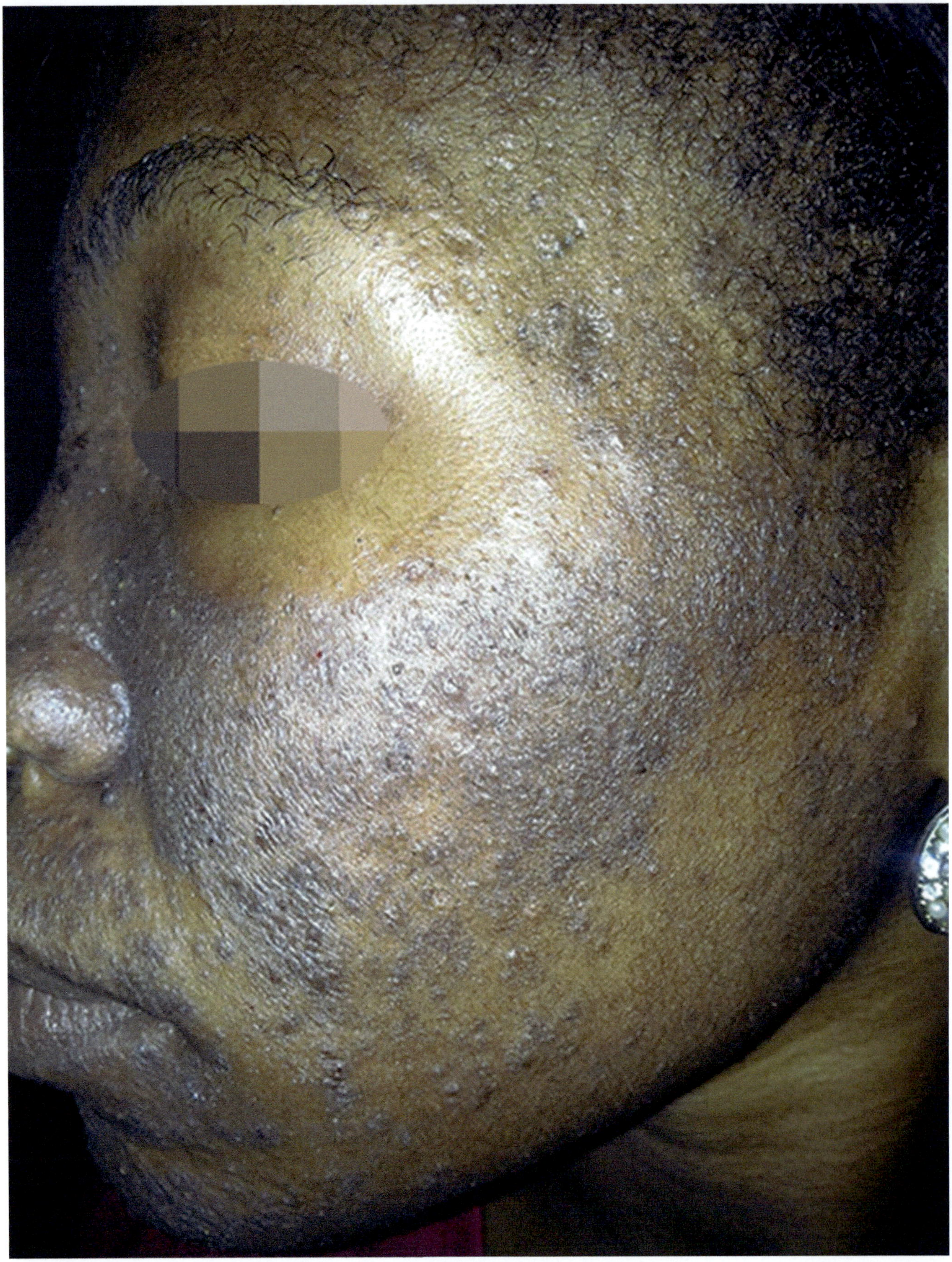

Fig. 20.2 Rosacea in Nigeria: (**a**) erythematous rosacea with lid margin involvement in a female

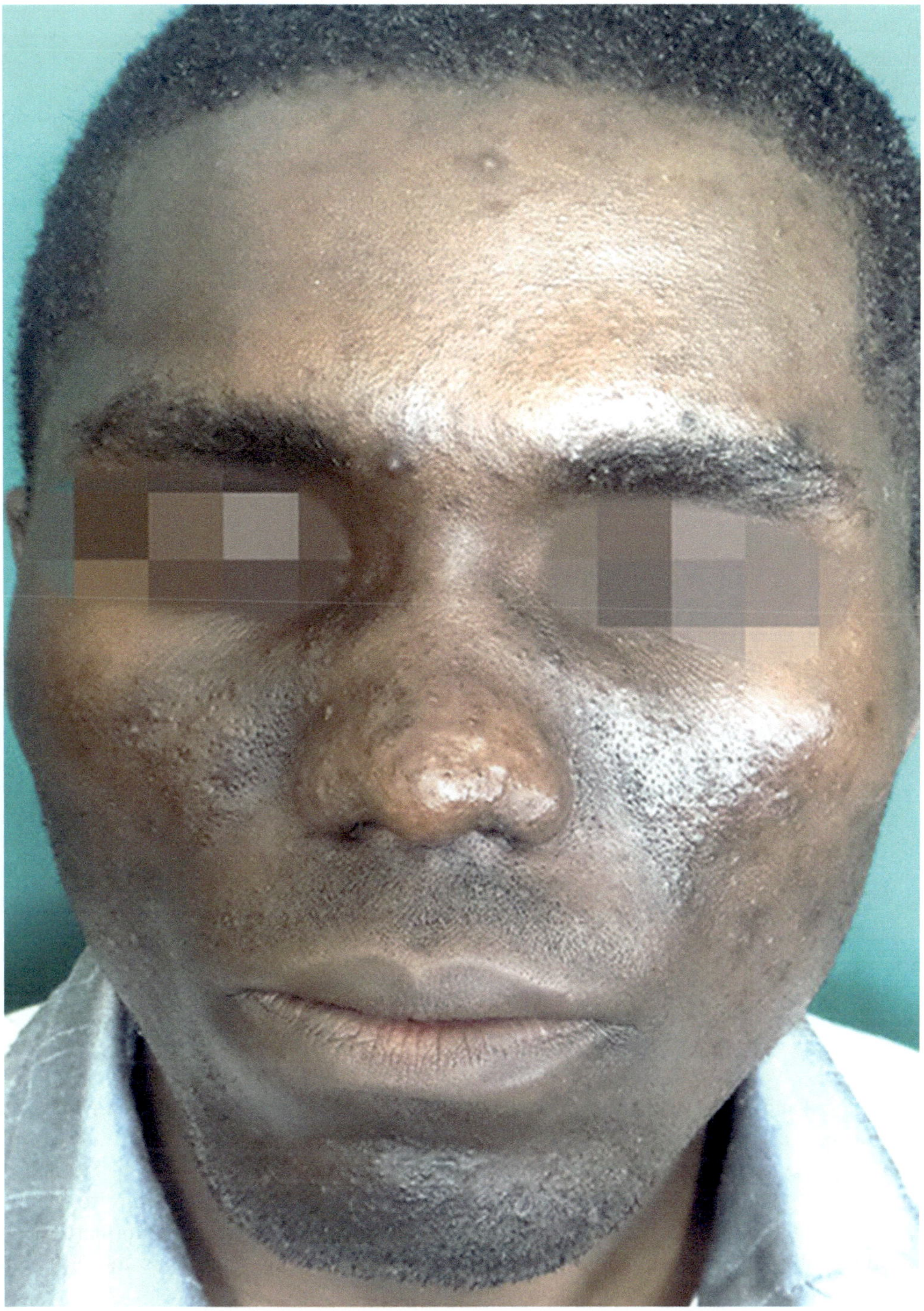

Fig. 20.3 *Erythematous rosacea* with *glandular rhinophyma* in a Nigerian male

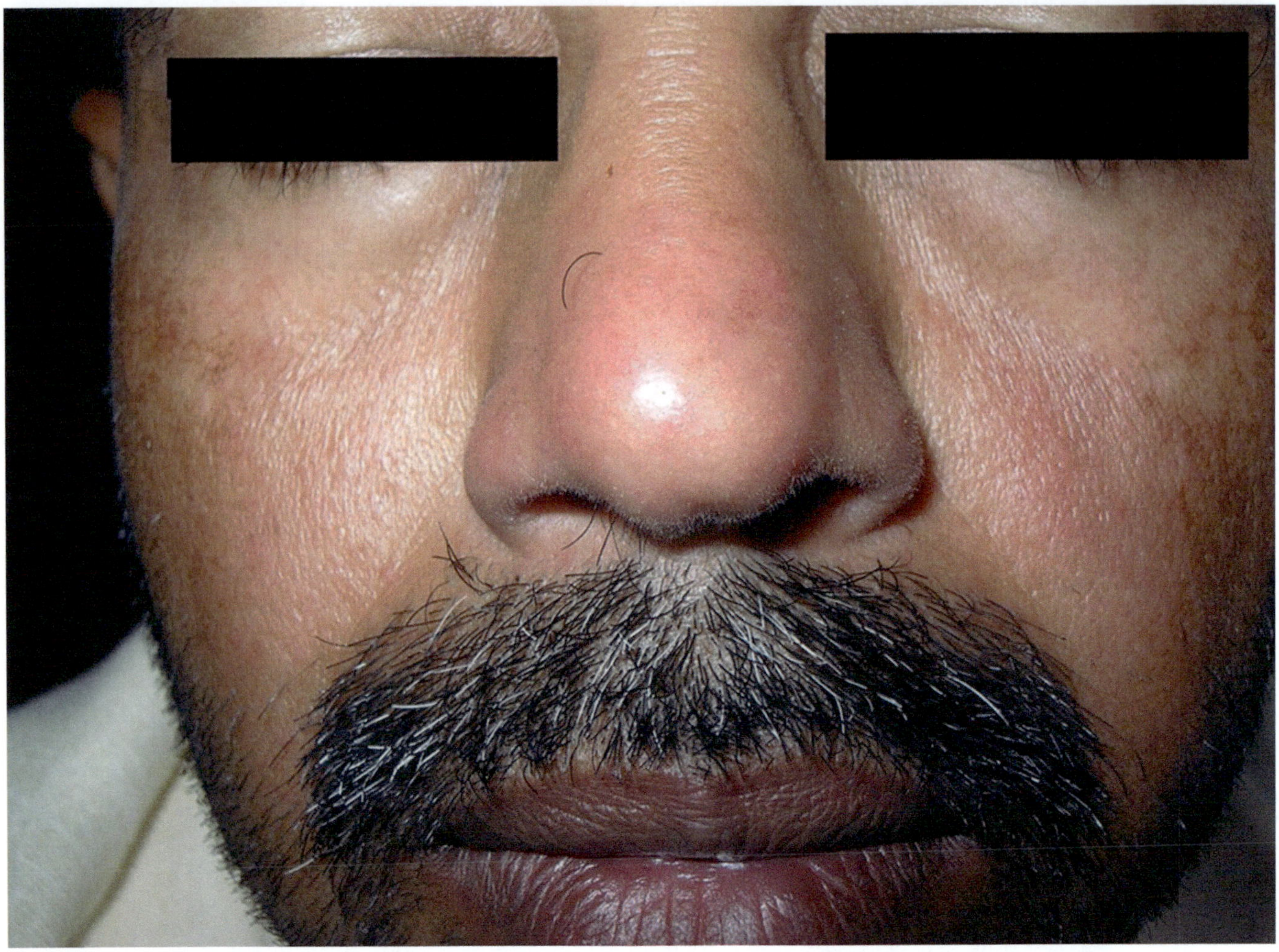

Fig. 20.4 *Erythematous rosacea* in an Indian male

skin type VI. On the other hand, the severity of rosacea subtypes was not significantly associated with the skin type. Interestingly, pruritus was the leading subjective symptom in dark skin with rosacea (92%) and not burning or stinging as in Caucasians in Northern Europe and the Americas. Furthermore, postinflammatory hyper- or hypopigmentation was completely absent [7]. Ocular rosacea has been reported in Saudi Arabia [29].

In the Far East (Korea, China, Taiwan, Japan), sun exposure, hot baths, and physical exercise were the most common precipitating factors. Like in Northern Europe, the most frequent clinical presentation is the erythematotelangiectatic

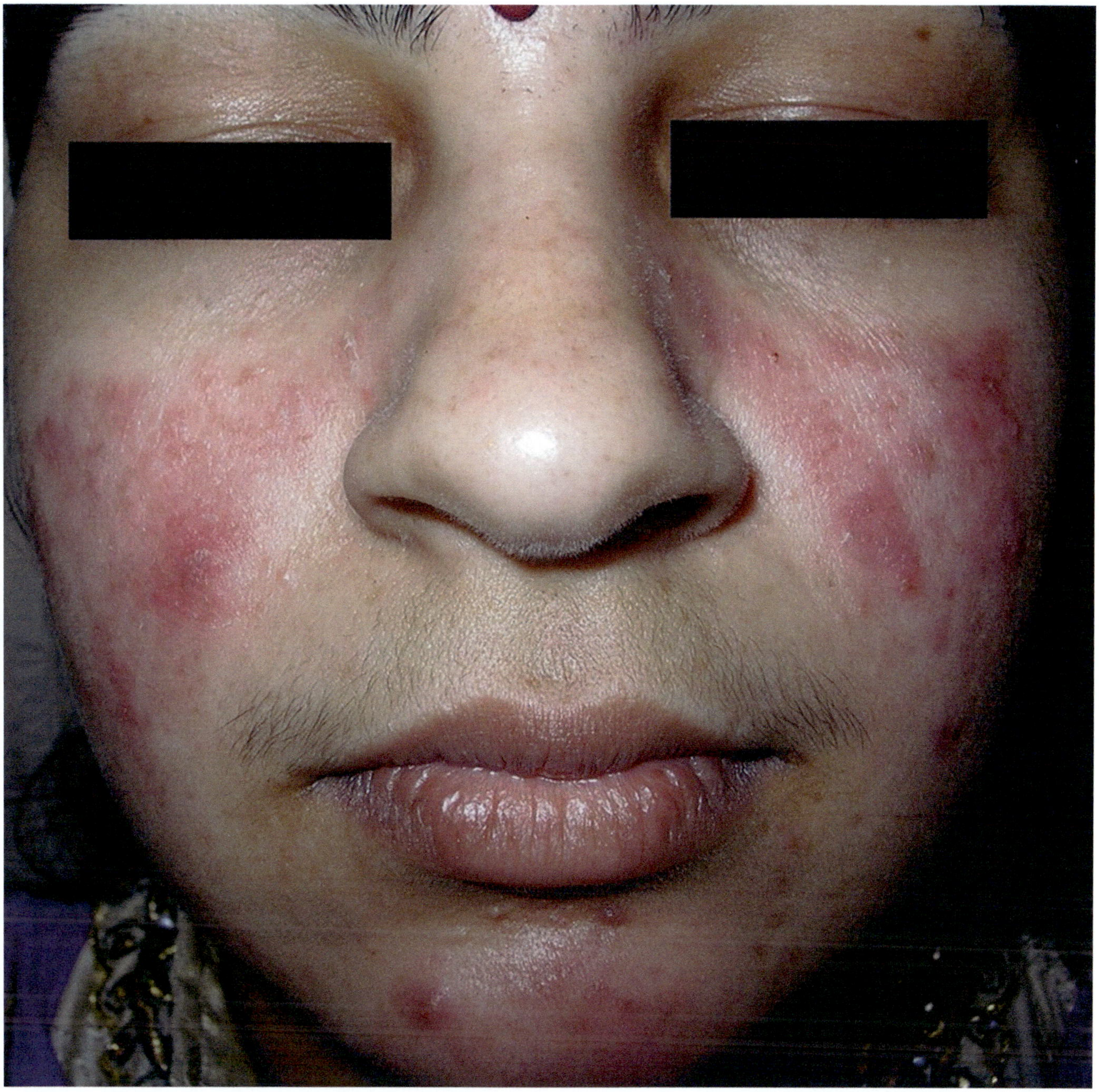

Fig. 20.5 *Papulopustular rosacea* in an Indian female

subtype (43–96%), whereas several patients present with a mixture of subtypes.

Phymatous rosacea occurs in less than 5–30% of the total number of patients [30, 31]. In India all types of rhinophyma (glandular, fibroangiomatous, pendulans) may be seen (Figs. 20.6, 20.7 and 20.8). In Japan, rhinophyma is extremely rare and manifests on the lower half of the nose only [32]. Papulopustular rosacea without remarkable centrofacial erythema shows a more favorable prognosis than other subtypes [33]. Partial or complete remission was recorded in 61.5% and 20.9% of the patients, respectively. The median time to complete remission was 56 months.

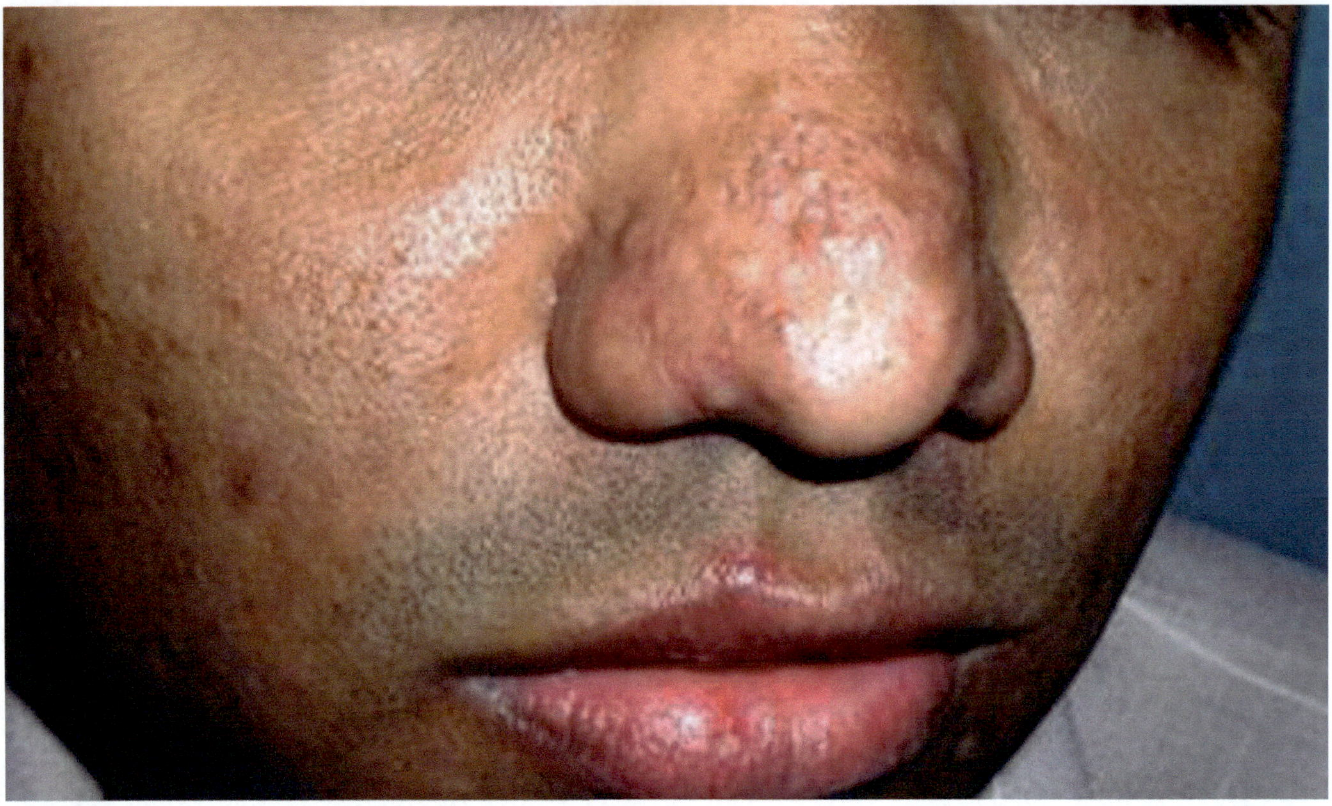

Fig. 20.6 *Glandular-type rhinophyma* in an Indian male. *From Wollina U, Verma SB. Rhinophyma: A Variation of Rosacea? In: Zouboulis CC, Katsambas AD, Kligman AM (editors). Pathogenesis and Treatment of Acne and Rosacea. Springer, Berlin, 2014; pp. 661–664*

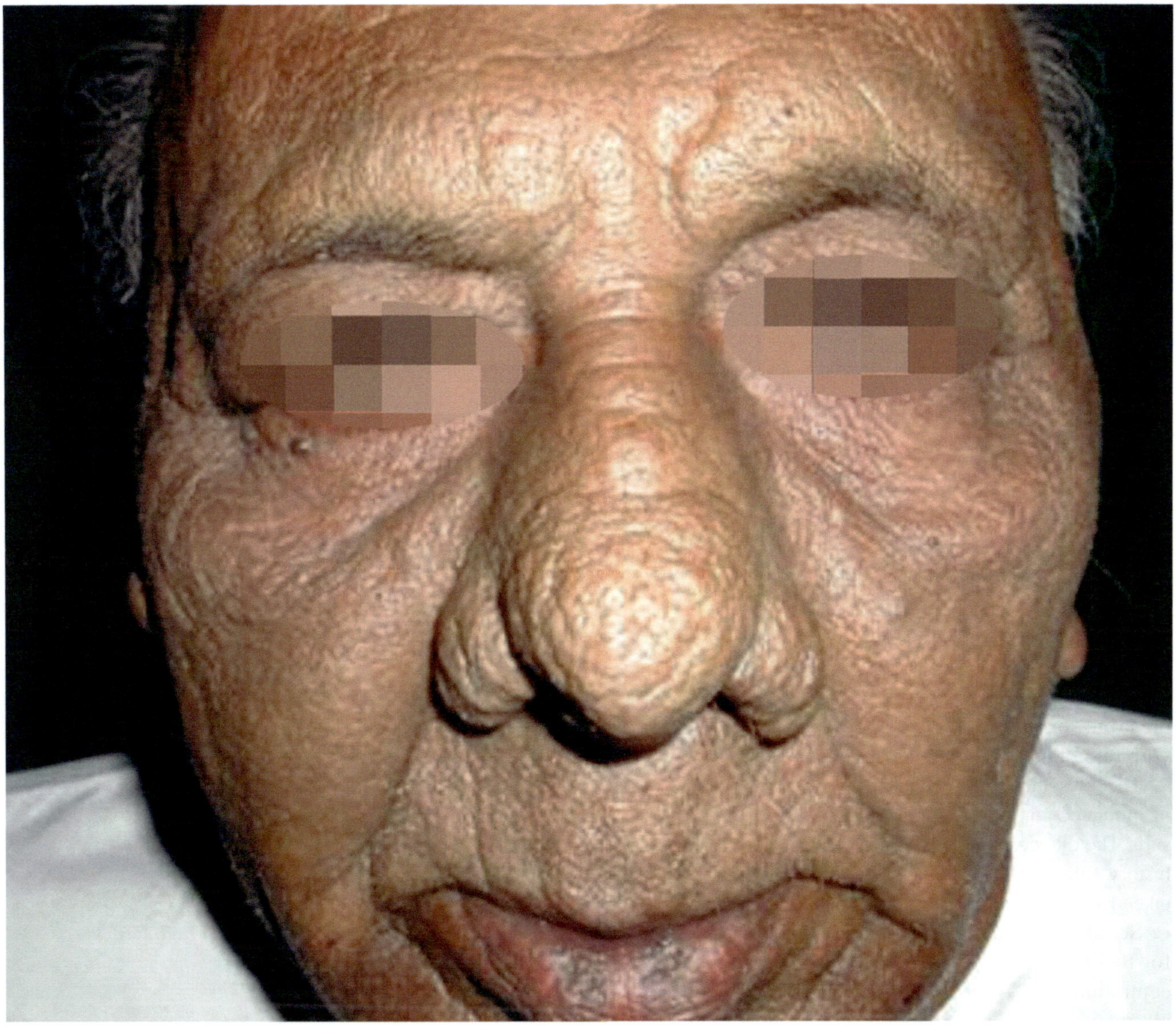

Fig. 20.7 *Fibroangiomatous rhinophyma* in combination with edematous rosacea of the cheeks in an Indian male. *From Wollina U, Verma SB. Rhinophyma: A Variation of Rosacea? In: Zouboulis CC, Katsambas AD, Kligman AM (editors). Pathogenesis and Treatment of Acne and Rosacea. Springer, Berlin, 2014; pp. 661–664*

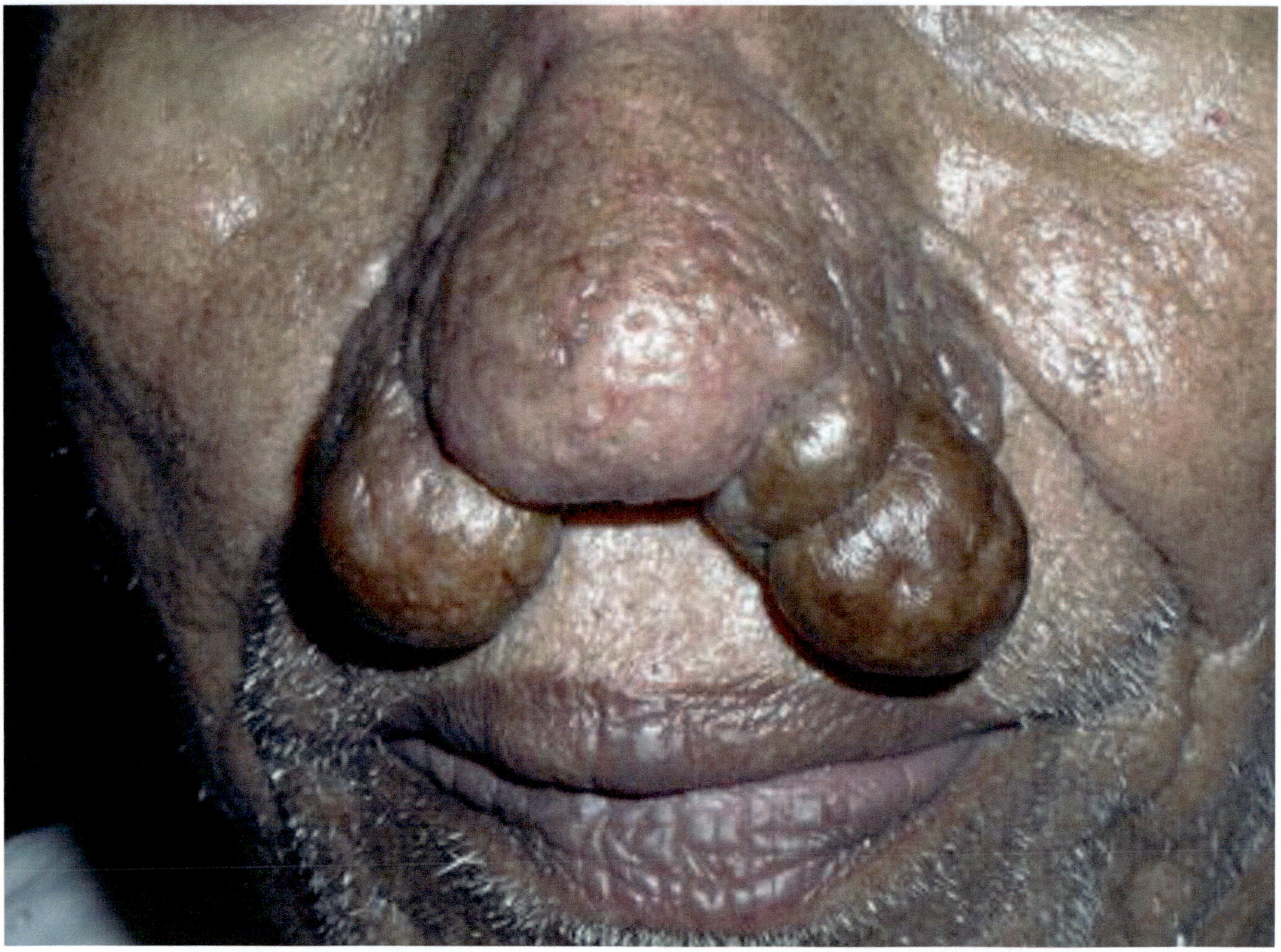

Fig. 20.8 *Actinic-type rhinophyma pendulans* in an Indian male. *From Wollina U, Verma SB. Rhinophyma: A Variation of Rosacea? In: Zouboulis CC, Katsambas AD, Kligman AM (editors). Pathogenesis and Treatment of Acne and Rosacea. Springer, Berlin, 2014; pp. 661–664*

20.4 Treatment

There is a lack of clinical trials in patients with dark skin; however, it seems that the treatment of rosacea in ethnic patients with dark skin does not differ from that of the Caucasians. Avoidance of irritants as well of triggering factors is mandatory as a general measure in all ethnic groups and subtypes [34] (Table 20.2). On the other hand, Limited availability of medical care and resources may delay diagnosis and treatment in many parts of the world. In rural areas, herbal remedies are used for topical treatment such as green tea, oatmeal, chamomile, and tea tree oil [35]. Topical metronidazole is a first-line medical management for inflammatory rosacea independent from the skin type. In patients with skin types V and VI, erythematotelangiectatic rosacea is less common. These patients will benefit not as much from topical brimonidine tartrate gel as Caucasians do.

Oral doxycycline (40 mg 1x/d to 100 mg 2x/d p.o.) is the most widely used as an oral drug for treating rosacea, being effective and safe in all patients irrespective of their skin type [36].

Table 20.2 Treatment of rosacea [35]

Management	Drugs/procedure	Subtype
Topical, registered	Metronidazole	Papulopustular
	Azelaic acid	Papulopustular
	Brimonidine	Erythematotelangiectatic
	Ivermectin	Papulopustular
Topical, off label	Retinoids	Papulopustular
	Benzoyl peroxide	Papulopustular
	Cyclosporin A	Ocular
	Calcineurin inhibitors	Steroid-induced rosacea
	Permethrin	Rosacea-like demodex folliculitis
	Benzyl benzoate	Rosacea-like demodex folliculitis
Systemic, registered	Doxycycline	Papulopustular
	Isotretinoin	Papulopustular
Systemic, off label	Doxycycline	Ocular
	Tetracyclines	Papulopustular, ocular
	Macrolides (erythromycin, azithromycin)	Papulopustular, ocular
	Metronidazole	Papulopustular, rosacea-like demodex folliculitis
	Isotretinoin	Phymatous, extrafacial, rosacea fulminans, steroid-induced
	Dapsone	Phymatous, rosacea fulminans
	Beta-blockers (carvedilol)	Erythematotelangiectatic
	Ivermectin	Rosacea-like demodex folliculitis
Physical modalities	Lasers	Erythematotelangiectatic, phymatous
Surgical intervention	Dermabrasion, derma shaving	Phymatous

References

1. Wollina U. Classical clinical presentation of rosacea. In: Zouboulis CC, Katsambas AD, Kligman AM, editors. Pathogenesis and treatment of acne and rosacea. Berlin: Springer; 2014. p. 653–9.
2. Al-Dabagh A, Davis SA, McMichael AJ et al. Rosacea in skin of color: not a rare diagnosis. Dermatol Online J. 2014;20(10).
3. Rueda LJ, Motta A, Pabón JG, et al. Epidemiology of rosacea in Colombia. Int J Dermatol. 2017;56:510–3.
4. Li J, Li M, Chen Q, et al. Quality of life among patients with rosacea: an investigation of patients in China using two structured questionnaires. J Eur Acad Dermatol Venereol. 2016;30:e98–9.
5. Doe PT, Asiedu A, Acheampong JW, et al. Skin diseases in Ghana and the UK. Int J Dermatol. 2001;40:323–6.
6. Koffi-Aka V, Kouassi AA, D'Horpock FA, et al. Rhinophyma in a black African. Rev Laryngol Otol Rhinol (Bord). 2002;123:109–10.
7. Al Balbeesi AO, Halawani MR. Unusual features of rosacea in saudi females with dark skin. Ochsner J. 2014;14:321–7.
8. Khaled A, Hammami H, Zeglaoui F, et al. Rosacea: 244 Tunisian cases. Tunis Med. 2010;88:597–601.
9. Rathi SK, Kumrah L. Topical corticosteroid-induced rosacea-like dermatitis: a clinical study of 110 cases. Indian J Dermatol Venereol Leprol. 2011;77:42–6.
10. Steinhoff M, Schauber J, Leyden JJ. New insights into rosacea pathophysiology: a review of recent findings. J Am Acad Dermatol. 2013;69:S15–26.
11. Two AM, Hata TR, Nakatsuji T, et al. Reduction in serine protease activity correlates with improved rosacea severity in a small, randomized pilot study of a topical serine protease inhibitor. J Invest Dermatol. 2014;134:1143–5.
12. Fischer J, Meyer-Hoffert U. Regulation of kallikrein-related peptidases in the skin—from physiology to diseases to therapeutic options. Thromb Haemost. 2013;110:442–9.
13. Li N, Yamasaki K, Saito R, et al. Alarmin function of cathelicidin antimicrobial peptide LL37 through IL-36γ induction in human epidermal keratinocytes. J Immunol. 2014;193:5140–8.
14. Yamasaki K, Gallo RL. Rosacea as a disease of cathelicidins and skin innate immunity. J Investig Dermatol Symp Proc. 2011;15:12–5.
15. Wollina U. Rhinophyma—unusual expression of simple-type keratins and S100A in sebocytes and abundance of VIP receptor-positive dermal cells. Histol Histopathol. 1996;11:111–5.
16. Fimmel S, Abdel-Naser MB, Kutzner H, et al. New aspects of the pathogenesis of rosacea. Drug Discovery Today Dis Mech. 2008;5:e103–11.
17. Dajnoki Z, Béke G, Kapitány A, et al. Sebaceous gland rich skin is characterized by TSLP expression and distinct immune surveillance which is disturbed in rosacea. J Invest Dermatol. 2017;137:1114–25.
18. Sulk M, Seeliger S, Aubert J, et al. Distribution and expression of non-neuronal transient receptor potential (TRPV) ion channels in rosacea. J Invest Dermatol. 2012;132:1253–62.

19. Zhao YE, Peng Y, Wang XL, et al. Facial dermatosis associated with Demodex: a case-control study. J Zhejiang Univ Sci B. 2011;12:1008–15.
20. Hua TC, Chung PI, Chen YJ, et al. Cardiovascular comorbidities in patients with rosacea: a nationwide case-control study from Taiwan. J Am Acad Dermatol. 2015;73:249–54.
21. Tebbe B, Geilen CC, Orfanos CE. Nachweis von Helicobacter pylori bei Dermatosen. Klinischer Zufallsbefund oder pathologenetische Assoziation? Hautarzt. 1996;47:587–90.
22. El-Khalawany M, Mahmoud A, Mosbeh AS, et al. Role of Helicobacter pylori in common rosacea subtypes: a genotypic comparative study of Egyptian patients. J Dermatol. 2012;39:989–95.
23. Chen W, Plewig G. Are Demodex mites principal, conspirator, accomplice, witness or bystander in the cause of rosacea? Am J Clin Dermatol. 2015;16:67–72.
24. Wilkin J, Dahl M, Detmar M, et al. Standard classification of rosacea: report of the National Rosacea Society Expert Committee on the classification and staging of rosacea. J Am Acad Dermatol. 2002;46:584–7.
25. Egeberg A, Hansen PR, Gislason GH, et al. Exploring the association between rosacea and Parkinson disease: a Danish nationwide cohort study. JAMA Neurol. 2016;73:529–34.
26. Egeberg A, Hansen PR, Gislason GH, et al. Patients with rosacea have increased risk of dementia. Ann Neurol. 2016;79:921–8.
27. Del Rosso JQ. Advances in understanding and managing rosacea: part 1: connecting the dots between pathophysiological mechanisms and common clinical features of rosacea with emphasis on vascular changes and facial erythema. J Clin Aesthet Dermatol. 2012;5:16–25.
28. Bhargava R, Chandra M, Bansal U, et al. A randomized controlled trial of omega 3 fatty acids in rosacea patients with dry eye symptoms. Curr Eye Res. 2016;41:1274–80.
29. Al Arfaj K, Al Zamil W. Spontaneous corneal perforation in ocular rosacea. Middle East Afr J Ophthalmol. 2010;17:186–8.
30. Bae YI, Yun SJ, Lee JB, et al. Clinical evaluation of 168 Korean patients with rosacea: the sun exposure correlates with the erythematotelangiectatic subtype. Ann Dermatol. 2009;21:243–9.
31. Lee WJ, Lee YJ, Lee MH, et al. Prognosis of 234 rosacea patients according to clinical subtype: the significance of central facial erythema in the prognosis of rosacea. J Dermatol. 2016;43:526–31.
32. Furukawa M, Kanetou K, Hamada T. Rhinophyma in Japan. Int J Dermatol. 1994;33:35–7.
33. Lee WJ, Lee YJ, Won CH, et al. Clinical evaluation of 30 patients with localized nasal rosacea. J Dermatol. 2016;43:200–2.
34. Zouboulis CC, Schaller M, Gollnick HPM. Antimicrobial treatment of rosacea. In: Ólafsson JH, Hay RJ, editors. Antibiotic and antifungal therapies in dermatology. Berlin: Springer; 2016. p. 41–56.
35. Wu J. Treatment of rosacea with herbal ingredients. J Drugs Dermatol. 2006;5:29–32.
36. Alexis AF, Webster G, Preston NJ, et al. Effectiveness and safety of once-daily doxycycline capsules as monotherapy in patients with rosacea: an analysis by Fitzpatrick skin type. J Drugs Dermatol. 2012;11:1219–22.

Psoriasis in Skin of Color

21

Leah A. Cardwell, Chelsea Kesty, Steven R. Feldman, and Amy J. McMichael

21.1 Epidemiology

Psoriasis is a chronic inflammatory disease that affects approximately 3.2% of the adult population of the USA. Amongst this population, Caucasians have the highest prevalence rate at 3.6%, while in non-Caucasians or individuals with skin of color the prevalence is lower, 1.9%, 1.6%, and 1.4% in African Americans, Hispanics, and other non-Caucasians, respectively [1]. Based on these statistics, one might gather that psoriasis is less likely in skin of color [2]. One of the earliest review articles detailing psoriasis prevalence by ethnic origin highlights several groups including the specific categories: Caucasian, African American, black-skinned South African, Fiji Islands, American Indian, Latin American Indian, Japanese, and Indonesians [3]. The 1965 text perpetuates the idea that psoriasis is relatively common in Caucasians and much less frequent in skin of color while acknowledging that psoriasis may not be as rare in those of African descent as previously believed. It was proposed that in evaluating the incidence of psoriasis among different ethnic groups, the potential influence of variables such as genetics, climate, diet, degree of skin pigmentation, exercise, stress level, economic factors, social factors, and hygiene factors must be considered [3]. This study was subject to selection bias as the text concluded that psoriasis was uncommon in black-skinned individuals during a time period when black-skinned individuals with psoriasis were much less likely to visit the dermatologist than white Caucasians.

There is no agreement in the literature regarding severity of disease across different ethnic groups. In a study of psoriasis patients in Brazil, mixed ethnic and black-skinned people did not present with a more severe clinical form of the disease, and prevalence of psoriasis was nearly equal in these populations as in whites [4]. This is in contrast to studies completed in European and North American populations where the prevalence is especially high in Caucasians as compared to their black-skinned counterparts [1, 2]. These inconsistencies in the literature, regarding the severity of disease in various ethnic groups, continue to muddy the waters of psoriasis prevalence, especially across nations [2, 5].

Psoriasis prevalence varies based on geographic region; countries further from the equator are noted to have higher psoriasis prevalence rates [6]. Climate factors may also play a role in psoriasis prevalence variation. Patients report that their psoriasis condition improves in summer and worsens in winter as cold temperatures can lead to patient-perceived worsening of psoriasis [7]. A study on the natural history of psoriasis noted that, in the majority of subjects, hot weather and sunlight had a beneficial effect [8]. El Nino Southern Oscillation (ENSO), a climate phenomenon which occurs every 2–7 years characterized by fluctuations in ocean temperature and atmospheric pressure causing changes in weather patterns around the world, has been associated with a decrease in the reported cases of psoriasis [9]. These variations in psoriasis prevalence support the idea that psoriasis is a complex disease influenced by genetics, environment, and potentially other factors. While region-specific population studies have provided valuable insight regarding the worldwide burden of disease, international research using standardized methods would be beneficial in clarifying the broader epidemiology of psoriasis.

21.2 Clinical Picture

For providers with minimal experience in treating patients with skin of color, diagnosing psoriasis can be a clinical challenge [10–12]. Several differences in psoriasis clinical presentation have been noted; providers reported more dyspigmentation, thicker plaques, and less erythema in African American psoriasis patients [13] (Fig. 21.1). In fairer skin

L. A. Cardwell · C. Kesty · S. R. Feldman (✉) · A. J. McMichael
Department of Dermatology, Wake Forest University School of Medicine, Winston-Salem, NC, USA
e-mail: lcardwe@wakehealth.edu; ckesty@health.usf.edu; sfeldman@wakehealth.edu; amcmicha@wakehealth.edu

C. E. Orfanos et al. (eds.), *Pigmented Ethnic Skin and Imported Dermatoses*, https://doi.org/10.1007/978-3-319-69422-1_21

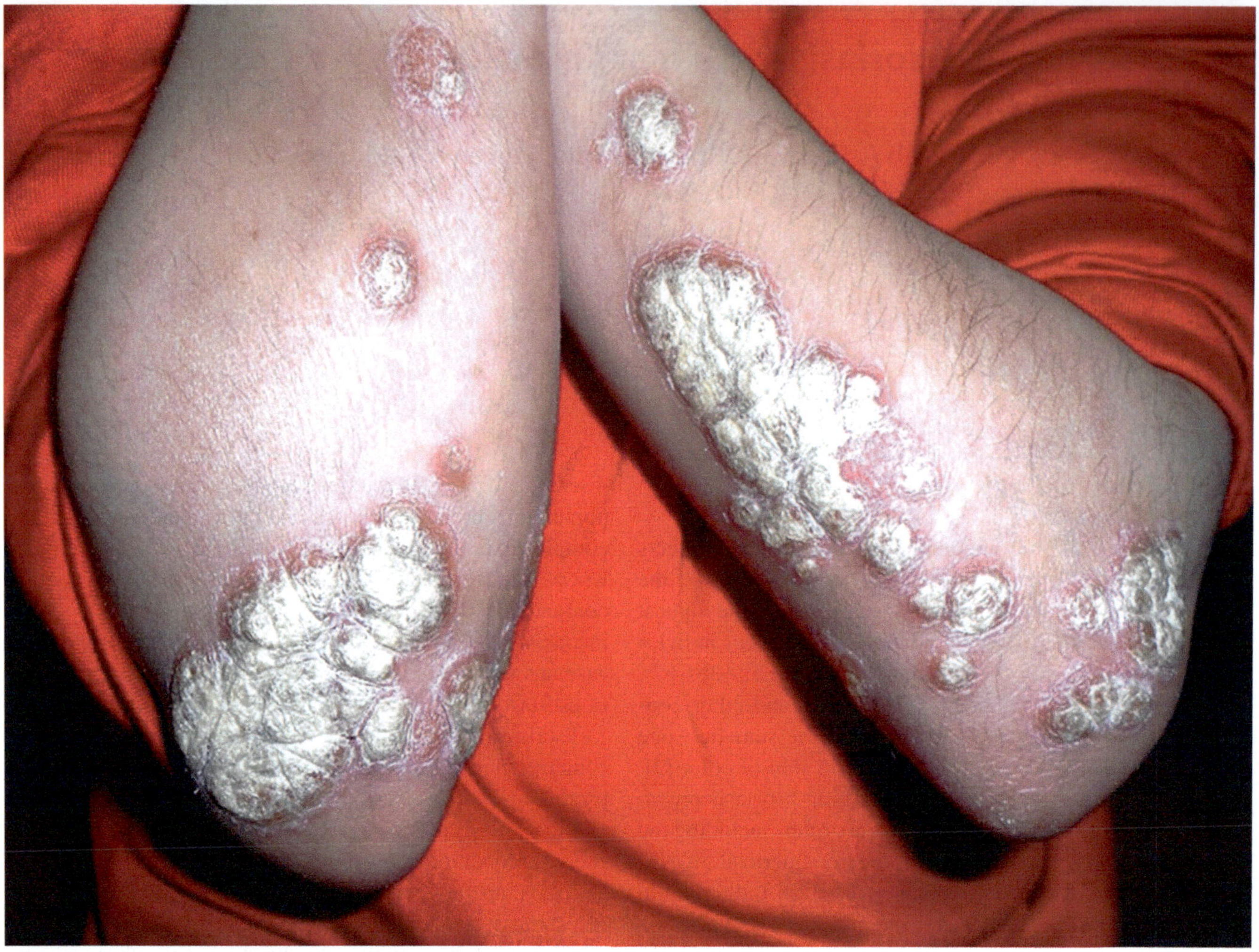

Fig. 21.1 Severe, hyperkeratotic psoriatic plaques in a Tanzanian female with typical localization (untreated; courtesy CEO)

types, psoriasis lesions are described as well-demarcated, red or salmon-colored papules or plaques with overlying silvery scales, while in darker skin types, the lesions tend to have more of a violaceous and dusky color with overlying silvery scale (Fig. 21.2). African Americans with psoriasis reported having greater body surface area involvement than Caucasian patients. Body surface area involvement was quantified by the amount of psoriasis that could be covered with the palm of the patient's hand. African Americans reported 3–10 palms of body surface involvement, while Caucasians reported 1–2 palms of body surface involvement [2]. Occasionally, erythrodermic psoriasis is seen, either spontaneously as an acute psoriatic erythroderma or following long-term treatment with corticosteroids (Fig. 21.3). In dark-skinned patients postpsoriatic hyperpigmentation (melanoderma) may occur after clinical recovery of the lesions due to increased production and deposition of melanin, in contrast to postpsoriatic leukoderma in Caucasians (Fig. 21.4). Post-inflammatory hyperpigmentation may last months to years and is the source of significant distress in patients with skin of color.

Diagnosing psoriasis in skin of color patients may also be challenging due to similarities in presentation to other dermatologic diseases. Differential diagnoses for psoriasis in skin of color includes atopic dermatitis, lichen planus, sarcoidosis, and cutaneous lupus. In order to rule out other diagnoses, a thorough skin, scalp, and nail (Fig. 21.5) examination is crucial, and a biopsy may be helpful. Through physical investigation one can identify psoriasis characteristics including nail changes, sharply demarcated scaly plaques, and typical distribution areas (the extensor surfaces, scalp, umbilicus, and intergluteal cleft). In assessing active psoriatic lesions, one must consider that erythema may be harder to detect in skin of color. In contrast to the red or salmon-colored lesions seen in fairer skin types, the lesions may appear dark brown or violaceous [14].

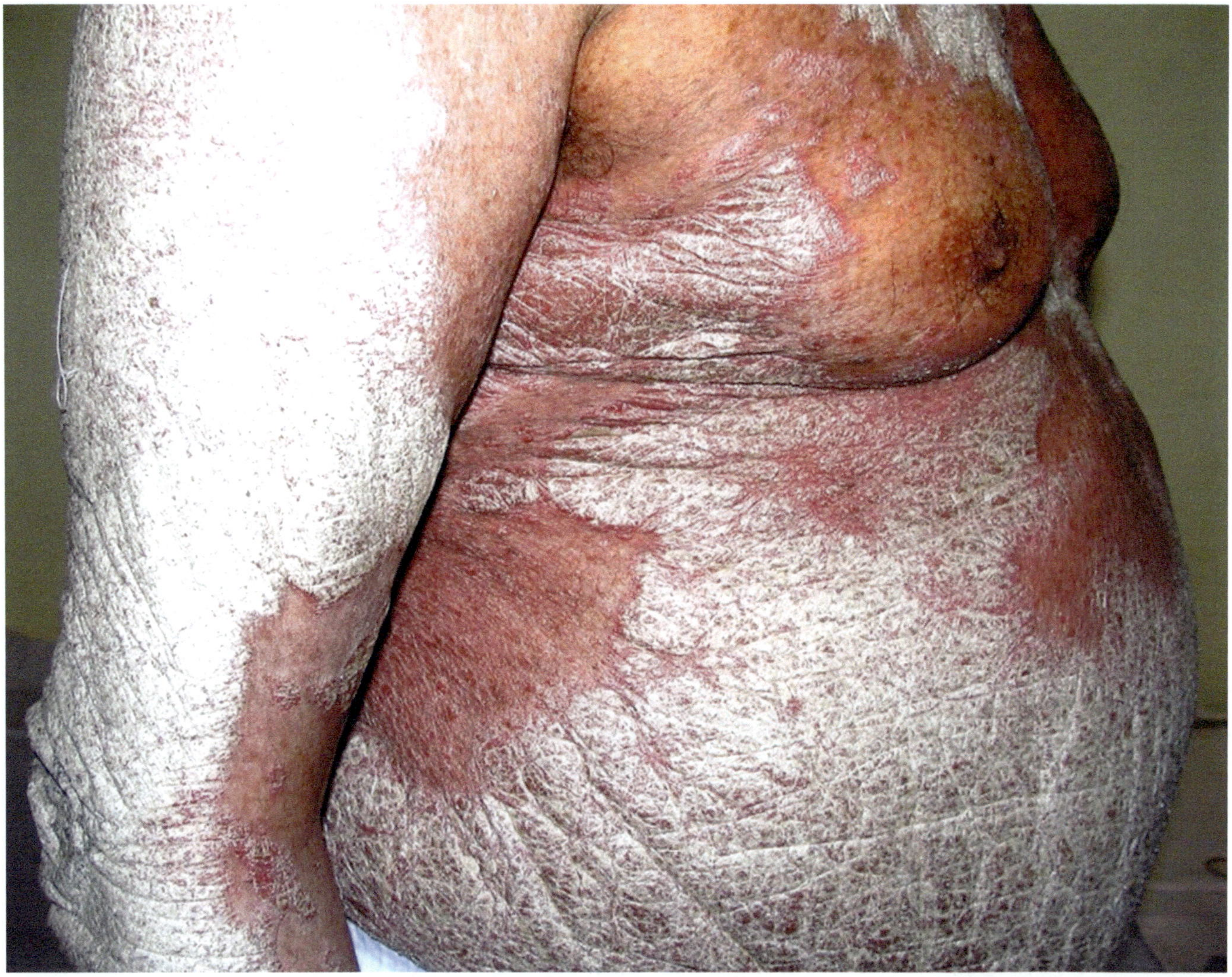

Fig. 21.2 Generalized *plaque-like psoriasis* in an Egyptian male (untreated; courtesy CEO)

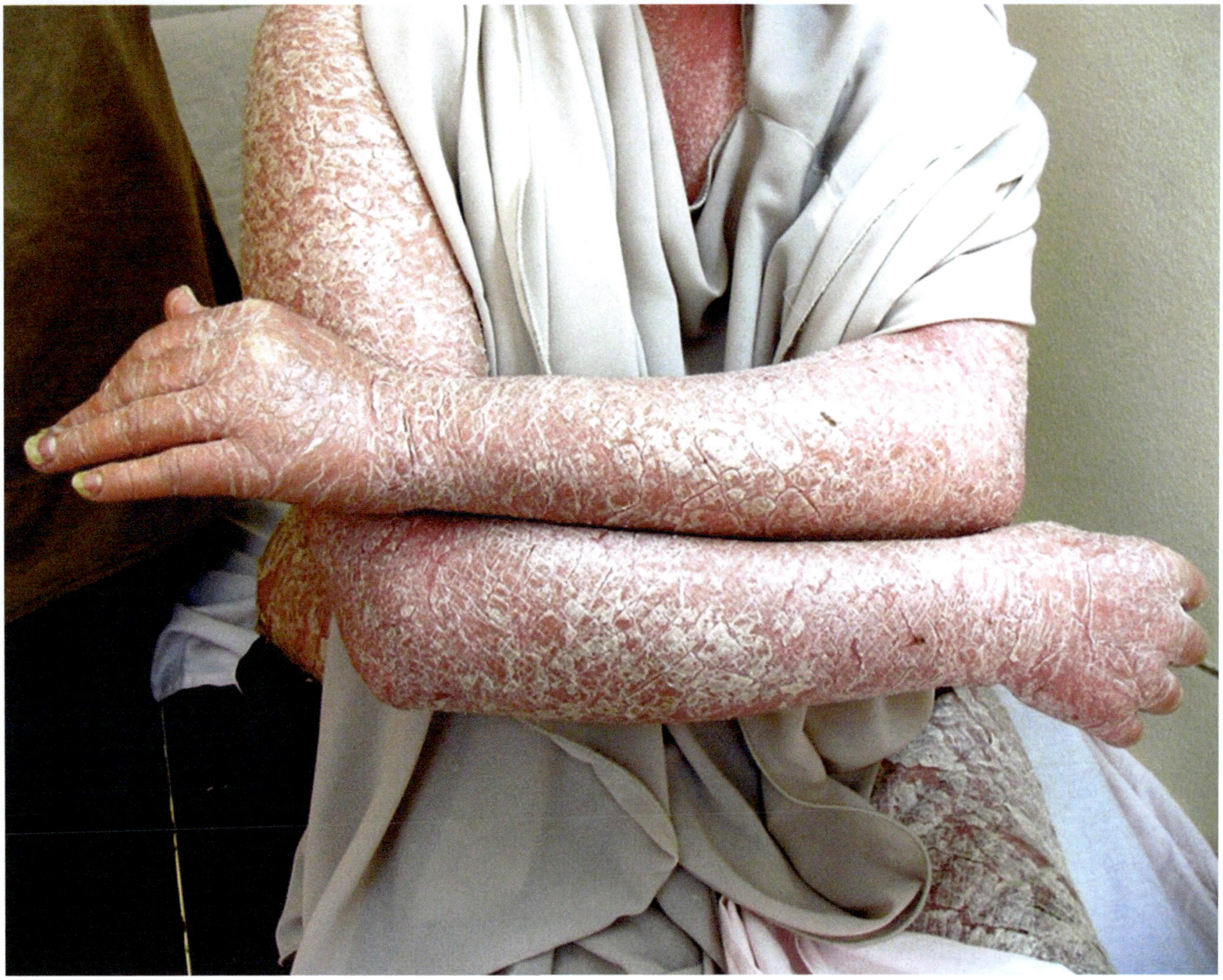

Fig. 21.3 *Erythrodermic psoriasis* in an Egyptian female, after previous long-term treatment with potent topical corticosteroids (courtesy CEO)

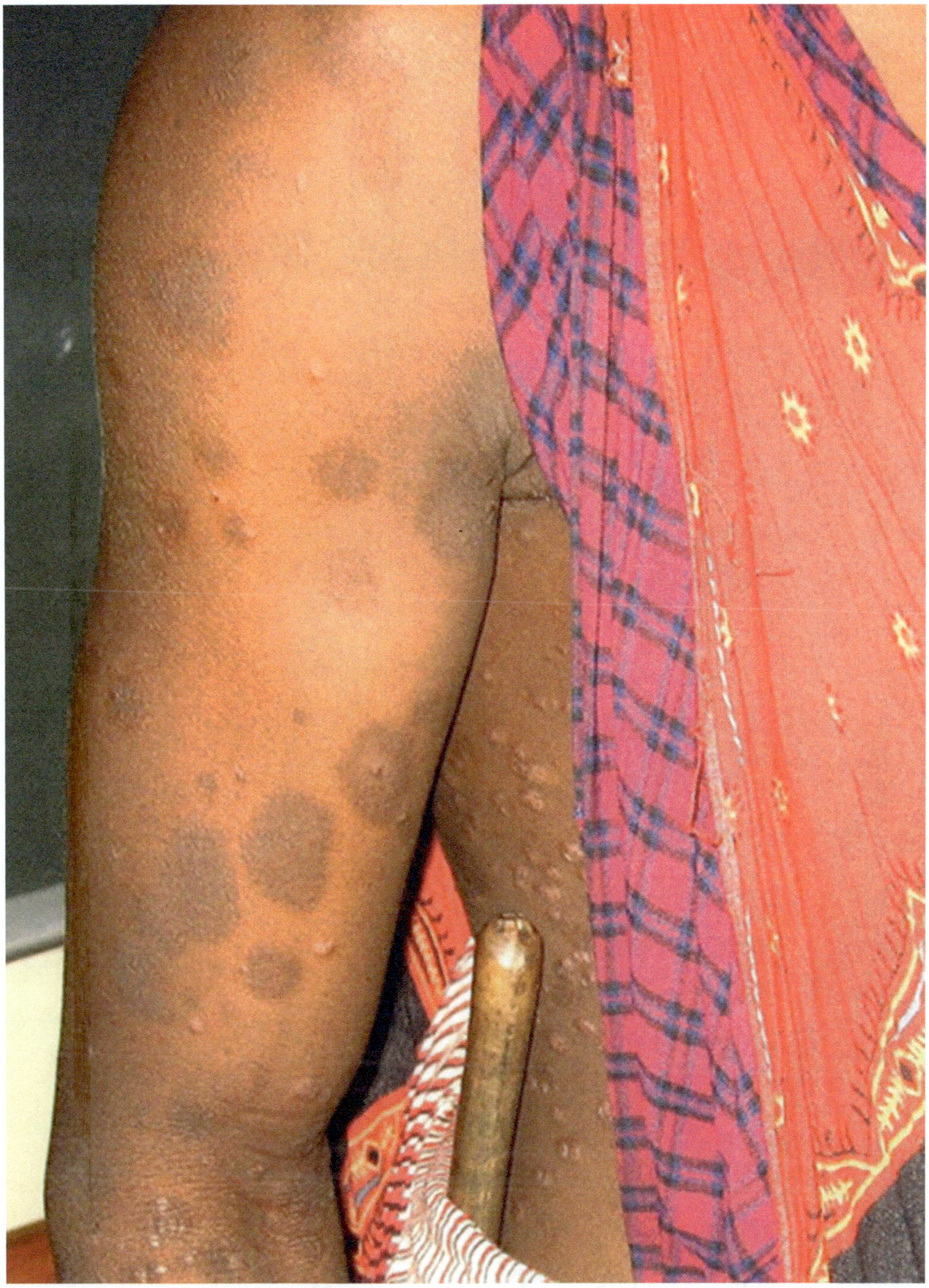

Fig. 21.4 Postpsoriatic hyperpigmented macules (melanoderma) in an African Maasai after long-term treatment with methotrexate. A few remaining scaling lesions are seen on his trunk (courtesy CEO)

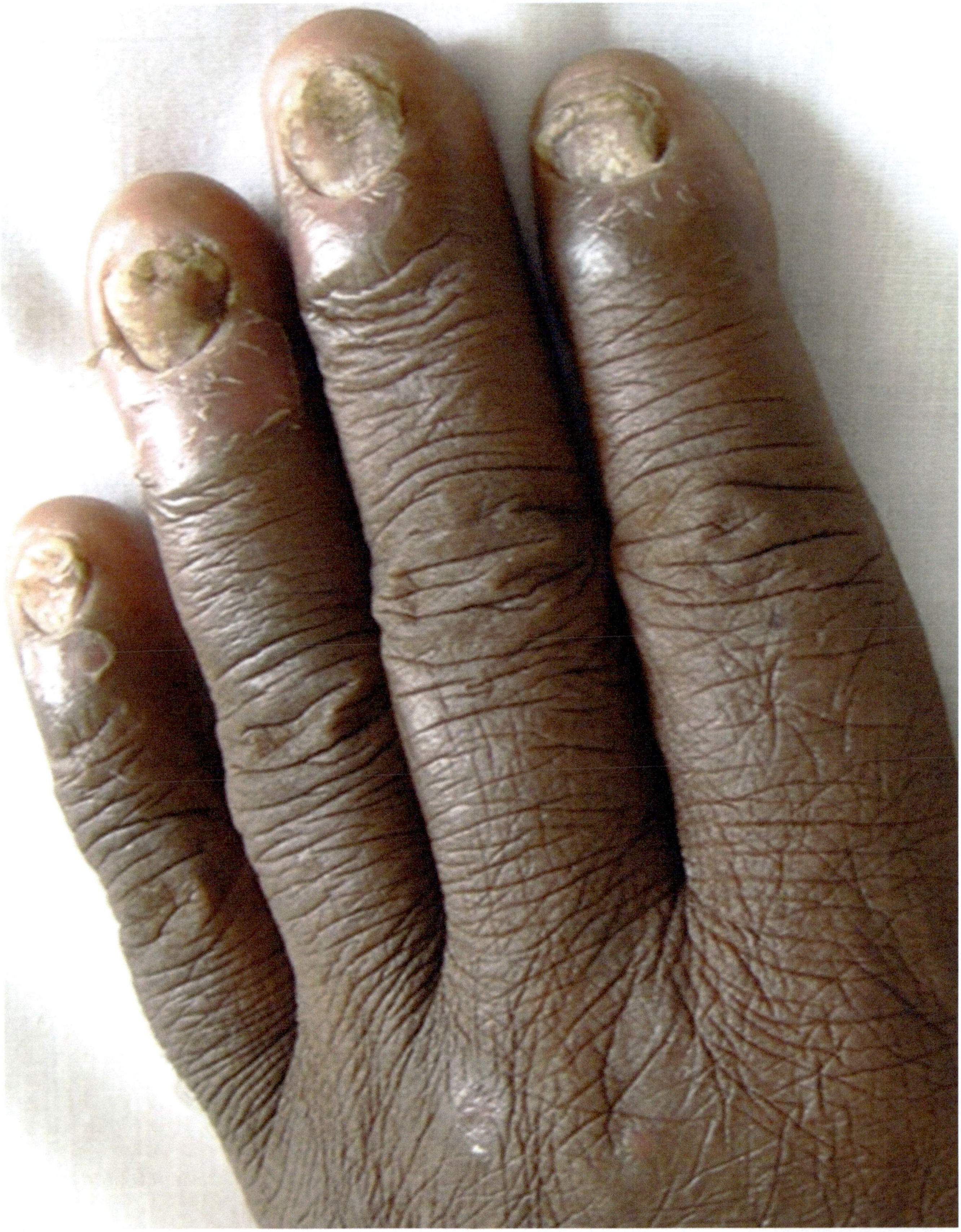

Fig. 21.5 Involvement of the nails in psoriasis

21.3 Etiology/Pathogenesis

As the understanding of immunology and genetics becomes more sophisticated, the full picture of psoriasis is better elucidated. Psoriasis is a complex disease with environmental, genetic, and immunological factors contributing to initiation and maintenance of skin lesions. It seems that keratinocyte hyperproliferation occurs due to dysregulation of the immune system. Cytokine release in the epidermis contributes to the inflammatory nature of disease. Nine chromosomal loci have been identified as having statistically significant linkage to psoriasis; one of these is PSORS1, which is the main genetic determinant of psoriasis [15]. Genetic investigation into psoriasis has identified T cells and dendritic cells as principal cells involved in the pathogenesis, while type I interferons, interferon gamma, and TNF-α are key cytokines involved [16, 17]. Plasmacytoid dendritic cells, producers of interferon-α, are abundant in the skin of patients with psoriasis activated to produce this cytokine at sites of the disease [18]. Keratinocytes in psoriatic epidermis have antimicrobial peptides which play a chemotactic role and facilitate the inflammatory process [19]. T cells translocate from the dermis to the epidermis and secrete cytokines including interferon-γ and IL-17. Type 17 helper T cells produce IL-17 as well as IL-22. IL-22 induces hyperproliferation of the epidermis manifesting as well-demarcated papules or plaques with overlying silvery scale [20, 21].

Studies have identified genomic factors related to psoriasis risk in patients with skin of color. TNFAIP3 and TNIP1 are polymorphisms which confer increased risk for psoriasis in South Indian Tamils [22]. In Europeans LCE3C and LCE3B gene deletion is a common susceptibility factor but also confers increased risk in Chinese and Mongolian populations [23]. Polymorphisms in the CCHCR1 and HLA-C genes of North Indians were associated with psoriasis risk; two haplotypes were revealed to be high risk for psoriasis in the North Indian population [24].

21.4 Management

Psoriasis treatment options include topical and systemic medications as well as phototherapy (Table 21.1). Topical medications indicated for psoriasis include corticosteroids of varying potency, vitamin D analogs, calcineurin inhibitors, anthralin, salicylic acid, and coal tar (Table 21.2). Systemic medications include methotrexate, acitretin, cyclosporine, apremilast, and various biologics such as etanercept, adalimumab, secukinumab, ustekinumab, infliximab, and ixekizumab (Tables 21.3 and 21.4). Generally, topical medications are favored in localized mild-to-moderate psoriasis, while

Table 21.1 Overall schedule of treatment

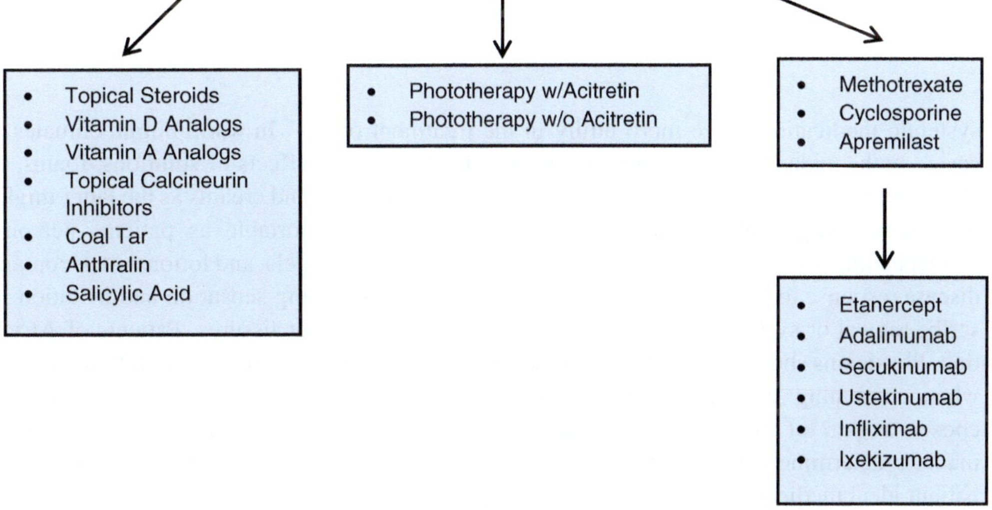

Table 21.2 Modalities for topical treatment

Medication	Mode of action	Dosing	Comments
Topical corticosteroids (i.e. clobetasol propionate, betamethasone dipropionate)	Anti-inflammatory, antiproliferative	Twice daily for up to 4 weeks	Keep a close eye on clinical improvement, and taper when this occurs to avoid irreversible skin atrophy
Topical vitamin D3 analogs (i.e. calcipotriene, calcitriol)	Epidermal antiproliferative effect, induces apoptosis of inflammatory cells	Once or twice daily for up to 8 weeks	May be irritating. Typically prescribed in combination with topical steroids to expedite results and limit duration of use
Topical vitamin A analogs (i.e. tazarotene)	Decreases epidermal hyperproliferation	Once daily (evening)	Avoid use in women of child-bearing age due to risk of teratogenicity
Topical calcineurin inhibitors (i.e. tacrolimus, pimecrolimus)	Decreases the release of inflammatory cytokines	Twice daily for up to 8 weeks	For use in intertriginous areas and face
Coal tar	Unknown	Once daily for at least 12 weeks duration	Poor adherence due to unfavorable smell and clothing-staining capability
Anthralin	Anti-inflammatory and antiproliferative effect via suppression of IL-6, IL-8, and TNF-alpha [25]	Once daily for at least 8 weeks duration	Poor adherence due to staining capability
Salicylic acid	Keratolytic action	Once daily, may occlude the area at night	If combined with topical corticosteroids, penetration and efficacy are increased

Table 21.3 Systemic medications

Medication	Mode of action	Dosing	Comments
Methotrexate	Inhibits folate production which in turn inhibits T-cell proliferation and induces T-cell apoptosis; increases adenosine, an anti-inflammatory molecule	Evaluate renal function, hematologic data, and liver function for signs of toxicity Subsequent doses 7.5–25 mg weekly. Supplementation of folate recommended	Available as oral and intramuscular formulation; Intramuscular administration limits gastrointestinal side effects
Vitamin A derivatives (etretinate, acitretin)	Reduces hyperproliferation of keratinocytes by binding to nuclear receptors responsible for gene transcription	Up to 50 mg per day, may start at lower dose and escalate as tolerated; may start at higher dose and then de-escalate for rapid improvement and to avoid side effects	Avoid use in women of child-bearing age due to risk of teratogenicity; Can be used in combination with phototherapy to reduce the risk of skin cancer
Cyclosporine	Interacts with calcineurin to reduce IL-2 and other cytokines produced by T lymphocytes	2.5–4 mg/kg divided into two doses	Risk of renal toxicity
Apremilast	Inhibits phosphodiesterase-4 thereby preventing the breakdown of cAMP; its levels rise and thereby reduce cytokine production	Up to 30 mg 2×/day and may be increased gradually to reach this dose	Relatively safe medication but lower success rate than biologics; Pregnancy category C

systemic medications have more utility in the treatment of cases with widespread moderate-to-severe involvement. However, topical medications may also be used as adjuvant management in patients with moderate-to-severe psoriasis.

Depending on disease severity, patient preference, and disease response to prior therapies, providers may opt to prescribe topical or systemic medications alone or in combination. Physicians should be mindful of medication side effects when combining medications. If topical medications are chosen as part of the treatment regimen, effort should be made to determine patient preferred topical vehicle. Use of patient ideal medication vehicles can increase patient adherence to treatment regimens.

In warm humid climates, patients may prefer the cooling effects of solutions, foams, gels, and lotions over ointments and creams as the latter might prove to be greasy and uncomfortable as patients perspire. However, solutions, foams, gels, and lotions often contain alcohol which can cause stinging sensation and irritation in patients with skin breakdown or fissures. Patients of African American origin may prefer ointments and lotions over gels, foams, and creams for the treatment of scalp conditions. In one study, African Americans were 12 times more likely to choose ointment preparations and 2.5 times more likely to choose lotion preparations than Caucasians and tended to choose vehicles based on similarity to products already used [28]. Therefore,

Table 21.4 Systemic treatment of moderate-to-severe psoriasis with biologic medications

Medication	Mode of action	Dosing	Comments
Etanercept	Acts as a receptor fusion protein decoy, binds free TNF-alpha and decreases TNF activity, decreases inflammation	50 mg twice weekly for 3 months and then 50 mg once weekly	Targets the immune system, so may increase the risk of infection or malignancy
Adalimumab	Monoclonal antibody against TNF-alpha, decreases inflammation	80 mg initially and then 40 mg every other week	Targets the immune system, so may increase the risk of infection or malignancy
Secukinumab	Monoclonal antibody against IL-17A, decreases the inflammation and epidermal changes evident in psoriasis	300 mg once weekly for 5 weeks and then 300 mg every 4 weeks	May increase the risk of infection. May exacerbate inflammatory bowel disease
Ustekinumab	Monoclonal antibody against IL-12 and IL-23, inhibits the downstream inflammatory signaling pathway	45 mg at 0 and 4 weeks and then 45 mg every 12 weeks	Targets the immune system, so may increase the risk of infection or malignancy
Infliximab	Monoclonal antibody against TNF-alpha, decreases inflammation	5 mg/kg at 0, 2, and 6 weeks and then 5 mg/kg every 8 weeks	Targets the immune system, so may increase the risk of infection or malignancy
Ixekizumab	Humanized IL-17A antagonist	160 mg at week 0; 80 mg at weeks 2, 4, 6, 8, 10, and 12; and then 80 mg every 4 weeks	May increase the risk of infection. May exacerbate inflammatory bowel disease

it is beneficial to interview patients regarding current hair and skin care regimens.

Phototherapy, another psoriasis treatment option, is typically reserved for patients with moderate-to-severe psoriasis. This option has relatively low side effect and contraindication profiles as compared to oral psoriasis medications. Types of phototherapy effective for psoriasis include narrow-band ultraviolet B (Nb-UVB), broad-band ultraviolet B (Bb-UVB), psoralen plus ultraviolet A (PUVA), and excimer laser. The proposed mechanism of action of light management is through apoptosis of T lymphocytes and local immunosuppression which plays a role in curtailing the immunologic component of disease pathogenesis. Phototherapy is contraindicated in photosensitive patients. The main side effect of phototherapy is increased risk for inducing non-melanoma and/or melanoma skin cancers. Nb-UVB regimens are designed based on minimal erythema dose (MED), a measure of shortest amount of Nb-UVB required to induce erythema at 24 hours. PUVA regimens are designed based on skin type; home phototherapy and outpatient phototherapy options are available [29]. PUVA management increases the risk of non-melanoma and melanoma skin cancer, though these skin cancer risks are greater in white skin than in darker skin types [29]. The carcinogenic risks of PUVA indicate that its use should be limited to those patients where the benefits outweigh the risks of management [30]. Skin of color patients contend with greater risk of hyperpigmentation with PUVA management because skin types IV–VI are melanocompetent (skin tans well, rarely burns) [31]. In patients with skin types III–V, there was no significant difference in Psoriasis Area Severity Index (PASI) in patients treated with 100% of MED of Nb-UVB and 70% of MED of Nb-UVB. This suggests that suberythemogenic dosing of Nb-UVB in skin of color patients could minimize side effects without sacrificing efficacy [32]. Mediation of health system barriers to phototherapy may promote patient use, improve disease outcomes, and reduce healthcare costs [33].

21.5 Course and Further Monitoring

There are many medications in our armamentarium for psoriasis treatment, but these medications have varying efficacy and tolerability. Regardless of which treatment option is chosen, patients should be monitored periodically for clinical improvement, side effects, and tolerability. Patients may become frustrated when treatments have delayed results; they should be counseled about the importance of adherence to treatment regimens. Physicians should consider the importance of vehicle choice in promoting patient adherence. African Americans, and perhaps other patients with skin of color, prefer ointments and lotions. Just as treatment medication regimens should be individualized, so should vehicle regimens. If vehicle preference is not considered, patient compliance will undoubtedly suffer. Regarding systemic medication, methotrexate can be administered orally or intramuscularly. The latter route can bypass the gastrointestinal side effects caused by the oral route. Failure to educate patients regarding formulation options for a medication may lead to low adherence rates [29]. Compliance rates in skin of color patients seem to lag behind that of Caucasians. In a study assessing treatment expectations, medication compliance and treatment satisfaction in adult, and female acne patients, white patients reported using prescribed acne medications for a greater number of days compared to skin of color patients. The majority of the individuals across ethnic groups expected quick resolution of acne on their respective treatment regimens, but these "overnight results" were expected more frequently by non-white patients. Failure of treatment regimens to meet expectations, albeit unrealistic, may lead to patient frustration and poor medication compliance. In order to optimize patient compliance, physicians should prioritize building patient rapport and emphasizing patient education. Written instructions are a good strategy to ensure that patients understand the treatment regimen. Other beneficial tactics include utilization of fixed-dose combination therapies to decrease the complexity of the regimen and scheduling more frequent visits for a short period after a treatment change to reinforce instructions [34]. Patients should be encouraged to join the National Psoriasis Foundation (NPF), a patient advocacy group for patients with psoriasis and psoriatic arthritis. The sense of community imparted by the NPF may play a supportive role in the lives of psoriasis patients.

References

1. Rachakonda TD, Schupp CW, Armstrong AW. Psoriasis prevalence among adults in the United States. J Am Acad Dermatol. 2014;70:512–6.
2. Gelfand JM, Stern RS, Nijsten T, et al. The prevalence of psoriasis in African Americans: results from a population-based study. J Am Acad Dermatol. 2005;52:23–6.
3. Farber EM, Grauer FZF. Racial incidence of psoriasis. Cesk Dermatol. 1965;40:289–97.
4. Porto Ferreira C, Martins CJ, Issa PR, et al. Psoriasis affects individuals of African descent and white Brazilians similarly. Actas Dermosifiliogr. 2010;101:230–4.
5. Leder RO, Farber EM. The variable incidence of psoriasis in sub-Saharan Africa. Int J Dermatol. 1997;36:911–9.
6. Parisi R, Symmons DPM, Griffiths CEM, et al. Global epidemiology of psoriasis: a systematic review of incidence and prevalence. J Invest Dermatol. 2012;133:377–85.
7. Balato N, Di Costanzo L, Patruno C, et al. Effect of weather and environmental factors on the clinical course of psoriasis. Occup Environ Med. 2013;70:600.
8. Farber EM, Nall ML. The natural history of psoriasis in 5,600 patients. Dermatology. 1974;148:1–18.
9. Andersen LK, Davis MDP. The effects of the El Nino southern oscillation on skin and skin-related diseases: a message from the International Society of Dermatology Climate Change Task Force. Int J Dermatol. 2015;54:1343–51.
10. Barlow RJ, Schulz EJ. Chronic subcorneal pustulosis with vasculitis: a variant of generalized pustular psoriasis in black South Africans. Br J Dermatol. 1991;124:470–4.
11. Curtis AR, Yosipovitch G. Erythrodermic verrucous psoriasis. J Dermatolog Treat. 2012;23:215–8.
12. Delaney TA, Smith NP. Lichen planus mimicking and coexisting with psoriasis in a black patient. Australas J Dermatol. 1993;34:59–62.
13. McMichael AJ, Vachiramon V, Guzmán-Sánchez DA, Camacho F. Psoriasis in African-Americans: a caregivers' survey. J Drugs Dermatol. 2012;11:478–82.
14. Petit A. Skin semiology and grading scales. In: Dadzie OE, Petit A, Alexis A, editors. Ethnic dermatology principles and practice. Chichester: Wiley-Blackwell; 2013. p. 5–17.
15. Bowcock AM, Krueger JG. Getting under the skin: the immunogenetics of psoriasis. Nat Rev Immunol. 2005;5:699–711.
16. Yao Y, Richman L, Morehouse C, et al. Type I interferon: potential therapeutic target for psoriasis? PLoS One. 2008;3:e2737.
17. Haider AS, Lowes M, Suàrez-Fariñas M, et al. Cellular genomic maps help dissect pathology in human skin disease. J Invest Dermatol. 2008;128:606–15.
18. Funk J, Langeland T, Schrumpf E, et al. Psoriasis induced by interferon-alpha. Br J Dermatol. 1991;125:463–5.
19. Büchau AS, Gallo RL. Innate immunity and antimicrobial defense systems in psoriasis. Clin Dermatol. 2007;25:616–24.
20. Nestle FO, Kaplan DH, Barker J. Psoriasis. N Engl J Med. 2009;361:496–509.
21. Nickoloff BJ, Xin H, Nestle FO, et al. The cytokine and chemokine network in psoriasis. Clin Dermatol. 2007;25:568–73.
22. Indhumathi S, Rajappa M, Chandrashekar L, et al. TNFAIP3 and TNIP1 polymorphisms confer psoriasis risk in South Indian Tamils. Br J Biomed Sci. 2015;72:168–73.
23. Riveira-Munoz E, He S-M, Escaramís G, et al. Meta-analysis confirms the LCE3C_LCE3B deletion as a risk factor for psoriasis in several ethnic groups and finds interaction with HLA-Cw6. J Invest Dermatol. 2011;131:1105–9.
24. Gandhi G, Buttar BS, Albert L, et al. Psoriasis-associated genetic polymorphism in North Indian population in the CCHCR1 gene and in a genomic segment flanking the HLA-C region. Dis Markers. 2011;31:361–70.
25. Mrowietz U, Jessat H, Schwarz A, et al. Anthralin (dithranol) in vitro inhibits human monocytes to secrete IL-6, IL-8 and TNF-alpha, but not IL-1. Br J Dermatol. 1997;136:542–7.
26. Lowenthal KE, Horn PJ, Kalb RE. Concurrent use of methotrexate and acitretin revisited. J Dermatolog Treat. 2008;19:22–6.
27. van de Kerkhof PC, Cambazard F, Hutchinson PE, et al. The effect of addition of calcipotriol ointment (50 micrograms/g) to acitretin therapy in psoriasis. Br J Dermatol. 1998;138:84–9.
28. Fisher EJ, Adams BB. African American and Caucasian patients' vehicle preference for the scalp. J Am Acad Dermatol. 2008;58(Suppl 1):1–6.
29. Farhangian ME, Anderson KL, Feldman S. Practical psoriasis management. Create Space Independent Publishing Platform; 2015.
30. Archier E, Devaux S, Castela E, et al. Carcinogenic risks of psoralen UV-A therapy and narrowband UV-B therapy in chronic plaque psoriasis: a systematic literature review. J Eur Acad Dermatol Venereol. 2012;26(Suppl 3):22–31.
31. Syed ZU, Hamzavi IH. Role of phototherapy in patients with skin of color. Semin Cutan Med Surg. 2011;30:184–9.
32. Youssef RM, Mahgoub D, Mashaly HM, et al. Different narrowband UVB dosage regimens in dark skinned psoriatics: a preliminary study. Photodermatol Photoimmunol Photomed. 2008;24:256–9.
33. Yeung H, Wan J, Van Voorhees AS, et al. Patient-reported reasons for the discontinuation of commonly used treatments for moderate to severe psoriasis. J Am Acad Dermatol. 2013;68:64–72.
34. Rendon MI, Rodriguez DA, Kawata AK, et al. Acne treatment patterns, expectations, and satisfaction among adult females of different races/ethnicities. Clin Cosmet Investig Dermatol. 2015;8:231–8.

Parapsoriasis

22

Constantin E. Orfanos

There are no accurate data on the prevalence and incidence of the clinically multifaceted group of parapsoriasis. The clinical variables in this group have a chronic course with only few clinical symptoms, if any; they may remain underreported although patients with parapsoriasis have an increased risk of subsequent cancers and increased mortality [1]. The group of parapsoriasis comprises several inhomogeneous, chronic-intermittently developing skin diseases which may clinically mimic psoriasis but are unrelated to each other with respect to their pathogenesis, histopathology, and response to treatment. Their etiology is unknown and the pathogenetic mechanisms are not fully understood. A part of these entities present inflammatory features as a reactive T-cell skin disease with vasculitis, often arising following infections, and another part is considered as precursor or early lymphoproliferative disorder with long-term progression into cutaneous T-cell lymphoma (CTCL). The majority of the entities included are associated with male predominance.

Four major clinical variables are included in this group, which seemingly represent separate entities despite their overlapping:

- *Pityriasis lichenoides chronica*
- *Pityriasis lichenoides et varioliformis acuta,* showing a more benign, rarely another severe ulceronecrotic course
- *Parapsoriasis en plaques,* with two subsets showing small and large plaques, possibly with different prognosis
- *Parapsoriasis lichenoides*, a rare clinical variant described under different designations (parakeratosis variegata, poikiloderma vasculare atrophicans)

Another entity related to this group is *lymphomatoid papulosis,* seen as a link between the two major pathogenetic mechanisms involved in parapsoriasis, the inflammatory response on one hand and a lymphoproliferative reaction on the other. The condition is recently categorized as a part of the CD30+ lymphoma group (see Chap. 36). A generally accepted nomenclature and classification of the single disorders is in view of their overlapping features still under ongoing debate, also because historically grown designations complicate the overview.

C. E. Orfanos, M.D.
The Free University of Berlin, Medical School Charité,
Berlin, Germany
e-mail: corfanos@t-online.de

22.1 Pityriasis Lichenoides Chronica (Syn.: Juliusberg's Disease)

Pityriasis lichenoides chronica (PLC) is an uncommon skin disease seen predominantly in children and adolescents, with an overall good prognosis. Small maculopapular, symmetrically distributed erythematous lesions with glossy scaling ("marienglas") are seen on the trunk and the extremities, which slowly flatten and may disappear under subtle scarring. Subjective complaints are completely absent, even in the phase of dissemination. For pathogenesis a skin reactive pattern to a past or latent viral infection or other infectious agent is suggested. The condition follows a chronic course, whereby rushes are seemingly provoked or maintained by other concomitant infections or nonspecific stimuli leading to episodic recurrences. Long-term remissions may be registered; full spontaneous regression is to be expected in a few years. Clinical and histological overlapping with the acute varioliform type of parapsoriasis may occur and make it difficult to reliably diagnose and classify a single case. However, the lymphocytic cell infiltrate in PLC lesions has been shown polyclonal, in contrast to monoclonal lymphocytic infiltrates often detected in PLEVA, usually linked with unfavorable prognosis [2].

The clinical presentation may differ in black-skinned individuals: in a series of five patients, four children, and one young adult, extensive prominent facial involvement with hypopigmented macules and patches was found posing a diagnostic challenge, whereas in one patient concomitant mycosis fungoides was diagnosed, underscoring the potential of the disease to develop into early lymphoma [3].

C. E. Orfanos et al. (eds.), *Pigmented Ethnic Skin and Imported Dermatoses*, https://doi.org/10.1007/978-3-319-69422-1_22

22.1.1 Management

PLC usually responds well to topical application of mild emulsions and corticosteroid creams together with oral antibiotics both in children (erythromycin 20–50 mg/kg/d) and in adults (tetracyclines, doxycycline); local irritants of any type should be avoided and possible foci found and treated. Topical modalities are particularly effective in children and cases following infections. In recalcitrant patients phototherapies are usually administered (UVB, PUVA) and were shown beneficial, although there is a high rate of recurrences [4]. Recently, complete responses were reported with narrowband UVB [5].

22.2 Pityriasis Lichenoides et Varioliformis Acuta (PLEVA) (Syn.: Parapsoriasis Guttata; Mucha-Habermann's Disease)

There are no comprehensive data on the prevalence or incidence of PLEVA, the disease is not common, and studies on larger groups of patients are lacking. In pigmented ethnic skin and Asian populations, only a few reports were recently published [6, 7]; it seems that there are no differences compared to Caucasian white skin.

For pathogenesis a cutaneous host immune response toward a beta-hemolytic streptococcal infection [8] or viral reactivation due to associations with Epstein-Barr virus [9], parvovirus [10], etc. is discussed, and a paraviral exanthema has been assumed [11]; however, further evidence for a viral infection is lacking. The etiology and the pathogenetic mechanisms of the disease remain not well understood. Overall, PLEVA combines inflammatory features with lymphoproliferative tissue characteristics. Its recognition as a separate entity is a debatable matter, because its presentation overlaps to some extend with the clinical features of PLC and/or febrile episodes with ulceronecrotic lesions may occur, as a severe complication of the classical type. They all make it often difficult to establish a precise diagnosis and categorize the condition. PLC and PLEVA may represent clinical expressions of the same entity with chronic and acute course [12]. PLEVA is often seen in young individuals and merits indeed awareness also because it occasionally shows a variable degree of activated T-lymphocytes and cellular atypias with T-cell receptor clonal rearrangement, causing difficulties to differentiate toward lymphomatoid papulosis [13]. It has been assumed that PLEVA is a benign clonal T-cell disorder, in which the clone arises from a subset of T cells in lesions of PLC [2].

Clinically, multiple papulosquamous lesions and hemorrhagic vesicles with central necrosis and varioliform appearance are presented, preferably on the trunk and the proximal extremities. In some cases they are distributed all over the body (Fig. 22.1). Mucosal lesions are not or only rarely noticed. The asymptomatic lesions persist over several weeks or months and heal with mild hypo- or hyperpigmented scarring, while new lesions appear (Fig. 22.2). Patient's symptomatology is generally poor. In the rare *Mucha-Habermann* subset, fulminant courses with hemorrhagic papulovesicles and ulcerations with occasional lymphadenopathy become prominent in a sudden onset, accompanied by high fever, joint pain, constitutional symptoms, and malaise (Fig. 22.3). It may occur both in children and adults. In skin biopsies lymphocytic vasculitis and cell monoclonality are often detected. Rarely, systemic vasculitis has been reported. Differential diagnosis toward drug-induced necrotizing vasculitis may be difficult (Fig. 22.4). The overall prognostic outcome is variable; a part of the cases becomes associated or proceed to develop cutaneous T-cell lymphoma. The Mucha-Habermann subset may become uncontrolled and rarely be lethal.

22.2.1 Management

There is no standardized protocol for treating PLEVA; the therapeutic strategy will depend on the severity of the case. Side medications and any instances of possible provocation by drugs, food, or local remedies should be avoided. The lesions do not respond to topical treatment. Calamine lotion and local antiseptics are helpful to avoid bacterial super infection. Particularly in hot climate zones, brucellosis, toxoplasmosis, or gastrointestinal foci (*Yersinia*, amoeba, helminthes) are to detect and eliminate, and oral antibiotics (erythromycin 1–2 g/day in children, clindamycin 3× 400 mg/day in adults) should be consequently administered over 2–3 weeks.

Phototherapy with PUVA or narrowband UVB will be successful to induce remission as a first-line option, whereas long-term monitoring will be mandatory to control relapses. Systemic corticosteroids alone are usually not effective; they may be helpful in severe ulceronecrotic courses, if given together with antibiotics [14] or with methotrexate [15]. Cases responsive to methotrexate alone have been also reported [16, 17]. Recently infliximab and intravenous immunoglobulins [18] or infliximab alone [19] was successfully used, particularly in patients with severe course.

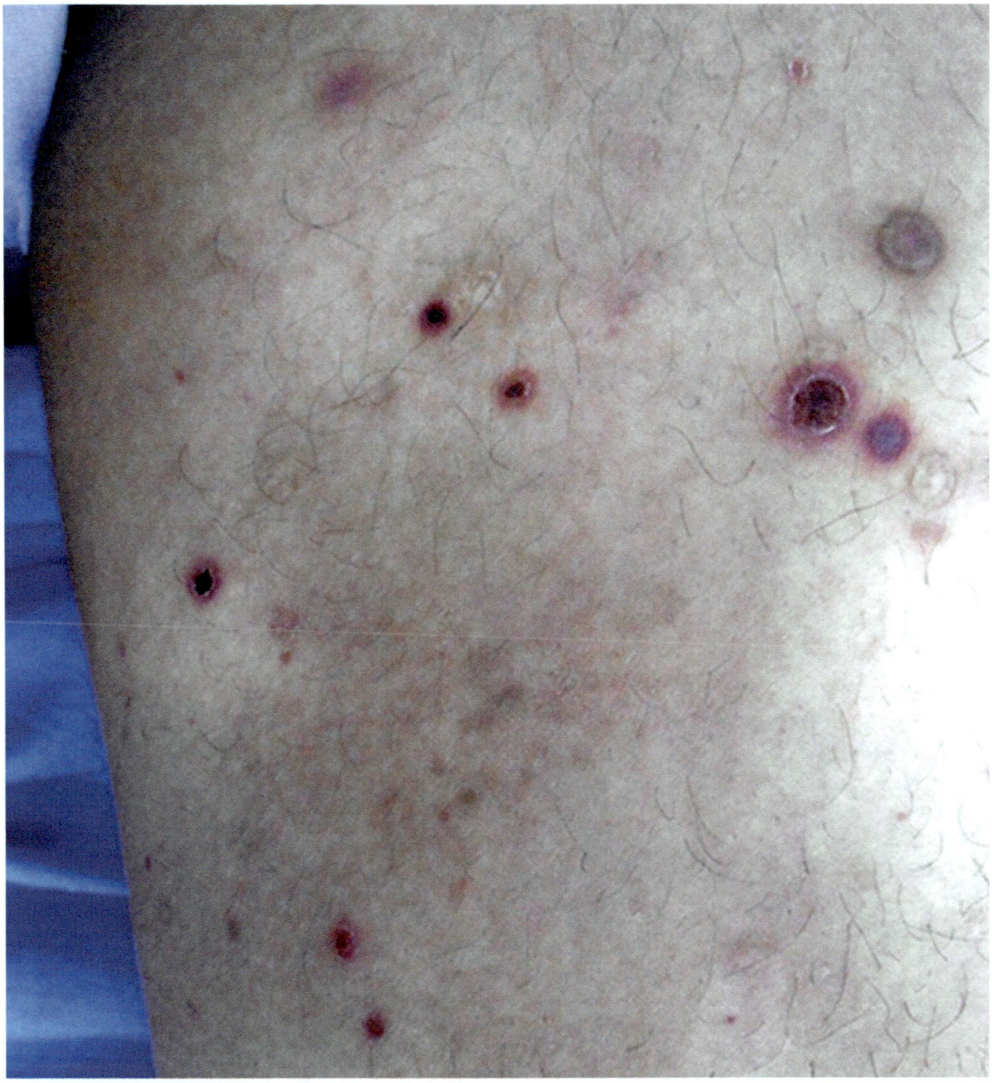

Fig. 22.1 *Pityriasis lichenoides varioliformis acuta* in the upper leg of a 17-year-old boy, 6 weeks after first onset

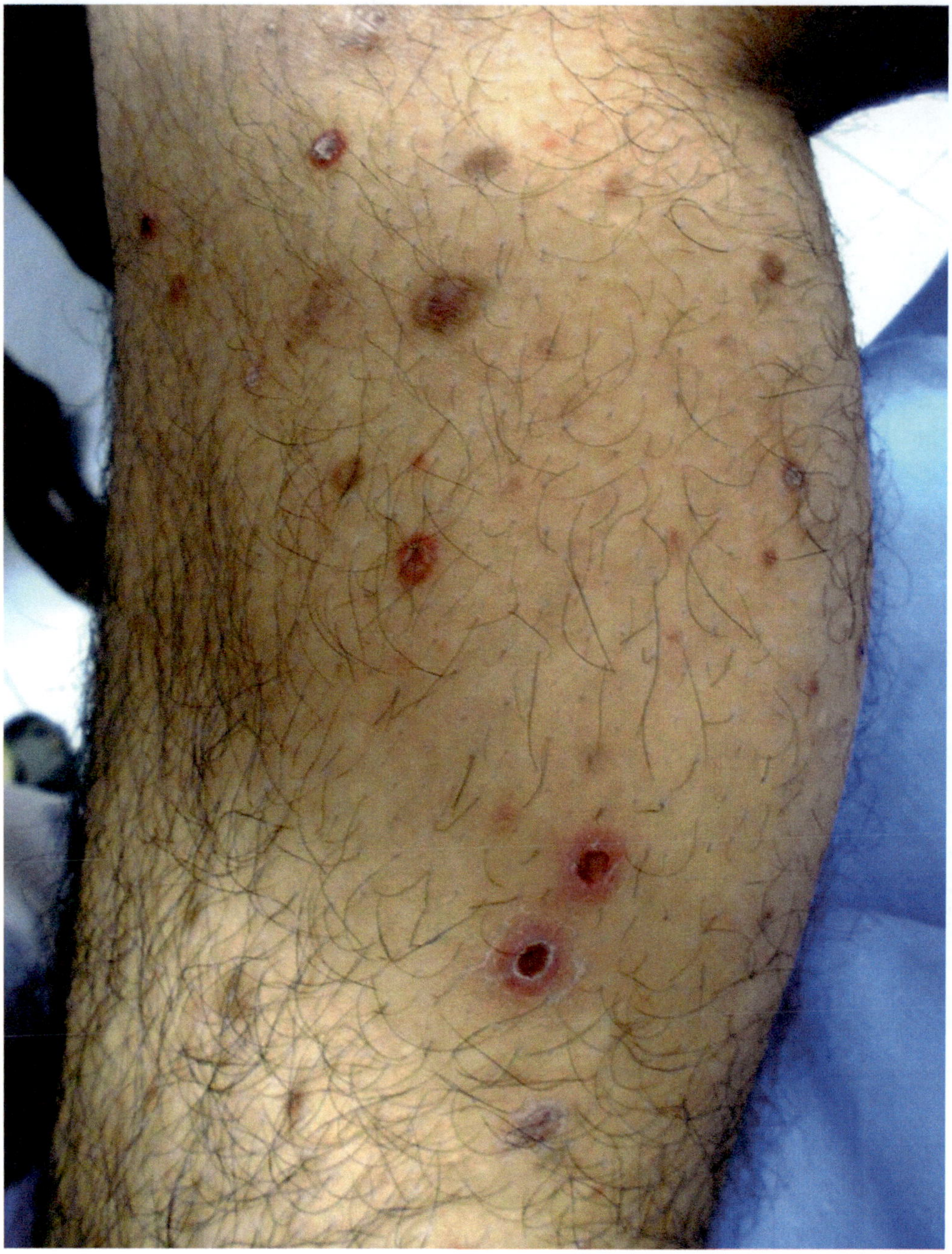

Fig. 22.2 Relapsing course of *pityriasis lichenoides varioliformis acuta* in a young adult male (Egypt) with new and old lesions

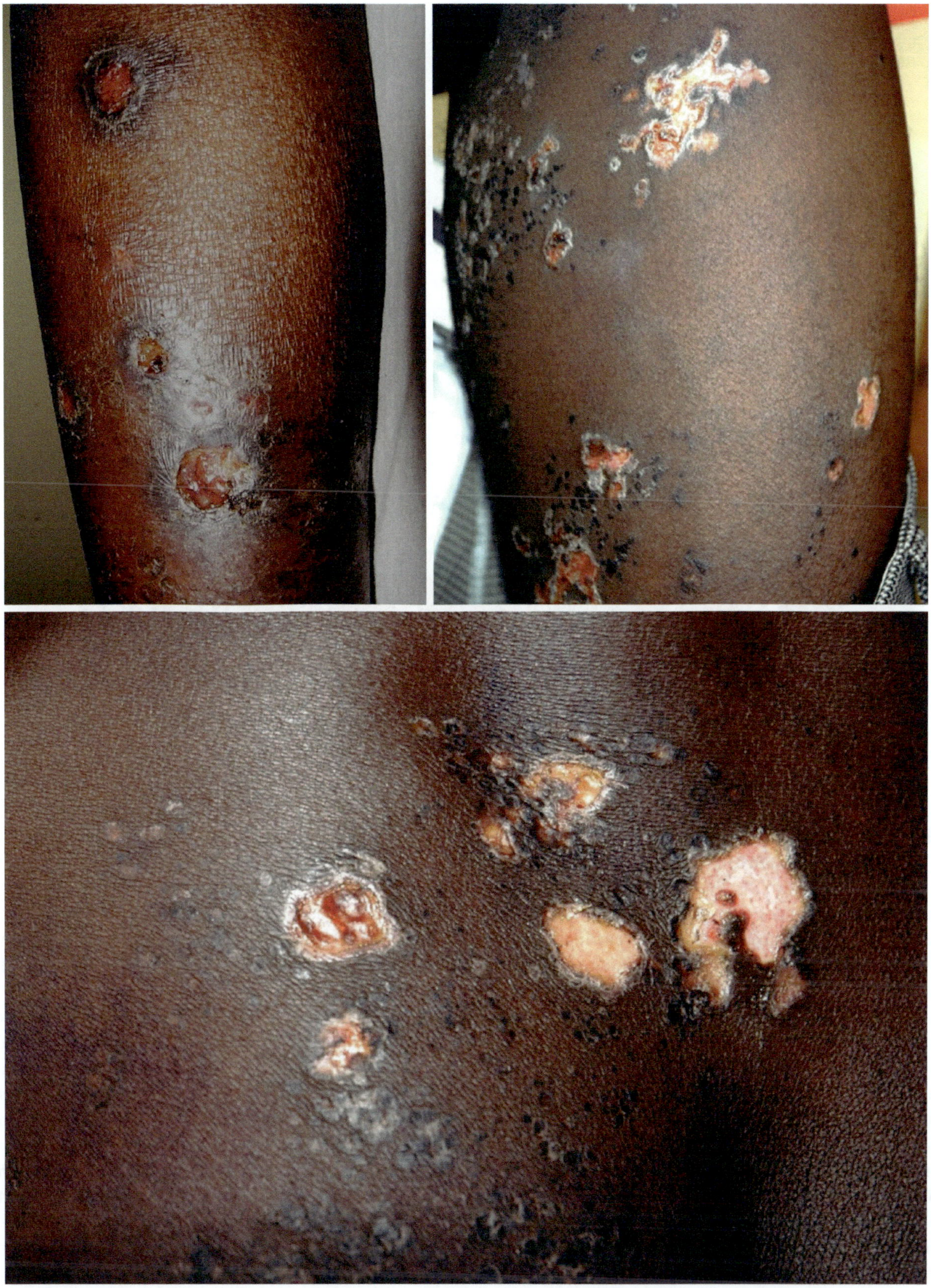

Fig. 22.3 Ulceronecrotic course of PLEVA, *Mucha-Habermann*'s disease in two African males

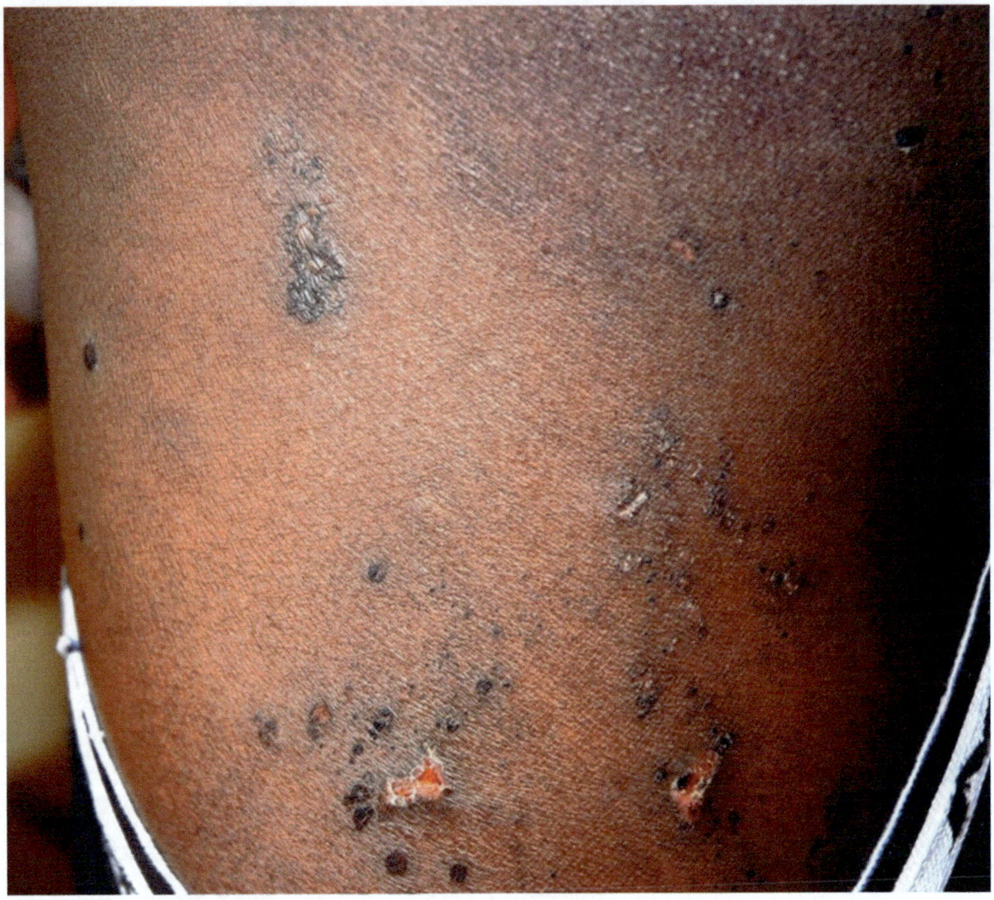

Fig. 22.4 Necrotizing vasculitis in an African male (Uganda), probably drug induced. DD: *Mucha-Habermann*'s disease

22.3 Parapsoriasis en Plaques (Syn.: Brocq's Disease)

Parapsoriasis en plaques (PP) is an erythemato-squamous disease with chronic course, commonly occurring in all geographic areas and ethnic groups. Middle-aged males are preferably affected, showing pruritic patches mostly on the trunk and upper extremities. PP is difficult to differentiate from early stages of mycosis fungoides, and data on its prevalence are striking sparse or not available.

Clinically, plaque parapsoriasis usually starts discreetly; the slightly erythematous lesions become gradually more visible and the itching more intense; infiltrated plaques are gradually manifested during the course of years. Cases of PP with 2–5 cm small lesions, occasionally linearly oriented along the skin lines (digitate dermatosis), and others with large lesions (10–15 cm) with similar morphology are seen. In African patients with dark pigmented skin, there is no erythema visible in PP; the lesions are hyperpigmented and not well demarcated; there is mild scaling, if untreated (Fig. 22.5). Facial lesions and epiphenomena due to scratching are seen. There is some controversy concerning the nature of the disease; some believe that particularly large plaque parapsoriasis should be classified as an early lymphoma; however, the evidence is rather poor. Undoubtedly, plaque parapsoriasis has a prolonged course, with around 15–30% of the cases progressing into mycosis fungoides/cutaneous T-cell lymphoma after a period of several years.

The early stage of CTCL cannot be differentiated from PP by clinical features, histopathologic characteristics, or immunophenotype [20]. It seems that both the small and the large plaque clinical variants have the potential to progress to cancer [21], even if the large plaque variant may do so more frequently or rapidly (6 toward 10 years in median). However, since there is no reliable prognostic marker to adapt to a given case, the individual outcome remains unpredictable.

22.3.1 Management

The management of plaque parapsoriasis requires a long-term strategy; the choice of treatment depends on the prog-

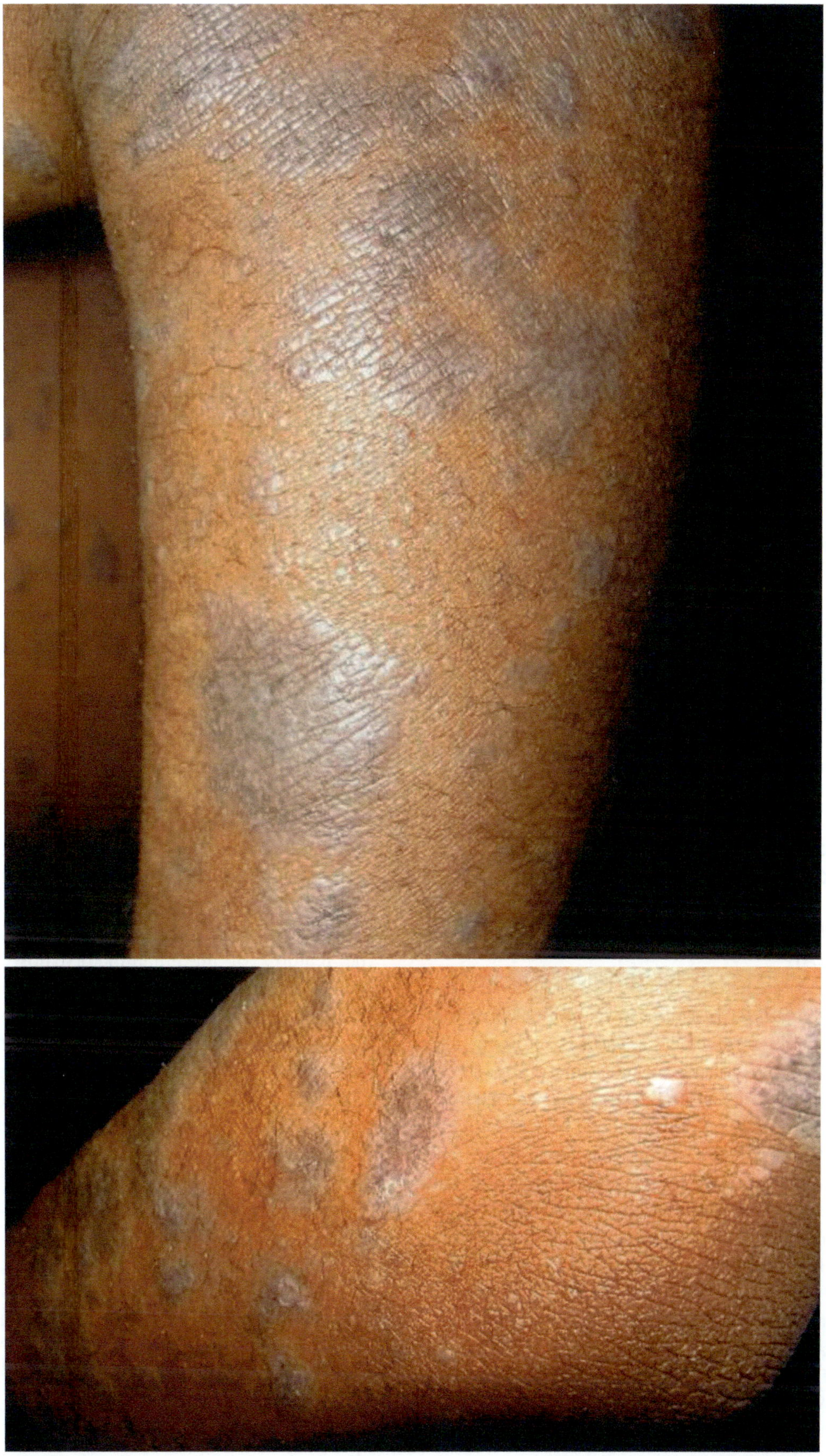

Fig. 22.5 *Plaque parapsoriasis* in an African male (Tanzania), slightly pruritic, after topical treatment with corticosteroids. DD: Early, plaque stage *mycosis fungoides*

Table 22.1 Clinical variables in the parapsoriasis group, characteristics, and recommendations for management

Clinical	Clinical course	Histology	Clonality	Progression to CTCL	Management
Pityriasis Lichenoides chronica (PLC)	Chronic, asymptomatic	Dermal inflammation (lymphocytic)	Polyclonal	Rarely seen	Mild emollients + antibiotics, nb-UVB[a]
Pityriasis Lichenoides et varioliformis acuta (PLEVA)	Chronic intermittent, remissions and relapses, asymptomatic	Vasculitis, often cellular atypicalities	Partly monoclonal	Possible	Calamine lotion, local antiseptics, antibiotics, nb-UVB[a], PUVA
Ulceronecrotic course (Mucha-Habermann)	Severe constitutional symptoms	Necrotizing vasculitis	In general polyclonal	None described	Systemic corticosteroids, MTX, TNF-α inhibitors (?)
Plaque parapsoriasis (PP)	Chronic progressive, pruritus	Dense epidermotropic cell infiltrate	Progressively monoclonal, CD4+, CD30+	15–30%	Mild emollients, PUVA, acitretin + PUVA
Parapsoriasis lichenoides (variegata, PV)	Chronic progressive	Not well studied	Not well studied	>30%	PUVA, acitretin + PUVA, MTX?

[a]Narrowband UVB

nostic assessment of the attending physician and varies considerably. Since the majority of patients are not likely to develop cancer, a sequential therapeutic schedule appears preferable to recommend. Local treatment with mild emollients and phototherapy with narrowband UVB or PUVA are helpful to induce remissions; addition of acitretin (0.3–0.5 mg/kg/day) may be considered (RePUVA). Local monitoring, staging, and control biopsies will be necessary to exclude progression to CTCL every year. The benefits of phototherapy are likely to remain equivocal in PP as far as progression to cancer is concerned [21]. Early aggressive treatment is not recommended.

22.4 Parapsoriasis Lichenoides (Syn.: Parapsoriasis Variegata, Parakeratosis Variegata, Poikiloderma Vasculare Atrophicans (Jacobi))

Parapsoriasis lichenoides is a rare, in its clinical presentation, highly variable form of parapsoriasis showing erythematous, only mildly pruritic macules intermingled with atrophic dyspigmented areas and telangiectasias. There is chronic course with male predominance. The variability of the clinical picture may be a source for controversies and lead to diagnostic misinterpretations. The prognostic outcome is not well studied; there are, however, observations on patients who developed lymph node enlargement and cutaneous T-cell lymphoma in a few years. Based on clinical experience, there is an overall agreement that the disease most likely represents a prelymphoma or even the first stage of poikilodermatous mycosis fungoides, with predominance of a CD8+ and CD4− T cells [22]; in other studies a predominant CD8+ CD56+ immunophenotype has been detected [23].

22.4.1 Management

The foremost therapeutic approach for this unusual phenotype of parapsoriasis/prelymphoma is early administration of phototherapy (PUVA), preferably in combination with an oral retinoid, acitretin, or isotretinoin (RePUVA). The prognostic outcome is generally good, in contrast to other cytotoxic MF variants with a CD 56+ immunophenotype known to pursue an aggressive course [24] (Table 22.1).

Conclusions

The group of parapsoriasis includes a series of rare entities with chronic course that occur in all geographic and climatic areas without ethnic preference. They have been described since long under varying designations, and their final classification is still open and debatable. The early stages are clinically discrete and often asymptomatic, difficult to recognize in pigmented skin, combining the features of an inflammatory host response to an unknown agent with a lymphoproliferative response in tissue, having the potential to progress into cutaneous T-cell lymphoma. The individual risk is unpredictable; overlapping clinical pictures and courses pose a challenge to the attending physician. Since most entities preferably affect children and younger adults, patients with parapsoriasis require long-term careful monitoring and supportive medical care.

References

1. Lindahl LM, Fenger-Grøn M, Iversen L. Subsequent cancers, mortality, and causes of death in patients with mycosis fungoides and parapsoriasis: a Danish nationwide, population-based cohort study. J Am Acad Dermatol. 2014;71:529–35.
2. Weinberg JM, Kristal L, Chooback L, et al. The clonal nature of pityriasis lichenoides. Arch Dermatol. 2002;138:1063–7.

3. Lane TN, Parker SS. Pityriasis lichenoides chronica in black patients. Cutis. 2010;85:125–9.
4. Maranda EL, Smith M, Nguyen AH, et al. Phototherapy for pityriasis lichenoides in the pediatric population: a review of the published literature. Am J Clin Dermatol. 2016;17:583–91.
5. Fernández-Guarino M, Aboin-Gonzalez S, Ciudad Blanco C, et al. Treatment of adult diffuse pityriasis lichenoides chronica with narrowband ultraviolet B: experience and literature review. Clin Exp Dermatol. 2017;42:303–5.
6. Koh WL, Koh MJ, Tay YK. Pityriasis lichenoides in an Asian population. Int J Dermatol. 2013;52:1495–9.
7. Ankad BS, Beergouder SL. Pityriasis lichenoides et varioliformis acuta in skin of color: new observations by dermoscopy. Dermatol Pract Concept. 2017;7:27–34.
8. English JC, Collins M, Bryant-Bruce C. Pityriasis lichenoides varioliformis acuta and group-a beta hemolytic streptococcal infection. Int J Dermatol. 1995;34:642–4.
9. Edwards BL, Bonagura VR, Valacer DJ, et al. Mucha Habermann's disease and arthritis: possible association with reactivated Epstein-Barr virus infection. J Rheumatol. 1989;16:387–9.
10. Nanda A, Alshalfan F, Al-Otaibi M, et al. Febrile ulceronecrotic Mucha-Habermann disease (pityriasis lichenoides et varioliformis acuta fulminans) associated with parvovirus infection. Am J Dermatopathol. 2013;35:503–6.
11. Fölster-Holst R, Zawar VP, Chuh A. Paraviral exanthems. Expert Rev Anti-Infect Ther. 2016;14:601–11.
12. Khachemoune A, Blyumin ML. Pityriasis lichenoides: pathophysiology, classification, and treatment. Am J Clin Dermatol. 2007;8:29–36.
13. Romaní J, Puig L, Fernández-Figueras MT, et al. Pityriasis lichenoides in children: clinicopathologic review of 22 patients. Pediatr Dermatol. 1998;15:1–6.
14. Yang CC, Lee JY, Chen W. Febrile ulceronecrotic Mucha-Habermann disease with extensive skin necrosis in intertriginous areas. Eur J Dermatol. 2003;13:493–6.
15. Sotiriou E, Patsatsi A, Tsorova C, et al. Febrile ulceronecrotic Mucha-Habermann disease: a case report and review of the literature. Acta Derm Venereol. 2008;88:350–5.
16. Suárez J, López B, Villalba R, et al. Febrile ulceronecrotic Mucha-Habermann disease: a case report and review of the literature. Dermatology. 1996;192:277–9.
17. Griffith-Bauer K, Leitenberger SL, Krol A. Febrile ulceronecrotic Mucha-Habermann disease: two cases with excellent response to methotrexate. Pediatr Dermatol. 2015;32:e307–8.
18. Meziane L, Caudron A, Dhaille F, et al. Febrile ulceronecrotic Mucha-Habermann disease: treatment with infliximab and intravenous immunoglobulins and review of the literature. Dermatology. 2012;225:344–8.
19. Kreuter A, Knispel S, Wieland U, et al. Complete resolution of febrile ulceronecrotic Mucha-Habermann disease following infliximab therapy. J Dtsch Dermatol Ges. 2016;14:184–6.
20. Kikuchi A, Naka W, Harada T, et al. Parapsoriasis en plaques: its potential for progression to malignant lymphoma. J Am Acad Dermatol. 1993;29:419–22.
21. Väkevä L, Sarna S, Vaalasti A, et al. A retrospective study of the probability of the evolution of parapsoriasis en plaques into mycosis fungoides. Acta Derm Venereol. 2005;85:318–23.
22. Bloom B, Marchbein S, Fischer M, et al. Poikilodermatous mycosis fungoides. Dermatol Online J. 2012;18(12):4.
23. Shiomi T, Monobe Y, Kuwabara C, et al. Poikilodermatous mycosis fungoides with a CD8+ CD56+ immunophenotype: a case report and literature review. J Cutan Pathol. 2013;40:317–20.
24. Wain EM, Orchard GE, Mayou S, et al. Mycosis fungoides with a CD56+ immunophenotype. J Am Acad Dermatol. 2005;53:158–63.

23 Lichen Planus and Lichenoid Disorders

Mohamed Badawy Abdel-Naser

Lichen is a rather common chronic inflammatory, immune-mediated disease which affects the skin and the mucous membranes; it occurs in Caucasian and in pigmented skin populations without ethnic predilection. The clinical manifestations represent a non-specific mucocutaneous reactive pattern, precipitating after diverse irritating factors and environmental conditions. It seems that individuals with heavily pigmented or black skin are predisposed to develop a lichenoid response after chronic irritation.

Several phenotypes of lichen occur; furthermore, there are several lichenoid dermatoses that clinically or histopathologically resemble lichen and represent a diagnostic challenge for the attending physician [1]. The reactive pattern of lichen may be also produced by a variety of drugs and chemicals in susceptible individuals. Cutaneous lichen often involves the extremities, characterized by flat polygonal papules and plaques and intense pruritus. Lesions of the oral mucosa can be the sole clinical presentation or be accompanied by cutaneous and/or other mucosal manifestations in the genital area and the eyes. Systemic mucosal involvement is rare.

23.1 Lichen Planus

23.1.1 Epidemiology

The prevalence of lichen planus varies in the range of 0.22–5% worldwide, with slight female predominance [1, 2]. Among dark-skinned individuals, the hypertrophic, actinic, and pigmented variants are more prevalent, and more children are involved in African-Americans [3, 4]. In addition, postinflammatory hyper- or hypopigmentation is a characteristic outcome of cutaneous lesions in dark-skinned populations. In African countries hepatitis C virus infection is more prevalent among patients with lichen planus, particularly in those with the erosive mucous membrane type [5].

23.1.2 Clinical Picture

Lichen planus is characterized by flat-topped polygonal papules often showing fine, whitish points or lacy lines on their surface, the Wickham striae. They are often symmetrically arranged on the extremities, affecting the distal volar aspects (Fig. 23.1a, b). If localized on the trunk, the lesions may follow the lines of Blaschko in a dermatomal zosteriform pattern or be linearly arranged along the lines of local friction as a Koebner phenomenon. The palms and the soles may be also involved showing symmetrical scaly lesions and, less frequently, hyperkeratotic plaques with prominent pruritus [6]. In some patients hyperkeratotic plaques with follicular accentuation predominate, corresponding to *lichen hypertrophicus*.

In hot climate zones, *lichen actinicus* (tropicalis) occurs frequently in sun-exposed areas, presenting nummular patches and plaques (Fig. 23.2), occasionally surrounded by hypopigmented halo. *Lichen annularis* is an uncommon asymptomatic form that classically involves the male genitalia and to a lesser extent the axilla, the groin, and the extremities. *Lichen pigmentosus* is a particular entity involving sun-exposed areas often seen on the face or the neck (Fig. 23.3), causing facial hyperpigmentation (see also Chap. 26). In biopsies hyperkeratosis, hypergranulosis, saw-toothed acanthosis, liquefaction degeneration of basal keratinocytes, and a band-like mononuclear dermal infiltrate of T lymphocytes at the dermoepidermal interface are characteristic features; melanin incontinence may occur.

The mucous membranes, especially the buccal mucosa, are frequently affected alone or together with cutaneous lesions (70%), being reticulate, atrophic, or erosive (ulcerative). Similar lesions may occur on the palate, the tongue, and the lips simulating leukoplakia (Fig. 23.4), sometimes caused by irritancy or contact allergy to dental metals [7]. The vulvovaginal area is also commonly affected, labia and anus;

M. B. Abdel-Naser
Department of Dermatology and Venereology, Ain Shams University, Cairo, Egypt

C. E. Orfanos et al. (eds.), *Pigmented Ethnic Skin and Imported Dermatoses*, https://doi.org/10.1007/978-3-319-69422-1_23

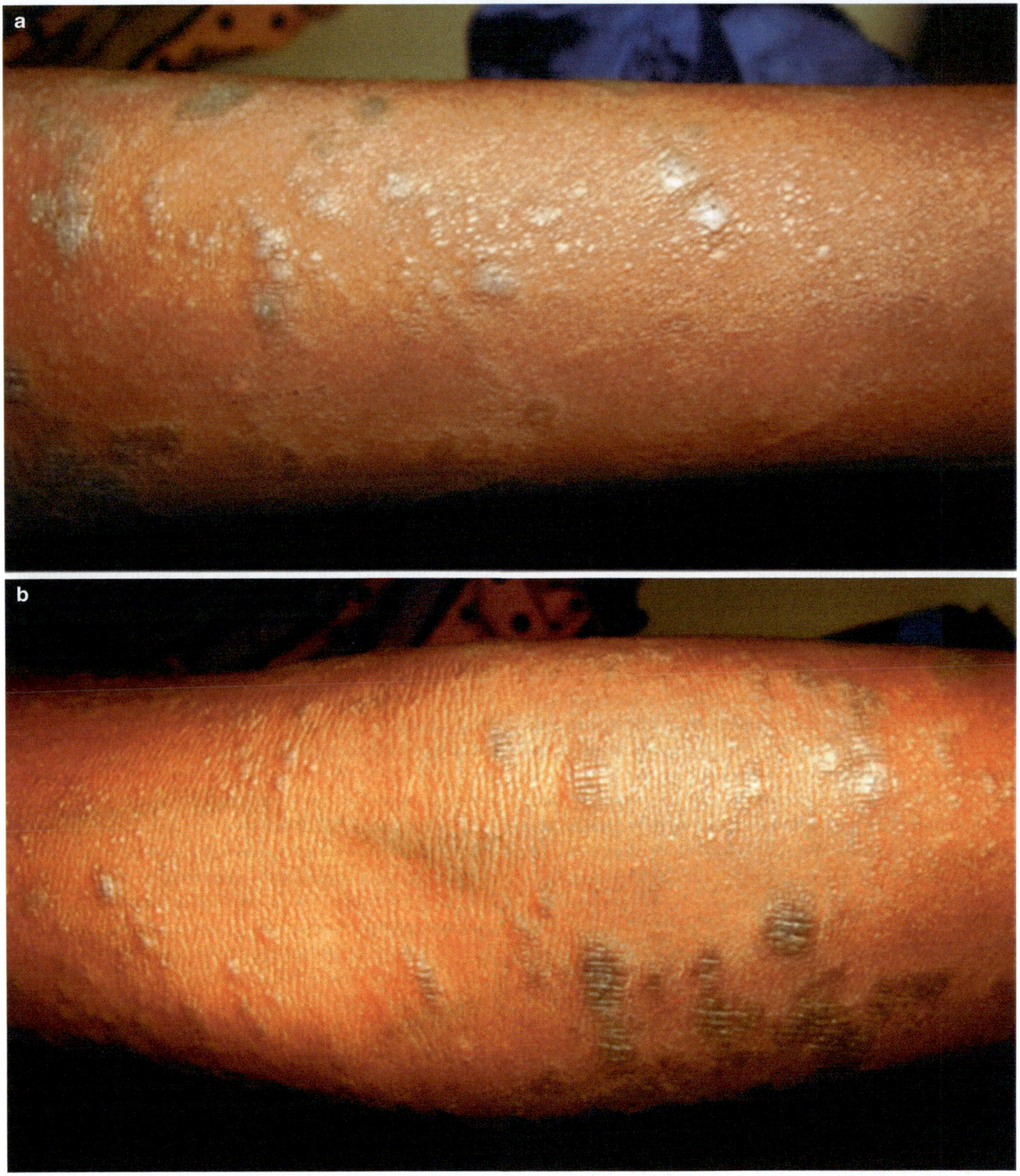

Fig. 23.1 (**a**, **b**) *Lichen planus*. Characteristic involvement of the extremities; some lesions are hyperpigmented due to melanin incontinence

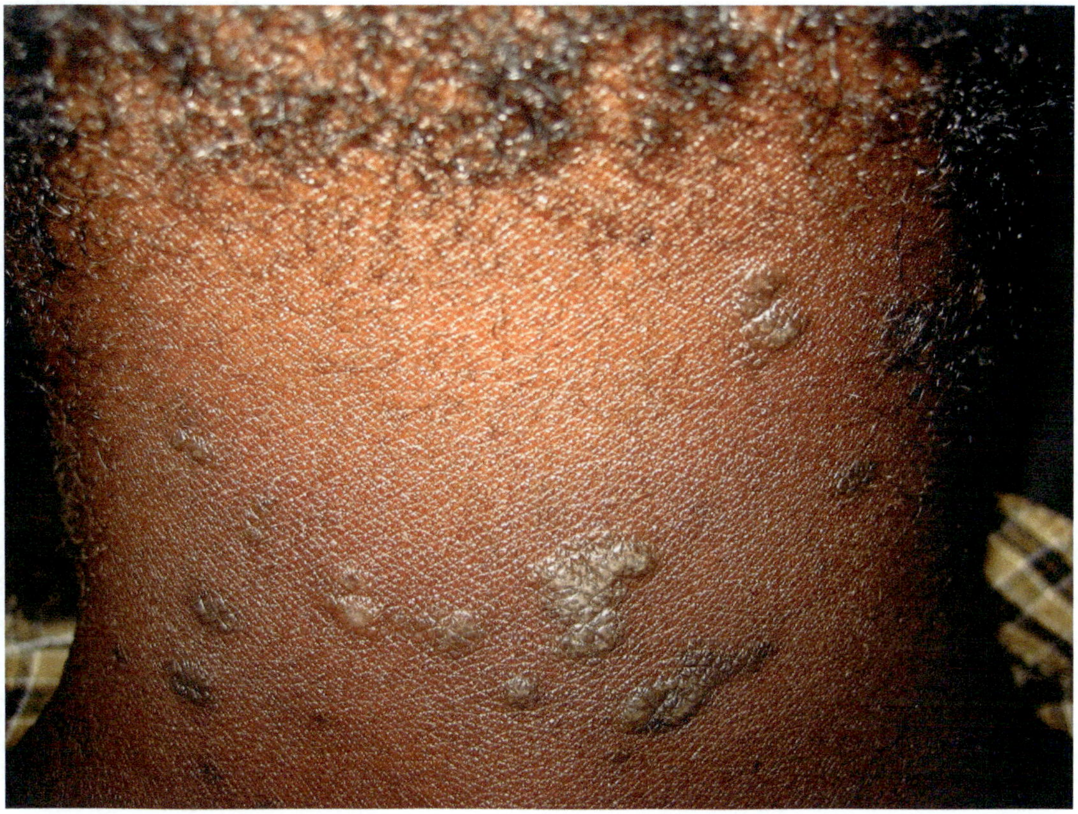

Fig. 23.2 *Lichen planus actinicus* (tropicalis) in sun-exposed area of the neck of a young Tanzanian male

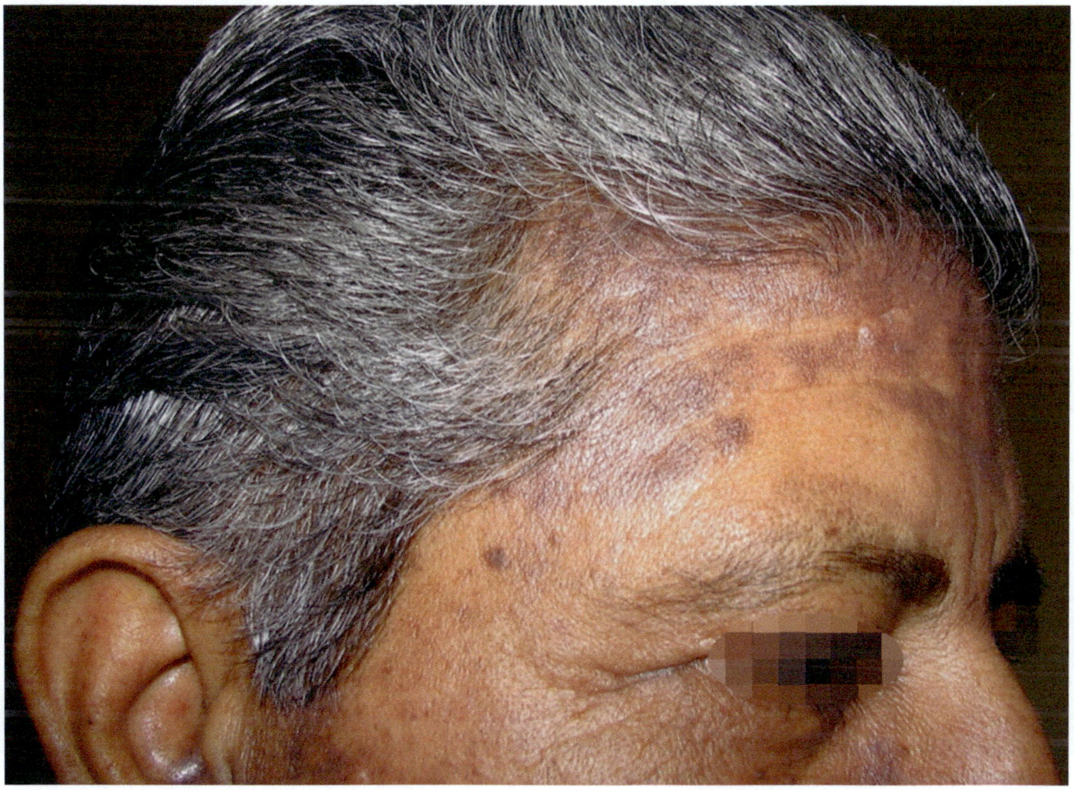

Fig. 23.3 *Lichen planus pigmentosus* on the face of an Egyptian male

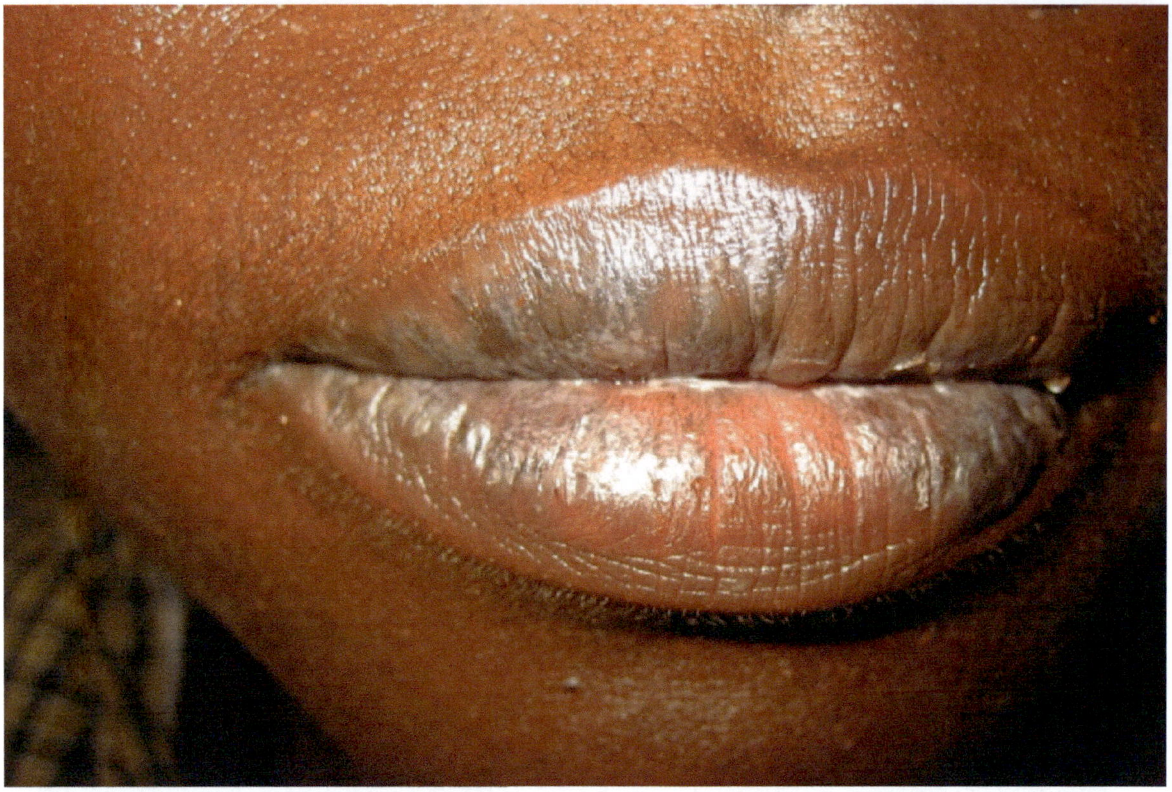

Fig. 23.4 *Lichen planus of the lip mucosa* mimicking leukoplakia

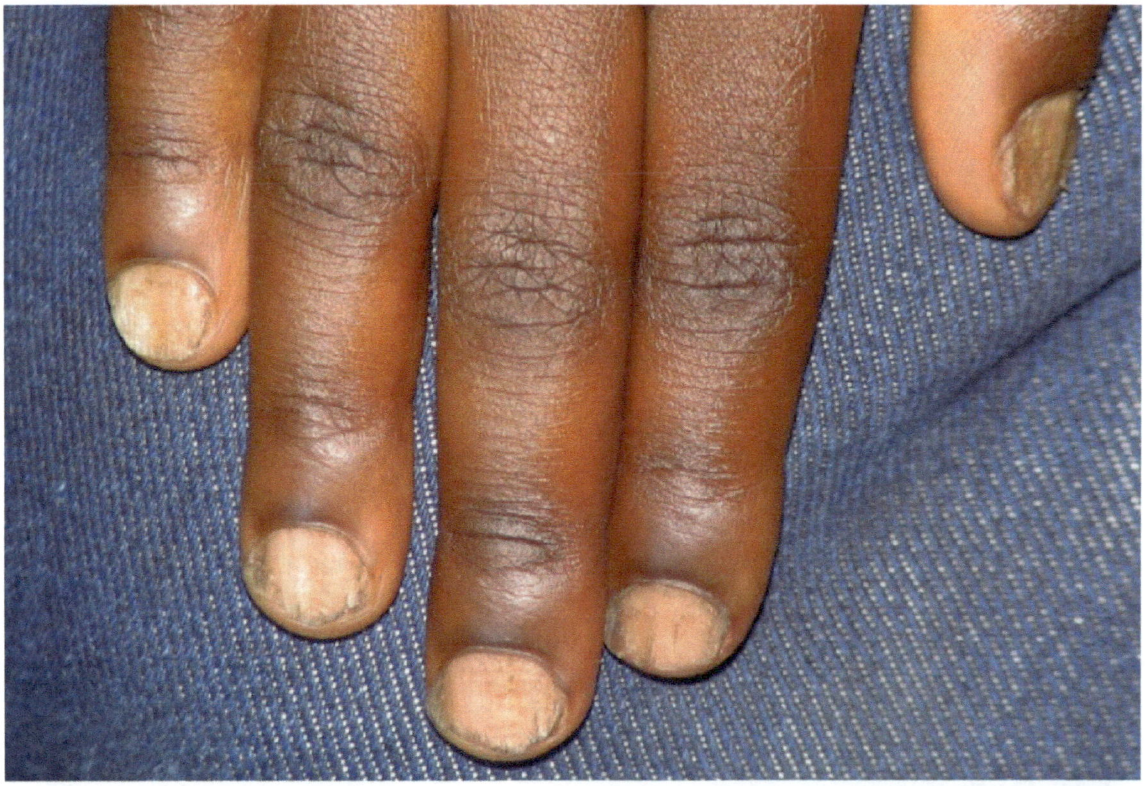

Fig. 23.5 Longitudinal fissuring and ridging of the nail plates in lichen planus; thickening above the proximal nail rim is visible, indicating involvement of the nail matrix

laryngeal, esophageal, and conjunctival involvement is rare [8]. Although there is no increased risk of malignancy in cutaneous lichen, 1–2% of the cases with oral involvement, particularly the erosive type, develop squamous cell carcinoma [9]. Lichenoid mucositis has been attributed to dental fillings, and patch testing may be indicated to identify the culprit.

Affection of the nails occurs in up to 10% of the cases in adults and may reach 19% in children [4, 10]. Fingernails are more commonly involved showing longitudinal fissuring and ridging of the nail plate (Fig. 23.5), occasionally resulting in destruction of the nail bed, onychorrhexis, and onycholysis. On the feet, erosions and ulcerations may occur, resulting in atrophic scarring and permanent loss of the toenails. Nail involvement is usually associated with cutaneous and oral lesions. *Twenty-nail dystrophy* is characterized by nail coarseness (*trachyonychia*) affecting all nails, as observed also in alopecia areata, psoriasis, and pemphigus vulgaris. Remarkable thickening may be noted mimicking *yellow nail syndrome*. Furthermore, erosive nail involvement rarely occurs with painful erosions and consequent scarring. In another rare variant, idiopathic atrophy of the nails can cause rapid diffuse nail atrophy and ultimately leads to permanent anonychia [10].

23.1.3 Management

Cutaneous lichen planus often resolves spontaneously within 1–2 years; mucosal lesions may be more resistant to therapeutic schedules and persist. Standard therapies include antihistaminics such as hydroxyzine to control pruritus, together with topical corticosteroid creams. Sprays or pellets of corticosteroids and triamcinolone as a gel are helpful for oral lesions; elixirs with diphenhydramine or tetracycline (3%) mouthwash should be held in the mouth for 10 min 3×/day. Intralesional corticosteroids are helpful in the management of hypertrophic and small localized persistent mucosal lesions [11], and likewise in hypertrophic skin lesions and lichen planus of the nails. Topical tacrolimus (0.1% ointment) and pimecrolimus (1% cream) were effective in mucosal involvement including oral lichenoid lesions in graft-versus-host disease (GVHD). Aloe vera gel was found safe and effective for patients with vulvar lichen [12]. For patients with severe acute involvement, 20 mg/day prednisolone is given orally, gradually tapering the dose over 3–6 weeks. Phototherapies with UVA1, narrowband UVB, and PUVA are also beneficial. Recalcitrant cases respond well to extracorporeal photopheresis [13].

For controlling the pruritic lesions, oral sulfasalazine may be administered in increasing dose 1.5–3 g/day for at least 4 weeks. As an alternative to systemic corticosteroids, acitretin was found effective at a dose of 30–50 mg/day for 8 weeks [14]. Mycophenolate mofetil has been successfully used for treatment of disseminated, erosive, hypertrophic, and bullous variants and may be preferred to other immune suppressants due to its safer side effect profile. Biologicals such as alefacept and efalizumab were found beneficial in a few severe cases with erosive mucosal involvement.

23.2 Other Lichen Variants

The Koebner phenomenon is an indicator for the susceptibility of the skin to develop a lichenoid reaction (Fig. 23.6). Secondary lichenification of contact eczema or atopic dermatitis is frequently seen after long-term duration (Fig. 23.7).

Lichen simplex chronicus Vidal is characterized by well-circumscribed, lichenified, and pruritic patches developing on any part of the body following chronic irritation (Fig. 23.8). The condition occurs preferably in adult females with no racial predilection, but is more commonly seen and prominent among individuals with pigmented and black skin. Preferred sites are the neck, the genital area, and the distal extremities. Persistent rubbing of the shins or upper back may result in dermal deposits of amyloid and development of macular or *lichen amyloidosus* [15]. Sites of atopic dermatitis, irritant or allergic contact dermatitis, insect bites, or other minor skin traumas are particularly prone to develop lichen simplex chronicus. Increased prevalence in patients with underlying anxiety and obsessive-compulsive disorders has been reported [16]. For treatment, potent topical corticosteroids are used under occlusion; for sensitive skin areas, topical tacrolimus and pimecrolimus are recommended. Avoidance of scratching is mandatory; topical application of aspirin/dichloromethane solution has an antipruritic effect [17]. Oral antihistaminics such as hydroxyzine and antianxiety preparations such as doxepin may also be helpful in selected cases.

Lichen striatus is a fairly common, self-limited pruritic linear eruption that primarily affects children and females. The condition starts as small erythematous papules forming a 1–3 cm-wide band that progress over a few weeks down the extremities or the trunk, often following the Blaschko lines [18]. Lesions involving the nail folds or nail matrix may result in onycholysis, splitting, and fraying, leading to total nail loss. The eruption usually appears suddenly and develops over days to weeks; however, it undergoes spontaneous resolution leaving postinflammatory hypopigmentations particularly in persons with darkly pigmented skin. Treatment is usually not needed, but mild topical corticosteroids under occlusion can be used to enhance spontaneous resolution.

Lichen nitidus is a chronic inflammatory condition, usually asymptomatic, characterized by minute, tiny flat-topped, pale uniform papules particularly conspicuous or prominent in dark-skinned populations (Fig. 23.9). Predilection sites include the lower abdomen, penis, and vulva, less commonly the inner surfaces of the thighs and the flexor aspects of wrists and forearms. Koebner phenomenon is often seen and nail affection may occur; as a rule, there is no mucosal involvement. A generalized form and hyperkeratotic variants have been described [19]. Actinic lichen nitidus has been reported

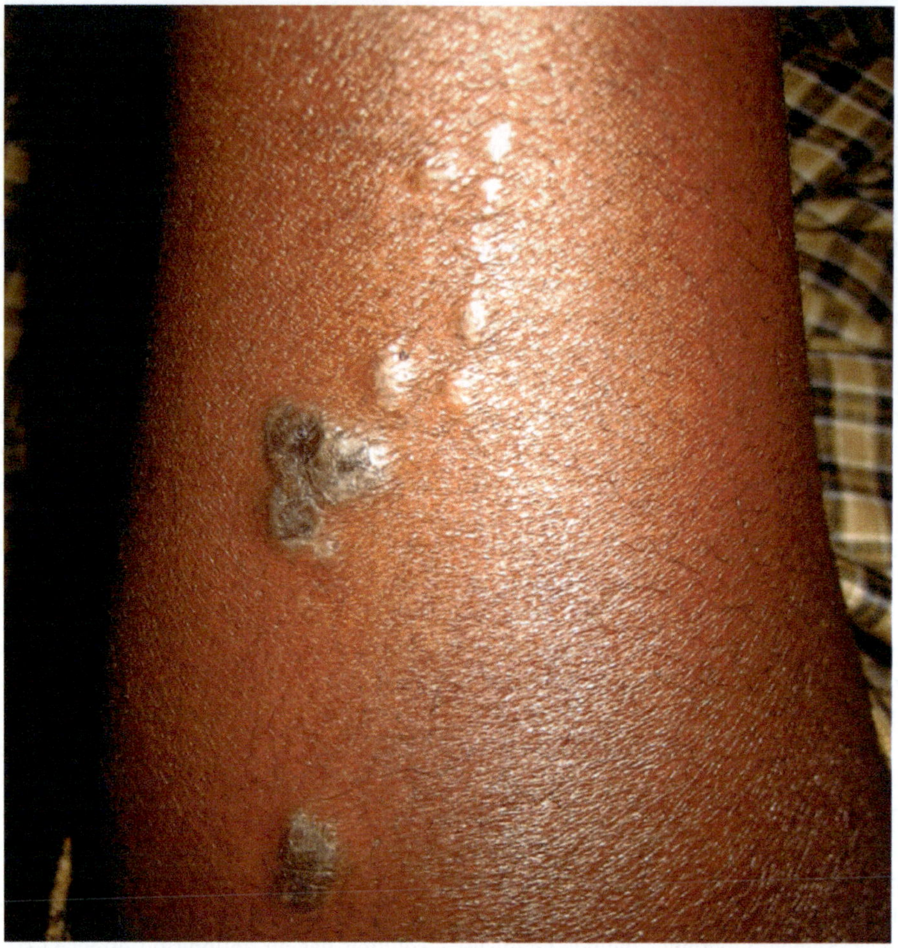

Fig. 23.6 *Koebner phenomenon* showing linearly arranged prominent lichen papules, partly hypertrophic

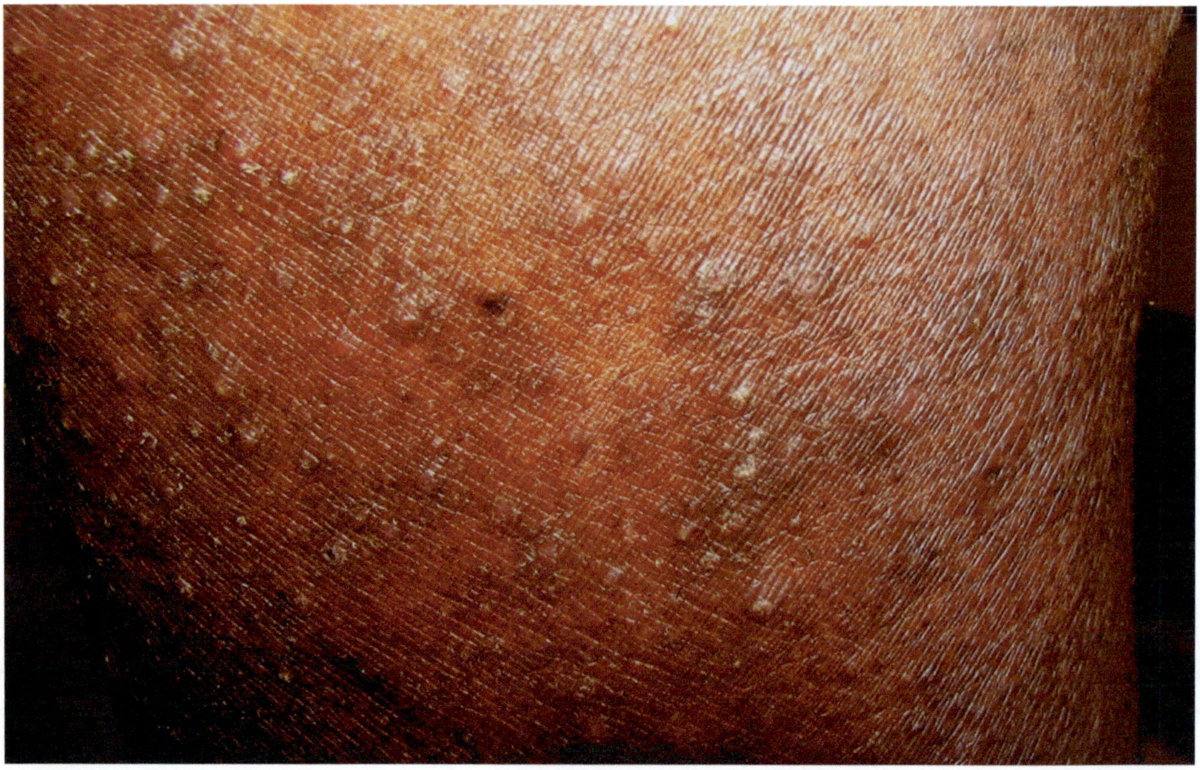

Fig. 23.7 *Lichenification of chronic eczema* showing a follicular pattern, characteristic in African skin

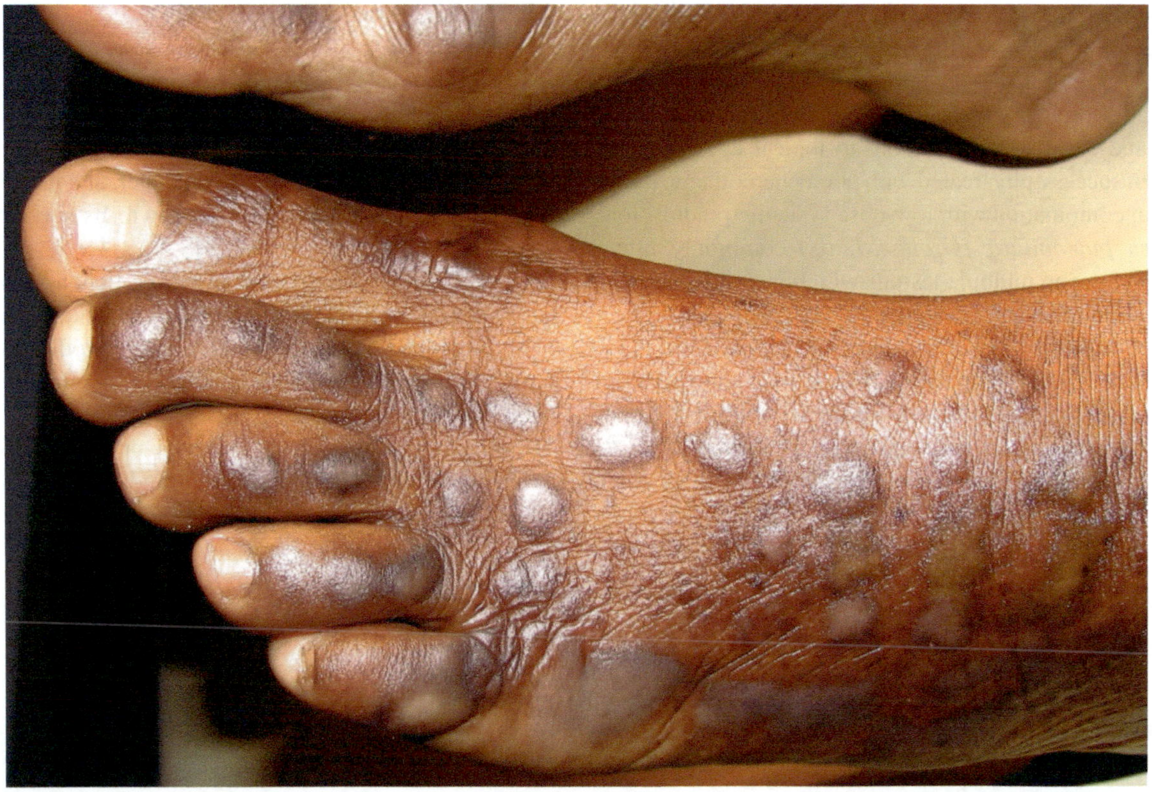

Fig. 23.8 *Lichen chronicus*, linearly arranged, on the feet of a young male, highly pruritic

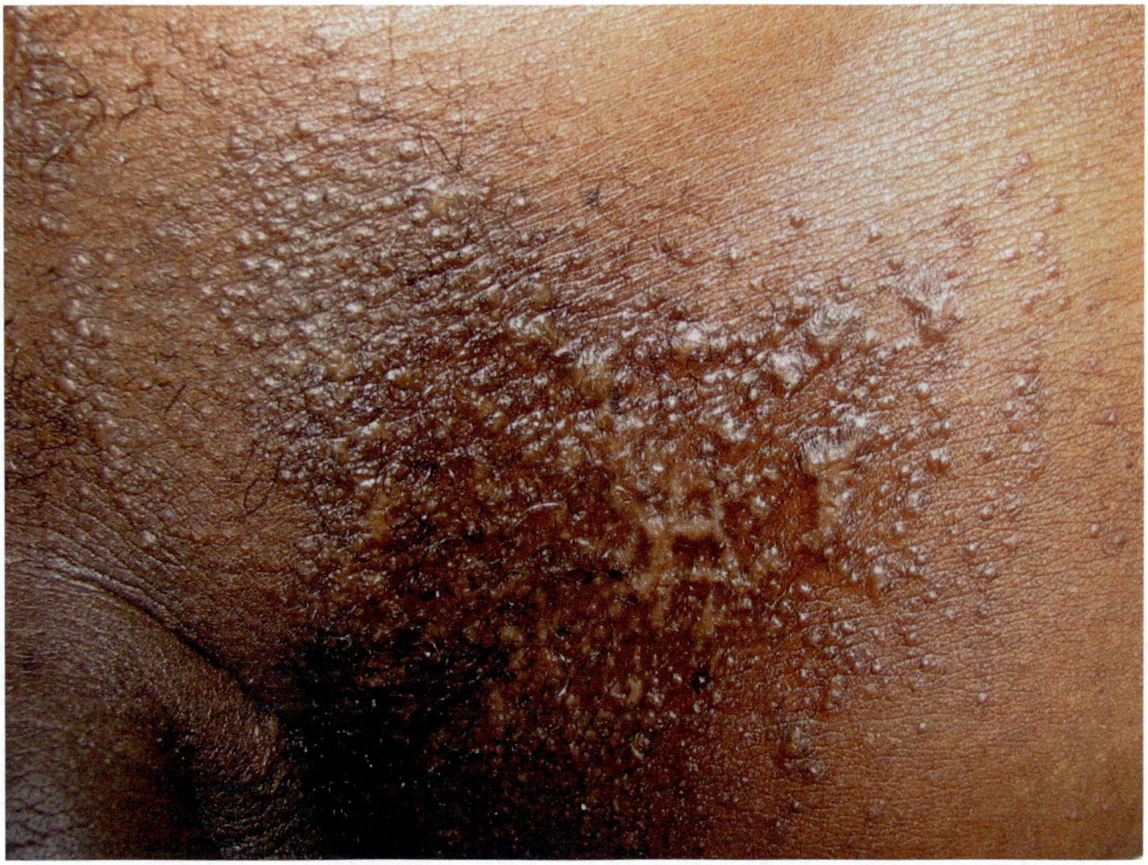

Fig. 23.9 *Lichen nitidus* in the genital area

in pigmented and black-skinned patients with lesions limited to sun-exposed areas and favorable response to sun protection. The condition is self-limited; topical tacrolimus was anecdotally proven effective in children. Widely spread lesions and cases non-responding to topical corticosteroids have been successfully treated with photochemotherapy alone [20] or in combination with low-dose systemic prednisolone.

Lichen planopilaris (Graham-Little) commonly affects the scalp showing multiple lesions with bilateral localization often leading to cicatricial alopecia (see Chap. 36).

Lichen-lupus erythematosus overlap syndrome refers to a heterogeneous group of patients with lesions showing clinically and histologically features characteristic for both dermatoses, indicating their coexistence. If localized on the scalp, scarring alopecia results [21]. Successful treatment with acitretin has been reported [22].

23.3 Lichenoid Disorders

Benign lichenoid keratosis is a common dermatosis consisting of a nonpruritic papule or slightly indurated plaque nearly always solitary on the trunk and the upper extremities. It usually measures 5–20 mm in diameter, and its color varies from bright red to violaceous to brown. Its surface may be smooth or slightly verrucous [23].

Lichenoid drug eruptions resemble lichen planus clinically, having macular and violaceous papular, often polygonal, pruritic lesions. They tend to be photodistributed and have confluent areas with a slightly eczematous nature (Fig. 23.10); there is less (if any) mucosal involvement. The eruption often appears weeks or months following exposure to the responsible agent and may take the same length of time to disappear following withdrawal of the

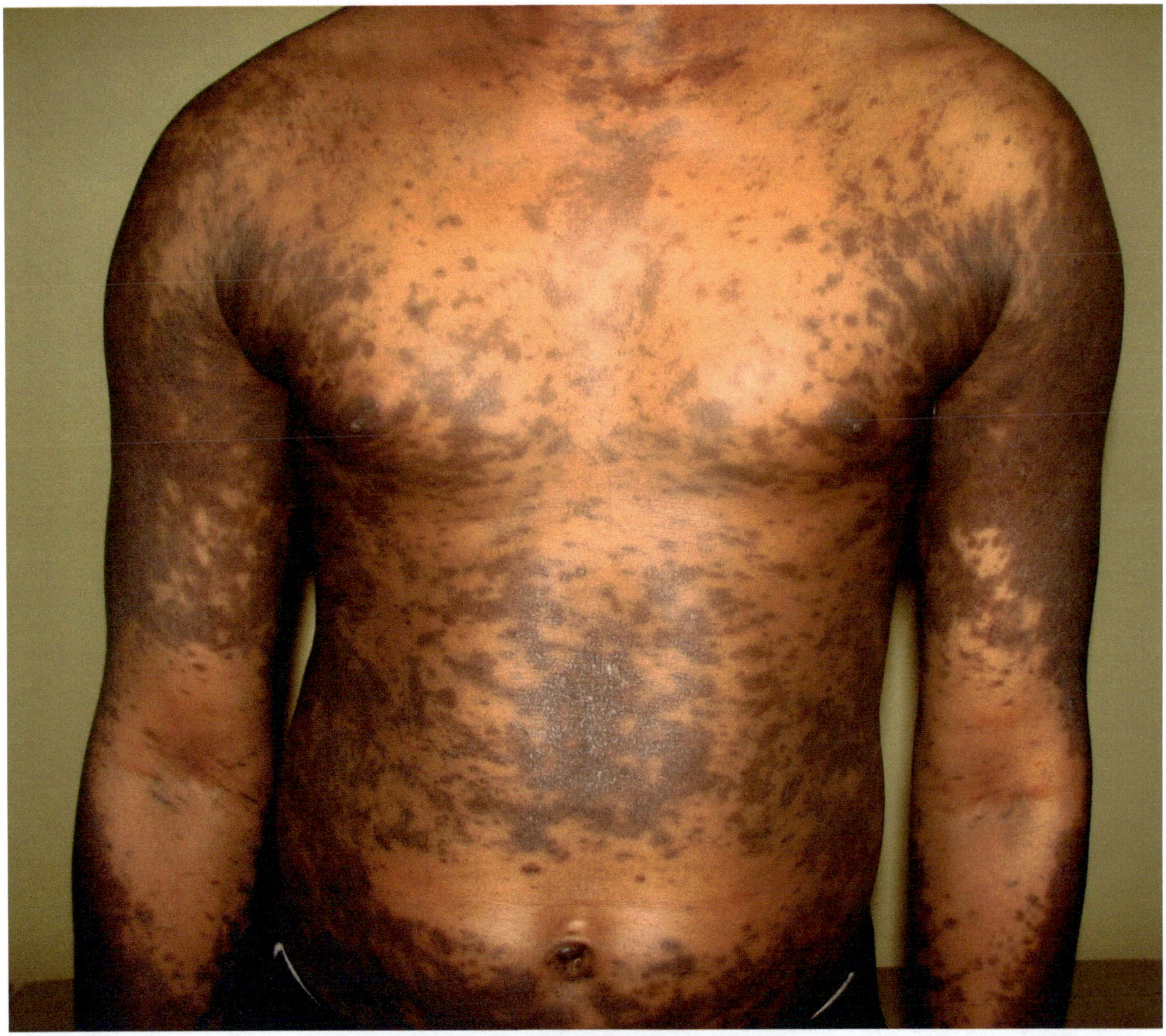

Fig. 23.10 *Lichenoid drug eruption* with confluent hyperpigmented macules after 2 months duration

drug. Lichenoid drug eruptions often leave postinflammatory hyperpigmentation, particularly in dark-complexioned individuals [24]. The most commonly implicated drugs are ACE inhibitors, thiazide diuretics, antimalarials, quinidine, beta-blockers, gold, penicillamine, and several others [25].

Graft-versus-host disease (GVHD) may be iatrogenic or rarely congenital in origin. The iatrogenic type usually follows bone marrow transplantation characterized by acute and chronic phases. In the chronic phase, an early lichenoid and a late sclerotic stage could be observed. The cutaneous and mucosal lesions of the early lichenoid stage resemble lichen planus not only clinically but also histologically; the skin may show extensive erythema and irregular hyperpigmentations. In the late stage, the skin becomes firm and inelastic with evident poikiloderma [26].

Chronic GVHD requires continued immunosuppressive management (1 mg/kg/day prednisolone) plus other immunosuppressive drugs such as ciclosporin A or mycophenolate mofetil. Extracorporeal photopheresis is effective in refractory chronic GVHD, whereas eczematoid GVHD responds well to PUVA [27, 28].

References

1. Le Cleach L, Chosidow O. Clinical practice. Lichen planus. N Engl J Med. 2012;366:723–32.
2. Gorouhi F, Davari P, Fazel N: Cutaneous and mucosal lichen planus: a comprehensive review of clinical subtypes, risk factors, diagnosis, and prognosis. Sci World J. 2014; Article ID 742826.
3. Alabi GO, Akinsanya JB. Lichen Planus in tropical Africa. Trop Geogr Med. 1981;33:143–7.
4. Nnoruka EN. Lichen planus in African children: a study of 13 patients. Pediatr Dermatol. 2007;24:495–8.
5. Ukonu AB, Augustine U. The prevalence of hepatitis C Virus (HCV) among lichen planus patients and its clinical pattern at the University of Abuja Teaching Hospital, Gwagwalada, Abuja, Nigeria. Glob J Health Sci. 2012;4:113–9.
6. Sanchez-Perez J, Buceta LR, Fraga J, et al. Lichen planus with lesions on the palms and/or soles: prevalence and clinicopathological study of 36 patients. Br J Dermatol. 2000;142:310–4.
7. Athavale PN, Shum KW, Yeoman CM, et al. Oral lichenoid lesions and contact allergy to dental mercury and gold. Contact Dermatitis. 2003;49:264–5.
8. Eisen D. The evaluation of cutaneous, genital, scalp, nail, esophageal, and ocular involvement in patients with oral lichen planus. Oral Surg Oral Med Oral Pathol Oral Radiol Endod. 1999;88:431–6.
9. Gonzalez-Moles MA, Scully C, Gil-Montoya JA. Oral lichen planus: controversies surrounding malignant transformation. Oral Dis. 2008;14:229–43.
10. Tosti A, Piraccini BM, Cambiaghi S, et al. Nail Lichen planus. In: Color atlas of nails. Berlin: Springer; 2010.
11. Cribier B, Frances C, Chosidow O. Treatment of lichen planus. An evidence-based medicine analysis of efficacy. Arch Dermatol. 1998;134:1521–30.
12. Rajar UD, Majeed R, Parveen N, et al. Efficacy of aloe vera gel in the treatment of vulval lichen planus. J Coll Physicians Surg Pak. 2008;18:612–4.
13. Becherel PA, Bussel A, Chosidow O, et al. Extracorporeal photochemotherapy for chronic erosive lichen planus. Lancet. 1998;14:805.
14. Abdel-Naser MB, Soehnchen R, Gollnick H. Linear lichen planus. Successful treatment with retinoids. Report of two cases. Eur J Dermatol. 1994;4:443–6.
15. Weyers W, Weyers I, Bonczkowitz M, et al. Lichen amyloidosus: a consequence of scratching. J Am Acad Dermatol. 1997;37:923–8.
16. Liao YH, Lin CC, Tsai PP, et al. Increased risk of lichen simplex chronicus in people with anxiety disorder: a nationwide population-based retrospective cohort study. Br J Dermatol. 2014;170:890–4.
17. Yosipovitch G, Sugeng MW, Chan YH, et al. The effect of topically applied aspirin on localized circumscribed neurodermatitis. J Am Acad Dermatol. 2001;45:910–3.
18. Muller CSL, Schmaltz R, Vogt T, et al. Lichen striatus and blaschkitis: reappraisal of the concept of blaschko linear dermatoses. Br J Dermatol. 2011;164:257–62.
19. Chen W, Schramm M, Zouboulis CC. Generalized lichen nitidus. J Am Acad Dermatol. 1997;36:630–1.
20. Szponar A, Borzęcki A, Sajdak-Wojtaluk A, et al. Lichen nitidus of the upper and lower limbs successfully treated with narrow-band UVB11 and PUVA phototherapy. Borgis-Nowa Medycyna. 2010;2:48–51.
21. Inaloz HS, Chowdhury MMU, Motley RJ. Lupus erythematosus/Lichen planus overlap syndrome with scarring alopecia. J Eur Acad Dermatol Venereol. 2001;15:171–4.
22. Lospinoso DJ, Fernelius C, Edhegard KD, et al. Lupus erythematosus/lichen planus overlap syndrome: successful treatment with acitretin. Lupus. 2013;22:851–4.
23. Morgan M, Stevens G, Switlyk S. Benign lichenoid keratosis: a clinical and pathologic reappraisal of 1040 cases. Am J Dermatopathol. 2005;27:387–92.
24. Bleicher PA, Dover JS, Arndt KA. Lichenoid dermatoses and related disorders. I. Lichen planus and lichenoid drug-induced eruptions. J Am Acad Dermatol. 1990;22:288–92.
25. Halevy S, Shai A. Lichenoid drug eruptions. J Am Acad Dermatol. 1993;29:249–55.
26. Wu PA, Cowen EW. Cutaneous graft-versus-host disease–clinical considerations and management. Curr Probl Dermatol. 2012;43:101–15.
27. Flowers ME, Apperley JF, van Besien K, et al. A multicenter prospective phase 2 randomized study of extracorporeal photopheresis for treatment of chronic graft-versus-host disease. Blood. 2008;112:2667–74.
28. Creamer D, Martyn-Simmons CL, Osborne G, et al. Eczematoid graft-vs-host disease: a novel form of chronic cutaneous graft-vs-host disease and its response to psoralen UV-A therapy. Arch Dermatol. 2007;143:1157–62.

Urticaria and Angioedema in Skin of Color

24

Uwe Wollina, Shyam B. Verma, and Karalikkattil T. Ashique

Urticaria and angioedema are common multifactorial skin reactions. They occur worldwide with all age groups and classes of the population affected. The lifetime prevalence rate for all types of urticaria in Europe was found 8.8%; for chronic urticaria it has been estimated 1.8%, with a predominance of females [1, 2]. Exact data in skin of color are lacking. In Americans with Asian ancestry or Pacific Islanders, urticaria is among the five top dermatological diagnoses [3]. In elderly African-Americans, self-reported urticaria was noted in 4.9% [4]. A nationwide study from China analyzing chronic urticaria (n = 2710) showed that the most frequent was the idiopathic subtype (68.1%), followed by physical urticaria (29.3%). Females were more commonly affected than males [5].

The prevalence of food-dependent exercise-induced anaphylaxis (FDEIA) in Japan and Korea has been reported <0.02%. The triggering factor of the disease may be exercise-induced redistribution of blood from viscera to skeletal muscles and skin. Warm climate may be an additional factor [6]. The disease is characterized by anaphylaxis with urticaria after exercise preceded by food ingestion. As a cause, various foods had been identified including nuts and wheat. In the latter case, the ω-5 gliadin prick test may represent an important diagnostic tool [7]. Hereditary angioedema (HAE) type I is the most common phenotype in Japanese population (57.8%), followed by type II (5.3%) (Table 24.1). The remaining cases were unclassified HAE [8]. In Taiwan, about 58% of the cases with the HAE type I were clinically symptomatic.

African-Americans have a 4.5-fold increased risk to develop angiotensin inhibitor-associated angioedema compared to white-skinned Americans [9]. In a genome-wide association study, *rs989692* in the gene encoding neprilysin (MME), an enzyme which metabolizes bradykinin and substance P, was significantly associated with angioedema in African-Americans [10].

24.1 Clinical Picture

Lesions of physical urticaria are slightly elevated pruritic papules, often skin colored (Fig. 24.1). Acute urticarial rashes are characterized by temporary flares of strongly pruritic, erythematous papules and plaques widely distributed over the entire skin, often involving the adjacent mucosa (Figs. 24.2 and 24.3a, b). They are clinically presented in a large number of varying clinical entities (Table 24.2). The clinical symptomatology of urticaria is in most cases not life-threatening; however, the quality of health-related life of the affected patients is reduced, particularly in chronic subtypes which require a comprehensive diagnostic workup. Apart from pure physical symptoms, patients experience restrictions in daily life activities and social life, sleep disturbances

Table 24.1 Clinical types of hereditary angioedema

Type	Frequency (%)	Characteristics
I	85	Functional and antigenic C1-esterase inhibitor insufficiency
II	14	Normal or elevated C1-esterase inhibitor levels but lack of functional activity
III	<1	Normal C1-esterase inhibitor levels, factor XII mutation, primarily in females

U. Wollina (✉)
Department of Dermatology and Allergology, Hospital Dresden-Friedrichstadt, Teaching Hospital of the Technical University of Dresden, Dresden, Germany
e-mail: wollina-uw@khdf.de

S. B. Verma, MBBS, DVD, FAAD, FRCP
Nirvana Skin Clinic, Vadodara, Gujarat, India

K. T. Ashique, M.B.B.S., D.D.V.L.
Department of Dermatology, Kims Alshifa Hospital, Malappuram, Kerala, India

C. E. Orfanos et al. (eds.), *Pigmented Ethnic Skin and Imported Dermatoses*, https://doi.org/10.1007/978-3-319-69422-1_24

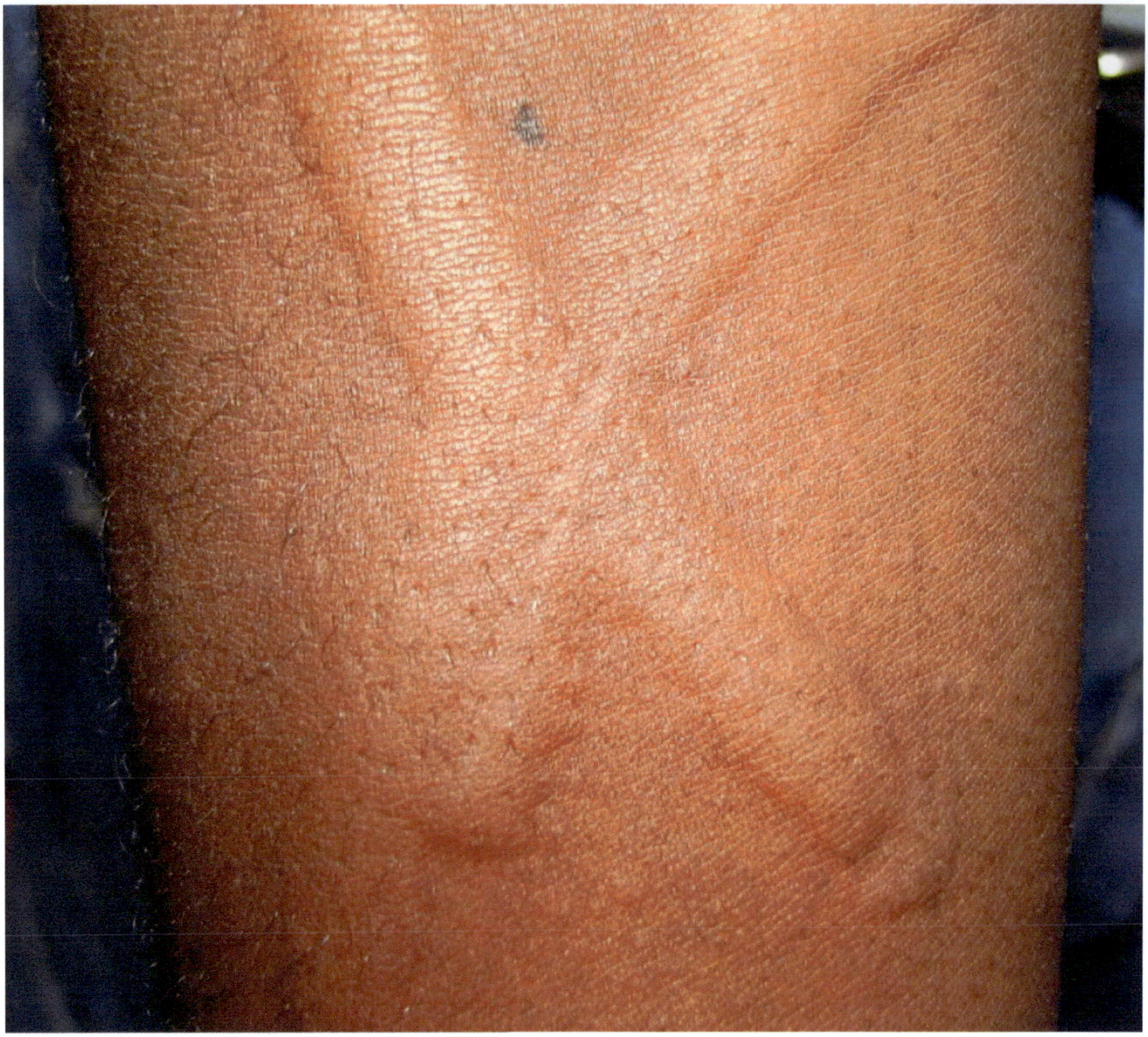

Fig. 24.1 *Urticarial dermographism* as a prototype of physical urticaria in skin of color

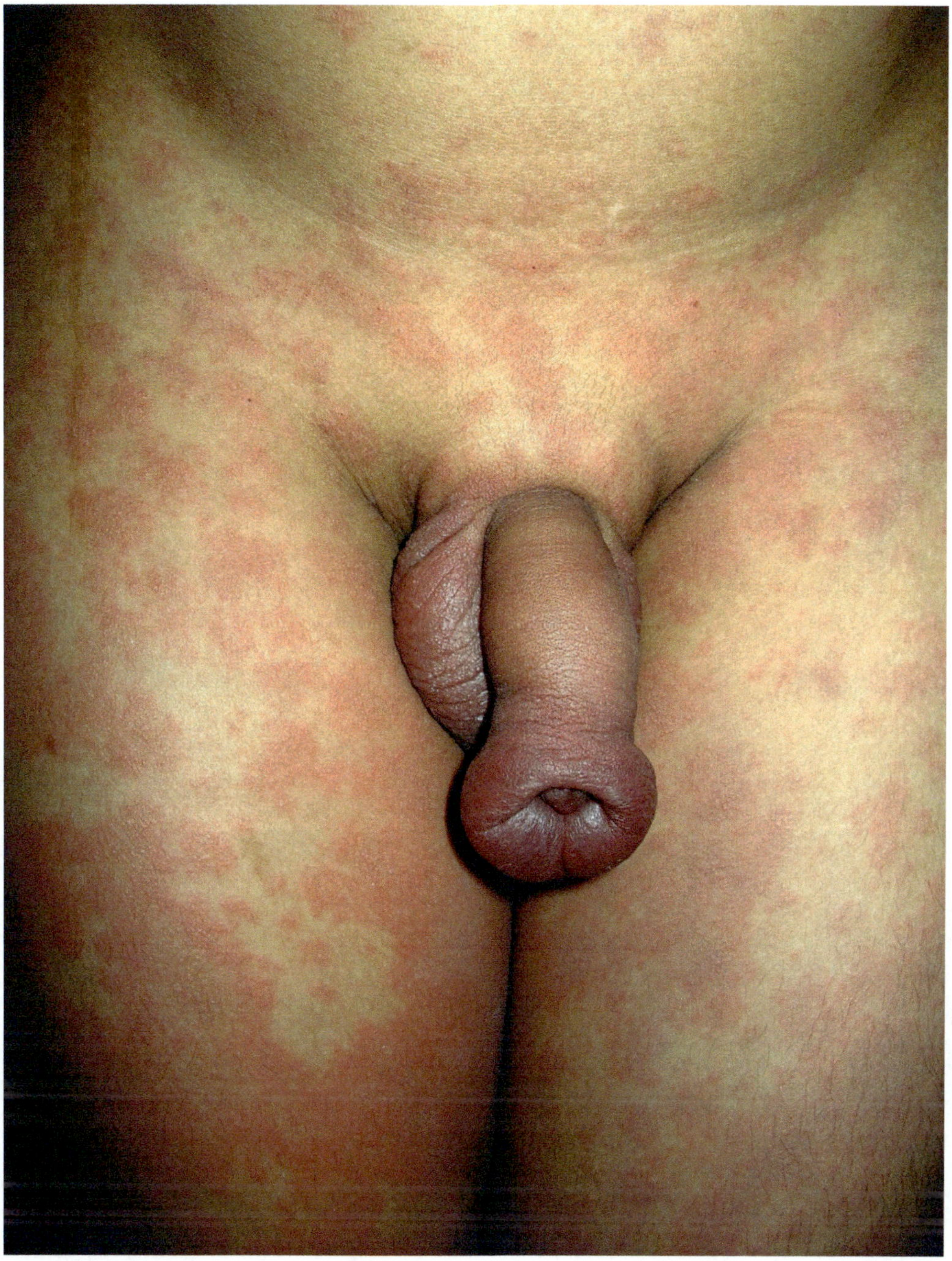

Fig. 24.2 *Acute urticaria* rush and penile edema in a young Indian boy

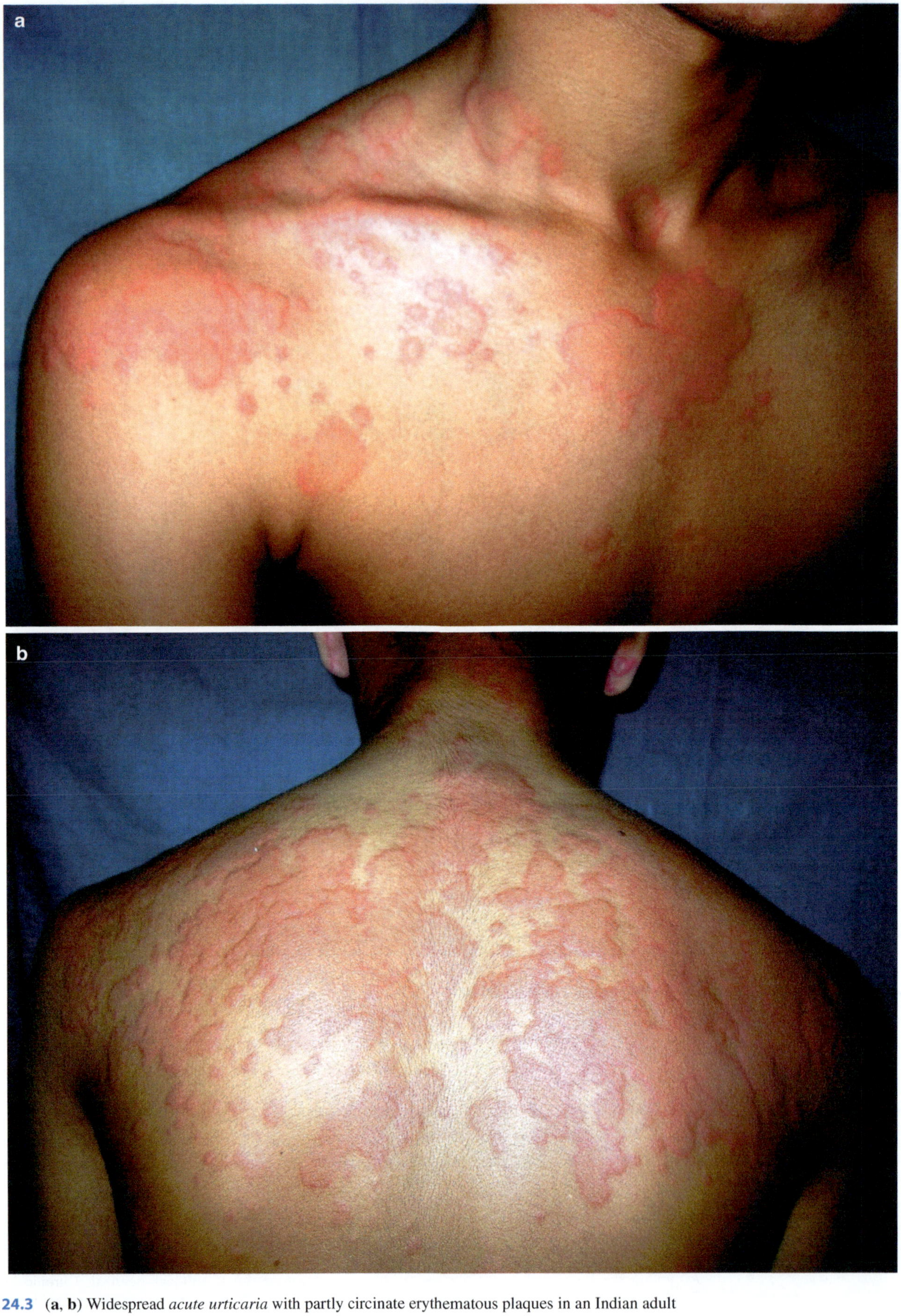

Fig. 24.3 (**a**, **b**) Widespread *acute urticaria* with partly circinate erythematous plaques in an Indian adult

Table 24.2 Major clinical variants of urticaria and angioedema

Idiopathic urticaria
Physical urticaria
Urticarial dermographism
Delayed pressure urticaria
Vibratory urticaria
Heat contact urticaria
Cold contact urticaria
Solar urticaria
Aquagenic urticaria
Cholinergic urticaria
Urticarial vasculitis
Contact urticaria
Angioedema
Idiopathic
C1-esterase inhibitor deficiency
Angioedema with wheals

Syndromes: Gleich's syndrome, *Schnitzler*'s syndrome, *Muckle-Wells* syndrome, familial Mediterranean fever, food-dependent exercise-induced anaphylaxis (FDEIA) with urticaria

are common, and psychiatric comorbidities may occur. For management a differentiation between *acute* episodes and *chronic* relapsing types of urticaria is recommended, when the clinical symptoms last for at least 6 weeks or longer.

Angioedema describes edematous swellings of dermal, subcutaneous, or submucosal tissues, which are often non-pruritic, occasionally pale, and painful. The most affected areas are the oral cavity and, to a lesser degree, the gastrointestinal mucosa. Both angioedema and urticaria represent possible symptoms of anaphylactic reactions.

24.2 Etiology/Pathogenesis

24.2.1 Urticaria

As a rule, mast cells are the primary effector cells in urticaria by expressing high-affinity receptors for IgE. Activation of the IgE receptors leads to degranulation of mast cells and the clinical appearance of wheals. Degranulation can be provoked by autoimmune mechanisms such as autoantibodies against IgE or FcεRI, IgE-induced allergies, immune complexes, and complement or bradykinin and various other tissue kinins [11]. Other non-immunologic factors leading to urticarial tissue reactions include pseudo-allergic reactions (aspirin, etc.), angiotensin-converting enzyme (ACE) inhibitors, vasoactive toxins (like nettle stings), and direct mast cell-degranulating agents such as opiates. ACE inhibitors are more often associated with angioedema than with urticaria.

The major mediators leading to an urticarial reaction include histamine, heparin, and various proteases. The circumstance that antihistamines do not completely control wheals and flares points to further mediators including prostaglandins, cytokines, and leukotrienes [9]. Mast cell-independent urticaria may result from hereditary or acquired C1-esterase inhibitor deficiency. Features of molecular genetics in various countries also seem to be involved in mast cell activation and inflammatory pathways [12]; current knowledge is summarized in Table 24.3.

Table 24.3 Molecular genetics in chronic urticaria. Risk factors and genetic markers

Urticaria type	HLA/Gene(s)	Variation(s)	Country
Chronic	HLA DRB1*0901	–	China
	DRB1*12		
	TGFβ1	−509C > T	Iran
Aspirin intolerance	ADORA3	−1050G > T	Korea
	IL-10	−564C > T; −819 T > C	Korea
	ALOX5	−1708G > A; 270G > A; 1728A > G	Korea
	CysLTR1	−634C > T	Korea
	PTGER4	−1254A > G	Korea
	CYO2C9	−1188 T > C	Korea

24.2.2 Angioedema

Angioedema can be caused by various factors. It is a primarily clinical observation that adverse events related to ACE inhibitors are more common in African-Americans, sometimes with prolonged angioedema requiring tracheostomy [13, 14]. In particular, the frequency of ACE-induced angioedema is increased in patients with dark skin where the ACE-II genotype is predominant. In genetic studies a significant association of ACE-induced angioedema to bradykinin receptor B2–9 allele has been identified. However, this genotype was not more frequent among patients with black skin or mixed ancestry in a study from South Africa [15]. In sub-Saharan Africa, angioedema is 5× more frequent than in the rest of the world; lip swelling accounts for >4% of adverse drug-related reaction from cardiometabolic drugs compared to <1% in the rest of the world [16]. In Nigeria, the prevalence of ACE inhibitor-induced angioedema has been estimated 1.6/1000 patient/years [17].

A study from India analyzed drug-induced cutaneous reactions and found urticaria as the most common clinical manifestation with 64% [18]. In a study from Singapore, periorbital angioedema was the most common presentation, often associated with concomitant urticaria lesions. The most common causative factors were seafood crustaceans, mollusks, and bird's nests [19]. In Saudi Arabia, acute urticaria is the leading symptom of anaphylaxis (71%) and food the trigger in 2/3 of cases. The most important allergens are tree nuts (25.2%) followed by eggs (16.4%), sesame (14.7%), and milk (11.3%). Almost half of their patients were <18 years of life [20].

Other factors contributing to angioedema are herbal products used for self-treatment. In Thailand, *Andrographis paniculata* is widely used for self-medication. It occasionally leads to angioedema [21]. HAE in Chinese patients presented with swelling on the extremities in 83.5%, the laryngopharynx in 58.9%, the face in 55.1%, the gastrointestinal tract in 34.2%, the trunk in 18.4%, and around the genital area in 15.3%. The frequency of gastrointestinal attacks seems to be lower in patients from the Far East compared to Western countries [23].

24.2.3 Parasitic Infections as a Cause of Urticaria/Angioedema Reactions

Loiasis caused by infestation with the African eye worm (*Loa loa*) is common in the rain forests of West and Central Africa, where up to 13 million people are affected. Most patients are asymptomatic. In case of adult worms migrating through the subcutaneous tissues, urticarial hypersensitivity reactions may occur, also manifesting as periodic angioedema [22]. Infestations with *Strongyloides stercoralis* are lifelong diseases affecting up to 100 million people worldwide. Estimated prevalence rates are of 5–50% in South and Central America, 25–45% in Cambodia, 41% in Laos, 28% in Australia, and 16% in China. *S. stercoralis* cause not only abdominal pain and diarrhea but also periodical urticarial symptoms in about 2/3 of all cases [24]. During treatment of *strongyloidiasis* and *schistosomiasis* with antihelminthic drugs, the *Mazzotti reaction* may occur, characterized by hypotension, tachycardia, angioedema, and acute urticaria [25].

Larvae of *Anisakis simplex* are parasites of sea fishes; by consumption of infected raw fish, *anisakiasis* can develop in humans. In the Far East, where raw fish is traditionally often consumed, anisakiasis is observed. The most common manifestations of the disease are urticarial rashes, abdominal pain, and anaphylaxis. Patients demonstrate high serum-specific IgE levels [26].

Urticaria was also reported as a possible symptom of *malaria*. In an Indian study on 320 hospitalized patients with malaria, acute urticaria was seen in nearly 6% of the cases [27].

24.3 Management

After excluding any possible causes of flares, the mainstay of urticaria treatment is oral antihistamines and/or short courses of oral corticosteroids. In a double-blind randomized, placebo-controlled crossover study, one dose of 5 mg levocetirizine was compared with 2× 60 mg fexofenadine in histamine-induced wheal and flare reactions of Caucasians and Japanese volunteers. No clinically significant ethnic differences in the responsiveness to these drugs were observed [28].

Patients with chronic relapsing urticaria nonresponsive to antihistamines will benefit from monoclonal IgG antibodies against IgE (omalizumab, Xolair®, 150–300 mg sc every 2–4 weeks) over 6–9 months or the administration of classical systemic immunosuppressants such as cyclosporine A and mycophenolate mofetil [29]. For cold-associated urticaria and various urticarial syndromes, a IL-1βrec antagonist is recommended (canakinumab, Illaris® 150 mg sc. at 1, 6, 12 weeks). In India, a combination of human immunoglobulins and histamine dihydrochloride (histaglobulin) was investigated in a prospective trial on patients with chronic urticaria. One milliliter was injected subcutaneously once a week for 8 weeks. This treatment reduced the urticarial activity score by almost 90% [30]. Mast cell-driven angioedema is treated by antihistamines, oral or intravenous corticosteroids, and epinephrine. ACE-induced angioedema does need airway assistance. While icatibant and fresh frozen plasma may be beneficial, drugs used for mast cell-driven angioedema are not beneficial or bear harms [31]. The treatment of choice for severe HEA attacks is human plasma-derived C1-esterase inhibitors such as Berinert® or Cynrize®.

Other compounds recently introduced for the same indication are a kallikrein inhibitor Kalbitor®, the bradykinin 2-receptor antagonist icatibant (Firazyr®), or conestat alfa, a human recombinant human C1rec-inhibitor (Ruconest®, Rhucin®) [32, 33]. The clinical efficacy of these new drugs is still under ongoing clinical research.

24.4 Course and Further Monitoring

Genetic studies are needed to explain different clinical presentations and epidemiological data in urticaria/angioedema. Pharmacogenetics may help to tailor more specific treatment of these conditions in various ethnic groups.

References

1. Weller K, Altrichter S, Ardelean E, et al. Chronic urticaria. Prevalence, course, prognostic factors and impact. Hautarzt. 2010;61:750–7.
2. Zuberbier T, Balke M, Worm M, et al. Epidemiology of urticaria: a representative cross-sectional population survey. Clin Exp Dermatol. 2010;35:869–73.
3. Davis SA, Narahari S, Feldman SR, et al. Top dermatologic conditions in patients of color: an analysis of nationally representative data. J Drugs Dermatol. 2012;11:466–73.
4. Caretti KL, Meregan DR, Mehregan DA. A survey of self-reported skin disease in the elderly African-American population. Int J Dermatol. 2015;54:1034–8.
5. Zhong H, Song Z, Chen W, et al. Chronic urticaria in Chinese population: a hospital-based multicenter epidemiological study. Allergy. 2014;69:359–64.

6. Jo E-J, Yang M-S, Kim Y-J, et al. Food-dependent exercise-induced anaphylaxis occurred only in a warm but not a cold environment. Asia Pac Allergy. 2012;2:161–4.
7. Thalayasingam M, Allameen NA, Soh JY, et al. Wheat-dependent exercise-induced anaphylaxis: a retrospective case review from a tertiary hospital. Postgrad Med J. 2014;90:488–92.
8. Ohsawa I, Honda D, Nagamachi S, et al. Clinical manifestations, diagnosis, and treatment of hereditary angioedema: survey data from 94 physicians in Japan. Ann Allergy Asthma Immunol. 2015;114:492–8.
9. Brown NJ, Ray WA, Snowden M, et al. Black Americans have an increased rate of angiotensin converting enzyme inhibitor-associated angioedema. Clin Pharmacol Ther. 1996;60:8–13.
10. Pare G, Kubo M, Byrd JB, et al. Genetic variants associated with angiotensin-converting enzyme inhibitor-associated angioedema. Pharmacogenet Genomics. 2013;23:470–8.
11. Moolani Y, Lynde C, Sussman G. Advances in understanding and managing chronic urticaria. F1000Res. 2016;5. pii: F1000 Faculty Rev-177.
12. Losol P, Yoo H-S, Park H-S. Molecular genetic mechanisms of chronic urticaria. Allergy Asthma Immunol Res. 2014;6:13–21.
13. Peacock ME, Park DS, Swiec GD, et al. Perioral angioedema associated with angiotensin-converting enzyme inhibitor. J Peridontol. 2005;76:651–4.
14. Kupfer Y, Ramachandran K, Tessler S. ACE inhibitor-induced angioedema in elderly African American females requiring tracheostomy. J Natl Med Assoc. 2010;102:529–30.
15. Moholisa RR, Rayner BR, Owen EP, et al. Association of B_2 receptor polymorphism and ACE activity with ACE inhibitor-induced angioedema in black and mixed-race south Africans. J Clin Hypertens. 2013;15:413–9.
16. Berhe DF, Juhlin K, Star K, et al. Adverse drug reaction reports for cardiometabolic drugs from sub-Saharan Africa: a study in VigiBase. Tropical Med Int Health. 2015;20:797–806.
17. Aiavi AAL, Adiqun AQ. Angioedema and cough in Nigerian patients receiving ACE inhibitors. Br J Clin Pharmacol. 2000;50:81–2.
18. Doshi K, Yegnanarayan R, Gokhale N. A retrospective study of drug induced cutaneous adverse reactions (CADR) in patients attending tertiary care hospital. Curr Drug Saf. 2017;12: 46–50.
19. Thong BYH, Cheng YK, Leong KP, et al. Immediate food hypersensitivity among adults attending a clinical immunology/allergy centre in Singapore. Singap Med J. 2007;48:236–40.
20. Sheikh F, Amin R, Rehan Khaliq AM, et al. First study of pattern of anaphylaxis in a large tertiary care hospital in Saudi Arabia. Asia Pac Allergy. 2015;5:216–21.
21. Suwankesawong W, Saokaew S, Permsuwan U, et al. Characterization of hypersensitivity reactions reported among *Andrographis paniculata* users in Thailand using health Product Vigilance Center (HPVC) database. BMC Complement Altern Med. 2014;14:515.
22. Ali S, Fisher M, Juckett G. The African eye worm: a case report and review. J Travel Med. 2008;15:50–2.
23. Xu YY, Jiang Y, Zhi YX, et al. Clinical features of hereditary angioedema in Chinese patients: new findings and differences from other populations. Eur J Dermatol. 2013;23:500–4.
24. Khieu V, Srey S, Schär F, et al. *Strongyloides stercoralis* is a cause of abdominal pain, diarrhea and urticaria in rural Cambodia. BMC Res Notes. 2013;6:200.
25. Olson BG, Domachowske JB. Mazzoti reaction after presumptive treatment for schistosomiasis and stronglyloidiasis in a Liberian refugee. Pediatr Infect Dis. 2006;25:466–8.
26. Choi S-J, Lee J-C, Kim M-J, et al. The clinical characteristics of *Anisakis* allergy in Korea. Korean J Intern Med. 2009;24:160–3.
27. Deshwal R. Clinical and laboratory profile of hospitalized malarial patients: an Agra-based study. J Assoc Physicians India. 2016;64:44–7.
28. Schoepke N, Church MK, Maurer M. The inhibition by levocetirizine and fexofenadine of the histamine-induced wheal and flare response in healthy Caucasians and Japanese volunteers. Acta Derm Venereol. 2013;93:286–93.
29. Fine LM, Bernstein JA. Guideline of chronic urticaria. Allergy Asthma Immunol Res. 2016;8:396–403.
30. Rajesh G, Keerthi S, Karthikeyan K, et al. Weekly injections of histaglobulin produces long-term remission in chronic urticaria: a prospective clinical trial. Indian J Pharm. 2016;48:292–7.
31. Curtis RM, Felder S, Borici-Mazi R, et al. ACE-I angioedema: accurate diagnosis may prevent epinephrine-induced harm. West J Emerg Med. 2016;17:283–9.
32. Lei W-T, Shyur S-D, Huang L-H, et al. Type I hereditary angioedema in Taiwan—clinical, biological features and genetic study. Asian Pac J Allergy Immunol. 2011;29:327–31.
33. Craig T, Pürsün EA, Bork K, Bowen T, Boysen H, Farkas H, Grumach A, Katelaris CH, Lockey R, Longhurst H, Lumry W, Magerl M, et al. WAO guideline for the management of hereditary angioedema. Arerugi. 2015;64:1215–41.

25 Vitiligo and Leukodermas

Mohamed Badawy Abdel-Naser
and Constantin E. Orfanos

Although most dermatoses inducing changes of the content and distribution of melanin discoloring the skin are not life-threatening, they have a tremendous psychological and socioeconomic impact among people with skin of color, particularly in African populations with darkly pigmented or black skin. There is a plethora of genetic and/or acquired diseases associated with various types of leukoderma; postinflammatory hypo- and hyperpigmentations are most common in African populations as secondary response after various dermatoses, burns, injuries, surgical interventions, injections, and action of chemicals [1]. They are all disfiguring and cause major psychological discomfort to the patients, with vitiligo being the most prevalent cause of deep concern [2].

25.1 Vitiligo

25.1.1 Epidemiology

Vitiligo is a common acquired skin disorder leading to loss of melanin in the skin, partly also of mucous membranes, affecting a considerable number of the world population. The pooled prevalence of vitiligo in population- or community-based studies was 0.1–0.2% and in hospital-based studies 1.4–2.1% [3]. In India the incidence of vitiligo has been reported in the range of 0.5–2.5% with a high prevalence of 8.8% in Gujarat and Rajasthan [4]. High prevalence is also reported in African populations with female preference [3, 5]; however, accurate records are lacking and increased awareness among dark-skinned individuals may influence the data. The incidence varies considerably depending on geographic region and ethnicity.

Vitiligo may appear at any time from birth to senescence, although the onset is most commonly observed in persons aged 10–30 years, frequently following stressful events and/or associated with other diseases of autoimmune origin. Coexistence of vitiligo with Hashimoto's thyroiditis, diabetes mellitus (type 1), lupus erythematosus, alopecia areata, pernicious anemia, Addison's disease, and several others is occasionally registered. If widely spread and localized in visible skin areas, the lesions of vitiligo are disfiguring; they indicate loss of inherited skin color as a marker of identity and cause psychosocial implications, emotional trauma, and stigmatization for the individuals affected.

25.1.2 Etiology/Pathogenesis

The pathogenesis of vitiligo is still a subject of ongoing research; several etiologic theories offer controversial views [6]. However, there is convincing evidence that complex autoimmune mechanisms of unknown etiology induced by stress, possibly of multifactorial origin, lead to the destruction of genetically predisposed epidermal melanocytes. Follicular melanocytes are less frequently affected. The exogenous precipitating factors which ultimately trigger the autoimmune response that targets the melanin-producing cells and drives to progressive depigmentation are mostly non-specific, including physical or chemical trauma, any conditions with overproduction of reactive oxygen species (ROS). Thus, interplay of oxidative stress and immune responses is likely to be a primary event in vitiligo [7]. Low levels of antioxidants, disturbed antioxidant pathways, and

M. B. Abdel-Naser
Department of Dermatology and Venereology,
Ain Shams University, Cairo, Egypt

C. E. Orfanos (✉)
The Free University of Berlin, Medical School Charité,
Berlin, Germany
e-mail: corfanos@t-online.de

C. E. Orfanos et al. (eds.), *Pigmented Ethnic Skin and Imported Dermatoses*, https://doi.org/10.1007/978-3-319-69422-1_25

polymorphisms of ROS-associated genes may play a contributory role [8], with autoimmune cell-mediated and antibody-dependent cellular cytotoxicity responses leading to melanocyte destruction. In addition, an intrinsic defect of melanocytes with genetic predisposition, multiple susceptibility loci, and neurotoxic effects has been suggested to be implemented in the pathogenesis of the disease [4, 9].

25.1.3 Clinical Picture

Vitiligo is clinically classified into *segmental* and widely spread *non-segmental* types. In general, any skin site can be affected, such as the trunk and genitalia; however, feet and face, particularly the perioral and periocular areas, the forearms, and hands, are the most commonly affected (Figs. 25.1 and 25.2). Initial lesions often first appear in areas of friction, local injury, or exposure to chemicals; the oral cavity may be also involved. Segmental vitiligo is characterized by one or more well-defined lesions in a dermatomal pattern, seen often in the distribution of the trigeminal nerve, together with white hair (poliosis). Non-segmental vitiligo is manifested as scattered white patches of varying size, sometimes symmetrically localized (Fig. 25.3); acrofacial lesions are frequent. Mixed features of segmental and acrofacial types occur. Koebner phenomenon often leads to development of vitiligo at sites of mechanical pressure, friction and trauma (wounds), burn, or abrasion, particularly in active disease (Fig. 25.4). Universal vitiligo refers to almost complete depigmentation of the body usually associated with syndromic endocrinopathies. Other organ affections, such as eyes and ears, are of little clinical impact [10].

The lesions appear as round, oval, or linear in shape, well-demarcated milky white macules and patches. Occasionally, elevated erythematous lesions are seen in sun-exposed areas that can be mildly pruritic (*inflammatory vitiligo*; Fig. 25.5). The borders are characteristically convex and the lesions range in size from millimeters to several centimeters. The course is unpredictable, the loss of skin pigment may progress and the lesions enlarge centrifugally.

Other clinical variants include *trichrome vitiligo*, showing lesions with intermediate zones of hypochromia between the depigmented and normally pigmented skin also showing perifollicular accentuation and *quadrichrome vitiligo*, which additionally shows dark-brown zone at sites of perifollicular repigmentation (Figs. 25.6 and 25.7). Vitiligo also develops in patients with melanoma, whereby the sites of depigmentation may or may not be near the tumor; both in common and *melanoma-associated vitiligo*, the oral mucosa, the eyes (iritis, uveitis), and the hair (poliosis) can be affected, accompanying the skin lesions.

25.1.4 Diagnosis

The diagnosis of vitiligo is usually made on the basis of clinical features. Wood's light is helpful to distinguish vitiligo from other hypopigmented macules particularly among patients with less pigmented skin. Rarely, skin biopsies are needed to exclude coexisting inflammatory dermatosis (i.e., lupus erythematosus); a complete absence of melanocytes with total loss of epidermal pigment favors vitiligo. In early progressive lesions, superficial perivascular and perifollicular lymphocytic infiltrates of predominantly T-cytotoxic cells may be observed at the margins close to normal skin. Degenerative changes in keratinocytes and melanocytes, increased numbers of Langerhans cells, and epidermal vacuolization may also be observed at the borders between lesions and adjacent skin [11].

Discolorations of the skin and the oral cavity due to drugs (quinine, quinacrine, chloroquine, chlorpromazine, minocycline, zidovudine among others) and heavy metals (amalgam, mercury, lead) may be confused with common vitiligo and genetic pigment abnormalities in black-skinned individuals.

25.1.5 Management

The response of vitiligo to therapeutic measures is remarkably slow and highly variable. Avoidance of any exogenous triggers or aggravating factors is mandatory for any successful procedure for management (see overview Table 25.1).

Topical modalities: Potent corticosteroids such as mometasone 0.1% or clobetasol 0.05% are applied 1–2×/day for at least 3 months with satisfactory response, particularly on progressive lesions in sun-exposed areas. For vitiligo lesions in the face, genitals, axillae, and breasts, less potent steroid compounds are recommended, to be applied every other week for avoiding skin atrophy and hypertrichosis. Topical *calcineurin inhibitors* such as 0.1% tacrolimus (2×/day) also deliver good therapeutic results and can be used on alternative weeks. Combinations of tacrolimus cream 0.1% with excimer laser, pimecrolimus cream 1% with narrowband UVB, or microdermabrasion were shown beneficial. The combination of topical calcipotriol and narrowband UVB or PUVA or 4% khellin ointment with excimer laser showed better response than monotherapy.

Phototherapies: Topical PUVA can be successfully used in localized or widespread vitiligo with application of 8-MOP (0.001% to be gradually increased up to 0.1–0.3%) 30 min prior to UVA radiation (0.1–0.3 J/cm^2 UVA) or sun exposure 2–3×/week. In hot climate zones, sunscreens (SPF 15 or higher) are recommended for daily use to minimize risk of sunburn and solar damage. The patients should be also assured that increased tanning of the normal skin surrounding the lesions is not permanent.

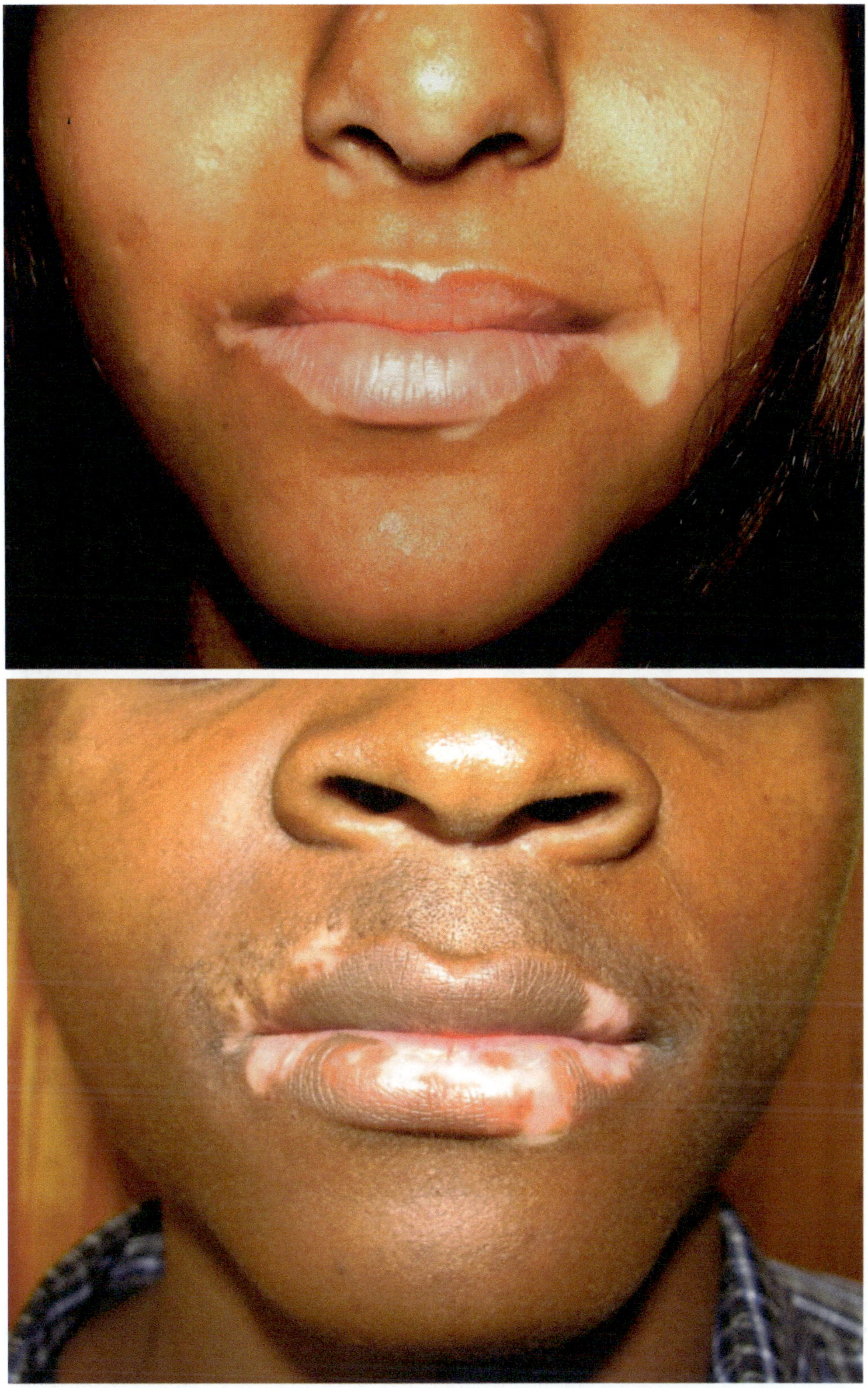

Fig. 25.1 Early facial vitiligo involving the lip mucosa and perioral region in an Egyptian female and a young African adolescent

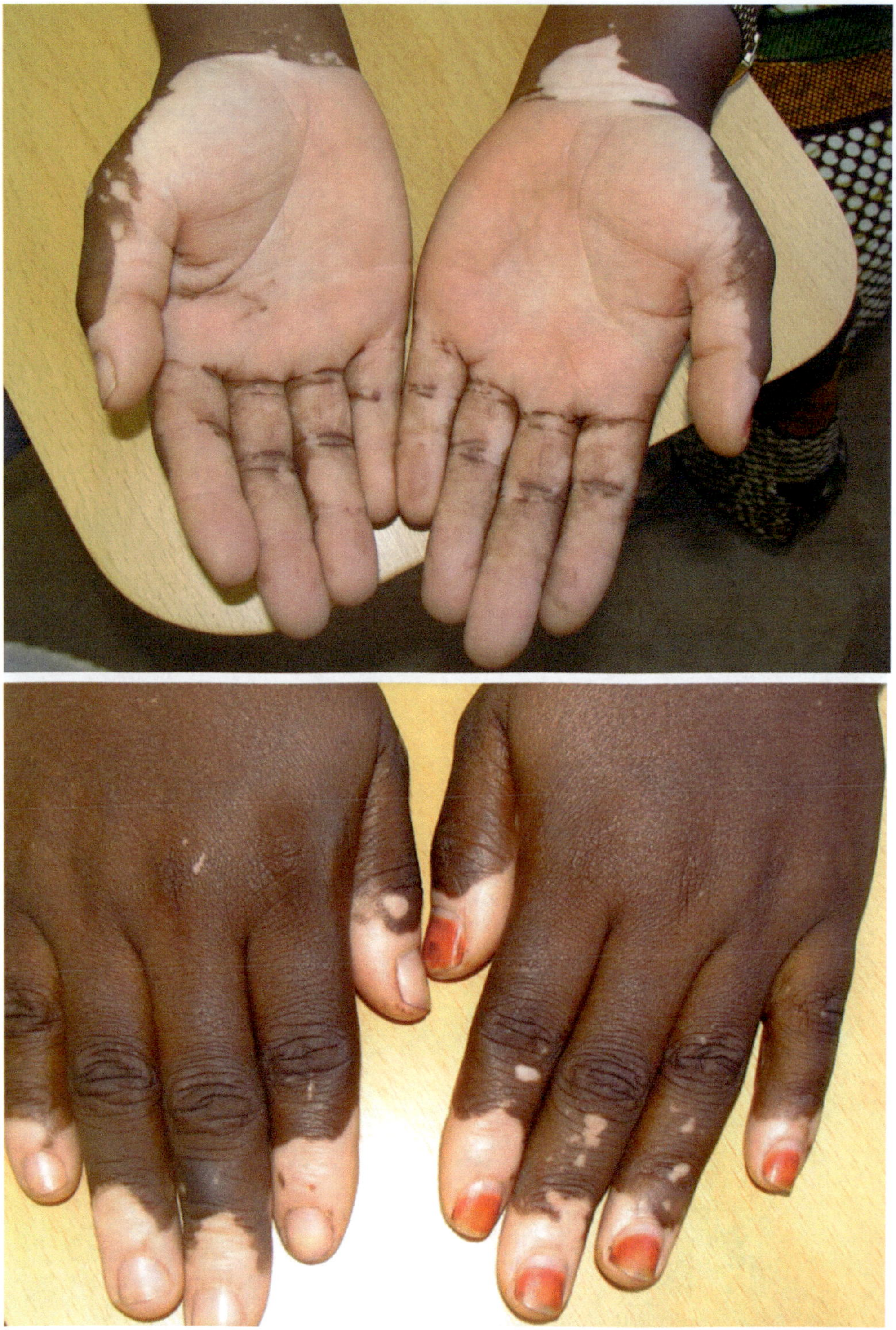

Fig. 25.2 Sharply demarcated involvement of the palms and fingertips in an African female. Note the pigmented skin of the interphalangeal creases

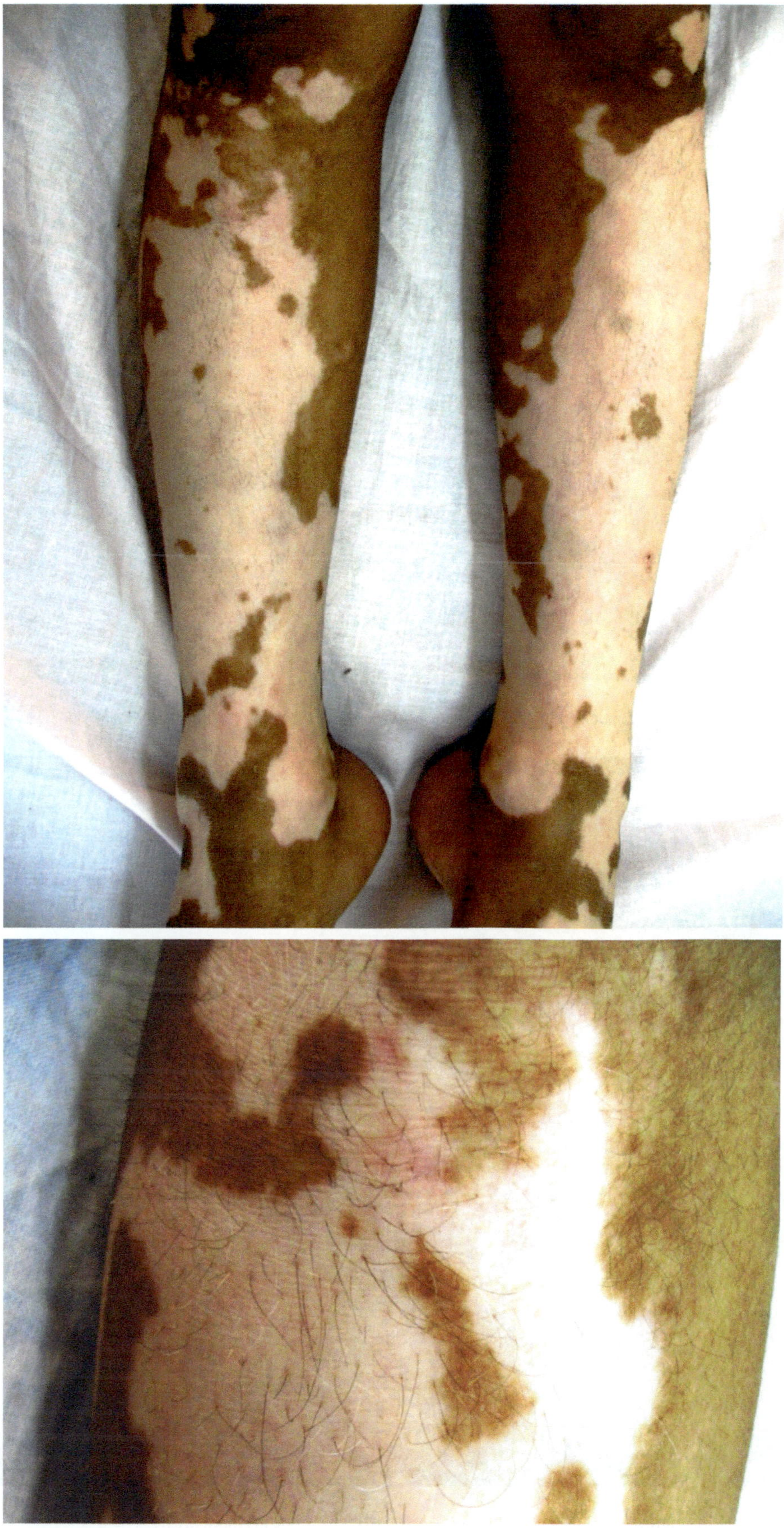

Fig. 25.3 Symmetrical vitiligo of the lower legs (up) in the lesions growing hairs remain pigmented (down)

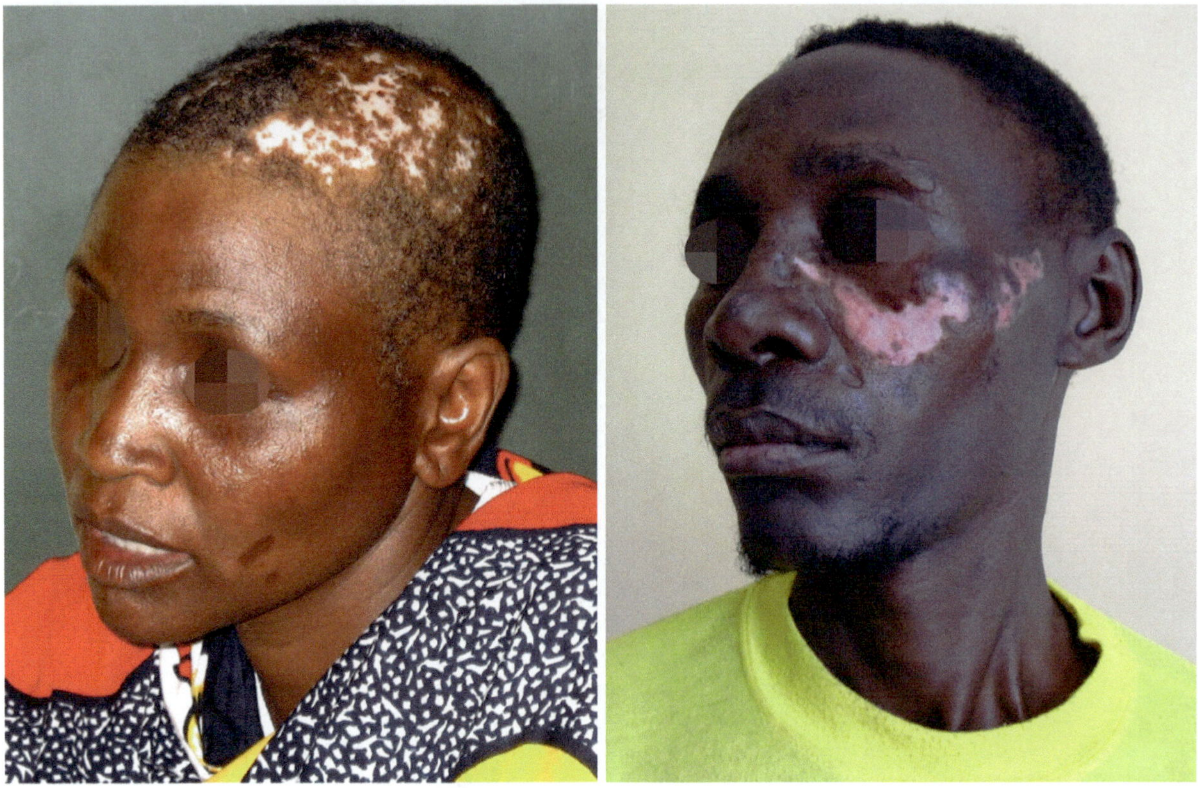

Fig. 25.4 Vitiligo lesions triggered by Koebner phenomenon in areas of previous scarring dermatosis

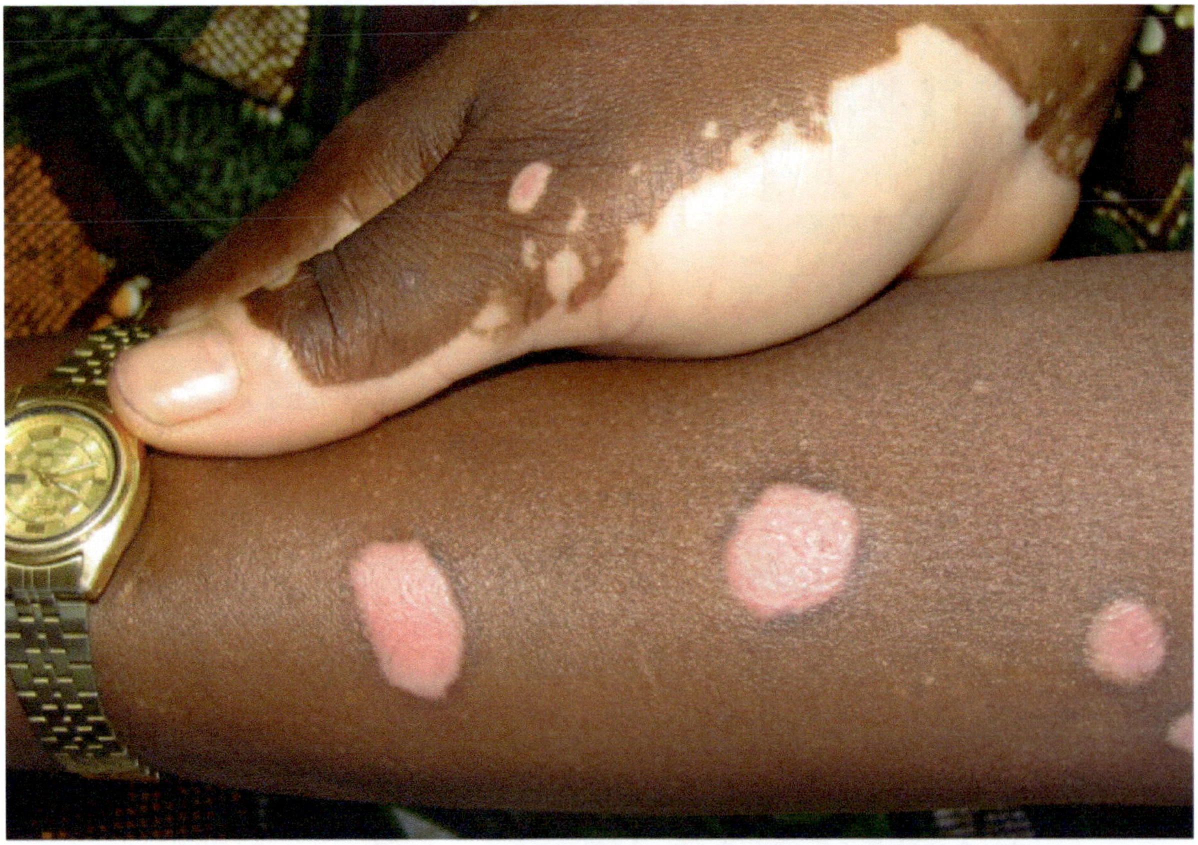

Fig. 25.5 Lesions of *inflammatory vitiligo* localized in sun-exposed areas. DD: Lupus erythematosus

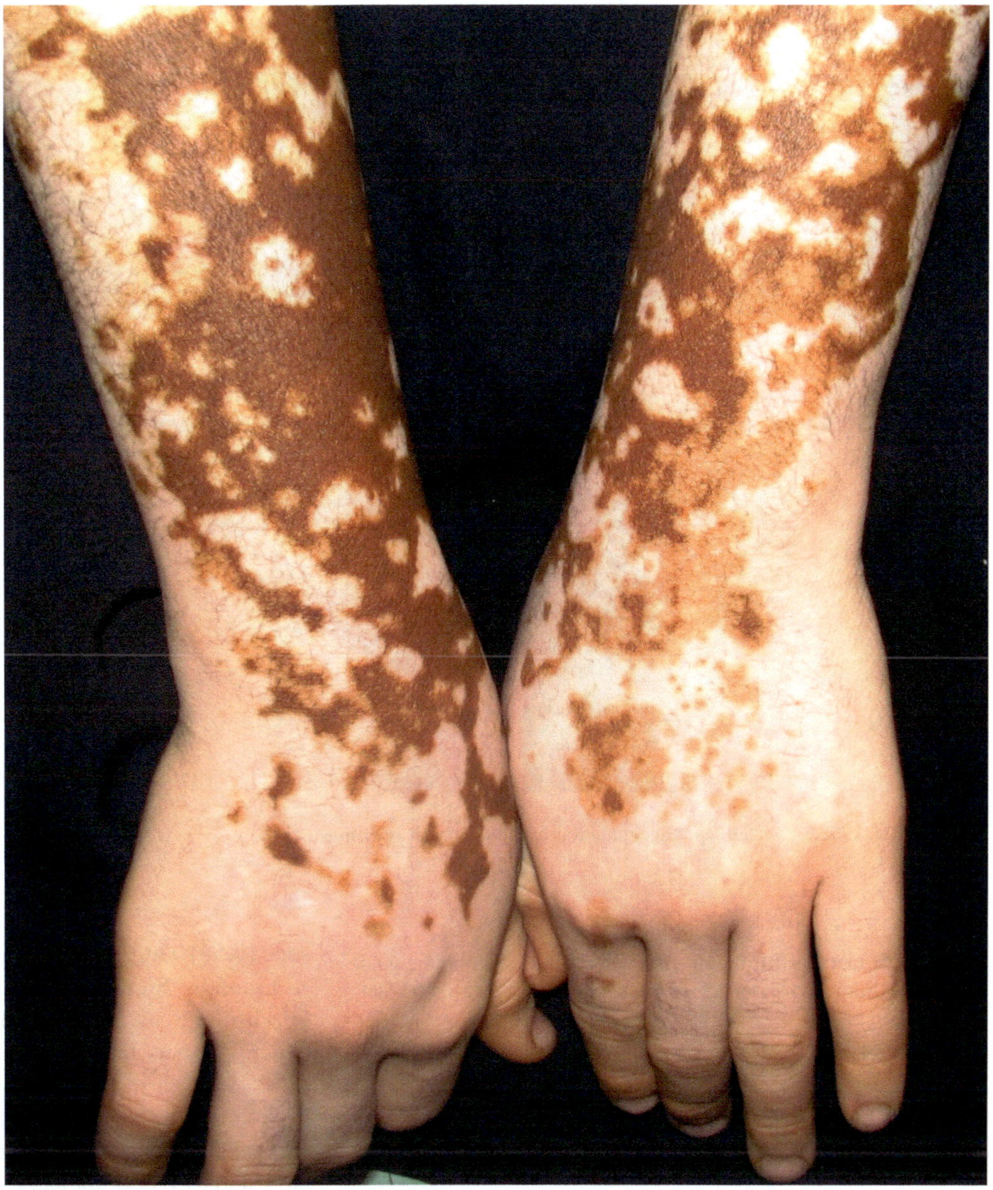

Fig. 25.6 Characteristic *trichrome vitiligo*, symmetrically involving the forearms and hands

Systemic PUVA (8-MOP 0.6–0.8 mg/kg; 5-MOP 1.2–1.8 mg/kg; trimethylpsoralen 0.6 mg/kg) followed by exposure to artificial UVA or natural sunlight after 1–3 h is commonly implemented in patients with skin types IV–VI. Several months (2–3 sessions/week) are required before perifollicular and marginal skin repigmentation merges to produce confluent repigmentation (Fig. 25.8); acral regions remain highly unresponsive. Patients are instructed to use UVA-protective eyeglasses during daytime. PUVA is contraindicated below the age of 12; those with history of skin malignancy, photosensitivity, and renal and liver diseases; and in pregnant and lactating women.

Topical KUVA (3–5% khellin cream) may be used with natural sunlight due to its safety, though its efficacy has not been yet established. Khellin is not recommended for oral use.

Narrowband UVB applied 2–3 times/week is particularly safe in children and pregnant or lactating women with only few side effects such as pruritus and xerosis. It has several advantages over PUVA such as shorter treatment times, no drug costs, no adverse GI effects, and no need for subsequent photoprotection. It has become the first choice of management for adults and children with generalized vitiligo.

Systemic drugs: Systemic corticosteroids as a short course (minipulse) have been used occasionally in progressing and early-onset vitiligo. Betamethasone (5 mg) or dexametha-

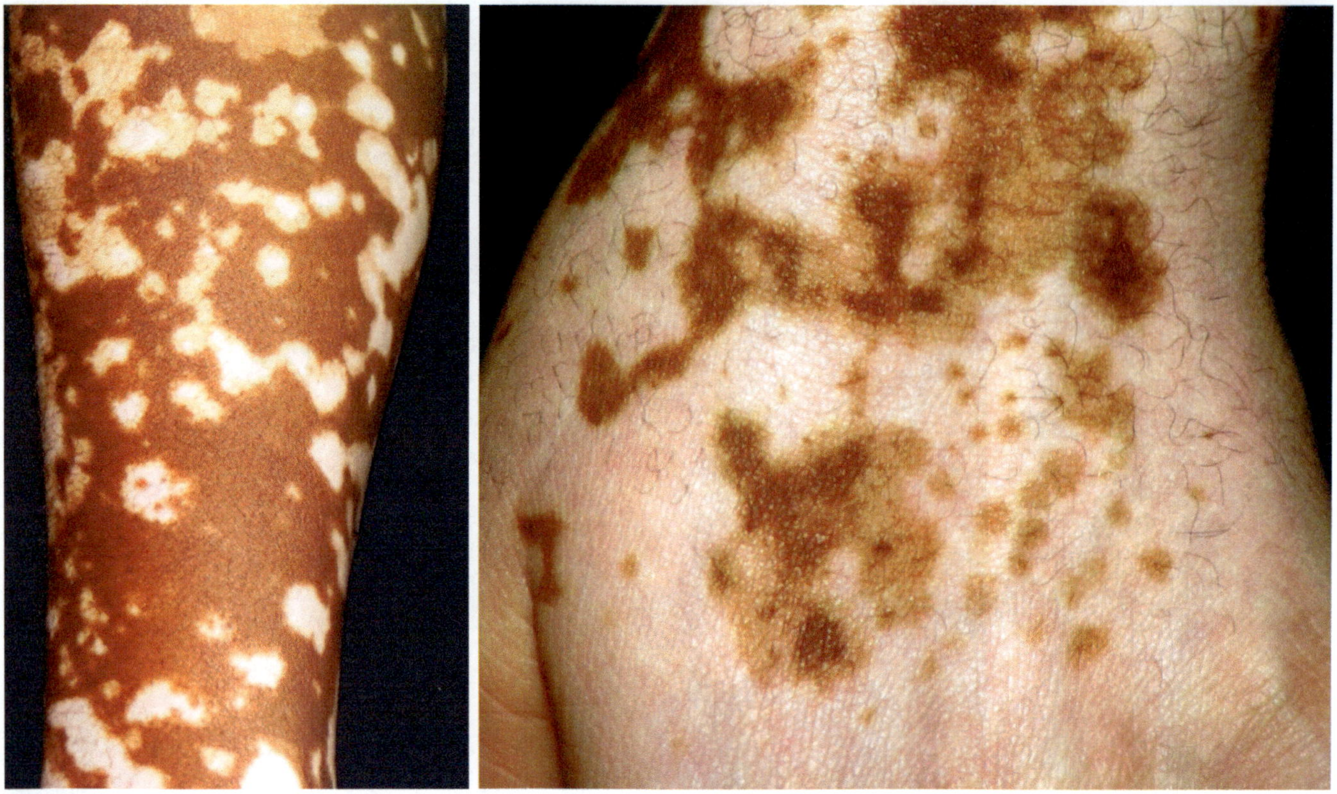

Fig. 25.7 *Trichrome vitiligo* with accentuation of the follicular openings

Table 25.1 Outlines for management of vitiligo based on the guidelines of the European Dermatology Forum Consensus [12]; modified

Clinical type		Management
Segmental or limited *Non-segmental* (<2–3% body surf.)	I. Line	Topical corticosteroids, topical calcineurin inhibitors (tacrolimus, pimecrolimus)
	II. Line	Narrowband UVB, excimer monochromatic lamp
Non-segmental vitiligo	I. Line	Stabilization with narrowband UVB (>3 months up to 9 months if there is a response). Combination with topical therapies, including reinforcement with UVB sessions Topical or, preferably, systemic PUVA
	II. Line	Systemic corticosteroids (over 3–4 months minipulse). If rapidly progressing or no stabilization under narrowband UVB, addition of immunosuppressants
	III. Line	Stabilization and grafting in non-responding areas with high cosmetic impact[a]
	IV. Line	Depigmentation (hydroquinone monobenzylether or 4-methoxyphenol alone or associated with Q-switched ruby laser) in non-responding widespread (> 50%) or visible recalcitrant vitiligo (face/hands)

[a]Koebner phenomenon may limit repigmentation; grafting is not recommended in acral localization (dorsum of hands, etc.)

sone (7.5–10 mg) is given on two successive days weekly for 1–3 months. Steroids seem to reliably arrest the progression of vitiligo with limited efficacy on repigmentation. The benefits versus the overall toxicity must be weighed carefully. In non-responding progressive cases, addition of immunosuppressants is possible. Recently, various biologicals such as tofacitinib [13], topical ruxolitinib (1.5% cream) [14], and MSH (afamelanotide) [15] have been used, but evidence is still incomplete.

Laser therapies: Excimer lasers (monochromatic at 308 nm) can be used to treat limited stable patches of vitiligo; the treatment is well tolerated and safe. However, it is expensive as it is applied twice weekly for an average of 24–48 sessions [16]. Combination of laser sessions with topical 0.1% tacrolimus and short-term systemic steroids is more effective, particularly in nonsegmental vitiligo [17].

Depigmentation: Depigmenting procedures are usually recommended for patients with widespread vitiligo (>80% of body area) particularly after failure or unsatisfactory efforts to induce repigmentation. The long-term social and emotional consequences of depigmentation must be considered, and consultation with a mental health professional is recommended. Depigmentation may be achieved by topical application of hydroquinone monobenzylether (20% cream 2×/day for 3–12 months); also 4-methoxyphenol, 88% phenol, and physical modalities such as cryotherapy and lasers are often

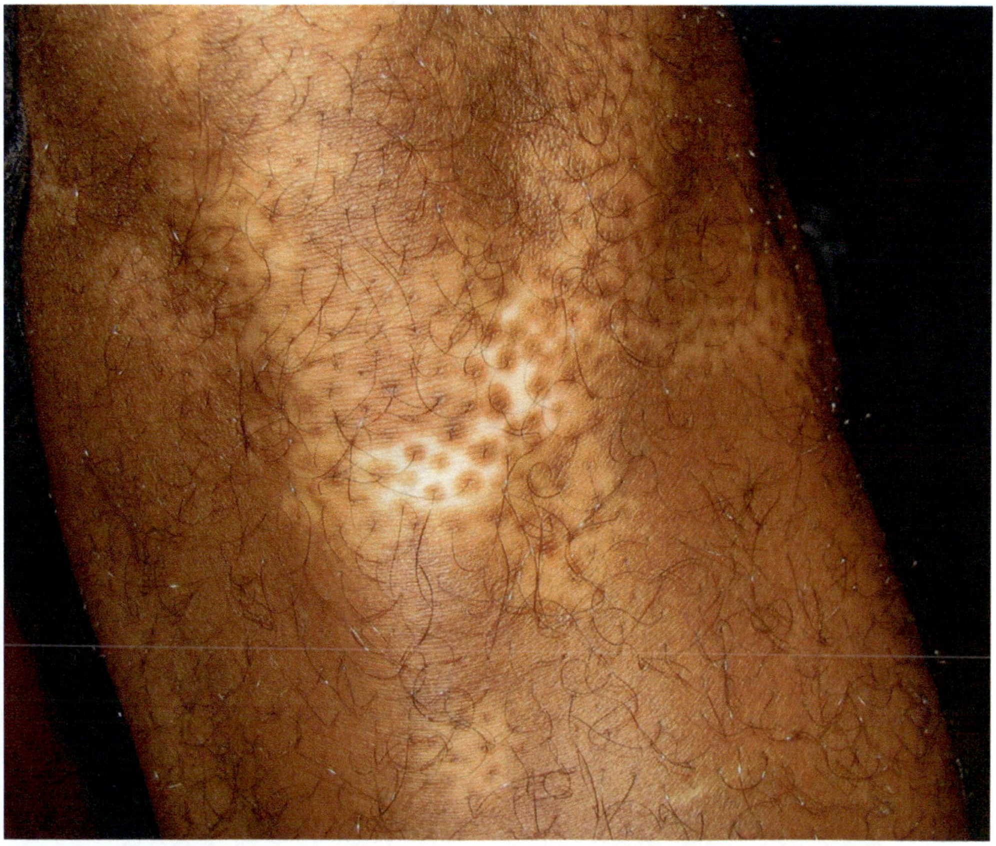

Fig. 25.8 Repigmentation of vitiligo lesion with accentuation of the follicular openings after management with PUVA

successfully used for depigmentation [18]. Burning, itching, allergic contact dermatitis, and other side effects may occur and be considered.

Cosmetic procedures: Camouflage may be helpful but is difficult due to the difficulties of skin color matching. There are several commercial preparations that provide an acceptable cosmetic coverage and can be used supportively during other therapeutic measures. Micropigmentation (tattooing) is not recommended, since the disease usually progresses and the lesions enlarge (Fig. 25.9).

Surgical interventions: Surgical techniques of transferring autologous melanocytes from pigmented skin are suitable for localized and small areas of vitiligo not responding to other modalities. They can be recommended only in selected stabilized cases; in active disease a cell-mediated immune response with cytotoxic T-lymphocytes and LFA-1-positive infiltrating cells may take place toward the grafted melanocytes [19]. Punch grafting rarely delivers satisfactory results (cobblestone appearance); suction blister grafting offers better results, but is suitable only for small areas. Ultrathin epidermal sheet grafting requires skill and experience covering larger areas; also epidermal cell suspensions may be applied. Transplants of pure cultured melanocytes or mixed cultures of melanocytes and keratinocytes are suitable for large areas, but the procedure is expensive, is time-consuming, and requires specialized facilities and staff.

Overall, surgical procedures are efficacious in most anatomic locations, being of little value for acral areas; unilateral vitiligo responds well in a high proportion of patients, and bilateral disease may also respond, when stable [20].

25.2 Leukodermas Due to Other Pigmentary Skin Disease

Besides vitiligo several genetic and acquired skin disorders occur, presenting hypo-and/or depigmented lesions (leukodermas) as a prominent feature, mimicking vitiligo (Table 25.2).

Postinflammatory hypopigmentation is attributed to loss of function of the melanocytes due to inflammatory cell dysregulation. It frequently follows common dermatoses in heavily pigmented or black skin. *Pityriasis alba* is more often seen on the face in children with dry skin and is manifested as multiple ill-defined irregular hypopigmented patches with fine scaling and mild erythema. Atopic predisposition and excessive sun exposure are precipitating factors for the development of such lesions. It is a self limiting

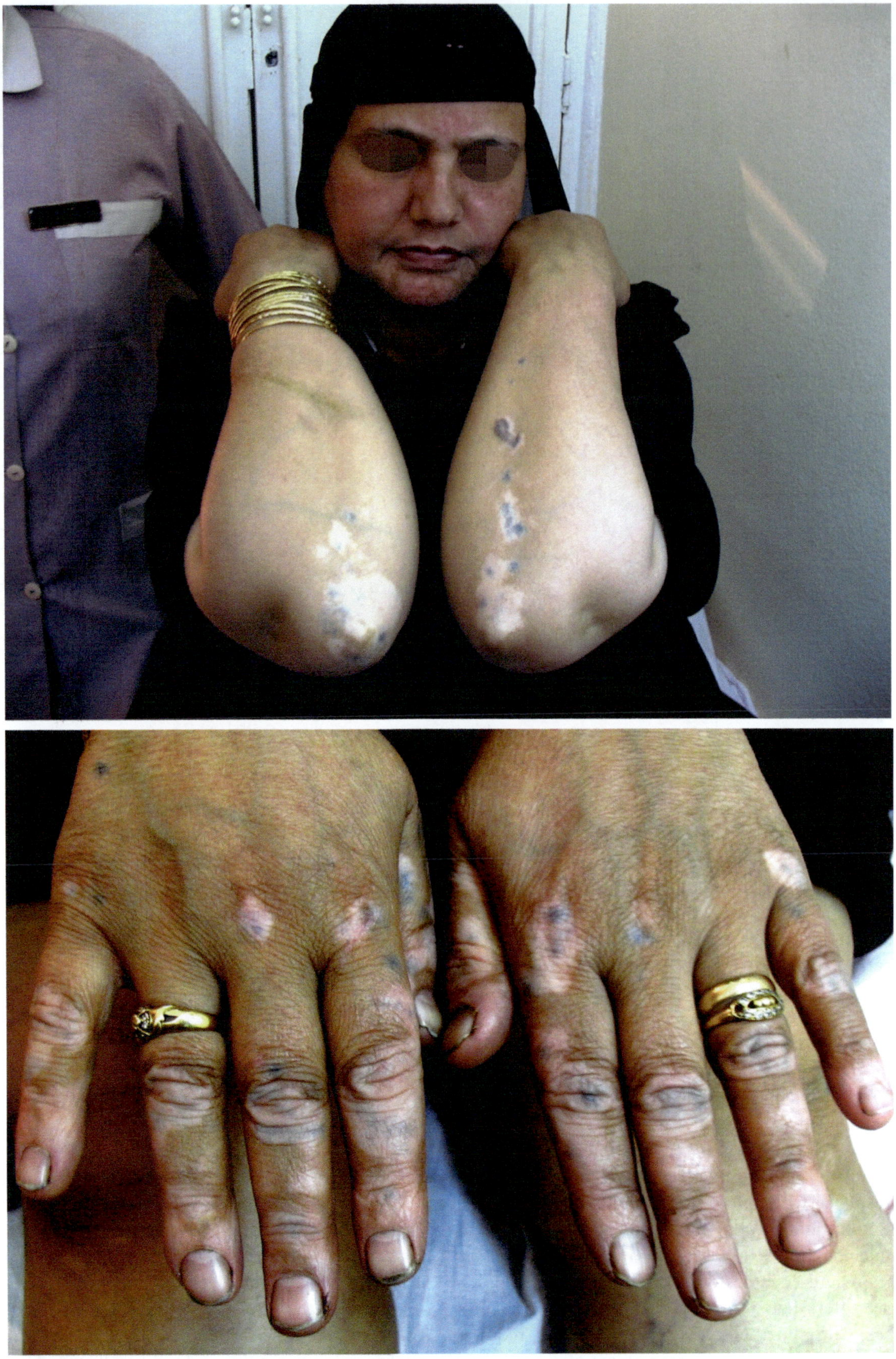

Fig. 25.9 Tattooing for minor lesions causing Koebner phenomenon in progressive vitiligo

Table 25.2 Skin disorders and syndromes with leukodermas

Postinflammatory Pityriasis alba, atopic dermatitis, psoriasis (pseudoleukoderma), parapsoriasis (achromians), chronic discoid lupus erythematosus, halo nevus, secondary syphilis, leprosy, onchocerciasis, treponematoses
Congenital/hereditary N. Depigmentosus, N. Anemicus, hypomelanosis of Ito, tuberous sclerosis, albinism, piebaldism, *Waardenburg* syndrome, phenylketonuria
Other conditions Pityriasis versicolor, idiopathic guttate hypomelanosis, hypopigmented mycosis fungoides, *Vogt-Koyanagi-Harada* syndrome, *Alezzandrini* syndrome
Chemically induced: Hydroquinone monobenzylether, *p*-tertiary butyl phenol, arsenic *(partly occupational)* intoxication, among others

condition, though sun protection with mild emollients and low-potency topical steroids provides rapid improvement. In psoriasis *pseudoleukoderma* often results due to increased keratinocytic turnover during or after treatment of plaques. The hypopigmented lesions of *parapsoriasis achromians* are morphologically similar to lesions of pityriasis alba. In *discoid lupus erythematosus*, hypopigmentation is characterized by epidermal atrophy and the characteristic distribution in sun-exposed areas with some follicular plugging and telangiectasias. True vitiligo may coexist with lupus erythematosus. *Halo nevus* (*Sutton*) is a depigmented halo around a preexisting pigmented lesion more commonly seen in children and young adults. Following exclusion of melanoma, no specific treatment is required as the lesion gradually resolves. Also in leprosy sharply demarcated oval or round hypopigmented macules with dry scaly center and erythematous borders may occur. Loss of superficial sensation and thickened cutaneous nerves give clues to the diagnosis.

25.2.1 Hereditary and Congenital Disorders

Nevus depigmentosus is a leukoderma typically seen on the trunk, easily confirmed by Wood's light. *Nevus anemicus* is a congenital vascular anomaly presenting as a hypopigmented macule or patch since birth that persists throughout life. It is characterized by irregular margins and becomes indistinguishable from surrounding skin on pressure (diascopy test) or with Wood's light.

Hypomelanosis of Ito (*incontinentia pigmenti achromians)* is characterized by mosaic distribution of hypopigmented macules and bands of speckled or mottled, grayish-brown to blue-black patches involving the skin, conjunctiva, sclera, tympanic membrane, and oral and nasal mucosa. Genetic mosaicism is the most likely explanation for its inheritance [21]. The skin lesions are present from birth, are asymptomatic, and can be associated with neurological, skeletal, hair, and dental defects. Wood's lamp examination enhances the pattern.

Tuberous sclerosis (epiloia) is an autosomal dominant neurocutaneous disorder characterized by typical ash-leaf-shaped hypomelanotic macules mimicking vitiligo, seizures, angiofibromas, and mental retardation. The macules are the earliest lesions seen at birth, occur predominantly on the thorax and legs, can be multiple, and become prominent when examined under Wood's lamp. They resemble the café au lait spots in neurofibromatosis 1 (*von Recklinghausen*'s disease). A decreased activity of the sweat glands with a modified starch-iodine test may be helpful for differential diagnosis [22].

Albinism is partial or complete congenital absence of melanin in the eyes alone or in the eyes, skin, and hair (oculocutaneous albinism, OCA) that is autosomal recessively inherited. The lack of melanin results in a pale skin and increased risk of skin cancer (see Chap. 41). The eyes should be protected in all types of albinism by dark UV-blocking sunglasses [23]. OCA is further divided into several subtypes depending on the particular genetic mutation, with or without associated syndromes:

(a) *Chediak-Higashi syndrome* with immunologic deficiency and characterized by fever, hepatosplenomegaly, lymphadenopathy, pancytopenia, and infiltration of the nervous system. Systemic steroids and intrathecal methotrexate are effective, but recurrence is common and bone marrow transplantation is lifesaving.
(b) *Hermansky-Pudlak syndrome* with hemorrhagic diathesis and accumulation of ceroid-like material with development of atypical nevi, acanthosis nigricans, trichomegaly, and other skin lesions of solar damage.
(c) *Griscelli syndrome* is similar to *Chediak-Higashi* syndrome but with prominent neurologic features and absence of the characteristic giant intracytoplasmic inclusion bodies in granulated cells. Patients with OCA should be advised to apply broad-spectrum sunscreens (SPF $\geq$ 30), together with other methods that provide sun protection.

Piebaldism is a rare autosomal dominant syndrome with variable phenotype presenting at birth and is due to the absence of melanocytes. The condition is typically manifested by white forelock and multiple symmetrical hypopigmented or depigmented macules affecting the face, trunk, and proximal extremities. *Waardenburg syndrome* comprises the cutaneous features of piebaldism in addition to bilateral congenital deafness, heterochromic irides, and a broadened nasal root. Congenital leukodermas are frequently seen on the face, trunk, or limbs [24].

Phenylketonuria is an autosomal recessive disorder caused by deficiency of phenylalanine hydroxylase in the liver, clinically characterized by hypopigmentation of the skin and hair and mental retardation; affected children are blue eyed with blond hair and fair skin with severe photosensitivity. Epilepsy, phenylpyruvic acid in urine, hypopigmentation, pseudoscleroderma, and atopic dermatitis occur. Low-phenylalanine diet given shortly after birth has been recommended for treatment [25]; currently, gene therapies are underway.

25.2.2 Miscellaneous

Pityriasis versicolor may lead to hypopigmented macules as a result of inhibition of tyrosinase by dicarboxylic acids released by *Malassezia furfur*. Wood's lamp examination shows yellow fluorescence. After treatment with topical preparations or systemic antifungals, repigmentation may require several weeks or months to resolve and the recurrence rate is high. Other infections that may cause hypopigmentations include syphilis, other treponematoses (pinta), and onchocerciasis.

Idiopathic guttate hypomelanosis is a common acquired disorder more frequently affecting women after the age of 40. The lesions chiefly occur on the shins and less commonly forearms as multiple small (6–8 mm) irregular in shape but sharply demarcated depigmented macules [26]. The pathogenesis of the disease is controversially discussed; recently excimer laser has been reported beneficial for management [27].

Hypopigmented mycosis fungoides is a unique variant of mycosis fungoides characterized by gradually progressive hypopigmented macules and patches with skin atrophy. The lesions are commonly seen in the trunk, mostly among patients with dark skin [28]. Pruritus may be a clinical feature. Multiple and repeated skin biopsies may be needed to reach the diagnosis. Hypopigmented mycosis fungoides responds well to UVA and UVB, resulting in long-term remissions [28, 29].

Vogt-Koyanagi-Harada syndrome may occur in Africa [30] characterized by vitiligo together with uveitis, aseptic meningitis, dysacusis, tinnitus, poliosis, and alopecia. The condition responds well to topical and systemic steroids which are crucial in preventing blindness. Also *Alezzandrini syndrome* is a rare condition characterized by a unilateral gradual loss of visual acuity due to degenerative uveitis [31]. The condition is followed by ipsilateral appearance of facial vitiligo, poliosis of the eyebrows and eyelashes, and other abnormalities after some years.

Some chemicals and drugs (Table 25.2) in addition to others, such as liquid nitrogen, steroids (intralesional, intraarticular and to a lesser extent potent topical preparations) and bleaching agents may also induce hypopigmentation.

Conclusions

Vitiligo is a rather common chronic skin disease leading to loss of the inherited skin color based on a dysfunction and finally full destruction of melanocytes. Particularly ethnic populations with heavily pigmented or black skin are affected. The disease manifests itself early in life and may progress causing severe discomfort, stigmatization, and socioeconomic implications to the affected individuals. It has to be differentiated from hereditary or acquired leukodermas. Despite all efforts, the etiology of vitiligo is unknown and the pathogenetic mechanisms are not clearly understood. Triggers of multifactorial origin may manifest progressive depigmentation via autoimmune cytotoxic mechanisms targeting predisposed melanocytes. Currently, there is increasing interest of the international medical community [32] to better define core outcome measures in future trials introducing emerging treatments for vitiligo, also assessing quality of life.

References

1. Berthe S, Faye O, Bagayogo B, et al. Etiology of acquired hypochromic patches in dermatological area in Mali. Mali Med. 2012;27:6–9.
2. Osman AM, Elkordufani Y, Abdullah MA. The psychological impact of vitiligo in adult Sudanese patients. Afr J Psychiatry (Johannesburg). 2009;12:284–6.
3. Zhang Y, Cai Y, Shi M, et al. The prevalence of vitiligo: a meta-analysis. PLoS One. 2016;11:e0163806.
4. Shajil EM, Chatterjee S, Agrawal D, et al. Vitiligo: pathomechanisms and genetic polymorphism of susceptible genes. Indian J Exp Biol. 2006;44:526–39.
5. Kiprono S, Chaula B. Clinical epidemiological profiles of vitiligo. East Afr Med J. 2012;89:278–81.
6. Schallreuter KU, Bahadoran P, Picardo M, et al. Vitiligo pathogenesis: autoimmune disease, genetic defect, excessive reactive oxygen species, calcium imbalance, or what else? Exp Dermatol. 2008;17:139–40; discussion 141–60.
7. Laddha NC, Dwivedi M, Mansuri MS, et al. Vitiligo: interplay between oxidative stress and immune system. Exp Dermatol. 2013;22:245–50.
8. Xie H, Zhou F, Liu L, et al. Vitiligo: how do oxidative stress-induced autoantigens trigger autoimmunity? J Dermatol Sci. 2016;81:3–9.
9. Spritz RA. The genetics of generalized vitiligo. Curr Dir Autoimmun. 2008;10:244–57.
10. Ayanlowo O, Olumide YM, Akinkugbe A, et al. Characteristics of vitiligo in Lagos, Nigeria. West Afr J Med. 2009;28:118–21.
11. Abdel-Naser MB, Krueger S, Krasagakis K, et al. Further evidence for involvement of both cell mediated and humoral immunity in generalized vitiligo. Pigment Cell Res. 1994;7:1–8.
12. Taieb A, Alomar A, Böhm M, et al. Guidelines for the management of vitiligo. The European Dermatology Forum Consensus. Br J Dermatol. 2013;168:5–19.
13. Craiglow BG, King BA. Tofacitinib citrate for the treatment of vitiligo: a pathogenesis-directed therapy. JAMA Dermatol. 2015;151:1110–2.
14. Rothstein B, Joshipura D, Saraiya A, et al. Treatment of vitiligo with the topical Janus kinase inhibitor ruxolitinib. J Am Acad Dermatol. 2017;76:1054–60.e1.

15. Lim HW, Grimes PE, Agbai O, et al. Afamelanotide and narrowband UV-B phototherapy for the treatment of vitiligo: a randomized multicenter trial. JAMA Dermatol. 2015;151:42–50.
16. Chimento SM, Newland M, Ricotti C, et al. A pilot study to determine the safety and efficacy of monochromatic excimer light in the treatment of vitiligo. J Drugs Dermatol. 2008;7:258–63.
17. Abdel Latif AA, Ibrahim SM. Monochromatic excimer light versus combination of topical steroid with vitamin D3 analogue in the treatment of nonsegmental vitiligo: a randomized blinded comparative study. Dermatol Ther. 2015;28:383–9.
18. Grimes PE, Nashawati R. Depigmentation therapies for vitiligo. Dermatol Clin. 2017;35:219–27.
19. Abdallah M, Abdel-Naser MB, Moussa MH, et al. Sequential immunohistochemical study of depigmenting and repigmenting minigrafts in vitiligo. Eur J Dermatol. 2003;13:548–52.
20. Falabella R. Surgical approaches for stable vitiligo. Dermatol Surg. 2005;31:1277–84.
21. Ream M. Hypomelanosis of Ito. Handb Clin Neurol. 2015;132:281–9.
22. Gualandri L, Boccardi D, Menni S. A different approach for identifying hypomelanotic macules in tuberous sclerosis complex. G Ital Dermatol Venereol. 2015;150:501–3.
23. Manga P, Kerr R, Ramsay M, et al. Biology and genetics of oculocutaneous albinism and vitiligo—common pigmentation disorders in southern Africa. S Afr Med J. 2013;103:984–8.
24. Milunsky JM. Waardenburg syndrome type I. In: Pagon RA, Adam MP, Ardinger HH, et al., editors. Gene reviews® [Internet]. Seattle: University of Washington, Seattle; 1993–2017.
25. Viecelli HM, Harbottle RP, Wong SP, et al. Treatment of phenylketonuria using minicircle-based naked-DNA gene transfer to murine liver. Hepatology. 2014;60:1035–43.
26. Juntongjin P, Laosakul K. Idiopathic guttate hypomelanosis: a review of its etiology, pathogenesis, findings, and treatments. Am J Clin Dermatol. 2016;17:403–11.
27. Gordon JR, Reed KE, Sebastian KR, et al. Excimer light treatment for idiopathic guttate hypomelanosis: a pilot study. Dermatol Surg. 2017;43:553–7.
28. Hassab-El-Naby HM, El-Khalawany MA. Hypopigmented mycosis fungoides in Egyptian patients. J Cutan Pathol. 2013;40:397–404.
29. Bisherwal K, Singal A, Pandhi D, et al. Hypopigmented mycosis fungoides: clinical, histological, and immunohistochemical remission induced by narrow-band Ultraviolet B. Indian J Dermatol. 2017;62:203–6.
30. Oluleye TS, Rotimi-Samuel AO, Adenekan A, et al. Two cases of Vogt-Koyanagi-Harada's disease in sub-Saharan Africa. Int Med Case Rep J. 2016;9:373–6.
31. Gupta M, Pande D, Lehl SS, et al. Alezzandrini syndrome. BMJ Case Rep. 2011. https://doi.org/10.1136/bcr.04.2011.4052. pii: bcr0420114052.
32. Gan EY, Eleftheriadou V, Esmat S, et al. Repigmentation in vitiligo: position paper of the Vitiligo Global Issues consensus conference. Pigment Cell Melanoma Res. 2017;30:28–40.

Facial Pigmentary Disorders

26

Marwa Abdallah

Skin hyperpigmentation results from increased number of epidermal melanocytes, increased synthesis of melanin, or both. Occasionally, deposition of melanin or other exogenous pigments in the deeper dermis causes changes of skin color. Facial pigment disorders include various dermatologic entities; they may also reflect organ dysfunction or metabolic conditions (e.g., pellagra, porphyria), result from deposition of metals (argyria, mercury intoxication), or be a side effect of chemicals and drugs. Postinflammatory hyperpigmentations of different origin may occur and overlap.

Facial hyperpigmentations are clearly more common in populations with darker skin due to the higher activity of the melanocytes. They are visible and have a strong impact on the quality of life of the individuals affected [1]. Particularly females are more prone to get involved than males and feel psychosocial discomfort [2]. Hyperpigmentations of the face require careful diagnosis, management, and treatment.

26.1 Clinical Entities

26.1.1 Melasma

Melasma consists of well-defined patches of light or dark brown cutaneous hyperpigmentation with irregular borders showing centro-facial, malar, and mandibular localization (Fig. 26.1). The lesions get darker after exposure to the sun. The centro-facial pattern is the most common, leading to involvement of the forehead, nose, cheeks, upper lip, and chin [3]. In skin biopsies increased melanin synthesis and deposition rather than increased number of melanocytes are found. The pathogenesis of melasma is complex. Pregnancy, oral contraceptive pills, family history, and dark skin types remain among the major predisposing factors, while UV exposure has a major role in its induction and frequent relapses [4]. Interestingly, visible light, especially that in the blue light range, can increase skin pigmentation adding to the burden of melasma relapse [5]. Although melasma is usually diagnosed clinically, Wood's light or confocal laser microscopy helps in localizing melanin level. Modified MASI (Melasma Area and Severity Index) score helps in assessing disease severity and follow-up of treatment success [6].

26.1.2 Lichen Planus Pigmentosus

The pigmented variant of lichen planus is rather rare in Caucasians, more commonly seen in heavily pigmented skin. It affects primarily the forehead and temples and presents by slate gray, gray-brown, blue-brown color due to the dermal location of melanin (Fig. 26.2). The border of the lesions is ill-defined and mild pruritus may be present. Diffuse, reticular, and blotchy patterns have been observed on the face and neck [7]. Lichen planus pigmentosus has been associated with lichen planus elsewhere [8], frontal fibrosing alopecia [9], and hepatitis C virus infection [10]. Dermoscopy may help for diagnosis [9].

26.1.3 Riehl's Melanosis

Riehl's melanosis presents as gray-brown to blue-brown pigmentation of the face, often in a reticulate pattern. Occasionally, it occurs on other parts of the body, especially if the contact allergen is in textiles [2]. Riehl's melanosis represents a low-grade contact or photo-contact dermatitis to different cosmetic, textile, occupational, or airborne allergens (Fig. 26.3), which lead to delayed hypersensitivity reactions with vacuolation of basal keratinocytes and pigmentary incontinence. Ultraviolet light may play a role, since the lesions are found often in a photo-distributed manner, and some allergens are known to be photosensitizers [11]. Patch tests are positive in many cases [12].

M. Abdallah
Department of Dermatology and Venereology,
Ain Shams University, Cairo, Egypt
e-mail: marwa.abdallah@med.asu.edu.eg

C. E. Orfanos et al. (eds.), *Pigmented Ethnic Skin and Imported Dermatoses*, https://doi.org/10.1007/978-3-319-69422-1_26

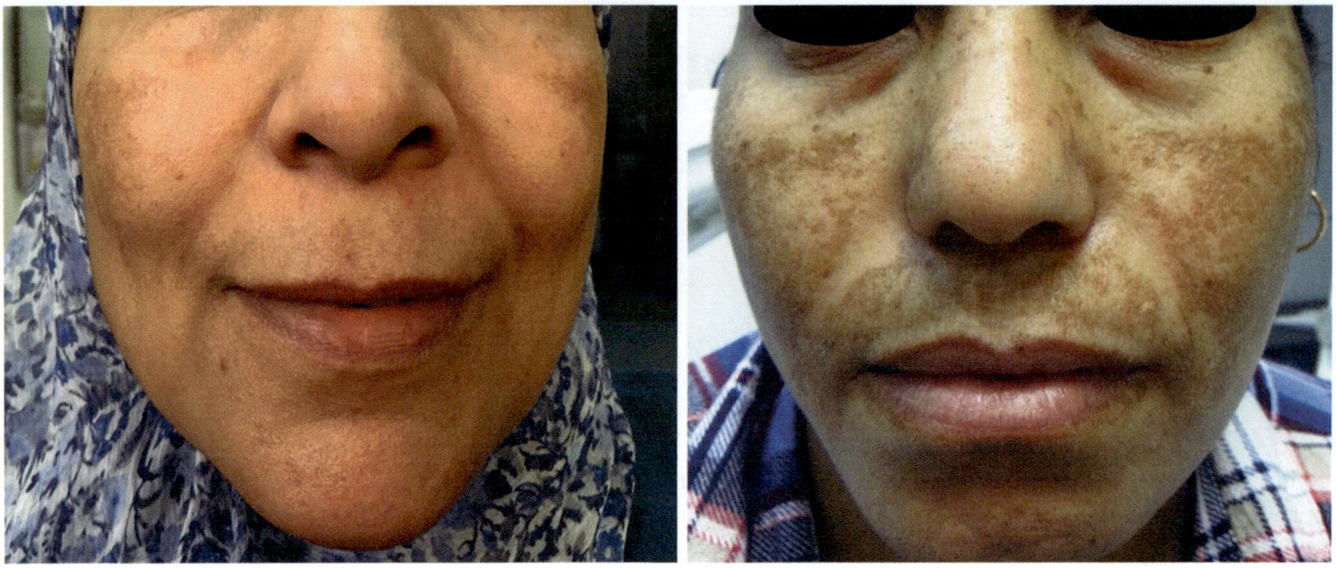

Fig. 26.1 *Melasma* on the cheeks and the upper lips in females

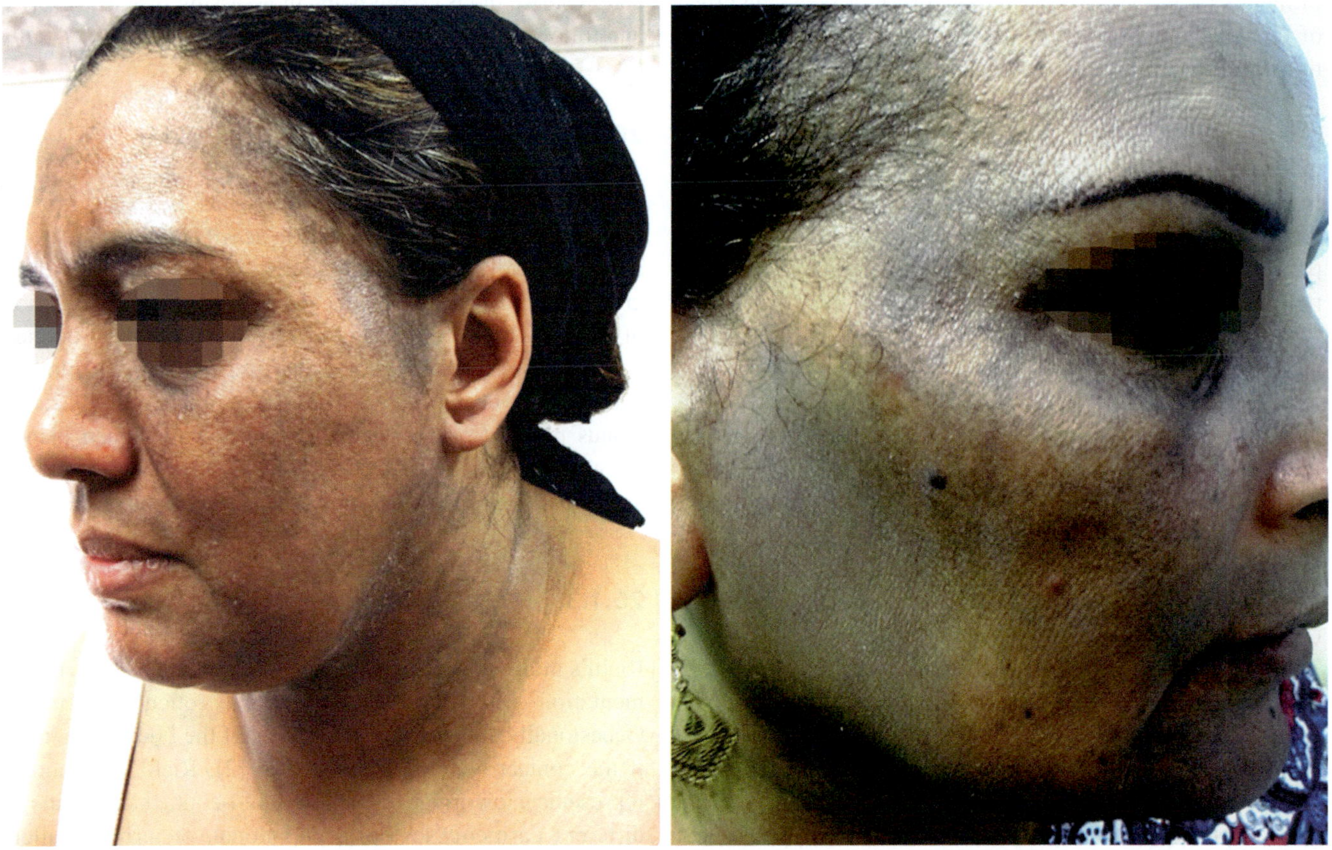

Fig. 26.2 *Lichen pigmentosus* in Egyptian females with sun-exposed face and neck (left) and on the whole face, mostly expressed on forehead and temples (right)

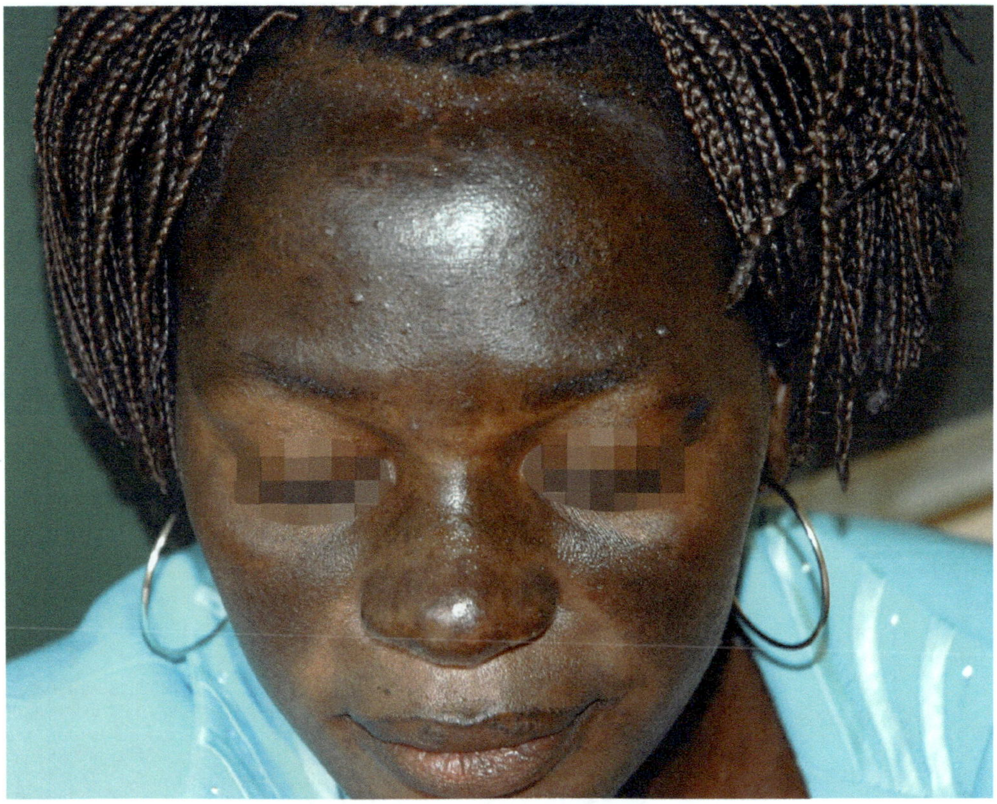

Fig. 26.3 *Riehl's melanosis*, most likely due to topical application of cosmetics containing phototoxic compounds (RDTC Moshi, Tanzania; courtesy Dr. M. Ketema)

26.1.4 Erythema Dyschromicum Perstans

This rare entity presents as ashy-colored macular dyspigmentations, slowly progressive, favoring the face, neck, trunk, and the upper extremities, seen mostly in patients with pigmented ethnic skin (Fig. 26.4). Early lesions may show a rim of inflammation. In a Korean study, the face was affected in 32%, the trunk in 69.1%, and the neck in 39.7% of the cases. The disease is usually asymptomatic, but some patients may complain of some itching [13]. The etiology is not known; a delayed type hypersensitivity reaction may play a role [14]. Its clinical and histopathological discrimination from pigmented lichen and Riehl's melanosis is sometimes difficult. History of cosmetics, erythematous borders, or patch tests may help in discriminating the three entities [8, 12].

26.1.5 Congenital Pigment Disorders

Melanocytic nevi appear either shortly after birth or at the age of puberty. *Nevus of Ota* was first described in Asians but is seen also in Africans and other ethnic groups. Due to the deep dermal location of pigmented melanocytes, the lesions clinically appear blue in color. Lesions are unilateral and tend to be composed of multiple tiny macules that coalesce together giving a mottled appearance. Sites of predilection are the ophthalmic and maxillary branches of the trigeminal nerve (Fig. 26.5). Concomitant eye affection is frequently seen. A bilateral location is seen in 5–15% of the cases [15].

26.1.6 Other Rare Conditions

Erythromelanosis follicularis usually starts in childhood or adolescence and consists of a triad of follicular hyperkeratosis, ill-defined erythema, and pigmentation in the preauricular area extending to the cheeks, temples, and neck. The lesions do not show atrophy and are usually asymptomatic, but some patients may complain of burning or itching sensation [16]. Keratosis pilaris of other body sites is almost always an accompanying finding. The etiopathogenesis remains to be elucidated; a genetic background and an environmental role with sun exposure and xerosis are precipitating factors [17]. *Poikiloderma of Civatte* is seen in middle-aged women and is characterized by reddish-brown reticulated pigmentation with atrophy and telangiectasias on the lateral cheeks and side of the neck with no follicular papules [2]. *Erythrose peribuccale pigmentaire Brocq* occurs in females and is characterized by scaling and orange-yellow-brown to erythematous discoloration around the nose and chin [14].

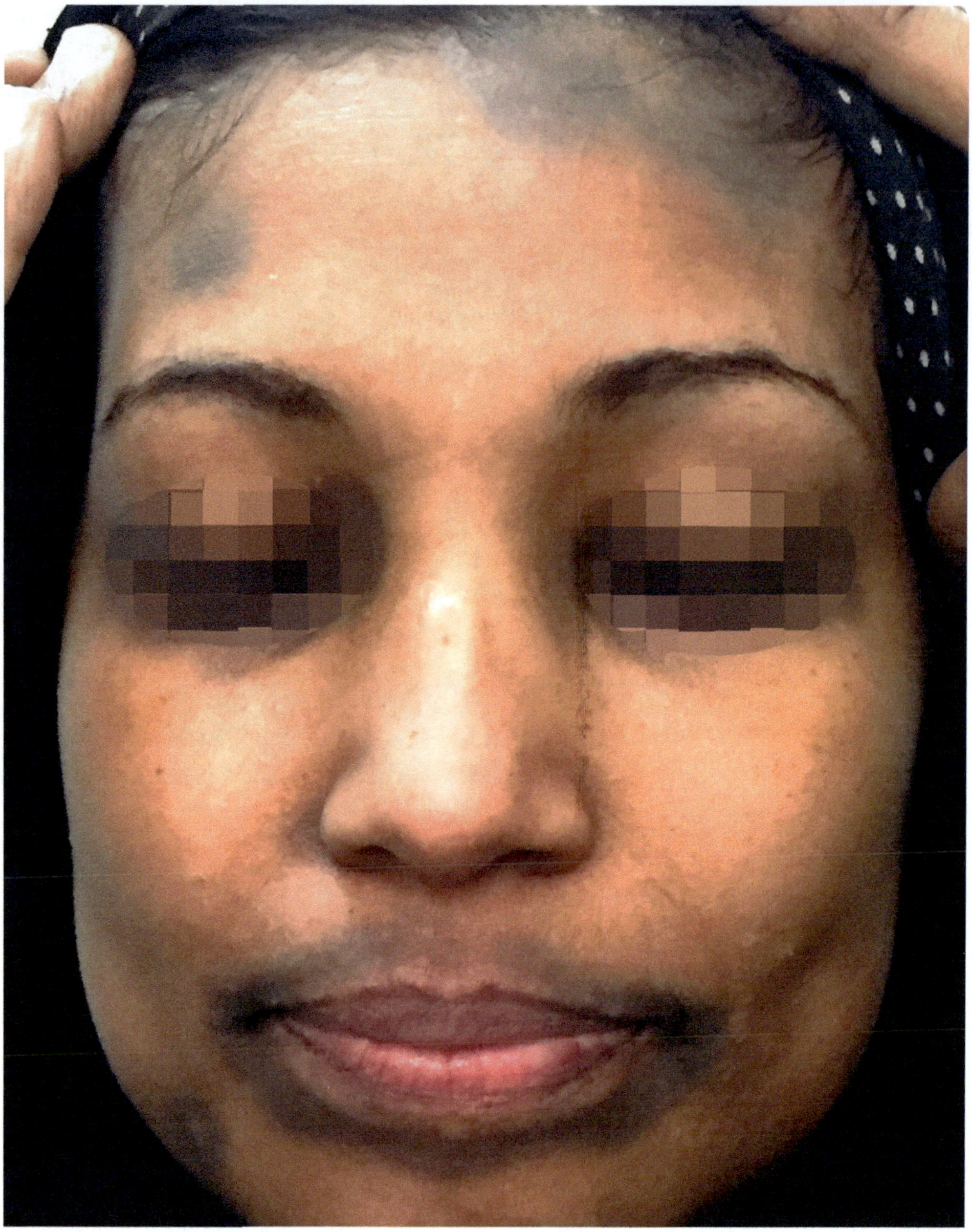

Fig. 26.4 *Erythema dyschromicum perstans*. Ashy-colored facial macular dyspigmentations in an Egyptian female (lesions also on the trunk)

26.2 Postinflammatory Hyperpigmentations on the Face

Postinflammatory hyperpigmentations of the face may follow acne, folliculitis, pseudofolliculitis, fixed drug eruptions, lichen planus, wounds, and abrasions; they follow the shape and distribution of the original disease. However, patients do not always recall a cause [18]. In addition, they may be iatrogenic, following chemical peeling, laser, or other procedures, especially in people of pigmented ethnic skin [19]. Inflammatory mediators such as cytokines, leukotrienes, and prostaglandins produced during the pathogenesis of inflammatory conditions stimulate melanocyte function resulting in hyperpigmentation. In addition, basal damage of keratinocytes leads to dropping off of melanin into the deeper dermis and accumulation of melanophages [20]. Tetracyclines, doxycycline, thiazide diuretics, salicylanilides, amiodarone, piroxicam, chlorpromazine among others may induce

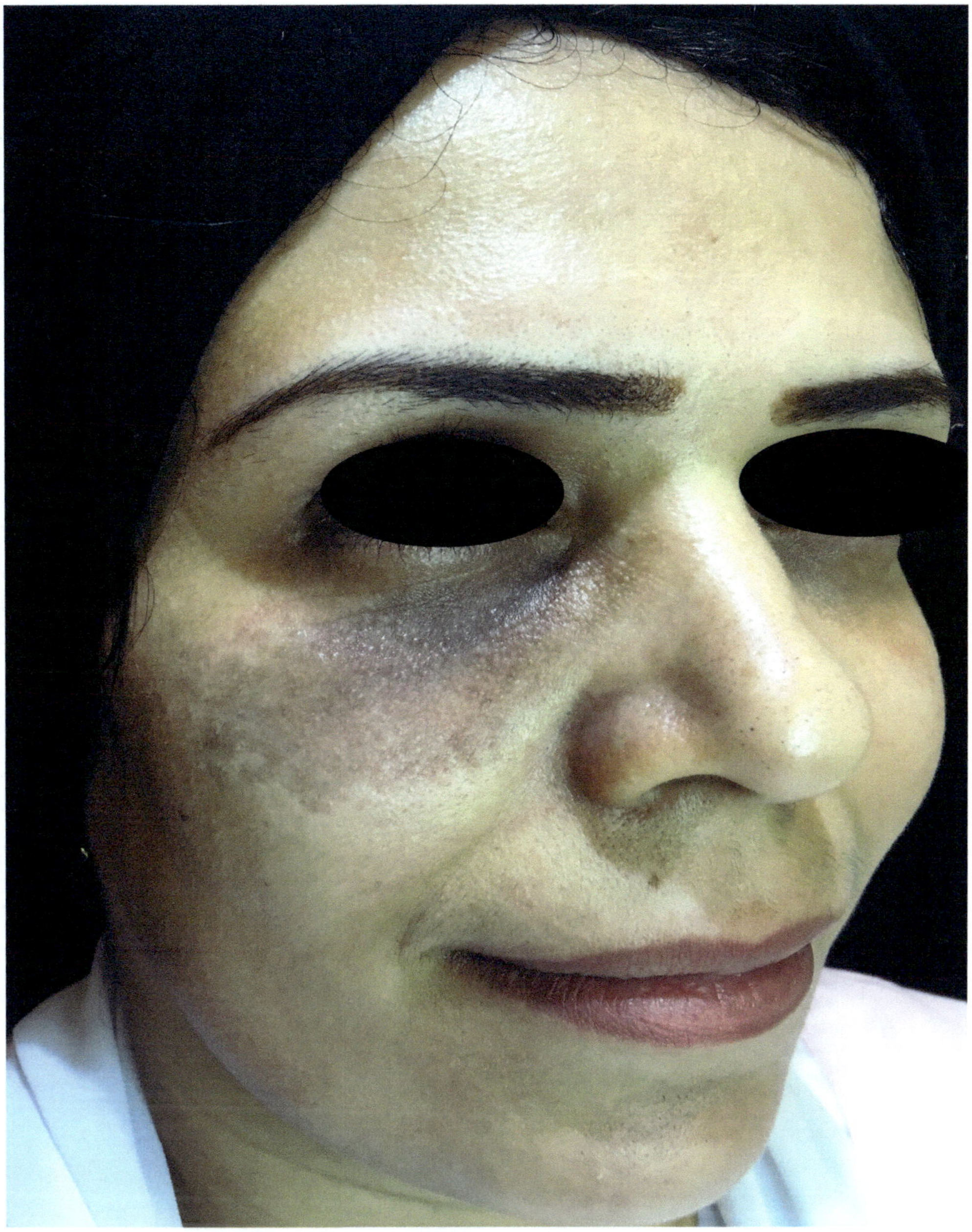

Fig. 26.5 *Nevus of Ota*, maxillary type

phototoxic reactions in the sun-exposed facial skin (Fig. 26.6), and the topical application of perfumes containing psoralens may show exaggerated sunburn reactions; they often subside leaving diffuse or localized facial hyperpigmentations. Berloque dermatitis is an example of a localized phototoxic reaction [21]. A good history and proper physical examination are of great value for diagnosis. Postinflammatory hyperpigmentations slowly resolve, but in many cases they persist for months or years necessitating medical intervention [18].

26.3 Idiopathic Facial Pigment Disorders

Idiopathic facial pigmentations may occur and be sometimes strongly expressed in the face of patients with heavily pigmented ethnic skin.

Pigmentary demarcation lines are borders of abrupt transition between hyperpigmented skin and lighter areas first reported on the trunk, designated A–E, and then described on the face, designated F, G, H. They usually appear around the age of puberty [22, 23]. Types F (temporo-zygomatic area

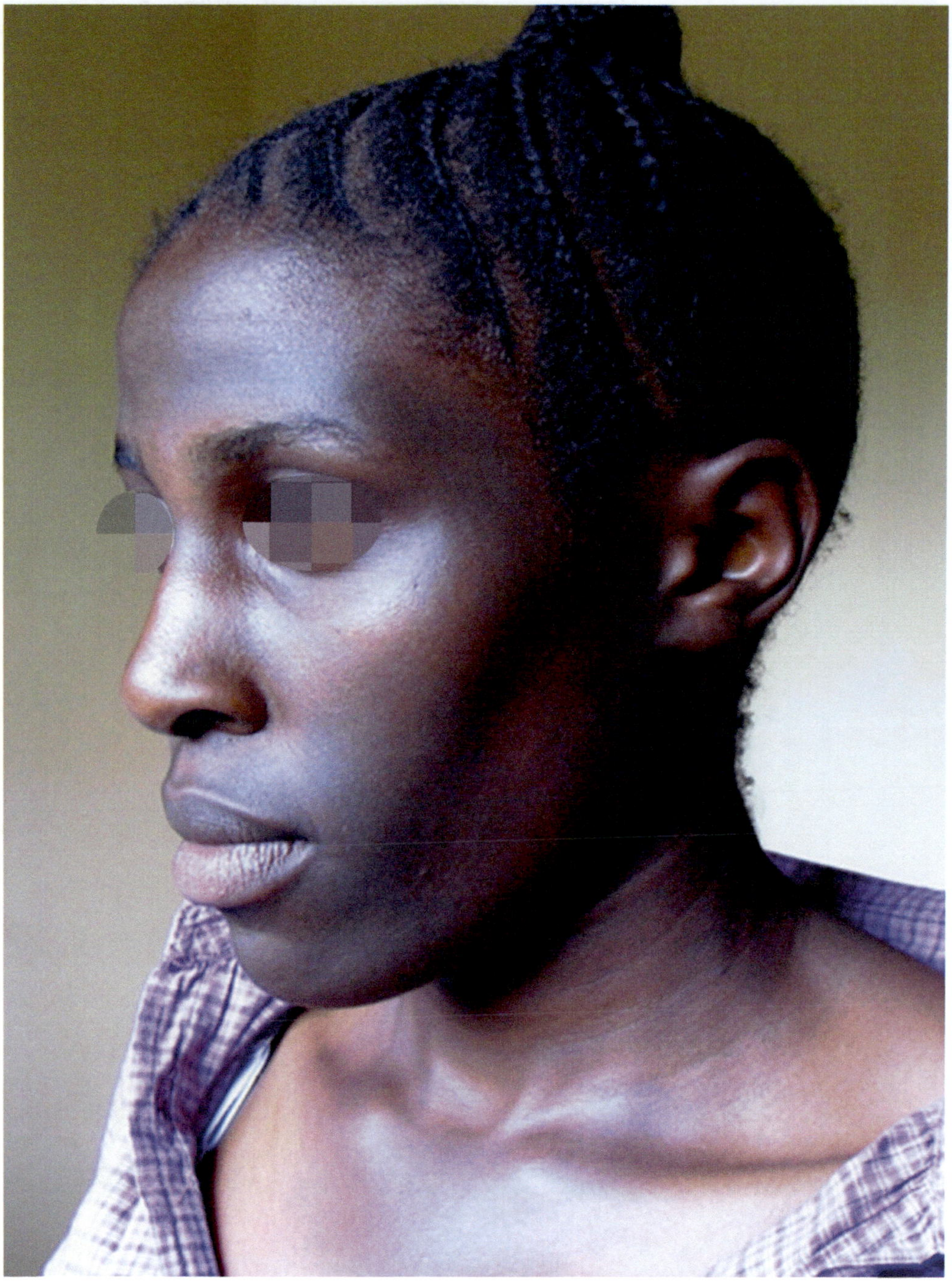

Fig. 26.6 *Drug-induced melanosis* of the face and neck, most likely due to oral intake of doxycycline (courtesy CEO)

ending in a V-pattern) and H (perioral area) are more common than G (temporo-zygomatic area ending in a W-pattern); different combinations thereof have been observed. Clinically, the lesions have a diffuse, light to dark gray, or slate gray to brownish color. Their margins are sharp at some areas and blurred in others, often developing freckles on the surface [23].

Periorbital melanosis is possibly an idiopathic variant, since types F and G often extend around the eyes (Fig. 26.7). Other causes of periorbital pigmentation include visible venules, shadowing from wrinkles, deep tear trough, or overhanging tarsal muscle, postinflammatory hyperpigmentation due to atopic or contact dermatitis, or edema. A mixture of the different types is often encountered [24].

Besides, *maturational dyschromia* appears as a diffuse darkening on the lateral forehead and cheekbones of elderly people. It results from chronic sun exposure and is a troubling condition [14].

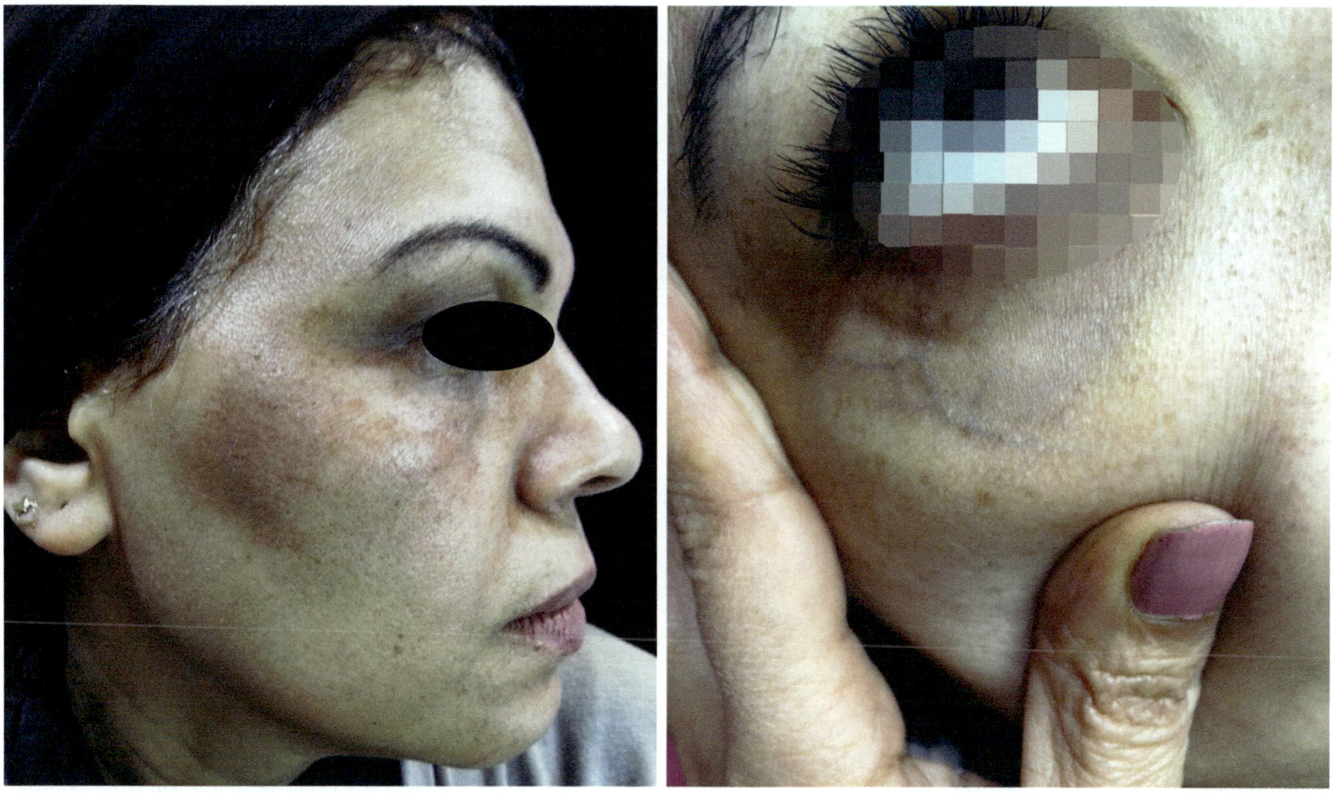

Fig. 26.7 *Idiopathic periorbital melanosis* with infraorbital pigment demarcation line F (left), vascular type infra-orbital pigmentation, by stretching the skin, the vessels become more prominent (right)

26.4 Other Causes of Facial Hyperpigmentation

Seborrheic keratoses are considered among the signs of aging in dark-skinned people [25]. *Solar lentigines* are often encountered with seborrhoeic keratoses and seem to be related. They are regarded as clinical signs of photoaging, and their number and size increase with age. *Dermatosis papulosa nigra* is a variant of seborrhoeic keratosis, often seen on the cheeks and temples of dark-skinned individuals. It appears as multiple, hyperpigmented, sessile, smooth-surfaced 1–5 mm papules [26].

Pellagra results from niacin deficiency, due either to decreased intake or to metabolic interferences (alcoholism, drugs, *Hartnup* disease). The condition is generally rare but is occasionally encountered in developing countries exposed to prolonged war or famine [27]. Clinically it presents as a phototoxic reaction especially on the neck (Casal's necklace) and the dorsa of the upper and lower limbs. In addition, mucositis and painful fissures of the palms and soles are observed [28].

Exogenous ochronosis is a paradoxical hyperpigmentation of the skin after prolonged use of hydroquinone-containing bleaching creams, especially when used in high concentrations (≥4%). It appears in a diffuse macular pattern in sun-exposed areas, often around the eyes. In histopathology banana-shaped yellow deposits are found in the dermis. The condition is frustrating to the patient and to the physicians treating melasma and other facial hyperpigmentations [29].

Argyria is a rare condition due to the ingestion of silver compounds. Silver salt deposits occur in the skin, nails, and mucous membranes, leading to blue or blue-gray uniform pigmentation, especially in the face and other sun-exposed areas [30]. Localized argyria usually develops by accidental exposure to silver compounds such as jewelers, local disinfectants, manufacturers among others [31].

26.5 Treatment

Treatment protocols of different hyperpigmentary disorders depend on the cause and site of pigment present. Epidermal hyperpigmentation responds to bleaching creams, peeling, fractional ablative and non-ablative lasers, or intense pulsed light (Table 26.1). Dermal hyperpigmentation is more difficult to treat; Q-switched lasers, which reach the dermis, should be considered. Sun avoidance, sun protection (caps, umbrella), and sunscreens against UVA and UVB are essential in all cases. Treating the underlying condition helps to stop the progress of the disease and may lead to decreased pigmentation. When using topical and oral therapies, the

Table 26.1 Overview of modalities for treating facial hyperpigmentation

Suppression of melanogenesis	Removal of pigmentation
Inhibition of melanin synthesis Hydroquinone Azelaic acid Kojic acid Ascorbic acid Retinoids, among others *Preparations recently used:* Dioic acid, *N*-acetyl glucosamine, Tranexamic acid, metformin, oligopeptides Mulberry extracts, resveratrol, Silymarin, other botanicals	*Peeling* Glycolic acid, Trichloroacetic acid (TCA) among others *Q-switched Lasers* Ruby (694 nm), alexandrite (755 nm) Nd-YAG* (1064 nm), Frequency-doubled Nd-YAG (532 nm) *Ablative lasers* CO_2 (10,600 nm), erbium (2940 nm) *Fractional lasers* Fractional non-ablative Fractional ablative (CO_2 and erbium) Fractional Q-switched ruby laser *Pulsed dye laser* (585 and 595 nm)
Inhibition of melanin transfer: Niacinamide, soy	*Intense pulsed light*
Treatment of facial hyperpigmentation due to clinical entities: *Lichen pigmentosus*: Topical corticosteroids or calcineurin inhibitors; oral antimalarials, low-dose isotretinoin, dapsone *Erythema dyschromicum*: Topical corticosteroids or calcineurin inhibitors; oral corticosteroids, clofazimine, dapsone, antimalarials, or narrow-band UVB *Erythromelanosis*: Topical keratolytics (salicylic acid), retinoids alone or with hydroquinone, and other bleaching agents *Acanthosis nigricans*: Oral metformin, topical keratolytics, urea, calcipotriol, bleaching agents *Pellagra:* Supplementation of niacin	

duration of treatment usually takes 12 weeks to show results. With energy-based devices (lasers and IPL), it requires multiple sessions spaced 2, 4, or 8 weeks apart, according to different regimens [1]. *Idiopathic facial pigmentation* and *erythromelanosis follicularis* tend to show temporary response to treatment [2]. Deeply localized nevi of Ota require up to ten sessions of Q-switched laser to show a cosmetically acceptable response [18].

Conclusions

Facial pigmentary disorders are a heterogeneous group of conditions often seen in populations with heavily pigmented skin. Many of the described conditions show considerable overlap and await consensus in their diagnosis. Treatments with bleaching agents, chemical peelings, and energy-based devices should be cautiously applied in patients with skin of color, since these tools incite some kind of inflammation that often leads to postinflammatory hyperpigmentation. Patients must be warned to keep away from the sun; use protective clothing and sunscreen creams of high protection factors to avoid any stimulation of melanin synthesis. In conditions like melasma, a tinted sunscreen is recommended, since visible light lead to increased pigmentation.

References

1. Chang MW. Disorders of hyperpigmentation. Chapter 67. In: Bolognia JL, Jorizzo JL, Schaffer JV, editors. Dermatology. 3rd ed. Amsterdam: Elsevier; 2012. p. 1049–74.
2. Khanna N, Rasool S. Facial melanoses: Indian perspective. Indian J Dermatol Venereol Leprol. 2011;77:552–63.
3. Kang WH, Yoon KH, Lee ES, et al. Melasma: histopathological characteristics in 56 Korean patients. Br J Dermatol. 2002;146:228–37.
4. Ortonne JP, Arellano I, Berneburg M, et al. A global survey of the role of ultraviolet radiation and hormonal influences in the development of melasma. J Eur Acad Dermatol Venereol. 2009;23:1254–62.
5. Duteil L, Cardot-Leccia N, Queille-Roussel C, et al. Differences in visible light induced-pigmentation according to wavelengths: a clinical and histological study in comparison with UVB exposure. Pigment Cell Melanoma Res. 2014;27:822–6.
6. Pandya AG, Hynan LS, Bhore R, et al. Reliability assessment and validation of the Melasma Area and Severity Index (MASI) and a new modified MASI scoring method. J Am Acad Dermatol. 2011;64:78–83.
7. Kanwar AJ, Dogra S, Handa S, et al. A study of 124 Indian patients with lichen planus pigmentosus. Clin Exp Dermatol. 2003;28:481–5.
8. Ghosh A, Coondoo A. Lichen planus pigmentosus: the controversial consensus. Indian J Dermatol. 2016;6:482–6.
9. Pirmez R, Duque-Estrada B, Donati A, et al. Clinical and dermoscopic features of lichen planus pigmentosus in 37 patients with frontal fibrosing alopecia. Br J Dermatol. 2016;175:1387–90.
10. Al-Mutairi N, El-Khalawany M. Clinicopathological characteristics of lichen planus pigmentosus and its response to tacrolimus ointment: an open label, non-randomized, prospective study. J Eur Acad Dermatol Venereol. 2010;24:535–40.
11. Nakayama H. Pigmented contact dermatitis and chemical depigmentation. In: Rycroft R, Menne T, Frosch P, Lepoittevin J, editors. Textbook of contact dermatitis. 3rd ed. New York: Springer; 2001. p. 319–33.
12. Tienthavorn T, Tresukosol P, Sudtikoonaseth P. Patch testing and histopathology in Thai patients with hyperpigmentation due to erythema dyschromicum perstans, lichen planus pigmentosus, and pigmented contact dermatitis. Asian Pac J Allergy Immunol. 2014;32:185–92.
13. Chang SE, Kim HW, Shin JM, et al. Clinical and histological aspect of erythema dyschromicum perstans in Korea: a review of 68 cases. J Dermatol. 2015;42:1053–7.
14. Vashi NA, Kundu RV. Facial hyperpigmentation: causes and treatment. Br J Dermatol. 2013;169(suppl 3):41–56.
15. Rabinovitz HS, Barnhill R. Benign melanocytic neoplasms. Chapter 115. In: Bolognia JL, Jorizzo JL, Schaffer JV, editors. Dermatology. 3rd ed. Amsterdam: Elsevier; 2012. p. 1851–80.
16. Rather S, Yaseen A, Mukhija M. Erythromelanosis follicularis faciei et colli—a cross-sectional, descriptive study. Indian J Dermatol. 2016;61:308–13.
17. Augustine M, Jayaseelan E. Erythromelanosis follicularis faciei et colli: relationship with keratosis pilaris. Indian J Dermatol Venereol Leprol. 2008;74:47–9.

18. Nouveau S, Agrawal D, Kohli M, et al. Skin hyperpigmentation in indian population: insights and best practice. Indian J Dermatol. 2016;61:487–95.
19. Davis EC, Callender VD. Postinflammatory hyperpigmentation: a review of the epidemiology, clinical features, and treatment options in skin of color. J Clin Aesthet Dermatol. 2010;3:20–31.
20. Lacz NL, Vafaie J, Kihiczak NI, et al. Postinflammatory hyperpigmentation: a common but troubling condition. Int J Dermatol. 2004;43:362–5.
21. Kutlubay Z, Sevim A, Engin B, et al. Photodermatoses, including phototoxic and photoallergic reactions (internal and external). Clin Dermatol. 2014;32:73–9.
22. Malakar S, Dhar S. Pigmentary demarcation lines over the face. Dermatology. 2000;200:85–6.
23. Somani VK, Razvi F, Sita VV. Pigmentary demarcation lines over the face. Indian J Dermatol Venereol Leprol. 2004;70:336–41.
24. Roh MR, Chung KY. Infraorbital dark circles: definition, causes, and treatment options. Dermatol Surg. 2009;35:1163–71.
25. Rajesh G, Thappa DM, Jaisankar TJ, et al. Spectrum of seborrheic keratoses in south Indians: a clinical and dermoscopic study. Indian J Dermatol Venereol Leprol. 2011;77:483–8.
26. Niang SO, Kane A, Diallo M, et al. Dermatosis papulosa nigra in Dakar, Senegal. Int J Dermatol. 2007;46(suppl 1):45–7.
27. Seal AJ, Creeke PI, Dibari F, et al. Low and deficient niacin status and pellagra are endemic in postwar Angola. Am J Clin Nutr. 2007;85:218–24.
28. Wan P, Moat S, Anstey A. Pellagra: a review with emphasis on photosensitivity. Br J Dermatol. 2011;164:1188–200.
29. Levin CY, Maibach H. Exogenous ochronosis: an update on clinical features, causative agents and treatment options. Am J Clin Dermatol. 2001;2:213–7.
30. Molina-Hernandez AI, Diaz-Gonzalez JM, Saeb-Lima M, et al. Argyria after silver nitrate intake: case report and brief review of literature. Indian J Dermatol. 2015;60:520.
31. García-Martínez P, López Aventín D, Segura S, et al. In vivo reflectance confocal microscopy characterization of silver deposits in localized cutaneous argyria. Br J Dermatol. 2016;175:1052–5.

Erythema Multiforme and Stevens-Johnson Syndrome

27

Mohamed Badawy Abdel-Naser

Erythema multiforme (EM) is an acute, self-limited, occasionally recurring skin disease considered to be a type IV hypersensitivity reaction to certain infections, medications, and other triggering factors. The skin disease may present within a wide spectrum of severity: *EM minor* is characterized by pathognomonic target- or iris-like cutaneous lesions with minimal or no mucosal involvement, whereas *EM major* shows extensive involvement of the mucosal membranes and frequently systemic symptoms. The timely affection of skin and mucous membranes in EM has created confusion with other severe dermatoses, such as *Stevens-Johnson syndrome* (SJS) and *toxic epidermal necrolysis* (TEN). In recent years, evidence has been provided that EM major and SJS/TEN are separate entities clinically manifested with similar cutaneous and mucosal involvement differing not only in severity but also in several demographic characteristics and causes [1, 2].

27.1 Erythema Multiforme (Minor/Major)

27.1.1 Epidemiology/Etiology

Erythema multiforme is rather uncommon, particularly in pigmented skin. It affects all ages, predominantly young adults without racial predilection. Several causes have been implicated in the etiology of the disease: in nearly 90% of the cases, an underlying infection with herpes simplex virus types I and II is found as an antigen triggering factor [3, 4], less often an infection with mycoplasma pneumonia, mostly in children [5]. Other infections such as EBV, CMV, HCV virus, influenza virus among others have been also registered. Occasionally drug-induced EM occurs, precipitated by nonsteroidal anti-inflammatory drugs (NSAIDs), sulfonamides, antiepileptics, and antibiotics [6, 7]. Recurrent or persistent EM has been also reported in patients with hematologic and solid organ malignancies.

M. B. Abdel-Naser
Department of Dermatology and Venereology,
Ain Shams University, Cairo, Egypt

27.1.2 Pathogenesis

Genetic susceptibility can be a predisposing factor for the disease [8]. However, it is not known why only a small proportion of patients with recurrent HSV infection develops EM. Incomplete fragmentation of viral DNA by phagocytic cells, increased number of CD34+ cells and abnormal response to *pol* protein, or a combination of these factors has been proposed as a cause [4]. Epithelial cell expression of viral DNA fragments that have been transported by circulating macrophages and CD34+ Langerhans cell progenitors recruits helper T cells that release effector cytokines; both are responsible for the epithelial damage and the dermal perivascular infiltrate. In drug-induced EM, epithelial damage is caused by cytotoxic T cells, TNF-α, perforin, and granzyme B [4, 9].

EM classically develops 9–14 days after first exposure to the infectious agent or the offending drug. On subsequent challenge, the cutaneous reaction occurs within several hours to 1–2 days [8].

27.1.3 Clinical Picture

As a rule, *EM minor* shows clinically edematous papules intermingled with typical target lesions disseminated over the trunk and the extremities; in *EM major* the skin lesions and their distribution are similar, but one or more mucous membranes with epidermal detachment are also involved. History of previous or current infection, in most cases of viral origin, prodromi or use of medications within 2 months before onset may be helpful for diagnosis in both types, but they often lack in the *minor* type of the disease. The onset of the rash is abrupt; it fully develops within 3 days on the extremities with centripetal spreading. On examination, initial lesions are purpuric macules, or urticarial

C. E. Orfanos et al. (eds.), *Pigmented Ethnic Skin and Imported Dermatoses*, https://doi.org/10.1007/978-3-319-69422-1_27

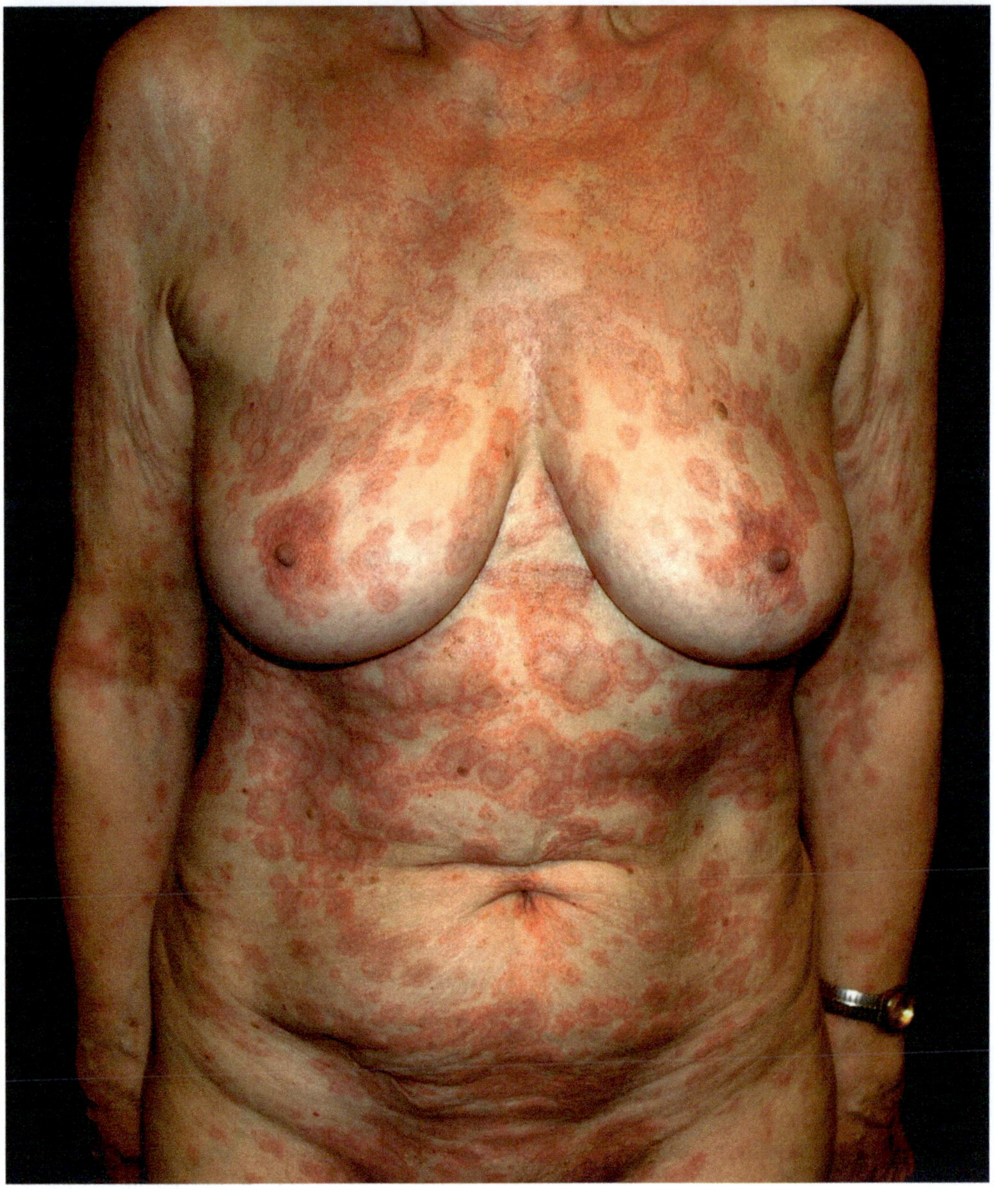

Fig. 27.1 *Erythema multiforme minor* disseminated on the trunk and the upper extremities without mucosal involvement (courtesy of Department of Dermatology and Venereology, HELIOS Klinikum Krefeld; photo ChA)

papules are seen on the trunk and the upper extremities that expand to a maximum of 2 cm over 24–48 h, often developing vesicles or bullae in their center (Fig. 27.1). The periphery gradually changes to become cyanotic or violaceous forming a typical concentric, target or iris lesion, as the hallmark of the disease (Fig. 27.2). Polycyclic or arcuate forms may occur. Pruritus or burning sensation is occasionally reported [6]. In pigmented or black skin, vesicle or bulla formation may predominate, and the color characteristics of the lesion are not easy to recognize. The palms, neck, and face are frequently involved; lesions of the soles and flexural aspects of the extremities are less common. A zosteriform distribution may be present. Koebner phenomenon may be observed but the Nikolsky's sign is negative. Although EM does not lead to scarring, postinflammatory hyperpigmentation may persist after disease resolution, particularly in patients with pigmented skin.

In *EM major* 50% of the patients experience influenza-like prodromi that precede the rash by 1 or 2 weeks. The skin lesions are usually more prominent, and the involvement of the oral mucosa is more severe, causing difficulties to open the mouth, eat, or drink. Conjunctival involvement may cause lacrimation, photophobia, burning eyes, or visual impairment. Genital lesions are painful and may lead to urinary retention. Shortness of breath or difficulty in breathing may occur due to tracheobronchial epithelial involvement. *Recurrent* or *persistent EM* is a rare variant showing repeated or continuing development of widespread typical and atypical EM lesions, with or without mucosal affection. Associations with various viral infections, inflammatory bowel disease, and internal neoplasms have been reported [8]. *Oral EM* is another unique subset which affects mainly the oral mucosa in which the lips and portions of the oral

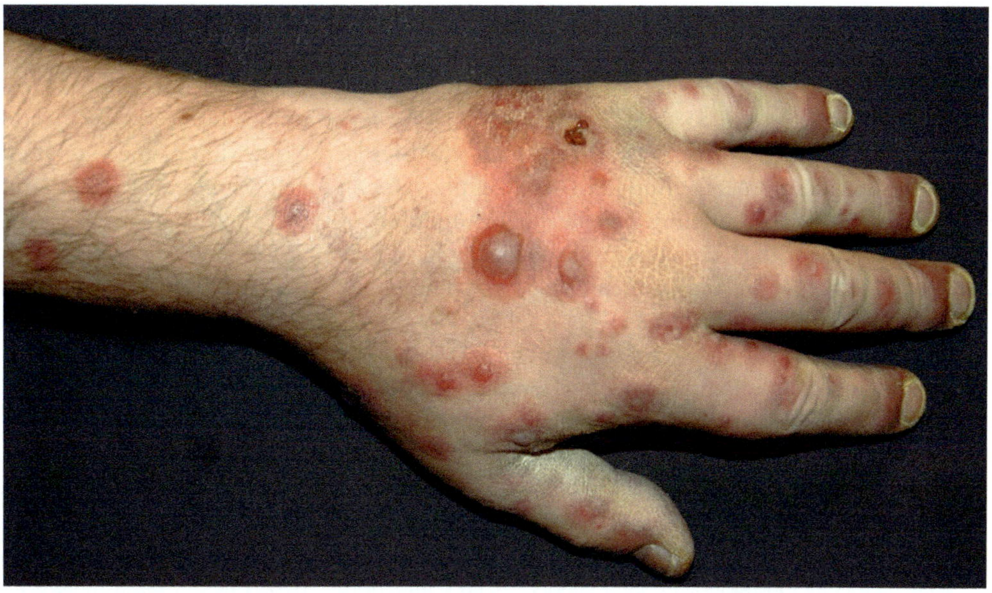

Fig. 27.2 Characteristic target lesion in *erythema multiforme major* with acral bulla formation

cavity are involved. The tongue, gingiva, and buccal mucosa are usually severely affected.

Diagnosis of EM is based on clinical findings as no specific tests are available. Histopathology and direct immunofluorescence of cutaneous and mucosal EM are similar but nonspecific; they can be useful in ruling out differential diagnoses, when necessary. Biopsies reveal a vacuolar interface dermatitis showing lymphocytic infiltrate along the dermoepidermal junction with hydropic degeneration and dyskeratosis of the basal keratinocytes; perivascular lymphocytic infiltrates are sparse. Serum antinuclear antibody tests may be helpful in cases in which cutaneous lupus erythematosus is suspected (*Rowell's syndrome*, *urticarial vasculitis*). Patients with idiopathic recurrent or persistent EM and oral EM require selected laboratory testing to rule out underlying infections and other inflammatory, autoimmune, or malignant disorders.

27.1.4 Management

Mild asymptomatic EM cases do not require treatment. Oral antihistamines and topical steroids in addition to analgesics, local skin care, and soothing mouthwashes (e.g., oral rinsing with warm saline or solutions of diphenhydramine, xylocaine, etc.) can be used to provide relief. The use of liquid antiseptics (0.05% chlorhexidine) during bathing helps to prevent superinfection. Local supportive care for eye involvement is important including topical lubricants for dry eyes, sweeping of conjunctival fornices, and removal of fresh adhesions. In such cases, an ophthalmologist should be consulted. In patients with coexisting or recent HSV infection, early treatment with oral acyclovir may lessen the number and duration of cutaneous lesions [10, 11]. The use of prednisolone 40–80 mg/day for 1–2 weeks is controversial. Continuous oral acyclovir 400 mg 2×/day is effective in suppressing recurrent EM even if HSV is not an obvious precipitating factor [3, 11]. Valaciclovir 500–1000 mg/day and famciclovir 125–250 mg/day have greater oral bioavailability and can be tried as an alternative. The dosage of the antiviral may be reduced or discontinued once the patient is recurrence-free for 4 months [12]. Several other medications have been tried in patients with recurrent EM, such as dapsone, antimalarials, azathioprine, cyclosporine, thalidomide among others. Although these medications have shown benefit in some patients, the evidence to support their use is limited.

27.2 Stevens-Johnson Syndrome/Toxic Epidermal Necrolysis (SJS/TEN)

Stevens-Johnson syndrome and *toxic epidermal necrolysis* (SJS/TEN) are clinical manifestations of a single entity characterized by severe muco-epidermolytic reaction, differing from EM major in the extent of its skin involvement and its unfavorable prognosis. The mucosal involvement is prominent. SJS is mostly drug-induced, involving <10% of the total body surface area, whereas TEN seems exclusively drug-induced, involving >30%. SJS may overlap with TEN in some cases [13].

27.2.1 Epidemiology/Etiology

SJS/TEN is a rare condition, accounting for an incidence rate of 1.2–6/million and a mortality rate of 1–5% for SJS and incidence of 0.4–1.2/million and mortality rate of 25–30% for TEN. SJS/TEN affects all ages and races [13, 14]. In an Asian population, anticonvulsants, especially carbamazepine, were the most frequently implicated drugs, followed by antibiotics, and NSAIDs [15], whereas, in a teaching hospital in Lomé, Togo, nevirapine was highlighted as a major cause in 89 patients [16]. Saka et al. (2013) collected and evaluated 177 cases with SJS/TEN from four countries in sub-Saharan Africa (Benin, Burkina Faso, Central African Republic, and Togo), pointing out the high proportion of patients infected with HIV; in this group antibacterial sulfonamides, nevirapine, and antituberculosis drugs were identified as frequent SJS/TEN causes [17].

TEN is one of the most serious and often lethal bullous drug reactions. As notorious drugs to cause TEN in Caucasians were allopurinol, carbamazepine, lamotrigine, nevirapine, oxicam NSAIDs, phenobarbital, phenytoin, sulfamethoxazole, and other sulfur antibiotics and sulfasalazine [18]. In African populations, antimalarials and antiretroviral drugs are often the cause.

Risk factors include slow acetylator genotypes, HIV infection, lymphoma, and patients with brain tumors who are undergoing concomitant radiotherapy and treatment with antiepileptics.

27.2.2 Pathogenesis

Predisposed individuals develop a specific immune response to the culprit drug or its metabolite which results in a strong expression of the cytolytic molecule FasL on keratinocytes and secretion of granulysin from cytotoxic T cells and NK cells and annexin A1 from monocytes. This induces FasL- and granulysin-mediated apoptosis and/or annexin-dependent necroptosis of keratinocytes with subsequent epidermal cell death and detachment.

27.2.3 Clinical Picture

SJS is characterized by epidermal detachment with extensive bulla formation and profound erosive mucosal lesions similar to but worse than those in EM major. The skin lesions present only two zones of color: a central, dusky purpura or a central bulla with a surrounding macular erythema, often not seen in heavily pigmented or black skin (Figs. 27.3 and 27.4). The mucosal

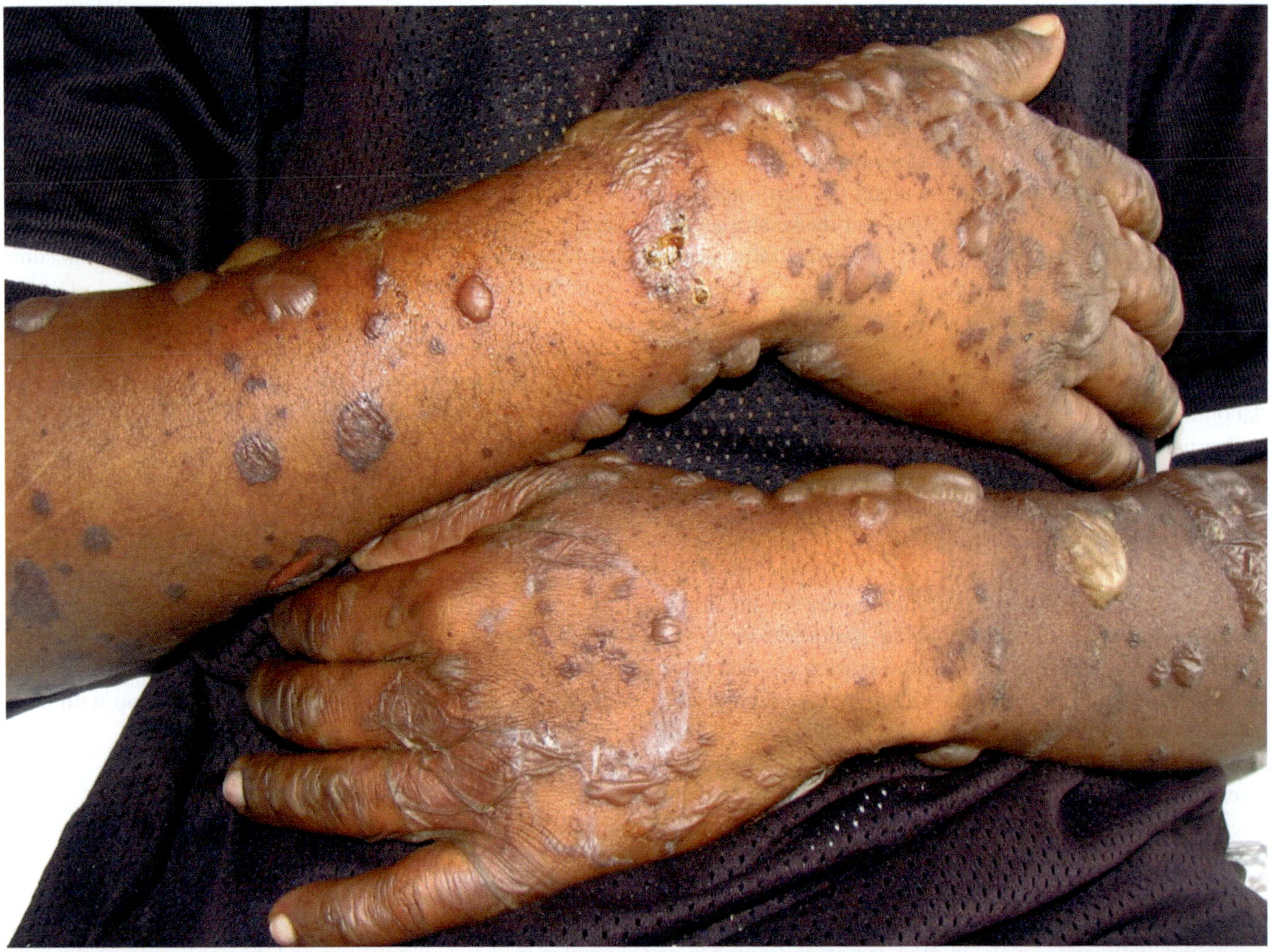

Fig. 27.3 *Stevens-Johnson syndrome* with typical lesions and multiple blister formation on the dorsal aspect of the arms and hands of a young man with pigmented skin (Tanzania); third day after onset, most likely caused by oral intake of antimalarials

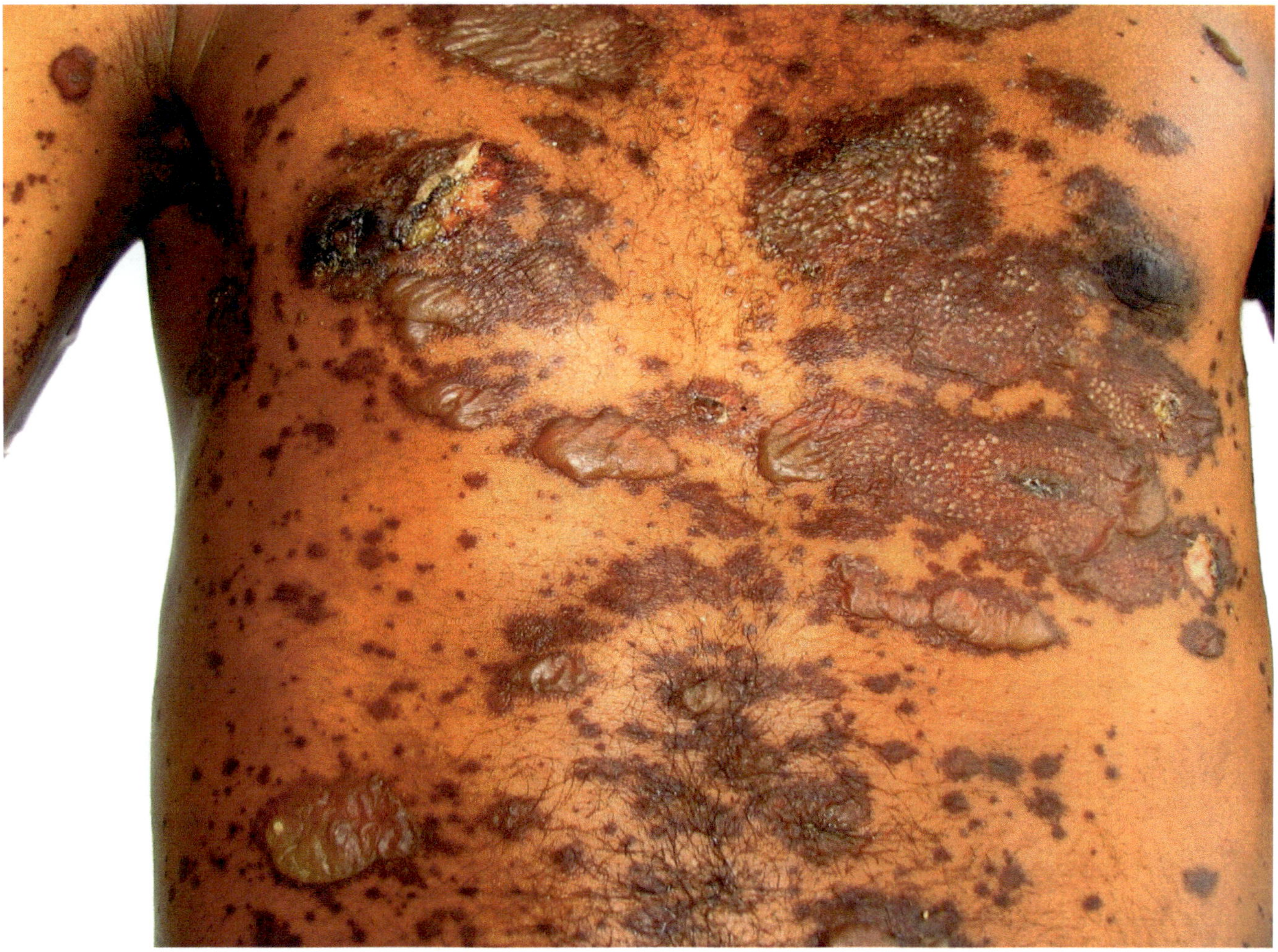

Fig. 27.4 Widespread lesions on the trunk showing purpuric target-like lesions and extensive blister formation in *Stevens-Johnson syndrome* in pigmented skin

involvement is prominent, including stomatitis, conjunctivitis, or affection of other mucosal areas (Fig. 27.5). At confluence, the initial purpuriform maculae show a positive Nikolsky's sign. Other manifestations are fever and involvement of at least one internal organ, such as the liver, kidney, or gastrointestinal tract. Genetic susceptibility has been reported [13].

The disease starts with painful erythema that develops into tense blisters rapidly extending. The affection of the mucous membranes is prominent and debilitating. Oral erosions are painful, manifested by severe crusting of the lips, increased salivation, and impaired alimentation. Other mucous membranes, such as the oropharynx, tracheobronchial tree, esophagus, gastrointestinal tract, genitalia, and anus, express symptoms related to these particular sites. The conjunctivae are erythematous and painful, and the lids are edematous and often stuck together. Adhesions between the eroded conjunctiva and eyelids may occur, and keratitis, corneal erosions, and a sicca-like syndrome may develop [19]. After healing postinflammatory hypo- and hyperpigmentations are seen.

27.2.4 Management

The fatal nature of SJS/TEN requires early transfer to an intensive care or a burn unit, coupled with early withdrawal of any offending drug, and followed by prompt supportive management with fluid and electrolyte balance adjustment. Drug elimination might be enhanced by using plasmapheresis and *N*-acetylcysteine. Meta-analysis studies supported a significant benefit of i.v. immunoglobulin [20] at doses greater than 2 g/kg; [13, 14] several centers have incorporated this schedule into their treatment protocols. Combination with other modalities, such as pulse therapies with corticosteroids, has shown better results; [20, 21] however, the use of systemic steroids in SJS/TEN is controversial when considering the risk of gram-negative sepsis [22]. Most authors do not recommend indiscriminate use of steroids in the management of TEN.

Cyclosporine may induce fast cessation of blister formation and rapid reepithelialization in TEN (3–5 mg/kg/day every 12 h for 8–24 days). The tendency to develop sepsis is

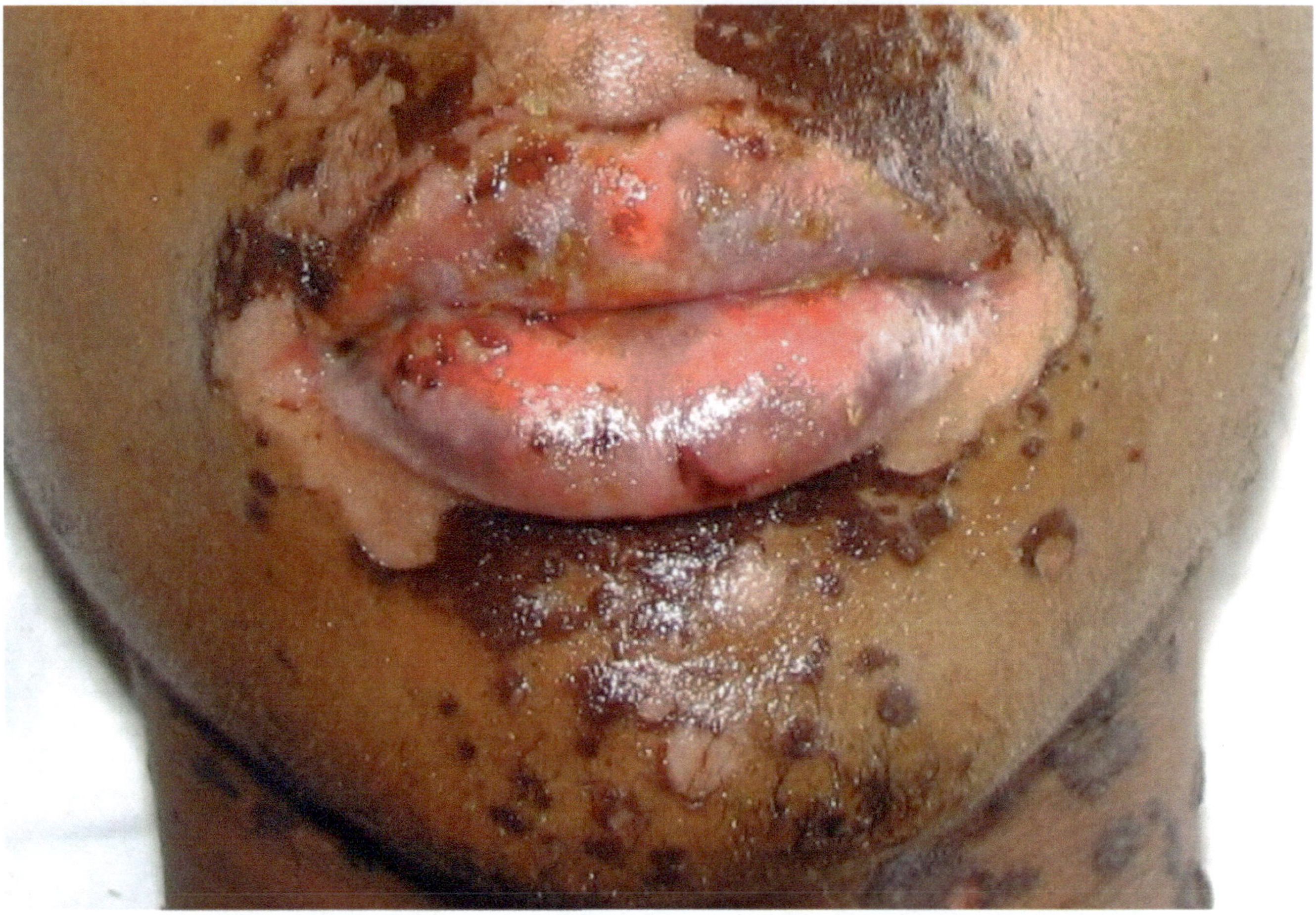

Fig. 27.5 Perioral and lesions of the lip mucosa in *Stevens-Johnson syndrome*

the main concern of its use. In comparison with a series of historical controls, cyclosporine treatment was found more effective [23]. For other medications implemented in the treatment of TEN such as cyclophosphamide and etanercept [24], additional data are required. Denuded skin and wounds should be treated conservatively; blistered skin acts as a natural biological dressing which likely favors reepithelialization. Nonadhesive wound dressings are used where required. Nanocrystalline silver dressings showed satisfactory results due to the ease of application, antimicrobial properties, and low frequency of change [25].

References

1. Bastuji-Garin S, Rzany B, Stern RS, et al. Clinical classification of cases of toxic epidermal necrolysis, Stevens-Johnson syndrome, and erythema multiforme. Arch Dermatol. 1993;129:92–6.
2. Auquier-Dunant A, Mockenhaupt M, Naldi L, et al. Correlations between clinical patterns and causes of erythema multiforme majus, Stevens-Johnson syndrome, and toxic epidermal necrolysis: results of an international prospective study. Arch Dermatol. 2002;138:1019–24.
3. Huff JC. Erythema multiforme and latent herpes simplex infection. Semin Dermatol. 1992;11:207–10.
4. Aurelian L, Ono F, Burnett J. Herpes simplex virus (HSV)-associated erythema multiforme (HAEM): a viral disease with an autoimmune component. Dermatol Online J. 2003;9:1.
5. Langley A, Anooshiravani N, Kwan S, et al. Erythema multiforme in children and Mycoplasma pneumoniae aetiology. J Cutan Med Surg. 2016;20:453–7.
6. Huff JC. Erythema multiforme. Dermatol Clin. 1985;3:141–52.
7. Joseph TI, Vargheese G, George D, et al. Drug induced oral erythema multiforme: a rare and less recognized variant of erythema multiforme. J Oral Maxillofac Pathol. 2012;16:14514–8.
8. Sokumbi O, Wetter DA. Clinical features, diagnosis, and treatment of erythema multiforme: a review for the practicing dermatologist. Int J Dermatol. 2012;51:889–902.
9. Kokuba H, Aurelian L, Burnett J. Herpes simplex virus associated erythema multiforme (HAEM) is mechanistically distinct from drug-induced erythema multiforme: interferon-gamma is expressed in HAEM lesions and tumor necrosis factor-alpha in drug-induced erythema multiforme lesions. J Invest Dermatol. 1999;113:808–15.
10. Lemak MA, Duvic M, Bean SF. Oral acyclovir for the prevention of herpes-associated erythema multiforme. J Am Acad Dermatol. 1986;15:50–4.

11. Tatnall FM, Schofield JK, Leigh IM. A double-blind, placebo-controlled trial of continuous acyclovir therapy in recurrent erythema multiforme. Br J Dermatol. 1995;132:267–70.
12. Kerob D, Assier-Bonnet H, Esnault-Gelly P, et al. Recurrent erythema multiforme unresponsive to acyclovir prophylaxis and responsive to valacyclovir continuous therapy. Arch Dermatol. 1998;134:876–7.
13. Harr T, French LE. Toxic epidermal necrolysis and Stevens-Johnson syndrome. Orphanet J Rare Dis. 2010;5:39. https://doi.org/10.1186/1750-1172-5-39.
14. Creamer D, Walsh SA, Dziewulski P, et al. UK guidelines for the management of Stevens-Johnson syndrome/toxic epidermal necrolysis in adults 2016. J Plast Reconstr Aesthet Surg. 2016;69: e119–53.
15. Tan SK, Tay YK. Profile and pattern of Stevens-Johnson syndrome and toxic epidermal necrolysis in a general hospital in Singapore: treatment outcomes. Acta Derm Venereol. 2012;92:62–6.
16. Saka B, Kombaté K, Mouhari-Toure A, et al. Stevens-Johnson syndrome and toxic epidermal necrolysis in a teaching hospital in Lomé, Togo: retrospective study of 89 cases. Med Trop (Mars). 2010;70:255–8.
17. Saka B, Barro-Traoré F, Atadokpédé FA, et al. Stevens-Johnson syndrome and toxic epidermal necrolysis in sub-Saharan Africa: a multicentric study in four countries. Int J Dermatol. 2013;52:575–9.
18. Mockenhaupt M, Viboud C, Dunant A, et al. Stevens-Johnson syndrome and toxic epidermal necrolysis: assessment of medication risks with emphasis on recently marketed drugs. The EuroSCARstudy. J Invest Dermatol. 2008;128:35–44.
19. Yip LW, Thong BY, Lim J, et al. Ocular manifestations and complications of Stevens-Johnson syndrome and toxic epidermal necrolysis: an Asian series. Allergy. 2007;62:527–31.
20. Lissia M, Figus A, Rubino C. Intravenous immunoglobulins and plasmapheresis combined treatment in patients with severe toxic epidermal necrolysis: preliminary report. Br J Plast Surg. 2005;58:504–10.
21. Yamane Y, Matsukura S, Watanabe Y, et al. Retrospective analysis of Stevens-Johnson syndrome and toxic epidermal necrolysis in 87 Japanese patients—treatment and outcome. Allergol Int. 2016;65:74–81.
22. Hirahara K, Kano Y, Sato Y, et al. Methylprednisolone pulse therapy for Stevens-Johnson syndrome/toxic epidermal necrolysis: clinical evaluation and analysis of biomarkers. J Am Acad Dermatol. 2013;69:496–8.
23. Valeyrie-Allanore L, Wolkenstein P, Brochard L, et al. Open trial of ciclosporin treatment for Stevens-Johnson syndrome and toxic epidermal necrolysis. Br J Dermatol. 2010;163:847–53.
24. Paradisi A, Abeni D, Bergamo F, et al. Etanercept therapy for toxic epidermal necrolysis. J Am Acad Dermatol. 2014;71:278–83.
25. Smith SD, Dodds A, Dixit S, et al. Role of nanocrystalline silver dressings in the management of toxic epidermal necrolysis (TEN) and TEN/Stevens-Johnson syndrome overlap. Australas J Dermatol. 2015;56:298–302.

28 Bullous Diseases in Dark Skin

Anes Yang, Emily K. Kozera, and Dédée F. Murrell

Blisters are commonly caused by injuries, in particular by burns or specific skin irritation, and heal relatively rapidly without leaving scars. However, a series of autoimmune disorders affecting the skin and the mucous membranes initiate the formation of antibodies against adhesion proteins in skin and mucosal membranes causing chronic and consistent blistering, occasionally leading to scars. The presence of autoantibodies in tissue is visible by direct immunofluorescence (DIF), and circulating autoantibodies may also occur and be detected. Several clinical entities characterized by bulla formation may then arise and also overlap (Table 28.1). The management of these bullous disorders is difficult, and, if left untreated, life-threatening conditions may result.

The geographic distribution of bullous skin diseases is mostly variable; some of them are more common in Caucasians, and some others are frequent in populations with dark skin, being overrepresented in certain geographic areas. *Pemphigus vulgaris* is more common in India and Southeast Asia than in other geographic regions, whereas the second major pemphigus subtype, *pemphigus foliaceus*, has high prevalence in South America and is endemic in Brazil. This condition is more often diagnosed in dark-skinned populations than in Caucasians. Also *linear IgA dermatosis* appears more prevalent in North Africa. No clear evidence for skin color or ethnic predilection exists for *bullous pemphigoid, Hailey-Hailey disease*, and *mucous membrane pemphigoid*. Overall, it seems likely that genetic and environmental factors significantly contribute governing the autoimmune pathogenesis of blistering skin diseases.

A. Yang (✉) · E. K. Kozera · D. F. Murrell
Department of Dermatology, St. George Hospital, University of South Wales, Sydney, NSW, Australia
e-mail: Anes.Yang@unsw.edu.au; e.kozera@unsw.edu.au; D.Murrell@unsw.edu.au

28.1 Pemphigus Vulgaris

Pemphigus vulgaris (PV) is an autoimmune blistering skin disease characterized by acantholysis that results in development of intraepidermal and intraepithelial blisters in the skin and erosions on mucous membranes. PV has an incidence of around 1/100,000 people [1]. In white-skinned populations, PV affects preferably Jewish or Mediterranean descendants [2]; however, the prevalence of PV is higher in populations with dark skin. In the Arab world from the Middle East to the countries in North Africa, possibly also in Sudan and East Africa, both major pemphigus subtypes (vulgaris and foliaceus) are rather common, showing considerable variations in their frequencies [3]. Among the Asian countries, PV is reportedly the most common bullous disease in Malaysia [4], whereas in a clinic-based survey, 4.4 million people were assessed to have some clinical variant of pemphigus in Kerala, India. The large majority had PV, which is the most common bullous disease among the Indian population [5]. More than half of the patients diagnosed with PV were under the age of 40; this is in contrast to data from western studies where PV tends to occur in an older age group. Also children as young as 5 years were seen among the Indian population, which contradicts the majority of the western reports that PV rarely affects children and young adults [6].

28.1.1 Pathogenesis

Patients with PV develop autoantibodies to intercellular antigens found within the Malpighian epithelia, leading to loss of cell adhesion between neighboring keratinocytes. The mostly accepted target antigens are the calcium-dependent intercellular adhesion proteins of the desmosomes, desmogleins 1 and 3 [7]. The type of desmoglein affected has clinical significance, as the location of PV lesions depends on the specific desmoglein targeted by the immune response. Desmoglein 1 is most readily found within the superficial

C. E. Orfanos et al. (eds.), *Pigmented Ethnic Skin and Imported Dermatoses*, https://doi.org/10.1007/978-3-319-69422-1_28

Table 28.1 Common bullous diseases and their immunophenotypes

Focus of pathogenetic process	Clinical entity	Gene/target protein	DIF/histology
Intraepidermal	*Pemphigus foliaceus*	Desmoglein 1	Suprabasal acantholysis; lesional and perilesional intercellular IgG deposits
	Pemphigus vulgaris	Desmoglein 1, 3	Suprabasal and basal acantholysis; lesional and perilesional intercellular IgG deposits
	Other pemphigus subtypes (P. vegetans, erythematosus, herpetiformis, eosinophilic, paraneoplastic)	Desmoglein 1, 3; Desmocollin 1, 2, 3 laminin γ-1, envoplakin, periplakin	Malpighian acantholysis
	Benign familial chronic pemphigus (Hailey-Hailey)	ATP2C1 gene	Suprabasal clefting
Basal membrane zone (BMZ)	*Bullous pemphigoid (in adults and childhood)*	180 and 230 kDa proteins (upper lamina lucida)	Linear IgG and C3 deposits in BMZ; subepidermal bulla formation
	Mucous membrane pemphigoid	180 and 230 kDa proteins, laminin 332, α6-integrin, β4-integrin	Linear IgG, IgA, C3 deposits in BMZ; subepithelial bulla formation
	Dermatitis herpetiformis (Duhring)	Epidermal transglutaminase 3	Granular IgA deposits within the dermal papillae; subepidermal bulla formation
	Linear IgA bullous disease	97 and 120 kDa proteins	Linear IgA deposits in BMZ; subepidermal bulla formation
	Pemphigoid gestationis	180 and 230 kDa proteins	Linear IgG and C3, rarely IgM, IgA deposits in BMZ; subepidermal bulla formation
Subepidermal	*Epidermolysis bullosa acquisita*	Collagen VII	Linear IgG and C3, rarely IgM, IgA deposits in BMZ; subepidermal bulla formation

epidermal layers; in contrast, desmoglein 3 is predominant within nonkeratinized epithelia such as mucosal surfaces. The presence of other non-desmoglein antigens, i.e., anti-E-cadherin antibodies, keratinocyte, and acetylcholine receptors, has also been suggested. The increased incidence of PV in young Indian patients has been associated with a higher frequency of DSG3*TCCCC and DSG3*TCCTC, two different desmoglein 3 haplotypes [8]. It has also been reported that Indian patients with PV had largely increased incidence of certain MHC class alleles and haplotype frequencies, specifically DRB1*1404, DQA1*0101, and DQBI*0503.

28.1.2 Clinical Picture

PV often starts in the mucosa of the oral cavity before affecting the skin. Short-lived flaccid blisters burst quickly, leaving irregularly shaped, painful erosions and ulcerations in the oral cavity that only slowly heal. Most commonly affected sites include the buccal mucosa, lips, palate, and tongue. Besides the oral mucosa, bullous lesions develop on the skin affecting the scalp, face, neck and upper back, and chest. The Nikolsky sign is positive in PV. The lesions heal with crusting without scarring; in African black skin, they often cause depigmentations (Figs. 28.1 and 28.2). Involvement of the mucosa in the pharynx and larynx is manifested by hoarseness; also the eye, the conjunctiva, and esophagus as well as genital mucosa may be affected with painful erosions.

Diagnosis of PV is based on skin biopsies showing characteristic histological features such as suprabasal acantholytic blisters, together with findings with direct immunofluorescence (DIF) also demonstrating intercellular deposition of IgG in perilesional skin. ELISA for IgG antibodies to desmoglein 3 and/or desmoglein 1 may also be found [9]. Acantholytic blistering with painful mucocutaneous erosions resembling PV may occur in association with various neoplasms, most commonly lymphomas, sarcomas, thymomas, and Castleman's disease (*paraneoplastic pemphigus*).

28.1.3 Treatment

An optimal strategy for treating PV is not fully established. As a routine schedule, high doses of systemic corticosteroids are administered, often pulse dexamethasone, combined with methotrexate, or cyclophosphamide; the pulses control the rash, while the mucosal lesions may persist and new bullae may appear, often located at the extremities (Fig. 28.3). In recent years standard treatment has been enriched with the successful introduction of rituximab in treating pemphigus and other bullous dermatoses, also in patients with dark skin

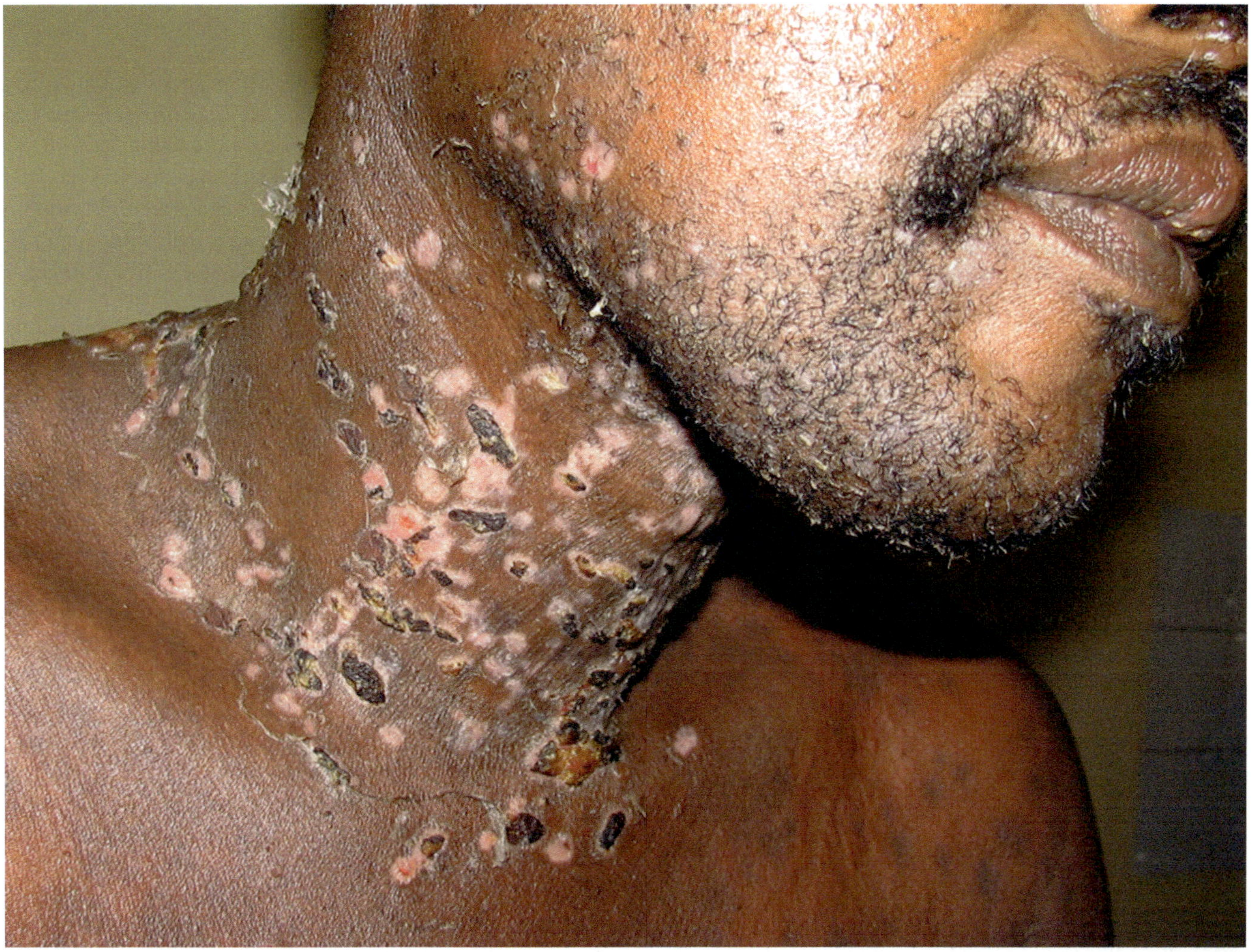

Fig. 28.1 *Pemphigus vulgaris* in a young African male. Treatment with prednisolone and methotrexate leads to satisfactory response with lesional depigmentation and crusting (courtesy PDTC Moshi, Tanzania; photo CEO)

[10]. Other options for PV broadly in use today include intravenous rituximab [11] or high doses of oral corticosteroids with or without addition of other immunosuppressive or immunomodulating drugs, such as adjuvant cyclophosphamide, mycophenolate mofetil, methotrexate, or azathioprine [12], based on the needs of the individual patient. Occasionally, intravenous immunoglobulins are used alone or in addition to the above [13]. In paraneoplastic pemphigus, detection and treatment of the underlying neoplasm are mandatory.

28.2 Pemphigus Foliaceus

Pemphigus foliaceus (PF) occurs in limited geographic areas, except for Brazil, where it is endemic known as *fogo selvagem* [14]. It is considered to be a more benign clinical variant of pemphigus vulgaris. The disease is an autoimmune disorder developing antibodies against desmoglein 1, leading to superficial erosions in the skin.

Brazilian PF has an incidence of almost 3% with several million patients involved each year [2]. The disease is in Brazil 20× more common than pemphigus vulgaris, primarily affecting children, adolescents, and young adult Amerindians between the ages 12 and 17, with an equal sex ratio. In contrast, middle-aged adults are affected among the Caucasian populations in Europe and North America. Genetic susceptibility may play a role in the pathogenesis of the disease; however, no specific genes have been yet identified. Individuals exposed to hematophagous insects are more susceptible to develop the disease [14]. Besides Brazil, PF occurs in other South American countries, such as in Peru, Paraguay, and Colombia, and has been also reported to be as common as or even more common than PV in African countries with large Arab populations such as Algeria, Libya [3], Morocco [3], Tunisia [15], and Mali [16]. PF has been registered in Africans with dark skin more frequently than in those with fair skin living in South Africa [17].

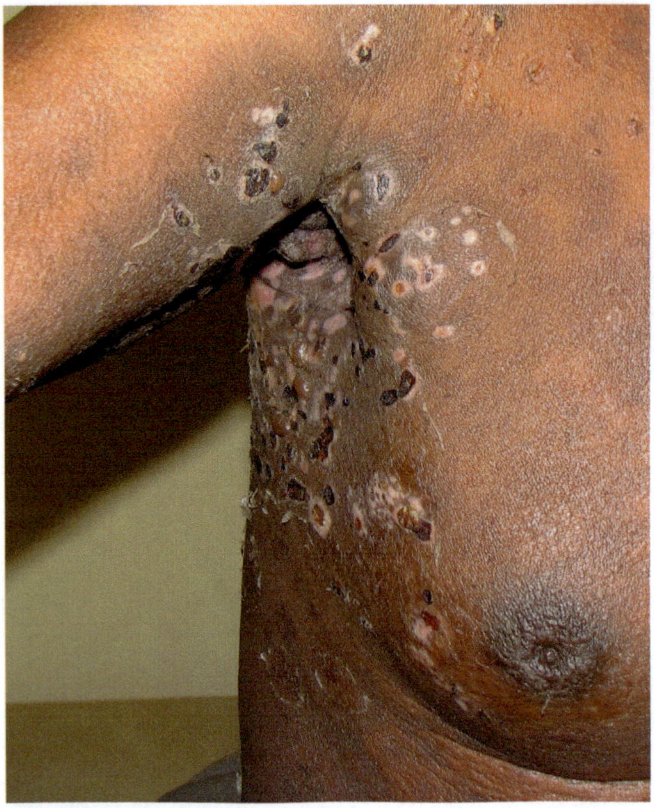

Fig. 28.2 *Pemphigus vulgaris*. Involvement of the axillary folds (undertreatment; courtesy CEO)

28.2.1 Clinical Picture

PF is clinically characterized by flaccid bullae with associated scaling and crusting. Initially, the seborrhoeic areas are affected; unlike pemphigus vulgaris, PF often involves the face, but the mucosal surfaces are usually spared [18]. A few classical cases were registered in Tanzania (Fig. 28.4). The lesions may later be widespread and generalized, presenting severe exfoliative dermatitis with severe oozing and crusting (Fig. 28.5). The Nikolsky sign is also positive in PF. Diagnosis is made by histological examination of skin biopsies showing acantholytic blisters in the superficial epidermal layers. A distinctive pattern with eosinophilic spongiosis has been found in cases seen in Mali [16]. Direct immunofluorescence on perilesional skin demonstrates intercellular deposition of IgG. ELISA for IgG antibodies to desmoglein 1 may also be positive.

As a rule, PF has a benign clinical course also because it remains restricted to the skin, although it can progress to a severe course and requires intensive medical care. The risk of mortality in patients with PF is not statistically increased relative to the general population [19].

In Europe single cases of *pemphigus erythematosus/Senear-Usher syndrome* may clinically and histologically correspond to PF.

28.2.2 Treatment

Treatment generally involves the administration of high-dose systemic corticosteroids in combination with other immunomodulators such as cyclosporine or azathioprine, to be slowly stepped down when remission appears; full recovery may take months to years [15]. Intravenous administration of immunoglobulins was reported as an effective treatment for PF, and also infliximab has been successful in a number of patients with refractory disease [20]. Recently, the efficacy of rituximab has been well documented both in adults and in juvenile PF, including refractory cases unresponsive to systemic corticosteroids [21].

28.3 Bullous Pemphigoid

Bullous pemphigoid (BP) is a common blistering disease of autoimmune origin occurring in all ethnic groups throughout the world. The disease affects equally both sexes, predominantly the elderly, with a majority of cases in people over the age of 60 and median age of presentation at the age of 80. The incidence of BP varies between 4 and 22 cases per million in Europe, where it is considered the most common autoimmune blistering disorder in the skin. However, in Asian countries such as Thailand and Malaysia, pemphigus vulgaris may be more common [22]. A rare subtype of the disease is *bullous pemphigoid in childhood*. In a recent analysis of US nationwide inpatient data on pediatric blistering disease, bullous pemphigoid of childhood was found associated with black skin and Hispanic ethnicity [23].

28.3.1 Pathogenesis

Generalized bullae develop in the subepidermal layer with mostly linear deposition of immunoglobulins and complement within the basement membrane zone at the lamina lucida. The binding of autoantibodies to BP antigen-180 kDa (BP 180) and BP antigen-230 kDa (BP 230) stimulates a destructive inflammatory cascade that leads to the separation of the epidermis from the dermis. BP often subsides spontaneously within several months or years. BP has been associated with neurological disorders and internal malignancies in several observational studies and case reports. Drug-induced BP has also been reported in several studies [24]. In Western literature, there are more than 50 pharmacological agents reported associated with bullous pemphigoid, the most common being a series of antibiotics, sulfonamides, diuretics, and ACE inhibitors [25].

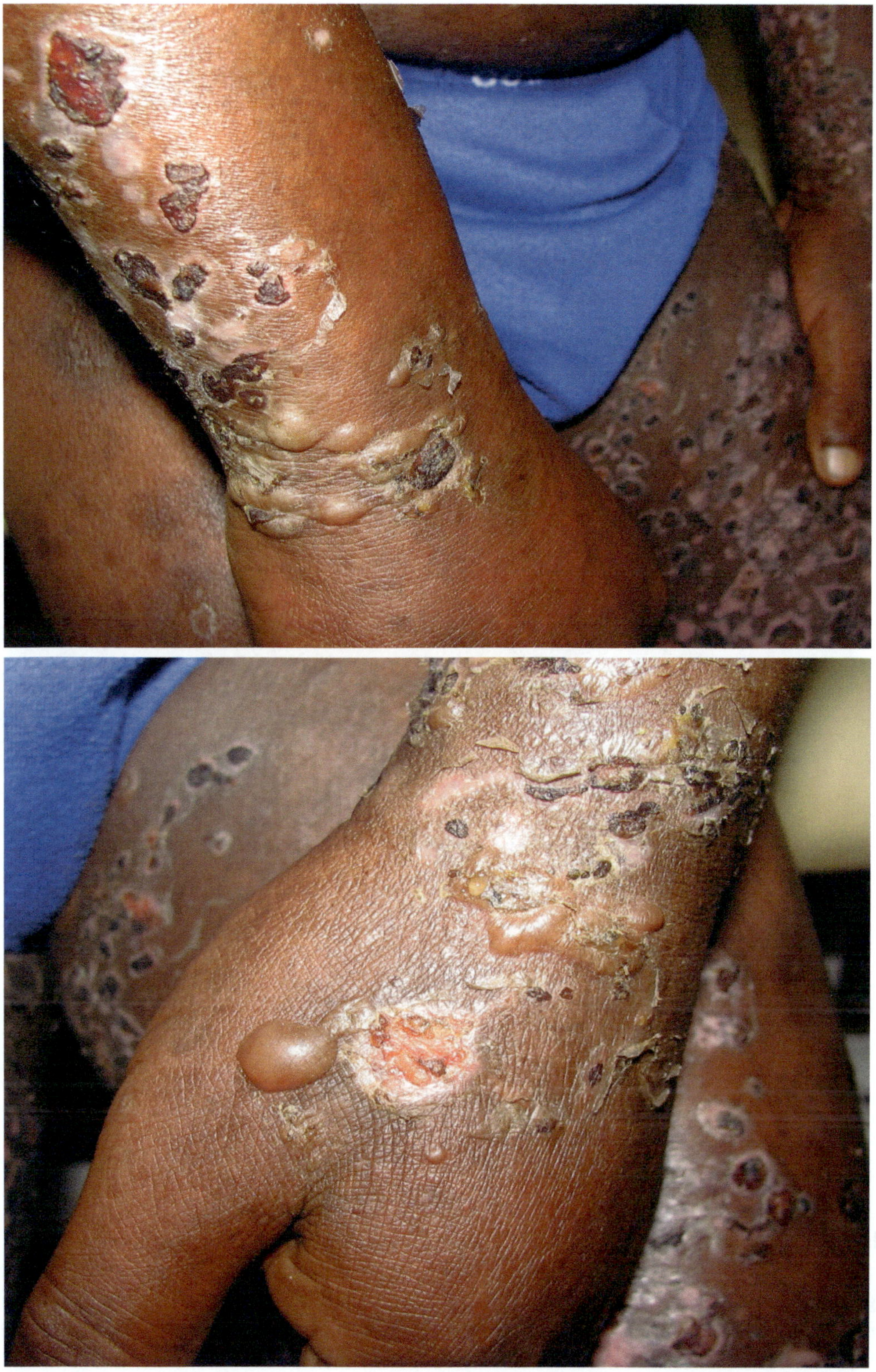

Fig. 28.3 *Pemphigus vulgaris* in an African male showing crusting after initiation of treatment; new blisters still arising at the extremities (courtesy CEO)

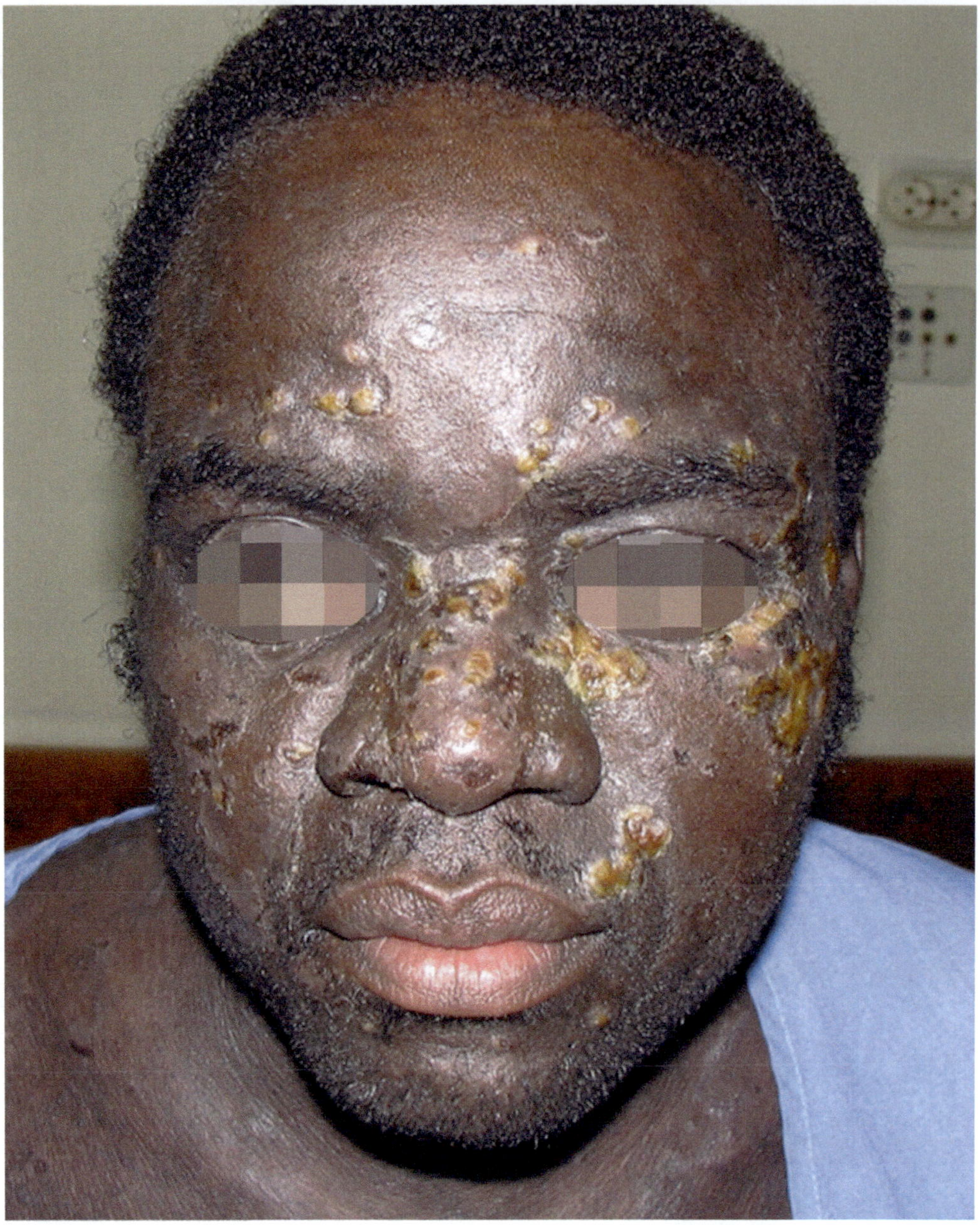

Fig. 28.4 *Pemphigus foliaceus* in a Tanzanian male from a rural area, Kilimanjaro District. Early localized involvement of the face (courtesy RDTC Moshi, Tanzania; photo CEO)

28.3.2 Clinical Picture

BP usually begins with a pruritic non-bullous phase that can persist for years before a polymorphic bullous phase follows. During the non-bullous phase, the manifestations are non-specific, with pruritus of variable severity, sometimes accompanied by excoriated eczematous, papular, and/or fixed urticarial-like lesions. The nonspecific presentation may persist for several months. Following the non-bullous phase, thin-walled tense haemoserous bullae often appear, preferably on the flexor surfaces of the arms and legs, in the axillae, abdomen, and groin. The Nikolsky sign is negative. BP rarely involves the oral mucous membranes. Rupturing of the bullae in BP creates pruritic erythematous erosions. Healing of the erosions is usually rapid with no atrophic scarring [24].

The infantile form of BP (*bullous pemphigoid of childhood*) presents the same characteristics as in adults with widespread tense bullous lesions, often involving the trunk, hands, and feet, with some mucosal involvement. Differential diagnosis toward linear IgA bullous disease is clinically difficult (Figs. 28.6 and 28.7).

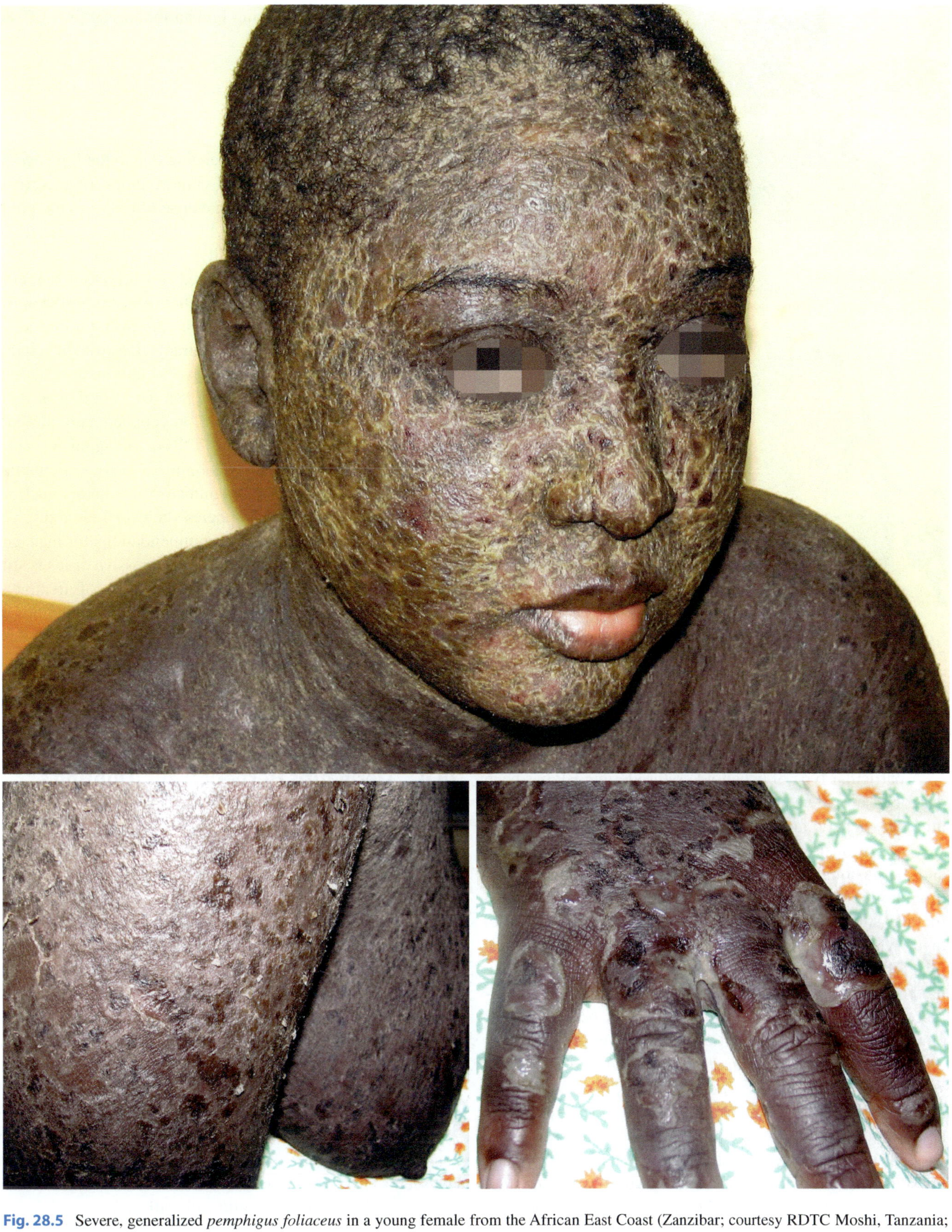

Fig. 28.5 Severe, generalized *pemphigus foliaceus* in a young female from the African East Coast (Zanzibar; courtesy RDTC Moshi, Tanzania; photos: CEO)

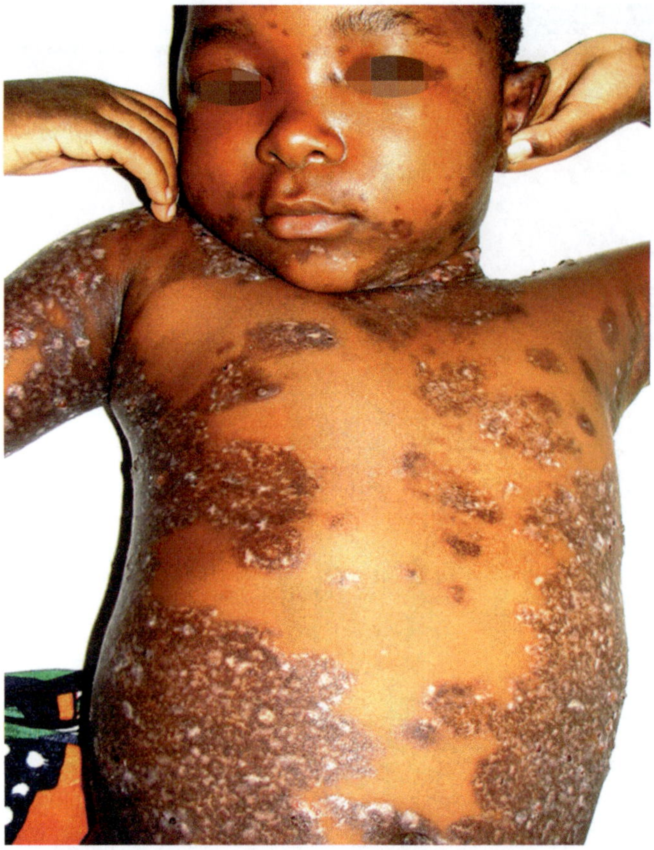

Fig. 28.6 Generalized bullous disease after several recurrences in a 2-year-old Arab boy from the East African Coast. DD: Bullous pemphigoid in childhood/linear IgA bullous disease (courtesy RDTC Moshi, Tanzania; photo CEO)

A particular type of lichenoid erythrodermic BP has been described in patients of African origin [26], probably determined by genetic factors.

The diagnosis of BP is made based on lesional biopsy and perilesional direct immunofluorescence and indirect immunofluorescence. Typical histopathological findings include subepidermal blister formation with lymphocytic, histiocytic, and eosinophilic cell infiltrates in the upper dermis. DIF will demonstrate linear IgG and C3 deposits along the basement membrane zone. Serum indirect immunofluorescence on salt-split skin will distinguish between other clinical immunobullous entities and rare varieties such as *epidermolysis bullosa acquisita*, *bullous lupus erythematosus*, *anti-laminin 332 pemphigoid*, and *anti-p200 pemphigoid*. Antibody deposition in BP is localized to the epidermal side of basement membrane zone-split skin, whereas the others are typically found on the dermal side. If possible, antigen-specific serologic testing with enzyme-linked immunosorbent assay (ELISA) can be performed and identify increased circulating IgG antibodies against BP180 and BP230 [9, 24].

28.3.3 Treatment

The management of BP is challenging due to the high age of the patients and the presence of comorbidities. Oral corticosteroids are effective and safe in a dose of 0.75–1.0 mg prednisolone/day per kg body weight; higher doses seem to be associated with higher mortality rates. As an alternative, administration of only topical remedies with ultrapotent corticosteroids (clobetasol propionate) has been advocated in BP [27]. In severe, recalcitrant patients, administration of corticosteroid-sparing agents such as tetracyclines (doxycycline), nicotinamide, or immunosuppressive or immunomodulating drugs is routinely recommended [28]. The addition of dapsone, azathioprine, methotrexate, mycophenolate mofetil, intravenous immunoglobulins, TNF-α antagonists, anti-CD20 agents, and of procedures aiming to remove circulating pathogenic antibodies and inflammatory mediators such as plasmapheresis and immunoapheresis may be required.

Overall, there are no valid recommendations for management of BP; the efficacy of immunosuppressive drugs is still under ongoing evaluation [29]. The choice of treatment depends on the severity and the presence of comorbidities in each particular case. Pediatric cases of BP respond well to topical corticosteroids and generally have a rather favorable prognosis; dapsone and mycophenolate mofetil may be further choices for treatment in infants.

28.4 Dermatitis Herpetiformis (Duhring's Disease)

Dermatitis herpetiformis (DH) is an autoimmune blistering disease most frequently diagnosed in individuals of northern European origin or heritage; it is a rare condition in populations with dark skin. The disease is caused by gluten sensitivity in genetically susceptible individuals, representing a cutaneous manifestation of celiac disease, whereby the responsible autoantigen in celiac disease is tissue transglutaminase (TG2) and epidermal transglutaminase (TG3) in DH [30]. Virtually all patients with DH carry the HLA-DQ2 or HLA-DQ8 haplotype [31]. It is estimated that the incidence of DH in Caucasians ranges between 0.1 and 3.5/100,000 people per year, with prevalence between 1.2 and 75.3/100,000 people, the highest rates registered in Scandinavia and parts of the USA. Today, the incidence of DH seems to be declining due to better detection and earlier treatment of subclinical or mild celiac disease.

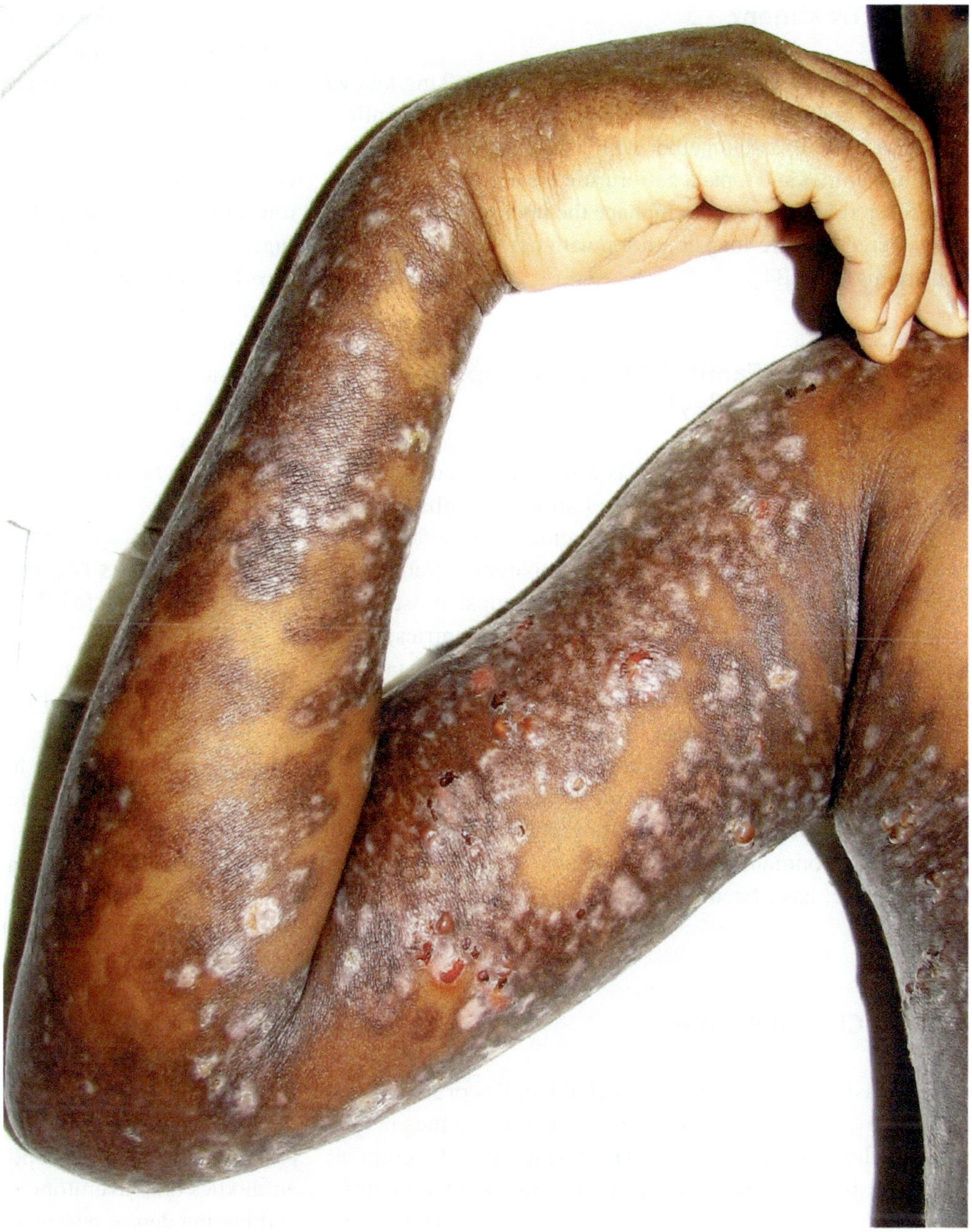

Fig. 28.7 Generalized bullous disease in childhood (pat. Fig. 28.3; photo CEO)

28.4.1 Clinical Picture

DH has a slow insidious onset often starting in early adulthood and affects more males than females by a ratio ranging between 1.1 and 1.9:1. It is characterized by intensely pruritic, symmetrical, grouped vesicles and papules, commonly distributed on the elbows, knees, scalp, buttocks, and shoulder blades. The severity of the disease varies widely, and the lesions often heal without atrophic scarring; however, post-inflammatory dyspigmentation may occur [32]. Approximately half of the patients affected develop hyperpigmentation in the areas where skin lesions were present. Occasionally, petechiae or purpura on acral surfaces are primary cutaneous manifestations of DH [33]. In 30% of the cases, gastrointestinal involvement may be detected (gluten-sensitive enteropathy).

The diagnosis is made based on skin biopsies and DIF showing granular subepidermal deposits of IgA within the dermal papillae as a key diagnostic feature, together with neutrophilic cell infiltrates in the upper dermis. Approximately 70% of patients also have circulating IgA antibodies against the smooth muscle cell endomysium [32].

28.4.2 Treatment

The treatment of DH consists of oral dapsone (1–2 mg/kg bw/day) as initial management to control the cutaneous manifestations of the disease together with life-long gluten-free diet. Antihistamines and topical antipruritic creams or low-potency corticosteroids are given to manage the intense itching. DH is considered as a life-long condition with occasional spontaneous remissions [34].

28.5 Benign Familial Chronic Pemphigus (Hailey-Hailey)

Hailey-Hailey disease (HHD) is a rare inherited skin disease leading to a chronic course of superficial blistering in regions of increased friction. Its incidence is 1/50,000 in the general population. There is no apparent difference in prevalence among the various ethnic groups; most cases have been described in European and Asian countries; more recently, a series of cases were reported from Tunisia [35]. HHD is caused by several mutations of the ATP2C1 gene, mostly identified in Chinese families, which is responsible for encoding the human secretory pathway Ca^{2+}/Mn^{2+}-ATPase protein-1 [36]. As a result, epidermal hyperplasia, dyskeratosis and suprabasal clefting develop [37]. A number of environmental conditions such as heat, moisture, friction, etc. have been identified as aggravating factors in HHD [38].

28.5.1 Clinical Picture

The classical clinical picture of HHD shows pruritic vesicles, scaly, well-demarcated, erythematous plaques resulting in flat painful erosions. The lesions mostly erupt at sites of friction, particularly at the anatomical flexures including the axillary, genitocrural, and submammary folds. Young individuals are affected, mostly 20–40 years in age, without gender predilection. The patients experience frequent relapses and significant impairment in their life quality. Secondary bacterial and candidal infections often occur. Diagnosis is made by histological examination of skin biopsies showing suprabasal acantholysis, while immunofluorescence studies would return a negative result [37].

28.5.2 Treatment

The management of HHD is challenging; it requires sufficient control of all precipitating factors or activities that may trigger the clinical manifestation of the disease (excessive sweating, obesity, local trauma, horse and bicycle riding, exposure to UV radiation among others), together with eliminating any aggravating factors such as secondary bacterial or fungal infections, often Candida intertrigo, causing koebnerization. Topical low-potency corticosteroids and steroid-sparing agents such as tacrolimus are used to control blistering and achieve partial clearing; alternatively, topical and/or systemic antibiotics (doxycycline, minocycline) are given. If topical management is ineffective, systemic administration of dapsone, isotretinoin/acitretin, methotrexate, cyclosporine, and thalidomide may be administered for management [39, 40]. In selected cases surgical interventions, cryotherapy, photodynamic sessions, and laser ablation are additional options that may be beneficial.

28.6 Mucous Membrane Pemphigoid (Cicatricial Pemphigoid)

The designation *mucous membrane pemphigoid* (MMP) characterizes a group of rare chronic autoimmune blistering conditions that affect the mucous membranes. There is no ethnic preference known. MMP may occur in any population throughout the world, affecting females twice as often as males. The average age of onset is in the sixth or seventh decade, although the disease can develop in any age. The incidence of MMP is roughly estimated to be two cases per million people per year [41].

28.6.1 Pathogenesis

Antibodies against BP180, BP230, laminin-332, α6β4-integrin, and type VII collagen have all been identified in patients with MMP around the basement membrane. These antibodies bind to epitopes located in the lower lamina lucida and lamina densa, possibly accounting for the increased risk of scarring in MMP compared to BP which has epitopes located in the upper lamina lucida. Ocular involvement is more commonly associated with β4-integrin subunit of α6β4, whereas antibodies to the α6 subunit have been linked to oral disease. MMP has an extended long time course, with frequent remissions and relapses [42].

28.6.2 Clinical Picture

MMP presents with blisters affecting the mucous membranes of the body, most commonly the mouth and eye; however, the nose, throat, genitalia, and anus may also be involved. Unlike BP, the blisters in MMP heal with scarring, and patients are left with reticulated, white striations of mucosal fibrosis. The clinical symptomatology often starts with erythema, bleeding, blistering, and eroding of the gingiva, palate, and buccal mucosa. Esophageal and laryngeal involvement may lead to dysphagia and dysphonia; progressive scarring and stenosis of the esophagus or larynx can cause other significant clinical complications [43].

Ocular involvement is presented with conjunctivitis or erosions forming on the conjunctiva. Usually, only one eye is first involved with the second becoming affected within the following 2 years. Initial symptoms are pain or grittiness in the eye, glaucoma, entropion, and trichiasis. Symblepharon, corneal opacity, vision impairment, and blindness may develop over time [42]. When MMP only involves the eyes or mouth, scarring is less severe than variants where other mucosal surfaces are also involved. In a fifth of cases, the skin of the face and neck may be affected, healing with scarring and dyspigmentation.

The diagnosis of MMP is made based on lesional skin biopsies, perilesional DIF, and serum indirect immunofluorescence (IIF). Typical histopathological findings are subepidermal blister formation with lymphocytic, histiocytic, neutrophilic, and eosinophilic cell infiltrates in the upper dermis. There may also be plasma cell infiltration and subepidermal fibrosis. DIF demonstrates linear IgG and/or IgA and/or linear C3 staining along the basement membrane zone; IIF on salt-split skin is useful to recognize patients at risk for malignancy-associated laminin-32 CP [42].

28.6.3 Treatment

The treatment of MMP is similar to that of BP, with additional therapies targeted at the specific sites involved. Early consultation and referral to oral specialists, ophthalmologists, and otolaryngologists are important [9]. Ocular involvement requires systemic immunosuppressive treatment to achieve remission and avoid scarring leading to blindness [44, 45].

28.7 Linear IgA Bullous Disease

Linear IgA bullous disease is a rare autoimmune skin disorder with incidence reports ranging from less than 0.5 to 2.3 cases per million individuals per year. The disease affects most commonly children aged 10 months to 6 years and adults over the age of 60 [46]. There has been no solid relationship established linking the disease with certain ethnic groups or gender [47]; however, linear IgA bullous dermatosis is frequently seen in Africa, particularly in children, in contrast to DH which is uncommon. Cases were reported from Mali [48], and the condition is considered in Tunisia as the most common autoimmune bullous disease in children [49].

28.7.1 Pathogenesis

The disease is characterized by linear deposition of IgA at the dermal-epidermal junction [50]. Many patients exhibit IgA antibodies, which target antigens within the basement membrane zone (97 and 120 kDa) that are transmembrane proteins responsible for epidermal-dermal adhesion [51]. An autoimmune vesiculobullous variant that mimics MMP, DH, or BP associated with linear deposition of IgA antibodies along the basement membrane is drug-induced; the most common responsible agent is vancomycin, clinically presented in a manner that closely imitates toxic epidermal necrolysis [52].

28.7.2 Clinical Picture

The clinical symptomatology of IgA-linear bullous disease presents some similarities to DH, without the presence of an underlying gluten-sensitive enteropathy. The classical presentation involves widespread, annular blisters that appear to be tense and filled with fluid [53]. Mucous membranes, most commonly the oral and eye mucosa, are frequently affected [46] (Fig. 28.8). Additional dermatologic manifestations can include erythematous plaques, blanching macules and papules, or targetoid erythema multiforme-like lesions [54]. Among the pediatric population, the blisters tend to be localized to the lower abdomen and anogenital areas, often involving the perineum (Fig. 28.9). Adults, however, tend to present with blisters on the trunk and the limbs.

Overall, the differential diagnosis of bullous disorders in infants based on clinical features only is difficult (Fig. 28.10); the gold standard for diagnosing linear IgA bullous disease are skin biopsies and DIF showing linear IgA deposition at the dermal-epidermal junction [50]. Circulating IgA antibodies against the basement membrane zone (97 and 120 kDa) can also be detected [51].

28.7.3 Treatment

It is important that any ruptured erosion are cleaned and then dressed with sterile materials. Some patients with infected lesions may require treatment with a topical antibiotic such as mupirocin. An ophthalmologist should also be consulted in order to thoroughly assess the ocular mucosa. The first-line ongoing treatment for linear IgA disease is monotherapy with oral dapsone [55]. If dapsone is contraindicated, the most appropriate alternatives are glucocorticoids, azathioprine, methotrexate, tetracyclines, erythromycin, and cyclosporine. The concurrent use of dapsone (50–100 mg/day) and mycophenolate mofetil (1 g/day) enabled the complete

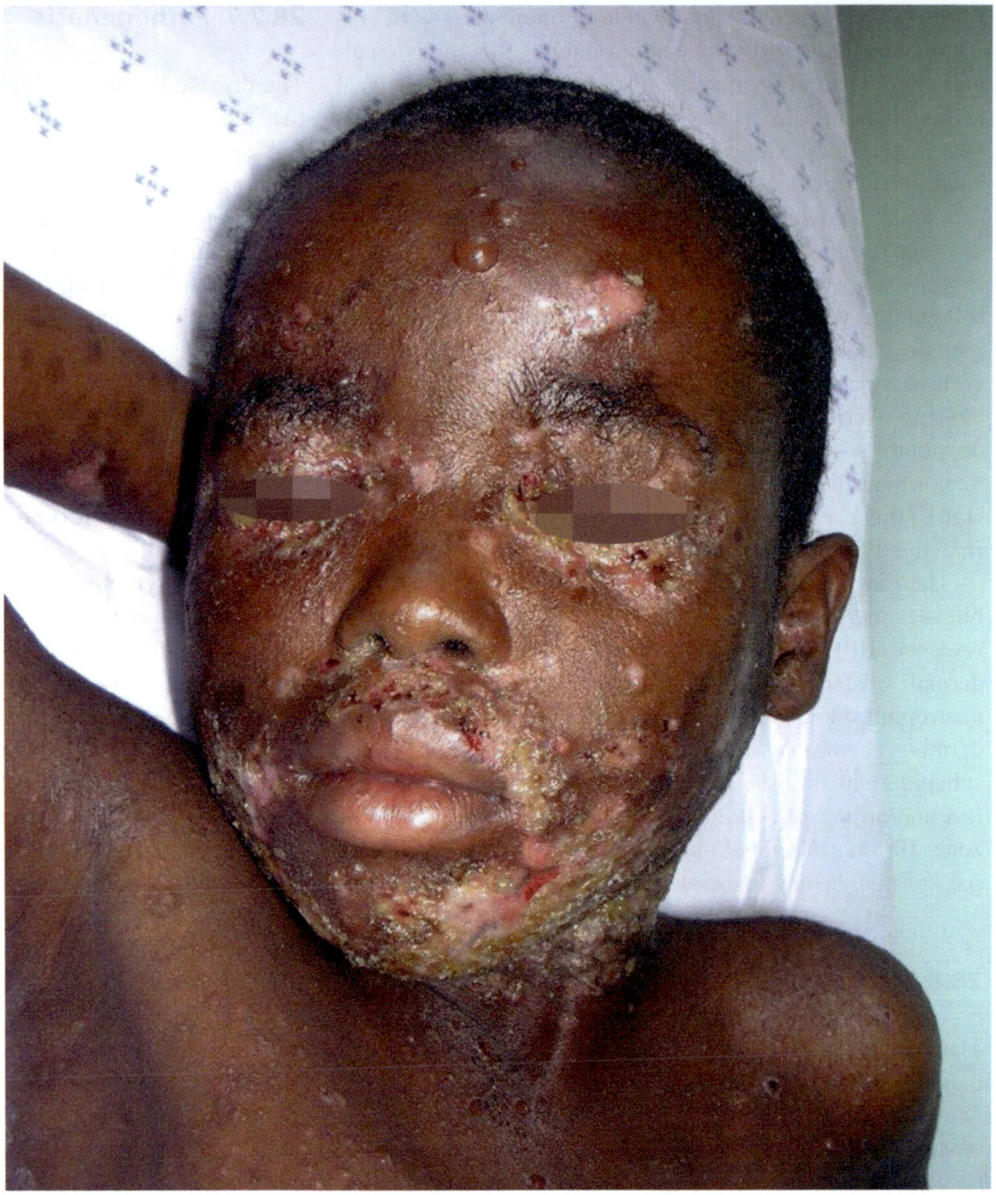

Fig. 28.8 *Linear IgA bullous disease*. Involvement of the perioral and periocular areas in an African young boy

remission of dermatological manifestations caused by linear IgA bullous disease in Brazil [56].

28.8 Pemphigoid Gestationis (Herpes Gestationis)

Pemphigoid gestationis (PG) is an autoimmune blistering disease associated with pregnancy, most commonly presenting in the second and third trimesters [57] and also during the immediate postpartum period. PG is reported to occur in approximately 1 in 50,000 pregnancies among the general population in the USA. It has been suggested that it is less common in females with dark skin compared to Caucasian females [58], possibly reflecting an association with specific HLA haplotypes. However, the disease has been recently reported in series of Tunisian [59] and Saudi females [60], mostly multigravidas.

28.8.1 Pathogenesis

PG is characterized by the deposition of complement (C3) in the lamina lucida of the cutaneous basement membrane, with or without IgG deposition. Patients develop antibodies for hemidesmosomal proteins (BP180 and BP230), which belong to the immunoglobulin G1 subclass. The binding of IgG to the basement membrane will trigger an autoimmune

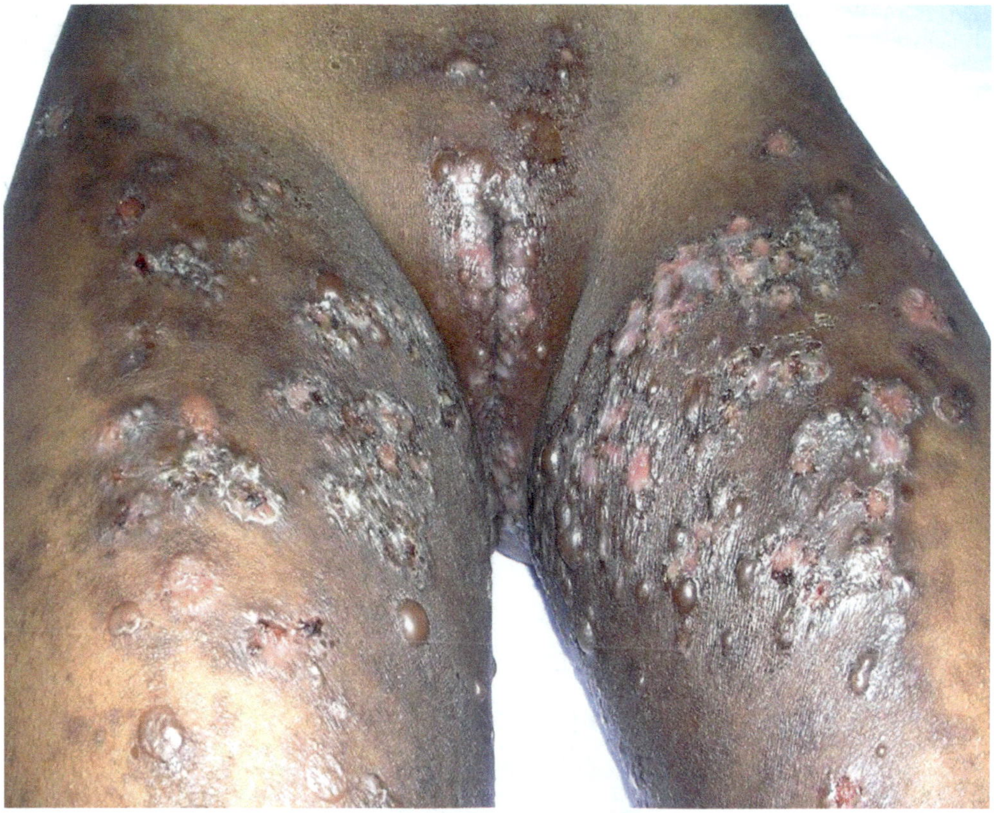

Fig. 28.9 *Linear IgA bullous disease* in the genital area of a young African female, also involving the upper legs, perigenital area, and labia majora

response, provoking the formation of subepidermal vesicles and blisters [61].

28.8.2 Clinical Picture

PG presents extremely pruritic and erythematous plaques which tend to start around the periumbilical region and then spread to cover the trunk and extremities. Over time, the rash evolves from plaques to become vesiculobullous. The disease resolves weeks to months after delivery. Histological examination shows junctional blistering and predominant eosinophilic cell infiltrate; keratinocytic necrosis and dermal edema are often but not always observed [58]. Direct immunofluorescence demonstrates a linear band of C3 deposition with or without deposition of IgG along the basement membrane.

28.8.3 Treatment

There is no standard treatment for PG although it is generally considered to revolve under the application of ultrapotent topical corticosteroids [61]. In more severe or resistant cases, systemic immunosuppressants, such as prednisone, may also be necessary to manage the disease, as well as the use of antihistaminic agents [57].

28.9 Epidermolysis Bullosa Acquisita

The *acquired variant of epidermolysis bullosa* (EBA) is a rare cutaneous vesiculobullous disorder affecting 0.2 cases per 1 million people, with only minimal or no mucosal involvement [62]. It occurs mostly in adults, showing a recurrent course with skin fragility, milia formation, and mild scarring, reminiscent to the dystrophic type of the inherited epidermolysis bullosa [63]. Gastrointestinal involvement and dysphagia may occur. Crohn's disease is associated with ¼ of all cases with EBA. Histological examination shows subepidermal bulla formation with linear IgG deposits at the dermoepidermal junction; however, in only a part of the EBA cases, published autoantibodies to type VII collagen were identified, leading to a decrease of functioning anchoring fibrils; in a few BP180 has been detected. Overrepresentation in patients with dark skin of African origin with atypical clinical presentations has been reported; high EBA frequencies were also registered in American blacks associated with the HLA-DR2 [64, 65].

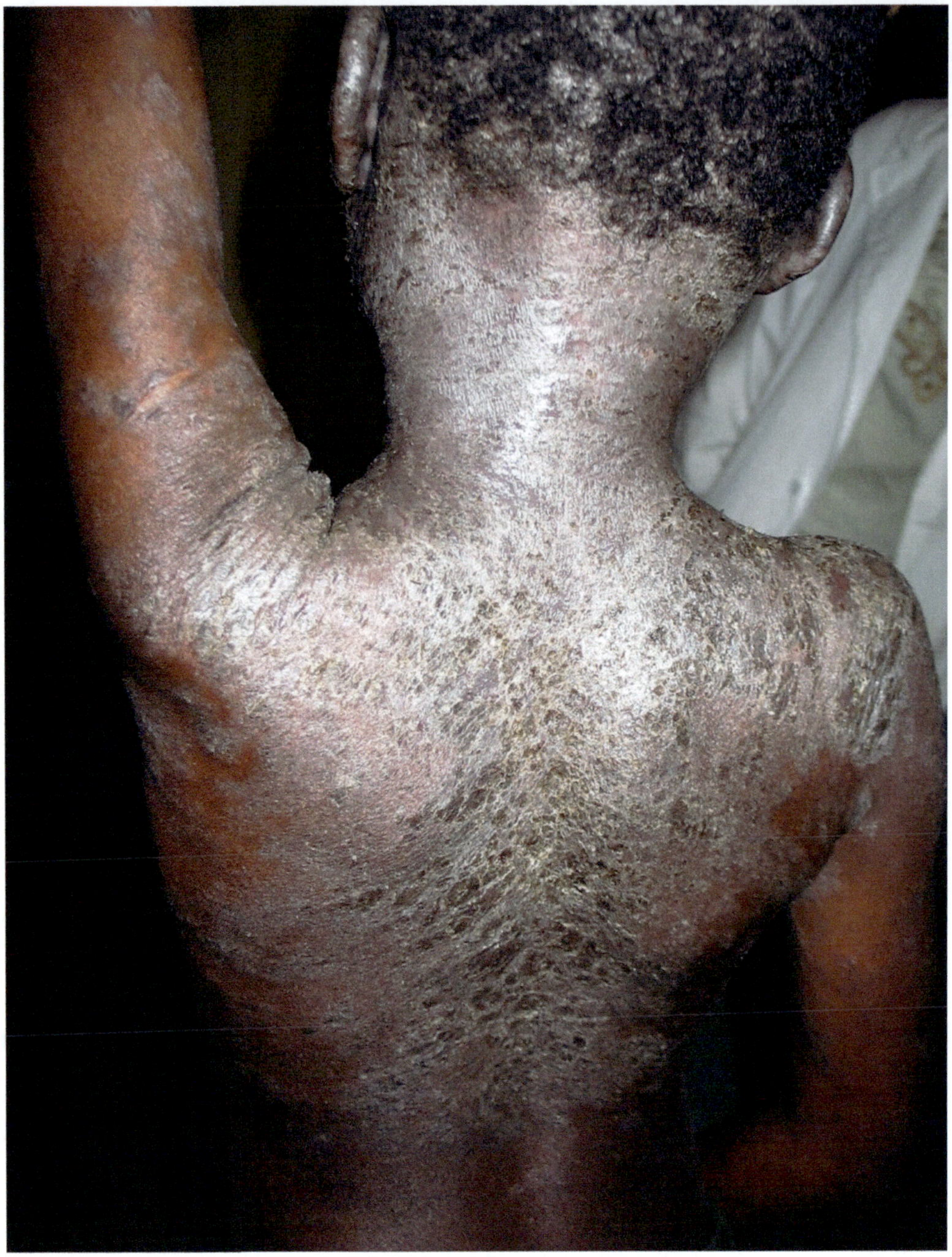

Fig. 28.10 Widespread bullous disease in an 8-year-old African boy (topical calamine lotion); DD: Pemphigus foliaceus/linear IgA bullous disease (courtesy RDTC Moshi, Tanzania; photo CEO)

Management is often unsatisfactory; colchicine, dapsone, infliximab, administration of immunoglobulins, and similar drugs and modalities were only partially successful [66].

Conclusions

Bullous dermatoses are worldwide common autoimmune disorders caused by autoantibodies targeted toward epidermal and mucosal structures responsible for cell and tissue adhesion. Their geographic distribution varies significantly, whereas the clinical symptomatology of the arising entities is multifaceted. The occurrence of conditions with acantholytic blister formation has endemic character in part, focused in India for pemphigus vulgaris, Brazil for pemphigus foliaceus, and North Africa/Tunisia for both subtypes. The varying geographic occurrence of bullous dermatoses is possibly related to the effect of genetic polymorphisms governing the susceptibility of predisposed individuals for autoimmune processes. In addition, populations living in rural areas are often affected suggesting that antigenic mimicry may be initiated via environmental agents or stimuli and become pathogenic. Physicians should be aware of the worldwide peculiarities of bullous skin diseases to ensure correct diagnosis and enable better treatment for the affected populations.

References

1. Venugopal SS, Murrell DF. Diagnosis and clinical features of pemphigus vulgaris. Dermatol Clin. 2011;29:373–80.
2. Alpsoy E, Akman-Karakas A, Uzun S. Geographic variations in epidemiology of two autoimmune bullous diseases: pemphigus and bullous pemphigoid. Arch Dermatol Res. 2015;307:291–8.
3. Saleh MA. Pemphigus in the Arab world. J Dermatol. 2015;42:27–30.
4. Adam BA. Bullous diseases in Malaysia: epidemiology and natural history. Int J Dermatol. 1992;31:42–5.
5. Kanwar AJ, De D. Pemphigus in India. Indian J Dermatol Venereol Leprol. 2011;77:439–95.
6. Singh R, Pandhi R. A clinicopathological study of pemphigus. Indian J Dermatol Venereol Leprol. 1973;39:126.
7. Patel F, Wilken R, Patel FB, et al. Pathophysiology of autoimmune bullous diseases: nature versus nurture. Indian J Dermatol. 2017;62:262–7.
8. Capon F, Bharkhada J, Cochrane N, et al. Evidence of an association between desmoglein 3 haplotypes and pemphigus vulgaris. Br J Dermatol. 2006;154:67–71.
9. Murrell DF. Blistering diseases: clinical features, pathogenesis, treatment. Berlin: Springer; 2015.
10. Kanwar AJ, Tsuruta D, Vinay K, et al. Efficacy and safety of rituximab treatment in Indian pemphigus patients. J Eur Acad Dermatol Venereol. 2013;27:e17–23.
11. Anandan V, Jameela WA, Sowmiya R, et al. Rituximab: a magic bullet for pemphigus. J Clin Diagn Res. 2017;11:WC01–6.
12. Shaik F, Botha J, Aboobaker J, et al. Corticosteroid/cyclophosphamide pulse treatment in South African patients with pemphigus. Clin Exp Dermatol. 2010;35:245–50.
13. Zhao C, Murrell DF. Pemphigus vulgaris: an evidence-based treatment update. Drugs. 2015;75:271–84.
14. Aoki V, Rivitti EA, Diaz LA. Cooperative Group on Fogo Selvagem Research: update on fogo selvagem, an endemic form of pemphigus foliaceus. J Dermatol. 2015;42:18–26.
15. Morini JP, Jomaa B, Gorgi Y, Saguem MH, Nouira R, Roujeau J-C, Revuz J. Pemphigus foliaceus in young women: an endemic focus in the Sousse area of Tunisia. Arch Dermatol. 1993;129:69–73.
16. Mahé A, Flageul B, Cissé I, et al. Pemphigus in Mali: a study of 30 cases. Br J Dermatol. 1996;134:114–9.
17. Aboobaker J, Morar N, Ramdial PK, Hammond MG. Pemphigus in South Africa. Int J Dermatol. 2001;40:115–9.
18. Orne CM, Hale CS, Meehan SA, Leger M. Pemphigus foliaceus. Dermatol Online J. 2014;20(12). pii: 13030/qt9bf1p1pc.
19. Kridin K, Zelber-Sagi S, Bergman R. Pemphigus vulgaris and pemphigus foliaceus: differences in epidemiology and mortality. Acta Derm Venereol. 2017;97:1095-9.
20. Green MG, Bystryn J-C. Effect of intravenous immunoglobulin therapy on serum levels of IgG1 and IgG4 antidesmoglein 1 and antidesmoglein 3 antibodies in pemphigus vulgaris. Arch Dermatol. 2008;144:1621–4.
21. Loh TY, Paravar T. Rituximab in the management of juvenile pemphigus foliaceus. Dermatol Online J. 2017;23(6). pii: 13030/qt0415n1r5.
22. Lo Schiavo A, Ruocco E, Brancaccio G, et al. Bullous pemphigoid: etiology, pathogenesis, and inducing factors: facts and controversies. Clin Dermatol. 2013;31:391–9.
23. Ren Z, Hsu DY, Silverberg NB, et al. The inpatient burden of autoimmune blistering disease in US children: analysis of nationwide inpatient sample data. Am J Clin Dermatol. 2017;18:287–97.
24. Schmidt E, della Torre R, Borradori L. Clinical features and practical diagnosis of bullous pemphigoid. Dermatol Clin. 2011;29:427–38.
25. Stavropoulos PG, Soura E, Antoniou C. Drug-induced pemphigoid: a review of the literature. J Eur Acad Dermatol Venereol. 2014;28:1133–40.
26. Joly P, Tanasescu S, Wolkenstein P, et al. Lichenoid erythrodermic bullous pemphigoid of the African patient. J Am Acad Dermatol. 1998;39:691–7.
27. Bernard P, Charneux J. Bullous pemphigoid: a review. Ann Dermatol Venereol. 2011;138:173–81.
28. Spivey J, Nye AM. Bullous pemphigoid: corticosteroid treatment and adverse effects in long-term care patients. Consult Pharm. 2013;28:455–62.
29. Kirtschig G, Middleton P, Bennett C, et al. Interventions for bullous pemphigoid. Cochrane Database Syst Rev. 2010;(10):CD002292.
30. Collin P, Salmi TT, Hervonen K, et al. Dermatitis herpetiformis: a cutaneous manifestation of coeliac disease. Ann Med. 2017;49:23–31.
31. Salmi TT, Hervonen K, Kautiainen H, et al. Prevalence and incidence of dermatitis herpetiformis: a 40-year prospective study from Finland. Br J Dermatol. 2011;165:354–9.
32. Bolotin D, Petronic-Rosic V. Dermatitis herpetiformis. Part I. Epidemiology, pathogenesis, and clinical presentation. J Am Acad Dermatol. 2011;64:1017–24.
33. Tu H, Parmentier L, Stieger M, et al. Acral purpura as leading clinical manifestation of dermatitis herpetiformis: report of two adult cases with a review of the literature. Dermatology. 2013;227:1–4.
34. Zone JJ, Meyer LJ. Dermatitis herpetiformis. Immunol Ser. 1989;46:565–82.
35. Benmously-Mlika R, Bchetnia M, Deghais S, et al. Hailey-Hailey disease in Tunisia. Int J Dermatol. 2010;49:396–401.
36. Meng L, Gu Y, Du XF, et al. Two novel ATP2C1 mutations in patients with Hailey-Hailey disease and a literature review of sequence variants reported in the Chinese population. Genet Mol Res. 2015;14:19349–59.
37. Thompson LD. Hailey-Hailey disease. Ear Nose Throat J. 2016;95:370.
38. Burge SM. Hailey–Hailey disease: the clinical features, response to treatment and prognosis. Br J Dermatol. 1992;126:275–82.
39. D'Errico A, Bonciani D, Bonciolini V, et al. Hailey-Hailey disease treated with methotrexate. J Dermatol Case Rep. 2012;6:49–51.
40. Nanda KB, Saldanha CS, Jacintha M, et al. Hailey-Hailey disease responding to thalidomide. Indian J Dermatol. 2014;59:190–2.
41. Bertram F, Brocker EB, Zillikens D, et al. Prospective analysis of the incidence of autoimmune bullous disorders in Lower Franconia, Germany. J Dtsch Dermatol Ges. 2009;7:434–40.
42. Chan LS, Ahmed AR, Anhalt GJ, et al. The first international consensus on mucous membrane pemphigoid: definition, diagnostic criteria, pathogenic factors, medical treatment, and prognostic indicators. Arch Dermatol. 2002;138:370–9.
43. Fleming TE, Korman NJ. Cicatricial pemphigoid. J Am Acad Dermatol. 2000;43:571–91.
44. Queisi MM, Zein M, Lamba N, et al. Update on ocular cicatricial pemphigoid and emerging treatments. Surv Ophthalmol. 2016;61:314–7.
45. Sobolewska B, Deuter C, Zierhut M. Current medical treatment of ocular mucous membrane pemphigoid. Ocul Surf. 2013;11:259–66.
46. Wojnarowska F, Marsden R, Bhogal B, et al. Chronic bullous disease of childhood, childhood cicatricial pemphigoid, and linear IgA disease of adults: a comparative study demonstrating clinical and immunopathologic overlap. J Am Acad Dermatol. 1988;19:792–805.
47. Fortuna G, Marinkovich MP. Linear immunoglobulin A bullous dermatosis. Clin Dermatol. 2012;30:38–50.
48. Mahé A, Flageul B, Bobin P. Bullous IgA linear dermatosis of children in Mali. Ann Dermatol Venereol. 1996;123:544–8.

49. Kharfi M, Khaled A, Karaa A, et al. Linear IgA bullous dermatosis: the more frequent bullous dermatosis of children. Dermatol Online J. 2010;16(1):2.
50. Boccaletti V, Di Nuzzo S. Linear IgA bullous disease. N Engl J Med. 2014;370:2228.
51. Guide SV, Marinkovich MP. Linear IgA bullous dermatosis. Clin Dermatol. 2001;19:719–27.
52. Waldman MA, Black DR, Callen JP. Vancomycin-induced linear IgA bullous disease presenting as toxic epidermal necrolysis. Clin Exp Dermatol. 2004;29:633–6.
53. Chen S, Mattei P, Fischer M, et al. Linear IgA bullous dermatosis. Eplasty. 2013;13:ic49.
54. Billet SE, Kortuem KR, Gibson LE, et al. A morbilliform variant of vancomycin-induced linear IgA bullous dermatosis. Arch Dermatol. 2008;144:774–8.
55. Kenani N, Mebazaa A, Denguezli M, et al. Childhood linear IgA bullous dermatosis in Tunisia. Pediatr Dermatol. 2009;26:28–33.
56. Passos L, Rabelo RF, Matsuo C, et al. Linear IgA/IgG bullous dermatosis: successful treatment with dapsone and mycophenolate mofetil. An Bras Dermatol. 2011;86:747–50.
57. Cobo MF, Santi CG, Maruta CW, et al. Pemphigoid gestationis: clinical and laboratory evaluation. Dermatol Clin. 2009;64:1043–7.
58. Shornick JK, Bangert JL, Freeman RG, Gilliam JN. Herpes gestationis: clinical and histologic features of twenty-eight cases. J Am Acad Dermatol. 1983;8:214–24.
59. Boudaya S, Turki H, Meziou TJ, et al. Pemphigoid gestationis: a study of 15 cases. J Gynecol Obstet Biol Reprod (Paris). 2003;32:30–4.
60. Al-Saif F, Elisa A, Al-Homidy A, et al. Retrospective analysis of pemphigoid gestationis in 32 Saudi patients—clinicopathological features and a literature review. J Reprod Immunol. 2016;116:42–5.
61. Soutou B, Aractingi S. Skin disease in pregnancy. Best Pract Res Clin Obstet Gynaecol. 2015;29:732–40.
62. Hallel-Halevy D, Nadelman C, Chen M, Woodley DT. Epidermolysis bullosa acquisita: update and review. Clin Dermatol. 2001;19:712–8.
63. Gupta R, Woodley DT, Chen M. Epidermolysis bullosa acquisita. Clin Dermatol. 2012;30:60–9.
64. Zumelzu C, Le Roux-Villet C, Loiseau P, et al. Black patients of African descent and HLA-DRB1* 15:03 frequency overrepresented in epidermolysis bullosa acquisita. J Invest Dermatol. 2011;131:2386–93.
65. Howard T, Brunner WC. Epidermolysis bullosa acquisita in an 18-year-old African-American male: a case report. S D Med. 2009;62:50–1.
66. Ishii N, Hamada T, Dainichi T, et al. Epidermolysis bullosa acquisita: what's new? J Dermatol. 2010;37:220–30.

Noninfectious Granulomas in Pigmented Skin

29

Nour Kibbi and Abdul-Ghani Kibbi

Granulomatous skin diseases are a diverse group of disorders resulting from a chronic inflammatory responses to infectious and noninfectious antigens and/or other organic or inorganic materials that the immune system is unable to eliminate. The diagnosis of granulomatous diseases relies heavily on clinical and pathological examination. The unifying finding is an inflammatory infiltrate predominantly composed of histiocytes, macrophages, and giant cells, sometimes showing collagen degeneration and caseation necrosis. In this chapter, we review the clinical and pathological presentation of these diseases, with a special focus on pigmented skin.

29.1 Cutaneous Sarcoidosis

Sarcoidosis is a multisystem granulomatous disease of unknown etiology shown to affect individuals of any race, age, or gender, though it has a well-described predilection for skin of color [1]. The lifetime risk of sarcoidosis is estimated at 2.7% for black-skinned women compared with only 1% in women with white skin. The incidence follows a bimodal distribution, with one peak occurring between the ages of 25 and 35 and the other between 45 and 65. Individuals with pigmented skin typically develop sarcoidosis at a later age [2]. Moreover, in patients with pigmented skin, in general, and African Americans in particular, the sarcoidosis phenotype appears to be more acute and severe [3]. Though poorly understood, the disease is thought to result from hyperactivation of the cell-mediated immune response resulting in B-cell stimulation and immunoglobulin production. Monocytes are then attracted which transform into epithelioid histiocytes and multinucleated giant cells thus leading to granuloma formation. It is not well-understood whether an infectious antigen or autoimmune process acts as a triggering event for granuloma formation. In addition, a few haplotype associations have been described which suggests a genetic susceptibility.

29.1.1 Clinical Picture

The lesions of cutaneous sarcoidosis present as red-brown well-circumcised papules on the face, lips, neck, chest, and extremities (Fig. 29.1). Beyond the skin, the lung, lymph nodes and eyes are most often involved. Skin lesions may take on other morphologies such as flat topped papules and plaques without scale or ulceration; these generally portend a good prognosis [4]. Hypopigmented patches are more common in black-skinned patients. By contrast, erythema nodosum, a feature of a subacute, transient type of sarcoidosis (Löfgren syndrome), is less frequently seen in skin of color [5, 6]. Other rare findings include ichthyosis, alopecia, discrete micropapular skin lesions, or even erythroderma. Nail changes can be present including clubbing, subungual hyperkeratosis, and onycholysis. Skin lesions are common and often are the first sign of systemic sarcoidosis, occuring in 1/3 of all patients. As with some inflammatory conditions, *sarcoidal granulomas* home to pre-existing scars or areas of prior trauma (Fig. 29.2). Unlike in lighter skin types, diascopy is not helpful for diagnosis in heavily pigmented skin. Histologically superficial and deep dermal epithelioid cell granulomas are seen. As they are without lymphocytic infiltrate, they are referred to as "naked tubercles." Hilar lymphadenopathy is often present along with granulomatous infiltration of the small airways, ultimately resulting in lung fibrosis. Fevers, weight loss, and pulmonary infiltrates are more common in Indian patients. Granulomas may occur in any other organ as well, including the liver, spleen, heart, eye, and bone. An increased incidence has been reported in patients starting anti-retroviral management for HIV [7], as well as in patients receiving interferon-α and ribavirin for chronic hepatitis C virus infection [8].

N. Kibbi (✉)
Department of Dermatology, Yale University, New Haven, CT, USA
e-mail: nour.kibbi@yale.edu

A.-G. Kibbi
Department of Dermatology, American University of Beirut Medical Center, Beirut, Lebanon
e-mail: agkibbi@aub.edu.lb

C. E. Orfanos et al. (eds.), *Pigmented Ethnic Skin and Imported Dermatoses*, https://doi.org/10.1007/978-3-319-69422-1_29

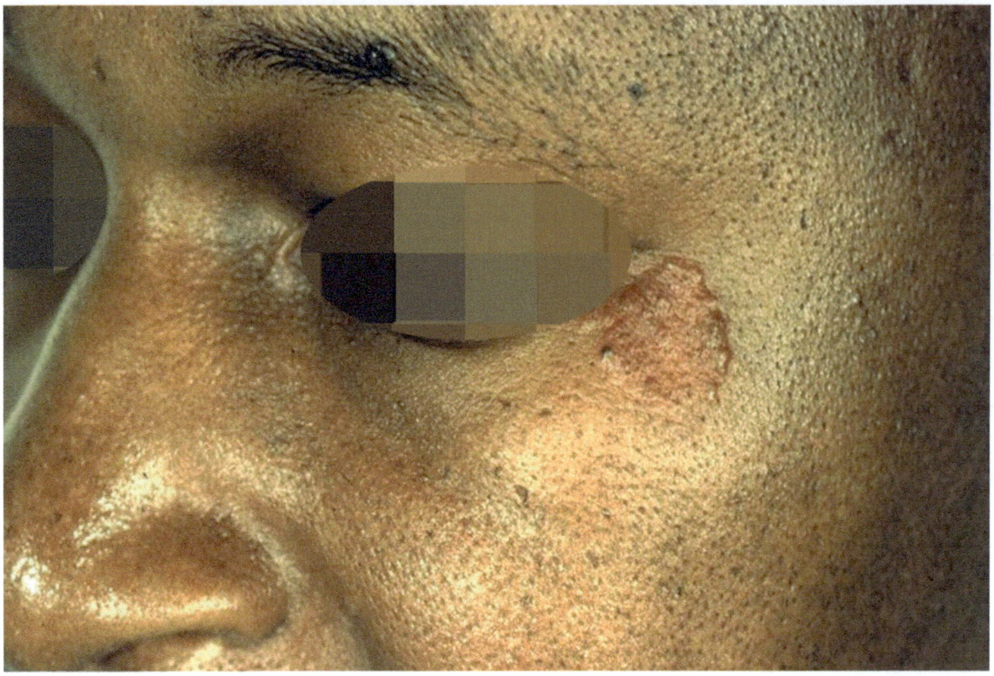

Fig. 29.1 *Cutaneous sarcoidosis* (courtesy Prof. S.W. Wassilew)

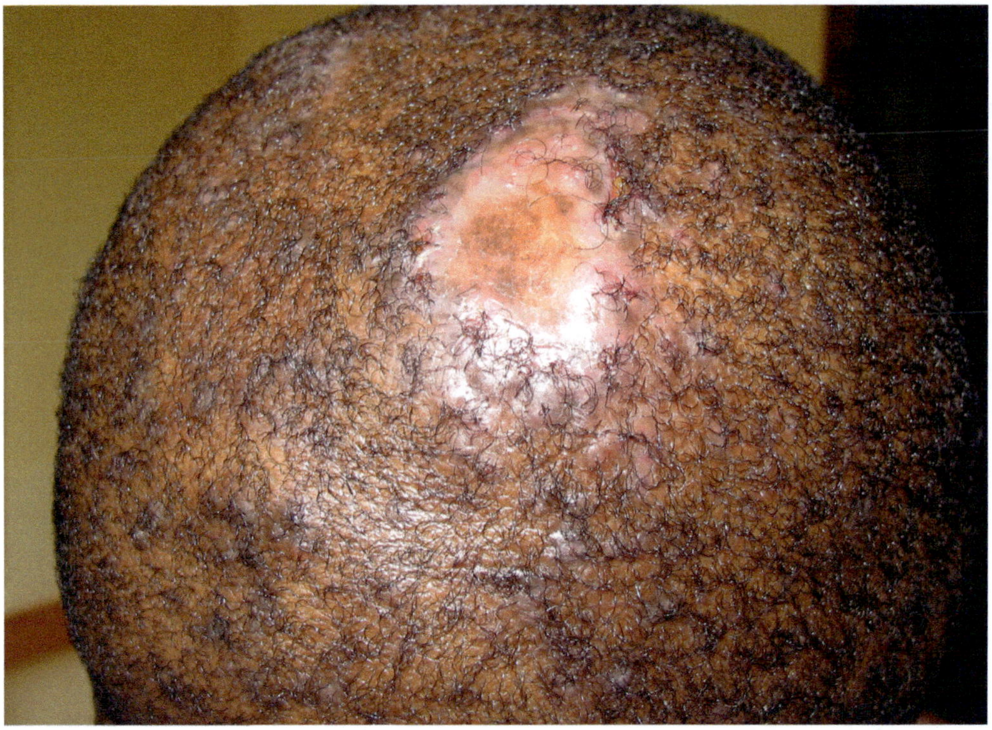

Fig. 29.2 *Sarcoidal granuloma* appearing in a traumatic scar on the scalp of a young African male possibly as an exaggerated reaction to ruptured hair follicles

29.1.2 Management

Topical, intralesional, or systemic corticosteroids are the mainstay of treatment. Oral prednisolone at 1 mg/kg/day for 4–6 weeks with a slow taper over months is used to treat systemic involvement. Antimalarials such as hydroxychloroquine 200–400 mg/day or chloroquine 250–500 mg/day [9] may be added as steroid-sparing drugs. Caution is required with these medications in pigmented skin where G6PD deficiency (and subsequent agranulocytosis) is more common. Ophthalmologic monitoring is recommended. In recalcitrant cases, methotrexate 10–25 mg/

week with or without corticosteroids may be helpful. Other medications reported to be effective include thalidomide 50–300 mg/day [10], isotretinoin 1 mg/kg/day for 3–8 months [11], and TNF-α inhibitors. The latter may be problematic as there are reports that TNF-a inhibitors may precipitate sarcoidosis [12]. PUVA has been reported as an effective treatment for cutaneous lesions [13].The long-term prognosis of the disease varies depending on the degree of any systemic involvement. Though ethnicity may influence the type of cutaneous involvement, it did not appear to influence prognosis [14].

29.2 Granuloma Annulare

Granuloma annulare (GA) is a rare, benign, and self-limited disorder usually affecting young individuals under the age of 30, with a female/male ratio of 2:1. Viral infections, insect bite reactions, and sun exposure have been proposed as precipitating pathogenetic factors [15], and associations with thyroid disease, diabetes [16], dyslipidemia [17], and various malignancies have been reported [18, 19].

29.2.1 Clinical Picture

GA presents with arciform or annular pink-red papules and plaques located on the extremities, most commonly the hand and arms (Fig. 29.3). Generalized superficial, deep subcutaneous and, rarely, perforating GA subtypes may occur (Fig. 29.4). In perforating variants, the papules may look prominent and umbilicated mimicking other perforating dermatosis, papulonecrotic tuberculid, or molluscum contagiosum. Deep dermal or subcutaneous granuloma annulare presents with large, painless nodular lesions that resemble rheumatoid nodules [20]. Periocular GA is a rare subtype that mimics lupus miliaris disseminatus faciei, granulomatous perioral dermatitis, or sarcoidosis. This type has a predilection for African-Americans, and while the course remains mostly asymptomatic, in some cases, it may precipitate ptosis [21].

29.2.2 Management

The disease is benign and spontaneously resolves within 2 years in 50% of the cases. If necessary, topical and intralesional steroids may be considered for management. In

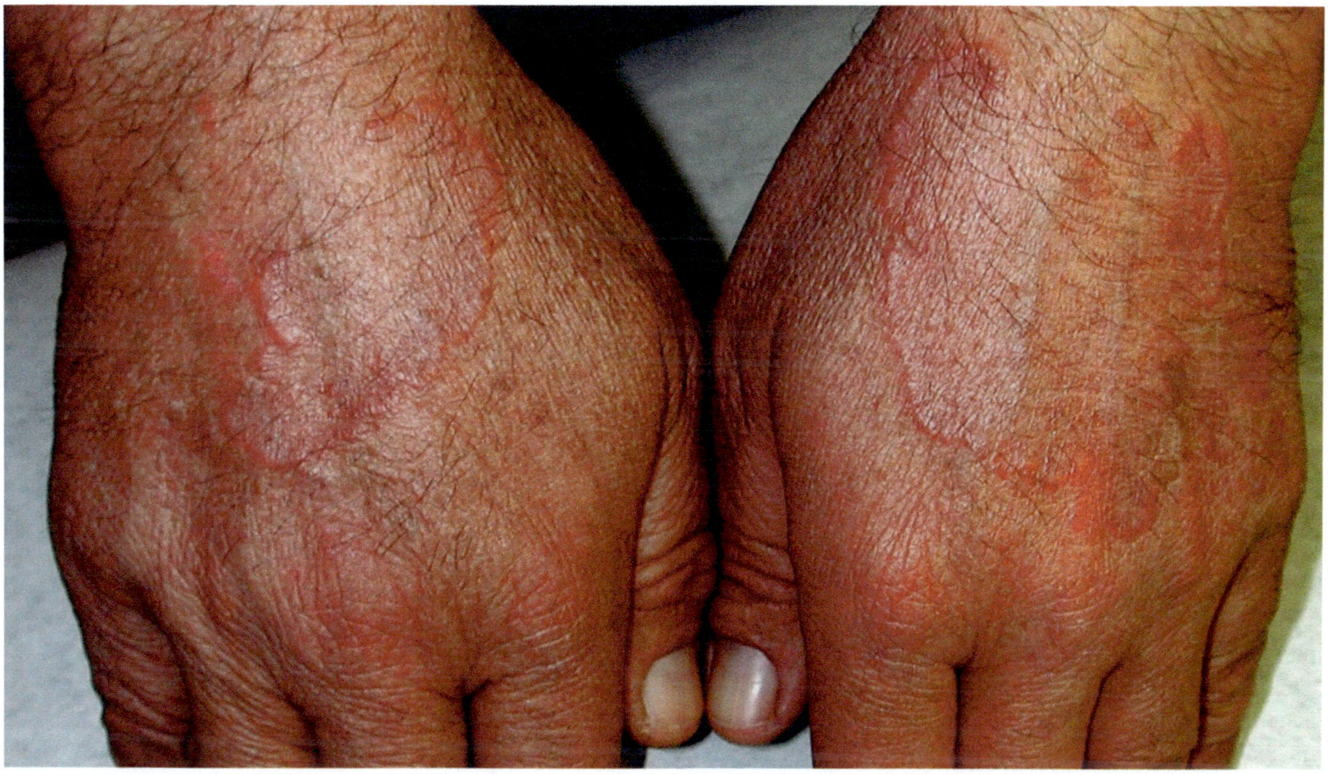

Fig. 29.3 *Granuloma annulare* (courtesy Prof. S. T. Zaynoun, Beirut, Lebanon)

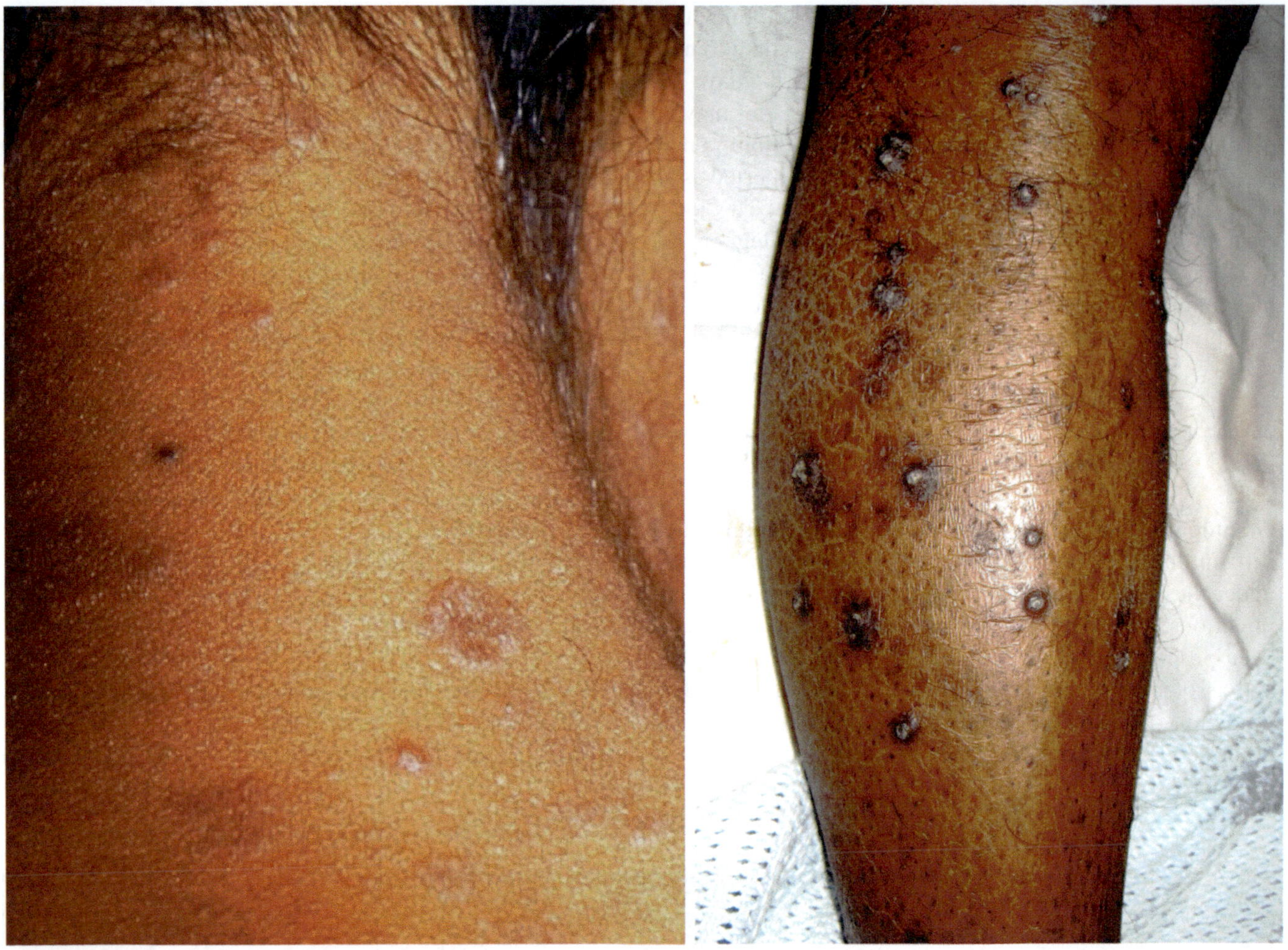

Fig. 29.4 Left: *Disseminated granuloma annulare* (courtesy Prof. S.W. Wassilew); Right: *Perforating granuloma annulare*; DD: Perforating folliculitis

patients with widely spread or generalized lesions, isotretinoin [22], antimalarials [23], and cyclosporine [24] have been used with varying degrees of success.

29.3 Necrobiosis Lipoidica

Necrobiosis lipoidica is a rare granulomatous disease, occurring in females with an estimated female/male ratio of 3:1. Though the disease is reported in conjunction with diabetes, skin lesions of necrobiosis lipoidica were found in only 0.3–1.2% of patients with diabetes [25], but were associated with poorer outcomes [26]. Etiology and pathogenesis are unclear. The presence of immunoreactants in the vessel wall of lesional and uninvolved skin suggests an immunological mechanism [27]. Histologically, it presents as palisaded and interstitial granulomas alternating with tiers of degenerated collagen with stark lack of mucin.

29.3.1 Clinical Picture

Clinically, necrobiosis lipoidica presents with multiple yellow-brown, atrophic plaques with elevated rim and telangiectasias, often located in the pretibial region of both legs (Fig. 29.5). In severe cases the lesions may ulcerate. Less commonly, the face and the upper extremities are involved, where lesions tend to be more annular or serpiginous. Within the plaques, the sensation to pinprick or to fine touch may be reduced, and hypohidrosis and alopecia are common. Rarely, squamous cell carcinomas within lesions of necrobiosis lipoidica have been reported [28].

29.3.2 Management

No treatment has proven to be effective in the treatment of necrobiosis lipoidica. Topical steroids for early lesions, intralesional steroids into active borders, oral corticosteroids [29], or UVA1

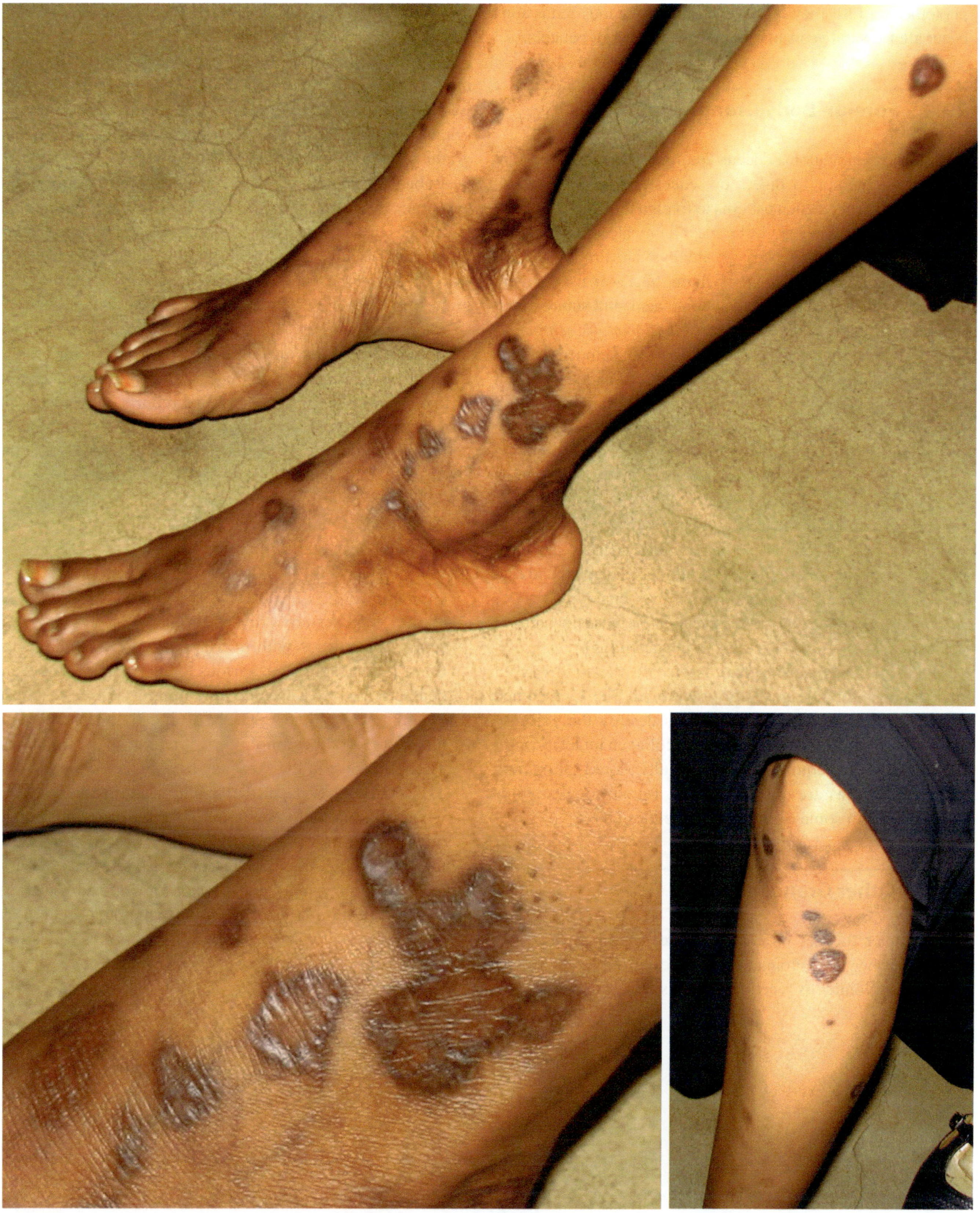

Fig. 29.5 *Necrobiosis lipoidica* (non-diabeticorum) in two young Tanzanian females

phototherapy [30] may be beneficial. Spontaneous remissions occur after several years in a significant number of patients.

29.4 Foreign Body Granulomas

Foreign body granulomas occur commonly as they represent the body's attempt to digest or sequester foreign material. Though different reaction patterns to foreign material have been described, such as lichenoid, chronic inflammatory, and pseudolymphomatous, foreign body granulomas are the most common. Tattoo ink, zirconium, beryllium, talc, soft tissue fillers such as bovine collagen and hyaluronic acid, and suture material are frequent inciting materials. *Granulomatous ochronosis* may develop from topical cosmetics in black-skinned patients [31]. Histologically, foreign material is surrounded by giant cells. Though typically confined to the skin, the development of tattoo granuloma may be associated with and lead to a diagnosis of sarcoidosis, as tattoo granulomas may be a presenting sign for sarcoidosis [32, 33]. In addition, inoculation of infectious agents (*M. fortuitum*) by tattooing may cause mixed-type granulomas [34]. Clinically the lesions appear within a few weeks of placement of a tattoo, but some reactions occur years later. Nodules or plaques are seen with or without tenderness and erythema. Pigment can also migrate into the regional lymph nodes and remain a chronic low-grade irritant. In rare cases, squamous cell carcinoma may develop in a red-ink tattoo [35].

Total surgical excision and lasers are the mainstay of management for foreign body granuloma. The Q-switched ruby, alexandrite, and Nd:YAG lasers destroy the chromophores in a tattoo leaving the adjacent collagen intact. Several wavelengths are required to treat a multicolored tattoo, and multiple sessions are often necessary. Intralesional steroids may be used in some cases for inflamed lesions.

29.5 Other Granulomatoses

This chapter focuses on commonly reported and relatively well-described granulomatous diseases in pigmented skin. Other granulomatous reactions such as *rheumatoid nodules*, *granulomatous cheilitis (Melkersson-Rosenthal)*, and *Crohn's disease*, are not well-described in pigmented skin. For instance, rheumatoid nodules, though poorly described in dark skin, are reportedly highly prevalent in Brazilian women with rheumatoid arthritis [36]. Moreover, interstital granulomatous dermatitis and palisaded neutrophilic and granulomatous dermatitis are two entities that have well-described associations with rheumatoid arthritis, lupus, and systemic vasculitis in fair-skinned indivudals, but remain poorly described in pigmented skin. Lastly, though the granulomatous disease of cutaneous Crohn's is not described in skin of color, the neutrophilic dermatosis, pyoderma gangrenosum is (Fig. 29.6), particularly in Tunisia [37].

Therapies for these entities include intralesional or systemic corticosteroids and immunomodulators such as oral dapsone, mesalazine, clofazimine, hydroxychloroquine, and/or thalidomide. There are occasional reports of cyclosporine A, azathioprine, mycophenolate mofetil, TNF-α inhibitors, and other biologics being used successfully [38]. In the absence of randomized clinical trials or consensus guidelines, management for these rare diseases should be tailored to the individual patient, with consideration given to disease severity and host risk factors.

Conclusions

Granulomatoses are a diverse group of localized or disseminated entities with overlapping clinical manifestations in the skin and various other organs. They are characterized by a chronic inflammatory tissue response to unknown antigens. The unifying hallmark in these disorders is the pathological finding of granulomas. Their presence in the skin may be a sign of systemic disease. There was a particular emphasis in this chapter, when relevant and known, on the differences in clinical presentation in black populations. Why certain graunlomatous disorders, chiefly sarcoidosis, are more common in dark-skinned individuals is not known. More work is needed to explain this observation. Treatment in, in most cases, is symptomatic, and curative options are lacking at this time.

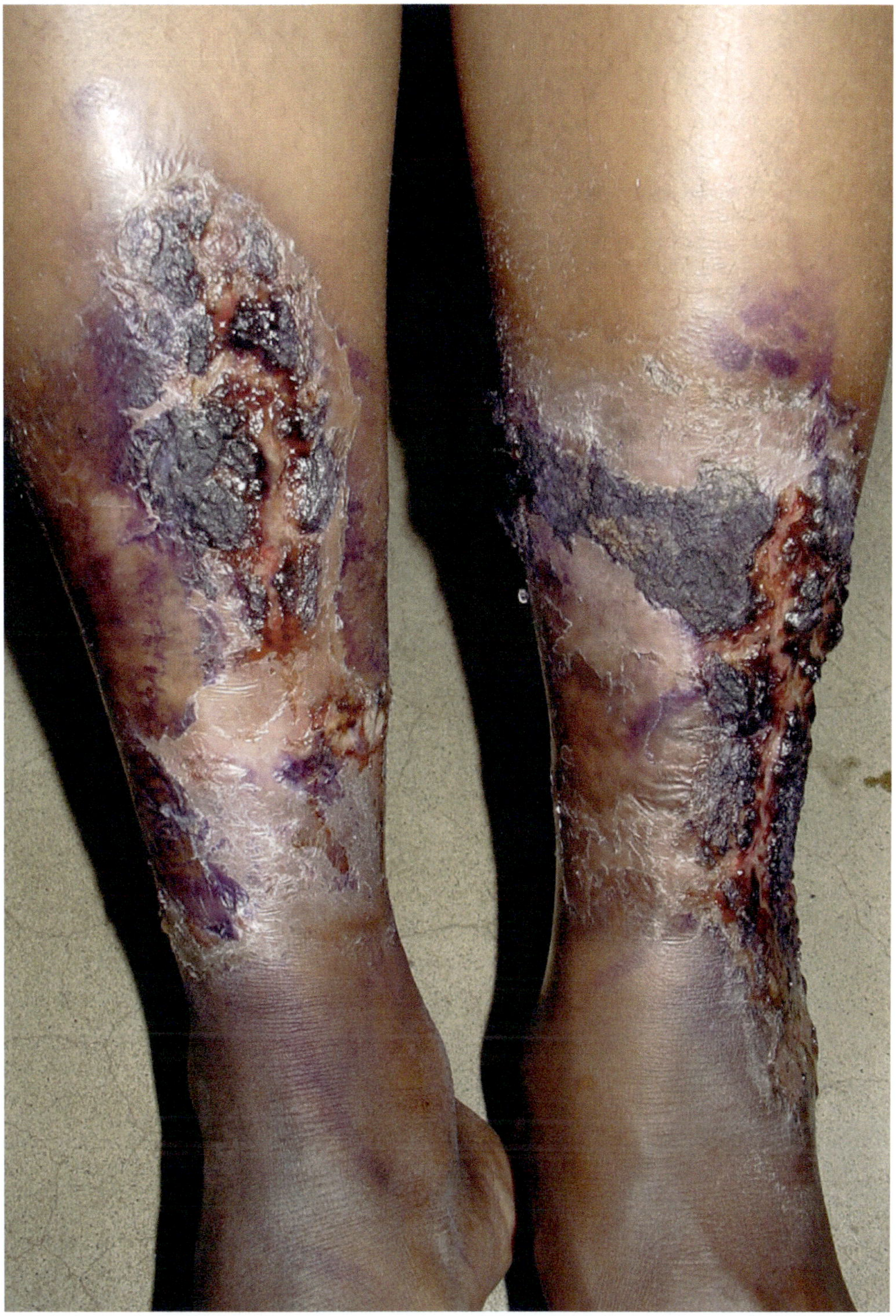

Fig. 29.6 *Pyoderma gangrenosum* in black skin

References

1. Rybicki BA, Major M, Popovich J, et al. Racial differences in sarcoidosis incidence: a 5-year study in a health maintenance organization. Am J Epidemiol. 1997;145:234–41.
2. Edmondstone WM, Wilson AG. Sarcoidosis in Caucasians, Blacks and Asians in London. Br J Dis Chest. 1985;79:27–36.
3. Jacyk WK. Cutaneous sarcoidosis in black South Africans. Int J Dermatol. 1999;38:841–5.
4. Marchell RM, Judson MA. Chronic cutaneous lesions of sarcoidosis. Clin Dermatol. 2007;25:295–302.
5. Minus HR, Grimes PE. Cutaneous manifestations of sarcoidosis in blacks. Cutis. 1983;32:361–3.
6. Sharma SK, Mohan A, Guleria JS. Clinical characteristics, pulmonary function abnormalities and outcome of prednisolone treatment in 106 patients with sarcoidosis. J Assoc Physicians India. 2001;49:697–704.
7. Roustan G, Yebra M, Rodriguez-Braojos O, et al. Cutaneous and pulmonary sarcoidosis in a patient with HIV after highly active antiretroviral therapy. Int J Dermatol. 2007;46:68–71.
8. Ramos-Casals M, Maña J, Nardi N, et al. Sarcoidosis in patients with chronic hepatitis C virus infection: analysis of 68 cases. Medicine (Baltimore). 2005;84(2):6.
9. Doherty CB, Rosen T. Evidence-based therapy for cutaneous sarcoidosis. Drugs. 2008;68:1361–83.
10. Lee JB, Koblenzer PS. Disfiguring cutaneous manifestation of sarcoidosis treated with thalidomide: a case report. J Am Acad Dermatol. 1998;39:835–8.
11. Georgiou S, Monastirli A, Pasmatzi E, et al. Cutaneous sarcoidosis: complete remission after oral isotretinoin therapy. Acta Derm Venereol. 1998;78:457–9.
12. Dhaille F, Viseux V, Caudron A, et al. Cutaneous sarcoidosis occurring during anti-TNF-alpha treatment: report of two cases. Dermatology. 2010;220:234–7.
13. Patterson JW, Fitzwater JE. Treatment of hypopigmented sarcoidosis with 8-methoxypsoralen and long wave ultraviolet light. Int J Dermatol. 1982;21:476–80.
14. Behbehani N, Jayakrishnan B, Khadadah M, et al. Long-term prognosis of sarcoidosis in Arabs and Asians: predictors of good outcome. Sarcoidosis Vasc Diffuse Lung Dis. 2006;23:209–14.
15. Studer EM, Calza AM, Saurat JH. Precipitating factors and associated diseases in 84 patients with granuloma annulare: a retrospective study. Dermatology. 1996;193:364–8.
16. Muhlemann MF, Williams DR. Localized granuloma annulare is associated with insulin-dependent diabetes mellitus. Br J Dermatol. 1984;111:325.
17. Wu W, Robinson-Bostom L, Kokkotou E, et al. Dyslipidemia in granuloma annulare: a case-control study. Arch Dematol. 2012;148:1131–6.
18. Li A, Hogan DJ, Sanusi ID, et al. Granuloma annulare and malignant neoplasms. Am J Dermatopathol. 2003;25:113–6.
19. Barksdale SK, Perniciaro C, Hailing KC, et al. Granuloma annulare in patients with malignant lymphoma: clinicopathologic study of thirteen new cases. J Am Acad Dermatol. 1994;31:42–8.
20. Evans MJ, Blessing K, Gray E. Pseudorheumatoid nodule (deep granuloma annulare) of childhood: clinicopathologic features of twenty patients. Pediatr Dermatol. 1994;11:6–9.
21. Chiang K, Bhalla R, Mesinkovska NA, et al. Periocular granuloma annulare: a case report and review of literature. Pediatr Dermatol. 2014;31:722–5.
22. Ratnavel RC, Norris PG. Perforating granuloma annulare: response to treatment with isotretinoin. J Am Acad Dermatol. 1995;32:126–7.
23. Simon M Jr, von den Driesch P. Antimalarials for control of disseminated granuloma annulare in children. J Am Acad Dermatol. 1994;31:1064–5.
24. Spadino S, Altomare A, Cainelli C, et al. Disseminated granuloma annulare: efficacy of cyclosporine therapy. Int J Immunopathol Pharmacol. 2006;19:433–8.
25. Peyri J, Moreno A. Marcoval: necrobiosis lipoidica. Semin Cutan Med Surg. 2007;26:87–9.
26. Boulton AJM, Cutfield RG, Abouganem D, et al. Necrobiosis lipoidica diabeticorum: a clinicopathologic study. J Am Acad Dermatol. 1988;18:530–7.
27. Quimby SR, Muller SA, Schroeter AL. The cutaneous immunopathology of necrobiosis lipoidica diabeticorum. Arch Dermatol. 1988;124:1364–71.
28. Uva L, Freitas J, Soares de Almeida L, et al. Squamous cell carcinoma arising in ulcerated necrobiosis lipoidica diabeticorum. Int Wound J. 2015;12:741–3.
29. Petzelbauer P, Wolff K, Tappeiner G. Necrobiosis lipoidica: treatment with systemic corticosteroids. Br J Dermatol. 1992;126:542–5.
30. Beattie PE, Dawe RS, Ibbotson SH, et al. UVA1 phototherapy for treatment of necrobiosis lipoidica. Clin Exp Dermatol. 2006;31:235–8.
31. Dogliotti M, Leibowitz M. Granulomatous ochronosis—a cosmetic-induced skin disorder in blacks. S Afr Med J. 1979;56:757–60.
32. Baumgartner M, Feldmann R, Breier F, et al. Sarcoidal granulomas in a cosmetic tattoo in association with pulmonary sarcoidosis. J Dtsch Dermatol Ges. 2010;8:900–2.
33. Collins P, Evans AT, Gray W, et al. Pulmonary sarcoidosis presenting as a granulomatous tattoo reaction. Br J Dermatol. 1994;130:658–62.
34. Suvanasuthi S, Wongpraparut C, Pattanaprichakul P, et al. Mycobacterium fortuitum cutaneous infection from amateur tattoo. J Med Assoc Thail. 2012;95:834–7.
35. Sherif S, Blakeway E, Fenn C, et al. A case of squamous cell carcinoma developing within a red-ink tattoo. J Cutan Med Surg. 2017;21:61–3. pii: 1203475416661311.
36. da Mota LM, Laurindo IM, dos Santos Neto LL. Demographic and clinical characteristics of a cohort of patients with early rheumatoid arthritis. Rev Bras Rheumatol. 2010;50:235–48.
37. Mebazaa A, Aounallah A, Naija N, et al. Dermatologic manifestations in inflammatory bowel disease in Tunisia. Tunis Med. 2012;90:252–7.
38. Wollina U, Haroske G. Pyoderma gangraenosum. Curr Opin Rheumatol. 2011;23:50–6.

30 Lupus Erythematosus in Pigmented and Black Skin

Evelina Buinsauskaitė and Constantin E. Orfanos

Lupus erythematosus (LE) is an autoimmune, chronic inflammatory, often multisystem disease, seen in all populations worldwide. It is characterized by a wide spectrum of clinical symptoms and immune serological parameters, with variable evolution and prognosis. The skin is the most frequent site of involvement, showing variable erythematous lesions and overlapping features which make the diagnosis by the physician often difficult, particularly in pigmented or black skin. There are various classifications and different variants and subtypes of the disease with three major forms: The *discoid or chronic cutaneous lupus* (DLE), the *subacute cutaneous lupus* (SCLE), and the *systemic* form of the disease with involvement of the joints or visceral organs (SLE).

30.1 Incidence

The incidence of LE and its clinical manifestations vary according to the characteristics of the population studied, race, ethnicity, sex group, the predominant age, and the period of time studied. The data given also change based on the classification used. There are only a few reports available on the incidence of cutaneous LE, contradictory in part, whereas, numerous epidemiological studies on SLE in skin of color were published. In general, DLE can affect any race, with some early reports suggesting that higher prevalence in populations with white skin [1–3]. DLE was found more common among African-Americans, whereas SCLE was more common among Caucasians [4]. In 2000 a retrospective epidemiological study performed in French Guiana revealed that the average annual incidence of DLE was 2.59 per 100,000 inhabitants, lower than expected from another study performed on African-Americans [5, 6].

For SLE evidence suggests that this type is more common in Asians and African-Americans than in Caucasians; its incidence and prevalence have been consistently found higher in people with black skin. Also the rates of age-adjusted incidence and prevalence of SLE were higher in Afro-Caribbean people than in whites [7]. In Nigeria, the incidence of both discoid and systemic LE was reported to increase over the years [8]. A similar trend was observed in the frequency of childhood DLE in Tunisia [9]. However, in Tunisia chronic lupus erythematosus is a relatively rare disorder when compared to other African countries, where prevalence is 7–10 times more frequent [10, 11].

30.2 Etiology/Pathogenesis

The precise etiology of the cutaneous LE still needs to be clarified as its pathogenesis involves multiple factors including genetic, hormonal, infectious, and environmental. Cutaneous LE is polygenic; however, no wide genome scans have been performed, whereas over 25 risk loci have been identified for SLE patients [4]. Immunogenetic studies showed that HLA-A1, HLA-B8, HLA-DR3, HLA-A3, HLA-B7, HLA-DR2, and HLA-C4A haplotypes are associated with a risk to develop LE [12]. The influence of sexual hormones is underlined by higher prevalence of the disease in females and during the postpubertal period; furthermore, in about 20% of the cases, reactivation of LE is triggered by pregnancy and oral contraceptives [13]. A number of viruses like the exogenous Epstein-Barr virus and human endogenous retroviruses (HERV), HRES-1, ERV-3, HERV-E 4–1, HERV-K10, HERV-K18 have been implicated to be linked to the pathogenesis of SLE. Cutaneous LE has been also reported associated to be with smoking, not with alcohol consumption [14].

E. Buinsauskaitė
Dermatovenerologist, Kaunas, Lithuania

C. E. Orfanos (✉)
The Free University of Berlin, Medical School Charité, Berlin, Germany
e-mail: corfanos@t-online.de

C. E. Orfanos et al. (eds.), *Pigmented Ethnic Skin and Imported Dermatoses*, https://doi.org/10.1007/978-3-319-69422-1_30

A large number of drugs are able to induce SCLE, such as hydralazine, hydrochlorothiazide, sulfasalazine, chlorpromazine, carbamazepine, terbinafine, angiotensin-converting enzyme inhibitors, and others. Exposure to ultraviolet light, both UVA and UVB, may induce and/or exacerbate skin involvement [15].

30.3 Clinical Picture

30.3.1 Discoid or Chronic Cutaneous Lupus (DLE)

DLE usually affects young women (28.5–42 years of age) with a prevalence of female/male ratio of 1.97–5.0:1 [10, 11, 16, 17]. One study demonstrated that African-Americans presented initially with greater disease damage than Caucasians and in conjunction with disease activity [17]. Severe, progressed DLE cases with mutilations are occasionally seen in sub-Saharan Africa.

In pigmented skin brownish-blackish macules and papules are seen in early stages of the disease. They are most commonly found on the sun-exposed areas, however, scalp, upper trunk and distal extremities can also be affected. On the face "butterfly" pattern is common, presented on both cheeks with possible impairment of the bridge of nose and lips. The lesions are slightly elevated, with hyperkeratotic scaling, mostly hypopigmented. Hyperpigmented borders and central atrophy evolve with the progression of the disease and the entire lesions may become fully depigmented (Fig. 30.1). On palpation, roughness of the surface or hyperesthesia may be observed and follicular keratoses are noted when surface scales are removed, for example with tweezers (carpet-tack sign). Long-term exposure to ultraviolet light in patients with heavily pigmented skin aggravates the lesions and causes severe dyspigmentations with an increase of local symptoms such as irritation and itch (Figs. 30.2 and 30.3). Variants of chronic DLE resembling vitiligo has been reported in West Africans [16]; they are commonly seen in African patients with black skin. Since true vitiligo may also occur together with LE, differential diagnosis will be difficult in some late cases (Fig. 30.4).

Hyperkeratotic scales and mutilation can be observed when the lesions affect the ears, the lips and the tip of the nose. In hair-bearing areas of black skin thinning of the hair and scarring alopecia are common features due to the tendency of coiled hair to revert to the skin when cut. A subtype of DLE in black skin shows elevated nodular lesions, partly hyperkeratotic, usually formed on the face and trunk (*tumidus*). In another subtype the inflammatory process is located in the lower dermis and the subcutaneous fat, showing painful nodules mainly in the areas with increased fat deposition (*LE profundus*). African patients with lupus when compared with other series comprising Asian and white Caucasians also show greater frequency of periorbital edema as an initial manifestation of the disease [18]. Once the regression starts, deeply depressed and ulcerated scarring lesions may occur. Review of the literature revealed that this subset of lupus profundus appears to have a more benign course. Any cutaneous site with predilection for the face, upper trunk, and proximal extremities, can have mucosal involvement. Clinically tense bullae can be then observed on erythematous or dark brown round macules and patches.

30.3.2 Subacute Cutaneous Lupus (SCLE)

This subtype is definitely less frequent in patients with strongly pigmented or black skin than in Caucasians. The patients with SCLE are often photosensitive; the skin lesions frequently occur on sun-exposed areas like the face and neck as well as disseminated on the chest, upper back, and shoulders (Fig. 30.5). They may be macular, papulosquamous, and/or annular and resolve without scarring. Annular SCLE lesions often demonstrate hypopigmented areas with central telangiectasias, which may remain for months or become permanent, in rare cases [19]. In the papulosquamous variant, numerous oval or round scaly plaques are seen with usually negative carpet tack sign.

30.3.3 Systemic Lupus (SLE)

Cutaneous manifestations also occur in SLE patients, often presenting butterfly rashes and lesions of the face. Diffuse facial hyperpigmentations, periungual telangiectasias, alopecia, and mucosal involvement are more common in SCLE and SLE than in DLE subtypes (Figs.30.6 and 30.7). The systemic manifestation mainly involves the joints, kidneys, pleura, the pericardium, and brain. Women are 9× more frequently affected than men, and African-Americans and Latin-American mestizos are much more frequently affected by SLE than Caucasians showing higher disease morbidity [20]. Criteria for classification were developed by the American Rheumatism Association in 1971, revised in 1982, and annotated in 1997. These criteria were developed and validated for the classification of patients with long-standing established disease and may exclude patients in early stages or disease limited to a few organs only. Thus, in spite of their excellent sensitivity (>85%) and specificity (>95%) for patients with established disease, their sensitivity for patients in early phases may be significantly lower [20].

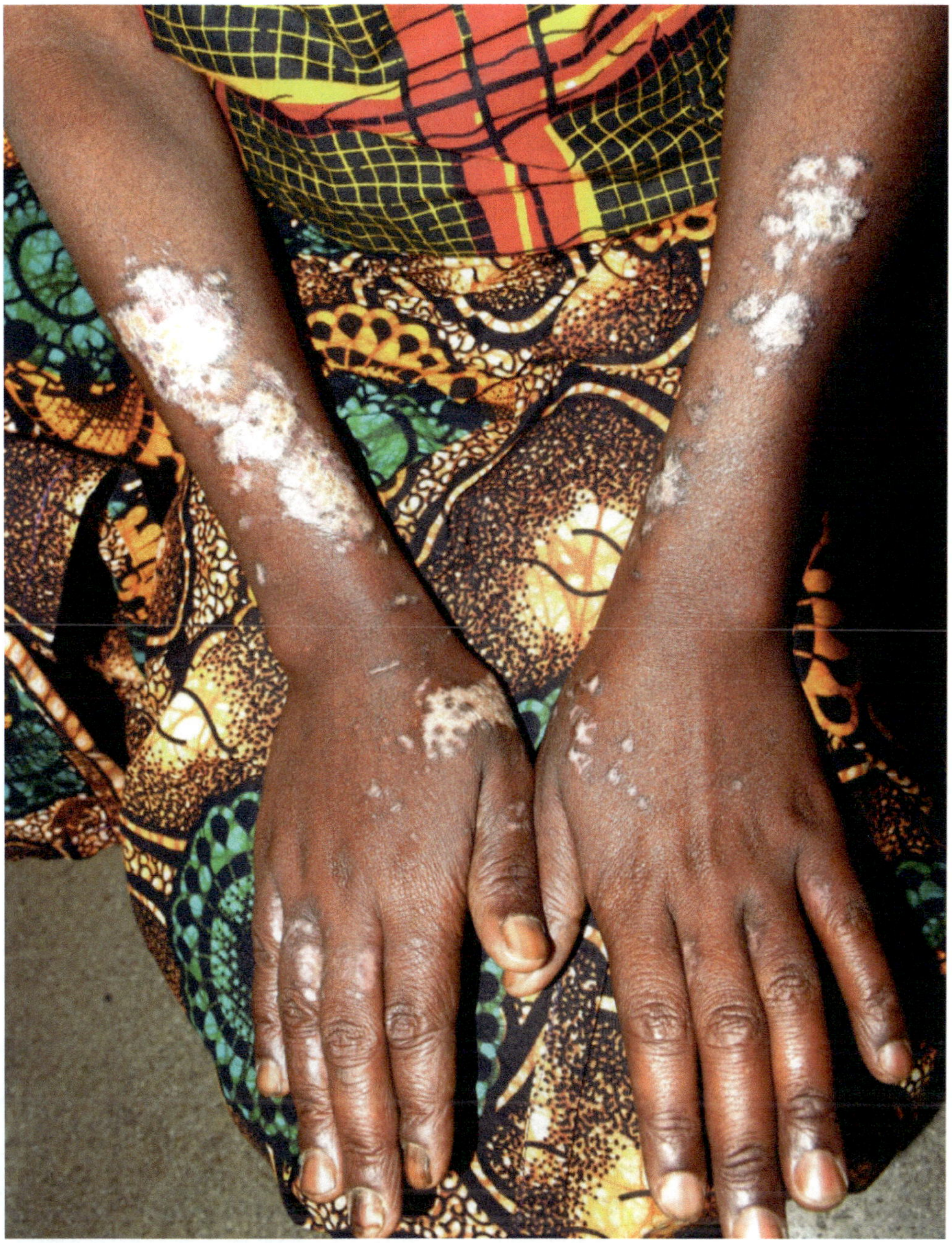

Fig. 30.1 Lesions of DLE in pigmented skin

30.4 Management

In all cases with cutaneous involvement, routine assessment for possible signs and findings indicating SLE should be performed, as 20% of the patients with generalized DLE and 5% of all patients with localized DLE progress to SLE [21].

Protection from exposure to ultraviolet light is obligatory for all patients, particularly for those with the SCLE subtype. Sun-protective clothing, sunglasses, and broad-spectrum sunscreens should be applied 20 min before any sun exposure and reapplied every 2–3 h continuously throughout the day. Cumulative low-dose UV exposure from indoor fluorescent light bulbs can worsen the disease; therefore, patients with cutaneous LE are recommended to use compact bulbs with the lowest UV irradiance. They should be also encouraged to address vitamin D insufficiency [22].

Three common antimalarials are currently used for treatment of cutaneous LE: hydroxychloroquine, chloroquine,

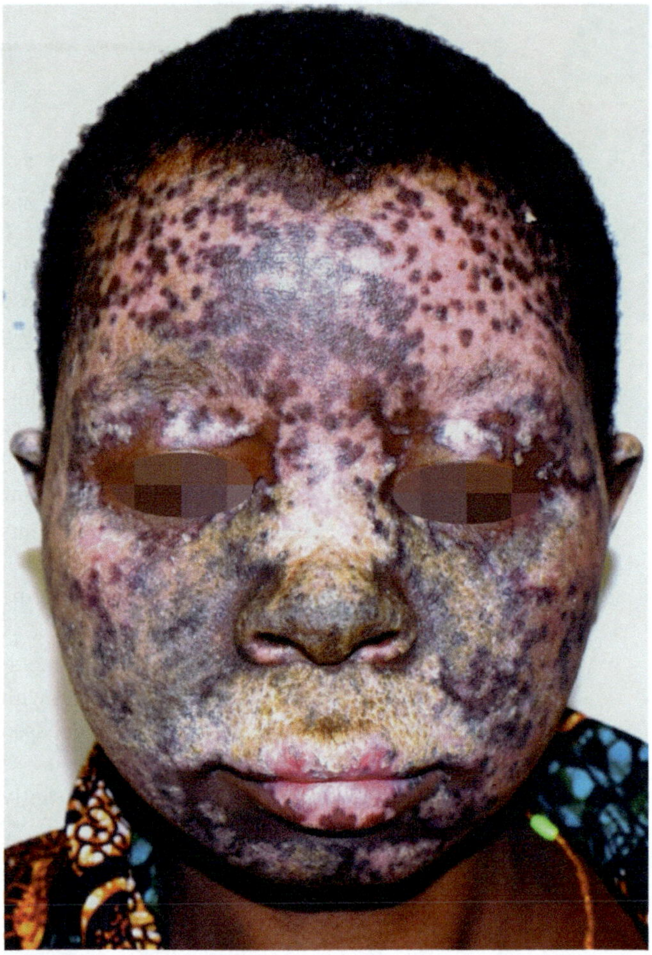

Fig. 30.2 Widespread, severe DLE with facial dyspigmentation and hyperkeratoses

and quinacrine. Administration of hydroxychloroquine is the worldwide first-line antimalarial management; quinacrine can only be obtained in compounding pharmacies, mostly used in combination with chloroquine or hydroxychloroquine [23]. The dosing of chloroquine and hydroxychloroquine is based on the ideal body weight: 3 mg/kg/day (250 mg/day) and <6.5 mg/kg/day (400 mg/day), respectively. Long-term maintenance requires ophthalmological controls yearly to avoid drug-induced retinopathy, and cumulative dosage of chloroquine should not exceed 500 g. Quinacrine is generally dosed at 100 mg/day. Patients should be warned against smoking; patients with cutaneous LE who smoke were reported to respond significantly less likely to antimalarials [24].

Alternatives include various immunomodulators such as dapsone (25–150 mg/day) or thalidomide (50–100 mg/day). Also, systemic retinoids such as acitretin (10–50 mg/day) and isotretinoin (0.2–0.5 mg/kg/day) may be helpful in recalcitrant cases.

Topical or intralesional corticosteroids may be successfully used for treatment of cutaneous lesions, their potency choice depending on their location. Low-potency corticosteroids (0.5–2% hydrocortisone) are advisable for the face and other thin skin areas, and mid-potency corticosteroids (0.5% triamcinolone, betamethasone) are often used for the trunk and extremities, while high-potency preparations (clobetasol) may be administered for the scalp and other thick skin regions. To avoid systemic absorption and suppression of the hypothalamic-pituitary axis, no more than 45 g per week of high potency or 100 g per week of low- to mid-potency topical steroid should be applied (without occlusion). Topical

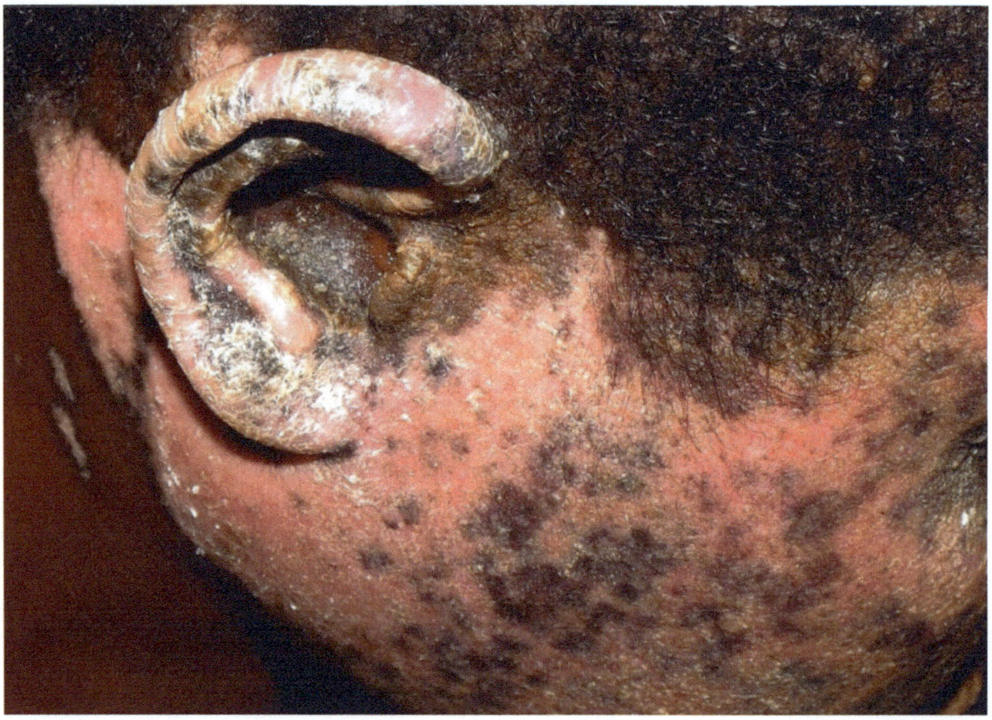

Fig. 30.3 Involvement of the ear with spotted dyspigmentations of the face

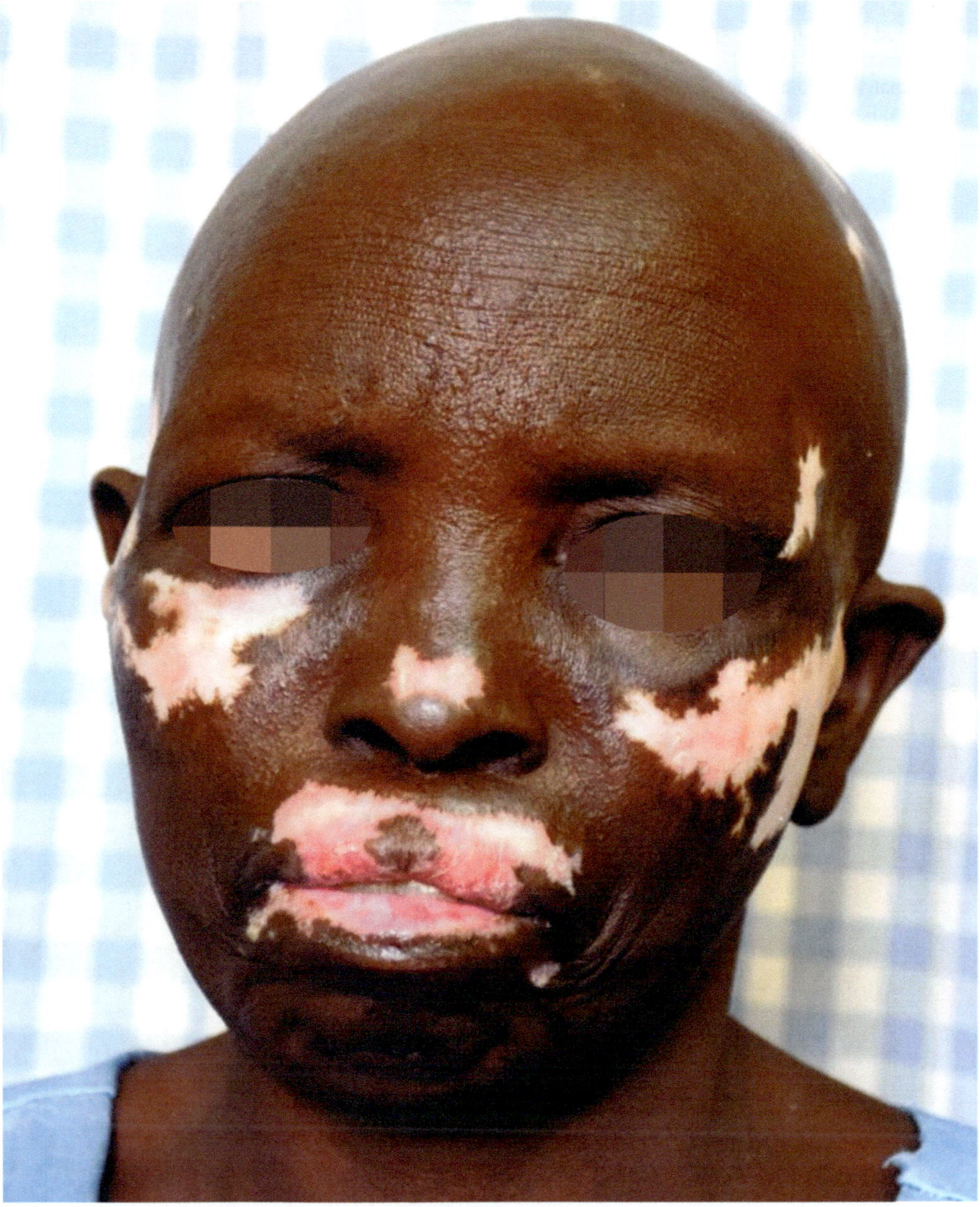

Fig. 30.4 Scarring DLE with depigmented, vitiliginous facial lesions and ectropion

calcineurin inhibitors (tacrolimus, pimecrolimus) are also given for topical treatment of the face and ears.

Short courses of systemic corticosteroids (50–80 mg/day, tapered down to 5–15 mg/day), together with or without azathioprine (50–100 mg/day), will help to control extensive cutaneous involvement and flares, before initiating treatment with antimalarials. Management of systemic LE is difficult and often requires high doses of corticosteroids on a longer term. Biologicals have been consistently ineffective in DLE, SCLE, and SLE. In contrast, recent controlled studies indicate that the BlyS inhibitor belimumab is beneficial in severe cases with organ involvement (Benlysta® i.v. inj.,10 m/kg, 3×/month). Concomitant administration of belimumab will suppress DSI (*disease severity index*) and will reduce the dose of oral corticosteroids required. Systemic steroids are not recommended for long-term management of LE; arthropathies respond to nonsteroidal anti-inflammatory drugs (ibuprofen, ketoprofen, naproxen, indomethacin).

Physical modalities (cryotherapy, dermabrasion, lasers, tattooing) were shown to be effective for hyperkeratotic scarring lesions; however, these treatment options increase the risk of developing post-inflammatory pigmentation disorders and hypertrophic scars and induce keloid formation in pigmented or black skin.

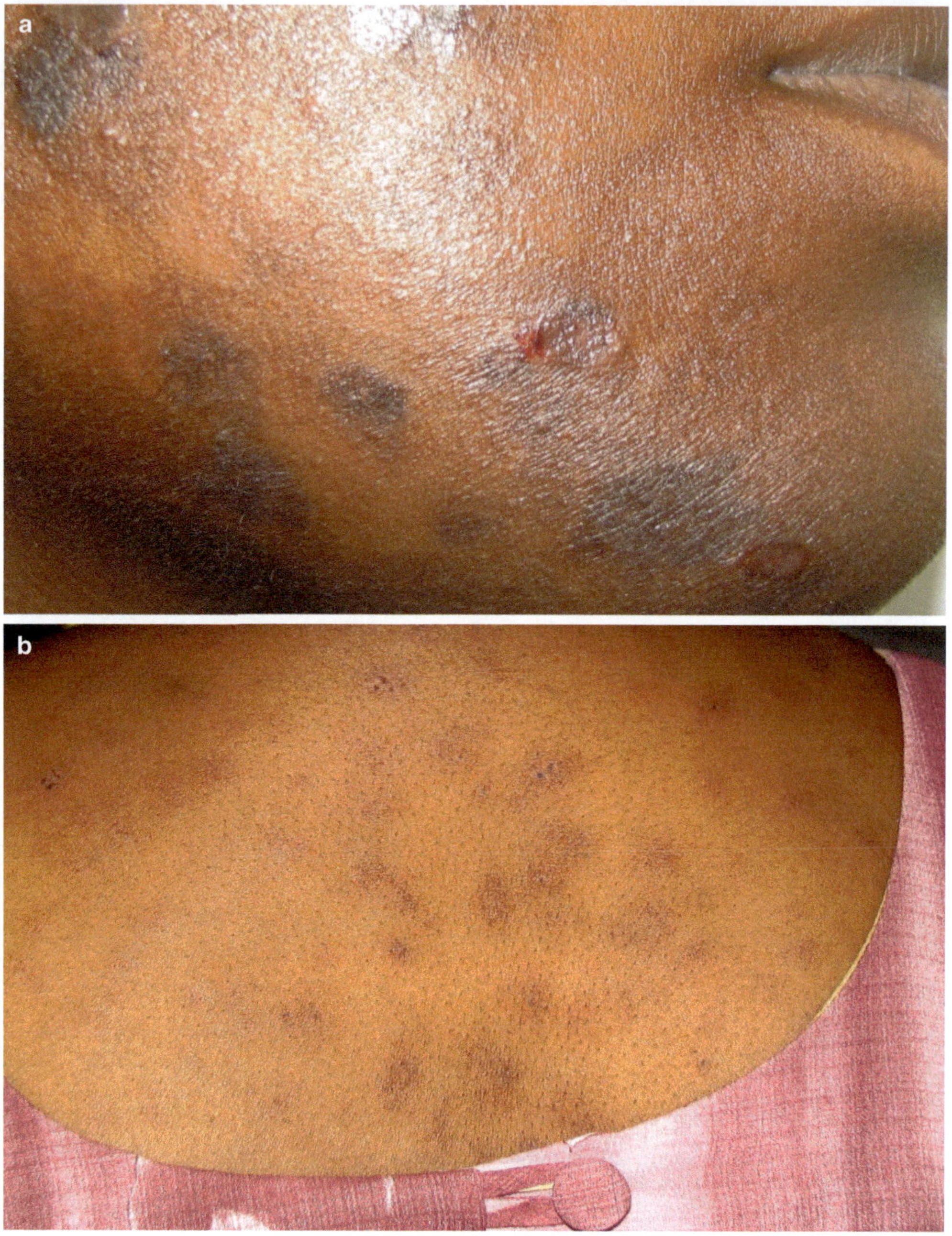

Fig. 30.5 SCLE in pigmented skin: annular lesions on the face (**a**) and disseminated macular lesions on the trunk (**b**)

30.5 Course

The course of DLE and SLE are difficult to predict, while the course of SCLE is rather long- lasting, showing relapsing flares interrupted by periods of improvement. The atrophic lesions with hyperpigmented borders in DLE patients with black/pigmented skin may end with permanent, hypopigmented scars. Repigmentation is slow or lacking. The classic rashes of SCLE heal without scarring; however, pigment alterations may also remain. These permanent alterations in pigmentation and scars are prevalent in colored skin and have a significant psychosocial effect, especially when present on the face [19].

Keloid formation is characterized by exaggerated response to injuries, frequently occurring in African populations. Patients with highly pigmented or black skin are more prone to develop hypertrophic scars or keloids due to LE lesions. However, evidence suggested that it is the activity of the disease and not the damage or its parameters of scarring and dyspigmentation that affect their quality of life [17].

DLE is known to be associated with nonmelanoma skin cancer. Lesions of the scalp, lips, ears and nose, which are chronically exposed to the sun and have become hypopigmented and scarred, are at the highest risk to develop squa-

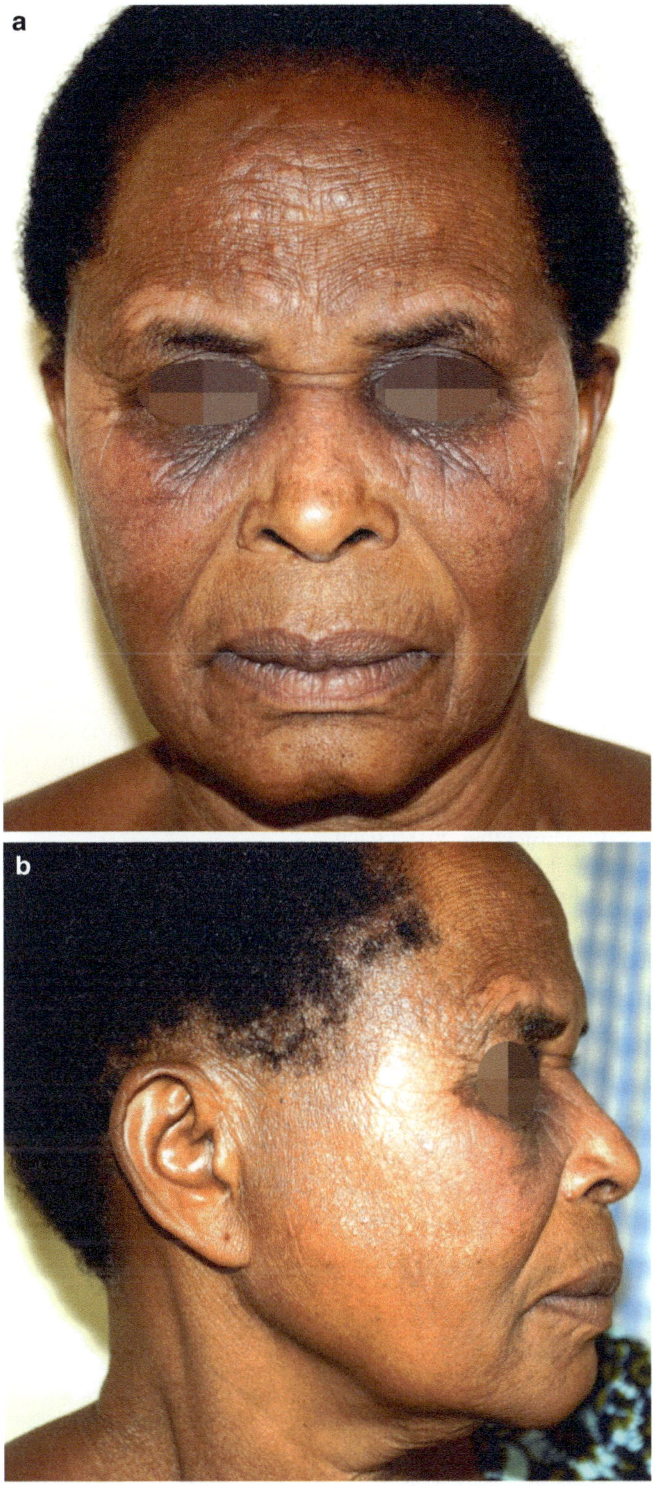

Fig. 30.6 (**a**, **b**) Diffuse generalized SCLE in pigmented skin

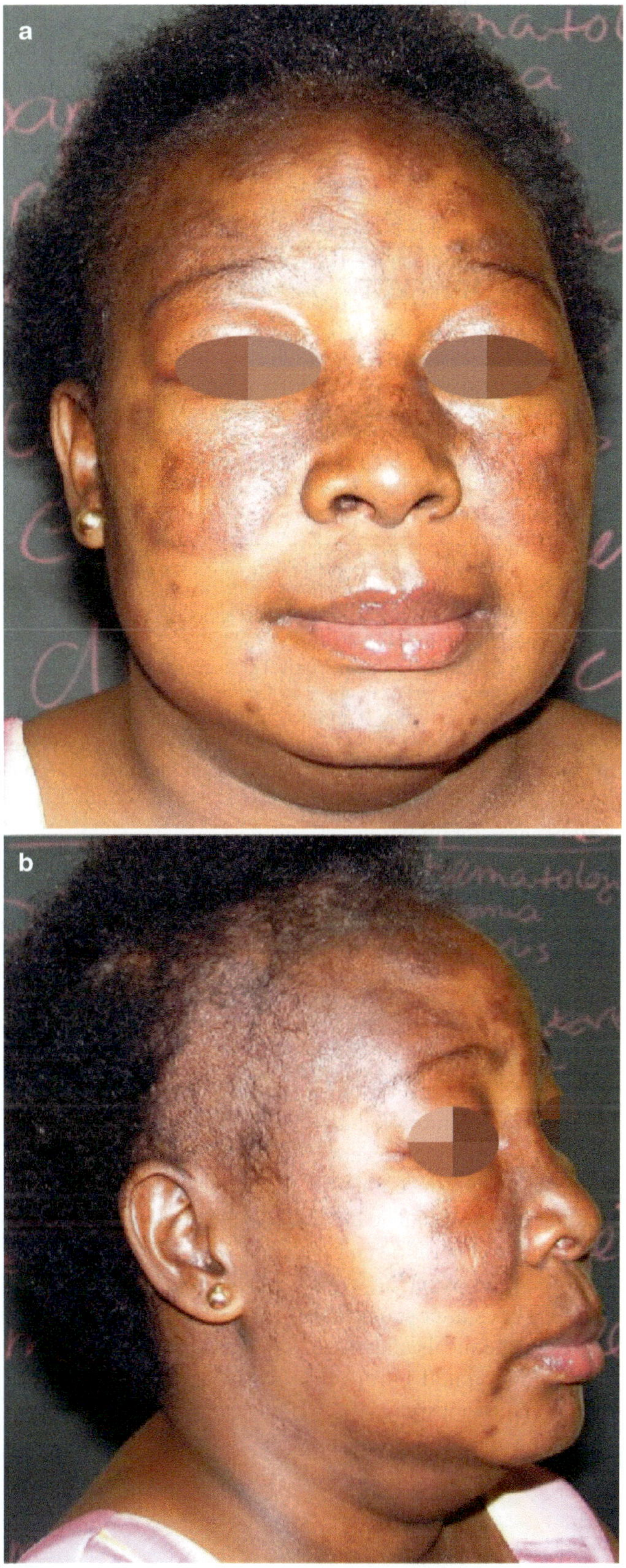

Fig. 30.7 (**a**, **b**) Cutaneous involvement in SLE with butterfly erythema, periorbital edema, and scarring alopecia in the frontoparietal area (see also Chap. 35)

mous cell carcinoma. Chronic scarring is an established risk factor for cutaneous SCC in black-skinned patients [25]. The morbidity and mortality rates for LE-associated carcinoma are higher in African-Americans than in Caucasians. The time for development of DLE-related carcinoma may vary between months and 20 years [26].

References

1. Findlay GH, Lups JG. The incidence and pathogenesis of chronic discoid lupus erythematosus. An analysis of 191 consecutive cases from the Transvaal. S Afr Med J. 1967;41:694–8.
2. Tebbe B, Orfanos CE. Epidemiology and socioeconomic impact of skin disease in lupus erythematosus. Lupus. 1997;6:96–104.
3. Ng PP, Tan SH, Koh ET. Epidemiology of cutaneous lupus erythematosus in a tertiary referral centre in Singapore. Australas J Dermatol. 2000;41:229–33.
4. Grönhagen CM, Nyberg F. Cutaneous lupus erythematosus: an update. Indian Dermatol Online J. 2014;5:7–13.
5. Callen JP. Chronic cutaneous lupus erythematosus: clinical, laboratory, therapeutic, and prognostic examination of 62 patients. Arch Dermatol. 1982;118:412–6.
6. Deligny C, Clyti E, Sainte Marie D, et al. Incidence of chronic cutaneous lupus erythematosus in French Guiana: a retrospective population-based study. Arthritis Care Res. 2010;62:279–82.
7. Johnson AE, Gordon C, Palmer RG, et al. The prevalence and incidence of systemic lupus erythematosus in Birmingham, England. Relationship to ethnicity and country of birth. Arthritis Rheum. 1995;38:551–8.
8. Ogunbiyi AO, Daramola OO, Alese OO. Prevalence of skin diseases in Ibadan, Nigeria. Int J Dermatol. 2004;43:31–6.
9. Cherif F, Mebazaa A, Mokni M, et al. Childhood discoid lupus erythematosus: a Tunisian retrospective study of 16 cases. Pediatr Dermatol. 2003;20:295–8.
10. Mahfoudh A, Khaled A, Chtourou O, et al. Chronic lupus erythematosus: 104 Tunisian cases. Tunis Med. 2010;88:742–5.
11. Deligny C, Marie DS, Clyti E, et al. Pure cutaneous lupus erythematosus in a population of African descent in French Guiana: a restrospective population-based description. Lupus. 2012;21:1467–71.
12. Graham RR, Ortmann WA, Langefeld CD, et al. Visualizing human leukocyte antigen class II risk haplotypes in human systemic lupus erythematosus. Am J Hum Genet. 2002;71:543–53.
13. Fabbri P, Cardinall C, Giomi B, et al. Cutaneous lupus erythematosus. Orphanet Encyclopedia, October 2004.
14. Boeckler P, Cosnes A, Frances C, et al. Association of cigarette smoking but not alcohol consumption with cutaneous lupus erythematosus. Arch Dermatol. 2009;145:1012–6.
15. Wenzel J, Zahn S, Tüting T. Pathogenesis of cutaneous lupus erythematosus: common and different features in distinct subsets. Lupus. 2010;19:1020–8.
16. Jacyk WK, Damisah M. Discoid lupus erythematosus in the Nigerians. Br J Dermatol. 1979;100:131–5.
17. Verma SM, Okawa J, Propert KJ, et al. The impact of skin damage due to cutaneous lupus on quality of life. Br J Dermatol. 2014;170:315–21.
18. Jacyk WK, Bhana KN. Lupus erythematosus profundus in black South Africans. Int J Dermatol. 2006;45:717–21.
19. Nozile W, Adgerson CN, Cohen GF. Cutaneous lupus erythematosus in skin of color. J Drugs Dermatol. 2015;14:343–9.
20. Bertsias G, Cervera R, Boumpas D. Systemic lupus erythematosus: pathogenesis and clinical features. In: EULAR textbook on rheumatic diseases. Geneva, Switzerland: European League against Rheumatism; 2012. p. 476–505.
21. Lee HJ, Sinha AA. Cutaneous lupus erythematosus: understanding of clinical features, genetic basis, and pathobiology of disease guides therapeutic strategies. Autoimmunity. 2006;39:433–44.
22. Word AP, Perese F, Tseng LC, et al. 25-OH vitamin D levels in African American and Caucasian/Hispanic cutaneous lupus subjects. Br J Dermatol. 2012;166:372–9.
23. Chang AY, Werth VP. Treatment of cutaneous lupus. Curr Rheumatol Rep. 2011;13:300–7.
24. Jewell ML, McCauliffe DP. Patients with cutaneous lupus erythematosus who smoke are less responsive to antimalarial treatment. J Am Acad Dermatol. 2000;42:983–7.
25. Motswaledi MH, Khammissa RA, Wood NH, et al. Discoid lupus erythematosus as it relates to cutaneous squamous cell carcinoma and to photosensitivity. SADJ. 2011;66:340–3.
26. Molomo EM, Bouckaert M, Khammissa RA, et al. Discoid lupus erythematosus-related squamous cell carcinoma of the lip in an HIV-seropositive black male. J Can Res Ther. 2015;11:1036.

Dermatomyositis

31

Peter B. Chansky, Lavanya Mittal, Cord Sunderkötter, and Victoria P. Werth

Dermatomyositis (DM), in addition to *polymyositis* (PM) and inclusion body myositis, is categorized as an autoimmune inflammatory myopathy. This group of disorders is characterized by the notable features of symmetric proximal skeletal muscle weakness and laboratory findings consistent with muscle inflammation. DM, unique among the group of inflammatory myopathies, also exhibits a set of distinctive and bothersome cutaneous findings and may present with other systemic symptoms such as interstitial lung disease, arthritis, dysphagia, and an increased risk for internal malignancy. Classic DM presents with skin findings, proximal muscle weakness, and laboratory or radiologic evidence of myositis. When DM occurs in the complete absence of muscular symptoms and muscle inflammation, it is known as *amyopathic DM* (formally DM sine myositis). The presence of DM-related skin signs with subclinical myopathy and borderline evidence of muscle inflammation is known as hypomyopathic DM [1].

While DM and PM were originally thought to share the same disease pathogenesis, there is recent evidence to suggest that they each represent different pathogenic processes [2]. However, despite these etiologic differences and the presence of skin predominant disease only in DM, it is important to note that DM and PM can both present with a confusing clinical picture due to overlapping symptoms with several other connective tissue disorders and autoimmune diseases. Given the chronic course and multi-system involvement of DM, it is essential for dermatologists to recognize and accurately diagnose this disease to implement proper screening and initiate treatment.

31.1 Epidemiology

DM is quite rare in the general population but is found in countries and climates all over the world. A variety of epidemiological studies performed in several countries and specific subpopulations provide the only data available on this uncommon disease; nonetheless, they are markedly limited by a paucity of affected individuals and limited geographical diversity and, thus, may not be easily generalized outside of their original study domain. Also, DM and PM were not always assessed separately. Many of the best epidemiological studies for inflammatory myopathies were conducted in the United States or with a predominantly Caucasian population. Regardless, a summary of the data to date is presented below.

DM exhibits a bimodal age distribution with a large incidence peak in the elderly, known as adult-onset DM, and a smaller peak during childhood, known as juvenile DM. A few notable studies are responsible for our current understanding of the age distribution in DM.

In an early 15-year retrospective study of 153 patients with PM or DM seen at the University of California Los Angeles Medical Center, the average age of incidence was between the ages of 40 and 50 years old with a female to male ratio of 2:1

P. B. Chansky and L. Mittal are first coauthors of this chapter.

P. B. Chansky · L. Mittal
Corporal Michael J. Crescenz Veterans Affairs Medical Center, Philadelphia, PA, USA

Department of Dermatology, Perelman School of Medicine, University of Pennsylvania, Philadelphia, PA, USA

C. Sunderkötter
Department of Dermatology, Martin-Luther-University of Halle Wittenberg, Halle, Germany

Department of Dermatology and Venerology, Universitätsklinikum Münster, Münster, Germany
e-mail: cord.sunderkoetter@ukmuenster.de

V.P. Werth, M.D. (✉)
Department of Dermatology, Perelman Center for Advanced Medicine, Philadelphia, PA, USA
e-mail: werth@pennmedicine.upenn.edu

C. E. Orfanos et al. (eds.), *Pigmented Ethnic Skin and Imported Dermatoses*, https://doi.org/10.1007/978-3-319-69422-1_31

[3]. This female gender predominance was further confirmed in a 1996 large-scale US epidemiological study [4], whereas the combined incidence of DM and PM was estimated at 2 per 100,000 and the combined prevalence at 5 per 100,000. Juvenile DM and PM occurred in 7% of patients with an average age of incidence of 8.7 years old. In a retrospective French study of 79 patients with PM and DM seen at the University of Lille and Rouen medical centers, the median age of diagnosis was 52 years old with a range of 5–86 years old [5]. In this study, 29% of patients developed DM or PM after the age of 65 years old, and 9% of patients developed disease at less than 25 years old. In this patient population, the percentage of new cases progressively increased with age, with the highest number of cases seen in the age ranges 45–64 years old and older than 65 years old. Numerous population-based studies have been completed and give a range for the incidence and prevalence of the inflammatory myopathies. In particular, a landmark study in Olmstead County, Minnesota, shed light on the epidemiology of the amyopathic subset of DM. Published in 2010, this 31-year retrospective population-based study found the mean age of diagnosis of DM to be 57.4 years old with a range of 30.5–95 years old after excluding three juvenile cases. The majority of patients were female (76%) and white (83%). After adjusting for age and sex, the overall incidence of all subtypes of DM was 9.63 per 1 million persons, and the prevalence was 21.42 per 100,000 persons. Clinically amyopathic DM represented approximately 21% of all cases of DM with an adjusted incidence of 2.08 per 1 million persons.

A recent systematic review published in 2015 best summarizes international epidemiological literature on inflammatory myopathies to date [6]. Forty-six original articles published between 1966 and 2013, reporting the incidence and prevalence of inflammatory myopathies across five continents, were reviewed. The combined incidence of inflammatory myopathies was estimated at 7.98 cases per million per year between 1951 and 2010, and the prevalence was estimated at 14 cases per 100,000 between 1982 and 2010. While differences were observed in the reported results, this systematic review failed to show significant geographical discrepancy in the epidemiological results. Of note, the incidence of DM showed an increasing latitudinal gradient in the countries of the northern hemisphere with a rate of 28% in Singapore (+1.36 latitude), 17.3% in Allegheny County (+38.0 latitude), and 13.8% in Gavleborg County (+58.41 latitude). This finding is in agreement with a prior study which demonstrated that the prevalence of DM increased significantly in nine European countries with increasing latitude and further identifies UV radiation as an immunological aggravator [7].

In terms of DM disease type, Caucasians account for a larger proportion of clinically amyopathic DM (ranging from 70 to 86%), with African-American patients only comprising a very small percentage (<1%); for patients with classic DM seen at a large tertiary medical center, 18% were African-American [8–10]. Although there is no concrete data to support this concept, it is generally believed among rheumatologists and dermatologists that DM patients with darker skin often present with classic DM with muscle involvement, while DM patients with Caucasian skin are more frequently amyopathic.

Overall, specific epidemiological studies of DM in patients with pigmented ethnic skin are lacking, and, consequently, there is a need for larger studies with broader geographic and racial diversity to highlight potential epidemiological trends and underlying genetic and environmental determinants of this disease.

31.2 Clinical Picture

Adult-onset DM encompasses classic DM and clinically amyopathic DM, which includes both *amyopathic* and *hypomyopathic* DM. Classic DM presents with signs of proximal muscle weakness, laboratory evidence of muscle inflammation (such as elevated creatinine kinase or aldolase, abnormal electromyogram, biopsy, or MRI), and the characteristic cutaneous manifestations. Amyopathic DM describes individuals with cutaneous symptoms without signs of muscle weakness or myositis or of Lupus Erythematosus. Lastly, hypomyopathic DM refers to the appearance of typical skin findings with no signs of muscle weakness but subclinical laboratory evidence of muscle inflammation, which may be seen after the resolution of myositis with treatment [11].

The skin findings in DM are characterized by particular anatomic distributions of active lesions or scarring damage. Activity is represented by increasing degrees of erythema, scale, and erosion/ulceration, while damage is represented by poikiloderma and calcinosis cutis. Erythema, a sign of skin inflammation, ranges in severity from livid or pink to red to dark red and is usually the first cutaneous finding in DM. Scale is also a marker of activity. Pruritus can become excessive and induce rubbing or scratching, subsequently forming lichenification or crust. Poikiloderma, also commonly seen in patients with cutaneous lupus, refers to the presence of hyperpigmentation, hypopigmentation, telangiectasias, and epidermal atrophy and often occurs in a sun-exposed pattern.

The signs of cutaneous DM readily occur in particular anatomic locations that are almost pathognomonic for the disease. The "heliotrope" rash refers to a pink-violet patch of erythema around the eyelids with periorbital edema. Facial erythema is readily seen (Fig. 31.1), as well as erythematous scaly psoriasiform-like plaques on the scalp. Photodistributed erythema and poikiloderma on the upper chest and upper back are known as the "V sign" (Fig. 31.2) and the "shawl sign" (Fig. 31.3). Papular erythematous discoloration of the knuckles of the hand is the textbook presentation known as

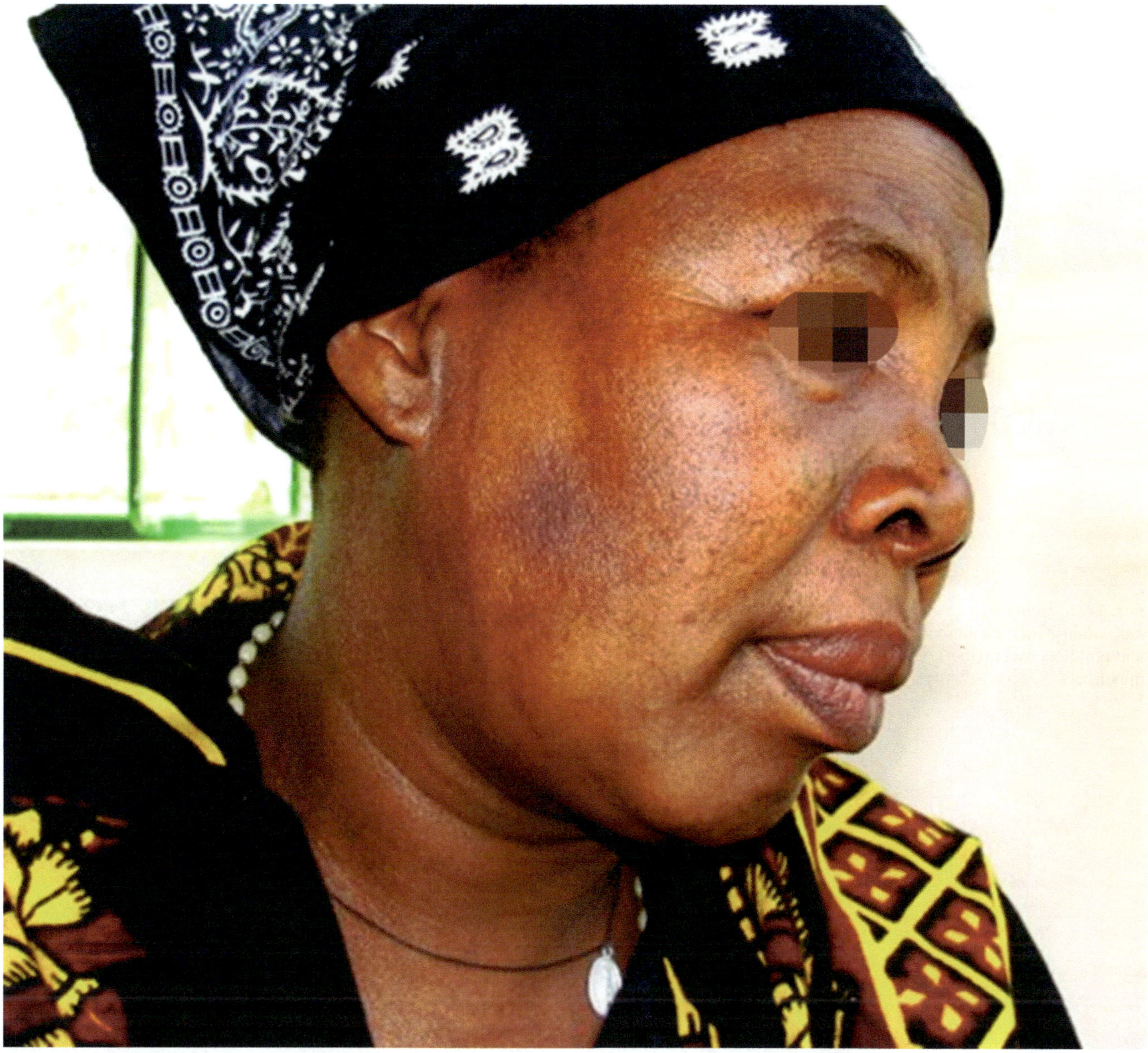

Fig. 31.1 *Dermatomyositis* in a Tanzanian female (Photo: CEO)

"Gottron's papules" (Fig. 31.4). When erythema and scale are visible on the extensor surfaces of the elbows, knees, or ankles, it is known as "Gottron's sign." Poikiloderma and erythema on the lateral thighs is known as the "holster sign" (Fig. 31.5). The presence of scale, lichenification, and erythema on the lateral and palmar sides of the fingers is known as "mechanic's hands." Lastly, the presence of nail fold changes, such as cuticular dystrophy ("ragged" cuticles) and visible telangiectasias (capillary changes), are also characteristic [12, 13]. Overall, the skin findings in DM are quite irritating and pruritic and can lead to a significantly impaired quality of life. Although pruritus can be generalized, it often has a predilection for the scalp in DM.

Given the frequency of DM and a lack of large-scale research studies, clinical presentation among DM patients with pigmented ethnic skin has been rarely investigated. While well-known differences in skin properties exist between Caucasian and pigmented skin, it is not clear that they contribute to differences in the clinical presentation of DM in most patients [14]. Darker skin types, however, may exhibit hyperpigmentation that can obscure underlying erythema. This is best documented in a study measuring minimal perceptible erythema (MPE) after the addition of dinitrochlorobenzene to the skin of the back, which found MPE to be significantly lower in Caucasian compared to African-American skin [15, 16]. Further studies are needed

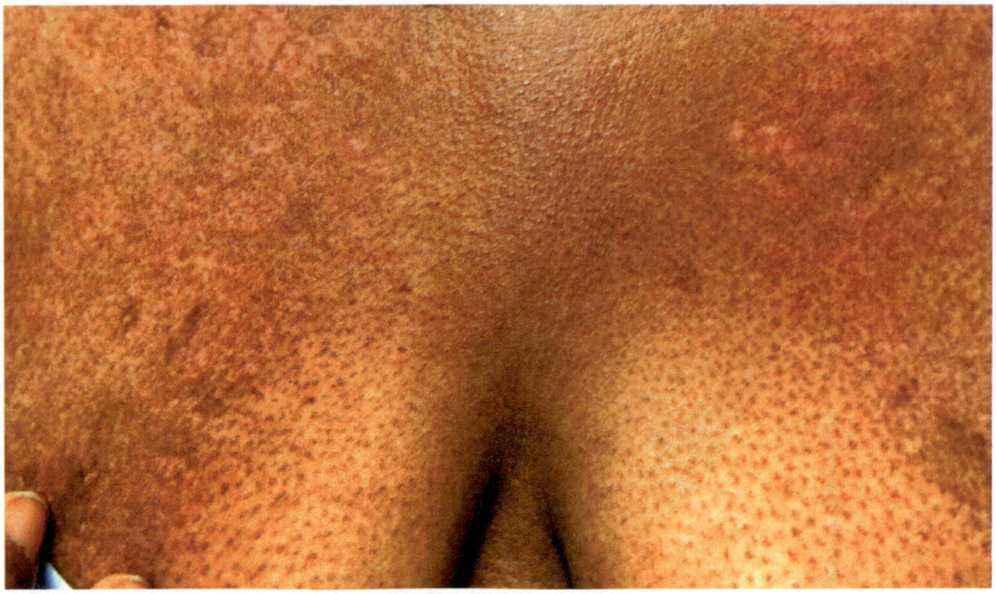

Fig. 31.2 *V sign in dermatomyositis:* Photodistributed poikilodermatous erythema on the chest

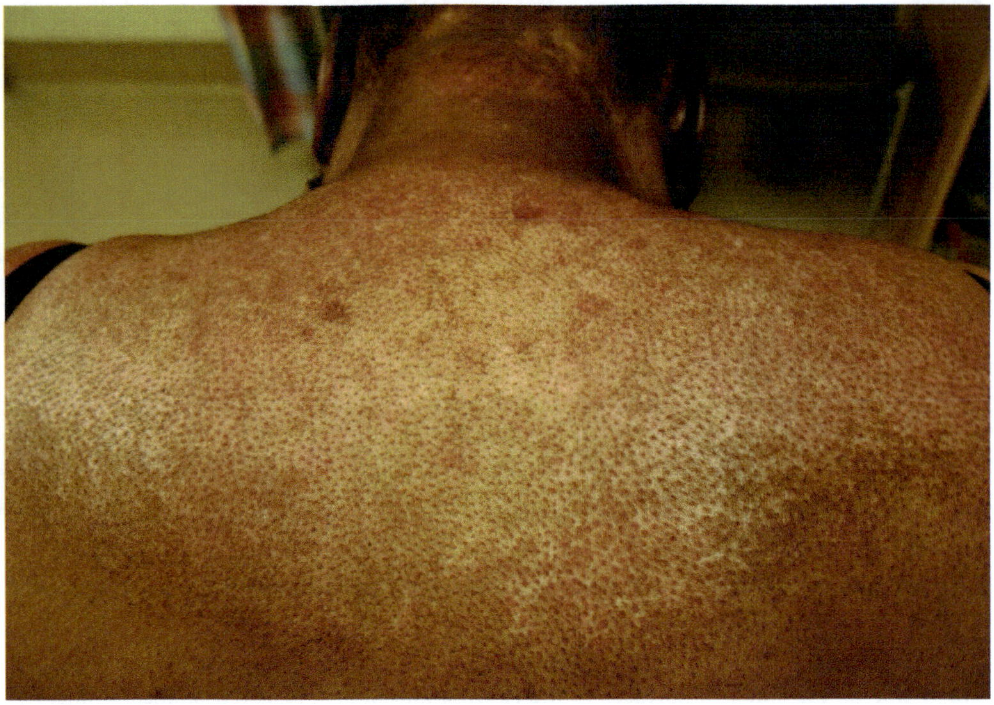

Fig. 31.3 *Shawl sign in dermatomyositis*: erythema and poikiloderma on the upper back

to specifically address a potential innate difficulty in assessing variation in erythema in DM patients with skin of color. Additionally, the dyspigmentation seen in poikiloderma is more obvious in DM patients with pigmented skin due to the visual contrast of decreased pigmentation against their native skin tone. Thus, signs of damage are more obvious than activity in some skin of color DM patients.

A biopsy of affected skin is critical in generating an accurate diagnosis. DM is a chronic multisystem disease and can also present with systemic symptoms. Patients often complain of generalized fatigue and a feeling of "low energy."

Due to the involvement of muscles in classic DM, patients exhibit symmetric proximal muscle weakness with preserved reflexes and may describe difficulty in performing normal activities such as combing one's hair or standing from a seated position. Moreover, it is essential to perform a complete physical exam because DM can affect the pulmonary, gastrointestinal, and cardiovascular systems, leading to interstitial lung disease, dysphagia, and cardiac conduction abnormalities. Raynaud's phenomenon and polyarthritis can also occur. Dermatologists should be vigilant of overlapping symptoms of other autoimmune connective tissue disorders

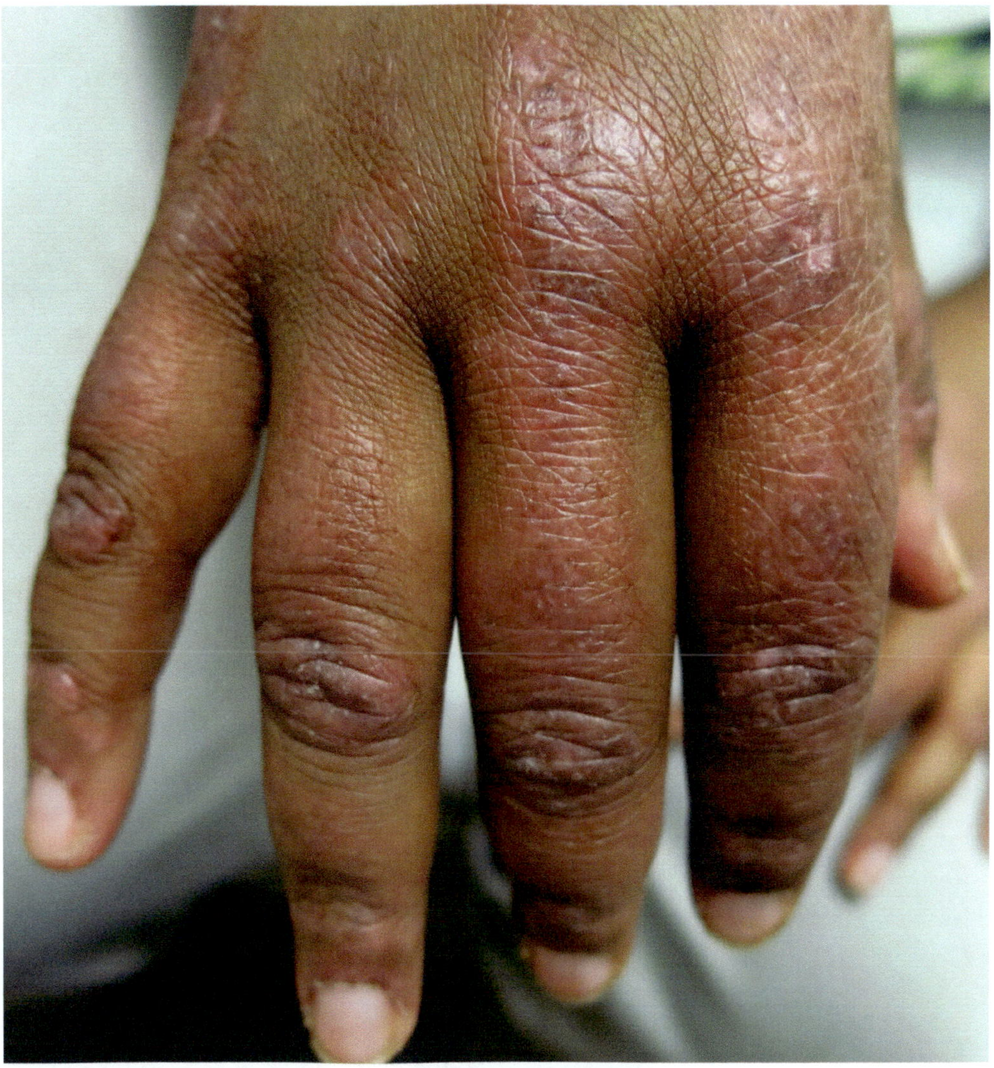

Fig. 31.4 *Gottron's papules in dermatomyositis*: erythematous papules with some scaling on the dorsal knuckles

that can contribute to a confusing clinical picture. Manifestations of rheumatoid arthritis, mixed connective tissue disease, systemic sclerosis, Sjögren's syndrome, and subacute cutaneous lupus erythematosus can be seen in patients with DM as well as in patients with PM [1].

Overall, there is a dearth of relevant literature and evidence for specific variation in clinical presentation in DM patients with pigmented skin. There is a critical need for further research in this area to shed light on potential differences in clinical presentation and treatment in DM patients with skin of color.

31.3 Etiology and Pathogenesis

The etiology of DM remains uncertain. To date, it is understood to be an idiopathic immune-mediated process that may be triggered in the genetically predisposed by a host of external factors. In PM, autoreactive cytotoxic T cells cause muscle fiber necrosis via the perforin pathway [11]. DM, in contrast, involves complement deposition and activation, which results in vasculopathy, endomysial capillary lysis, and muscle ischemia. Although autoantibodies may be present in patients with DM, it is unclear whether they serve a pathogenic role or primarily represent an epiphenomenon [2]. There do not appear to be pathophysiological differences among various ethnicities.

In skin biopsies, typical skin lesions in active DM show epidermal atrophy, vacuolar degeneration of the basal keratinocytes, interface dermatitis with lymphocytic infiltration, and mucin accumulation [1, 11]. Careful clinical-pathologic correlation is required as these pathologic changes are often impossible to distinguish from findings in systemic lupus erythematosus. Muscle biopsy specimens classically demonstrate a perifascicular and perivascular lymphocytic infiltrate with type II muscle fiber atrophy, necrosis, regeneration, and hypertrophy [17]. A muscle biopsy is not mandatory in patients with unequivocal clinical and laboratory signs of proximal myositis and skin symptoms typical for DM. In patients with moderate or subclinical myopathy, P magnetic

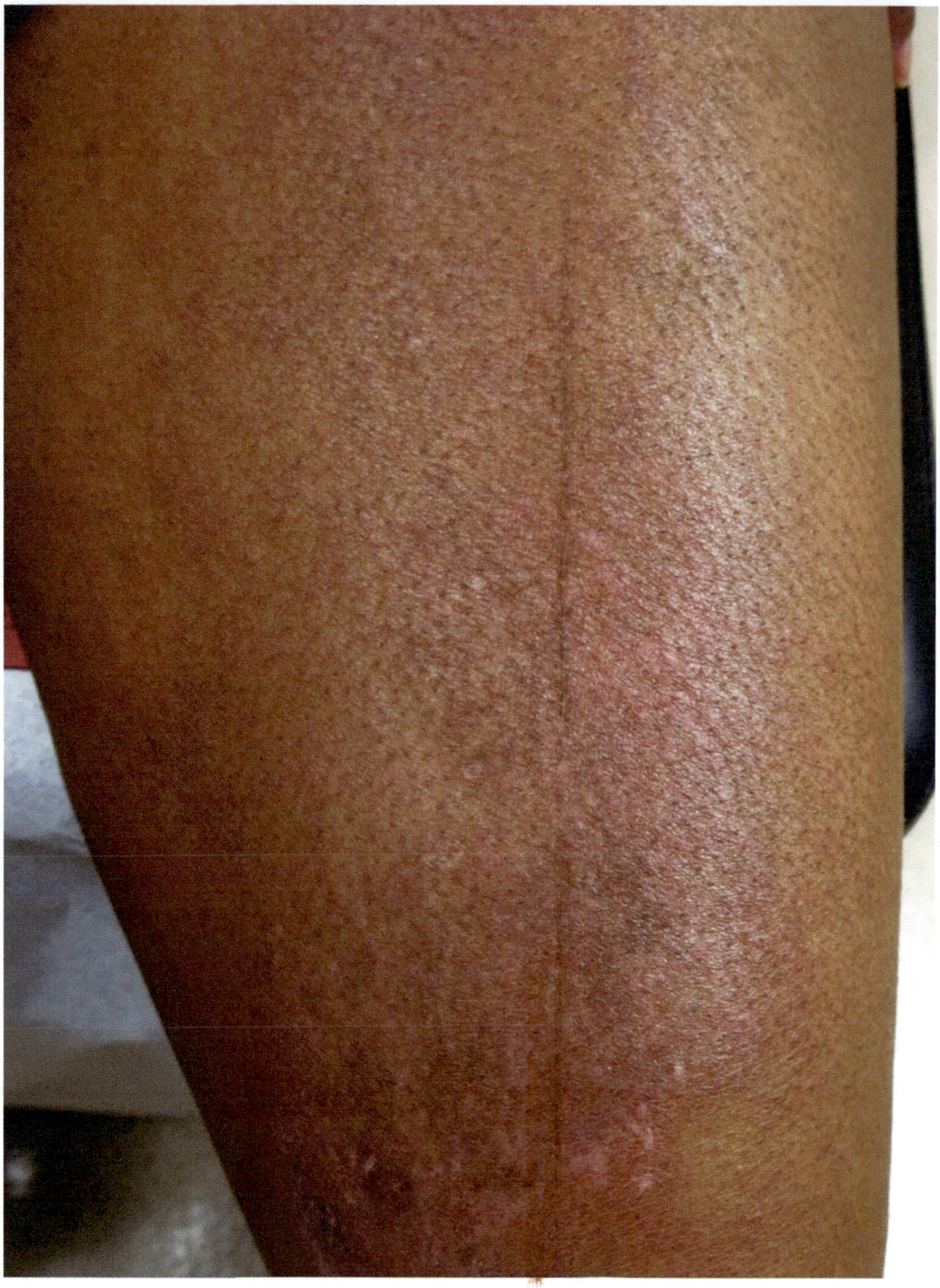

Fig. 31.5 *Holster sign* in dermatomyositis: poikiloderma and erythema on the thigh

resonance spectroscopy has been demonstrated to be useful for evaluating and quantifying metabolic disturbances in DM after standardized exercises [18].

Autoantibodies in DM have nuclear or cytoplasmic targets that serve a role in nucleic acid strand separation (nuclear helicase), translational transport (signal recognition particle complex), or protein synthesis (tRNA synthetase). These antibodies are likely to become clinically useful for identifying certain disease subtypes, especially once testing is standardized [2, 19]. In Asians, anti-MDA5 autoantibodies mark an amyopathic form of DM with rapidly progressive interstitial lung disease (ILD), increased serum ferritin, and poor prognosis. Whereas the anti-MDA5 titer correlates with disease severity in Asians, this correlation is weaker in Caucasians [20]. The presence of anti-melanoma differentiation-associated gene 5 antibodies (anti-MDA5) marks a subtype of DM associated with variable presentations in Caucasians but severe disease in Asians [21, 22]. International genome-wide association studies on DM are ongoing, and results are pending [23]. External triggers in the genetically predisposed may include malignancy, drugs such as anti-TNF biologic agents, endotheliotropic viral infections, and bacterial proteins with sequence homology to myosin [11, 17, 24].

There is an increased relative *risk of malignancy* in both DM and PM, but the risk is higher for DM. Although the risk of malignancy is increased in all genders and age-groups, the risk is higher in males and in patients 45 years of age or older as compared to their younger counterparts [25]. The tumor may be present prior to or concurrent with the onset of myositis, but in the majority of cases, it is diagnosed within 1 year after the myositis presentation [26]. Tumors can also appear up to 5 years later. In general, any type of tumor can induce *paraneoplastic DM* including ovarian, breast, bronchial, pancreas, gastric, and colon cancer, and non-Hodgkin lymphoma. In individuals of Asian descent, nasopharyngeal carcinoma is also common [26, 27]. Among patients with paraneoplastic DM, skin and muscle symptoms are usually more severe and less responsive to management, the disease onset is more acute, and involvement of pharyngeal and diaphragmatic muscles as well as those of the distal extremities is more common relative to presentations associated with non-paraneoplastic forms [28, 29].

Certain infections may potentially trigger DM, and this possibility must be considered in immigrants and refugees. HIV infection can be associated with DM in patients from endemic areas, and HIV seroconversion may be the initial presentation of this disease [30–32]. Moreover, parasitic infections must be ruled out when evaluating immigrants, refugees, and the immunocompromised. In previous reports, leishmaniasis induced a DM-like cutaneous eruption, and toxoplasmosis was concomitant with some cases of classic DM, which responded to treatment of the underlying parasitic infection [33, 34].

31.4 Management

Skin and muscle disease demonstrate a diverging response to management in that cutaneous lesions and debilitating pruritus may persist despite improvement and resolution of myositis [35]. There is a lack of double-blind placebo-controlled trials for DM, and available therapies for its skin manifestations are inadequate. The main difference between those with amyopathic disease versus those with classic DM is that skin disease in the absence of muscle involvement frequently does not require treatment with systemic corticosteroids [36].

In managing skin symptoms, it is important to counsel patients regarding the importance of sun protection and sun avoidance for the prevention of cutaneous flares, given the increased sensitivity to ultraviolet light in DM [35]. Initial pharmacologic treatments include topical corticosteroids, which may alleviate the frequency of associated pruritus, and lesions have demonstrated improvement on topical immunomodulators such as pimecrolimus (1%) and tacrolimus (0.03–0.1%) in a few cases [36, 37]. Systemic treatments include antimalarials either as monotherapy (hydroxychloroquine <6.5 mg/kg/day) or in combinations, i.e., hydroxychloroquine with quinacrine or chloroquine with quinacrine [38, 39]. Of note, myositis does not seem to improve on hydroxychloroquine alone.

If cutaneous symptoms persist, systemic immunosuppressants may be given. Of the drugs used, the following have shown efficacy: corticosteroids for severe cases (up to 1 mg/kg/day), weekly methotrexate (5–25 mg/week) [40], intravenous immunoglobulins (2 g/kg/month) [41], mycophenolate mofetil (1–1.5 g twice daily) [35, 42], and rituximab [43, 44]. Leflunomide [45] and antiestrogens [46] may also be beneficial. Although skin symptoms improved after stem cell transplantation, they alone do not warrant it.

Cutaneous calcinosis, frequently occurring in children, may be avoided by systemic corticosteroids (pulse management) [47]. Existent cutaneous calcinoses have in some cases been shown to respond to diltiazem (5 mg/kg/day), pamidronate (4 mg/kg/day) ([48]; case series), or local application of sodium thiosulfate. For treatment of the sometimes excruciating pruritus or burning sensation, gabapentin may present a good option (no studies, personal experience).

Treatment of myositis: For systemic and muscle disease in DM, systemic corticosteroids (1 mg/kg/day) with a prolonged taper are the standard treatment. The highest dose is maintained for at least 2–4 weeks and until there is evidence of clinical improvement. If the disease responds rapidly, corticosteroids can be tapered to half of the initial dose by 6 months. With this approach, 75% of patients become clinically disease-free by 2–3 years. In the setting of advanced or recalcitrant disease, pulse prednisone, split-dose prednisone in doses above 1 mg/kg/day, or steroid-sparing agents may be initiated.

For relapse prevention or acute treatment of steroid refractory disease, steroid-sparing agents may be added in combination with corticosteroids and can include azathioprine (2–3 mg/kg/day), methotrexate (10–25 mg/week) [49, 50], mycophenolate mofetil (1–1.5 g/kg twice daily), and cyclosporine (3–5 mg/kg/day) [51, 52]. Methotrexate has a more rapid response than azathioprine (which has a therapeutic latency of 3–6 months) but also poses a greater risk of toxicity with occasional pneumonitis that is hard to distinguish from pulmonary involvement of DM. It should be started as a single dose of 5 mg/week, which, after 1 week, may be increased by 5 mg/week increments up to a target dose of 10–25 mg/week, depending on clinical symptoms [51, 53, 54]. Cyclosporine management requires regular monitoring of serum levels and renal function tests due to variable absorption and dose-dependent nephrotoxicity, which usually only occurs at doses greater than 5–6 mg/kg/day [55]. Although it is the preferred second-line management in childhood DM, a recent study on its safety profile and steroid-sparing effect would favor methotrexate. If patients do not respond to these immunosuppressants, rituximab (1000 mg IV given twice at 14-day intervals) may be effective. Refractory patients may also benefit from a trial of intravenous immunoglobulins (1 g/kg/day for 2 days/month), which may demonstrate improvement [41]. Other agents that have shown therapeutic promise for myositis include leflunomide, tacrolimus (1–3 mg twice daily), and cyclophosphamide (1–2 mg/kg per day PO or 0.5–1.0 g/m^2 intravenously) for severe refractory cases that have failed conventional management or for severe pulmonary disease, as can be seen with anti-MDA5 or antisynthetase syndrome [53, 54]. Previous studies have shown no benefit of plasmapheresis in DM [56].

For *maintenance management*, low-dose corticosteroids may be continued depending on therapeutic response, but a reduction in dose should be sought. Additional agents may be added if this reduction is difficult to achieve due to risk of relapse. Long-term management may include low-dose corticosteroid management, sometimes in combination with an immunosuppressive, for a period of 1–3 years or longer. During long-term corticosteroid management, renewed muscle weakness with normal or unchanged creatinine kinase (CK) activity may signal steroid-induced myopathy, which, aggravated by the effects of immobilization and concomitant systemic disease, may be difficult to distinguish from initial myositis symptoms. In such cases, corticosteroid reduction under careful clinical observation should be considered. Elevated CK and C-reactive protein (CRP) levels as well as pathological spontaneous activity on electromyography (EMG) argue against steroid-induced myopathy. Additionally, steroid-induced myopathy is unlikely in the absence of other signs and symptoms concerning for iatrogenic Cushing's syndrome. Considering the significant risks of long-term steroid management and immobilization, osteoporosis prevention and adjunctive physical management for improving muscle strength and endurance are critical aspects of management.

Regional and ethnic considerations in management: There are regional differences in the treatment practices for DM. In developing countries, physicians may not have access to certain costly therapies such as intravenous immunoglobulins or rituximab and favor adjuvants with fewer side effects as compared to immunosuppressants. Antimalarials were more frequently prescribed in Singapore, whereas methotrexate and rituximab were used only in the United States [57]. It is important to tailor management and management to ethnic differences in the clinical presentation and lab findings. Given the rapidly progressive interstitial lung disease and poor prognosis associated with anti-MDA5 antibody positive DM in Asian patients, this group must be treated with aggressive and early immunosuppression [21, 58]. Moreover, there is often an immune imbalance in autoimmune rheumatic diseases, and their treatment with immunosuppressants further increases the risk of serious infection. Among immigrants and refugees, the clinician must be alert to the risk of HIV or parasitic infection associated with DM and the possibility that pulmonary and extrapulmonary tuberculosis is comorbid with rheumatic disease [59, 60].

31.5 Course

With systemic corticosteroid and immunosuppressive drugs, patients have an excellent prognosis except adults with refractory myositis and systemic disease with associated advanced malignancy. Major causes of death in DM include ischemic heart disease, interstitial lung disease, and cancer. Other factors associated with poor prognosis include older age, progressive disease, initiation of management after 2 years of muscle symptoms, dysphagia, and cutaneous involvement of the trunk. The prevalence of interstitial lung disease associated with myositis can range from 5 to 40%, whereby pulmonary involvement is resistant to systemic corticosteroids and may be subclinical, rapidly progressive, or fatal. Also, there is a correlation between the presence of certain antibodies (anti-Jo-1, anti-PL-7, anti-PL-12, anti-DJ, and anti-EJ) and the development of pulmonary disease [61–63]; patients with anti-PL7/PL12 antibody-associated antisynthetase syndrome had a prevalence of ILD as high as 90%. However, it is crucial to regularly screen all DM patients for interstitial lung disease, also in the absence of these antibodies, considering the high incidence of pulmonary involvement.

References

1. Bolognia J, Schaffer JV, Duncan KO, et al. Dermatology essentials. Oxford: Saunders/Elsevier; 2014.
2. Dalakas MC, Hohlfeld R. Polymyositis and dermatomyositis. Lancet. 2003;362:971–82.
3. Bohan A, Peter JB, Bowman RL, et al. Computer-assisted analysis of 153 patients with polymyositis and dermatomyositis. Medicine (Baltimore). 1977;56:255–86.
4. Jacobson DL, Gange SJ, Rose NR, et al. Epidemiology and estimated population burden of selected autoimmune diseases in the United States. Clin Immunol Immunopathol. 1997;84:223–43.
5. Marie I, Hatron PY, Levesque H, et al. Influence of age on characteristics of polymyositis and dermatomyositis in adults. Medicine (Baltimore). 1999;78:139–47.
6. Meyer A, Meyer N, Schaeffer M, et al. Incidence and prevalence of inflammatory myopathies: a systematic review. Rheumatology (Oxford). 2015;54:50–63.
7. Hengstman GJ, van Venrooij WJ, Vencovsky J, et al. The relative prevalence of dermatomyositis and polymyositis in Europe exhibits a latitudinal gradient. Ann Rheum Dis. 2000;59:141–2.

8. Bendewald MJ, Wetter DA, Li X, et al. Incidence of dermatomyositis and clinically amyopathic dermatomyositis: a population-based study in Olmsted County, Minnesota. Arch Dermatol. 2010;146:26–30.
9. Gerami P, Schope JM, McDonald L, et al. A systematic review of adult-onset clinically amyopathic dermatomyositis (dermatomyositis sine myositis): a missing link within the spectrum of the idiopathic inflammatory myopathies. J Am Acad Dermatol. 2006;54:597–613.
10. Klein RQ, Teal V, Taylor L, et al. Number, characteristics, and classification of patients with dermatomyositis seen by dermatology and rheumatology departments at a large tertiary medical center. J Am Acad Dermatol. 2007;57:937–43.
11. James WD, Elston DM, Berger TG, et al. Andrews' diseases of the skin: clinical dermatology. 11th ed. London: Saunders Elsevier; 2011.
12. Klein-Weigel PF, Sunderkotter C, Sander O. Nailfold capillaroscopy microscopy - an interdisciplinary appraisal. Vasa. 2016;45:353–64.
13. Sander O, Sunderkotter C, Kotter I, et al. Capillaroscopy. Procedure and nomenclature. Z Rheumatol. 2010;69:253–62.
14. Wesley NO, Maibach HI. Racial (ethnic) differences in skin properties: the objective data. Am J Clin Dermatol. 2003;4:843–60.
15. Weigand DA, Gaylor JR. Irritant reaction in Negro and Caucasian skin. South Med J. 1974;67:548–51.
16. Zhao CYHE, Hao EY, Oh DD, et al. A comparison study of clinical-related atopic dermatitis outcome measures for intermediate- to dark-skinned patients. Br J Dermatol. 2017;176:985–92.
17. Krathen MS, Fiorentino D, Werth VP. Dermatomyositis. Curr Dir Autoimmun. 2008;10:313–32.
18. Pfleiderer B, Lange J, Loske KD, et al. Metabolic disturbances during short exercises in dermatomyositis revealed by real-time functional 31P magnetic resonance spectroscopy. Rheumatology (Oxford). 2004;43:696–703.
19. Targoff IN. Laboratory testing in the diagnosis and management of idiopathic inflammatory myopathies. Rheum Dis Clin N Am. 2002;28:859–90. viii
20. Parronchi P, Radice A, Palterer B, et al. MDA5-positive dermatomyositis: an uncommon entity in Europe with variable clinical presentations. Clin Mol Allergy. 2015;13:2.
21. Murase C, Muro Y, Akiyama M. Rapid increase of serum anti-MDA-5 antibodies and exacerbation of clinically amyopathic dermatomyositis/interstitial lung disease. J Eur Acad Dermatol Venereol. 2017;31:e43–4.
22. Fujimoto M, Watanabe R, Ishitsuka Y, et al. Recent advances in dermatomyositis-specific autoantibodies. Curr Opin Rheumatol. 2016;28:636–44.
23. Chinoy H, Lamb JA, Ollier WE, et al. An update on the immunogenetics of idiopathic inflammatory myopathies: major histocompatibility complex and beyond. Curr Opin Rheumatol. 2009;21:588–93.
24. Niklas K, Niklas AA, Majewski D, et al. Rheumatic diseases induced by drugs and environmental factors: the state-of-the-art - part two. Reumatologia. 2016;54:165–9.
25. Qiang JK, Kim WB, Baibergenova A, et al. Risk of malignancy in dermatomyositis and polymyositis: a systematic review and meta-analysis. J Cutan Med Surg. 2017;21:131–6.
26. Hill CL, Zhang Y, Sigurgeirsson B, et al. Frequency of specific cancer types in dermatomyositis and polymyositis: a population-based study. Lancet. 2001;357:96–100.
27. Chen YJ, CY W, Huang YL, et al. Cancer risks of dermatomyositis and polymyositis: a nationwide cohort study in Taiwan. Arthritis Res Ther. 2010;12:R70.
28. Andras C, Ponyi A, Constantin T, et al. Dermatomyositis and polymyositis associated with malignancy: a 21-year retrospective study. J Rheumatol. 2008;35:438–44.
29. Fardet L, Dupuy A, Gain M, et al. Factors associated with underlying malignancy in a retrospective cohort of 121 patients with dermatomyositis. Medicine (Baltimore). 2009;88:91–7.
30. Rajadhyaksha A, Baheti TG, Mehra S, et al. Dermatomyositis: a rare presentation of HIV seroconversion illness. J Clin Rheumatol. 2012;18:298–300.
31. Manie M. Meeting the challenges in the diagnosis of inflammatory myopathies. S Afr Med J. 2015;105:1076.
32. Ogoina D, Umar A, Obiako OR. Dermatomyositis associated with HIV-1 infection in a Nigerian adult female: a case report. Afr Health Sci. 2012;12:74–6.
33. Dauden E, Penas PF, Rios L, et al. Leishmaniasis presenting as a dermatomyositis-like eruption in AIDS. J Am Acad Dermatol. 1996;35:316–9.
34. Harland CC, Marsden JR, Vernon SA, et al. Dermatomyositis responding to treatment of associated toxoplasmosis. Br J Dermatol. 1991;125:76–8.
35. Lam C, Vleugels RA. Management of cutaneous dermatomyositis. Dermatol Ther. 2012;25:112–34.
36. Sunderkotter C, Nast A, Worm M, et al. Guidelines on dermatomyositis--excerpt from the interdisciplinary S2k guidelines on myositis syndromes by the German Society of Neurology. J Dtsch Dermatol Ges. 2016;14:321–38.
37. Hollar CB, Jorizzo JL. Topical tacrolimus 0.1% ointment for refractory skin disease in dermatomyositis: a pilot study. J Dermatolog Treat. 2004;15:35–9.
38. Woo TY, Callen JP, Voorhees JJ, et al. Cutaneous lesions of dermatomyositis are improved by hydroxychloroquine. J Am Acad Dermatol. 1984;10:592–600.
39. Ang GC, Werth VP. Combination antimalarials in the treatment of cutaneous dermatomyositis: a retrospective study. Arch Dermatol. 2005;141:855–9.
40. Kasteler JS, Callen JP. Low-dose methotrexate administered weekly is an effective corticosteroid-sparing agent for the treatment of the cutaneous manifestations of dermatomyositis. J Am Acad Dermatol. 1997;36:67–71.
41. Dalakas MC, Illa I, Dambrosia JM, et al. A controlled trial of high-dose intravenous immune globulin infusions as treatment for dermatomyositis. N Engl J Med. 1993;329:1993–2000.
42. Edge JC, Outland JD, Dempsey JR, et al. Mycophenolate mofetil as an effective corticosteroid-sparing therapy for recalcitrant dermatomyositis. Arch Dermatol. 2006;142:65–9.
43. Oddis CV, Reed AM, Aggarwal R, et al. Rituximab in the treatment of refractory adult and juvenile dermatomyositis and adult polymyositis: a randomized, placebo-phase trial. Arthritis Rheum. 2013;65:314–24.
44. Aggarwal R, Loganathan P, Koontz D, et al. Cutaneous improvement in refractory adult and juvenile dermatomyositis after treatment with rituximab. Rheumatology (Oxford). 2017;56:247–54.
45. Boswell JS, Costner MI. Leflunomide as adjuvant treatment of dermatomyositis. J Am Acad Dermatol. 2008;58:403–6.
46. Sereda D, Werth VP. Improvement in dermatomyositis rash associated with the use of antiestrogen medication. Arch Dermatol. 2006;142:70–2.
47. Paller AS. The use of pulse corticosteroid therapy for juvenile dermatomyositis. Pediatr Dermatol. 1996;13:347–8.
48. Oliveri MB, Palermo R, Mautalen C, et al. Regression of calcinosis during diltiazem treatment in juvenile dermatomyositis. J Rheumatol. 1996;23:2152–5.
49. Ruperto N, Pistorio A, Oliveira S, et al. Prednisone versus prednisone plus ciclosporin versus prednisone plus methotrexate in new-onset juvenile dermatomyositis: a randomised trial. Lancet. 2016;387:671–8.
50. Bunch TW. Prednisone and azathioprine for polymyositis: long-term followup. Arthritis Rheum. 1981;24:45–8.
51. Newman ED, Scott DW. The use of low-dose oral methotrexate in polymyositis and dermatomyositis. J Clin Rheumatol. 1995;1:99–102.

52. Oddis CV. Update on the pharmacological treatment of adult myositis. J Intern Med. 2016;280:63–74.
53. Moghadam-Kia S, Aggarwal R, Oddis CV. Treatment of inflammatory myopathy: emerging therapies and therapeutic targets. Expert Rev Clin Immunol. 2015;11:1265–75.
54. Oddis CV, Sciurba FC, Elmagd KA, et al. Tacrolimus in refractory polymyositis with interstitial lung disease. Lancet. 1999;353: 1762–3.
55. Faulds D, Goa KL, Benfield P. Cyclosporin. A review of its pharmacodynamic and pharmacokinetic properties, and therapeutic use in immunoregulatory disorders. Drugs. 1993;45:953–1040.
56. Miller FW, Leitman SF, Cronin ME, et al. Controlled trial of plasma exchange and leukapheresis in polymyositis and dermatomyositis. N Engl J Med. 1992;326:1380–4.
57. Yosipovitch G, Tan A, LoSicco K, et al. A comparative study of clinical characteristics, work-up, treatment, and association to malignancy in dermatomyositis between two tertiary skin centers in the USA and Singapore. Int J Dermatol. 2013;52:813–9.
58. Nakashima R, Hosono Y, Mimori T. Clinical significance and new detection system of autoantibodies in myositis with interstitial lung disease. Lupus. 2016;25:925–33.
59. MC L, Lai CL, Tsai CC, et al. Increased risk of pulmonary and extra-pulmonary tuberculosis in patients with rheumatic diseases. Int J Tuberc Lung Dis. 2015;19:1500–6.
60. PH W, Lin YT, Yang YH, et al. The increased risk of active tuberculosis disease in patients with dermatomyositis - a nationwide retrospective cohort study. Sci Rep. 2015;5:16303.
61. Kim SH, Park IN. Acute respiratory distress syndrome as the initial clinical manifestation of an antisynthetase syndrome. Tuberc Respir Dis (Seoul). 2016;79:188–92.
62. Mathai SC, Danoff SK. Management of interstitial lung disease associated with connective tissue disease. BMJ. 2016;352:h6819.
63. Marie I, Josse S, Decaux O, et al. Comparison of long-term outcome between anti-Jo1- and anti-PL7/PL12 positive patients with antisynthetase syndrome. Autoimmun Rev. 2012;11:739–45.

Drug Eruptions in Pigmented Skin

32

Baraka M. Chaula

Cutaneous adverse reactions to drugs are not uncommon. Clinical presentations on the skin are highly variable and can lead to serious clinical complications, be even lethal. The main challenge in managing these conditions is identifying the responsible drug. Currently, there is no definitive diagnostic test that can be applied to the wide range of the entities arising due to drug intolerance; the experienced physician has to reach clinical diagnosis.

32.1 Incidence

Adverse drug reactions caused by immune and nonimmune mechanisms are a major cause of morbidity and mortality worldwide. They are the most common iatrogenic illness, complicating 5–15% of therapeutic drug courses [1]. It has been reported that photodermatoses occur regularly in dark-skinned individuals despite higher melanin content and better photoprotection and that certain cutaneous reactions such as polymorphous light eruption are more common in African-Americans, as compared to Caucasians [2]. A multicentric study in sub-Saharan Africa showed that patients with cutaneous drug reactions leading to *Stevens-Johnson syndrome* (SJS) and *toxic epidermal necrolysis* (TEN) were associated with human immunodeficiency virus (HIV) and the antiretroviral drugs taken to treat the HIV infection [3]. Drug hypersensitivity syndromes with eosinophilia and systemic symptoms (DRESS) have been associated with mutations in genes that encode drug detoxification enzymes. The individuals carrying these mutations are at higher risk to develop DRESS [4]. In African populations, the allele frequency of HLA-B*5701, which is associated with abacavir sensitivity, is lower compared to Caucasians [5]. Abacavir, together with stavudine, nevirapine, and other medications of antiretroviral therapy (ART) often used in sub-Saharan Africa, and the incidence of severe drug-induced implications is rather high in the continent.

B. M. Chaula
Dermatology Unit, Department of Internal Medicine,
Mbeya Zonal Referral Hospital, Mbeya, Tanzania

32.2 Etiology

Drug eruptions are in most cases unpredictable in their severity and course. Both T-helper type 2 cells and CD8+ T-cells seem to be involved by playing different roles. The pathogenesis of drug eruptions with eosinophilia and systemic symptoms is complex and not completely understood. Several hypotheses have been put forward such as accumulation of toxic drug metabolites resulting from genetic enzymatic deficiency [6] or predisposition of certain HLA halotypes such as HLA-B*5701 for abacavir and HLA-B*5801 for allopurinol [7]. Also, viral drug interactions and inflammatory immune recovery reaction secondary to immune suppression induced by drugs have been considered [8, 9]. A genetic susceptibility to SJS/TEN may be a cause for adverse reactions to nevirapine.

32.3 Clinical Pictures

Adverse drug eruptions in the skin are multifaceted, showing eczematous, lichenoid, psoriasiform, or bullous appearances. For the physician, it is mandatory to recognize the responsible drug, if possible, and withdraw medication. Some clinical phenotypes are known to occur frequently in pigmented skin.

Drug-induced erythroderma can be dry, non-exfoliative, or exfoliative. The exact pathophysiological mechanisms leading to erythroderma are not completely known. Interactions among several cytokines and cellular adhesion molecules in erythroderma result into increase in the rate of epidermal turnover [10]. *Exfoliative dermatitis* mostly occurs in elderly. It appears to affect generally more men than women and has no racial preference. Clinically it presents

C. E. Orfanos et al. (eds.), *Pigmented Ethnic Skin and Imported Dermatoses*, https://doi.org/10.1007/978-3-319-69422-1_32

with generalized scaling of a large part of the body, with few areas where the skin is spared such as the nose. Accompanying signs and symptoms include itchiness, fever, and chills. The skin may become thickened. Chronic cases may present skin color changes with hyperpigmentation being more frequent than hypo- or depigmentation. Other features include palmoplantar keratoderma, shiny nails, and diffuse non-scarring alopecia. Extracutaneous features include lymphadenopathy, which can be prominent even in absence of an underlying malignancy [11]. The drugs most commonly implicated to cause erythroderma and exfoliative dermatitis in black skin are sulfa-containing compounds, antiretrovirals given for HIV infection [12], the antituberculosis drugs widely used in sub-Saharan Africa because of tuberculosis coexisting with HIV [13], and anticonvulsants [14].

Stevens-Johnson syndrome (SJS) and ***toxic epidermal necrolysis*** (TEN) are life-threatening mucocutaneous disorders. SJS is characterized by widespread sloughing of the skin and mucosal surface of the oral cavity and the eyes, sometimes involving the gut, kidneys, eye, genitalia, and/ or the lungs (Fig. 32.1). Occasionally, transitional features into TEN are seen (Fig. 32.2). Clinically, in SJS, epidermal necrosis and detachment amount to <10% of body surface area; when 10–30% of the area surface is affected, there is SJS/TEN overlap; and when >30% of the skin surface area is involved, TEN is diagnosed, the most severe form of the disease [15]. The epidermal detachment is characterized by confluence of purpuric macules or flat targetoid lesions which may be atypical. Lesions may be preceded by prodromes such as fever, malaise, headaches, and a morbilliform, maculopapular exanthema [16]. Systemic manifestations of TEN include erosions, necrosis and severe dysfunction of the eye, pulmonary, cardiovascular, gastrointestinal, renal, as well as hematopoietic system [15]. A genetic variant HCP5 was found in a sub-Saharan African country land population which induced susceptibility of developing SJS/TEN to nevirapine, commonly used for treatment of HIV infection in hot climate zones [17]. There is a considerable risk of nevirapine-associated SJS among HIV-infected pregnant women [18]. A retrospective multicenter study in sub-Saharan Africa

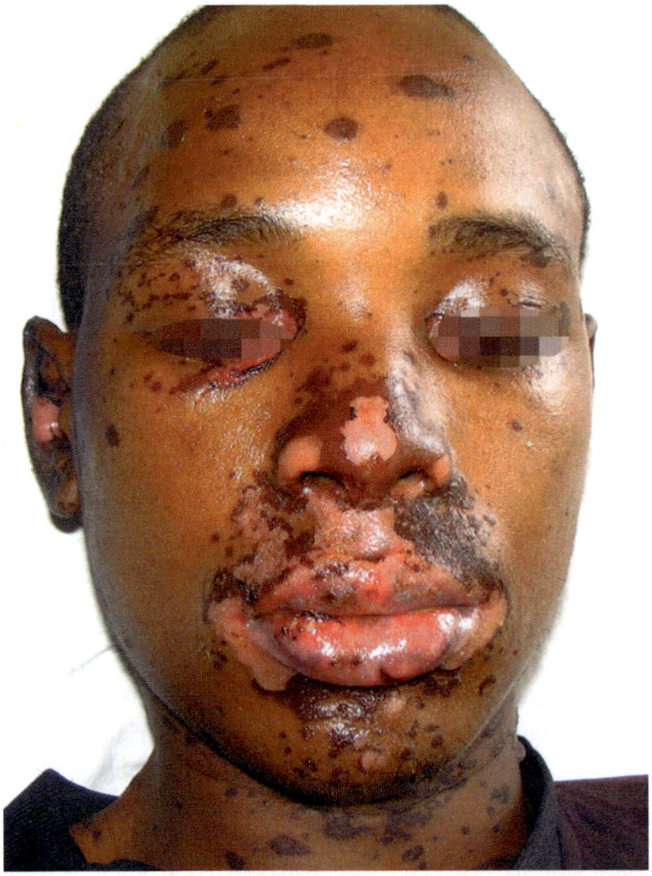

Fig. 32.1 *Stevens-Johnson syndrome* due to oral intake of antimalarials

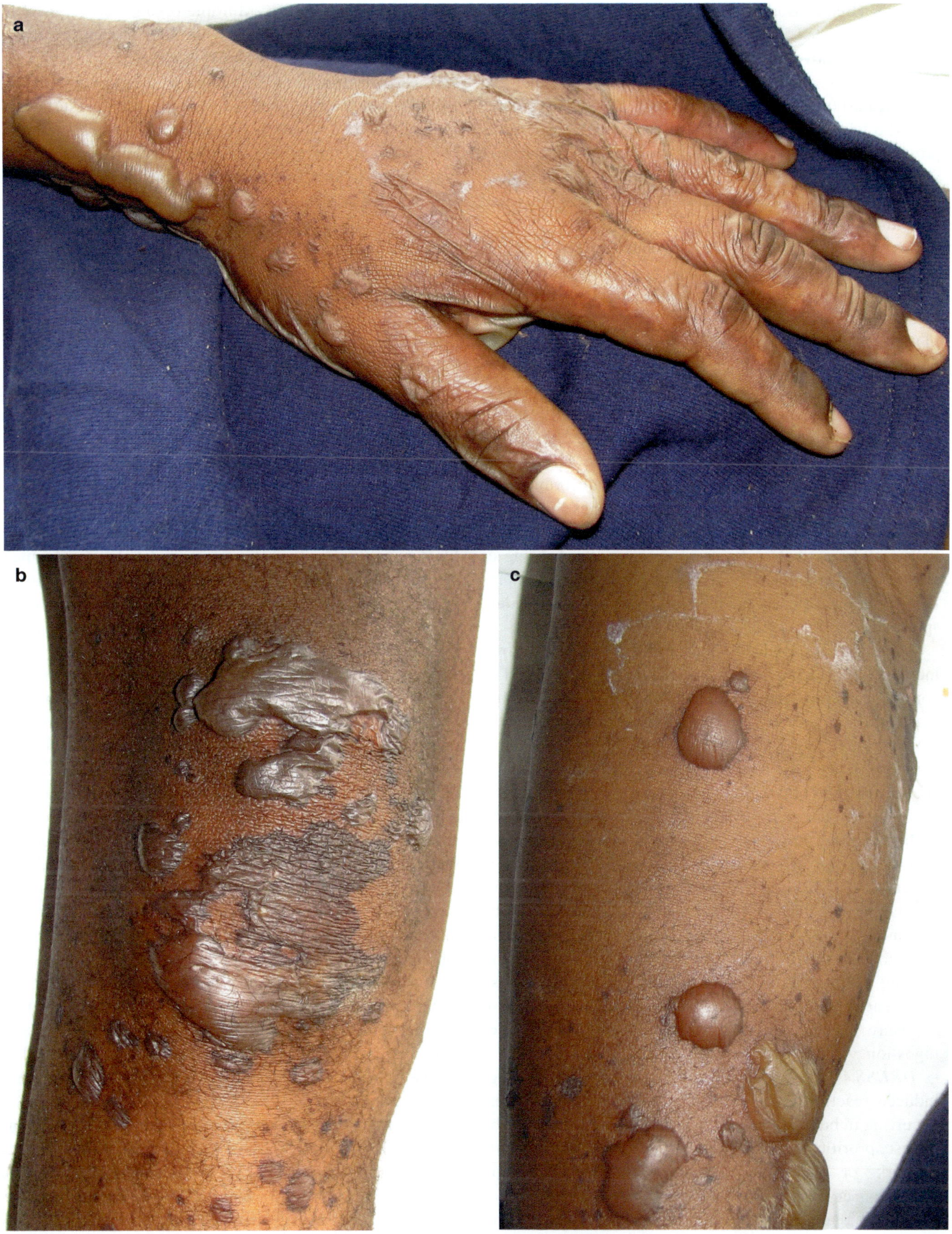

Fig. 32.2 *Stevens-Johnson syndrome*, partly with necrolytic lesions on the hands (**a**) and large bullae on the extremities (**b**, **c**)

countries (Benin, Burkina Faso, Central African Republic, and Togo) reported 54.8% of the registered SJS/TEN patients to be HIV positive and that the commonest drugs to cause SJS/TEN were antibacterial sulfonamides, nevirapine, and drugs against tuberculosis, respectively [3]. Healthcare workers, who take antiretrovirals despite being HIV negative as prophylaxis because of accidental exposure to blood, are also at high risk to develop SJS/TEN. Poor prognosis and mortality rate are high in Africa because of the various coexisting opportunistic infections.

Fixed drug eruptions (FDE) are characterized by recurrence of lesion(s) at the same site on re-administration of the offending drug. Both men and women are equally affected regardless of their age. Common morphologic feature of FDE is a single or a few erythematous or pigmented macules which may rapidly evolve into an edematous plaque or occasionally vesicles or blisters. In darkly pigmented skin, erythema is not recognized clinically, instead brownish-bluish hyperpigmentation is commonly seen (Fig. 32.3a, b). Morphological variations including urticarial, eczematous, morbilliform, scarlatiniform, nodular, and multiform lesions have also been reported. When the acute phase is over, a dark-bluish skin hyperpigmentation is the hallmark feature. FDE may be asymptomatic or accompanied by burning or pruritus and prominent local or systemic manifestations. After repeated recurrences, fixed drug eruptions may widely spread and present necrolytic features (Fig. 32.4).

The list of drugs implicated in FDE is endless; a true incidence will depend on the frequency of their use. The commonest drugs causing FDE in the tropics are in first place sulfa-containing antimalarials such as pyrimethamine with sulfadoxine which are widely used in tropical countries especially in sub-Saharan Africa where malaria is endemic. The population is frequently at risk for developing FDE. Second, sulfamethoxazole in combination with trimethoprim (co-trimoxazole) commonly used as a prophylaxis for opportunistic infections in HIV patients is the cause of FDE, due to their widespread use. Also metronidazole together with its derivative tinidazole may be the cause, being widely used for the treatment of helminth infections in the tropics. Worm infestations are rampant, making metronidazole an important cause for adverse drug reactions. FDEs will subsequently relapse on repeat exposure to the offending drug within hours after ingestion.

DRESS is a potentially life-threatening adverse drug-induced reaction involving the skin and internal organs, occurring in both adults and children [19]. The rash can be diffuse, pruritic, macular, or erythrodermatous exanthema. In dark- or black-skinned patients, hyperpigmentation rather than erythroderma is seen. Commonly affected areas include the face, upper trunk, upper limbs, and lower limbs. Bullae, vesicles, atypical targetoid plaques, and purpura may be present. Multiple organ systems involvement also occurs in DRESS syndrome. The most affected include renal, pulmonary, hematologic, hepatic, lymphatic, and cardiac function. Commonest drugs for inducing DRESS in pigmented skin include tetracyclines, sulfa-containing compounds such as trimethoprim-sulfamethoxazole, and also quinine, which is widely used against malaria in Africa. Abacavir and nevirapine are implicated and are also well known to cause severe TEN (Figs. 32.5 and 32.6). Other drug groups responsible for DRESS are anticonvulsants such as carbamazepine and phenobarbitone. In many less developed countries, there are no strict medical prescription regulations; almost all medications can be purchased over the counter. It has been reported that minocycline-induced DRESS presents mainly in patients of African or West Indian origin and that in heavily pigmented skin, DRESS has a prolonged course lasting several months after the suspected drug has been withdrawn [20].

32.4 Management

Identifying the responsible cause is the key for management of drug-induced skin eruptions. In most cases, this may be difficult; one may consider the possibility to discontinue all drugs, except those essential for the care of the patient. Substitution of a similarly acting but of different chemical structure drug may be helpful. Management and prognosis of SJS/TEN involve several factors such as extent of the skin affected, involvement of the mucosa, and the systemic condition of the patient. Team approach including multispecialty is essential, especially when exfoliative drug reaction occurs. Patients with extensive body involvement should be taken to intensive care burn units, where sterile environment can be accessed. This approach is not easily feasible in countries with limited resources. Central venous access should be obtained as early as possible, together with vital signs monitoring. Nasogastric tube is indicated for nutrition in case mucositis is present that can impair nutrition. Ophthalmologists and gynecologists should be consulted to prevent complications such as conjunctivitis with squamous metaplasia, trichiasis, symblepharon, and punctate keratitis. Vaginal phimosis and synechiae can be avoided by the use of Foley catheter [21]. Ocular complications can be reduced by the use of artificial tears, ophthalmic cyclosporine, and moisture chamber eyewear [21].

Fluid hydration should be started within the first 24 h, and fluids such as Ringer's lactate 1–2 ml/kg/% of body surface area involved can be given [22]. Nutrition should be initiated earlier to compensate for increased catabolic state. Anticoagulation management can be provided with low molecular weight heparin to prevent deep venous thrombosis.

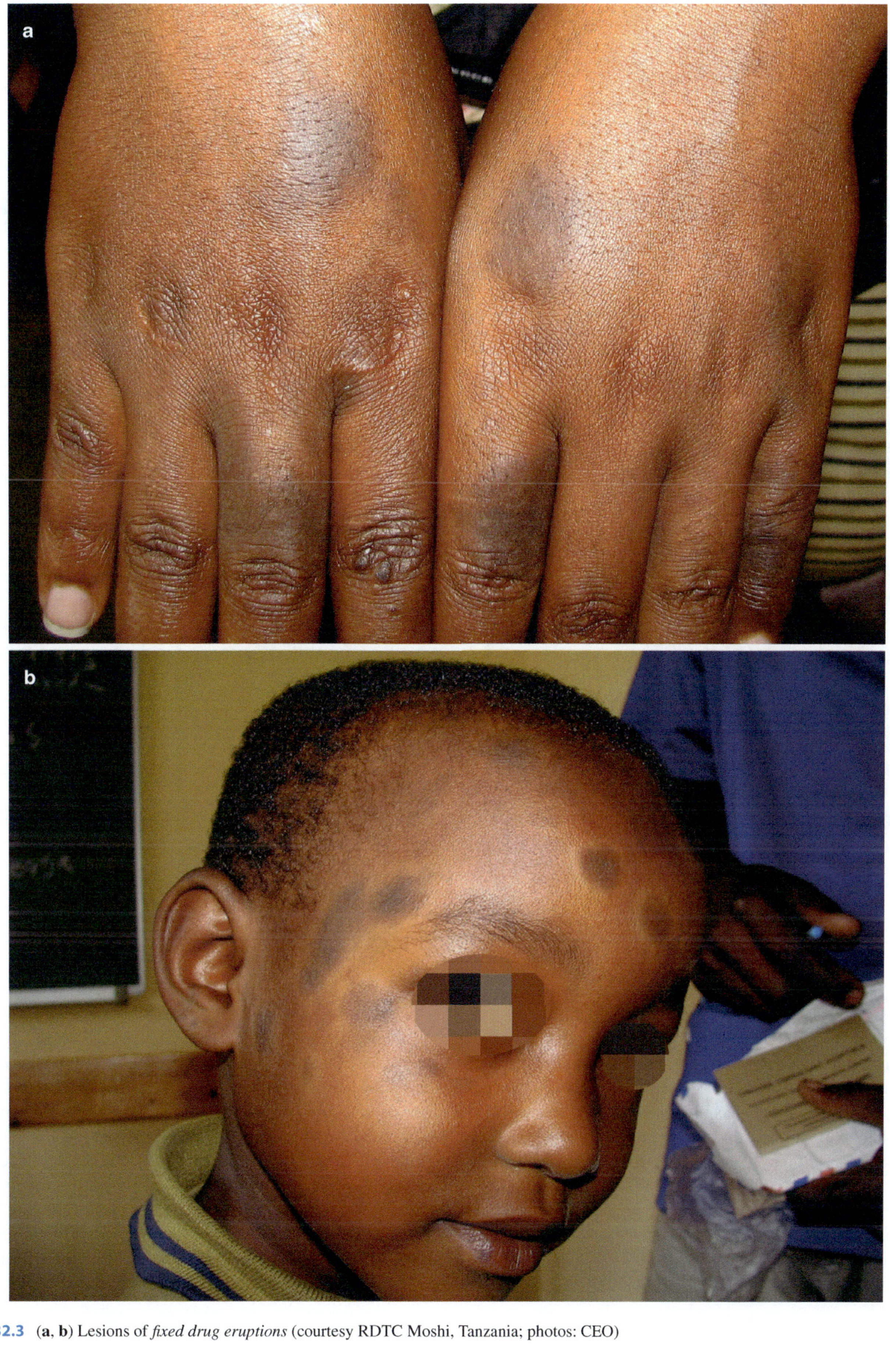

Fig. 32.3 (**a**, **b**) Lesions of *fixed drug eruptions* (courtesy RDTC Moshi, Tanzania; photos: CEO)

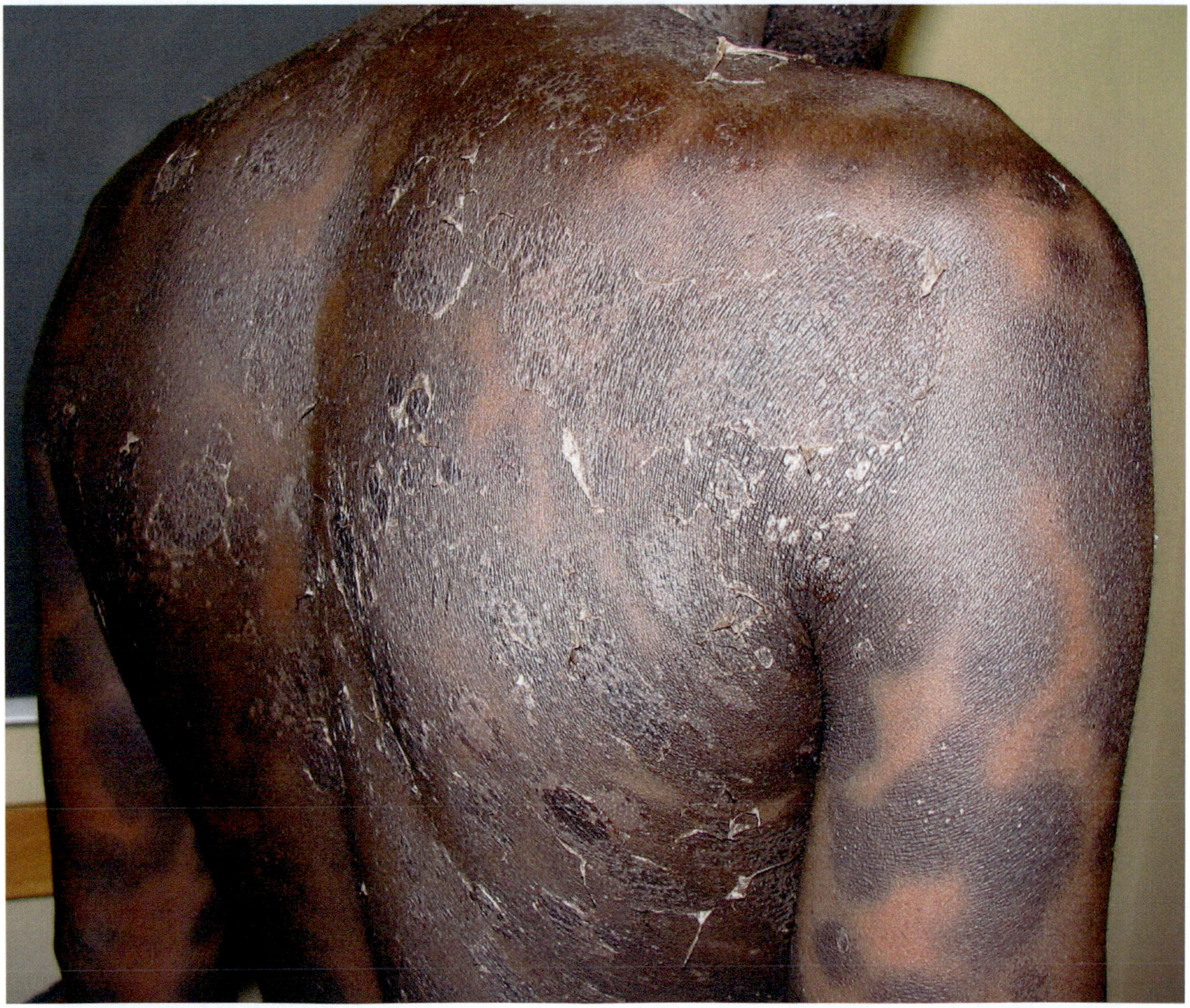

Fig. 32.4 *Recurrent fixed drug eruption*, widely spread, showing transition into necrolysis

Antibiotic management should be used if there is evidence of positive culture samples. Broad-spectrum antibiotics can be used if there is no evidence of source of infection. Prophylactic use of antibiotic is not recommended [21]. Coverage of the detached skin can be achieved by the use of paraffin gauze. Intravenous immune globulin (IVIG) has been used to treat TEN without firm conclusion and variable outcomes [23].

A generally accepted strategy on the use of high-dose corticosteroids in TEN patients has not been reached. Other therapies that have been used in TEN include TNF-α inhibitors, granulocyte colony-stimulating factor (GCSF), N-acetylcysteine, and cyclosporine. For DRESS, prompt removal/withdrawal of any suspected drugs is mandatory. Systemic administration of corticosteroids is initiated at a dosage of 1–2 mg/kg/day, tapering the dose over the course of 2–3 months after clinical and laboratory stabilization has been achieved. Other therapeutic schedules include high parenteral doses of immunoglobulins, plasmapheresis, cyclophosphamide, cyclosporine, mycophenolate mofetil, and rituximab. Prognostically, most patients with DRESS will recover completely if the causative drug is withdrawn. Mortality is around 10%, and death is commonly related to hepatic necrosis [4].

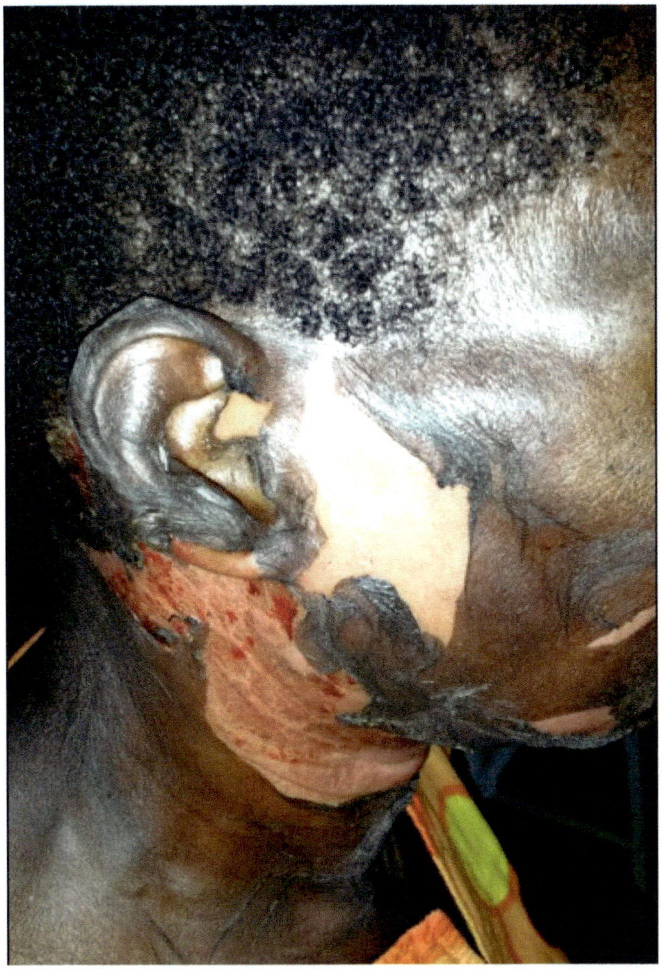

Fig. 32.5 *Toxic epidermal necrolysis*. Extensive skin peeling in a HIV-infected patient due to ART with nevirapine

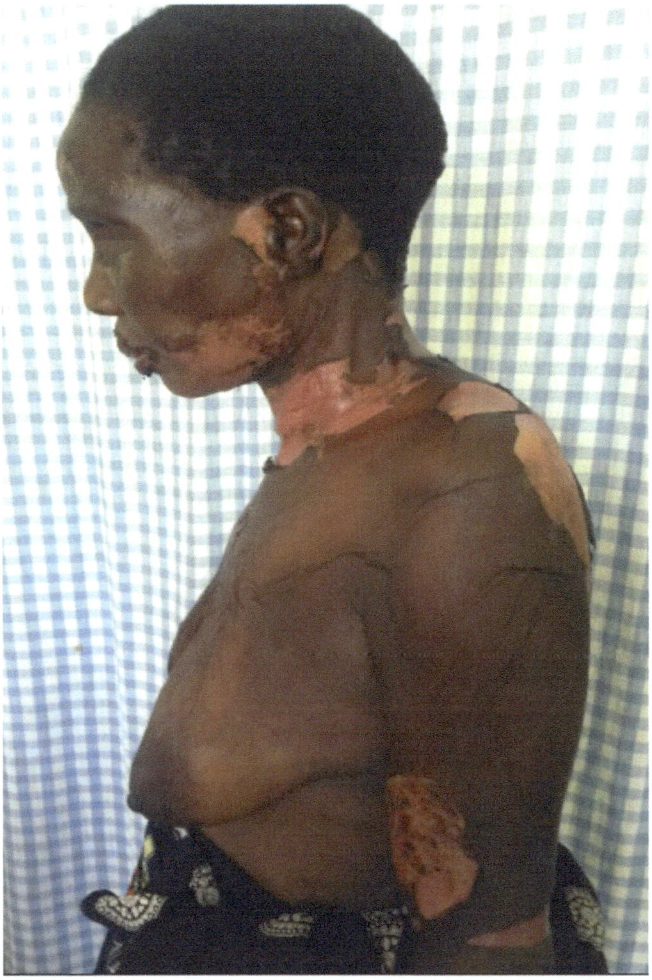

Fig. 32.6 Toxic epidermal necrolysis due to nevirapine (same patient as in Fig 32.5)

Conclusions

With increasing access to drugs such as antimalarials, antihelminthics, and antiretrovirals in developing countries, the rate of side effects induced by drugs also increases. Only a few of HIV/AIDS patients treated with ART experienced no adverse effects. It seems that increased susceptibility of dark- or black-skinned populations to develop SJS and TEN may be a cause for the frequency of the entities in dark-skinned African populations, including their prolonged course. These implications should be known by the attending physicians and health workers and be considered in schedules for patient care and monitoring.

References

1. Ditto AM. Drug allergy. In: Grammer LC, Greenberger PA, editors. Patterson's allergic disease. 6th ed. Philadelphia: Lippincott Williams & Wilkins; 2002. p. 295.
2. Nakamura M, Henderson M, Jacobsen G, et al. Comparison of photodermatoses in African-Americans and Caucasians: a follow-up study. Photodermatol Photoimmunol Photomed. 2014;30:231–6.
3. Saka B, Bauro-Traore F, Atadokpele FA, et al. Stevens-Johnson syndrome and toxic epidermal necrolysis in sub-Saharan Africa: a multicentric study in four countries. Int J Dermatol. 2013;52:575–9.
4. Husain Z, Reddy BY, Schwartz RA. DRESS syndrome. J Am Acad Dermatol. 2013;68:693–719.
5. Aihara M. Pharmacogenetics of cutaneous adverse drug reactions. J Dermatol. 2011;38:246–54.
6. Shear NH, Spielberg SP. Anticonvulsant hypersensitivity syndrome: in vitro assessment of risk. J Clin Invest. 1988;82:1826–32.
7. Chung WH, Hung SI, Chen YT. Human leukocyte antigens and drug hypersensitivity. Curr Opin Allergy Clin Immunol. 2007;7:317–23.
8. Descamps V, Valence A, Edlinger C, et al. Association of human herpes virus 6 infection with drug with drug reaction with eosinophilia and systemic symptoms. Arch Dermatol. 2001;137:301–4.
9. Kano Y, Inaoka M, Shiohara T. Association between anticonvulsant hypersensitivity syndrome and human herpes 6 reactivation and hypogammaglobulinemia. Arch Dermatol. 2004;140:183–8.
10. Freedberg IM, Eisen AZ, Wolff K, et al. Fitzpatrick dermatology in general medicine. 5th ed. New York, NY: McGraw-Hill; 1999. p. 534–7.

11. Sterry W, Steinhoff M. Erythroderma. In: Bologna J, Jorizzo JL, Shaffer JV, editors. Dermatology. 3rd ed. Philadelphia: Elsevier-Saunders; 2012. p. 171–81.
12. Salami TA, Enahoro Oziegbe O, Omeife H. Exfoliative dermatitis: patterns of clinical presentation in a tropical rural and sub-urban dermatology practice in Nigeria. Int J Dermatol. 2012;51:1086–9.
13. Lehloenya RJ. Outcomes of reintroducing anti-tuberculosis drugs following cutaneous adverse drug reactions. Int J Tuberc Lung Dis. 2011;15:1649–57.
14. Akhyani M, Ghoshi ZS, Toosi S, et al. Erythroderma: a clinical study of 97 cases. BMC Dermatol. 2005;5:5.
15. Schwartz RA, McDonough PH, Lee BW. Toxic epidermal necrolysis: part I. Introduction, classification. Clinical features, systemic manifestations, etiology, immunopathogenesis. J Am Acad Dermatol. 2013;69:173–81.
16. Schwartz RA, McDonough PH, Lee BW. Toxic epidermal necrolysis: part II prognosis, sequelae, diagnosis, differential diagnosis, prevention and treatment. J Am Acad Dermatol. 2013;69:187.
17. Borgiani P, Di Fusco D, Erba F, et al. Eur J Clin Pharmacol. 2014;70(3):275–8.
18. Dube N, Adewusi E, Summers R. Risk of nevirapine-associated Stevens-Johnson syndrome among HIV-infected pregnant women: the Medunsa National Pharmacovigilance Centre, 2007–2012. S Afr Med J. 2013;103:322–5.
19. Newell BD, Monifar M, Mancini AJ, et al. Retrospective analysis of 32 pediatric patients with anticonvulsant hypersensitivity syndrome (ACHSS). Pediatr Dermatol. 2009;26:536–46.
20. Covin JH, Sheth AP. Minocycline hypersensitivity syndrome with hypotension mimicking septic shock. Pediatric Dermatol. 2001;18:295–8.
21. Downey A, Jackson C, Harun N, et al. Toxic epidermal necrolysis: review of pathogenesis and management. J Am Acad Dermatol. 2012;66:995–1003.
22. Shiga S, Cartotto R. What are the fluid requirements in toxic epidermal necrolysis? J Burn Care Res. 2010;31:100–4.
23. Trent JT, Kirsner RS, Romanelli P, et al. Analysis of intravenous immunoglobulin for the treatment of toxic epidermal necrolysis using SCORTEN: the University of Miami experience. Arch Dermatol. 2003;139:39–43.

Behçet's Disease

Erkan Alpsoy

33

Behçet's disease (BD) is a chronic, relapsing inflammatory multisystem disease of unknown aetiology with the clinical features of mucocutaneous lesions and ocular, vascular, articular, neurologic, gastrointestinal, urogenital, pulmonary, and cardiac involvement [1, 2]. Mucocutaneous lesions are in the clinical presentation and can be considered the hallmarks of the disease. Their knowledge and recognition will permit earlier diagnosis and introduction of treatment with beneficial prognostic results for those affected. In most patients, the diagnosis can be made clinically on the basis of the mucocutaneous symptoms [2]. Since there is no pathognomonic test, multinational data have been recently revised, and International Criteria for Behçet's Disease (ICBD) have been proposed by an international team as a guide for BD diagnosis and classification [3].

33.1 Incidence

Behçet's disease (BD) has a global distribution. However, BD is more prevalent in populations along the Silk Road, extending from Japan to countries in the Middle East and the Mediterranean. The prevalence in these regions is 14–20 per 100,000 [4], and the highest is registered in Turkey; Azizlerli et al. [5] from Istanbul reported the prevalence to be 421 per 100,000 of the population aged 12 or older. Assaad-Khalil et al. [6] reported the prevalence as 7.6 per 100,000 in Egypt. Only a few cases were reported in sub-Saharan Africa [7]. The disease is rarely seen in European countries with decreasing frequency south to north; in the United Kingdom, the prevalence has been found to be 0.64 per 100,000, similar to 0.38 per 100,000 population in the United States [8]. In a cross-sectional prevalence study in the suburbs of Paris, Mahr et al. [9] reported the frequency of BD as 7.1/100,000. BD among immigrants of North African (34.6/100,000) or Asian ancestry (17.5/100,000) is significantly higher than that in the population of European descent (2.4/100,000).

33.2 Etiology/Pathogenesis

BD can affect all sizes and types of blood vessels, and endothelial cells are believed to be the primary target. The histopathologic features of BD are characterized by mainly vasculitis and thrombosis. The vasculitis may be a leukocytoclastic vasculitis or a neutrophilic vascular reaction. Although several immunological abnormalities have been demonstrated, the exact mechanism of the inflammatory changes occurring remains to be elucidated. Neutrophil activity is increased in BD, and the affected organs show a significant neutrophil and lymphocyte infiltration. It is believed that the stimulated lymphocytes contribute to neutrophil and endothelial cell activation in these patients. Recent studies indicate that Th17 and IL-17 pathways are also active in BD patients and play an important role particularly in acute attacks of the disease. Increased neutrophil activity and neutrophil infiltration in the affected organs might be caused by increased IL-17 response [10].

Genetic factors have been investigated extensively. Association with HLA-B51 is known as the strongest genetic susceptibility factor for BD. In a meta-analysis, de Menthon et al. [11] showed that subjects carrying HLA-B51/B5 have an increased risk of developing BD with an odds ratio of 5.78 compared to non-carriers of this antigen. It is thought to play a role in neutrophil activation. In a recent multicenter study, Hughes et al. [12] tried to localize the genetic association between HLA-B51 and BD and explored additional susceptibility loci in the HLA region. Over 8000 variants in the extended HLA locus were genotyped, and imputation and meta-analysis of almost 25,000 variants were carried out in two independent BD cohorts. The most significant association

E. Alpsoy
Department of Dermatology and Venereology,
Akdeniz University School of Medicine, Antalya, Turkey
e-mail: ealpsoy@akdeniz.edu.tr

C. E. Orfanos et al. (eds.), *Pigmented Ethnic Skin and Imported Dermatoses*, https://doi.org/10.1007/978-3-319-69422-1_33

was with rs116799036, which is located between HLA-B and MICA. In pairwise conditional analysis, the genetic association at rs116799036 remained significant independent of HLA-B-5101 in Turkish and Italian cohorts. Notably, the genetic association with HLA-B-51 completely disappeared when controlling for the genetic association with this SNP. This data strongly suggest that the association between HLA-B51 and BD can be explained by this SNP. Besides this study, six recent GWAS, with an exception of the study by Fei et al. [13], have confirmed the association of BD with HLA-B51 and reported new susceptibility genes on the remaining part of HLA class I region and several non-HLA genes for the disease [14–18]. Two of them, conducted in Turkey [18] and Japan [17], reported association between SNP of IL-10 and IL-23R/IL-12RB2 genes and BD. The disease-associated variants were located in the IL23R side of the hot spot suggesting the association with BD is more likely to be with IL23R rather than IL12RB2. IL23 which shares the p40 subunit with IL12 acts to induce T cell activation to produce IL17 and therefore is one of the main Th17 pathway activators.

33.3 Clinical Picture

Lesions are initially seen around the third or fourth decade of life, showing male predominance in Middle Eastern and Mediterranean countries and women predominance in Japan and Korea. Because of the lack of a universally recognized pathognomonic test, the diagnosis is primarily based on clinical criteria considering the mucocutaneous manifestations of the disease such as oral ulcers (OU), genital ulcers (GU), and cutaneous vasculitic lesions and the skin pathergy test (SPT).

Although some mucocutaneous lesions may vary in different ethnic groups, the presence of characteristic oral and genital ulcerations is the leading symptom in all affected individuals, regardless the color of their skin. OU start as erythematous, slightly raised vesiculopustular lesions evolving within 2–3 days into oval or round ulcerations with rolled borders and grayish-yellow necrotic base. They are recurrent and painful, mimicking aphthae, but usually multiple with relapses more frequent than in aphthous stomatitis [19]. An erythematous halo surrounds the ulcers (Fig. 33.1). Preferred

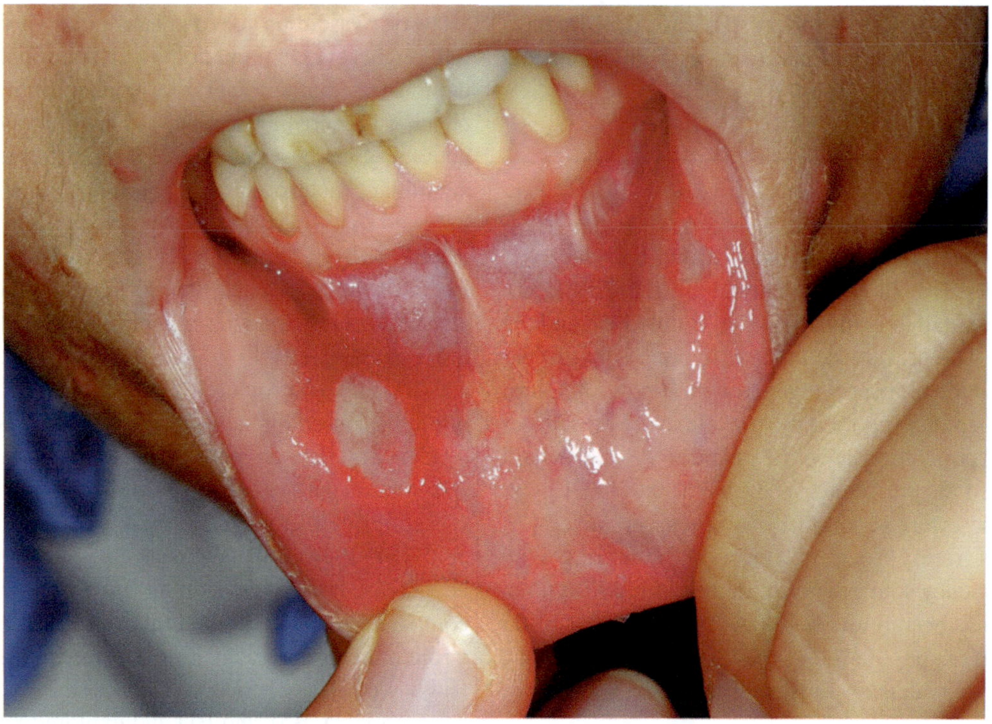

Fig. 33.1 Oral ulcers on the labial mucosa with erythematous rolled borders and a grayish-yellow necrotic base

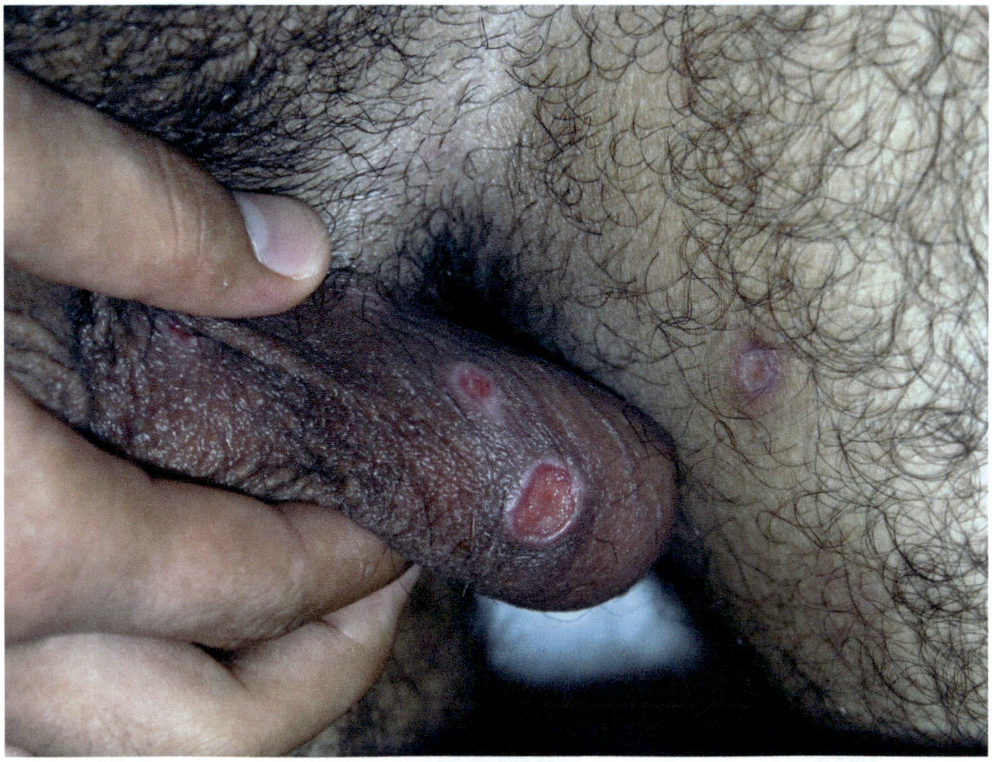

Fig. 33.2 Genital ulcers are similar in appearance and course to oral ulcers; the scrotum is the most commonly involved site in males

localizations are the mucous membranes of the lips, buccal mucosa, tongue, and soft palate. OU often subside spontaneously within 1–4 weeks and recur at intervals from days to months. Local trauma can induce new mucosal lesions. GU are similar in appearance and course to OU but may not recur as often. They are usually deeper than the OU and heal within 10–30 days with a tendency to leave scar. The labia majora is the most frequently involved site in females, but the labia minora, vaginal mucosa, and rarely cervix can also be affected. The scrotum is the most commonly involved site in males (Fig. 33.2). Ulcers can also be observed on the shaft and glans penis. Ulcers in the urethral orifice have also been reported. GU may occur in both genders in the groin, perineal, and perianal area [1, 20].

Various cutaneous vasculitic lesions have been described during the course of BD. The cutaneous lesions include mainly erythema nodosum (EN)-like lesions, papulopustular lesions (PPL), superficial thrombophlebitis (TFB), and the skin pathergy reaction (SPR). Other cutaneous vasculitic lesions such as extragenital ulceration, Sweet's syndrome-like lesions, pyoderma gangrenosum-like lesions, erythema multiforme-like lesions, pernio-like cutaneous lesions, palpable purpura, bullous necrotizing vasculitis, subungual infarctions, hemorrhagic bullae, furuncles, abscesses, and acral purpuric papulonodular lesions are rarely seen [20].

EN-like lesions are mostly seen in females and occur in about one-third of all patients. They have a typical clinical presentation with bilateral, pretibial, painful, hot, and erythematous nodules. In pigmented or black skin, because of the overlying pigmentation, erythema is not easily visible. Therefore, palpation is especially important for the examination of EN-like lesions. They do not ulcerate and resolve spontaneously within 2–3 weeks in pigmented or black-skinned patients with residual pigmentation (Fig. 33.3); however, recurrence is common [1, 21]. PPL are sterile, folliculitis or acne-like lesions on erythematous base which appear as a papule and in the course of 24–48 h become pustule. The trunk, buttocks, and the lower limbs (Fig. 33.4) are the most common locations [2]. In many cases, erythema in PPL is hardly noticeable on pigmented or black skin, and postinflammatory hyperpigmentation is more common. Superficial TFB is more common in males and frequently confused with EN-like lesions. The patients usually present with erythematous, tender subcutaneous nodules arranged in a linear fashion. The vein can be palpated as a string-like hardening because of thrombosis leading to vessel sclerosis with reddening of the

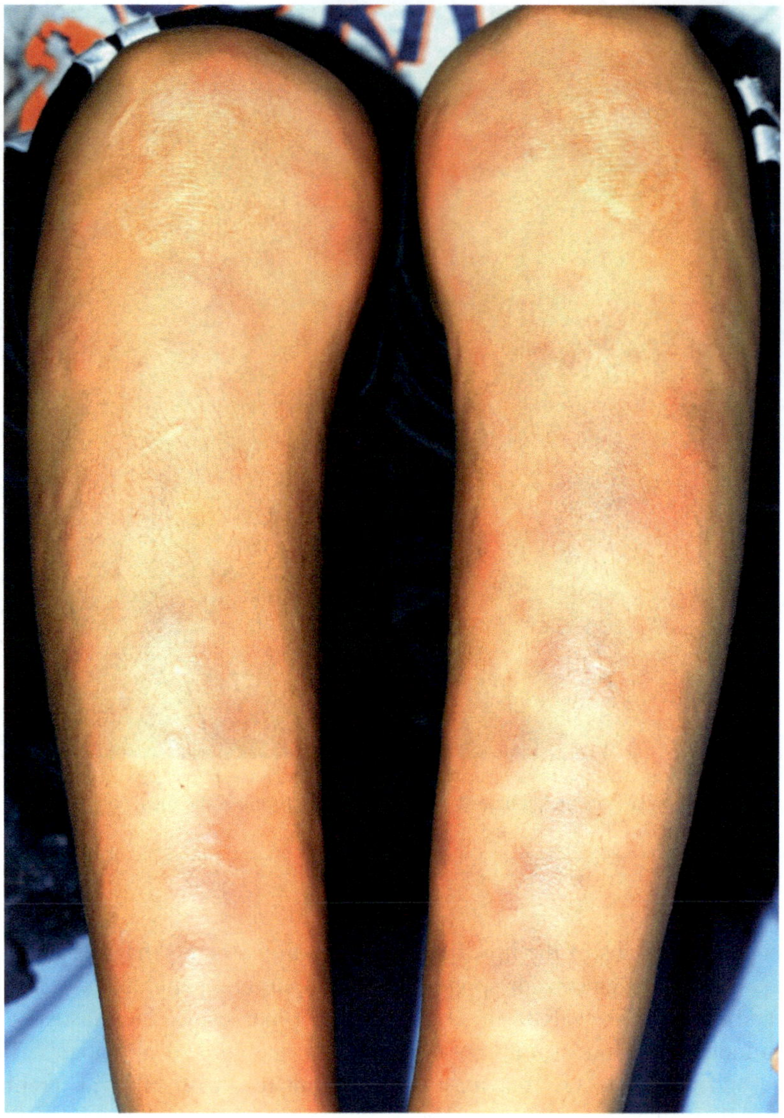

Fig. 33.3 Erythema nodosum-like lesions; painful, hot, erythematous nodules on the pretibial region

overlying skin. Erythematous nature of TFB can be very conspicuous in pigmented (Fig. 33.5) or black-skinned individuals. The location of nodules shows a tendency to change from day to day because multiple segments of the vein might be involved [2]. TFB is clinically important since it could frequently be associated with other forms of vascular disease, deep venous thrombosis and dural sinus thrombosis in the central nervous system [22]. SPT is a nonspecific skin hyper-reactivity, induced by needle prick. The test positivity is defined as the development of a papule or pustule at the needle-prick site at 48 h (Fig. 33.6). It is similar to the spontaneously occurring PPL of the disease, and more strongly positive among males. This test is applied to hairless part of the avascular volar forearm after cleansing the skin with alcohol swabs. A 20-gauge sterile needle is inserted at an angle of 45° to a depth of 5 mm. We use three pricks for each arm. The test is considered positive if an indurated erythematous small papule or pustule formation of ≥2 mm in diameter is observed. The SPT positivity varies between geographic areas, and it is considered highly sensitive and specific for BD in patients from Turkey, some from the Mediterranean, the Middle Eastern countries, and Japan [2].

33.4 Management

Treatment of BD has become much more effective in recent years, because of advances in understanding the pathogenesis of the disease and availability of a wide spectrum of therapeutic agents. Treatment is mainly based on the suppression

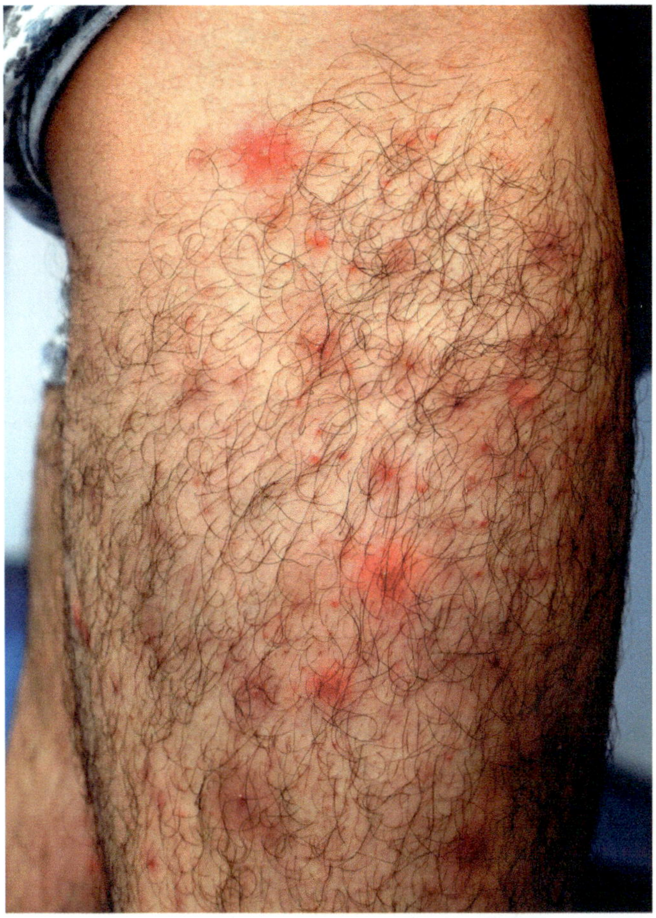

Fig. 33.4 Numerous papulopustular lesions on the right leg

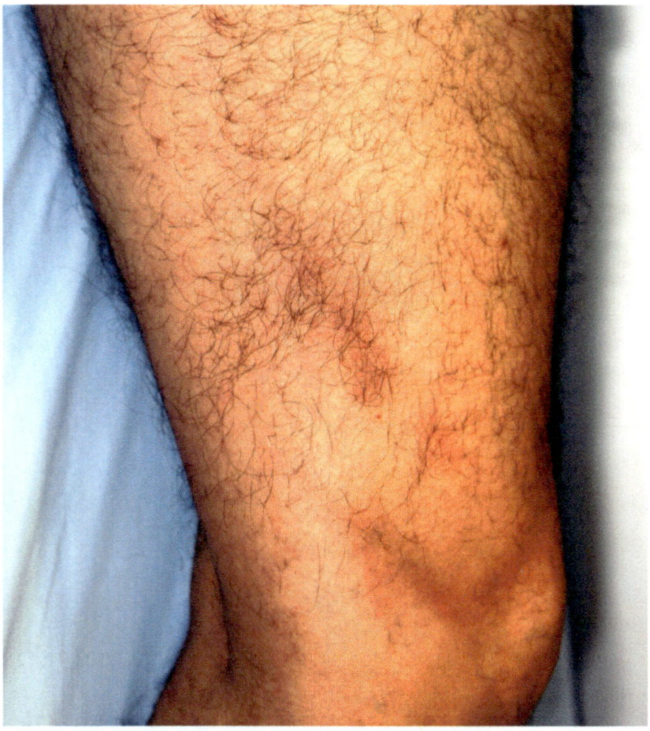

Fig. 33.5 Superficial thrombophlebitis; slightly erythematous, tender subcutaneous nodules arranged in a linear fashion on the leg

of inflammatory attacks of the disease using immunomodulatory and immunosuppressive agents. Treatment of BD depends on a number of factors such as involved organs and severity of these involvements, frequency of recurrences, disease duration, patient's age at disease onset, and patient's gender. However, the main aim of the treatment should be the prevention of irreversible organ damage, especially, during the early active phase of the disease.

33.5 Topical Treatment of Mucocutaneous Lesions

Corticosteroids (triamcinolone acetonide in oral paste t.i.d. or dexamethasone 0.1% in oral paste q.i.d.) suppress the inflammation associated with the formation of aphthae. Corticosteroids alone or in conjunction with antiseptics are effective on both OU and GU especially when they are used in the early stage of these lesions. They reduce pain severity and healing duration. Antimicrobial agents (Listerine mouth rinse and chlorhexidine gel, 2–4×/day) are used to control microbial load. They are effective on pain severity and duration in OU. Sucralfate (5 mL solution, 4×/day) decreases significantly the frequency, healing time, and pain of OU and the healing time and pain of GU. This compound binds to ulcerated tissue, forms a barrier, and augments ulcer healing. Amlexanox (5% in oral paste, 4×/day) accelerates the healing and decreases pain severity of OU. It has anti-inflammatory and antiallergic activities. 5-aminosalicylic acid 5% cream, 3×/day, increases the healing process and decreases pain of OU. Pimecrolimus cream, 2×/day, a topical immunomodulator, seems to be safe and efficient in the treatment of GU, by accelerating the healing process and shortening the pain duration. In addition to the abovementioned treatment approaches to OU, patients should be advised to maintain good daily oral hygiene. These patients should avoid irritating agents such as acid; crusty, hard, spicy, or salty nutrients; and alcoholic beverages. EN-like lesions are treated topically like those of classic EN. Wet dressings such as aluminum acetate 3–5% (Burow's solution) can be applied in the early stage of these lesions. This approach is also helpful for the treatment of superficial TFB. All management should be combined with rest in bed. For the clinician, it is very important to be aware that the topical treatment of the disease has only local effects [2].

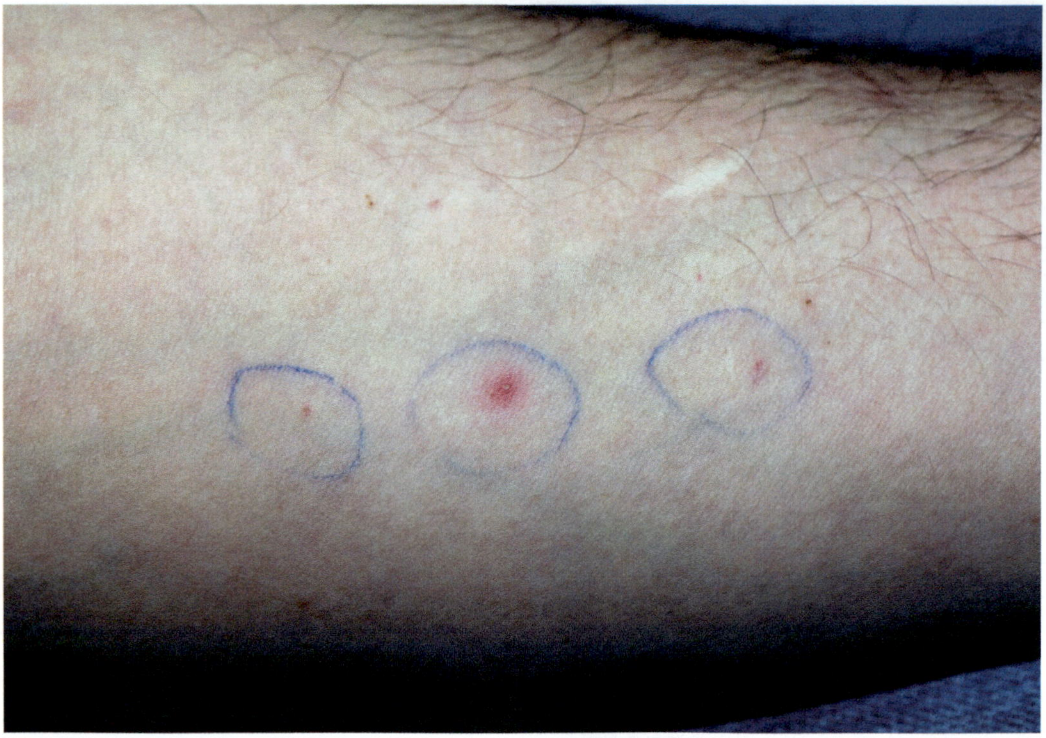

Fig. 33.6 The skin pathergy test positivity (middle prick)

33.6 Systemic Treatment of Mucocutaneous Lesions

The number of randomized controlled studies in systemic treatment of mucocutaneous BD is higher as compared with topical treatment, and their number has been increasing day by day. Following algorithmic approach for the systemic treatment of mucocutaneous BD is mainly based on randomized controlled studies and our clinical practice. In the treatment of OU, GU, EN-like lesions, and PPL, colchicine (1–2 mg/day, p.o.) should be the first choice. If this is not effective, colchicine can be combined with benzathine penicillin (1.2 MU/3–4 weeks, i.m.). Short-term corticosteroids (prednisolone, initial dose 40–60 mg/day p.o. for at least 4 weeks) in combination with other drugs such as colchicine can be used as an alternative in the treatment of acute attacks of OU, GU, EN-like lesions, and superficial TFB. Dapsone (100–150 mg/day p.o.) can also be used at this stage as an effective compound. Patients with severe mucocutaneous disease or those who are unresponsive to the respected treatments can be treated with azathioprine (2–2,5 mg/kg/day, p.o.). Thalidomide (100–300 mg/day) is also an effective choice. However, because of potential side effects, it should be used cautiously in selected patients. It is wise to keep in mind that EN-like lesions worsen during thalidomide treatment. Cyclosporin (5 mg/kg/day, p.o.), apremilast (30 mg/day, 2×/day), IFN alpha (3–12 MU/day, 3×/week, s.c.), and anti-TNF-α agents (etanercept 25 mg/day, 2×/week and infliximab and adalimumab in their usual dosages) are other alternatives to control the disease in unresponsive cases.

33.7 Course

BD runs a chronic course with unpredictable exacerbations and remissions. Current literature and our experience indicate that BD usually starts with relatively milder manifestations and severe involvements, in general, appear later. In most cases, OU are the most common manifestation followed by GU, PPL, EN-like lesions, and articular and ocular involvement. OU are also the most common onset manifestation which is followed by GU, EN-like lesions, and ocular involvement. In about 15% of the patients, more than one symptom appear at the same time as the onset manifestation. OU and GU are the most common combination among the simultaneous occurrence of symptoms. Therefore, relapsing bipolar oral and genital ulcers are strongly evocative of BD, and OU/GU precede other manifestations [20, 23].

Each or any combination of mucocutaneous, articular, and ocular symptoms of the disease may have significant pain or loss in function, or both. Besides considerable morbidity, the disease confers an increased mortality, mainly because of pulmonary as well as large vessel involvement, neurologic involvement, and bowel perforation. Mortality ratios as well as mucocutaneous and articular manifestations usually tend to decrease significantly with the passage of time [24]. Both the onset and the greatest damage of ocular involvement are usually within the first few years of the disease onset. However, recent data indicate that neurological, gastrointestinal, and large vessel involvements are exceptions and can have their onsets later (5–10 years) during the course of the disease [20, 22, 24, 25]. Higher frequency of serious manifestations, such as ocular, vascular, and neurological involvement, has been reported in male patients. On the other hand, EN-like lesions and articular involvement are more common in female patients [20, 22, 26, 27].

In summary, careful follow-up is mandatory since BD shows a continuous activity. Male gender, younger age of onset, and increased number of organ involvement at diagnosis are associated with a more severe disease and, therefore, require more aggressive treatment.

Conclusions

BD is a chronic, relapsing, inflammatory multisystem disease of unknown aetiology. OU, GU, cutaneous lesions (mainly EN-like lesions, PPL), superficial TFB, SPT, and ocular and articular involvement are the most frequent features. Mucocutaneous lesions are considered hallmarks of the disease and often precede other manifestations. Therefore, their recognition may permit earlier diagnosis and treatment with beneficial results for prognosis. BD is particularly prevalent in "Silk Route" populations but has a global distribution. The disease usually starts around the third or fourth decade of life. Gender distribution is roughly equal. The diagnosis is based on clinical criteria, as there is no pathognomonic test. Genetic factors have been investigated extensively, and association with HLA-B51 is still known as the strongest genetic susceptibility factor. Th17 and IL-17 pathways are active and play an important role, particularly in acute attacks of BD. Neutrophil activity is increased in BD, and the affected organs show a significant neutrophil and lymphocyte infiltration. HLA-B51 association and increased IL-17 response are thought to play a role in neutrophil activation. Treatment is mainly based on the suppression of inflammatory attacks of the disease using immunomodulatory and immunosuppressive agents. Although treatment has become much more effective in recent years with the introduction of newer drugs, BD is still associated with considerable morbidity and increased mortality. BD runs a chronic course with unpredictable exacerbations and remissions. Male gender, younger age of onset, and increased number of organ involvement at diagnosis are associated with a more severe disease and, therefore, require more aggressive treatment.

References

1. Behçet H. Uber rezidivierende aphthöse, durch ein Virus verursachte Geschwure, am Mund, am Auge, und an den Genitalien. Dermatol Wochenschr. 1937;105:1152–7.
2. Alpsoy E. Behçet's disease: a comprehensive review with a focus on epidemiology, etiology and clinical features, and management of mucocutaneous lesions. J Dermatol. 2016;43:620–32.
3. International Team for the Revision of the International Criteria for Behçet's Disease (ITR-ICBD). The international criteria for Behçet's disease (ICBD): a collaborative study of 27 countries on the sensitivity and specificity of the new criteria. J Eur Acad Dermatol Venereol. 2014;28:338–47.
4. Alpsoy E, Donmez L, Onder M, et al. Clinical features and natural course of Behcet's disease in 661 cases: a multicentre study. Br J Dermatol. 2007;157:901–6.
5. Azizlerli G, Kose AA, Sarica R, et al. Prevalence of Behcet's disease in Istanbul, Turkey. Int J Dermatol. 2003;42:803–6.
6. Assaad-Khalil SH, Kamel FA, Ismail EA. Starting a national registry for patients with Behçet's disease in North West Nile Delta region in Egypt. In: Hamza M, editor. Behçet's disease. Tunis (Tunisia): Pub Adhoua; 1979. p. 173–6.
7. Meda JR, Seni J, Mpondo B, Peck RN, Jaka H, Kilonzo SB. Behcet's disease presenting with recurrent ocular, oral, and scrotal inflammatory lesions in a young Tanzanian man: a case report. Clin Case Rep. 2014;2:133–6.
8. Calamia KT, Wilson FC, Icen M, Crowson CS, Gabriel SE, Kremers HM. Epidemiology and clinical characteristics of Behçet's disease in the US: a population-based study. Arthritis Rheum. 2009;61(5):600–4.
9. Mahr A, Belarbi L, Wechsler B, et al. Population-based prevalence study of Behçet's disease differences by ethnic origin and low variation by age at immigration. Arthritis Rheum. 2008;58: 3951–9.
10. Ekinci NS, Alpsoy E, Karakas AA, Yilmaz SB, Yegin O. IL-17A has an important role in the acute attacks of Behçet's disease. J Invest Dermatol. 2010;130:2136–8.
11. de Menthon M, Lavalley MP, Maldini C, Guillevin L, Mahr A. HLA-B51/B5 and the risk of Behcet's disease: a systematic review and meta-analysis of case-control genetic association studies. Arthritis Rheum. 2009;61:1287–96.
12. Hughes T, Coit P, Adler A, et al. Identification of multiple independent susceptibility loci in the HLA region in Behçet's disease. Nat Genet. 2013;45:319–24.
13. Fei Y, Webb R, Cobb BL, Direskeneli H, Saruhan-Direskeneli G, Sawalha AH. Identification of novel genetic susceptibility loci for Behcet's disease using a genome-wide association study. Arthritis Res Ther. 2009;11:R66.
14. Hou S, Yang Z, Du L, et al. Identification of a susceptibility locus in STAT4 for Behcet's disease in Han Chinese in a genome-wide association study. Arthritis Rheum. 2012;64:4104–13.
15. Kirino Y, Bertsias G, Ishigatsubo Y, et al. Genome-wide association analysis identifies new susceptibility loci for Behcet's disease and epistasis between HLA-B-51 and ERAP1. Nat Genet. 2013;45:202–7.
16. Lee YJ, Horie Y, Wallace GR, et al. Genome-wide association study identifies GIMAP as a novel susceptibility locus for Behcet's disease. Ann Rheum Dis. 2013;72:1510–6.
17. Mizuki N, Meguro A, Ota M, et al. Genome-wide association studies identify IL23R-IL12RB2 and IL10 as Behcet's disease susceptibility loci. Nat Genet. 2010;42:703–6.
18. Remmers EF, Cosan F, Kirino Y, et al. Genome-wide association study identifies variants in the MHC class I, IL10, and IL23R-IL12RB2 regions associated with Behcet's disease. Nat Genet. 2010;42:698–702.

19. Oh S, Han EC, Lee JH, Bang DT. Comparison of the clinical features of recurrent aphthous stomatitis and Behçet's disease. Clin Exp Dermatol. 2009;34:e208–12.
20. Alpsoy E, Zouboulis CC, Ehrlich CE. Mucocutaneous lesions of Behçet's disease. Yonsei Med J. 2007;48:573–85.
21. Kim B, LeBoit PE. Histopathologic features of erythema nodosum-like lesions in Behcet disease: a comparison with erythema nodosum focusing on the role of vasculitis. Am J Dermatopathol. 2000;22:379–90.
22. Tunc R, Saip S, Siva A, Yazici H. Cerebral venous thrombosis is associated with major vessel disease in Behçet's syndrome. Ann Rheum Dis. 2004;63:1693–4.
23. Ugurlu N, Bozkurt S, Bacanli A, Akman-Karakas A, Uzun S, Alpsoy E. The natural course and factors affecting severity of Behçet's disease: a single-center cohort of 368 patients. Rheumatol Int. 2015;35:2103–7.
24. Kural-Seyahi E, Fresko I, Seyahi N, et al. The long-term mortality and morbidity of Behcet syndrome: a 2-decade outcome survey of 387 patients followed at a dedicated center. Medicine (Baltimore). 2003;82:60–76.
25. Ideguchi H, Suda A, Takeno M, Ueda A, Ohno S, Ishigatsubo Y. Behçet disease: evolution of clinical manifestations. Medicine (Baltimore). 2011;90:125–32.
26. Bonitsis NG, Luong Nguyen LB, LaValley MP, et al. Gender-specific differences in Adamantiades-Behçet's disease manifestations: an analysis of the German registry and meta-analysis of data from the literature. Rheumatology (Oxford). 2015;54:121–33.
27. Yazici H, Tuzun Y, Pazarli H, et al. Influence of age of onset and patient's sex on the prevalans and severity of manifestations of Behçet's syndrome. Ann Rheum Dis. 1984;43:783–9.

Nail Disorders in Dark Skin

34

Moetaz El-Domyati and Noha H. Moftah

The *nail unit* is a skin appendage produced by the skin. Its major function is mechanical protection of the distal digit, also representing a part of the overall cosmetic appearance of the body. Genetic disorders, infections, various dermatoses, senility, tumors, etc. may result in a series of changes of the nail showing alterations of growth, color, thickness, and contour of the nail plate. Thus, examination of the digits and nails often provides diagnostic clues for underlying cutaneous or systemic disease. Alterations and deformities of the nails may be characteristic and helpful for the physician to support his diagnosis; others are not specific but still provide valuable clues for targeted medical investigation. Major differences of nail pathology between Caucasians and dark-skinned ethnic populations are not known or prominent; however, environmental exposure and socioeconomic circumstances in populations living in hot climate zones differ and cause differences in the clinical presentation and medical assistance. In addition, pigment lability in dark skin easily causes diffuse or striate melanonychia [1].

34.1 Infections of the Nail

34.1.1 Bacterial and Viral Infections

Nail infections are usually due to bacteria that invade damaged nails through the seal between the nail plate and the surrounding tissue and enter and cause inflammation in the hyponychium and swelling of the surrounding nail folds (*paronychia*). The most common causative agents are *Staphylococcus* spp., followed by pseudomonas and some streptococci; in rare cases herpes viruses may be the causative agent. In advanced cases discoloration of the nail plate and painful paronychia result, occasionally, with pus-filled small abscesses. Chronic paronychia may be painful and show periodic flare-ups in labor workers, after exposure to chemicals and other irritants, etc. Treatment is by warm soaks with water, liquid antibacterial soaps, and topical antibiotics; in severe cases oral antibiotics may be required. If a paronychial abscess is diagnosed, surgical drainage is indicated [2].

34.1.2 Fungal Infections

Infection of the nails with *dermatophytes*, *Tinea* (*T.*) *unguium* is common both in white Caucasians and in populations with darkly pigmented skin. The average prevalence in fair skin populations in Europe and North America is approximately 4% [3, 4] and up to 5.5–10% in populations with dark skin [5]. The prevalence of onychomycosis is clearly higher (>10%) in patients with diabetes, disturbances of blood circulation, peripheral neuropathies, immunocompromised individuals, and the elderly. In populations with dark skin, onychomycosis represents 20–40% of all onychopathies and about 30% of cutaneous fungal infections [5]. Tinea unguium represents 7.7% of all dermatophyte infections [6], whereby *T. interdigitale*, *T. rubrum*, and *T. verrucosum* are the most common agents [7]. Rarely, *T. soudanense* may be detected.

The clinical picture includes:

(a) *Distal and lateral subungual onychomycosis* (DLSO) which is the commonest pattern of fungal nail infection in most populations (Fig. 34.1a)
(b) *White superficial onychomycosis* (WSO) seen primarily on the toes, in which fungi invade the nail plate surface, with formation of small, well-delineated, opaque, white, powder-like, transverse coalescing islands
(c) *Proximal subungual onychomycosis* (PSO) which is the least common pattern, could be considered as the presenting sign of acquired immunodeficiency syndrome

M. El-Domyati (✉) • N. H. Moftah
Department of Dermatology, STDs and Andrology, Minia University, Al-Minya, Egypt

C. E. Orfanos et al. (eds.), *Pigmented Ethnic Skin and Imported Dermatoses*, https://doi.org/10.1007/978-3-319-69422-1_34

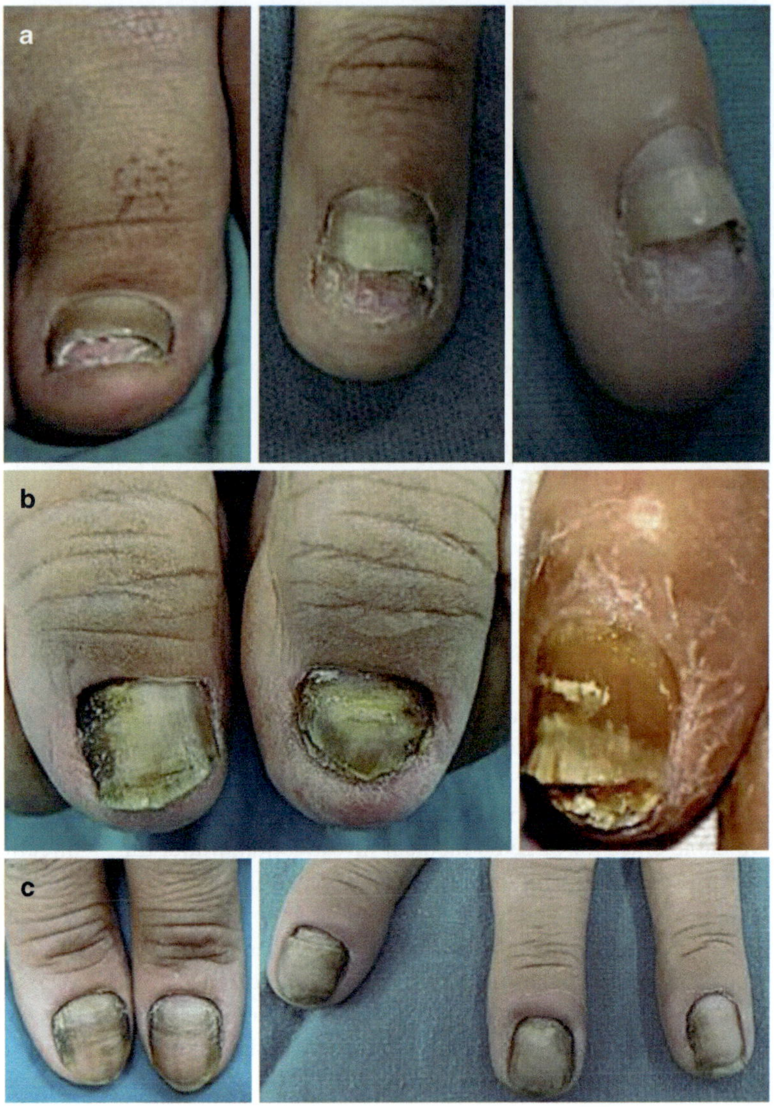

Fig. 34.1 (**a**) *Distal subungual onychomycosis* with distal onycholysis and subungual hyperkeratosis. (**b**) *Total dystrophic onychomycosis* with thickened, rough, friable, and hyperkeratotic nail plates. (**c**) *Candidal onychomycosis* with swollen proximal nail folds, loss of cuticle, patent proximal nail groove, and total dystrophic nails

(d) *Total dystrophic onychomycosis* (TDO) occurs as the result of progression of any of the three previous forms of onychomycosis with nail matrix involvement with rough, friable, hyperkeratotic, and crumbling nails (Fig. 34.1b)

Infections with *Candida* spp. commonly occur in hot climate zones and fingernails of females due to frequent handling of water and soap during household work leading to rough, irregular, convex, and dystrophic nails with loss of cuticle and proximal nail groove. *Candida albicans* can infect the nail as a primary or secondary pathogen (18–20%); however, secondary appearance is more common, especially after nail onycholysis and candidal paronychia. Nail matrix infection results in transverse depressions in the nail plate known as Beau's lines. In candidal onychomycosis, there is no subungual hyperkeratosis, and the nail does not crumble away as in TDO [5, 8] (Fig. 34.1c).

Infections with *non-dermatophytic molds* account for 1.5–6% of all onychomycoses that fall into two categories, causative agents which are isolated from affected nails, in particular *Scytalidium dimidiatum* and *Scytalidium hyalinum*, or opportunistic fungi that may be isolated as contaminants, e.g., *Scopulariopsis brevicaulis* and *Aspergillus sydowii* [8]. In tropical zones with moist environment, *Scytalidium* is often detected.

Diagnosis of onychomycosis is primarily based upon direct microscopy after scraping of hyperkeratotic nail bed and mounting in 10–30% KOH with warming to emulsify lipids or adding 36% dimethyl sulfoxide instead of heating.

Table 34.1 Commonly prescribed medications for onychomycosis

Treatment	Indications	Active agent	Dosing schedule	Cure rate (%)		Organism	Adverse effects	Comments
				Clinical	Mycotic			
Topical	– WSO – Mild DLSO – <50% of nail surface – <3 fingers – No matrix involvement	Ciclopirox 8% lacquer	Daily for 48 weeks	6–9	29–36 (77% with debridement)	DF, NDM, yeasts	– Periungual erythema	– Patients should not bathe for 8 h when applied – Damaged nail should be removed using scissors or nail clippers – Application to nail plate, nail bed, and hyponychium
		Amorolfine 5% lacquer	Weekly for 48 weeks	1	16	DF, NDM, yeasts	– Periungual erythema – Discoloration	
		Terbinafine solution	Daily for 48 weeks	1	16	DF, NDM, yeasts		
		Efinaconazole 10% solution	Daily for 48 weeks	16–17	53–55	DF, NDM, yeasts	– Local reaction	
		Tavaborole 5% solution	Daily for 48 weeks	7–9	31–36	DF, NDM, yeasts		
Systemic	– PSO – >50% of nail surface – >3 fingers	Terbinafine	250 mg 1×/day	66	76	DF, NDM	– GIT disturbances – Asymptomatic liver enzyme elevation	– Liver and renal function tests are required
		Itraconazole	*Pulse:* 200 mg 2×/day for 1 week/month	70	63	DF, NDM, yeasts	– GIT disturbances – Hypokalemia – Elevated transaminase and triglycerides	– Liver function tests are required especially with preexisting hepatic dysfunction – Contraindicated in patients with ventricular dysfunction or congestive heart failure
			Continuous: 200 mg 1×/day	70	69			
		Fluconazole	150–300 mg 1×/week	41	48	Candida, limited in DF	– GIT disturbances	– Liver function tests and potassium levels are required – Not FDA-approved in onychomycosis
Surgical debride-ment	Partial in: – Lateral nail involvement – Onycholytic pocket on nail undersurface				0		– Infection – Distal nail embedding	

WSO white superficial onychomycosis, *DLSO* distal lateral subungual onychomycosis, *PSO* proximal superficial onychomycosis; *DF* dermatophytes; *NDM* non-dermatophytic molds; *GIT* gastrointestinal; *FDA* Food and Drug Administration

Drug interactions: *Terbinafine*: antiarrhythmic agents, beta-blockers, SSRIs, tricyclic antidepressants, and warfarin; *Itraconazole*: benzodiazepines, calcium channel blockers, proton pump inhibitors, statins, and warfarin; *Fluconazole:* benzodiazepines, calcium channel blockers, statins, and terfenadine

The nail is examined for fungal hyphae, arthrospores, or yeast forms; however, direct microscopy cannot always identify the specific fungus. Cultures from nail bed or nail plate debris are performed for confirming diagnosis and ascertaining the exact etiologic fungus. Different media are used, including primary medium containing cycloheximide, which is directed against most NDM and bacteria, e.g., DTM mycosel (BBL), mycobiotic (DIFCO), and cycloheximide-free secondary media, but with addition of antibiotics to eliminate bacterial contamination, e.g., Sabouraud glucose agar, Littman Oxgall medium, and potato dextrose agar [5].

Treatment of fungal nail infections varies depending on the responsible organism and the severity of the infection. Topical antifungal treatment is difficult to perform and often remains unsuccessful, while systemic treatment is effective but may be associated with side effects. The usual duration of treatment with oral antifungals is 6–8 weeks for fingernail involvement and 12 weeks or longer for toenail involvement (Table 34.1). Despite the number of available antifungal drugs, not all patients with onychomycosis are cured because of nonadherence to treatment, incorrect diagnosis, or advanced disease. Moreover, there are long-term recurrence rates, ranging from 10 to 53% [9].

34.2 Nail Abnormalities in Dermatoses

34.2.1 Eczematous Dermatitis

Chronic eczematous dermatitis of hands and feet may precede a variety of nail changes. The nail changes include roughness, thickening, coarse and irregular pitting or grooving, transverse ridging, furrowing, nail shedding, onycholysis, and subungual hemorrhage. Acute and chronic paronychial inflammation which affects nail matrix secondarily may lead to nail plate dystrophy. In hot climate zones, long-standing dyshidrotic eczema with dystrophic nail changes may develop. Reactions to artificial nails have included paronychia, onychodystrophy, and dermatitis at contact areas [10].

34.2.2 Psoriasis

Pitting of the nail plate is the most common sign in psoriasis in around 15% of all patients, ranging from small pits to large irregular furrows (Figs. 34.2 and 34.3); it occurs in up to 80–90% of patients with psoriatic arthritis [11]. Pitting results from defective keratinization of the proximal matrix cells, with falling out of small foci of parakeratotic cells on the nail plate. Pitting can be seen also in alopecia areata, eczema, trauma, and pityriasis rubra pilaris. *Salmon or oil-drop patches* are a specific diagnostic sign of psoriatic nail; it is a translucent, yellowish-red discoloration in the nail bed that appears like spots or drops of oil under the nail plate. The yellow color results from parakeratotic and acanthotic processes of nail bed, while the reddish tones occur due to presence of plaques on the nail bed. Crumbling and nail plate thickening are observed in psoriasis after a prolonged period of persisting disease activity leading to total nail matrix destruction [11]; also, leukonychia may occur (Fig. 34.4). Diagnosis is usually made by presence of cutaneous lesions of psoriasis elsewhere. Direct microscopic examination should be performed to exclude onychomycosis which may coexist. Matrix or nail bed biopsies show as a major criterion neutrophils, with parakeratosis, focal hypogranulosis, and psoriasiform hyperplasia of the nail bed as minor criteria [12].

Treatment of nail psoriasis requires consequent application of topical remedies, intralesional injections, and in severe cases systemic administration of drugs such as oral retinoids. Application of intralesional corticosteroids is a second step after unsuccessful topical formulations (Tables 34.2 and 34.3). Conventional systemic therapies are indicated in management-resistant nail psoriasis, with or without cutaneous and psoriatic arthritis [13]. Treatment of nail psoriasis is often a time-consuming challenge for the physician with variable outcome; relapses are common [14].

34.2.3 Pityriasis Rubra Pilaris

Nail changes are common in pityriasis rubra pilaris (PRP) involving roughly 80% of the patients [15]. They are associated with type I adult onset PRP, especially with affection of the palms and soles. The nails are thickened and discolored distally with splinter hemorrhages. Nail dystrophy is less common in juvenile type V PRP. Psoriasiform pitting can occur in circumscribed type IV PRP (Fig. 34.4). Wedge-shaped thickening has been reported in type VI disease associated with human immunodeficiency virus infection [15].

34.2.4 Lichen Planus

Lichen planus occurs in <1% of the population with a particularly high rate in India [16]. Nail involvement appears with cutaneous lichen planus in 3–15% in Caucasians with fair skin, reaching up to 18% in populations with dark skin, or even in absence of cutaneous lesions [17, 18]. The etiology of the disease is unknown; various potential triggers, such as viral or bacterial antigens, metal ions, drugs, or physical factors, could initiate the autoimmune process [16]. Lichen planus of the nail matrix can result in diverse morphological alterations of the nail plate. The commonest change is longitudinal fissuring and ridging of the nail plate (onychorrhexis) arising either alone or in combination with distal splitting and thinning; the area of the nail matrix may appear prominent (Fig. 34.5). Similar changes are seen in old age, Darier's disease, alopecia areata, and vitiligo. Pterygium, which is detected in 6% of the patients [18], occurs as a result of adhesion of cuticle and matrix leading first to a split nail and later to onychomadesis and possible complete loss of the nail plate [17] resembling *anonychia* (Fig. 34.6). Also trachyonychia may be present in lichen affecting several or all nails. The clinical diagnosis is confirmed by histopathological examination in biopsies taken from the nail matrix, especially if cases with isolated nail involvement.

Treatment of nail lichen is difficult and disappointing. Retinoids, especially acitretin, occasionally combined with PUVA can be administered (Table 34.4).

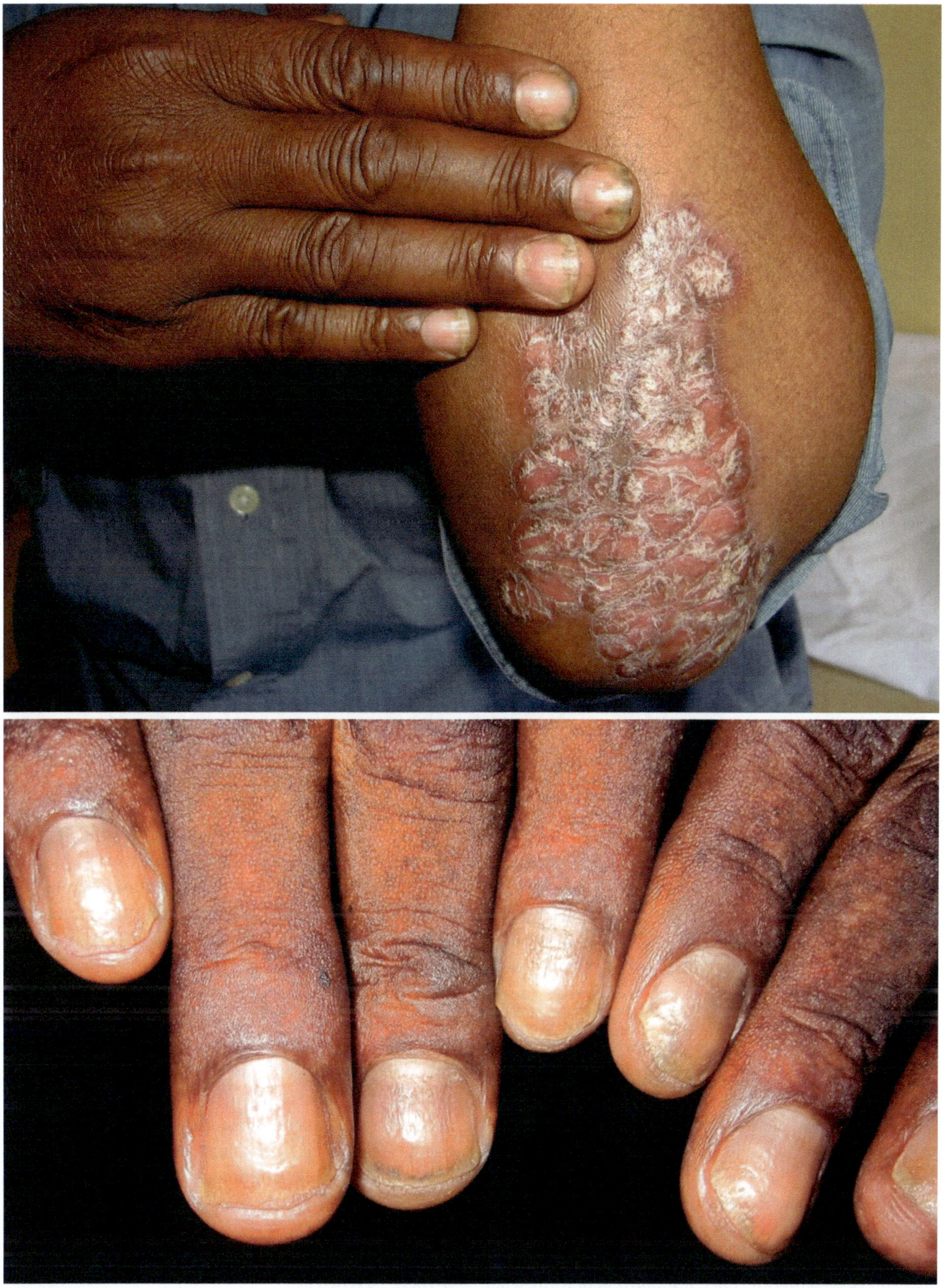

Fig. 34.2 Plaque-like psoriasis and *psoriatic nails* in African males showing thickening of the nail plate with irregular pitting (Uganda; courtesy CEO)

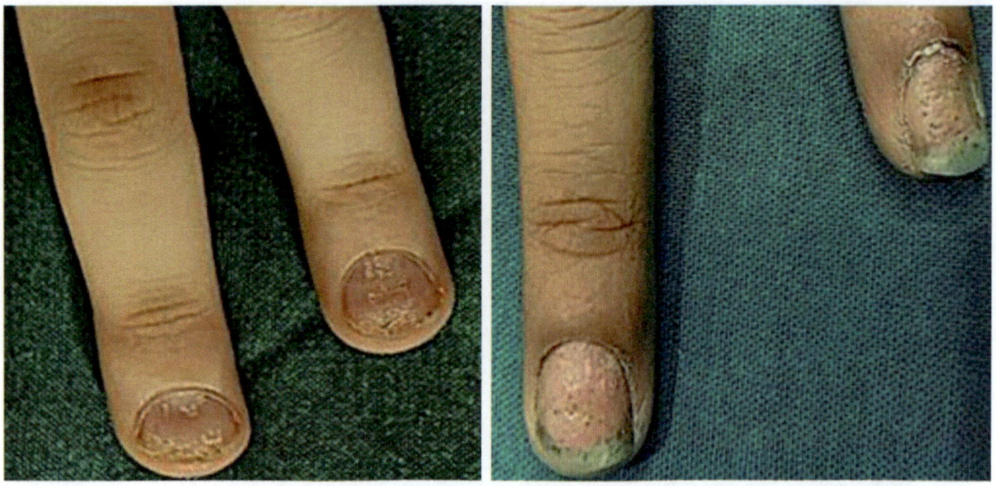

Fig. 34.3 *Nail psoriasis* in Egyptian young males showing pitting in the form of multiple irregular punctate depressions with random distribution

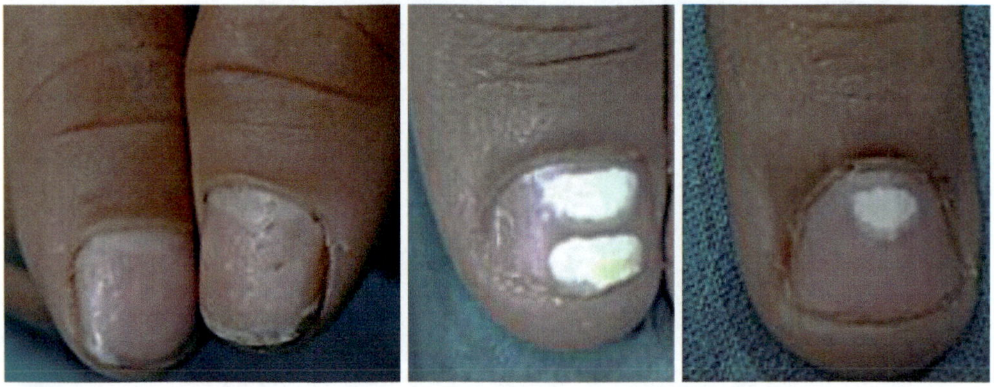

Fig. 34.4 Thickened nails and pitting of both thumbs in *pityriasis rubra pilaris* (left) and *secondary leukonychia* affecting nails of a patient with psoriasis (right)

34.2.5 Alopecia Areata

Involvement of the nail is regularly found in white Caucasians (7–66%) [15, 19] and is also common in dark skin populations with alopecia areata (44%) [20]. It seems that inflammatory cells targeting the hair follicles also interfere with keratinization in nails. Nail involvement in alopecia areata may either precede or follow the development of hairless patches on the scalp. Clinically, roughness and fine superficial pitting of the nail plate in a geometric pattern are seen, together with longitudinal ridging and sometimes red lunulae; trachyonychia and Beau's lines can also be seen in alopecia areata [19, 20], particularly in well-developed cases and long duration (Fig. 34.7). If the diagnosis of alopecia areata is not readily apparent, a biopsy of the nail matrix shows mild to moderate dense lymphocytic infiltrate associated with exocytosis and spongiosis.

For *treatment*, topical and intralesional administration of triamcinolone (2.5–3 mg/mL once a month) is helpful when spontaneous clearing of the nails does not occur. Nail changes may persist for a long period of time after complete hair regrowth [19].

34.2.6 Yellow Nail Syndrome

This rare clinical syndrome is a triad consisting of characteristic discoloration of the nails, lower limb lymphedema, and pulmonary manifestations such as bronchiectasia, chronic cough, and pulmonary effusion [21]. Chronic sinusitis is frequently associated and lymphatic impairment is often evoked. The syndrome has been also described in an Arab boy with facial dysmorphism and bilateral conjunctival pigmentation born to consanguineous parents [22] and also from India [23]. It is characterized by arrested nail growth, whereby fingernails and toenails are excessively hard and curved from side to side with diffuse pale yellow to dark yellow-green discoloration (Fig. 34.8). Absent cuticle and paronychia may be seen and secondary onycholysis is frequent. Treatment is symptomatic. Oral vitamin E alone or associated with triazole antifungals may achieve partial or total disappearance of nail discoloration [21].

34.2.7 Vitiligo

Vitiligo, an acquired pigmentary skin disorder, affects 0.1–4% of the population. Nail abnormalities are evident in up to

Table 34.2 Topical and intralesional treatment of nail psoriasis

Medication	Dosing	Prognosis	Potential adverse effects
Topical corticosteroids	Betamethasone dipropionate ointment 2×/day or clobetasol propionate 0.05% cream under occlusion for 12–20 weeks	– Equal efficacy on both nail matrix and bed signs	– Telangiectasias, cutaneous atrophy, tachyphylaxis, rebound flare, systemic absorption
Topical vitamin D3 derivatives	Calcipotriol ointment (50 g/m^2 per week) 2×/day for 20 weeks	– Signs of significant improvement of the nail bed – Combination of betamethasone dipropionate and calcipotriol ointment	– Local irritation, hypercalcuria, hypercalcemia
Tazarotene	Tazarotene 0.1% gel 1×/day for 12–24 weeks	– Significant improvement of onycholysis and pitting only – Improvement in hyperkeratosis and oil spots	– Local irritation, erythema, nail fold desquamation
Topical calcineurin inhibitors	Tacrolimus 0.1% ointment 1×/day at nail folds	– Equally effective on nail bed and nail matrix signs	
Anthralin	Dithranol in petrolatum 0.4–2% ointment to the affected nail bed and then washing after 30 min for 20 weeks	– Improvement of nail bed signs and, to a lesser extent, pitting	– Local irritation, staining of the nail plate, skin, and cloths
1% fluorouracil solution	2×/day for 24 weeks	– No or poor response	– Localized inflammation, infection, discoloration
Topical cyclosporine	70 mg/mL maize-oil-dissolved oral cyclosporine solution for 12 weeks	– Improvement of both nail bed and matrix – Not as effective as its systemic form due to its inability to penetrate the stratum corneum and instability in topical emulsion	– Yellowish discoloration
Intralesional injection of triamcinolone acetonide	– Injections of triamcinolone acetonide 5 mg/mL/month for 6 months in proximal nail fold and then 4 injections over the next 6 months and every 2 months for final 6–12 months – Injection of 10 mg/mL (0.1 mL in each of 4 periungual sites) every 2 months, for symmetrical delivery to nail matrix and nail bed	– Efficacy on nail bed psoriasis	– Short-term paresthesia, focal pain, hematoma, reversible nail fold atrophy

78% in fair skin populations and in 68% of patients with dark skin [24, 25]. The most common nail changes in vitiligo include longitudinal ridging and absent lunula. Other reported nail abnormalities are punctate leukonychia, pitting, flag sign, and Terry's nails [24, 25].

34.3 Nonspecific Nail Changes

Koilonychia or spooning of nails occurs when the free edge of the nail is averted with transverse and longitudinal concavity. It can be associated with some genetic diseases such as patella-nail syndrome and trichothiodystrophy, as well as iron-deficiency anemia, B12 deficiency, and endocrine conditions [26], or as a result from constant exposure to petrolatum-based solvents (Fig. 34.7c). Koilonychia may also be idiopathic in healthy toenails representing a normal variant in infancy.

Trachyonychia shows dull, rough, and fragile nail plate, with loss of luster and transparency (opaque, muddy, grayish-white discoloration) presenting the appearance of sandpaper nails. The term *twenty-nail dystrophy* is specifically used to describe trachyonychia involving all 20 nails. Trachyonychia can also be seen in lichen planus, alopecia areata, vitiligo, and Darier's disease. In psoriasis it exhibits a more thickened nail plate as opposed to the thinning noted in lichen planus [27].

Leukonychia is an abnormal, immature keratinization of the nail matrix resulting in white discoloration of the nail plate. It may occur as *primary*, true *leukonychia* due to

Table 34.3 Photochemotherapy, laser, and systemic drug treatment of nail psoriasis

Treatment	Dosing	Prognosis	Potential adverse effects	Laboratory Monitoring
PUVA	– Oral PUVA management, 2–3×/week, 8-methoxypsoralen (0.6 mg/kg) – Topical PUVA, 2–3×/week, using 1% solution 8-methoxypsoralen to proximal nail fold	– Effective in both nail bed and matrix signs	– No incidence of adverse effects	
Pulsed dye laser	– 1×/month session for 3 months	– Improvement in nail bed signs	– Temporary pain, resolving purpura	
Methotrexate	– 15 mg/week, in 2 divided doses for 24 weeks	– 43% improvement in nail matrix findings	– Hepatotoxicity, leucopenia, aplastic anemia ulcerative stomatitis, gastrointestinal disturbances	– Liver and renal function tests Complete blood count – Pregnancy test
Cyclosporine	– 3–5 mg/kg/day – Combination of calcipotriol (occlusive application at night) + oral cyclosporin (3–4.5 mg/kg/day) for 3 months	– More powerful and faster than other conventional systemic therapies – More efficacy in nail bed than nail matrix signs	– Renal dysfunction, hypertension, headache, paresthesia, hypertrichosis, gingival hyperplasia, gastrointestinal disorders, malignancies	– Blood pressure – Serum creatinine
Acitretin	0.2–0.3 mg/kg/day for 6–12 months	– Moderate efficacy (40–50%) particularly on nail bed signs	– Teratogenicity, hepatitis, hyperlipidemia, mucocutaneous dryness, progressive nail atrophy. So, it is used in thickened nails	– Liver function tests – Blood lipids – Pregnancy test
TNF-α inhibitors				
Infliximab	– i.v. infusions of 5 mg/kg infliximab at weeks 0, 2, and 6 and every 8 weeks	– 78–80% improvement at week 50	– Anaphylactic reactions (up to 1 h after intake), type IV delayed hypersensitivity reaction (3–12 days after intake). Rarely, demyelinating diseases, congestive heart failure, lymphoma, lupus-like syndrome	– Screening for tuberculosis – No vaccinations
Adalimumab	– s.c. injections of 80 mg, then 40 mg every other week	– Significant improvement at week 12 and complete resolution of nail signs at week 24	As infliximab	As infliximab
Etanercept	– s.c. injections 2 × 50 mg/week for 3 months and then 50 mg/week for 3 months	– 51% improvement after 54 weeks	As infliximab	As infliximab
Anti-IL monoclonal antibodies				
Ustekinumab	– s.c. injection 45 mg (or 90 mg if body weight >100 kg)	– 20% improvement of pitting, 30% of onycholysis	As infliximab	As infliximab
Secukinumab	– s.c. injection 150 mg at weeks 0, 1, 2, 4	– 19% improvement overall	As infliximab	As infliximab

involvement of the nail matrix in congenital defects, or as *secondary*, punctate, transverse, or striate leukonychia, being a result of trauma, onychomycosis, diabetes, systemic infections (measles, typhus, scarlet fever, diphtheria, and syphilis), and arsenic or lead poisoning. Diffuse type of leukonychia may be associated with leprosy, hemochromatosis, hypocalcemia, and acanthosis nigricans (Fig. 34.9). Transverse leukonychia occurs as Mees' lines, whereas white longitudinal bands are seen in candidiasis, Darier's disease, and after the use of quinacrine [28].

Pincer nail is a transverse over curvature of the nail plate. It may be inherited or acquired as it is associated with psoriasis, onychomycosis, nail tumors, systemic lupus erythematous, Kawasaki disease, and use of beta-blocker [29].

Beau's lines are horizontal grooves on the nail plate, involving several or all nails. They reflect an interruption of

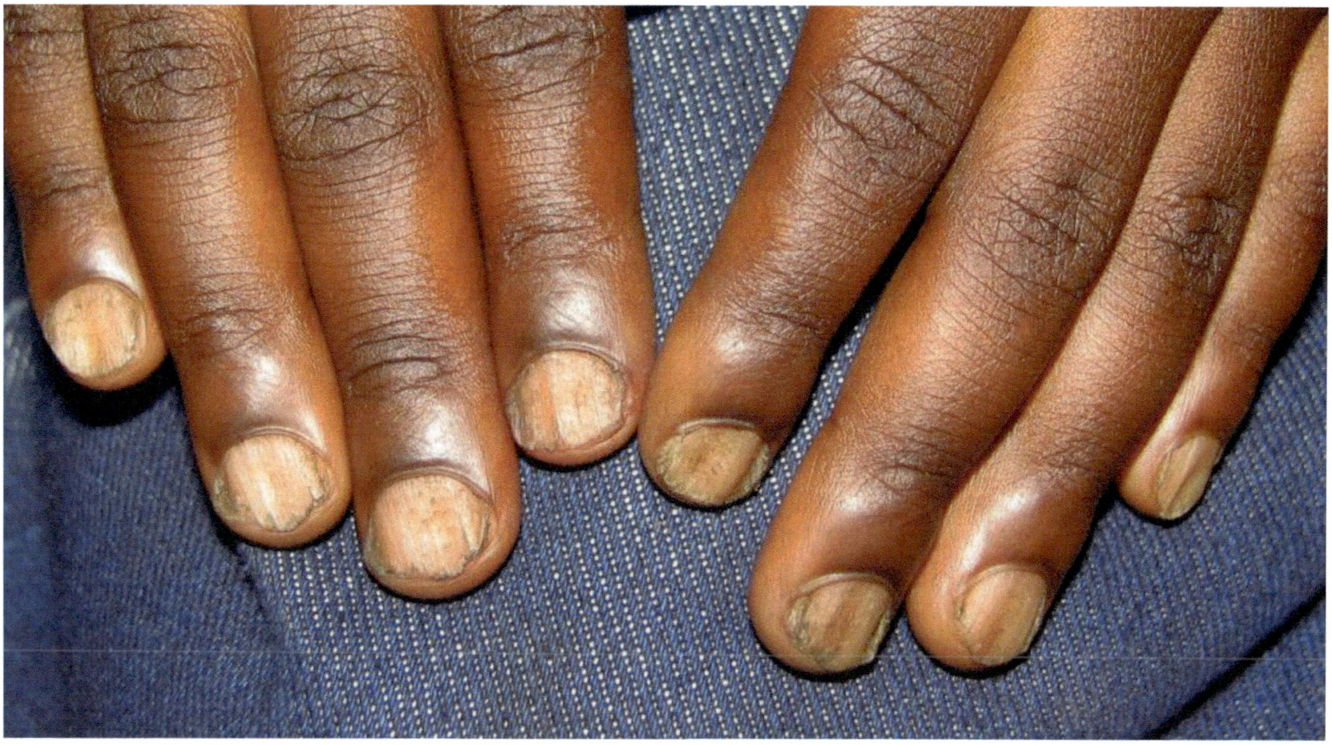

Fig. 34.5 *Lichen planus of the nails* in an African male showing linear fissuring, ridging, and irregular depressions resembling koilonychia. Note the swelling of the nail matrix (courtesy: CEO)

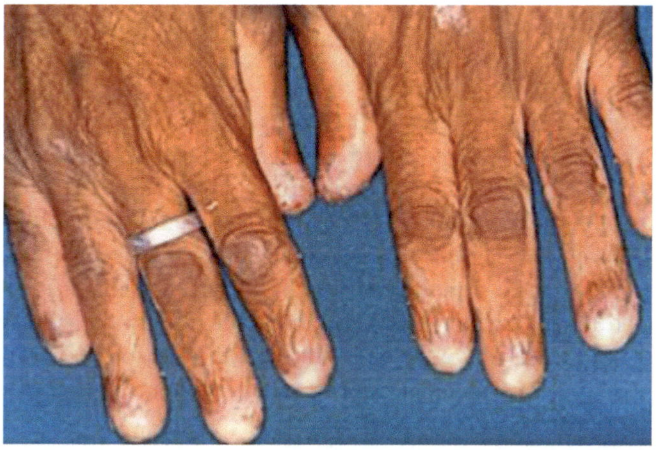

Fig. 34.6 *Anonychia* of all fingers resulting from scarring dystrophy in *acrodermatitis continua suppurativa Hallopeau*

nail bed mitosis. In dark skin populations, they are present particularly in poor nutritional status, severe illness, high fever, trauma, and sensitivity to drugs (Fig. 34.7b).

Digital clubbing is characterized by fibrovascular hyperplasia of the distal fingertip tissue presenting an increased longitudinal and horizontal curvature of the nail plate of both finger- and toenails. In clubbing, the angle of Lovibond (the angle between the nail plate and proximal nail fold when viewed from the side) is greater than 180°, whereas it is less than 160° in normal nails. Clubbing is seen occasionally in pulmonary or cardiovascular diseases, ulcerative colitis, and hepatic cirrhosis. It is assumed that digital clubbing may develop from increased blood flow within the microvasculature [30].

Onychocryptosis (ingrown nails) results when part of the nail plate pierces the lateral nail fold. Three major types are known: over-curvature of the nail plate (pincer nail), subcutaneous ingrowing toenail, and hypertrophy of the lateral nail fold. Clinically, onychocryptosis manifests as inflammation of the nail fold, often with granulation tissue formation causing considerable tenderness of the involved digit and pain [31].

Terry nails are characterized by a proximal white color that extends from proximal nail fold obscuring the lunula to narrow distal red/brown band (0.5–3 mm width). Some nails show white color only without reddish hue; pressing on the nail plate alters the color of the nail. Terry nails are represented in 30.6% of patients with chronic systemic diseases, especially with liver cirrhosis (80%), congestive heart failure (52%), diabetes mellitus (49%), and even aging. This condition may be caused by a decrease in vascularity and an increase of connective tissue in the nail bed (Fig. 34.10) [29, 32].

Half-and-half nails show proximal white half and distal red/brown half (20–60%) due to changes in nail bed color. It occurs as the most common sign of renal insufficiency, which shows also absent lunula and splinter hemorrhages

Table 34.4 Commonly prescribed medications for lichen planus

Medication	Dosing	Prognosis	Potential adverse effects
Topical steroids	– Daily application of high potent topical steroids	– Poor response to topical steroid	Telangiectasis, cutaneous atrophy, tachyphylaxis, rebound flare, systemic absorption
Topical calcineurin inhibitors	– Tacrolimus ointment, twice daily	– Improvement within 6 months	No side effects
Intralesional injection of triamcinolone acetonide	– Injections of 2.5–10/mL triamcinolone acetonide in proximal nail fold	– Complete cure after 2–6 months, but with recurrence	– Short-term paresthesia, transient focal pain, hematoma formation, reversible nail-fold atrophy, rupture of extensor tendon
Systemic corticosteroids	– Prednisolone (0.5–1 mg/kg daily orally) – Intramuscular injection of triamcinolone acetonide (0.5–1 mg/kg/month) was prescribed to children with typical nail lichen planus for 3–6 months until the proximal half of the nail was normal	– Complete cure after 2–6 months – Complete cure after 6–8 months (fingernails up to 8–12 months (toenails)	– No tolerance to the side effects of systemic corticosteroids. Recurrence was common
Methotrexate	– 10–20 mg/week, subcutaneously	Significant improvement of nail fold erythema, edema, and trachyonychia a few weeks after initiation of the treatment	
Biological therapies	– Subcutaneous injection of etanercept, 25 mg twice weekly for the first 6 months and 50 mg once weekly thereafter	– Marked improvement within 6–9 months	No side effects

[33] (Fig. 34.11). Roughly 60% of persons with chronic renal disease have nail manifestations [15].

Mees' lines are transverse white lines that may extend the complete width of the nail plate of single or multiple digits. Since the abnormality is in the nail plate and not the nail bed, Mees' lines migrate toward the distal end of the nail plate over time; they often indicate arsenic poisoning or renal failure [26].

Muehrcke lines are pairs of transverse white lines caused by edema within the nail bed, occasionally associated with hypoalbuminemia. They do not migrate distally as the nail grows since they originate in the nail bed and not the nail plate and disappear when pressure is applied to the nail plate [26].

Dilated periungual capillaries may be seen in the proximal nail folds in patients with rheumatoid arthritis, systemic lupus erythematosus, dermatomyositis, or scleroderma; examination with a magnifying glass may show irregular, twisted, and dilated vessels. These attributes give the area an injected, erythematous appearance when viewed with the naked eye. In addition, scleroderma shows pterygium inversum unguis especially with fingertip ulcerations and scarring. Nail affection ranges from 20% in systemic lupus erythematosus up to 80% in scleroderma [15].

Splinter hemorrhages appear as small linear structures, about 2–3 mm long, and are arranged at the distal end of the nail plate. They reflect rupture of wide caliber vessels and tracking of extravasated blood down the longitudinal furrows beneath the nail plate. The most common cause of splinter hemorrhage is trauma, followed by psoriasis, and then endocarditis if they are located in the proximal part on the nail plate, embolic events, and after certain medications. They may also occur in healthy individuals with increased capillary fragility and nail trauma.

Red lunula is nonspecific finding as it is present in alopecia areata, rheumatoid arthritis, congestive heart failure, pulmonary disorders, and carbon monoxide poisoning [26].

Subungual hematomas are painful red to black discolorations mostly caused by traumatic bleeding in the underlying vascular tissue of the nail bed. The faint reddish coloration of hemorrhage may not be easily identified in populations with dark skin and be misdiagnosed. If no nail bed laceration is suspected, treatment consists of drilling a hole through the nail with an electrocautery device or treatment with CO_2 laser to relieve the pressure.

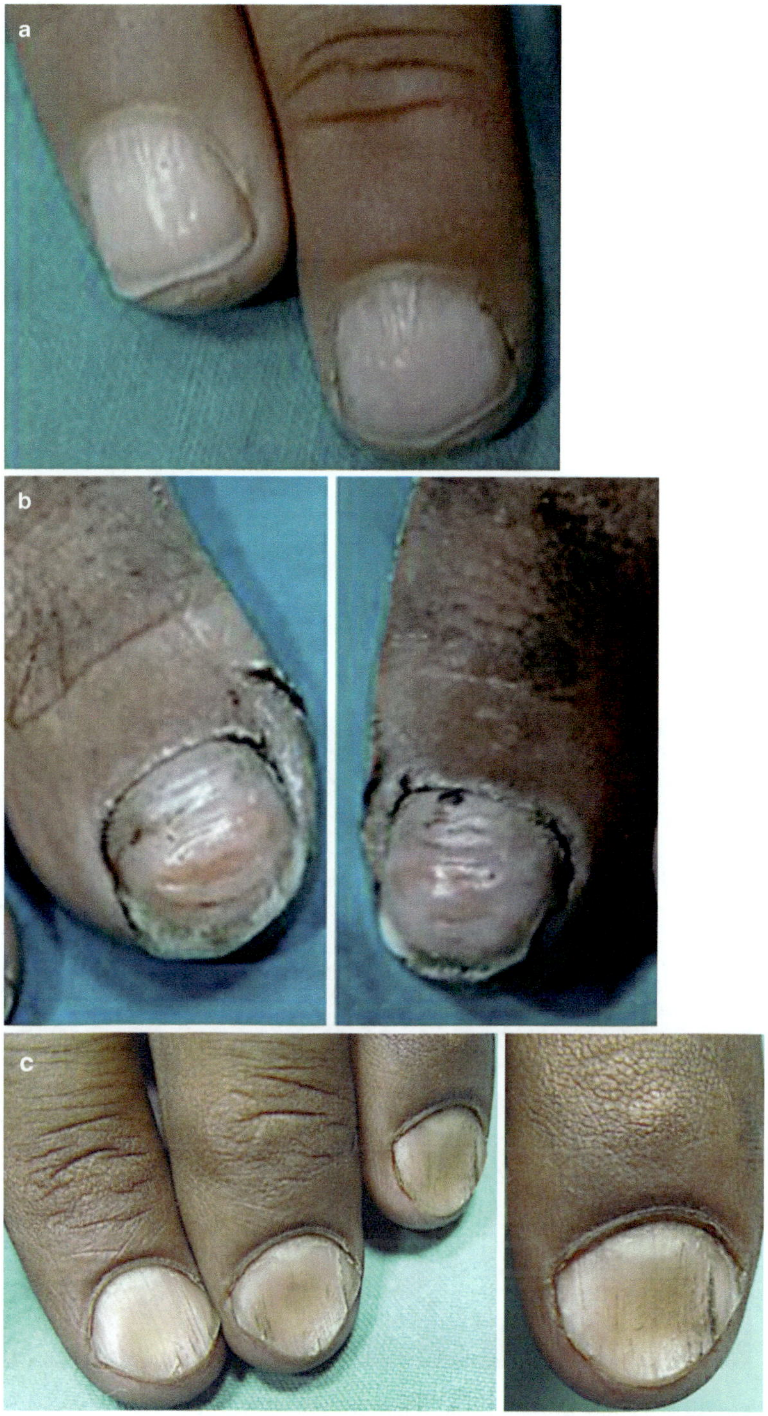

Fig. 34.7 (**a**) Superficial pitting and longitudinal ridging in *alopecia areata*. (**b**) Loss of cuticle and roughened nails with Beau's lines in *chronic eczema* of an aged patient. (**c**) *Koilonychia* showing the averted free edges of the nails with longitudinal and transverse concavities

Onycholysis is detachment of the nail plate from the nail bed along the distal margin of the nail plate that becomes white, often encircled by an erythematous border. Some possible causes of onycholysis are onychomycosis, psoriasis, hyperthyroidism, drug intake, or trauma. In so-called idiopathic cases of onycholysis, anemia and asymptomatic thyroid disease should be excluded.

34.4 Nail Disorders in Aging

In geriatric populations nail changes are due to impaired circulation and susceptibility of the senile nail apparatus to fungal infections, faulty biomechanics, neoplasms, concurrent cutaneous or systemic diseases, and related treatments. In populations with dark skin, nail changes range from 88% in

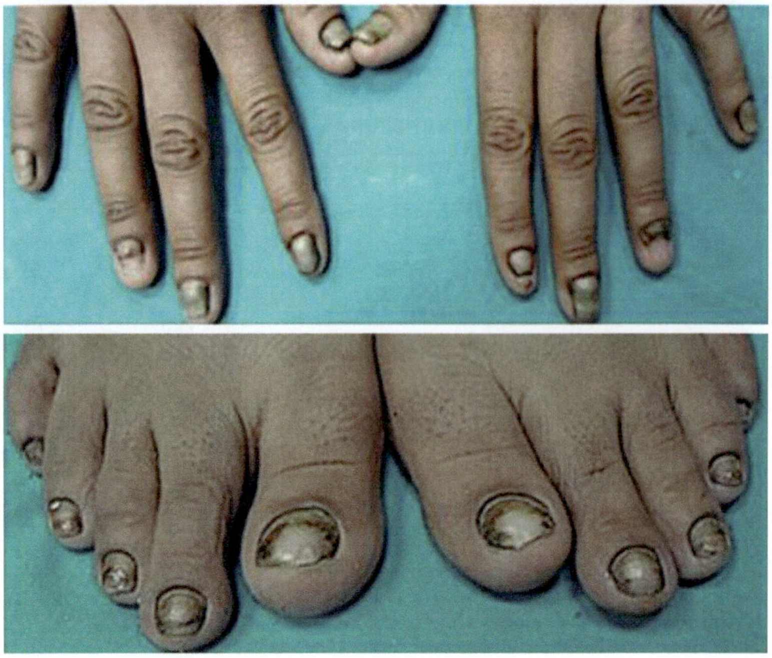

Fig. 34.8 *Yellow nail syndrome* with excessively hard curved fingernails and toenails showing pale to dark-yellow discoloration. Secondary onycholysis is seen in both ring fingers

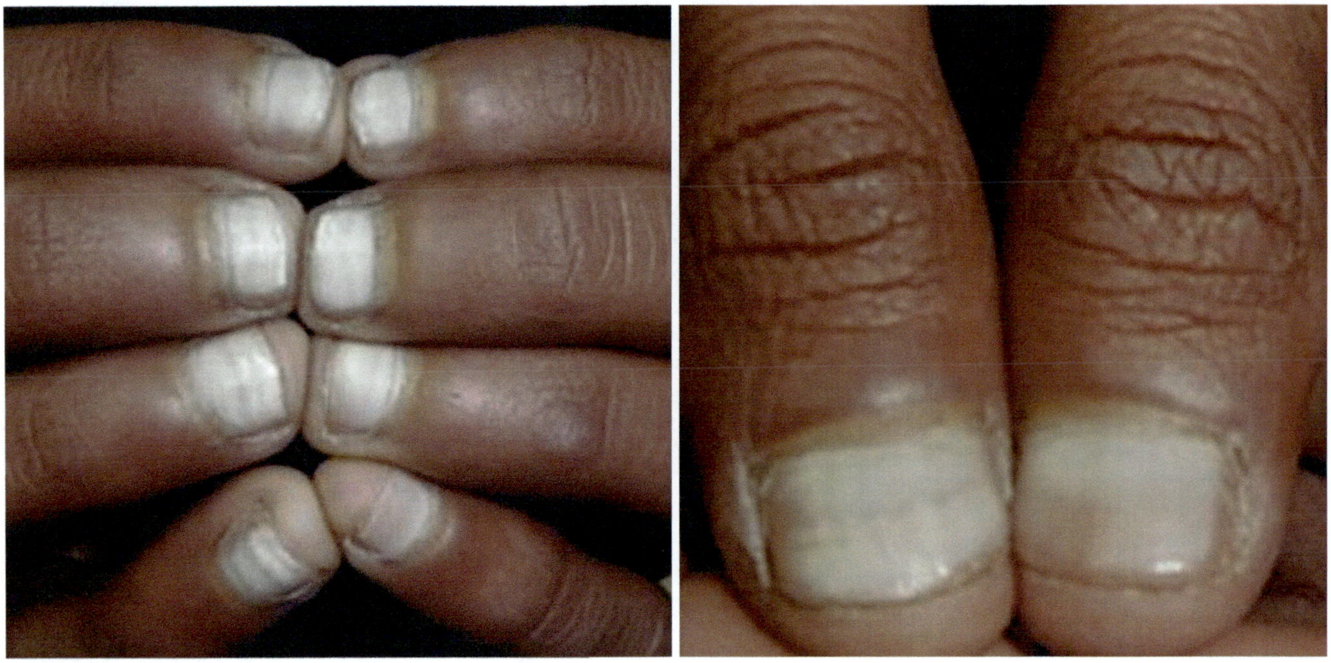

Fig. 34.9 Diffuse *leukonychia* in all fingers

Egypt [34] to 98% in India [35]. The commonest age-related nail changes seen were pale, dull, opaque, brittle, and lusterless nails, with decreased lunula visibility and onychorrhexis. The fingernails were more affected than the toenails [32]. It has been reported from India that among the age-related changes of the nail surface, prominent longitudinal ridges were the commonest (85%), followed by rough nails in 33% of the patients, transverse ridges in 23%, and lamellar split in 15% of cases [31]. Rough nails, transverse ridges (Beau's lines), and lamellar split were also reported in other aging populations [31]. Bony deformities of the digits, infrequent nail cutting, or ill-fitting shoes can cause faulty biomechanics leading to onychodystrophies such as *onychogryphosis*, *onychophosis*, *onychocryptosis*, *onycholysis*, and

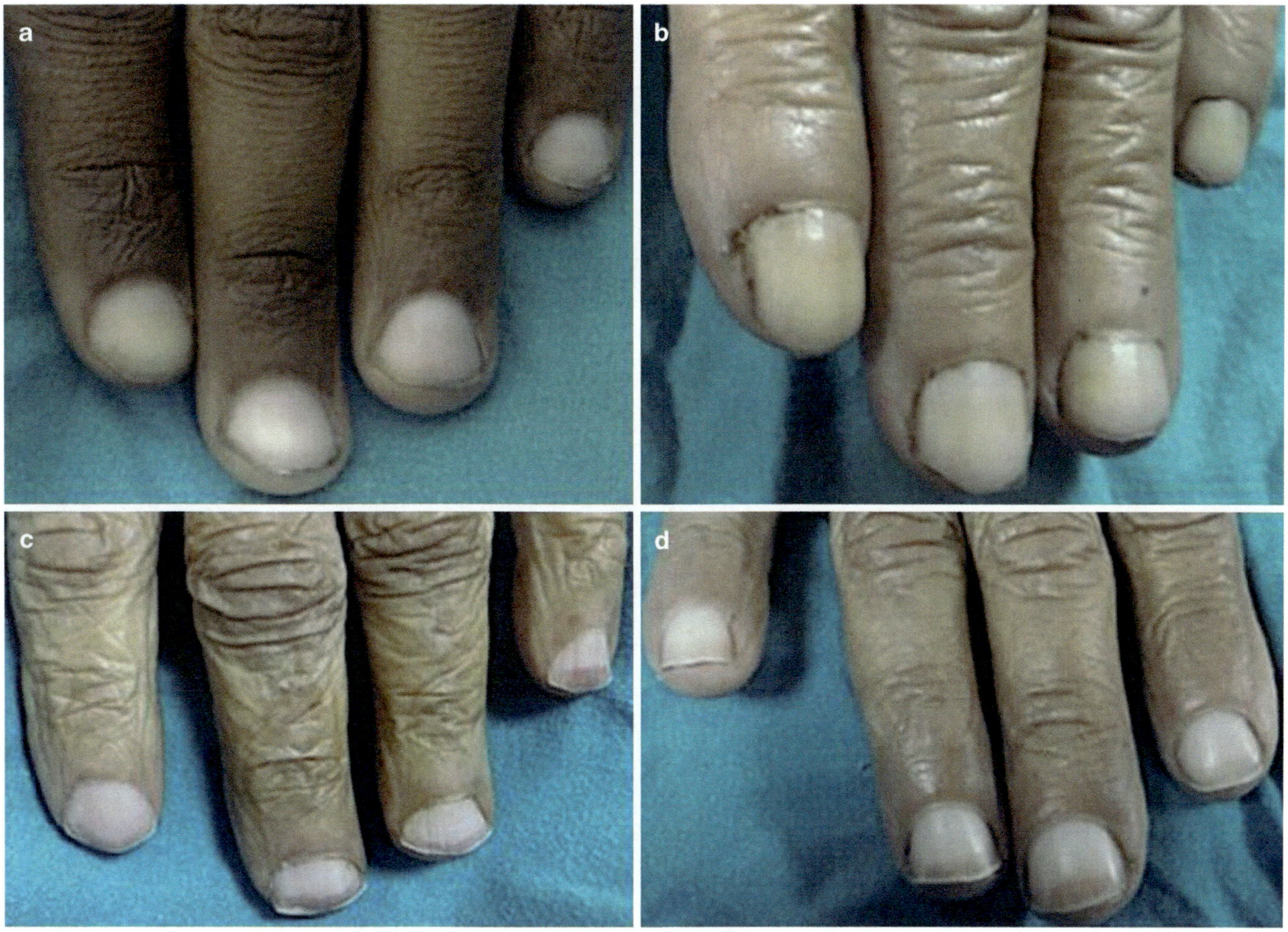

Fig. 34.10 *Terry nails.* White nail beds all over the whole nails (**a**, **b**) and proximal white nails with narrow distal red/brown band in liver cell failure (**c**, **d**)

Fig. 34.11 Half and half nail in a patient with renal failure

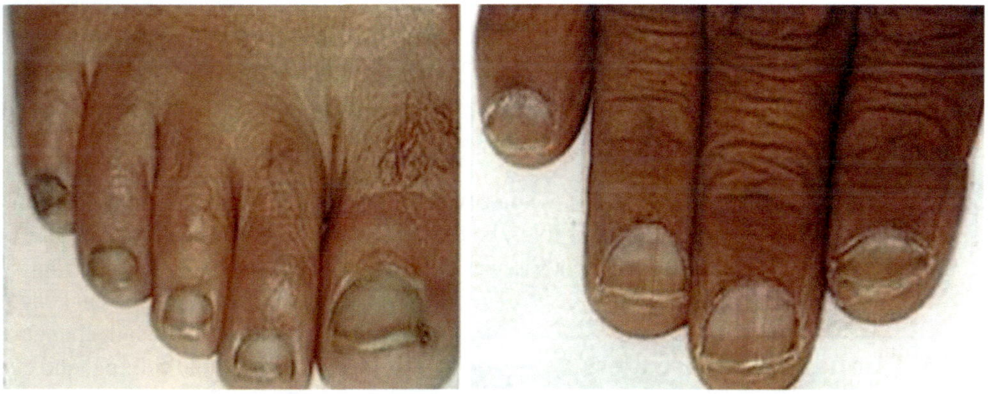

subungual hematomas. Onychogryphosis mostly involves the great toenail with enlargement, opacity, and thickening of the nail plate as well as hypertrophy of the underlying nail bed resulting in "ram hornlike" or "oyster-like." appearance. The nail plate initially grows upward and thereafter deviates laterally toward the other toes.

Treatment of nail disorders in the elderly includes conservative management by periodic trimming of the nail plate and use of appropriate footwear. Onychophosis can be treated by debridement of hyperkeratotic tissue by means of keratolytics (urea 20%, lactic acid 12%, or salicylic acid 6–20%), followed by application of emollients. In severe and intractable cases, sur-

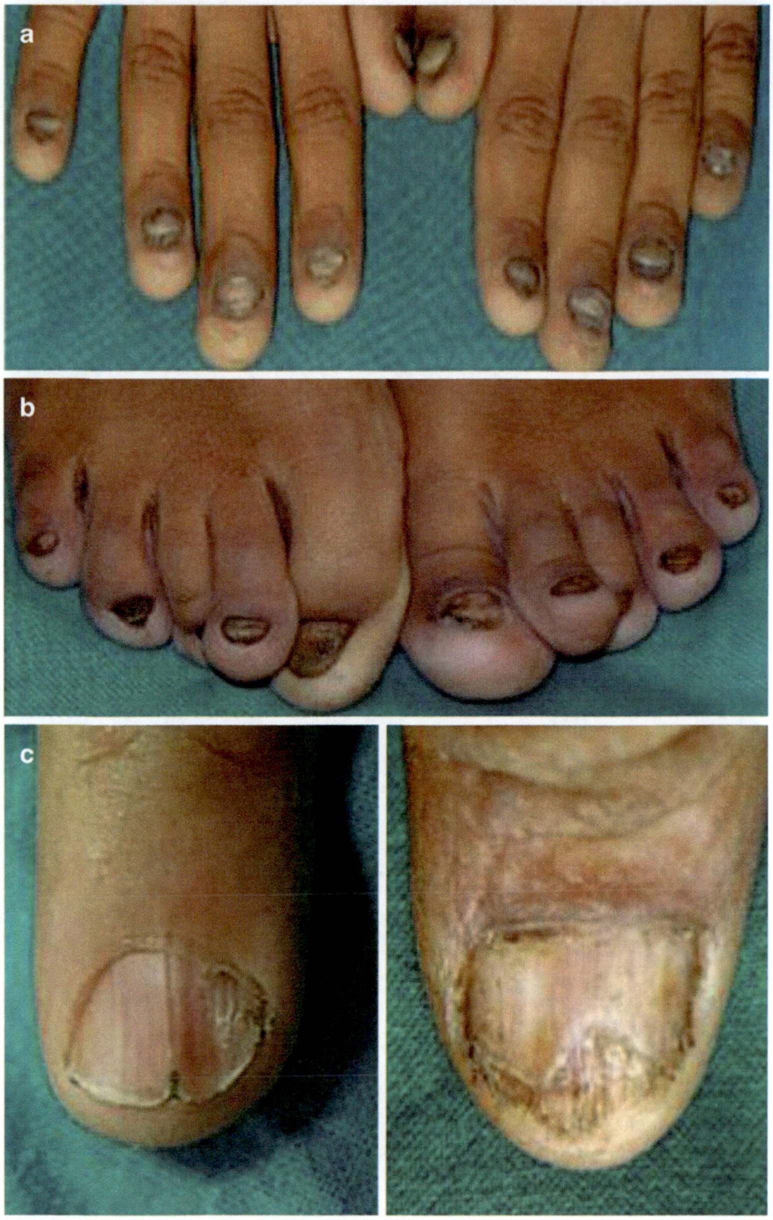

Fig. 34.12 Ridging and V-shaped notching of the free edges of some nail plates in *ectodermal dysplasia* (**a**, **b**) and small, ridged, discolored, and dystrophic nails in *Darier's disease* (**c**)

gical or chemical nail avulsion (phenol), with or without excision of the involved adjacent tissue (nail folds, bed, or matrix), can be employed in persons with sufficient vascular supply [31].

34.5 Genetic Nail Disorders

These include anonychia (absence of nails), koilonychia (concave curvature of the nail), *micronychia* (small nails), *polynychia* (more than one nail on a digit), and *brachyonychia* (racket nails) [36]. Some changes of the nails are clinical markers of an underlying multiorgan genodermatosis.

In *pachyonychia congenita*, massive thickening of the nail bed and brown discoloration of the nail plate with upward angulation of the distal free edge of the thickened nail plate occur. *Ectodermal dysplasias* present with nail disorders as anonychia or brittle, thin, ridged, and discolored nails. Nail dystrophy is an important component of the hidrotic type, in which nails are thickened, striated, and discolored [36] (Fig. 34.12). Nail changes such as pitting, transverse and longitudinal ridging, and even dystrophy manifest in *incontinentia pigmenti* [37].

Nail aplasia or dysplasias, particularly with presence of triangular lunulae, are characteristic for the *nail patella syndrome*, an autosomal dominant disorder caused by mutations in the LMX1B gene; the condition includes aplastic or hypoplastic patella and nephropathy, and onycholysis may occur with destruction of the underlying terminal phalanges [38, 39].

In another autosomal dominant entity, *epidermolysis bullosa simplex*, the nails may be normal early in life, but repeated traumas usually lead to scarring and dystrophy. In dystrophic type, there is scarring with mitten-like deformity of the digits due to loss of matrix. In junctional and acquired epidermolysis bullosa, the nails are thickened and dystrophic [40]. *Darier's disease* may show nail affection in 92% of patients. It presents with nail matrix (splitting, fragility, and red and white longitudinal streaks; Fig. 34.12) and distal nail bed signs such as subungual hyperkeratosis with overlying V-shaped notches at the free edge [41]. Also, twenty-nail dystrophy may occur [27].

34.6 Tumors of the Nail Apparatus

Nail-specific tumors may arise from all tissues of the nail apparatus; most of them are slowly growing neoplasms of low malignancy, also reported in patients with pigmented ethnic skin. Onychomatricoma, onychocytic matricoma, onychocytic carcinoma, and onychopapilloma all originate from the nail matrix, whereas onycholemmal cysts and proliferating onycholemmal tumors originate from the nail bed [42]. In particular, *onychomatricoma* has been recently described [43], often on the great toenail, while giant nail dystrophy may mask the tumor and be an obstacle for its surgical removal. Slowly growing onycholemmal carcinomas also occur.

Glomus tumor is a benign nail bed lesion, presenting with intense pinpoint throbbing pain, which is exacerbated by pressure or cold temperature. It is usually visible through the thin nail plate as a red or blue macule, although, when involving the matrix, it may not be visible. The treatment of choice is surgical excision [44]. *Digital fibrokeratoma* is another solitary lesion of few millimeters on the proximal nail fold, causing longitudinal grooves in the nail plate. Subungual and periungual fibromas, major diagnostic criteria for tuberous sclerosis complex, are multiple with variable sizes causing nail plate depressions. *Myxoid pseudocyst of digits* (digital mucous cyst) is the commonest benign tumor originating in the proximal nail fold compressing the matrix and causing depressed longitudinal grooves in the nail plate. Pseudocysts are formed by focal accumulations of mucin in the dermis without a defined cyst wall. They can be treated with intralesional injections of triamcinolone or surgical removal [44]. *Subungual exostosis* is not a true tumor but an outgrowth of the bone that occurs under the nail plate elevating it, resulting in inverted "U"-shaped nail plate with accentuation of dorsal interphalangeal joint skin crease and onychocryptosis. It may lead to pincer nail deformity. Subungual exostoses are more frequent on the toes after trauma. Treatment is by aseptic removal of the excess bone after radiographic confirmation.

Bowen's disease in the periungual area presents with periungual erythema, hyperkeratosis, fissures, and scaling with subungual involvement leading to onycholysis [45]. It can develop to invasive squamous cell carcinoma indicated by the occurrence of nodules, hemorrhage, and ulceration. It is more common on fingers (thumb and index) than toes with multiple finger involvement in immunocompromised carriers. Treatment is Mohs surgery or amputation of the digit for more deeply invasive lesions involving periosteum [46].

Acral lentiginous melanoma is a rare subtype of malignant melanoma but still the most common melanoma subtype in populations with pigmented skin (see Chap. 36). It arises usually with *longitudinal melanonychia* appearing as pigmented band of the nail plate, extending from the nail matrix to its periungual free edge [47]; dermoscopic examination may provide useful information to the dermatologist and facilitate the recognition of an underlying subungual melanoma [48]. In contrast to fair skin patients, melanonychia may also be presented in healthy persons with dark skin spontaneously or after drug intake (e.g., zidovudine, hydroxychloroquine), trauma of the nail matrix, or in presence of junctional melanocytic nevi [49].

References

1. Astur Mde M, Farkas CB, Junqueira JP, et al. Reassessing melanonychia striata in phototypes IV, V, and VI patients. Dermatol Surg. 2016;42:183–90.
2. Rockwell PG. Acute and chronic paronychia. Am Fam Physician. 2001;63:1113–6.
3. Rich P, Scher RK. An atlas of the diseases of the nail. London, UK: Parthenon Publishing Group; 2005. p. 61–77.
4. Sigurgeirsson B, Baran R. The prevalence of onychomycosis in the global population—a literature study. J Eur Acad Dermatol Venereol. 2014;28:1480–91.
5. Kaur R, Kashyap B, Bhalla P. Onychomycosis-epidemiology, diagnosis and management. Indian J Med Microbiol. 2008;26:108–16.
6. Abd Elmegeed AM, Ouf SA, Moussa TAA, et al. Dermatophytes and other associated fungi in patients attending to some hospitals in Egypt. Braz J Microbiol. 2015;46:799–805.
7. Yadav P, Singal A, Pandhi D, et al. Clinico-mycological study of dermatophyte toenail onychomycosis in New Delhi, India. Indian J Dermatol. 2015;60:153–8.
8. Singal A, Khanna D. Onychomycosis: diagnosis and management. Indian J Dermatol Venereol Leprol. 2011;77:659–72.
9. Westerberg DP, Voyack MJ. Onychomycosis: current trends in diagnosis and treatment. Am Fam Physician. 2013;88:762–70.
10. Kumar S, Shilpa K. Nail changes in other dermatological conditions. In: Sacchdanad S, Savitha AS, editors. Nail and its disorders. New Delhi: Jaypee; 2013. p. 105–17.
11. Tan ES, Chong WS, Tey HL. Nail psoriasis: a review. Am J Clin Dermatol. 2012;13:375–88.
12. Grover C, Reddy BS, Uma Chaturvedi K. Diagnosis of nail psoriasis: importance of biopsy and histopathology. Br J Dermatol. 2005;153:1153–8.
13. Pasch MC. Nail psoriasis: a review of treatment options. Drugs. 2016;76:675–705.
14. Sánchez-Regaña M, Sola-Ortigosa J, Alsina-Gibert M, et al. Nail psoriasis: a retrospective study on the effectiveness of systemic treatments (classical and biological therapy). J Eur Acad Dermatol Venereol. 2011;25:579–86.

15. Wollina U, Nenoff P, Haroske G, et al. The diagnosis and treatment of nail disorders. Dtsch Arztebl Int. 2016;113:509–18.
16. Lehman JS, Tollefson MM, Gibson LE. Lichen planus. Int J Dermatol. 2009;48:682–94.
17. Tosti A, Peluso AM, Fanti PA, et al. Nail lichen planus: clinical and pathologic study of twenty-four patients. J Am Acad Dermatol. 1993;28:724–30.
18. Anbar TS, Barakat M, Ghannam SF. A clinical and epidemiological study of lichen planus among Egyptians of AL-Minya province. Dermatol Online J. 2005;11:4.
19. Tosti A, Fanti PA, Morelli R, et al. Trachyonychia associated with alopecia areata: a clinical and pathologic study. J Am Acad Dermatol. 1991;25:266–70.
20. Gandhi V, Baruah MC, Bhattacharaya SN. Nail changes in alopecia areata: incidence and pattern. Indian J Dermatol. 2003;69:114–5.
21. Vignes S, Baran R. Yellow nail syndrome: a review. Orphanet J Rare Dis. 2017;12:42.
22. Nanda A, Al-Essa FH, El-Shafei WM, et al. Congenital yellow nail syndrome: a case report and its relationship to nonimmune fetal hydrops. Pediatr Dermatol. 2010;27:533–4.
23. Shetty S, Bhaskaranand N. Yellow nail syndrome. Indian Pediatr. 2016;53:1133.
24. Topal IO, Gungor S, Kocaturk OE, et al. Nail abnormalities with vitiligo. An Bras Dermatol. 2016;91:442–5.
25. Anbar TS, Abdel Hay R, Abdel-Rahman AT, et al. Clinical study of nail changes in vitiligo. J Cosmet Dermatol. 2013;12:67–72.
26. Fawcett RS, Linford S, Stulberg DL. Nail abnormalities: clues to systemic disease. Am Fam Physician. 2004;69:1417–24.
27. Sehgal VN. Twenty nail dystrophy trachyonychia: an overview. J Dermatol. 2007;34:361–36.
28. Holzberg M. Nail signs of systemic disease. In: Hordinsky MK, Sawaya ME, Scher RK, editors. Atlas of hair and nails. Philadelphia: Churchill Livingstone; 2000. p. 59–70.
29. Tully AS, Trayes KP, Studdiford JS. Evaluation of nail abnormalities. Am Fam Physician. 2012;85:779–87.
30. Gregoriou S, Argyriou G, Larios G, et al. Nail disorders and systemic disease: what the nails tell us. J Fam Pract. 2008;57:509–14.
31. Cohen PR, Scher RK. Ageing. In: Hordinsky MK, Sawaya ME, Scher RK, editors. Atlas of hair and nails. Philadelphia: Churchill Livingstone; 2000. p. 213–25.
32. Park KY, Kim SW, Cho JS. Research on the frequency of Terry's nail in the medical inpatients with chronic illnesses. Korean J Dermatol. 1992;30:864–70.
33. Dyachenko P, Monelise A, Shustak A, et al. Nail disorders in patients with chronic renal failure and undergoing haemodialysis treatment: a case control study. J Eur Acad Dermatol Venereol. 2007;23:340–4.
34. El-Domyati M, Abdel-Wahab H, Abdel-Azim E. Nail changes and disorders in elderly Egyptians. J Cosmet Dermatol. 2014;13:269–76.
35. Rao S, Banerjee S, Ghosh SK, et al. Nail changes and nail disorders in the elderly. Indian J Dermatol. 2011;56:603–6.
36. Irvine AD, Mellerio JE. Genetics and genodermatoses. In: Burns T, Breathnach S, Cox N, et al., editors. Rooks textbook of dermatology. 8th ed. Oxford: Wiley-Blackwell; 2010. p. 15.1–15.97.
37. Landy SJ, Donnai D. Incontinentia pigmenti (Bloch-Sulzberger syndrome). J Med Genet. 1993;30:53–39.
38. Bongers EM, Gubler MC, Knoers NV. Nail-patella syndrome. Overview on clinical and molecular findings. Pediatr Nephrol. 2002;17:703–12.
39. Figueroa-Silva O, Vicente A, Agudo A, et al. Nail-patella syndrome: report of 11 pediatric cases. J Eur Acad Dermatol Venereol. 2016;30:1614–7.
40. Tosti A, de Farias DC, Murrell DF. Nail involvement in epidermolysis bullosa. Dermatol Clin. 2010;28:153–7.
41. Burge SM, Wilkinson JD. Darier-White disease: a review of the clinical features of 163 patients. J Am Acad Dermatol. 1992; 27:40–50.
42. Haneke E. Important malignant and new nail tumors. J Dtsch Dermatol Ges. 2017;15:367–86.
43. Di Chiacchio N, Tavares GT, Tosti A, et al. Onychomatricoma: epidemiological and clinical findings in a large series of 30 cases. Br J Dermatol. 2015;173:1305–7.
44. Rich P, Scher RK. An atlas of diseases of the nail. London, UK: The Parthenon Publishing Group; 2005. p. 132–47.
45. Wollina U. Bowen's disease of the nail apparatus: a series of 8 patients and a literature review. Wien Med Wochenschr. 2015;165:401–5.
46. Kuschner SH, Lane CS. Squamous cell carcinoma of the perionychium. Bull Hosp Jt Dis. 1997;56:111–2.
47. Levit EK, Kagen MH, Scher RK, et al. The ABC rule for clinical detection of subungual melanoma. J Am Acad Dermatol. 2000;42:269–74.
48. Benati E, Ribero S, Longo C, et al. Clinical and dermoscopic clues to differentiate pigmented nail bands: an International Dermoscopy Society study. J Eur Acad Dermatol Venereol. 2017;31:732–6.
49. Zaias MN, Daniel CR. Nails in systemic disease. Dermatol Ther. 2002;15:99–106.

35 Disorders of the Scalp and Hair

Marwa Abdallah and Constantin E. Orfanos

Human hair my show different shapes: The hair shaft may be straight in Asians or curly in Negroid populations, in contrast to the straight and wavy hair of Caucasians. The short curly hair of black-skinned individuals grows slower and has a larger diameter than in whites. The hair shaft is rather irregular, often elliptically flattened; *trichonodosis* and *trichoptilosis* are often seen; and pair grouping occurs. The terminal follicles are large, partly curved, with a golf club-shaped bulb. Nevertheless, there are broad variations in number, size, and shape of the hair and the hair follicles between the different ethnics, tribes, and families. Some racial groups have clearly sparse beard and axillary hair; some others are more hypertrichotic.

Non-scarring hair loss such as *androgenetic alopecia* and *alopecia areata* are often seen in Caucasians. Their incidence in dark-skinned individuals is not clearly documented; *hypertrichosis* and *hirsutism* seem less frequent in black than in white skin. In contrast, disorders such as *scarring alopecias* are clearly more prevalent in Africans and more common in African-Americans, populations with short curly hair and increased susceptibility to damage [1, 2]. Scarring alopecias are often traumatically induced due to fancy hairstyles caused in women of color and curly hair by traction and the frequent use of chemical strengtheners, bleaching agents, hot combs, curlers, etc. Their misuse requires proper education [3]. Such techniques and cosmetic measures damage the hair shaft and traumatize the scalp skin and its hair follicles. Traction alopecia and exogenous *trichorrhexis nodosa* are more frequent in black children, and keloid scarring is more prevalent in individuals of African, Asian, and Hispanic descent [4].

35.1 Androgenetic Alopecia

Androgenetic alopecia (AGA) is the most common type of hair loss. It affects young males and females leading to decreased hair density over the crown in a patterned fashion. For the physician AGA appears a minor problem; nevertheless, for some of those affected, hair loss impacts their self-image and causes emotional distress and depression. The prevalence of AGA varies according to ethnicity, being highest in Caucasians and less in Asians and dark-skinned Africans. The incidence in all ethnic groups increases with age in both sexes, reaching up to 80% in Caucasian males and 46.6–60% in Asian males over 70 years of age, respectively [5–7]. The incidence in females is lower, being 29–42% over 70 years of age in the UK and USA [8, 9]. The prevalence in South Africans was reported to be 14.6% in males and 3.5% in females in a study group with median age of 36.1 years [10].

35.1.1 Pathogenesis

The cause of AGA is a polygenic genetic predisposition as a major requirement for the development of the characteristic clinical phenotype, obviously less common in dark-skinned populations. Polymorphisms of the androgen receptor gene (AR) were studied in white Caucasians as a potential risk factor. A locus on the X-chromosome has been described, and the importance of the X-chromosomal location of AR and the maternal line in the inheritance of AGA has been stressed (20p11, 3q26; [11, 12]). However, the results of genetic studies remained controversial. In a meta-analysis,

M. Abdallah
Department of Dermatology and Venereology,
Ain Shams University, Cairo, Egypt

C. E. Orfanos (✉)
The Free University of Berlin, Medical School Charité,
Berlin, Germany
e-mail: corfanos@t-online.de

C. E. Orfanos et al. (eds.), *Pigmented Ethnic Skin and Imported Dermatoses*, https://doi.org/10.1007/978-3-319-69422-1_35

no obvious association of triplet repeat polymorphisms of the AR gene with risk for AGA was found [13]. Today 12 genetic risk loci are known, but it is unclear which genes at these loci are relevant for AGA [14]. Genetic inheritance for the female pattern in women is even more complex [15]. A similar clinical phenotype is the androgen-dependent hair loss in females, preferably called *androgenic alopecia*, caused by excess of circulating androgens or increased peripheral metabolization of testosterone into dihydrotestosterone (DHT) via the 5α-reductase present in hair follicles. Clinical signs of peripheral hyperandrogenism and laboratory investigations should be helpful to the physician for differential diagnosis.

35.1.2 Clinical Features

Androgenetic hair loss starts in males usually with bitemporal recession and/or thinning of the hair density over the vertex and progresses up to complete baldness of crown and vertex in some (*male pattern* baldness; Fig. 35.1). Miniaturization of the hair and its follicle is the hallmark of AGA. As a rule, the condition is asymptomatic; a few patients may complain of itching and trichodynia accompanying or preceding the loss of hair. The end stage varies and may be typical for each family affected. In females the frontal hairline is preserved, and the thinning of hair density occurs usually over the crown, being more diffuse, also involving the occipital and temporal areas (*female pattern*). Frontal bitemporal recession is seen rarely in females (Fig. 35.2), and only a few males may show the female pattern of diffuse hair loss. Familial predisposition is often mentioned in history and pull tests (trichograms) show telogen shedding in periods of activity.

Particularly in females AGA should be differentiated from *chronic telogen effluvium* (increased shedding of hair over >6 months) due to other underlying causes such as anemia, iron deficiency, thyroid gland disorders, liver disease, chronic infections, malnutrition, dietary schedules, drug-induced, and possibly also long-standing emotional stress. Association of AGA with signs of hyperandrogenism such as the presence of seborrhea, acne, and hirsutism may accompany the loss of hair (SAHA syndrome, Fig. 35.3). Careful clinical examination, potential histology, and further laboratory investigations should exclude polycystic ovary, hormone, and metabolic disorders. Other types for differential diagnosis include rare cases of diffuse alopecia areata and *frontal fibrosing alopecia*.

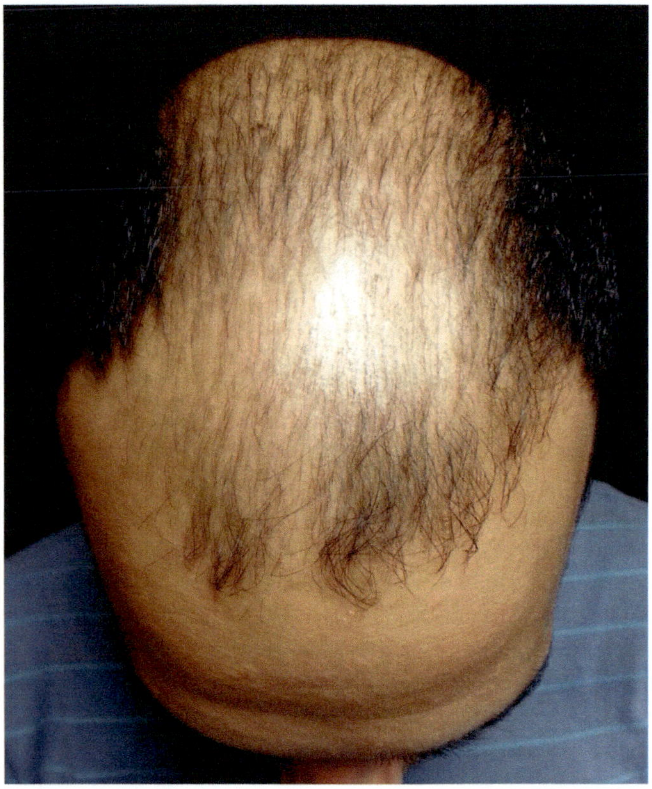

Fig. 35.1 *Androgenetic alopecia* (male pattern baldness) in an Egyptian male (type III skin)

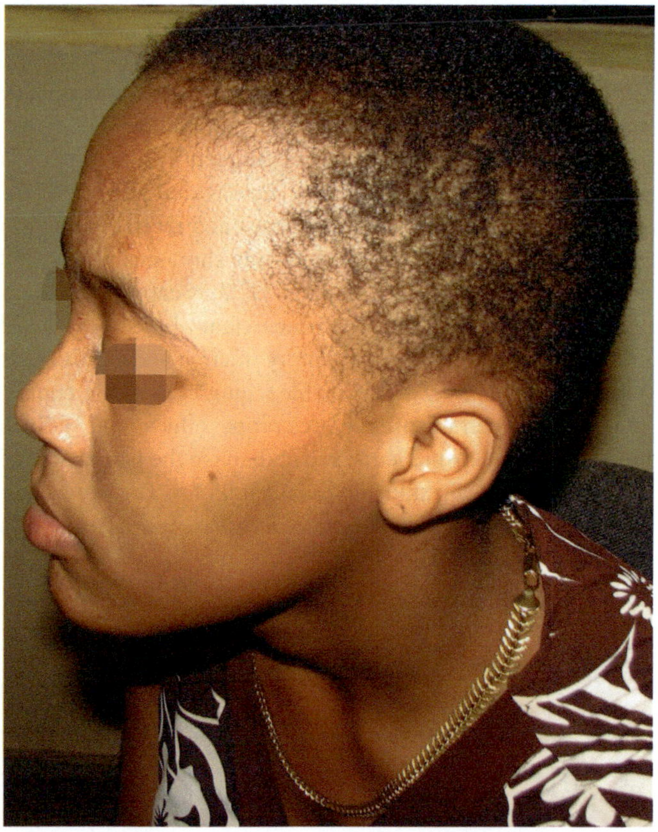

Fig. 35.2 Early *androgenetic alopecia* in an African female showing temporal bi-temporal recession and thinning of hair

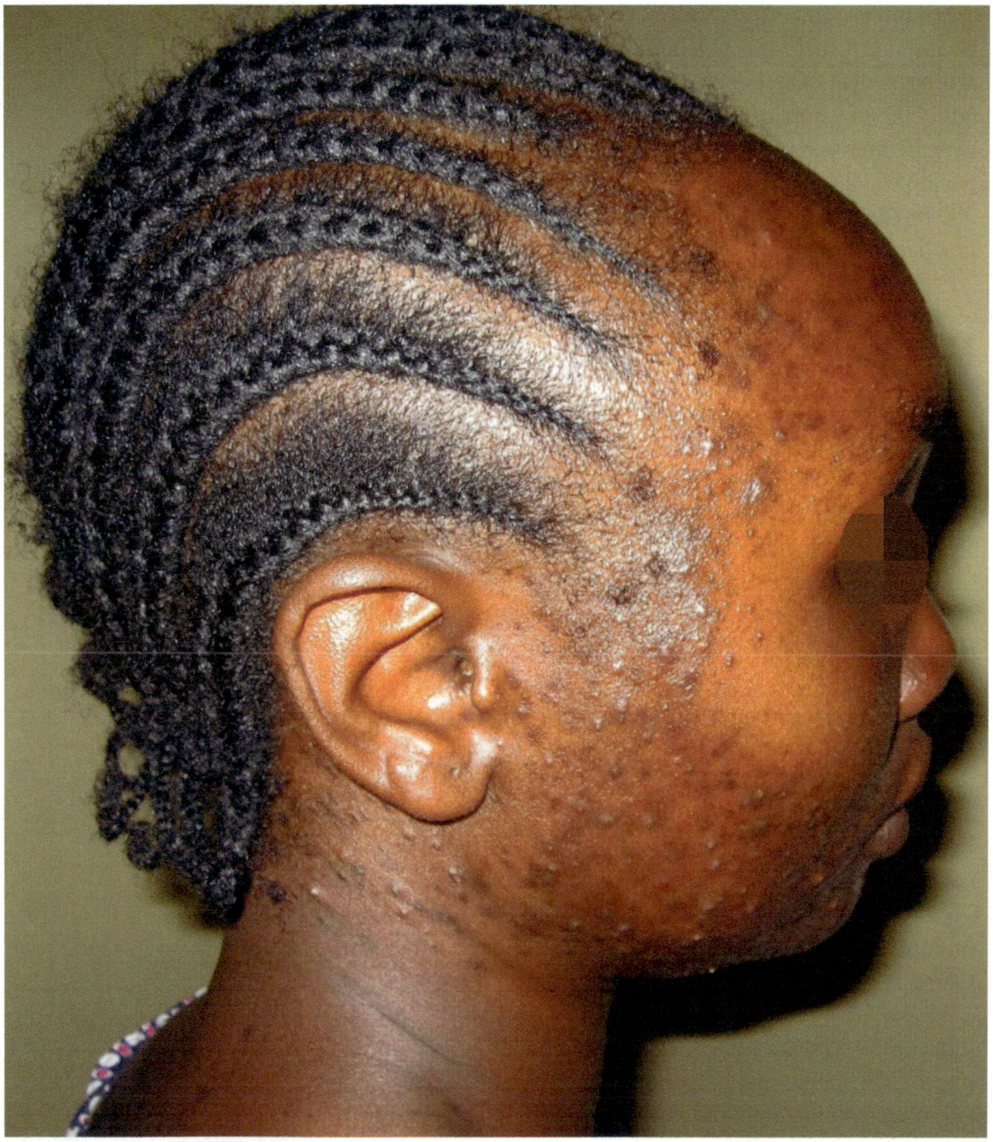

Fig. 35.3 *SAHA syndrome* (seborrhea, acne, hypertrichosis, androgenetic alopecia) together with *traction alopecia* (ethnic hair styling) in an African female

35.1.3 Management

AGA often affects quality of life, especially if it starts early in the 20s or teens, and is progressive associated with extensive rapid shedding. When AGA is diagnosed, the need for treatment depends on the personality of the individual affected. Males often consider AGA a physiologic process, while females are early alarmed and ask for correction. Topical preparations containing 2% and 5% minoxidil (1 mm 2×/day) may stimulate hair growth in 40–50% of the cases; after a year's use, there is measurable increase in hair density with moderate- to low-quality evidence and no difference in effect between 2% and 5% [16]. Side effects include scalp dryness and irritation. Allergic contact dermatitis is rarely encountered, mostly due to the vehicle. In women hypertrichosis of the face may be seen, especially with the higher concentration of the drug. In the future, agonists and antagonists of prostaglandins may be expected as candidates for treating AGA [17].

Oral treatment of males with *finasteride* (1 mg/day) shows 30% improvement if consequently continued over a year's period, being more effective on the vertex than on the frontal and parietal areas. As a side effect, erectile dysfunction may result. Since the drug decreases prostate-specific antigen (PSA) and may mask prostate cancer, the blood levels of PSA should be monitored before and during treatment. Higher doses of finasteride have been also applied in premenopausal and postmenopausal women with some success, especially in those with clinical hyperandrogenism. Strict contraception is necessary for avoiding male fetus feminization in those cases. *Dutasteride* is another possible oral candidate, found as effective as finasteride 1 and 5 mg, and its off-label use is not uncommon. Side effects were reported similar but more pronounced [18, 19]. As a potent antiandrogen, *cyproterone acetate* is given in females either in low dose (2 mg/day) combined with ethinyl estradiol as a contraceptive or at 50–100 mg/day over 10 days of each cycle. Also *spironolactone* has antiandrogenic properties and is widely used as an off-label drug (50–200 mg/day). Camouflage by dying the scalp skin and wigs are practical measures to cover the bald area, if necessary at all.

35.2 Hypertrichosis

Hypertrichosis entails growth of hair on follicle-containing non-androgen-dependent regions of the skin and is present from birth and more frequent in certain ethnic groups as *congenita* or acquired (*acquisita*).

Congenital hypertrichosis is found occasionally localized (nevoid) referring to atypical growth of lanugo or intermediate hair in a localized area of the body, at birth or early in life: *hypertrichosis cubiti* and *infrapatellar* or *anterior cervical hypertrichosis* [20–22]. It also occurs in hamartomas such as Becker's melanosis, plexiform neurofibromas, spinal dysraphism (faun tail sign), and congenital melanocytic nevi (Fig. 35.4). *Congenital generalized hypertrichosis* is rare, usually accompanied by other genetic disorders, characterized by the type of hair growing, mostly consisting of lanugo hair. Rare hereditary localized or generalized forms of hypertrichosis may manifest later in relation to genetic disorders (e.g., epidermolysis bullosa dystrophica, Hurler syndrome, Cornelia de Lange syndrome).

Acquired localized *or* generalized hypertrichosis may be induced by systemic diseases such as hypothyroidism, porphyria, dermatomyositis (children), celiac disease, anorexia nervosa, malnutrition, and marasmus or be a sign of malignancy. *Hypertrichosis lanuginosa acquisita* is often paraneoplastic, sometimes being overlooked [23]. It could even precede an underlying neoplasm. Localized types may occur in relation to friction, inflammation, or after topical application of corticosteroids, tacrolimus, and the prostaglandin analogues bimatoprost and latanoprost. The latter has been used to elongate eyelashes and thicken eyebrows [24]. Minoxidil used on the scalp for treatment of androgenetic alopecia may lead to local hypertrichosis of the face, especially when higher concentrations are used [25]. Minoxidil-induced generalized hypertrichosis has been reported in a 5-year-old child following the use of 5% solution after some months [26].

Drug-induced hypertrichosis after oral drug intake has been documented under acetazolamide, citalopram, corticosteroids, cyclosporine, diazoxide, metoclopramide, methyl-

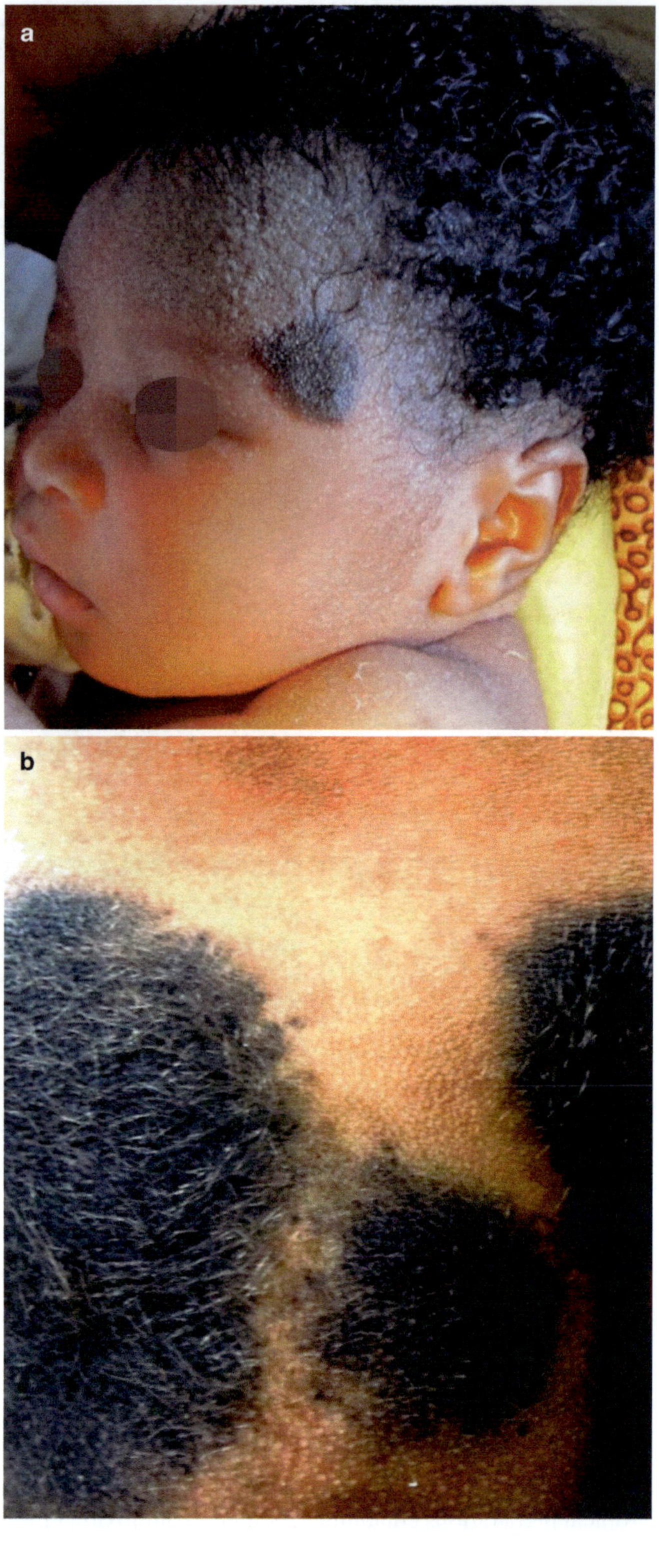

Fig. 35.4 Hypertrichosis in congenital melanocytic nevi: *Naevus pigmentosus pilosus* (**a**) in the forehead of a newborn and (**b**) in the lumbar area of a 26-year old Egyptian male

dopa, minoxidil, penicillamine, phenothiazines, phenytoin, reserpine, streptomycin, valproic acid, and others.

Paradoxical hypertrichosis has been reported after hair epilation with lasers, more often on the face and neck, in dark-skinned patients and in those with hormonal imbalance [27].

35.2.1 Management

Hair removal techniques, temporary by shaving and waxing or permanent by lasers, intense pulsed light, etc., are helpful for treating hypertrichosis (see below). Underlying causes should be investigated and treated if possible.

35.3 Hirsutism

Hirsutism is defined as increased growth of terminal hairs in a male distribution in females. In the majority of cases, it is caused by androgens derived from the ovary or the adrenal gland; only in a few hirsute women, the androgen levels are normal (*genetic* or *idiopathic hirsutism*). It is estimated that roughly 30% of all European women show some signs of hirsutism; however, only 10% of hirsute women require clinical investigations and treatment [28], showing ethnic differences in incidence. In Caucasians from Mediterranean countries with pigmented skin (types III and IV), hirsutism is more common compared to white Caucasians (types I and II), East Asian, and indigenous American and African women [29]. Not only the circulating levels of androgens play a pathogenetic role but also their metabolism into DHT and the number and sensitivity of the peripheral androgen receptors. Other hormones and cytokines may be involved in the transition of vellus into terminal hair; insulin has been reported to act synergistic with testosterone and influence the severity of hirsutism [30]. Different gene transcriptions are responsible for the transitional process, leading either to vellus-terminal transformation in androgen-dependent sites or, conversely, to terminal-vellus transformation on the scalp.

35.3.1 Clinical Features

The degree of hirsutism may vary from person to person and its localization on the body consisting of lanugo and intermediate or terminal hairs. For assessing its severity and the effectiveness of treatment, objective scoring indices have been introduced (Ferriman-Gallwey score; [31, 32].

Together with hirsutism varying degrees of seborrhea, acne, and androgenetic alopecia are often seen, posing severe psychological distress to the females affected. The resulting clinical phenotype is most characteristic to the dermatologist, known as *SAHA syndrome* [33], being a leading clinical phenotype indicating ovulatory dysfunction. An underlying PCO with oligo-/amenorrhea and anovulatory infertility is the most frequent cause of hirsutism. The prevalence of hirsutism in females with PCO ranges from 70 to 80%, vs. 4% to 11% in the general population [34]. In self-ratings the patients view their hirsutism as more severe than clinicians do, a critical fact for patient-centered care of hirsute patients [35]. Also, insulin resistance with type 2 (pre)diabetes, obesity, and acanthosis nigricans may rarely accompany the clinical picture (*HAIR-AN syndrome*).

The association of hirsutism with PCO and other metabolic syndromes was found more often in black women with PCO than in white women, with a significantly increased prevalence of low high-density lipoprotein and high glucose levels; the general cardiovascular risk was significantly increased in black adults [36].

Other underlying causes leading to hyperandrogenic hirsutism are adrenal hyperplasia or androgen-secreting tumors, showing a more rapidly progressive clinical course, up to full virilization. Galactorrhoea is a clinical symptom suggesting prolactinoma.

35.3.2 Management

Mild cases of hirsutism benefit from cosmetic measures removing excess hair by waxing, sugaring, plucking, threading, electrolysis, and intense pulsed light, in addition to shaving and depilatory creams containing thioglycolates available over the counter. Local application of creams containing eflornithine hydrochloride (Vaniqa®) decreases hair length and hair mass in around 70% of the cases after 2–3 months but is effective only as long as applied. Local irritation, induction of pseudofolliculitis, and mild acne may be seen as a side effect. Combinations with sessions with lasers lead to better outcome. In addition, eflornithine preparations are useful in cases of less pigmented blond hair, not treatable by lasers [37, 38].

Laser and intense pulsed light target anagen hairs and lead to hair reduction and permanent hair removal. Ruby (694 nm), alexandrite (755 nm), diode (880 nm), and Nd-YAG (1064 nm) lasers target melanin in the hair and aim at heating and destroying the dermal papilla and the bulge area where stem cells reside. Since melanin is present in the hair and its follicle, the best candidates for treatment with lasers are hirsute women with black, thick hair. Treatment with ruby and alexandrite lasers are more suited for fair-colored patients (types I–III), while Nd-YAG is more suited for dark skin colors (IV and V). Multiple sessions are needed to get a 80% reduction of hair growth. Sessions are spaced

4–6 weeks for the face and neck and 6–8 weeks for the rest of the body, depending on the hair cycle in each area. Patients with hyperandrogenism usually need more sessions, also requiring proper oral medication [39].

Oral medication of drugs is considered in severe cases of hyperandrogenic hirsutism, tailored to the underlying cause and any accompanying endocrinological disease together with a gynecologist or endocrinologist. Oral contraceptives are routinely administered in females in child-bearing period, particularly those containing gestagens with antiandrogenic action (dienogest, desogestrel, norgestimate, gestodene). They regulate the menstrual cycle, increase the level of circulating SHGB, and reduce endometrial hyperplasia in females with PCO. More potent are contraceptives containing cyproterone acetate (CPA, 2 mg), chlormadinone acetate (CMA, 2 mg), and drospirenone (3 mg). If the contraceptive treatment alone remains less effective over 6 months, oral spironolactone (50–200 mg/day), flutamide (250–500 mg/day), or finasteride (2.5–5 mg/day) could be added. In pooled data they were found more effective than placebo in reducing hirsutism [40]. Contraceptives combined with CPA in high dose (50–100 mg/day) over a limited period of the cycle exert a strong antiandrogenic action.

Insulin-sensitizing agents such as metformin and thiazolidinediones (e.g., pioglitazone) are used in females with PCO associated with insulin resistance. They improve hirsutism by increasing insulin sensitivity reducing insulin levels and, consequently, reduce the circulating free and biologically active androgens.

35.3.3 Course and Monitoring

Females with hirsutism should be monitored during treatment for any decrease of hair growth (density, thickness, and rate). FG scoring and patient self-assessment in intervals will help to follow up and adjust management, with hormonal evaluation in some cases. Lifelong treatment will be necessary. If pregnancy is desired, all medications should be stopped and drugs that may stimulate ovulation are given (clomiphene). Aromatase inhibitors (letrozole) and low-dose gonadotropins are also in use.

35.4 Alopecia Areata

Alopecia areata (AA) is an autoinflammatory disorder of unknown etiology with close relations to atopy, allergic rhinitis, vitiligo, juvenile diabetes, and autoimmune thyroiditis, leading to circumscribed hairless patches, mostly on the scalp, but also involving the eyebrows, the beard, and the entire body hair. The disease is observed in all races and also in dark-skinned patients.

The incidence of AA in Caucasians varies 0.5–2%, with frequent familiar predisposition (5–25%; [41]); however, the concordance of AA among identical twins is roughly 53%, not enough to be considered dominant. Also, there is a trend toward association with HLA-DR4 and HLA-DR5 profiles, but a clear genetic background is lacking. In races with pigmented or black skin, AA is reported to occur equally often as in Caucasians, although no exact data are available. Possibly the disease remains underdiagnosed. At hair clinics in Rio de Janeiro, 40% of AA patients were of skin phototypes V and VI [42]. In a Turkish population, a higher incidence was found in a military group than in a civil group, 5.4% vs. 1.7% [43].

35.4.1 Pathogenesis

The loss of hair in AA is due to cellular aggression toward the follicular keratinocytes and hair melanocytes, mediated by IFN-γ and CD4/CD8 cell populations [41]. The ongoing inflammatory reaction includes both the innate and acquired immune response via regulatory T-cells, Th17 cells, and also some NK cells; they accumulate around the peribulbar capillaries and invade the hair follicle. Cytotoxic $CD8^+NKG2D^+$ T-cells were found both necessary and sufficient for the induction of AA in mouse models of disease [44]. The cytotoxic T-cells inhibit the metabolic activity of the matrix cells above the apex of the dermal papilla and interrupt the growth of mature hair and melanogenesis in anagen IV. The hair bulb shrinks and remains inactive, whereas the inflammatory reaction moves toward the periphery, and hairless areas occur and enlarge. In these early phases, the number of catagen and resting telogen hairs is increased in hair-pull tests. If the hair follicles involved remain inactive over a time period longer than 5 years, the hair follicles are miniaturized, reduced in number, or disappear completely.

35.4.2 Clinical Features

The onset of the disease usually starts during early childhood showing well-demarcated, isolated, or multiple, roundish hairless lesions on the scalp. They usually occur at the age of 5 years with increasing incidence until the third decade (Figs. 35.5 and 35.6). Late manifestation of AA after the age of 50 is rather rare. Rapid courses, also showing diffuse hair loss, are sometimes observed, leading to generalized loss of hair (A. totalis, A. universalis). The lesions show thinning of the hair shafts and local circumscribed *poliosis* of hair, without erythema or scarring. The presence of cadaverized hairs (black dots), exclamation mark hairs, and vellus hairs indicates disease activity [45]. White dots regularly distributed among hair follicles and empty follicular units may also be observed. As a characteristic feature, rough abnormalities of the nail plate are

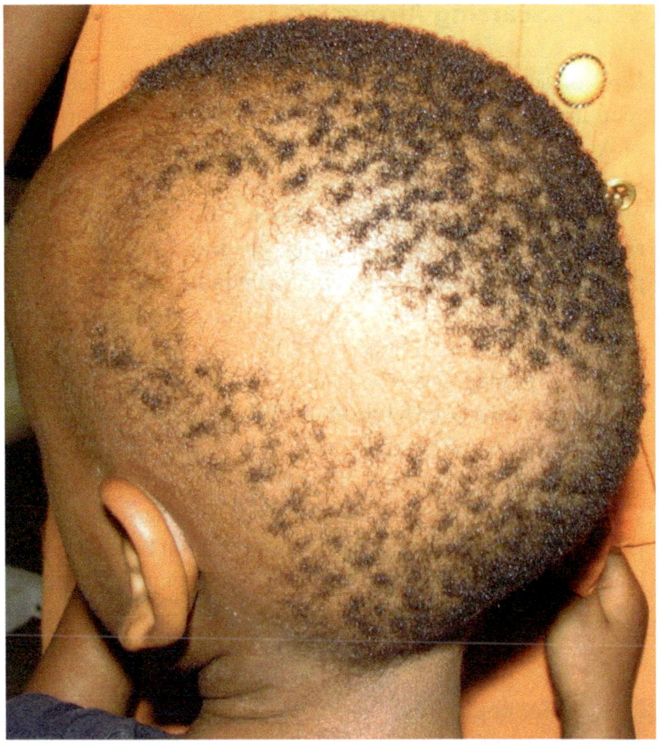

Fig. 35.5 Early onset of *alopecia areata* in a 6-year old African boy

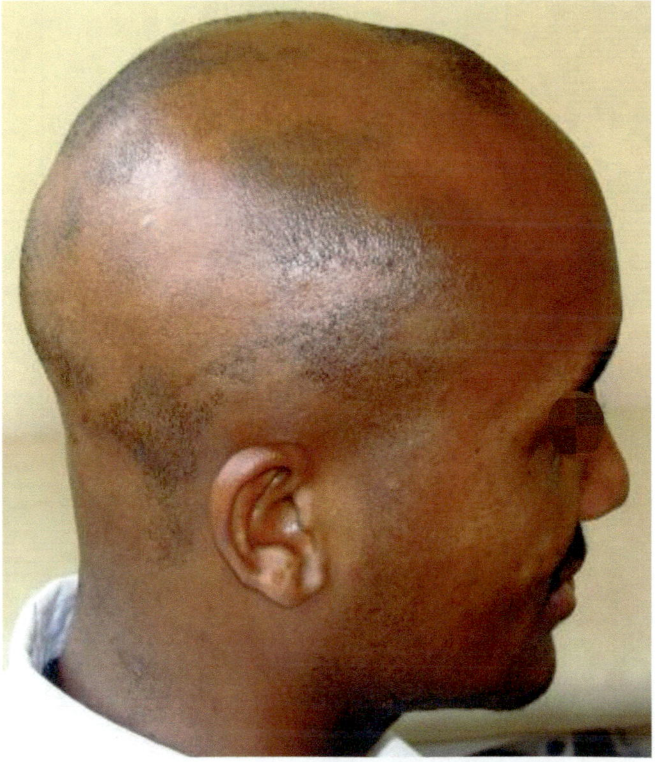

Fig. 35.6 Late stage of long-standing *alopecia areata* in an Ethiopian male

also seen in well-developed cases, underlining the disorder of keratinization in the nail matrix.

As a rule, physical examination and laboratory diagnostic procedures are required in patients with AA in order to assess concomitant atopic symptomatology and exclude any common association with other autoimmune diseases such as diffuse thyroiditis and juvenile diabetes.

35.4.3 Management

The treatment of AA is still not satisfactory. For localized patches on the scalp and beard, *corticosteroids* are mostly used, topically applied in creams or solutions (0.1% betamethasone, 0.1% mometasone, 0.05% clobetasol) and/or with intralesional injections of triamcinolone. Only marginal effects are seen with minoxidil and various topical irritants such as anthralin. In cases with multiple progressing lesions, prednisolone may be given orally (30–40 mg/day) reducing the dose to 5 mg/day over several weeks/months. In severe cases hair growth will be achieved after high pulse systemic administration of prednisolone (100–250 mg p.inf.) every 4 weeks over 6 months; however, relapses regularly occur after discontinuation of systemic corticosteroids.

Phototherapeutic schedules with *excimer laser* therapies and other light modalities, *narrowband UVB*, *high-strength UVA*, and *topical* and *systemic PUVA* or *RePUVA*, are well established in protocols for treatment of AA with varying results (regrowth of hair in 40–60%, several sessions required). Contact immunotherapies with *diphencyprone* (DPCP) in Europe and *dinitrochlorobenzene* (*DNCB*) and/or *squaric acid dibutylester* (SADBE) in Japan are administered in selected cases. Systemic immunomodulators and immunosuppressive drugs such as *chloroquine*, *dapsone*, *azathioprine*, and *cyclosporin A* are not helpful on a long term.

TNF-alpha blocking agents were applied recently in AA: *etanercept*, *efalizumab*, and *infliximab* had no consistent effect; they may even provoke lesions of AA which disappear after withdrawal [46–48]. While several authors have documented the occurrence of rapidly progressing AA under ongoing treatment with *adalimumab* [49, 50], others have reported its regression. *Tofacitinib*, a JAK inhibitor marketed for rheumatic arthritis and myelofibrosis (Xeljanz®), was found effective in severe AA (universalis) showing remarkable regrowth of hair after 4–5 months ([51–53]; 20 mg 2×/day). The topical application of Tofacitinib (2%) has also been reported effective [53]. Similarly, *ruxolitinib* (Jakavi®), another JAK inhibitor marketed for chronic idiopathic myelofibrosis, has been effective in AA [44, 54]. It seems that these two agents reduce the number of cytotoxic CD8 T-lymphocytes and NK cells attacking the hair follicle. Their overall safety and efficacy seem now promising but need further evaluation.

Regrowth of hairs in AA lesions is mostly seen in centrally located lesional areas; the new hair shafts may be thin with some variations of caliber and remain white until they grow longer. Interestingly, systemic steroid treatment leads regularly to immediate regrowth of pigmented hair.

35.4.4 Course and Prognosis

The course of AA is chronic, with a high rate of remissions and relapses. The prognosis is generally good on a long term, despite considerable interindividual variations. In the majority of cases, the patients recover completely after 3–8 years; there is progress into long-standing generalized alopecia only in <10%. Positive family history and early development or presence of *A. universalis* are associated with bad prognosis [55]. AA is not life-threatening, but its presence interferes with quality of life; nearly all patients need continuous psychological care, independent from the severity of the clinical picture.

35.5 Scarring Alopecias

Loss of scalp hair due to exogenous damage is frequently seen in black-skinned populations. The short and curly hair of Africans and/or African-Americans is more brittle, easily susceptible to exogenous damage; hair loss due to trauma is extremely common in black women [56]. It becomes scarring and irreversible when long-standing and results into patches of *cicatricial alopecia.* Traumatic alopecia may be due to customary causes such as local pressure and long-term friction in individuals wearing hair pieces and heavy huts or carrying heavy baskets or other weights on their heads [57]. Increased fibrosis ultimately leads to perifollicular fibrosis, scar formation, and miniaturization of the hair follicle. Traumatic hairstyling techniques are common in young African females and in African-American women [58], and physical trauma with severe traction bound to fancy hairstyles is a frequent cause of permanent alopecia (Fig. 35.7a, b).

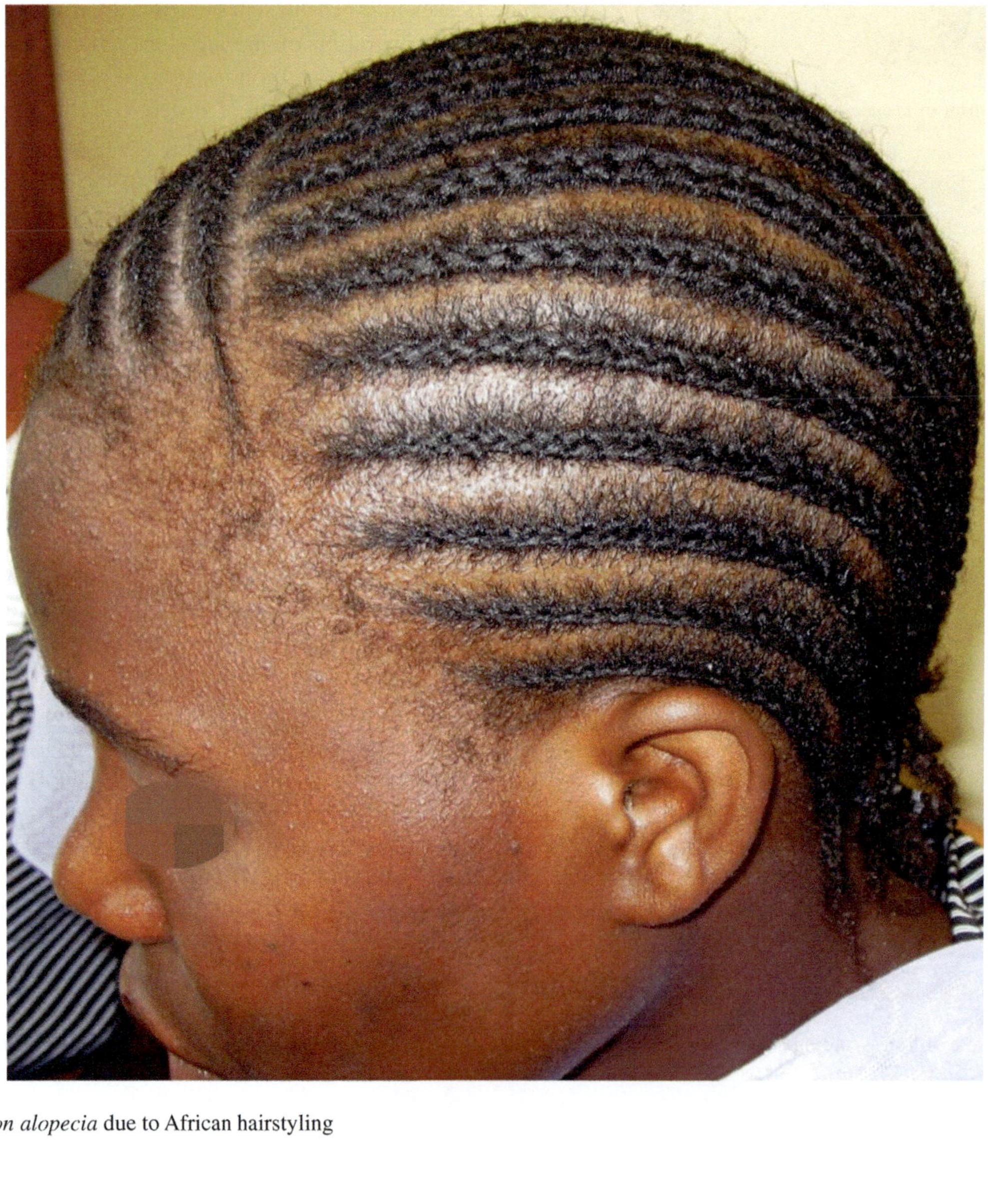

Fig. 35.7 *Traction alopecia* due to African hairstyling

Excess use of nylon-tufted hair brushes, hot combs, and various chemical hair relaxers and strengtheners (alkali solutions, thioglycolates, formaldehydes, etc.) leads to follicular damage, scar formation, and permanent hair loss, preferably in the central parietal areas of the scalp. Application of local concoctions or pomades is a regular practice among females with scarred alopecias in Nigeria [59], as it happens in other countries in Africa. Hot procedures with aggressive chemical agents that destroy the disulfide bonds of hair keratin may cause repeated burns and result in spotted dyspigmentations in black-skinned individuals, intermingled with scarring areas. In females such lesions are bizarrely demarcated, mostly localized in the central parietal area of the scalp (Fig. 35.8a, b). The term *central centrifugal cicatricial alopecia* has been recently coined and is widely used for females with genetic predisposition who practice traumatic hairstyling and for patients of African descent [60–62].

Permanent loss of hair is also seen in scalp lesions of dermatoses such as *keratosis pilaris*, *lichen planopilaris*, and *lichen follicularis*, showing follicular hyperkeratosis, papules, and pustules resulting in scarred patches (*pseudopelade* type of cicatricial alopecia; Fig. 35.9). They are often detected in late non-inflammatory stages; when the initial erythema has disappeared, follicular hyperkeratoses remain, and the disease follows a slow, progressive course of scarring (*Graham-Little syndrome*). In late stages the scalp lesions are irregularly scarred and hairless (Fig. 35.10a, b). In *fibrosing alopecia*, most likely a variant of cicatricial alopecia, recession of the frontotemporal hairline and loss of eyebrows may occur in females [60]. In *lupus erythematosus* (LE), diffuse alopecia without initial scarring often develops as a transitory finding in all forms of the disease with cutaneous involvement, including systemic LE [63]. In the chronic discoid subtype of LE, however, sharply demarcated scarring

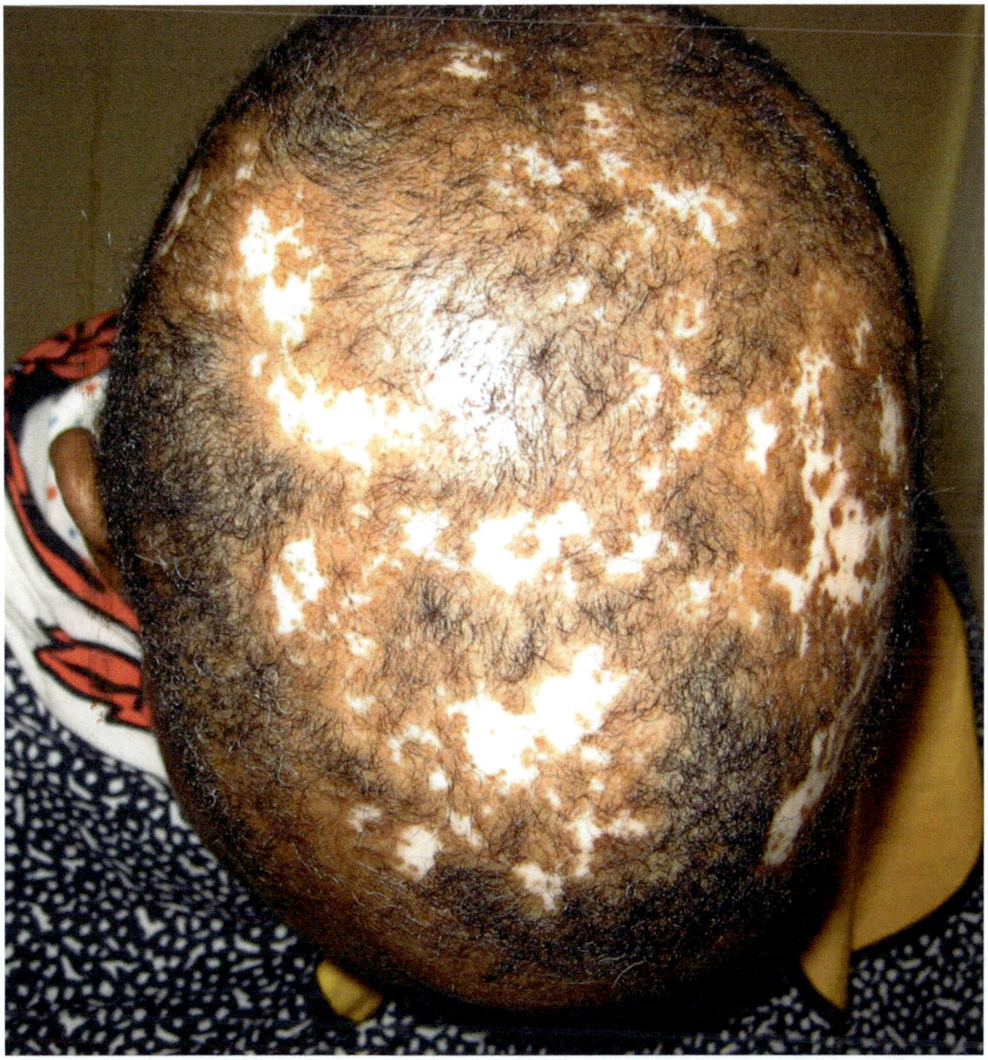

Fig. 35.8 *Central scarring alopecia* with dyspigmentations due to long-term damage of the scalp skin with cosmetic measures (hot combs, chemical strengtheners, burns etc.) in a 37-year old Tanzanian woman

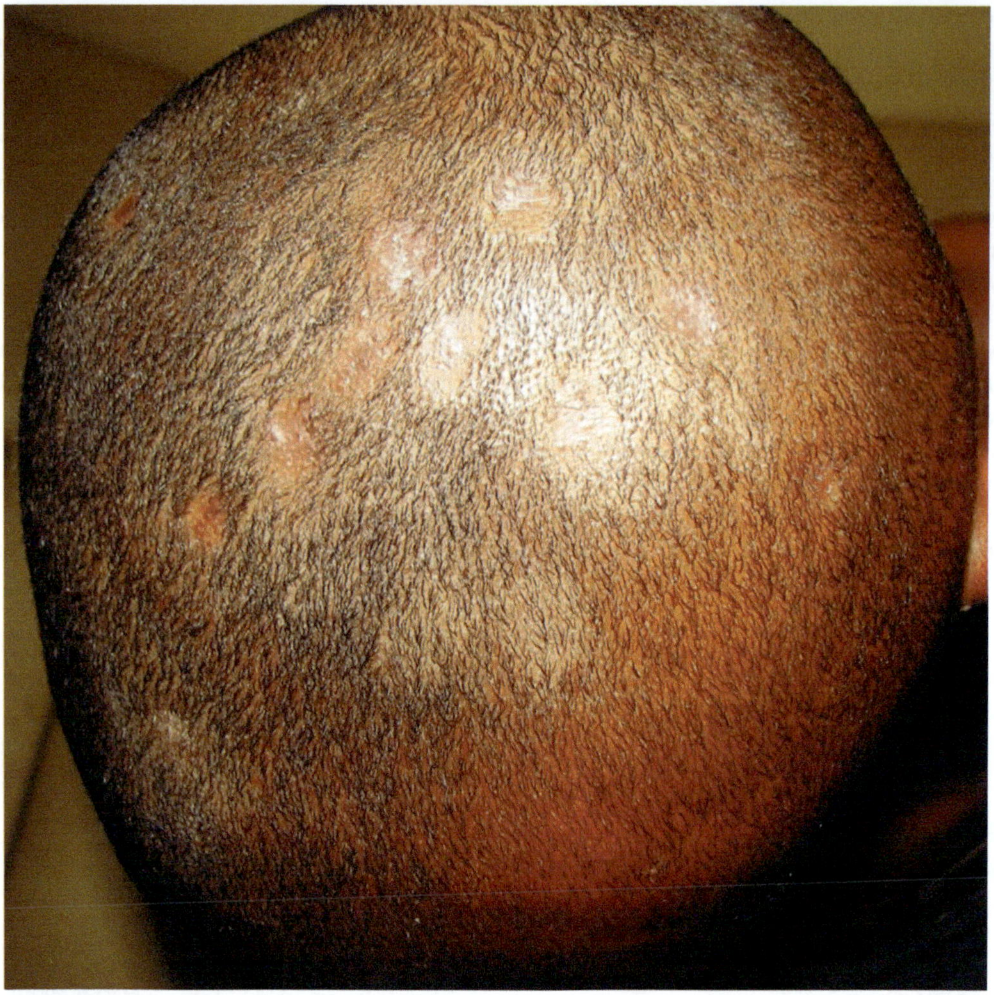

Fig. 35.9 Patches of scarring alopecia in a 16-year-old adolescent, *pseudopelade* type

lesions may occur on the scalp showing shifting or complete loss of pigment resembling vitiligo. Vitiligo-like hairless scalp lesions are a most characteristic feature in black-skinned patients with DLE (see Chap. 29). Another characteristic finding in black-skinned individuals is the occurrence of chronic *folliculitis decalvans* with inflamed papules and pustules mostly on the neck, rarely the beard, leading to the formation of multiple keloids (Fig. 35.11a, b). The lesions are occasionally pruritic and/or painful.

35.5.1 Management

Traumatic alopecias are reversible in early stages, if the exogenous trauma or other cause is recognized and eliminated. In long-standing cases, however, the hair follicles are miniaturized surrounded by fibrosis and will not completely recover. Local application of agents promoting vascularization may be helpful to stabilize the process of ongoing fibrosis and scarring. Mild topical corticosteroids and minoxidil can be used, with some promise for success. When the loss of hair is still progressing and the lesions clinically enlarge, potent topical (clobetasol) and/or intralesional corticosteroids (triamcinolone) are recommendable, together with oral treatment of any underlying disease with antibiotics, immunomodulators, and immunosuppressive drugs. In *folliculitis decalvans* clindamycin and rifampicin are often administered. Well-circumscribed scarring lesions may be surgically removed, and hair replacement surgery techniques may be applied in selected cases [64].

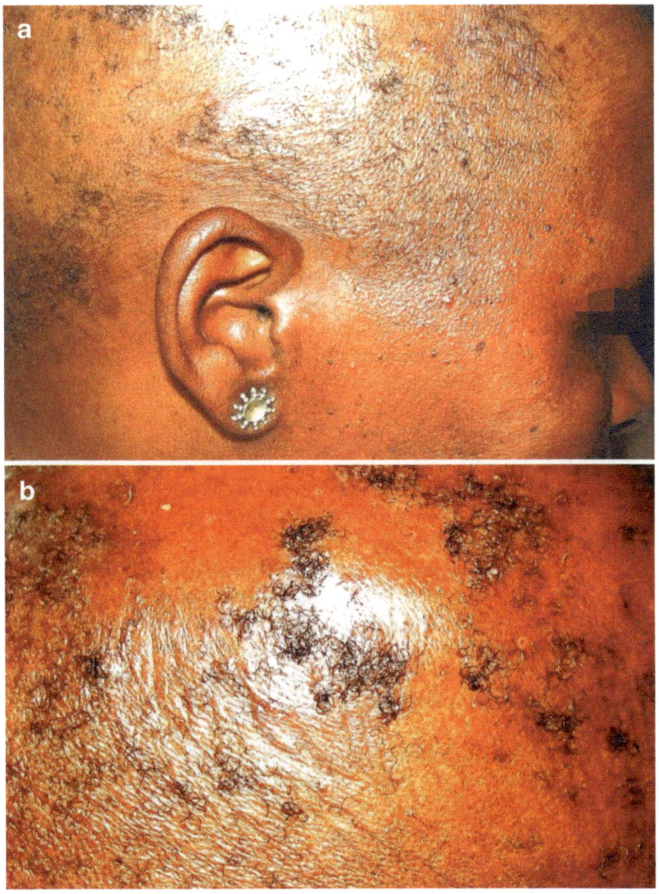

Fig. 35.10 (**a**, **b**) Scarring alopecia with resting follicular hyperkeratosis, papules, and pustules (*lichen follicularis*, *Graham-Little syndrome*)

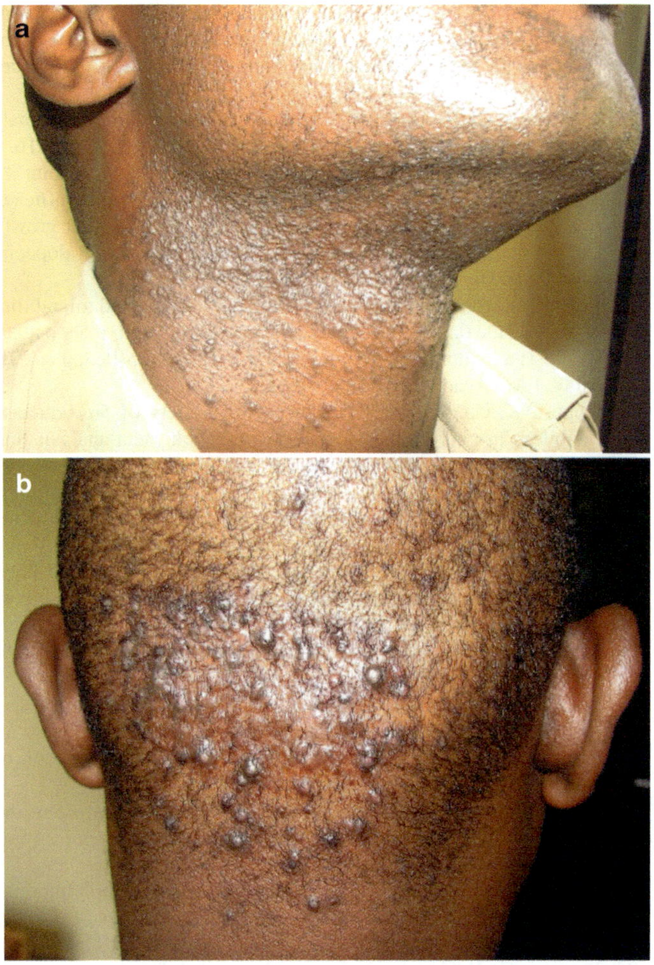

Fig. 35.11 Keloidal acne leading to alopecia, *Folliculitis keloidalis decalvans* (**a**) of the beard and (**b**) the neck

References

1. Lindsey SF, Tosti A. Ethnic hair disorders. Curr Probl Dermatol. 2015;47:139–49.
2. Semble AL, McMichael AJ. Hair loss in patients with skin of color. Semin Cutan Med Surg. 2015;34:81–8.
3. Fu JM, Price VH. Approach to hair loss in women of color. Semin Cutan Med Surg. 2009;28:109–14.
4. Madu P, Kundu RV. Follicular and scarring disorders in skin of color: presentation and management. Am J Clin Dermatol. 2014;15:307–21.
5. Paik JH, Yoon JB, Sim WY, et al. The prevalence and types of androgenetic alopecia in Korean men and women. Br J Dermatol. 2001;145:95–9.
6. Gan DC, Sinclair RD. Prevalence of male and female pattern hair loss in Maryborough. J Investig Dermatol Symp Proc. 2005;10:184–9.
7. Xu F, Sheng YY, Mu ZL, et al. Prevalence and types of androgenetic alopecia in shanghai, China: a community-based study. Br J Dermatol. 2009;160:629–32.
8. Birch MP, Messenger JF, Messenger AG. Hair density, hair diameter and the prevalence of female pattern hair loss. Br J Dermatol. 2001;144:297–304.
9. Norwood OT. Incidence of female androgenetic alopecia (female pattern alopecia). Dermatol Surg. 2001;27:53–44.
10. Khumalo NP, Jessop S, Gumedze F. Hairdressing and the prevalence of scalp disease in African adults. Br J Dermatol. 2007;157:981–8.
11. Hillmer AM, Hanneken S, Ritzmann S, et al. Genetic variation in the human androgen receptor gene is the major determinant of common early-onset androgenetic alopecia. Am J Hum Genet. 2005;77:140–8.
12. Hillmer AM, Flaquer A, Hanneken S, et al. Genome-wide scan and fine-mapping linkage study of androgenetic alopecia reveals a locus on chromosome 3q26. Am J Hum Genet. 2008;82:737–43.
13. Zhuo FL, Xu W, Wang L, et al. Androgen receptor gene polymorphisms and risk for androgenetic alopecia: a meta-analysis. Clin Exp Dermatol. 2012;37:104–11.
14. Chew EG, Tan JH, Bahta AW, et al. Differential expression between human dermal papilla cells from balding and non-balding scalps reveals new candidate genes for androgenetic alopecia. J Invest Dermatol. 2016;136:1559–67.

15. Nuwaihyd R, Redler S, Heilmann S. Investigation of four novel male androgenetic alopecia susceptibility loci: no association with female pattern hair. Arch Dermatol Res. 2014;306: 413–8.
16. van Zuuren EJ, Fedorowicz Z, Schoones J. Interventions for female pattern hair loss. Cochrane Database Syst Rev. CD007628, 2016.
17. Blume-Peytavi U, Lönnfors S, Hillmann K, et al. A randomized double-blind placebo-controlled pilot study to assess the efficacy of a 24-week topical treatment by latanoprost 0.1% on hair growth and pigmentation in healthy volunteers with androgenetic alopecia. J Am Acad Dermatol. 2012;66:794–800.
18. Eun HC, Kwon OS, Yeon JH, et al. Efficacy, safety, and tolerability of dutasteride 0.5 mg once daily in male patients with male pattern hair loss: a randomized, double-blind, placebo-controlled, phase III study. J Am Acad Dermatol. 2010;63:252–8.
19. Gupta AK, Charrette A. The efficacy and safety of 5α-reductase inhibitors in androgenetic alopecia: a network meta-analysis and benefit-risk assessment of finasteride and dutasteride. J Dermatolog Treat. 2014;25:156–61.
20. Tng VE, de Zwaan S. Hypertrichosis cubiti, a case report and literature review. Clin Case Rep. 2015;4:138–42.
21. Pavone V, Testa G, Falsaperla R, et al. Syringomyelia and bone malformations in the setting of hypertrichosis cubiti (hairy elbow syndrome). J Orthop Case Rep. 2015;5:32–4.
22. Megna M, Balato N, Patruno C, et al. Anterior cervical hypertrichosis: a case report and review of the literature. Pediatr Dermatol. 2015;32:252–5.
23. Slee PH, van der Waal RI, Schagen van Leeuwen JH, et al. Paraneoplastic hypertrichosis lanuginosa acquisita: uncommon or overlooked? Br J Dermatol. 2007;157:1087–92.
24. Coronel-Pérez IM, Rodríguez-Rey EM, et al. Latanoprost in the treatment of eyelash alopecia in alopecia areata universalis. J Eur Acad Dermatol Venereol. 2010;24:481–5.
25. Dawber RP, Rundegren J. Hypertrichosis in females applying minoxidil topical solution and in normal controls. J Eur Acad Dermatol Venereol. 2003;17:271–5.
26. Rampon G, Henkin C, de Souza PR, et al. Infantile generalized hypertrichosis caused by topical minoxidil. An Bras Dermatol. 2016;91:87–8.
27. Desai S, Mahmoud BH, Bhatia AC, et al. Paradoxical hypertrichosis after laser therapy: a review. Dermatol Surg. 2010;36:291–8.
28. Orfanos CE, Garbe C. Hypertrichose und hirsutismus. In: Eds, editor. Therapie der Hautkrankheiten. 2nd ed. Berlin: Springer; 2002. p. 1414–6.
29. Farrant P. Excessive growth of hair. In: Christopher EM, Griffiths CE, et al., editors. Rook's textbook of dermatology. 9th ed. New York: John Wiley & Sons Ltd; 2016. p. 89.64–8.
30. Landay M, Huang A, Azziz R. Degree of hyperinsulinemia, independent of androgen levels, is an important determinant of the severity of hirsutism in PCOS. Fertil Steril. 2009;92:643–7.
31. Ferriman DM, Gallwey JD. Clinical assessment of body hair growth in women. J Clin Endocrinol. 1961;21:1440–7.
32. Escobar-Morreale HF, Carmina E, Dewailly D, et al. Epidemiology, diagnosis and management of hirsutism: a consensus statement by the androgen excess and polycystic ovary syndrome society. Hum Reprod Update. 2012;18:146–70.
33. Orfanos CE, Adler YD, Zouboulis CC. The SAHA syndrome. Horm Res. 2000;54:251–8.
34. Spritzer PM, Barone CR, Oliveira FB. Hirsutism in polycystic ovary syndrome: pathophysiology and management. Curr Pharm Des. 2016;22:5603–13.
35. Pasch L, He SY, Huddleston H, et al. Clinician vs self-ratings of hirsutism in patients with polycystic ovarian syndrome: associations with quality of life and depression. JAMA Dermatol. 2016;152:783–8.
36. Hillman JK, Johnson LN, Limaye M. Black women with polycystic ovary syndrome (PCOS) have increased risk for metabolic syndrome and cardiovascular disease compared with white women without PCOS. Fertil Steril. 2014;101:530–5.
37. Wolf JE Jr, Shander D, Huber F, et al. Eflornithine HCl study group. Randomized, double-blind clinical evaluation of the efficacy and safety of topical eflornithine HCl 13.9% cream in the treatment of women with facial hair. Int J Dermatol. 2007;46:94–8.
38. Hamzavi I, Tan E, Shapiro J, et al. A randomized bilateral vehicle-controlled study of eflornithine cream combined with laser treatment versus laser treatment alone for facial hirsutism in women. J Am Acad Dermatol. 2007;57:54–9.
39. Somani N, Turvy D. Hirsutism: an evidence-based treatment update. Am J Clin Dermatol. 2014;15:247–66.
40. van Zuuren EJ, Fedorowicz Z. Interventions for hirsutism excluding laser and photoepilation therapy alone: abridged Cochrane systematic review including GRADE assessments. Br J Dermatol. 2016;175:45–61.
41. Gollnick H, Orfanos CE. Alopecia areata: pathogenesis and clinical picture. In: Orfanos CE, Happle R, editors. Hair and hair diseases. Berlin: Springer; 1990. p. 529–69.
42. de Moura LH, Duque-Estrada B, Abraham LS, et al. Dermoscopy findings of alopecia areata in an African-American patient. Patient J Dermatol Case Rep. 2008;27:52–4.
43. Şenel E, Doğruer Şenel S, Salmanoğlu M. Prevalence of skin diseases in civilian and military population in a Turkish military hospital in the central Black Sea region. J R Army Med Corps. 2015;161:112–5.
44. Xing L, Dai Z, Jabbari A, et al. Alopecia areata is driven by cytotoxic T lymphocytes and is reversed by JAK inhibition. Nat Med. 2014;20:1043–9.
45. Inui S, Nakajima T, Nakagawa K, et al. Clinical significance of dermoscopy in alopecia areata: analysis of 300 cases. Int J Dermatol. 2008;47:688–93.
46. Pelivani N, Hassan AS, Braathen LR, et al. Alopecia areata universalis elicited during treatment with adalimumab. Dermatology. 2008;216:320–3.
47. Le Bidre E, Chaby G, Martin L, et al. Alopecia areata during anti TNF-alpha therapy: nine cases. Ann Dermatol Venereol. 2011;138:285–93.
48. Tauber M, Buche S, Reygagne P, et al. Alopecia areata occurring during anti-TNF therapy: a national multicenter prospective study. J Am Acad Dermatol. 2014;70:1146–9.
49. Garcia Bartels N, Lee HH, Worm M, et al. Development of alopecia areata universalis in a patient receiving adalimumab. Arch Dermatol. 2006;142:1654–5.
50. Zschoche C, Bidier M, Hadaschik E. Alopecia areata during treatment with adalimumab: therapy with an alternative TNF-alpha inhibitor is possible. J Dtsch Dermatol Ges. 2013;11:450–3.
51. Craiglow BG, King BA. Killing two birds with one stone: oral tofacitinib reverses alopecia universalis in a patient with plaque psoriasis. J Invest Dermatol. 2014;134:2988–90.
52. Kennedy Crispin M, Ko JM, Craiglow BG, et al. Safety and efficacy of the JAK inhibitor tofacitinib citrate in patients with alopecia areata. JCI Insight. 2016;1:e89776.
53. Liu LY, Craiglow BG, King BA. Tofacitinib 2% ointment, a topical Janus kinase inhibitor, for the treatment of alopecia areata: A pilot study of 10 patients. J Am Acad Dermatol. 2018;78:403–4.e1.
54. Craiglow BG, Tavares D, King BA. Topical ruxolitinib for the treatment of alopecia universalis. JAMA Dermatol. 2016;152: 490–1.
55. Jang YH, Hong NS, Moon SY, et al. Long-term prognosis of alopecia totalis and alopecia universalis: A longitudinal study with more than 10 years of follow-up: Better than reported. Dermatology. 2017;233:250–6.

56. Tanus A, Caberlon Cruz Oliveira C, Villarreal Villareal DJ. Black women's hair: the main scalp dermatoses and aesthetic practices in women of African ethnicity. An Bras Dermatol. 2015;90:450–65.
57. Goerz G, Kind R, Lehmann P. Cicatricial alopecias. In: Orfanos CE, Happle R, editors. Hair and hair diseases. Berlin: Springer; 1990. p. 611–39.
58. Borovicka JH, Thomas L, Prince C, et al. Scarring alopecia: clinical and pathologic study of 54 African-American women. Int J Dermatol. 2009;48:840–5.
59. Nnoruka EN. Hair loss: is there a relationship with hair care practices in Nigeria? Int J Dermatol. 2005;44(suppl 1):13–7.
60. Moreno-Ramírez D, Camacho-Martínez F. Frontal fibrosing alopecia: a survey in 16 patients. J Eur Acad Dermatol Venerol. 2005;19:700–5.
61. Gathers RC, Lim HW. Central centrifugal cicatricial alopecia: past, present, and future. J Am Acad Dermatol. 2009;60:660–8.
62. Uhlenhake EE, Mehregan DM. Prospective histologic examinations in patients who practice traumatic hairstyling. Int J Dermatol. 2013;52:1506.
63. Ye Y, Zhao Y, Gong Y, et al. Non-scarring patchy alopecia in patients with systemic lupus erythematosus differs from that of alopecia areata. Lupus. 2013;22:1439–45.
64. Callender VD, McMichael AJ, Cohen GF. Medical and surgical therapies for alopecias in black women. Dermatol Ther. 2004;17:164–76.

36 Tumors in Pigmented Skin

Chalid Assaf, Alice U. Amani, Egemen Yildiz, and Sam T. Hwang

Skin cancer is worldwide the most common malignancy; non-melanoma skin cancer and malignant melanoma together represent 40% of all neoplasms in white Caucasians [1]. The worldwide incidence for basal cell carcinoma varies widely with highest rates in Australia >1000/100,000/person-year and lowest in parts of Africa <1/100,000/person-year. In the UK the average incidence rates were 76/100,000/person-year and 22/100,000 person-year for basal cell and squamous cell carcinoma, respectively [2]. In individuals with pigmented ethnic skin, the incidence of skin cancer is clearly lower as compared with white-skinned individuals, possibly as a result of the photoprotective effects of melanin [3], but skin cancer is often associated with greater mortality and morbidity in pigmented skin. This may be associated either with late diagnosis of the neoplasms in an advanced stage or with different tumor characteristics in populations with pigmented ethnic skin. It is important to further assess any differences of skin cancer between Caucasian and non-Caucasian populations and evaluate the etiology and risk factors in skin of color for developing cancer.

C. Assaf (✉)
Department of Dermatology and Venerology, HELIOS Klinikum Krefeld, Krefeld, Germany
e-mail: chalid.assaf@helios-kliniken.de

A. U. Amani
Service de Dermatologie, Centre Hospitalier Universitaire, Kigali, Rwanda
e-mail: chuk.hospital@chuk.rw

E. Yildiz
Department of Dermatology, University of California, Davis School of Medicine, Sacramento, CA, USA

Faculty of Medicine, Hacettepe University, Ankara, Turkey
e-mail: egemen.yildiz12@hacettepe.edu.tr

S. T. Hwang, M.D., Ph.D.
Department of Dermatology, University of California, Davis School of Medicine, Sacramento, CA, USA

36.1 Basal Cell and Squamous Cell Carcinoma

Basal cell carcinoma (BCC) and squamous cell carcinoma (SCC) are the most common cancers of the skin. BCC represents approximately 80% of the total, being the most common type in Caucasians, Asians, and Hispanics [4], while SCC is in second place accounting for 15–25% [5]. In contrast, SCC is the most common cutaneous malignancy in black-skinned individuals, representing 30% of all skin cancers. Hispanics are six times more likely to be diagnosed with BCC than with SCC and more likely to present multiple basal cell carcinomas [6]. Estimations revealed the total number of non-melanoma skin cancers in the US population in 2012 at 5.5 million and the total number of persons treated for non-melanoma skin cancers during the same time period at 3.3 million [7]. The overall incidence of BCC standardized in age, sex, and ethnicity during 1998–2012 was found slightly increased, with rates higher for whites than for persons of multiethnic origin [8].

36.1.1 Pathogenesis

Occupational or recreational exposure to the sun or UV light is the major cause for developing BCC, with increasing risk associated to increasing ambient radiation [9, 10]. The highest densities of tumors are on the most sun-exposed parts of the body and the lowest on the least exposed. In white Caucasians with histologically proven BCC, high socioeconomic status, red/blonde hair, and blue/green eyes were found related to BCC risk [11]. Other possible risk factors for BCC in black skin include albinism, scars, ulcers, chronic infections, sebaceous nevi, arsenic ingestion, immunosuppression, previous radiation treatment,

C. E. Orfanos et al. (eds.), *Pigmented Ethnic Skin and Imported Dermatoses*, https://doi.org/10.1007/978-3-319-69422-1_36

xeroderma pigmentosum, and physical or thermal trauma [5]. Metastatic BCC is rare in all ethnic groups; however, risk factors for metastasis include a tumor diameter greater than 2 cm, location on the central part of the face or ears, long-standing duration, incomplete excision, an aggressive histologic pattern of growth, and perineural or perivascular involvement [4].

Risk factors for developing SCC in skin of color are chronic scarring and inflammatory processes including hidradenitis suppurativa, LE, scars caused by chemical and thermal burns, skin ulcers, sites of previous radiation, and immunosuppression [12]. All non-healing lesions with scarring and inflammation should be biopsied. Chronic scarring and/or inflammatory processes were observed in 20–40% of the cases reported. UV light exposure may not be an important etiologic factor in the development of SCC in black skin [5].

Inappropriate activation of the hedgehog signaling pathway is found in sporadic and familial cases of multiple BCC. Secreted sonic hedgehog protein binds the tumor-suppressor protein patched homologue 1 (*Ptch1*), thereby abrogating *Ptch1*-mediated suppression of intracellular signaling by another transmembraneous protein. Loss-of-function mutations of *Ptch1* found in patients with *nevoid basal cell carcinoma* have been identified in 30–40% of sporadic cases of BCC. Other alterations in the hedgehog signaling pathway that have been implicated include gain-of-function mutations [4].

36.1.2 Clinical Picture

BCC arises in skin areas exposed to the sun, mostly on the head and neck (80%) followed by the trunk (15%), arms, and legs. The classical *nodular* BCC subtype usually presents as a pearly papule or nodule with overlying telangiectasias and rolled border, occasionally showing central ulceration and crusting. The *superficial* BCC subtype presents as a scaly erythematous patch or plaque; both may contain melanin, showing bluish or black color. *Sclerosing* BCCs appear as indurated, whitish, scar-like plaques with indistinct margins. The anatomic distribution of the tumor is similar for white Caucasians and African-Americans; in a study, 89% were found localized on the head and neck [13].

Nodular BCC is the most common subtype in all ethnic groups. Sclerosing BCCs are less frequently found in black-skinned patients than in Caucasians [5], whereas pigmentation is present in more than 50% of all BCCs in patients with dark or black skin and in Hispanics. In contrast, only 6% of BCCs are pigmented in Caucasians. In black skin, it may be hard to differentiate the tumor from other lesions such as pigmented seborrhoeic keratoses, melanocytic nevi, blue nevi, or even malignant melanoma (Fig. 36.1). Also SCC may be difficult to differentiate presenting patches or elevated plaques or nodules; lesions are usually erythematous with scales and crusts and could be confused with psoriasis, eczema, or trauma [14]; in pigmented skin strongly hyperkeratotic SCCs are occasionally seen (Fig. 36.2).

Nevoid basal cell carcinoma (Gorlin-Goltz syndrome) is an autosomal dominant disorder linked to 9q22.3-q31 and caused by mutations in *Ptch1*, the human homologue of the Drosophila patched gene. It comprises multiple BCCs, calcification of the falx cerebri, odontogenic cysts, and bifid ribs in patients with a clinical phenotype characterized by hypertelorism, broad nasal root, frontal bossing, palmar or plantar pits, and a short fourth metacarpal hand bone. Medulloblastomas and a variety of other internal neoplasms may occur. The syndrome has been also reported in black skin, yet the number of BCCs and the overall clinical expression are diminished compared with Caucasians [15, 16].

36.1.3 Management and Prevention

Total removal of the tumor using curettage and cautery or, preferably, with standard surgical excision with free surgical margins is the best option for management. A dermatoscope in the hands of experienced dermatologists/physicians will be of help to better recognize the borders of the lesion. Photodynamic therapies, Mohs micrographic surgery, and other techniques have to be considered for large tumors and difficult localizations in specialized centers.

Skin cancer awareness and behavior toward sun exposure varies significantly among countries, while sun protection is mandatory for prevention. A majority of 2100 Caucasian and Hispanic patients from different countries living in the USA believed there was a correlation between skin cancer and sun exposure; a minority associated skin cancer with "moderate" tanning [17]. Overall, 86% of the respondents claimed that they always took precautions against UV damage when in the sun, but only 26% applied sunscreens when exposed for more than one hour. The Anti-Cancer Council of Victoria, Australia, has been running sun protection programs such as "*Slip! Slop! Slap! and SunSmart*" for more than 20 years. Such programs changed knowledge and behavior by delivering a consistent and continuous message and decreased the frequency of skin cancer; there are positive changes in incidence and mortality trends [18]. Recent

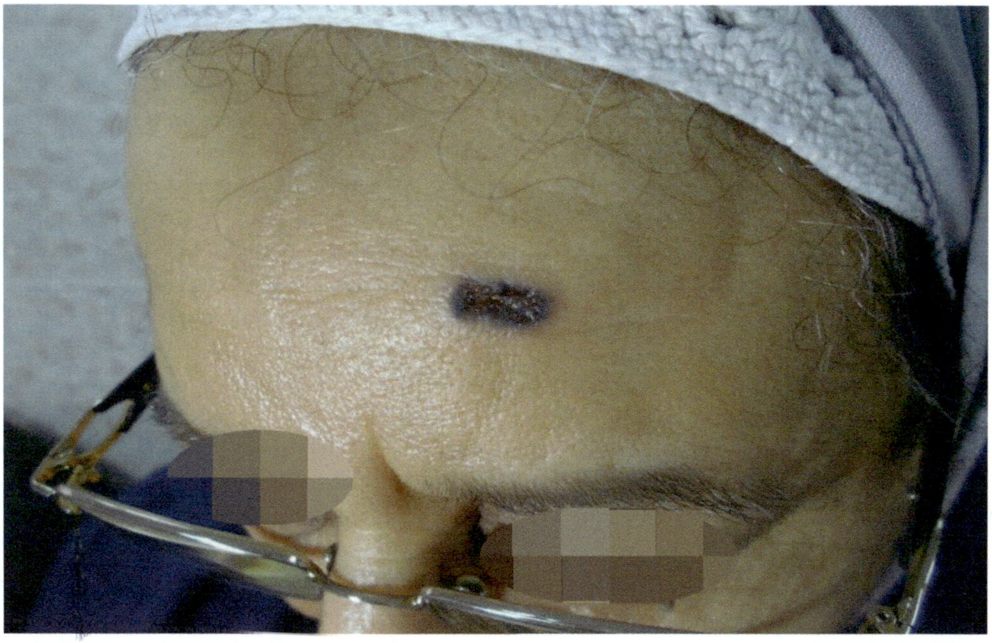

Fig. 36.1 *Pigmented basal cell carcinoma* on the forehead of an Egyptian female

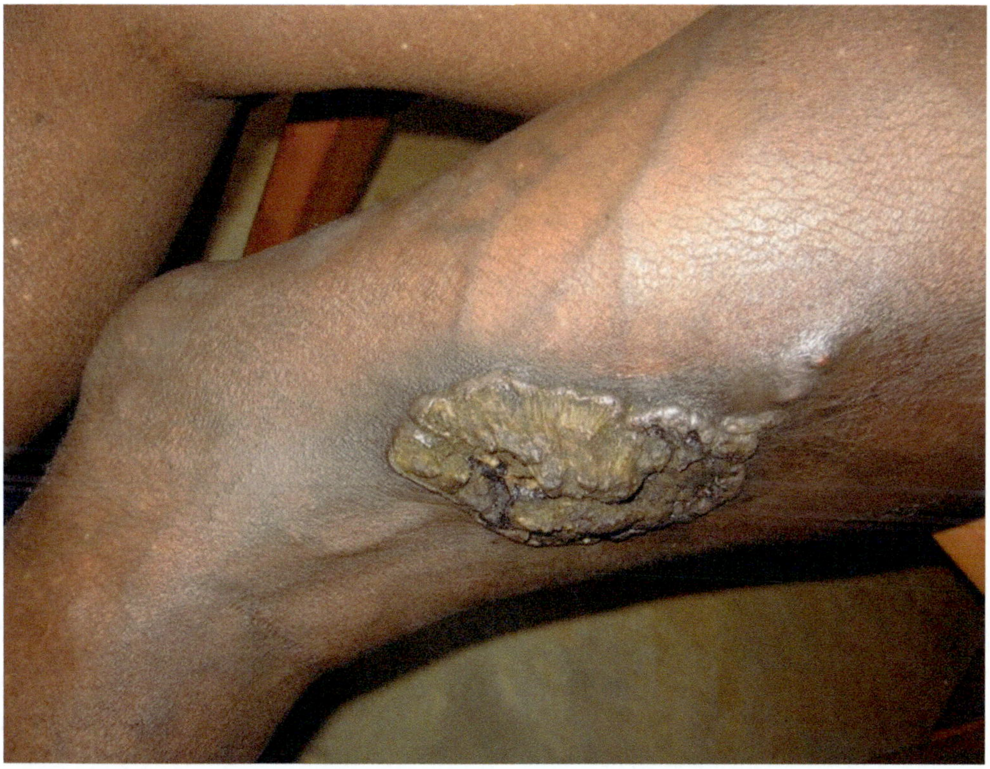

Fig. 36.2 Progressed hyperkeratotic *squamous cell carcinoma* of the leg in a Tanzanian male

technological advances should allow educational efforts to reach a larger part of the population. While black-skinned individuals, Asians, and Hispanics are less prone to develop skin cancer, the difficulty in making early diagnosis and a relative lack of effort to protect themselves from the sun make educational efforts important in these populations.

36.2 Malignant Melanoma

Melanoma is a malignant tumor (MM) that arises from melanocytes and leads to most skin cancer deaths. Despite a rising incidence rate observed worldwide in white Caucasians during the last four decades [19], the occurrence of MM in black-skinned populations has been stable. The incidence rates among black-skinned and Hispanic populations in the USA are far lower than in a white non-Hispanic population, 1.02 and 4.66 vs. 31.58/100,000, respectively [20]. Melanoma incidence rates were found increased in local US registries over the past two decades by 3.0–3.6% per year among non-Hispanic whites and 0.9–3.4% among white Hispanics while remaining relatively stable among the black-skinned population [21, 22]. However, significantly higher proportions of advanced MM are diagnosed in non-Hispanic black-skinned patients and in Hispanics than in non-Hispanic whites [23]. Overall, the number of new MM cases during 2009–2013 in the USA was 21.8/100,000 per year; an additional number of cases may remain unreported to cancer registries since MM is mostly diagnosed in hospital settings [24, 25]. Although the incidence of MM in pigmented dark or black skin is low as compared to Caucasians, it seems that MM is more likely to be late diagnosed in skin of color. A retrospective analysis on MM patients with known stage and ethnicity found that late-stage diagnosis was more common among Hispanic (26%) and non-Hispanic black-skinned patients (52%), as compared to patients with white skin (16%) [26]. Another analysis demonstrated that both males and females Hispanics had a larger proportion of thick lesions; tumors thicker than 1.5 mm accounted for 24.4% of the tumors among white males, but 35.4% among Hispanic males. The increase of incidence among Hispanic population was not a result of increased screening or changing classification [27].

Risk factors for developing MM are high exposure to sunlight, chronic cumulative dosages of UV radiation, and factors of the carrier such as family history of melanoma, increased number of nevi, presence of dysplastic nevi and freckling, fair skin complexion with light eyes and/or red hair, and number of sunburns [28]. In non-Caucasians some risk factors are controversial: in a large cohort study, the risk factors for MM were examined and showed that age, male sex, and susceptibility to sunburn phenotypes may be predictive of MM risk also in non-white populations [29]. In another study the incidence of MM was associated with increased UV index and lower latitude only in non-Hispanic whites, but not in black-skinned or Hispanic populations [30]. However, data from six US states that represented 73% of the total Hispanic and 77% of the total black population revealed a positive association of MM with UV exposure in whites, blacks, and Hispanics [31]. Individuals with skin type IV have more thymine dimers after repeated exposure to a minimal erythema dose (MED) than individuals with less pigmented skin type II; darker skin types also have better thymine dimer repair suggesting that a tan may not be a major factor in natural photoprotection [32].

In a study on 165 benign and malignant melanocytic skin tumors from a cohort of black-skinned Africans, low frequencies of BRAF and NRAS mutations were detected [33]. Nodular melanomas were found mutated for BRAF in 29%, SSMs in 24%, and LMMs in 15%; in contrast, only 8% of melanomas in black-skinned Africans showed mutations in different mutational localizations. No NRAS mutations were present in MM from black-skinned Africans [34]. In addition, 68% acral melanomas were found *cyclin D1* positive compared to 33% of non-acral tumors [35]. The melanocortin-1-receptor gene *(MC1R)* as a key regulator of skin pigmentation may also play a role, since darker pigmented Caucasians, i.e., subjects with no freckles, no red hair, and skin type III/IV and carriers of *MC1R*, had a 66% higher risk of developing melanoma [36].

Acral Lentiginous Melanoma (ALM) is the most common subtype of malignant melanoma in populations with pigmented skin, whereas the frequency of *superficial spreading melanoma* (SMM) clearly prevails among white Caucasians. ALM is a pigmented lesion localized on the extremities, particularly on palms and soles, characterized by lentiginous radial growth evolving into vertical invasive growth after months or years. Particularly its prolonged course indicates that ALM should be distinguished as a distinctive MM subtype. Overall, ALM accounts for less than 10% of all cutaneous MM in Caucasians, mostly in the elderly. This percentage is significantly higher in patients with black skin in Africa and a higher incidence is also registered in Asians [37]. Despite the fact that the overall MM incidence in populations with pigmented or black skin is low, ALM makes up a much higher proportion in MM patients with pigmented skin. ALM was diagnosed in 36% of all melanomas in black-skinned Africans, 18% in Asian Pacific islanders, and 9% in Hispanic whites but only 1% in non-Hispanic whites [38]. The prognosis of ALM is poor; some authors assume that ALM represents a biologically more aggressive melanoma [37]; however, it seems that the particular location is overlooked, and the tumor is late diagnosed. Non-white patients have thicker tumors at the initial presentation and are diagnosed at more advanced stages resulting in worse prognosis. In addition, ALM may mimic benign disease and be often misdiagnosed [39]. In a recent study in Mexico, the median Breslow Index of ALMs registered was 5.2 mm [40]; in another retrospective study on 15 melanoma cases in Nigeria, the lower limbs and feet were the most common anatomic site; the tumors were diagnosed at stage III or later, most of them in females [41]. Also in a retrospective analysis on 175 melanoma patients in South Africa, the overall prognosis of black-skinned MM patients was poor due to late presentation; only 30 patients survived longer than 3 years [42].

Particularly in hot climate zones, physicians serving populations with pigmented or black skin should carefully examine palms and soles to introduce early surgical intervention.

36.2.1 Pathogenesis

ALM often occurs in non-sun-exposed areas, with preferred localization in plantar skin. More than 60% of all ALMs are located on the feet followed by subungual sites, suggesting that trauma may be important in the pathogenesis since the sole of the foot is constantly exposed to pressure, friction, maceration, and irritation. In retrospective studies in which a trauma history was taken, a considerable number of patients reported prelesional trauma such as puncture wounds, stone bruises, friction blisters, contact dermatitis, etc. As an argument against the significance of trauma, it may be considered that the hand is exposed to more UV light and acute trauma. Another factor that may favor the frequent plantar location is that the higher density of melanocytes in the soles than in the palms. The classical risk factors for melanoma, such as fair skin type, sun exposure, blistering sunburn in infancy, and family or personal history of previous melanoma, seemed to be less important in patients with ALM [43]. No significant relation of the incidence of ALM to UV overexposure has been registered, and no correlation to genetic traits is presently known.

Nevertheless, ALM seems to harbor more and different genetic changes than other MM subtypes; KIT (18%), NRAS (14.5%), and BRAF (16%) mutations have been reported to be associated with acral lentiginous melanoma [44]. BRAF and NRAS mutations were significantly more common in females with ALMs located on the feet, compared with KIT mutated tumors which were more frequent at subungual sites. Clinicopathological features such as age at diagnosis, thickness, ulceration, histological subtype, and Clark's level showed no significant correlation with the mutational status.

36.2.2 Clinical Features

ALM is presented on the palms, soles, and subungual sites, predominantly in elderly patients 50–70 years old, showing slight female preponderance (Figs. 36.3 and 36.4). The hands are more often the location of subungual tumors with the first toe or finger most often involved. Foot tumors were usually found on weight-bearing surfaces, suggesting that pressure may play a pathogenetic role, possibly in relation with heat or repeated trauma. Recent reports on the pivotal role of the NUAK2 oncogene in ALM [45] might support this theory.

Subungual melanomas evolve slowly and often present as longitudinal melanonychia, being frequently misdiagnosed as benign malformation. Not all melanomas on volar and subungual localization are of the acral lentiginous type; SSMs and nodular or unclassifiable subtypes may also occur. In 124 subungual MM cases from the Sydney Melanoma Unit, 66% were of the acral lentiginous type, 25% on the great toe. Subungual melanoma in situ has been reported in a child, developed simultaneously on both thumbs and presented as longitudinal melanonychia. The finding of a parallel ridge pattern on dermoscopy may aid the diagnosis of early lesions of acral melanoma in situ. Also *melanomas of the nail matrix* can present as longitudinal melanonychia or as hyperpigmentation extending onto the hyponychium and beyond the proximal and lateral nail folds (*Hutchinson sign*).

Melanonychia is rare in Caucasians but is frequently seen in populations with pigmented ethnic skin as a manifestation of chronic trauma, onychomycosis, or after oral use of drugs, and pregnancy is a physiologic cause of longitudinal melanonychia in dark-skinned females. Nevertheless, the diagnosis of melanoma should be considered for all pigmented nail bands especially if they are heavily pigmented having irregular features and measure >3 mm in size.

36.2.3 Management

Aside from the availability in countries with dark-skinned populations, therapeutic options for MM depend upon the stage of the tumor at diagnosis. Self-awareness and education on examining suspicious moles and body areas including palms and soles are therefore important for early diagnosis and introduction of proper management in skin of color. Standard treatment for less invasive early-stage MM is the complete surgical excision with safety margins and further monitoring. Wide surgical excision is the preferred modality with safety margins established: 5 mm margin for surgical excision of melanoma in situ, 1 cm for all melanomas less than 2 mm thick, and 2 cm safety margin for thicker tumors [46]. Sentinel node biopsy in patients with tumors thicker than 1 mm is a common procedure and regional lymph node dissection may be necessary. Alternative surgical techniques like Mohs surgery may be an option in selected cases. Progressed stages of MM belong to specialized centers; stage IV cutaneous MM is considered incurable [47].

Today, new potent immunotherapies for advanced MM with CTLA-4 inhibitors (i.e., ipilimumab) and PD-1 inhibitors (i.e., nivolumab, pembrolizumab), as well as targeted therapies with BRAF and MEK inhibitors (i.e., vemurafenib and cobimetinib or dabrafenib and trametinib) for tumors

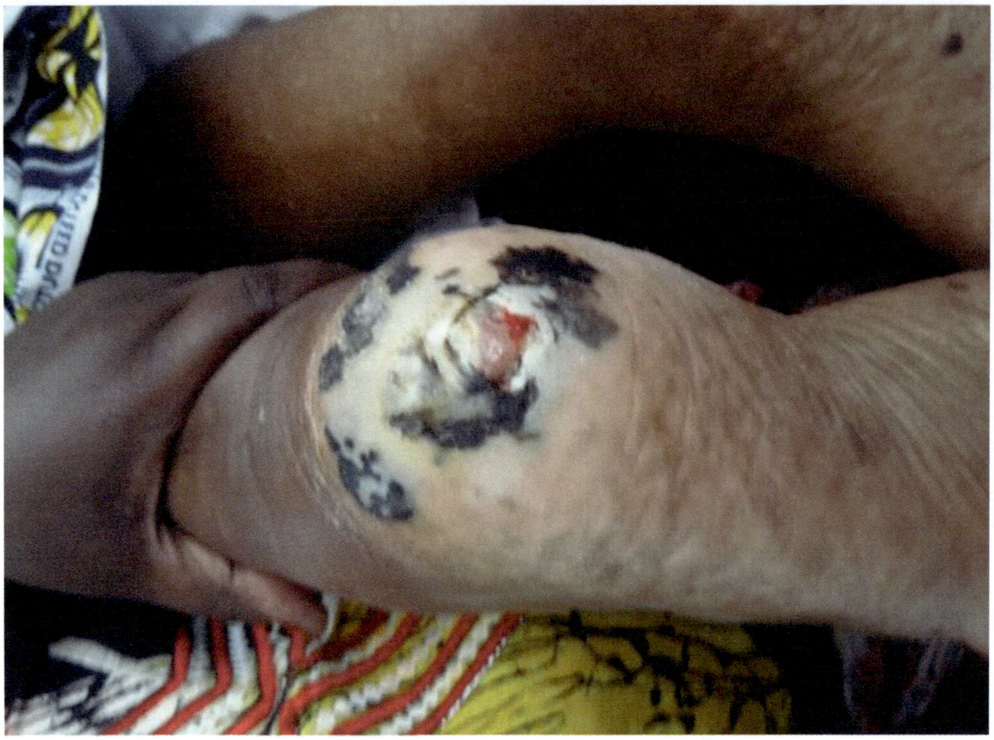

Fig. 36.3 Widely spreading *acrolentiginous malignant melanoma* (ALM) in an African female (Rwanda)

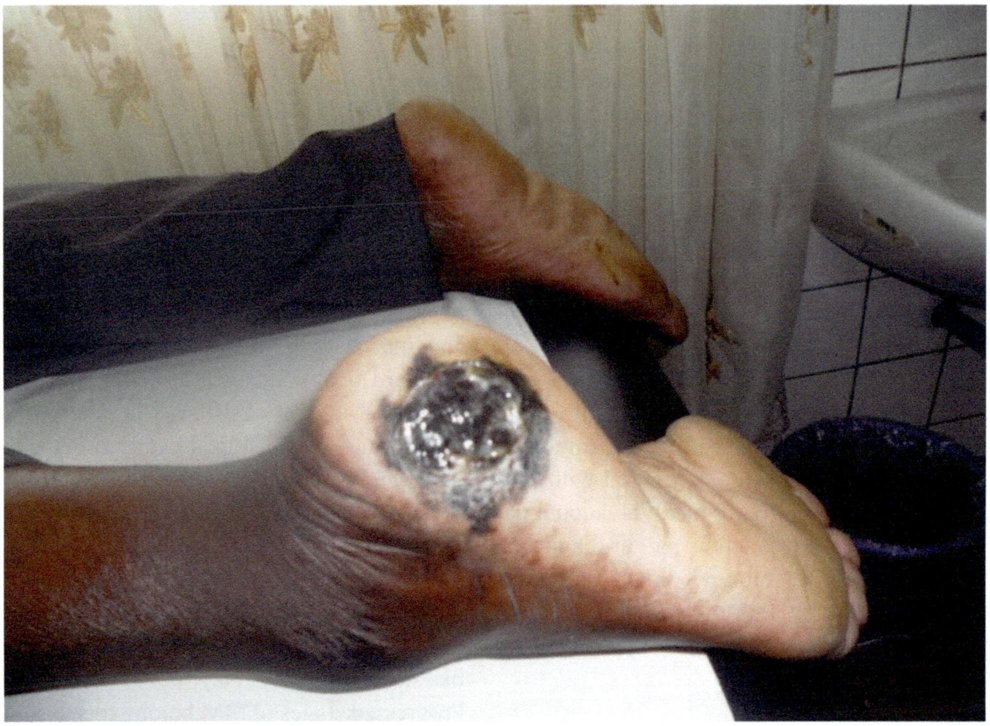

Fig. 36.4 Invasive, partly ulcerated *acrolentiginous malignant melanoma* (ALM) in a 58-year-old African male (Rwanda)

with BRAF mutations, have opened new horizons prolonging survival. These modalities have become a cornerstone in modern MM management.

36.3 Cutaneous Lymphoma

Cutaneous lymphomas represent clonal proliferations of neoplastic T or B lymphocytes and rarely of NK cells or plasmacytoid dendritic cells, recognized as heterogeneous groups of extranodal lymphomas with distinct variability in their clinical characteristics. Primary cutaneous lymphomas often show different clinical course and prognosis as compared to systemic lymphomas which may also involve the skin. Definition and classification of these entities are rapidly changing as knowledge grows. Lymphoid neoplasias are currently best classified by the WHO Classification of Neoplastic Diseases of the Hematopoietic and Lymphoid Tissues, which primarily categorizes the entities according to lineage and a combination of morphology, immunophenotype, genetic features, and clinical criteria [48].

The annual incidence of primary cutaneous lymphomas is estimated 0.5–1/100,000 [49]. Secondary cutaneous lymphomas are rarely seen, showing a clinically uniform picture despite their different histopathologic and morphologic features. Among ethnic groups, the age adjusted incidence rate was found highest for black-skinned individuals and lowest for Asians [50], with males twice as likely to get cutaneous lymphoma as females; this is a consistent finding among ethnic groups. Advanced age and black skin were found associated with poorer survival in patients with cutaneous lymphoma [51].

36.3.1 Pathogenesis

The group of cutaneous lymphomas is too heterogeneous to be pooled into a single pathogenetic concept. For many years, cutaneous T cell lymphomas (CTCL) were thought of as neoplasms following chronic antigen stimulation in which an initial inflammatory response leads to T-cell proliferation and to the emergence of a malignant clone [52]. However, the etiology remained unknown despite much effort given to identify a common causative antigen. A viral etiology for CTCL has been an attractive hypothesis given the similarities with adult T-cell lymphoma/leukemia associated with HTLV-1 infection. However, the results of studies to determine any association between cutaneous lymphoma and HTLV-1 remained contradictory. Epstein-Barr virus (EBV) has also been proposed as a pathogen based on its association with other lymphoproliferative disorders such as Burkitt's lymphoma. The possibility that EBV infection can lead to the proliferation and activation of T-cells in the epidermis has been suggested. Bacterial infections have also been implicated in the pathogenesis of CTCL, suggesting an association of *Staphylococcus aureus*; several studies suggested that *S. aureus* superantigen enterotoxins could provide or potentiate lymphocytic infiltration and chronic antigenic stimulation leading to T-cell clonal expansion.

Occupational risk factors may also play a causative role, since indolent dermatitis often precedes the diagnosis of skin lymphoma. Exposure to carcinogens in the professional environment could provide the chronic antigenic stimulation needed to initiate clonal expansion. Occupational exposure to chemicals considered hazardous was recorded in 30% of patients in a Mycosis Fungoides Study Group. Even though the hypothesis that cutaneous T-cell lymphoma is a disease due to chronic antigenic stimulation with ultimate emergence of a malignant T-cell clone still remains well established, the etiology of CTCL including the discovery of possible initiating events has yet to be determined [53].

36.3.2 Cutaneous T-Cell Lymphomas

Cutaneous T-cell lymphomas (CTCL) are non-Hodgkin malignancies characterized by a dominant skin-homing T-cell clone; they represent approximately 80% of all cutaneous lymphomas.

Mycosis fungoides: Mycosis fungoides (MF) is characterized by the development of patches progressing to plaques and tumors. Patients may simultaneously have more than one type of lesions [54]. In early patch stage MF, there are single or multiple, erythematous, well-defined scaly macules and patches of varying size, mostly in non-sun-exposed sites and intertriginous areas. The eruption may be asymptomatic or slightly pruritic; it occasionally regresses spontaneously without scarring. In history, a preceding "chronic dermatitis" is often mentioned, diagnosed as resistant contact dermatitis, atopic dermatitis, psoriasis, or eczema. Patches may last for months or years before progressing to sharply demarcated, scaly, and variably indurated plaques. Pruritus is often intense, resulting in excoriation, exudation, and secondary changes that may dominate the clinical picture. Hyper- and/or hypopigmented lesions and poikiloderma may occur; large plaques with annular, arcuate, or serpiginous borders are seen, developing into tumors. In progressed stages ulcerations occur (Figs. 36.5 and 36.6). Erythroderma may start de novo or follow, presenting as melanorythroderma in

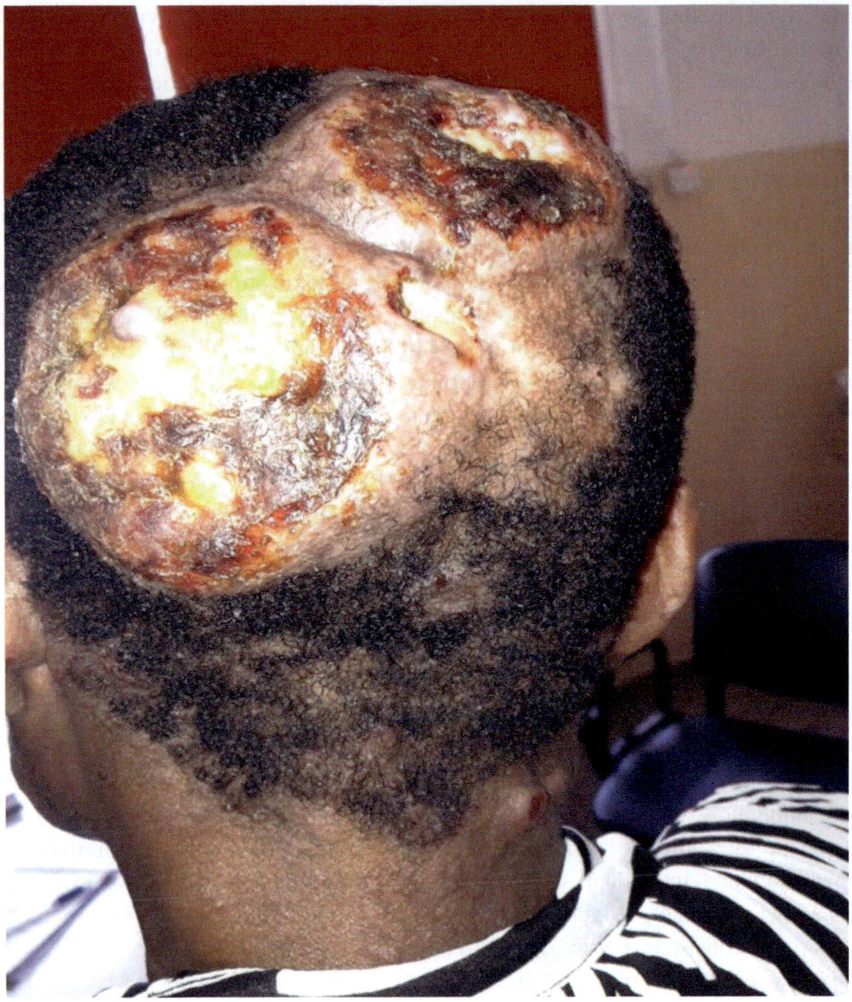

Fig. 36.5 Ulcerated *cutaneous T-cell lymphoma* (tumor stage mycosis fungoides) on the head of an African female patient (courtesy by Dr. J. Aryee-Boi, Ghana)

pigmented skin. The lesions are diffusely bright red with readily apparent scaling, but there may be characteristic symmetric islands of uninvolved skin. Constitutional symptoms such as fever, chills, weight loss, malaise, insomnia secondary to the overwhelming pruritus, and poor body temperature homeostasis occur with progressing disease. Hyperkeratosis, scaling and fissuring of palms and soles, alopecia, ectropion, nail dystrophy, and ankle edema may accompany the skin lesions. Differential diagnosis of classical MF toward Sézary syndrome is essential for treatment and prognosis [55].

Folliculotropic MF represents a distinct variant with preferential involvement of head and neck by folliculotropic T-cell infiltrates, with or without mucinous degeneration of the hair follicles. It occurs mostly in adults, but may occasionally affect children and adolescents. Patients present with grouped follicular papules, acneiform lesions, indurated plaques, and rarely tumors, which usually involve the head and neck region. The occurrence of alopecia, pruritus, and secondary bacterial infection is common. Infiltrated plaques in the eyebrows with concurrent alopecia are a common and highly characteristic finding. Involvement of the face may lead to leonine facies with marked accentuation of facial folds. Differential diagnosis includes lepromatous leprosy, sarcoidosis, and leishmaniosis. Unlike in classical MF, pruritus is often severe.

MF patients often develop hypopigmented lesions, a variant of early patch-type MF representing a most common feature of the disease in populations with pigmented ethnic skin. Responses to management introduce repigmentation [56].

Sézary syndrome: Sézary syndrome is a leukemic variant of CTCL, which occurs exclusively in adults. It is characterized by a triad consisting of diffuse erythroderma (melanoerythrodema

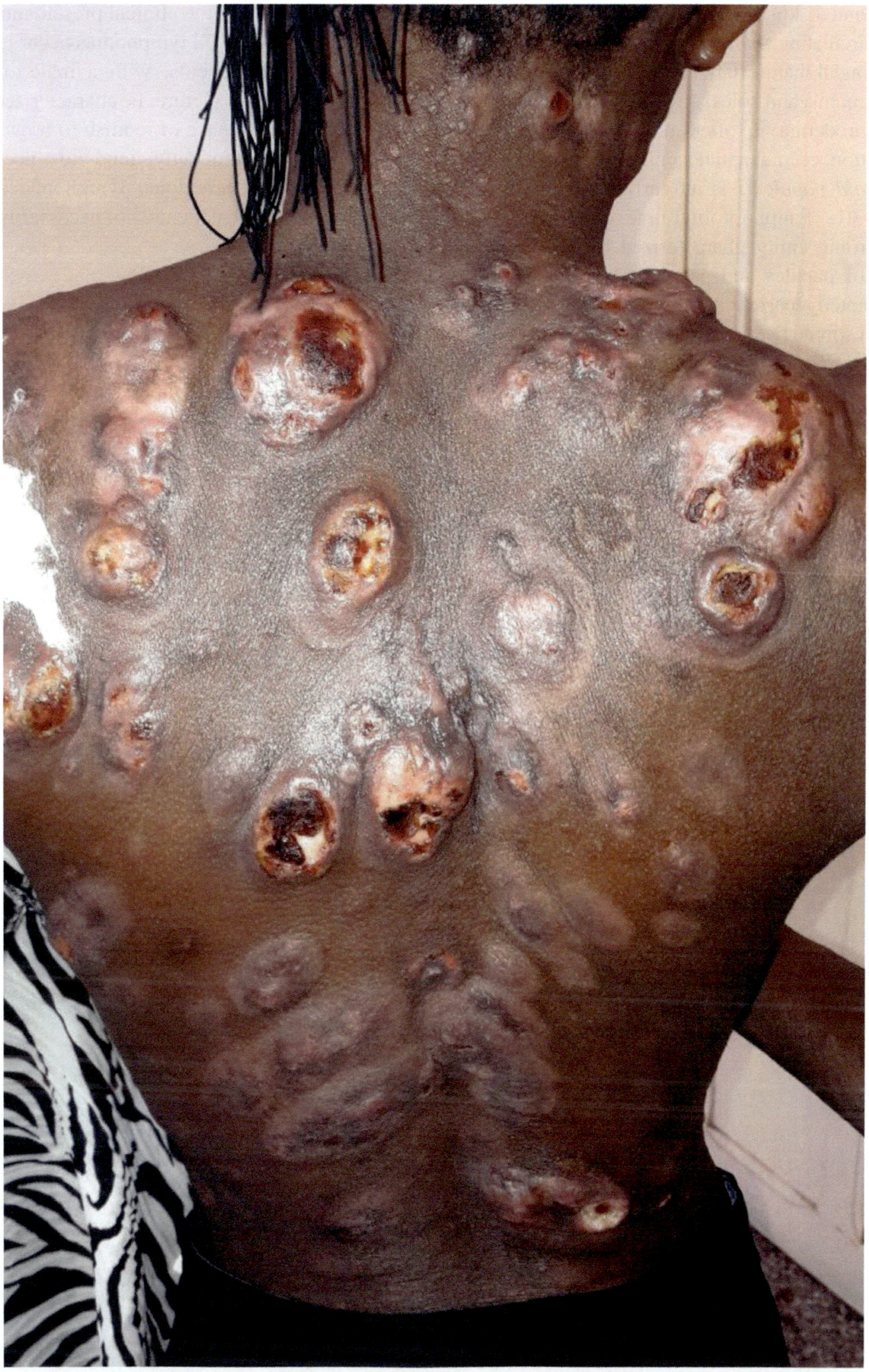

Fig. 36.6 Progressed *cutaneous T-cell lymphoma*: Tumor-stage *mycosis fungoides* on the back of an African female patient (courtesy by Dr. J. Aryee-Boi, Ghana)

in darker pigmented skin, Fig. 36.7), generalized lymphadenopathy, and circulating malignant T-cells with cerebriform nuclei [57]. Clinical manifestations include severe scaling or fissuring of the palms and soles, alopecia, and onychodystrophy. The erythroderma is often pruritic, associated with marked exfoliation, edema, and lichenification.

Lymphomatoid papulosis is an early described primary cutaneous CD30+ lymphoproliferative disorder [58], an uncommon chronic entity characterized by recurrent self-healing crops of papules and papulonodules. Clinically, it shows disseminated recurrent self-healing papules and papulonodules often spread over a period of months or years. The lesions typically involve the trunk and extremities and may be in various stages of evolution. The disease has a benign clinical course with a 10-year survival rate of nearly 100%. However, in 10–20% of the patients, lymphomatoid papulosis can precede, coexist with, or progressively develop into malignant lymphoma such as MF, Hodgkin, or nodal anaplastic large T-cell lymphoma.

Anaplastic large T-cell lymphoma consists of large tumor cells most of them expressing the CD30 antigen, with no evidence or history of MF or another CTCL type. Irrespective of the morphology of the tumor cells (anaplastic, immunoblastic, or pleomorphic), the clinical presentation and course are identical. CD30+ T-cell lymphomas occur in adults, rarely in children and adolescents, with a male-to-female ratio of 1.5:1. The clinical picture is characterized by solitary or locoregional occurrence of reddish to brownish nodules and tumors, which frequently tend to ulcerate. Secondary involvement of the regional lymph nodes is observed in roughly 25% of the patients, not necessarily associated with unfavorable prognosis.

36.3.3 Cutaneous B-Cell Lymphomas

B-lymphocyte-derived lymphomas (CBCL) may develop in the skin without systemic involvement at the time of diagnosis, comprising around 20% of all cutaneous lymphomas. They are mostly indolent in contrast to nodal B-cell malignancies [59].

Follicle center lymphoma is a neoplasm of clonal centrocytes and centroblasts with or without formation of follicular centers. Patients present non-scaling, solitary, or grouped papules, thick plaques, or tumors. Occasionally, annular erythema can be observed in the surrounding area. Typical localization is the head and neck region (Figs. 36.8 and 36.9).

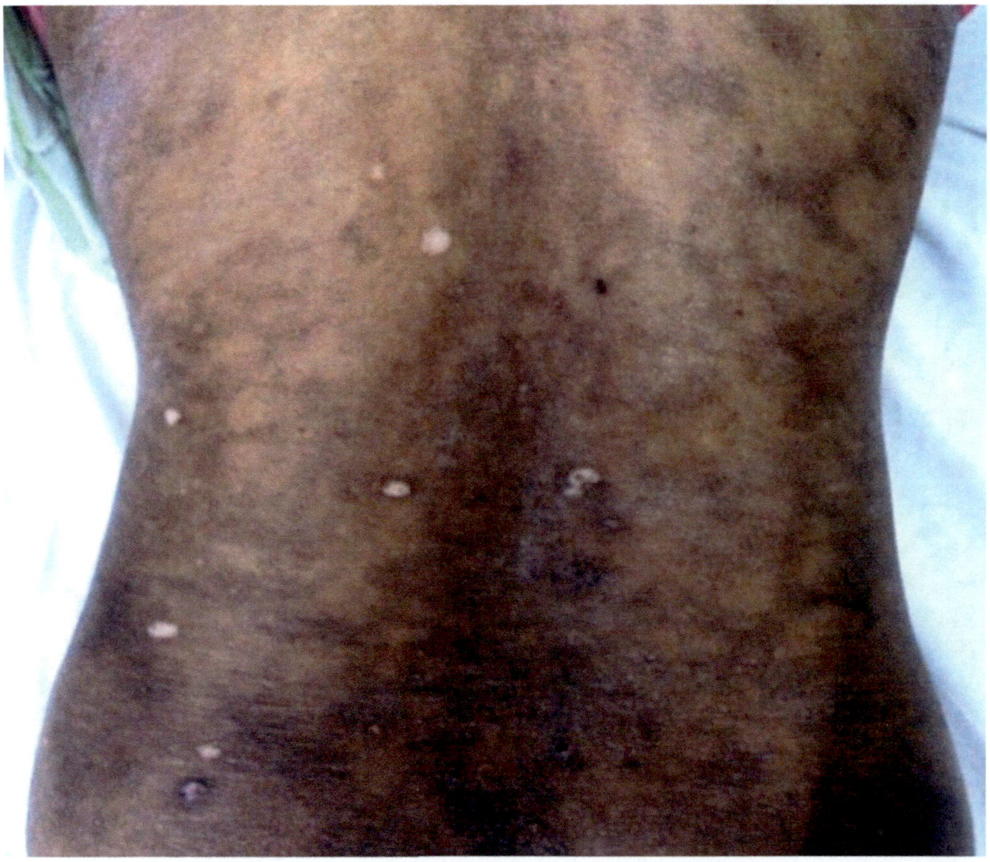

Fig. 36.7 Generalized *melanoerythroderma* in a patient with *Sézary syndrome*. Note several depigmented scars due to intractable pruritus

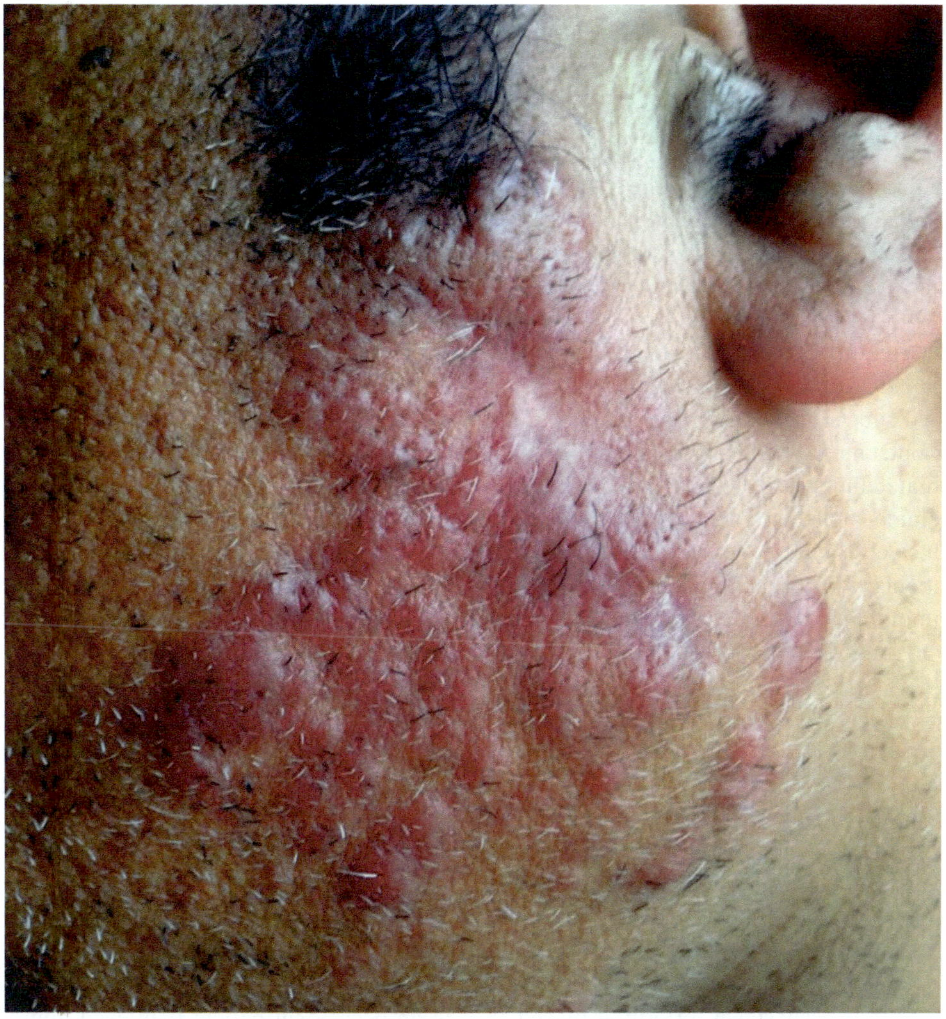

Fig. 36.8 Lesions of *primary cutaneous B-cell lymphoma (Primary cutaneous follicle center lymphoma, face)*

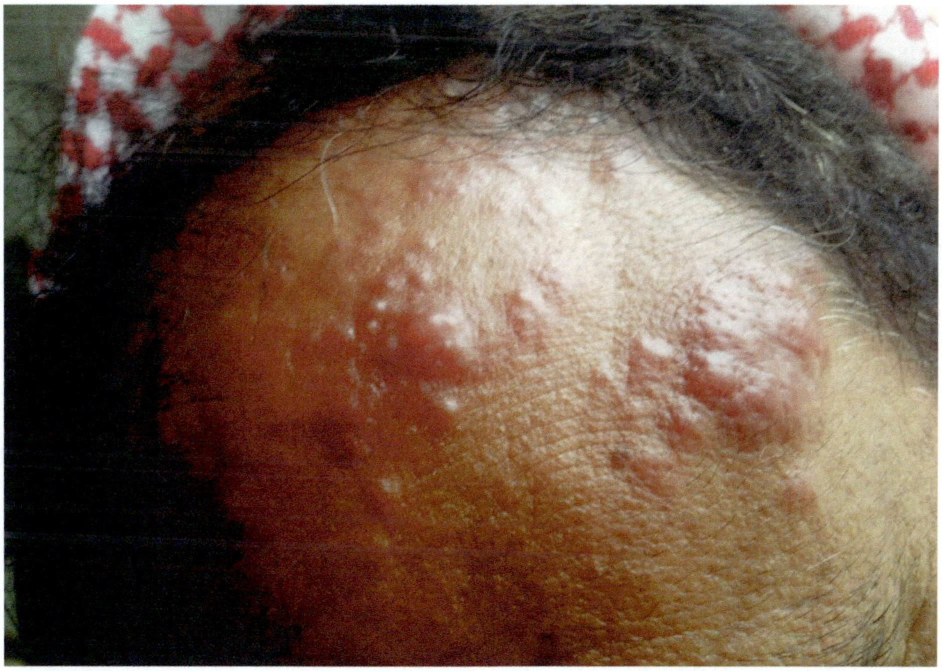

Fig. 36.9 *Primary cutaneous follicle center lymphoma* in a patient of Arab origin showing confluent papules and nodules on the forehead

The skin lesions increase in size over the years, but extracutaneous dissemination is uncommon, showing an estimated 5-year survival of 97%.

Marginal zone lymphoma is a neoplastic proliferation of small lymphocytes, lymphoplasmacytoid cells, and plasma cells, initially localized in the marginal zone of follicular centers, representing around 25% of all CBCL. The tumors commonly occur on the upper extremities or the trunk of adults with a median age of 55 years, preferably in females. Patients present with small red to violaceous papules, plaques, or nodules, frequently in multifocal localization.

Diffuse Large B-cell lymphoma, leg type: this type has been identified as a distinct clinical entity mainly because of its perceived poor outcome compared with other CBCL. It shows an intermediate clinical course with solitary or clustered bluish erythematous plaques and tumors composed of large B-cells exclusively localized on the legs. It usually affects elderly patients with a predominance of females. Ulceration is common. Only in rare cases other cutaneous sites than the legs are involved.

36.3.4 Management

In most cases a presumptive diagnosis can be made based on clinical examination. Histological, immunohistological, and, if available, molecular biological tissue investigations are required to define the exact type of lymphoma and introduce strategies for proper management [60, 61]. As a rule, treatment of CTCL is "stage-adapted," well distinguished from treatment of CBCL [62]. In early stages, priority is placed on local schedules such as topical corticosteroids, together with UVB or PUVA phototherapies. In patients with strictly localized disease, radiation management may also lead to long-term control. In advanced stages combinations of PUVA with retinoids or recombinant interferon-α are often successful. Monochemotherapy regimes with gemcitabine or liposomal doxorubicin are preferable to polychemotherapies [63].

36.4 Cutaneous Leiomyoma

Leiomyomas are benign soft tissue neoplasms that arise from smooth muscles. They can develop wherever a smooth muscle is present, both in Caucasians and in populations with darkly pigmented or black skin. Cutaneous localization is the second commonest after the uterus which accounts for 95% of all cases; cutaneous leiomyomas account for 75% of the extra-uterine leiomyomas [64]. Clinicopathologic data with special reference to multiple cutaneous leiomyomas and their relation to renal cell cancer are focused in the recent literature. It seems that both disorders result from heterozygous germline mutations in the fumarate hydratase gene [65, 66]. Cutaneous leiomyomas are relatively uncommon neoplasms; their exact incidence is not known [66]. Angioleiomyomas appear to occur more frequently than cutaneous of pilar origin [67], whereas genital leiomyomas are the least common variant. Comorbidity with uterine myomatosis may occur in females.

The exact pathogenesis of the tumor has yet to be determined. Cutaneous leiomyomas are thought to arise from the smooth muscle cells within the arrector pili of the pilosebaceous unit in the skin. Leiomyomas of the external genitalia are probably derived from the network of smooth muscles in the scrotum, vulva, and also areolae. Angioleiomyomas are believed to originate from the smooth muscle within the walls of arteries and veins.

Multiple pilar leiomyomas may occur sporadically or be inherited in an autosomal dominant fashion with variable penetrance, as a component of a cutaneous and uterine leiomyomatosis; they are also referred to as Reed's syndrome [68], a rare autosomal dominant disorder caused by mutations of the fumarate hydratase gene. Although the molecular basis of the syndrome is well known, it is not clearly understood how this translates into smooth muscle tumors.

36.4.1 Clinical Features

Cutaneous pilar leiomyomas can be solitary or multiple and in an occasional patient may even number in the hundreds. They present as firm, reddish-brown to skin-colored painful papules or nodules, 1–2 cm in diameter. Solitary pilar leiomyomas develop primarily during adulthood, both in men and women [69]; however, in a recent study on Indian population, male preference has been reported [70]. Most cutaneous leiomyomas usually develop solitary or multiple on the extremities and trunk, especially the shoulder (Fig. 36.10). Leiomyomas are often associated with spontaneous pain, pain induced by pressure or following cold exposure. Also rare congenital or pediatric cases in early childhood have been reported. When multiple, the distribution pattern is often clustered, linear, or along Blaschko's lines.

Since patients with multiple leiomyomas are predisposed to develop renal cell carcinoma, screening for excluding renal tumor is recommended. It is noted that dermatologists should be aware that correct evaluation of a patient with cutaneous leiomyomas involves a complete medical and family history, physical examination, and genetic counseling [71].

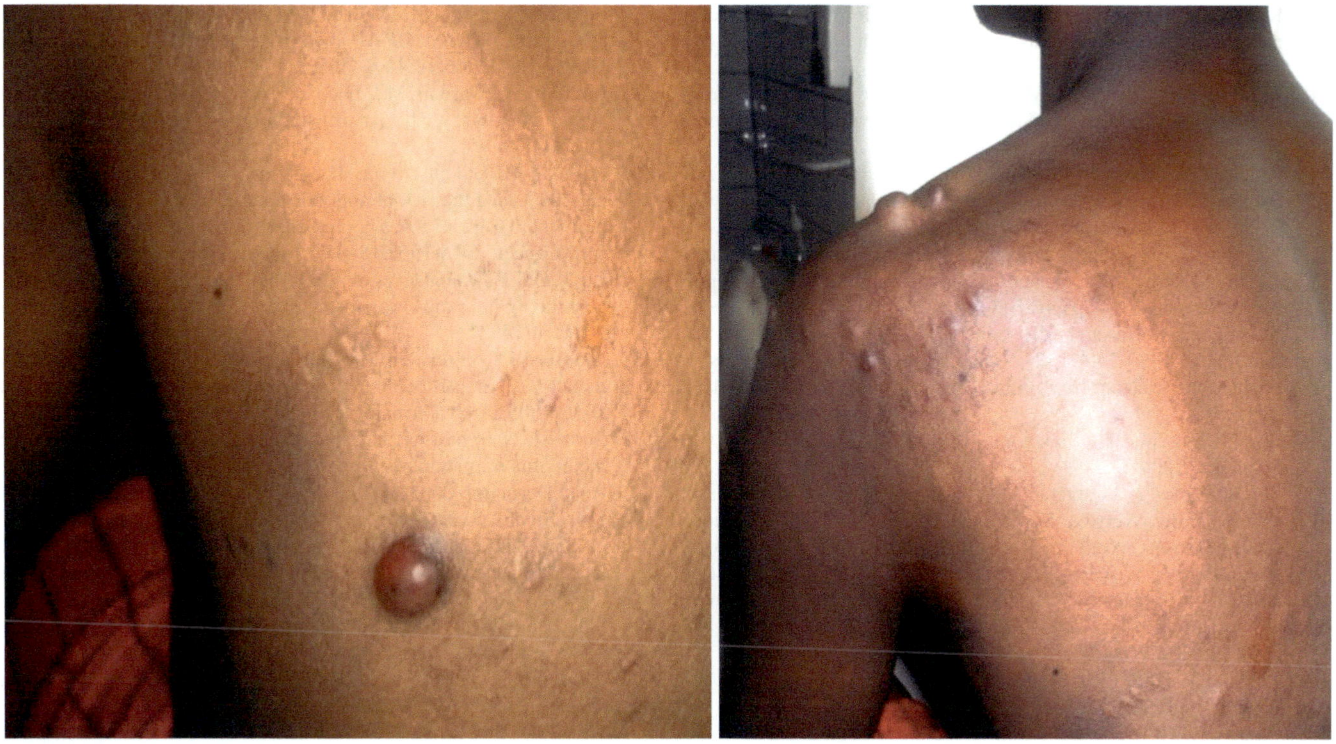

Fig. 36.10 Solitary *nodular cutaneous leiomyoma* (left); segmental pattern of *multiple, clustered cutaneous leiomyomas* on the left shoulder, also disseminated on the trunk in a Rwandan male (right)

36.4.2 Management

Surgical excision is usually curative for solitary or limited tumors. If not amenable to surgery because of number or location, treatment with gabapentin will provide relief from pain. Alternative medications that may reduce smooth muscle contraction are nifedipine, nitroglycerin, and doxazosin; also, cryotherapy or CO_2 laser ablation may be beneficial [72, 73]. The present experience with mitotically active leiomyomas is limited. There are no definitive criteria for distinguishing mitotically active leiomyomas from leiomyosarcomas, and there is significant overlap between the two entities. It would, therefore, appear prudent to completely excise mitotically active leiomyomas [74].

References

1. Ridky TW. Nonmelanoma skin cancer. J Am Acad Dermatol. 2007;57:484–501.
2. Lomas A, Leonardi-Bee J, Bath-Hextall F. A systematic review of worldwide incidence of non melanoma skin cancer. Br J Dermatol. 2012;166:1069–80.
3. Brenner M, Hearing VJ. The protective role of melanin against UV damage in human skin. Photochem Photobiol. 2008;84:539–49.
4. Rubin A, Chen EH, Ratner D. Basal-cell carcinoma. N Engl J Med. 2005;353:2262–9.
5. Gloster HM, Neal K. Skin cancer in skin of color. J Am Acad Dermatol. 2006;55:741–60.
6. Byrd-Miles K, Toombs EL, Peck GL. Skin cancer in individuals of African, Asian, Latin American, and American-Indian descent: differences in incidence, clinical presentation, and survival compared to Caucasians. J Drugs Dermatol. 2007;6:10–6.
7. Rogers HW, Weinstok MA, Feldman SR, et al. Incidence estimate of nonmelanoma skin cancer (keratinocyte carcinomas) in the U.S. population, 2012. JAMA Dermatol. 2015;151:1081–6.
8. Asgari MM, Moffet HH, Ray GT, et al. Trends in basal cell carcinoma incidence and identification of high-risk subgroups, 1998-2012. JAMA Dermatol. 2015;151:976–81.
9. Gallagher RP, Hill GB, Bajdik CD, et al. Sunlight exposure, pigmentary factors, and risk of non melanocytic skin cancer. I. Basal cell carcinoma. Arch Dermatol. 1995;131:157–63.
10. Armstrong BK, Kricker A. The epidemiology of UV induced skin cancer. J Photochem Photobiol B. 2001;63:8–18.
11. Lear JT, Tan BB, Smith AG, et al. Risk factors for basal cell carcinoma in the UK: case-control study in 806 patients. J R Soc Med. 1997;90:371–4.
12. Agbai ON, Buster K, Sanchez M, et al. Skin cancer and photoprotection in people of color: a review and recommendations for physicians and the public. J Am Acad Dermatol. 2014;70:748–62.
13. Halder RM, Bridgeman-Shah S. Skin cancer in African Americans. Cancer. 1995;75(suppl):667–73.

14. Kundu RV, Patterson S. Dermatologic conditions in skin of color: part I. Special considerations for common skin disorders. Am Fam Physician. 2013;87:850–6.
15. Kimonis VE, Goldstein AM, Pastakia B, et al. Clinical manifestations in 105 persons with nevoid basal cell carcinoma syndrome. Am J Med Genet. 1997;69:299–308.
16. Kulkarni P, Brashear R, Chuang TY. Nevoid basal cell carcinoma syndrome in a person with dark skin. J Am Acad Dermatol. 2003;49:332–5.
17. Halpern AC, Kopp LP. Awareness, knowledge and attitudes to nonmelanoma skin cancer and actinic keratosis among the general public. Int J Dermatol. 2005;44:107–11.
18. Montague M, Borland MR, Sinclair C. Slip! Slop! Slap! And SunSmart, 1980-2000: skin cancer control and 20 years of population-based campaigning. Health Educ Behav. 2001;28: 290–305.
19. Garbe C, Leiter U. Melanoma epidemiology and trends. Clin Dermatol. 2009;27:3–9.
20. SEER*Explorer: An interactive website for SEER cancer statistics [Internet]. Beta Version. Surveillance Research Program, National Cancer Institute. Available from http://seer.cancer.gov/explorer/.
21. Hu S, Parmet Y, Allen G, et al. Disparity in melanoma: a trend analysis of melanoma incidence and stage at diagnosis among whites, Hispanics, and blacks in Florida. Arch Dermatol. 2009;145:1369–74.
22. Rouhani P, Hu S, Kirsner RS. Melanoma in Hispanic and black Americans. Cancer Control. 2008;15:248–53.
23. Clairwood M, Ricketts J, Grant-Kels J, et al. Melanoma in skin of color in Connecticut: an analysis of melanoma incidence and stage at diagnosis in non-Hispanic blacks, non-Hispanic whites, and Hispanics. Int J Dermatol. 2014;53:425–33.
24. Watson M, Johnson CJ, Chen VW, et al. Melanoma surveillance in the United States: overview of methods. J Am Acad Dermatol. 2011;65(suppl 1):S6–16.
25. Cartee TV, Kini SP, .Chen SC: Melanoma reporting to central cancer registries by US dermatologists: an analysis of the persistent knowledge and practice gap. J Am Acad Dermatol, 2011; 65(suppl 1): S124–S325.
26. Hu S, Soza-Vento RM, Parker DF, et al. Comparison of stage at diagnosis of melanoma among Hispanic, black, and white patients in Miami-Dade County. Florida Arch Dermatol. 2006;142:704–8.
27. Cockburn MG, Zadnick J, Deapen D. Developing epidemic of melanoma in the Hispanic population of California. Cancer. 2006;106:1162–8.
28. Tucker MA, Goldstein AM. Melanoma etiology: where are we? Oncogene. 2003;22:3042–52.
29. Park SL, Le Marchand L, Wilkens LR, et al. Risk factors for malignant melanoma in white and non-white/non-African American populations: the multiethnic cohort. Cancer Prev Res (Phila). 2012;5:423–34.
30. Eide MJ, Weinstock MA. Association of UV index, latitude, and melanoma incidence in nonwhite populations-US surveillance, epidemiology, and end results (SEER) program, 1992 to 2001. Arch Dermatol. 2005;141:477–81.
31. Hu S, Ma F, Collado-Mesa F, et al. UV radiation, latitude, and melanoma in US Hispanics and blacks. Arch Dermatol. 2004;140:819–24.
32. Tadokoro T, Kobayashi N, Zmudzka BZ, et al. UV-induced DNA damage and melanin content in human skin differing in racial/ethnic origin. FASEB J. 2003;17:1177–8.
33. Akslen LA, Puntervoll H, Bachmann IM, et al. Mutation analysis of the EGFR-NRAS-BRAF pathway in melanomas from black Africans and other subgroups of cutaneous melanoma. Melanoma Res. 2008;18:29–35.
34. Saldanha G, Potter L, Daforno P, et al. Cutaneous melanoma subtypes show different BRAF and NRAS mutation frequencies. Clin Cancer Res. 2006;12:4499–505.
35. Ibrahim ZA, Narihan MZ, Ojep DN, et al. Cyclin D1 expression in acral melanoma: a case control study in Sarawak. Malays J Pathol. 2012;34:89–95.
36. Pasquali E, García-Borrón JC, Fargnoli MC, et al. MC1R variants increased the risk of sporadic cutaneous melanoma in darker-pigmented Caucasians: a pooled-analysis from the M-SKIP project. Int J Cancer. 2015;136:618–31.
37. Lu J, Dai B, Kong Y, et al. Acral melanoma in Chinese: a clinicopathological and prognostic study of 142 cases. Sci Rep. 2016;6(31432)
38. Bradford PT, Goldstein MA, Master ML, et al. Acral lentiginous melanoma: incidence and survival patterns in the United States, 1986-2005. Arch Dermatol. 2009;145:427–34.
39. Soon SL, Solomon AR Jr, Papadopoulos D, et al. Acral lentiginous melanoma mimicking benign disease: the Emory experience. J Am Acad Dermatol. 2003;48:183–8.
40. Lino-Silva LS, Domínguez-Rodríguez JA, Aguilar-Romero JM, et al. Melanoma in Mexico: clinicopathologic features in a population with predominance of acral lentiginous subtype. Ann Surg Oncol. 2016;23:4189–94.
41. Seleye-Fubara D, Etebu EN. Histological review of melanocarcinoma in Port Harcourt. Niger J Clin Pract. 2005;8:110–3.
42. Lodder JV, Simson W, Becker PJ. Malignant melanoma of the skin in black south Africans: a 15-year experience. S Afr J Surg. 2010;3:76–9.
43. Phan A, Touzet S, Dalle S, et al. Acral lentiginous melanoma: a clinicoprognostic study of 126 cases. Br J Dermatol. 2006;155:561–9.
44. Zebary A, Omholt K, Vassilaki I, et al. KIT, NRAS, BRAF and PTEN mutations in a Swedish sample with acral lentiginous melanoma. J Dermatol Sci. 2013;72:284–9.
45. Namiki T, Coelho SG, Hearing VJ. NUAK2: an emerging acral melanoma oncogene. Oncotarget. 2011;2:695–704.
46. Haigh P, DiFronzo L, McCready D. Optimal excision margins for primary cutaneous melanoma: a systematic review and meta-analysis. Can J Surg. 2003;46:419–26.
47. Agarwala SS. Current systemic therapy for metastatic melanoma. Expert Rev Anticancer Ther. 2009;9:587–95.
48. Willemze R, Jaffe ES, Burg G, et al. WHO-EORTC classification for cutaneous lymphomas. Blood. 2005;105:3768–85.
49. Criscione VD, Weinstock MA. Incidence of cutaneous T-cell lymphoma in the United States 1973-2002. Arch Dermatol. 2007;143:854–9.
50. Weinstock MA, Gardstein B. Twenty-year trends in the reported incidence of mycosis fungoides and associated mortality. Am J Public Health. 1999;89:1240.
51. Weinstock MA, Reynes JF. The changing survival of patients with mycosis fungoides: a population-based assessment of trends in the United States. Cancer. 1999;85:208–12.
52. Kim EJ, Hess S, Richardson SK, et al. Immunopathogenesis and therapy of cutaneous T cell lymphoma. J Clin Invest. 2005;115: 798–812.
53. Litvinov IV, Shtreis A, Kobayashi K, et al. Investigating potential exogenous tumor initiating and promoting factors for cutaneous T-cell lymphomas (CTCL), a rare skin malignancy. Oncoimmunology. 2016;5:e1175799.
54. Hwang ST, Janik JE, Jaffe ES, et al. Mycosis fungoides and Sézary syndrome. Lancet. 2008(9616); 371:945–57.
55. Vonderheid EC, Bernengo MG, Burg G, et al. Update on erythrodermic cutaneous T-cell lymphoma: report of the International Society for Cutaneous Lymphomas. J Am Acad Dermatol. 2002;46: 95–106.

56. Akaraphanth R, Douglass MC, Lim HW. Hypopigmented mycosis fungoides: treatment and a 6.5-year follow-up of 9 patients. J Am Acad Dermatol. 2000;42:33–9.
57. Möbs M, Knott M, Fritzen B, et al. Diagnostic tools in Sezary syndrome. G Ital Dermatol Venereol. 2010;145:385–91.
58. Macaulay WL. Lymphomatoid papulosis. A continuing self-healing eruption, clinically benign - histologically malignant. Arch Dermatol. 1968;97:23–30.
59. Bekkenk MW, Geelen FA, van Voorst Vader PC, et al. Primary and secondary cutaneous CD30(+) lymphoproliferative disorders: a report from the Dutch cutaneous lymphoma group on the long-term follow-up data of 219 patients and guidelines for diagnosis and treatment. Blood. 2000;95:3653–61.
60. Wilcox RA. Cutaneous B-cell lymphomas: 2016 update on diagnosis, risk-stratification, and management. Am J Hematol. 2016;91:1052–5.
61. Assaf C, Hummel M, Steinhoff M, et al. Early TCR-beta and TCR-gamma PCR detection of T-cell clonality indicates minimal tumor disease in lymph nodes of cutaneous T-cell lymphoma: diagnostic and prognostic implications. Blood. 2005;105:503–10.
62. Möbs M, Cerroni L, Flaig MJ, et al. Molecular diagnostics in cutaneous lymphomas. J Dtsch Dermatol Ges. 2013;11(suppl 4):25–35.
63. Trautinger F, Eder J, Assaf C, et al. European organisation for research and treatment of Cancer Consensus recommendations for the treatment of mycosis fungoides/Sézary syndrome - update 2017. Eur J Cancer. 2017;77:57–74.
64. Newman PL, Fletcher CD. Smooth muscle tumours of the external genitalia: clinicopathological analysis of a series. Histopathology. 1991;18:523–9.
65. Smit DL, Mensenkamp AR, Badeloe S. Hereditary leiomyomatosis and renal cell cancer in families referred for fumarate hydratase germline mutation analysis. Clin Genet. 2011;79:49–59.
66. Badeloe S, van Geel M, van Steensel MA, et al. From gene to disease; cutaneous leiomyomatosis. Ned Tijdschr Geneeskd. 2007;151:300–4.
67. Fletcher CDM. Soft tissue tumors. In: Fletcher CDM, editor. Diagnostic histopathology of tumors. 3rd ed. Philadelphia: Churchill Livingstone; 2007. p. 1527–93.
68. Badeloe S, Frank J. Clinical and molecular genetic aspects of hereditary multiple cutaneous leiomyomatosis. Eur J Dermatol. 2009;19:545–51.
69. Raj S, Calonje E, Kraus M, et al. Cutaneous pilar leiomyoma: clinicopathologic analysis of 53 lesions in 45 patients. Am J Dermatopathol. 1997;19:2–9.
70. Malhotra P, Walia H, Singh A, et al. Leiomyoma cutis: a clinopathological series of 37 cases. Indian J Dermatol. 2010;55:337–41.
71. Rongioletti F, Fausti V, Ferrando B, et al. A novel missense mutation in fumarate hydratase in an Italian patient with a diffuse variant of cutaneous leiomyomatosis (Reed's syndrome). Dermatology. 2010;221:378–80.
72. Thompson JA Jr. Therapy for painful cutaneous leiomyomas. J Am Acad Dermatol. 1985;13:865–7.
73. Christenson LJ, Smith K, Arpey CJ. Treatment of multiple cutaneous leiomyomas with CO2 laser ablation. Dermatol Surg. 2000;26:319–22.
74. Kim G. Multiple cutaneous and uterine leiomyomatosis (Reed's syndrome). Dermatol Online J. 2005;11:21.

HIV-Infection and Associated Dermatoses

37

Baraka M. Chaula

The skin as the largest body organ is an important marker for an underlying HIV infection. There is a broad spectrum of skin symptoms and diseases that can be seen arising as a result of the underlying infection and progressing severity of the disease, enabling the dermatologist to make early diagnosis. Depending on the immune status of the patient, various cutaneous manifestations occur. While the majority of them improve as the immune status stabilizes, some may present a paradox by either worsening or clinically becoming more apparent. Drugs used to treat HIV, such as the highly active antiretroviral management (HAART), can themselves lead to significant side effects that manifest on the skin.

37.1 Epidemiology

Since the beginning of the twenty-first century, significant progress has been made in saving millions of people dying from HIV/AIDS. A number of strategies have been put in place to end HIV/AIDS being a public health threat. In a global level, there are currently 36.7 million people living with HIV, and 1.8 million children less than 15 years are among them. In 2015 2.1 million people with 150,000 children were newly infected. AIDS-related deaths stood at 1.1 million with children constituting 110,000 deaths globally. The countries in sub-Saharan Africa with 25.5 million HIV-infected people living in this region remain the hardest hit area; among 5700 new HIV infections occurring every day, approximately 66% are in sub-Saharan Africa. There are 5300 adults aged 15 years and older, with women making around 47%, young people (15–24 years old) 35%, and young women (15–24 years old) 20% of the total [1]. The number of HIV-infected people on antiretroviral management between years 2010 and 2016, has increased from 7.5 million to 18.2 million, with approximately 12 million people living in sub-Saharan Africa. The United Nations targets by 2020 to have fewer than 500,000 new infections, with fewer than 500,000 AIDS-related deaths and zero discrimination [1]. Despite the tremendous efforts done so far, there are still challenges to be addressed. A significant number of countries still pose restrictions on HIV-related travels, while for others, same sex sexual relationship is considered a criminal offense. Combined efforts with adequate funding, social awareness, and political leadership willingness are crucial for effective prevention and treatment success to combat the deadly global HIV pandemic.

B. M. Chaula
Dermatology Unit, Department of Internal Medicine,
Mbeya Zonal Referral Hospital, Mbeya, Tanzania

37.2 Clinical Spectrum of HIV-Associated Dermatoses

The skin diseases arising in HIV-infected patients vary in their clinical picture and course. Their atypical clinical presentation is an important marker for the attending physician to suspect the underlying infection, take all necessary precautions and measures to confirm the diagnosis, and manage the patient, particularly in individuals with pigmented skin [2].

37.2.1 Inflammatory Dermatoses

One of the commonest skin manifestations in HIV-infected individuals is the *pruritic papular eruption* (PPE). In the tropics, the clinical presentation is that of papular lesions, intensely pruritic, often localized to the extremities [3]. Its pathogenesis is poorly understood and is thought to be a result of exaggerated immune response to arthropod bites [4]. Clinically it presents with monomorphic, hyperpigmented papules on the extensor surfaces of the extremities as well as the trunk; the face and mucous membranes are usu-

C. E. Orfanos et al. (eds.), *Pigmented Ethnic Skin and Imported Dermatoses*, https://doi.org/10.1007/978-3-319-69422-1_37

ally spared. PPE heals with hyperpigmented superficial scars, remaining as an important marker of an underlying HIV infection. Persisting or recurring PPE in patients being on HAART may indicate higher HIV viral load, as a marker of treatment failure [5]. Entities to consider mimicking PPE are *prurigo* and *eosinophilic folliculitis*. *Seborrheic dermatitis* is common in patients with HIV infection. In patients of African origin, it presents with extensive involvement to include the extremities, groin, and also axillae. In patients with short curled hair, greasy and thick yellow crusts are seen, often superinfected. In some cases it can lead to erythroderma and exfoliative dermatitis refractory to standard treatment [6]. *Psoriasis* associated with HIV is more common in white- than in black-skinned patients. It presents across all HIV stages, as frequent as in HIV-negative patients. In black-skinned Africans, psoriasis is one of the commonest causes of erythroderma and exfoliative dermatitis, where the typical erythematous silver scaling seen in white Caucasian skin is less developed. Patients of African descent and advanced HIV infection are more prone to develop papulosquamous *photodermatitis* [7]. It can be observed in up to 5% of all HIV patients with hyperpigmentation in sun-exposed areas. In addition, atypical lesions characterized by *leukoderma* or *vitiligo-like depigmentation*, some affecting the palms and soles, have also been reported [8]. *Xerosis* and *atopic dermatitis* can coexist in patients with HIV infection. Reduced skin lipid content resulting into increase in water is found in the dermis of both HIV and atopic dermatitis as compared to healthy individuals; excessive levels of epidermal carotenoids may potentially predispose HIV patients to premature skin aging [9].

37.2.2 Viral Infections

Infection with human papillomaviruses (HPV) is one of the most common sexually transmitted diseases in African countries. *Plane warts* are the commonest HPV presentation in dark-skinned patients, often seen early in HIV-infected individuals. Flat, hypopigmented papules are presented mostly on the head, face, and neck region (Fig. 37.1a, b). Most patients are unaware of a possible underlying HIV infection, being more concerned with the cosmetic outlook. *Vulgar warts* can be extensive and most disfiguring, presenting as papules or plaques, affecting mostly the extremities (Fig. 37.2). Widely spread disseminated plane and vulgar warts are seen in patients who present themselves late to a medical facility. Genital warts, *condylomata acuminata,* tend to present with fungating, exophytic masses on the genitalia (Fig. 37.3). They may occur across all stages of the disease. HPV infection of the genital mucosa such as the vulva may early present with vaginal discharge, and several patients give a history of having been treated with topical and oral antifungals. *Cervical, penile, and vulval/vaginal cancers* all are an increased risk for both treated and untreated HIV patients and may also arise under immune reconstitution [10]. HAART does not appear to diminish the frequency of premalignancies and malignancies. *Herpes simplex* virus (HSV) is another common viral infection in HIV patients especially with low CD4+ T-cell counts. The anogenital area is often the most affected; lesions tend to be extensive with ulceration and secondary infection in black-skinned patients. Hypertrophic, verrucous, and ulcerous lesions are atypical HSV presentations in HIV-infected individuals. When ulcerative, non-healing lesions of herpes simplex persist, the possibility of HIV association should be considered (Fig. 37.4). *Zoster* is seen due to reactivation of latent infection in patients with HIV. It presents with sudden eruption of painful, grouped vesicles in a single dermatome, preceded by painful non-vesicular rash. Although multidermatomal occurrence is possible, it is not often seen in dark-skinned African patients. Lesions present with vesicles and necrotic lesions with occasional superinfection. Postzosteric long-lasting pain, keloid formation, and skin depigmentation or hyperpigmentation are common sequelae of HIV-associated zoster. Pitting scars and skin depigmentation especially in exposed areas can be stigmatizing signs of an underlying HIV infection. *Mollusca contagiosa* are seen to affect more children than adults. Lesions are widely disseminated in HIV patients mostly on the face. They present as papules with umbilication, which clinically can be mistaken for warts or cryptococcosis. In adults, the lesions can be extensive and disfiguring sometimes covering the entire body.

37.2.3 Fungal Infections

Both superficial and disseminated infections are seen in HIV patients. Among the commonest mucocutaneous fungal infections is *oral candidiasis* (Fig. 37.5). It presents with whitish plaques on the oral cavity, especially the tongue, which on examination can be wiped using a spatula, in contrast to oral *hairy leukoplakia* which cannot be easily removed. Angular or lip cheilitis is an accompanying sign. In pigmented skin, skinfold intertrigo on submammary and inguinal areas characterized by whitish macerated plaques can be seen in immunosuppressed patients. Lesions of dermatophytic infections in HIV patients may be atypical, occasionally appearing as a result of *immune reconstitution inflammatory syndrome* (IRIS) showing extensive inflammatory and hyperpigmented progressive plaques with central desquamation. Paradoxically, such inflammatory lesions tend to occur in

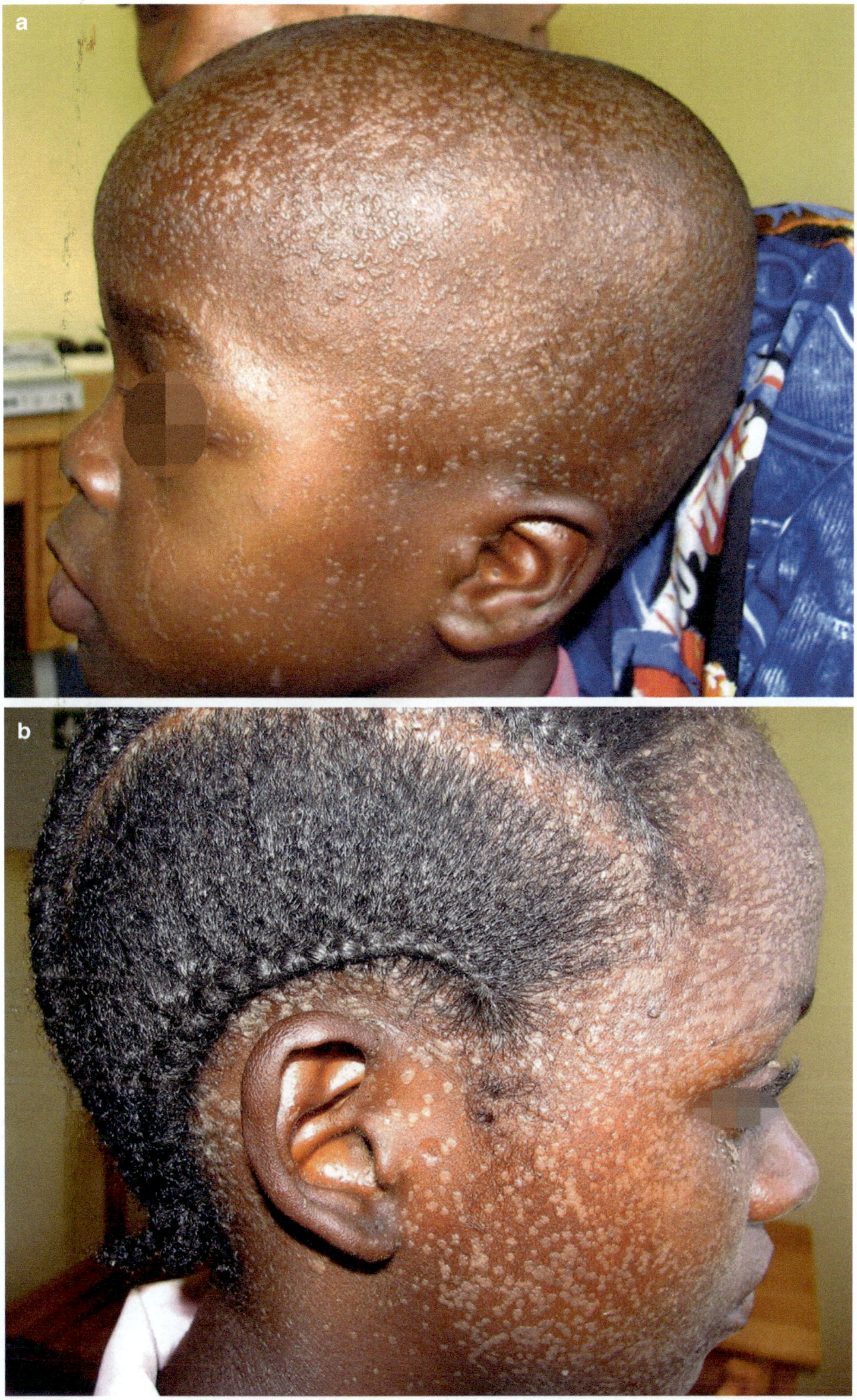

Fig. 37.1 (a, b) Disseminated plane warts in the face and scalp of a HIV-positive young boy and a HIV-positive young girl

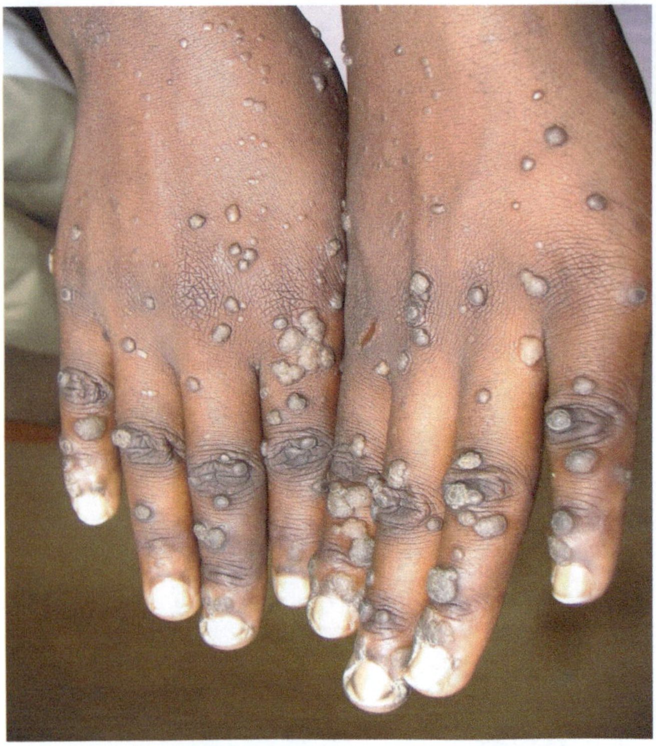

Fig. 37.2 Multiple, acrolocalized *vulgar warts* in an immune-suppressed male

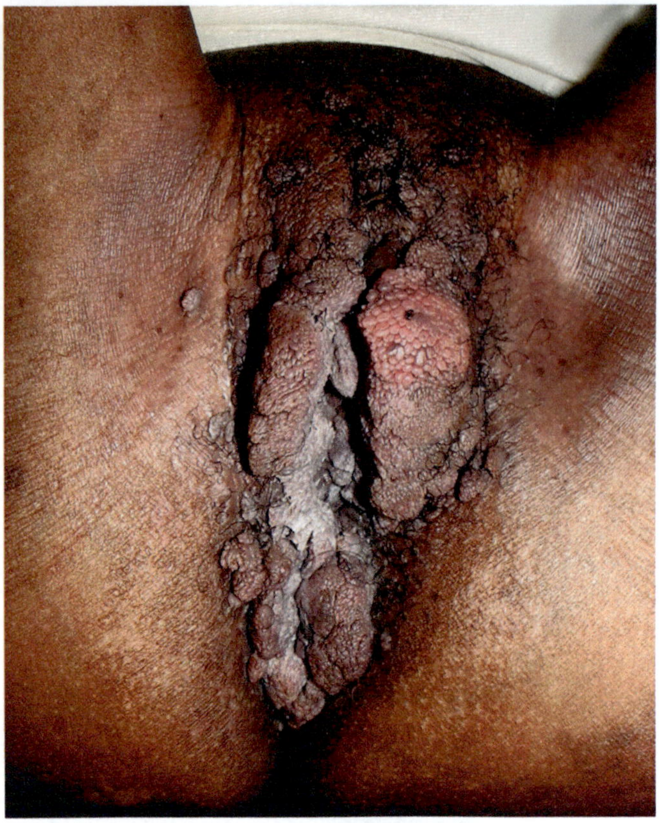

Fig. 37.3 *Giant genital warts* in a HIV-infected 19-year-old female

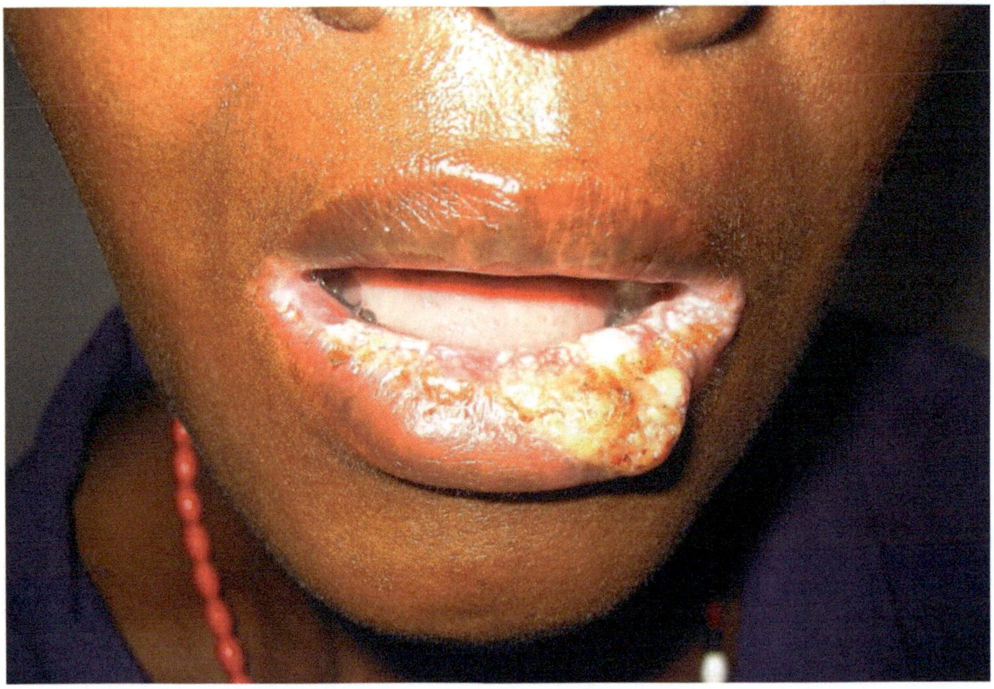

Fig. 37.4 Recurrent, *ulcerous herpes labialis* in a HIV-positive male

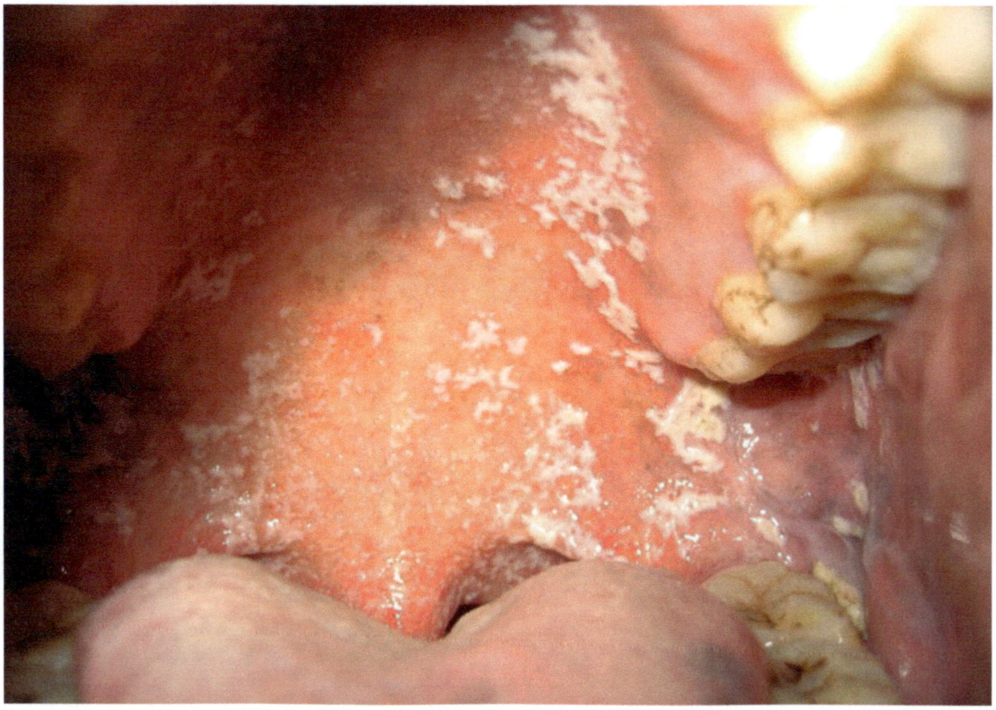

Fig. 37.5 Extensive *oral candidiasis* in early HIV infection

patients who started HIV management at a very low CD4 counts and weeks later unusual skin lesions appear [11]. Lymphocutaneous spread of *sporotrichosis* has been seen in HIV patients. Patients present with multiple nodular or ulcerating lesions on exposed areas such as the head and neck [12]. Opportunistic fungal infections with cutaneous presentation include *penicilliosis*, *cryptococcosis* (Fig. 37.6a, b), and *histoplasmosis* ([13]; Fig. 37.7). Although these organisms occur in geographically endemic areas, they can also be seen in non-endemic. Clinically nodular, dome-shaped, or umbilicated papules appear, mostly with systemic symptoms and fever. Cryptococcosis occurs in HIV patients with CD4+ counts <100/µl and is often lethal.

37.2.4 Bacterial Infections

Commonest presentations are skin infections with *Staphylococcus* and *Streptococcus* species. The clinical picture is diverse and includes impetigo, cellulitis, folliculitis, or abscesses. An important condition to consider in dark-skinned HIV-infected patients is *bacillary angiomatosis*, caused by *Bartonella* species, *B. henselae*, and *B. quintana* [14]. Clinically it presents as multiple, red to deep red or purplish dome-shaped papules and nodules which can be crusted, mostly on the face and extremities. Patient's CD4+ T-cells are usually <200/µl. Although not common, bacillary angiomatosis may clinically and histologically mimic Kaposi's sarcoma (Figs. 37.8 and 37.9). *Syphilis* has been reported to be on the rise coexisting with HIV infection. In contrast to Caucasians, syphilis may be atypical in pigmented skin, showing partly erythematous and/or pigmented macules and papules on the palms and soles (Fig. 37.10). Primary chancre which is usually painless can be painful, accompanied by extragenital chancres. Neurological involvement poses a greater risk in these patients [15, 16]. Clinicians should be aware that macular hyperpigmentation on the soles of dark-skinned patients may occur, not representing syphilis.

37.2.5 Mycobacterial Infections

The prevalence of *human tuberculosis* has clearly increased worldwide and is common in HIV-infected patients; however, cutaneous lesions of tuberculosis occur only rarely. If associ-

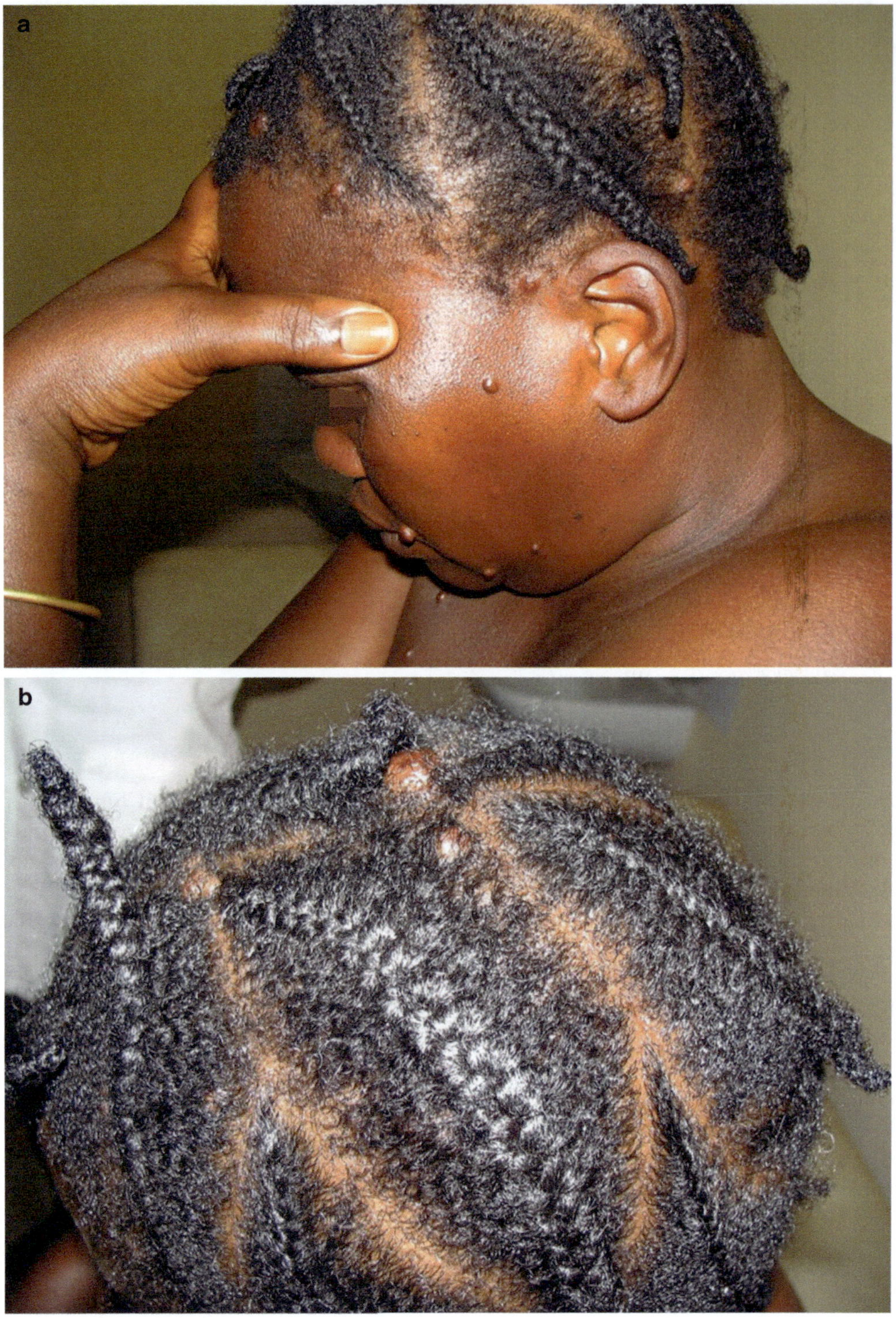

Fig. 37.6 (**a**, **b**) Disseminated nodular lesions of *cutaneous cryptococcosis* in a HIV-infected female (face, scalp)

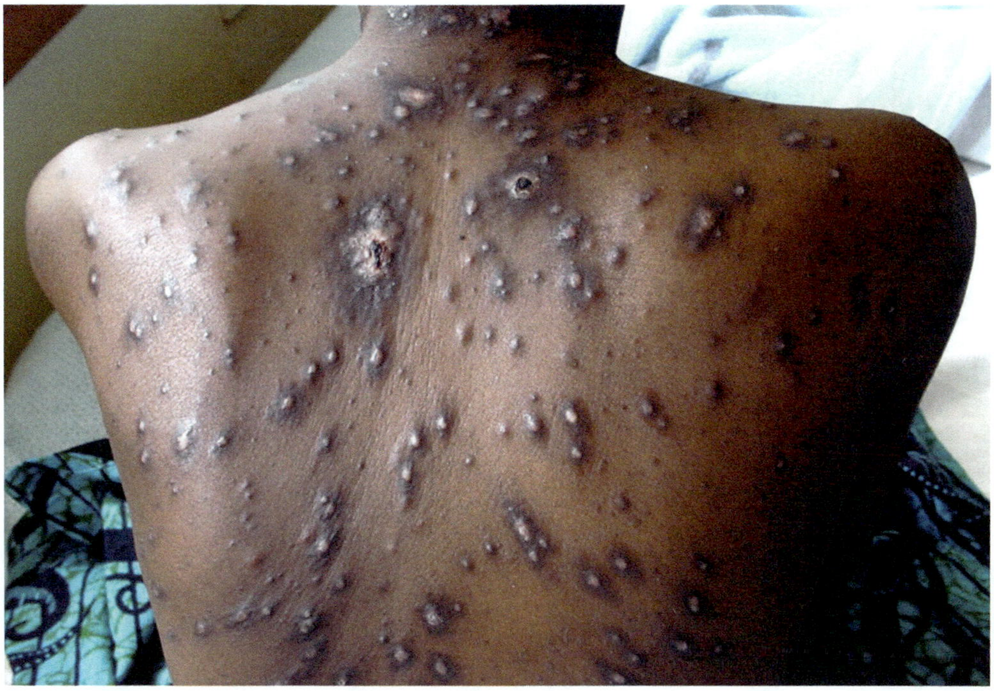

Fig. 37.7 Cutaneous lesions of progressed *histoplasmosis* in a HIV-infected female

ated with HIV, it can mimic other skin conditions. *Scrofuloderma* is the commonest clinical form of presentation, affecting mostly cervical and inguinal areas. Keratotic, hypertrophic, atrophic, ulcerative, or plane lupus vulgaris and other cutaneous manifestations are occasionally seen. Despite its rarity, clinicians in HIV-endemic areas should consider cutaneous tuberculosis in patients presenting atypical skin lesions. Also *leprosy* can coexist with HIV infection. However, HIV does not seem to increase the rate and course of leprosy in HIV-prevalent areas, as compared to tuberculosis. Leprosy may arise as a result of IRIS with type I lepra reaction. Patients present with multiple, well-defined, tender plaques widely distributed over the body, often accompanied by thickened peripheral nerves. In dark-skinned patients, the erythematous appearance is not often seen; instead, hyperpigmentation is the commonest presentation. Cutaneous tuberculosis usually responds to standard antituberculous drugs.

37.2.6 Protozoal Skin Infections

Leishmaniasis is a vector-borne disease in hot climate zones caused by protozoa belonging to the group of *Leishmania* species. It is classified as localized, cutaneous, mucocutaneous, diffuse cutaneous, and visceral leishmaniasis (see Chap. 8). Typical lesions begin as erythematous papules which enlarge to form nodules, undergoing ulceration and crusting. Atypical clinical presentations in HIV-infected patients may appear eczematoid, warty, sporotrichoid, or zosteriform; the diffuse cutaneous form is common. With impaired immunity in HIV, leishmaniasis can be reactivated, promoting HIV replication and thus leading to progression of AIDS [17].

37.2.7 Drug Reactions

In high prevalent areas, HIV-infected patients have increased risk for cutaneous side effects of drugs. Among the most frequent in HIV-infected are lipodystrophy, Stevens- Johnson syndrome, toxic epidermal necrolysis, and gynecomastia (Fig. 37.11a, b; [18]). Nevirapine, used in combination in HIV schedules, is the commonest culprit in causing adverse skin reactions [19].

37.2.8 Neoplasms

HPV-induced *anogenital cancer* is not rarely seen associated with progressed HIV infection, both in females and males (Fig. 37.12). Other body parts apart from the anogenital area may also develop squamous cell carcinomas in HIV-infected

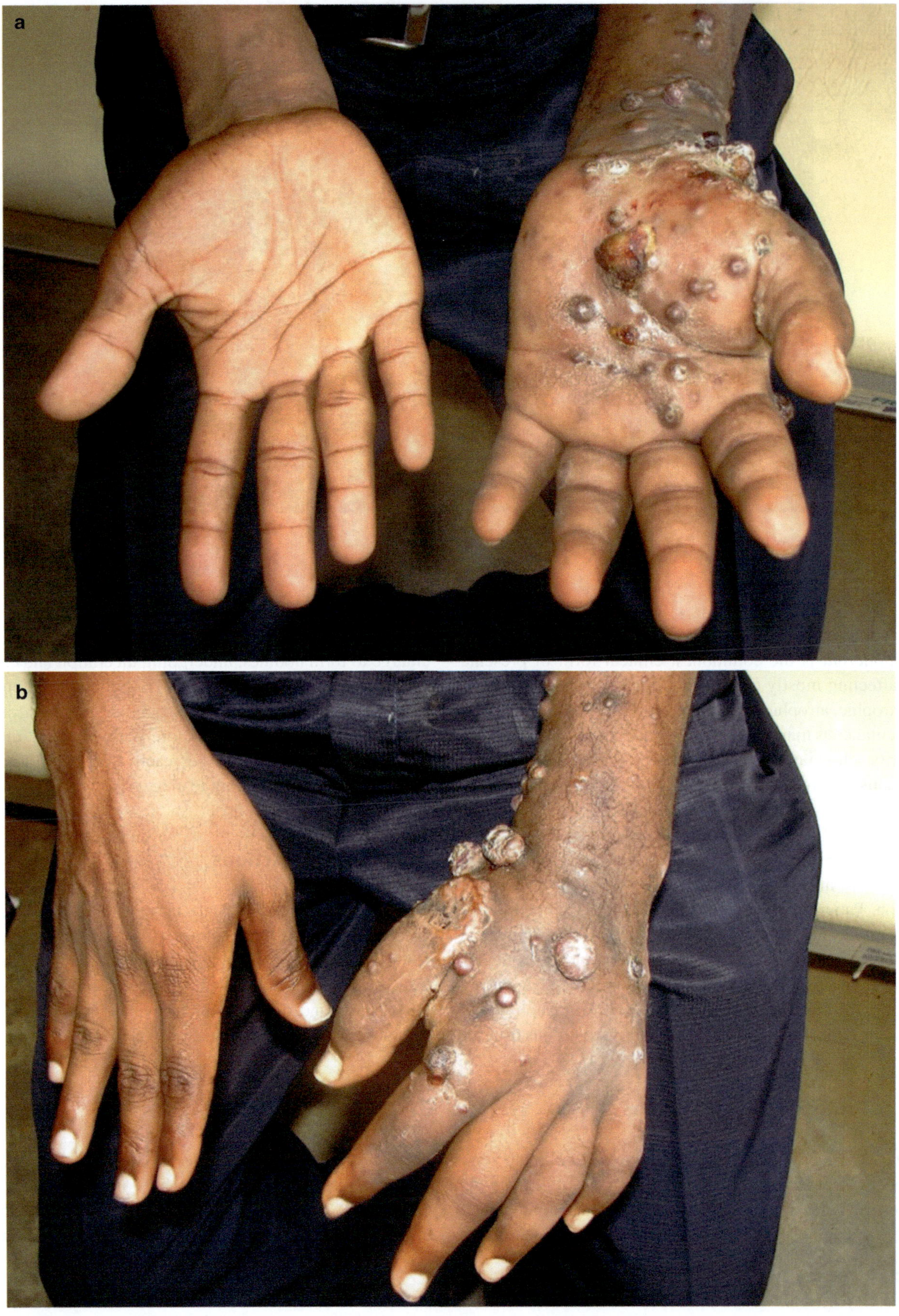

Fig. 37.8 *Acrolocalized, HIV-associated Kaposi's sarcoma* of the left hand with nodular lesions, most likely representing *bacillary angiomatosis*

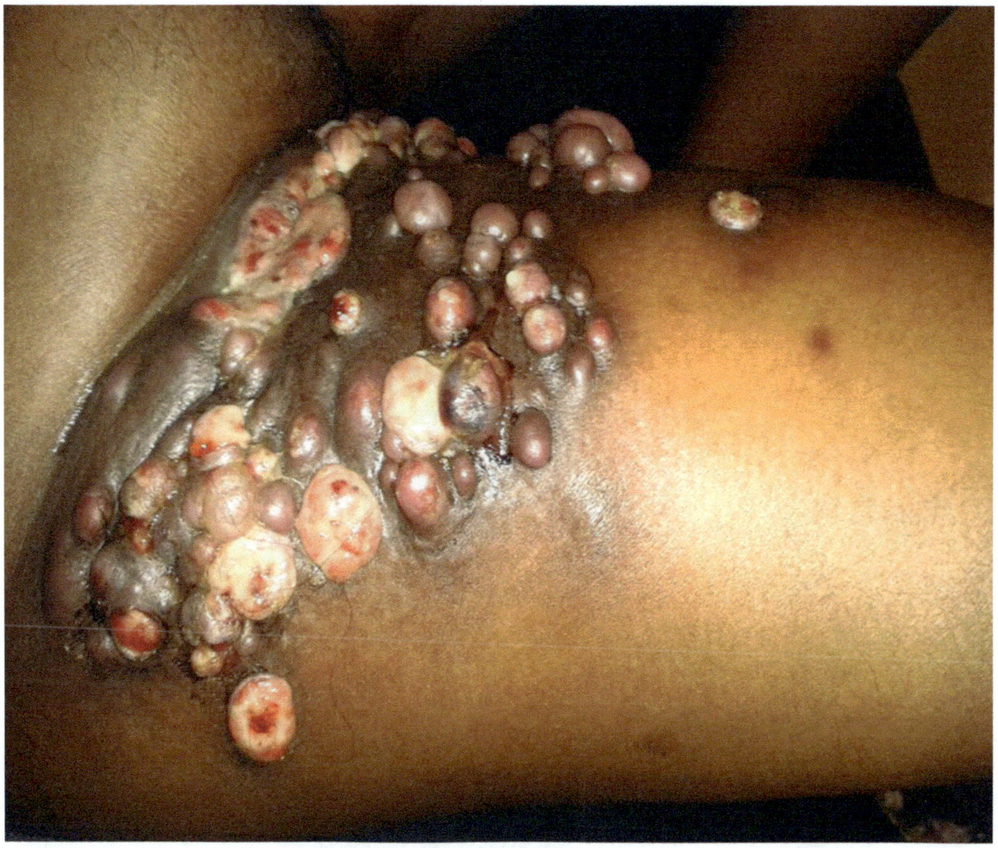

Fig. 37.9 Nodulated papules and plaques of *bacillary angiomatosis*, partly ulcerated, mimicking Kaposi's sarcoma (Courtesy of Dr. B. Sinishaw, Addis Ababa University)

patients [20, 21]. The risk of associated non-Hodgkin lymphoma is lower in Africa compared to that in developed countries [22]. *Kaposi's sarcoma* is the most common associated malignancy in African patients with HIV infection (see Chap. 38).

37.2.9 Disorders of Hair and Nails

Nail abnormalities are common in African patients with HIV infection. Infected patients with abnormal color such as gray/distal banded nails may be associated with low CD4+ T-cell counts [23]. Antiretroviral medications used to treat HIV infection such as zidovudine can result in nail pigmentation showing longitudinal melanonychia and/or bluish discoloration involving the nail plate. Alopecia universalis associated with HIV infection and spontaneous hair regrowth after HAART initiation has been reported in pigmented skin types [24]. Hair softening, straightening, and fracturing also occur.

37.3 Pathogenesis

HIV belongs to the genus *Lentivirus* of the *Retroviridae* family. It is made of enveloped RNA and uses an enzyme reverse transcriptase to produce DNA copies of the HIV RNA. The main modes of transmission are (a) sexual intercourse with an infected partner, (b) transmission during pregnancy from an infected mother to her unborn child, (c) through breastfeeding, and (d) via exposure to infected blood and its products. To a much lesser extent, there are means of acquiring the HIV infection via body fluids such as sputum, sweat, urine, saliva, nasal secretions, and also feces. During initial infection, the HIV virion binds to CD4+ T-lymphocytes, monocytes/macrophages, and dendritic cells in tissue. Initially, there is high viral load, followed by a decrease at the time of seroconversion, leading to a chronic phase of the infection. The cascade of the following mechanisms results in destruction of CD4+ homeostasis in lymph nodes and finally suppression of thymus CD4+ cell production. The decline in CD4+ T-cell/μl count in acute infection and con-

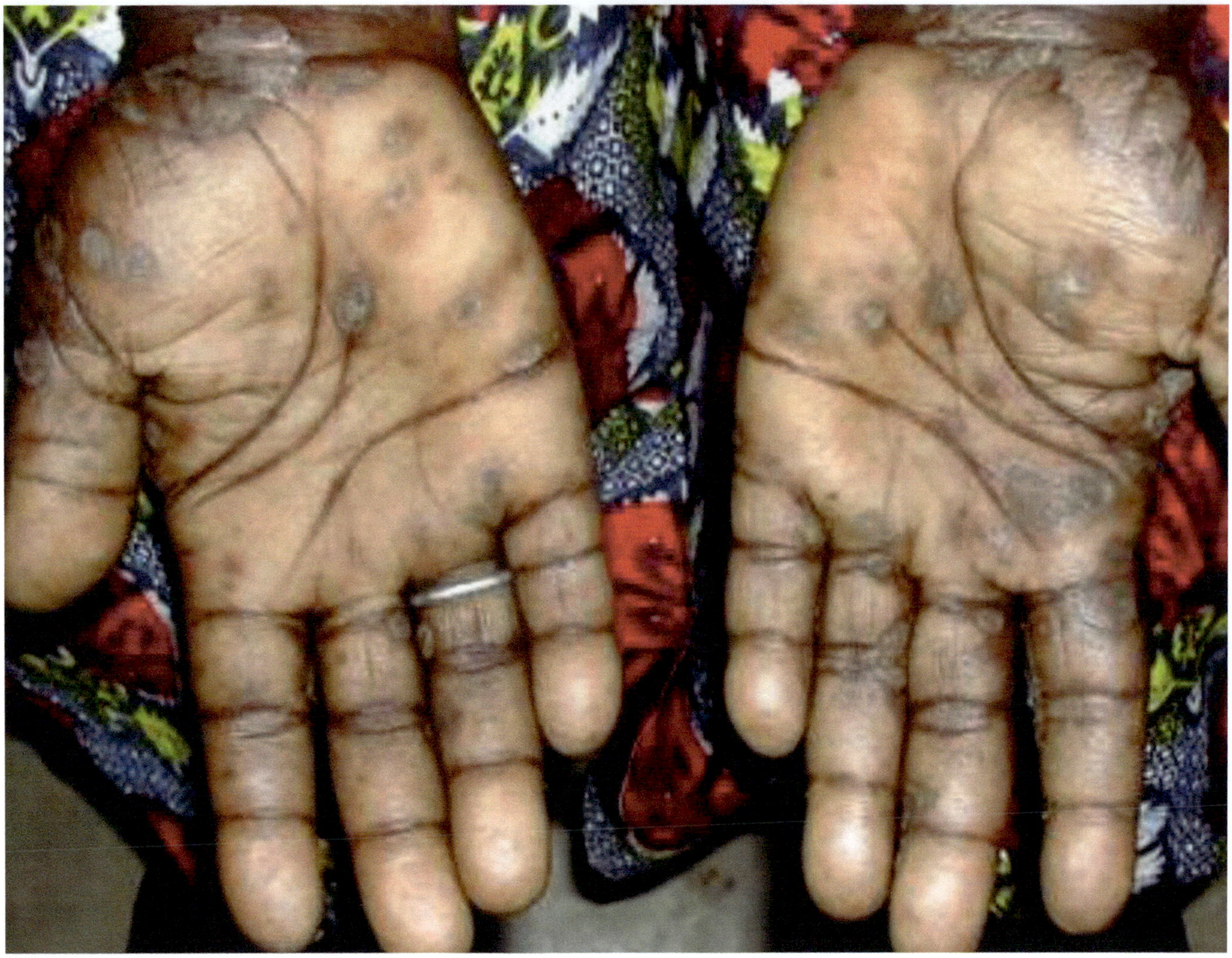

Fig. 37.10 Palmar pigmented macules and papules in *secondary syphilis* in a HIV-positive patient

tinuous drop during the chronic phase results in severe compromise of the immune system.

37.4 Management

There has been recent evidence that *early initiation* of antiretroviral treatment (ART) gives better outcomes compared with delayed treatment. Today, antiretroviral drugs are becoming easier available, more efficacious, and safer. In low- and middle-income countries with limited resources, newer classes of drugs such as integrase inhibitors are becoming affordable. New recommendations have made ART to be provided for lifelong regardless of CD4+ T-cell/µl counts to all pregnant and breastfeeding women. Viral load testing has been implemented in many countries as the appropriate means of monitoring patients who are taking ART. Clinical trials have provided evidence of the antiretroviral drug tenofovir disoproxil fumarate alone or combined with emtricitabine for use as *preexposure prophylaxis* (PrEP) to prevent HIV acquisition in a wide variety of settings and populations [1]. WHO recommends initiation of ART in all adults, pregnant and breastfeeding women, adolescents, and children living with HIV, regardless the clinical stage. As a matter of priority, patients with severe and clinically advanced HIV disease (WHO clinical stage 3 or 4 and with CD4+ count less than 350 T-cells/µl) should be considered first. First-line ART for adults should consist of two nucleoside reverse transcriptase inhibitors (NRTI) plus a non-nucleoside reverse transcriptase inhibitor (NNRTI) or an integrase inhibitor (INSTI). Different regimen modifications exist both for children <3 years old and for infants [1].

Topical antifungals are well established in the treatment of seborrheic dermatitis. Preparations easily available include ketoconazole 2% shampoo and terbinafine 1%

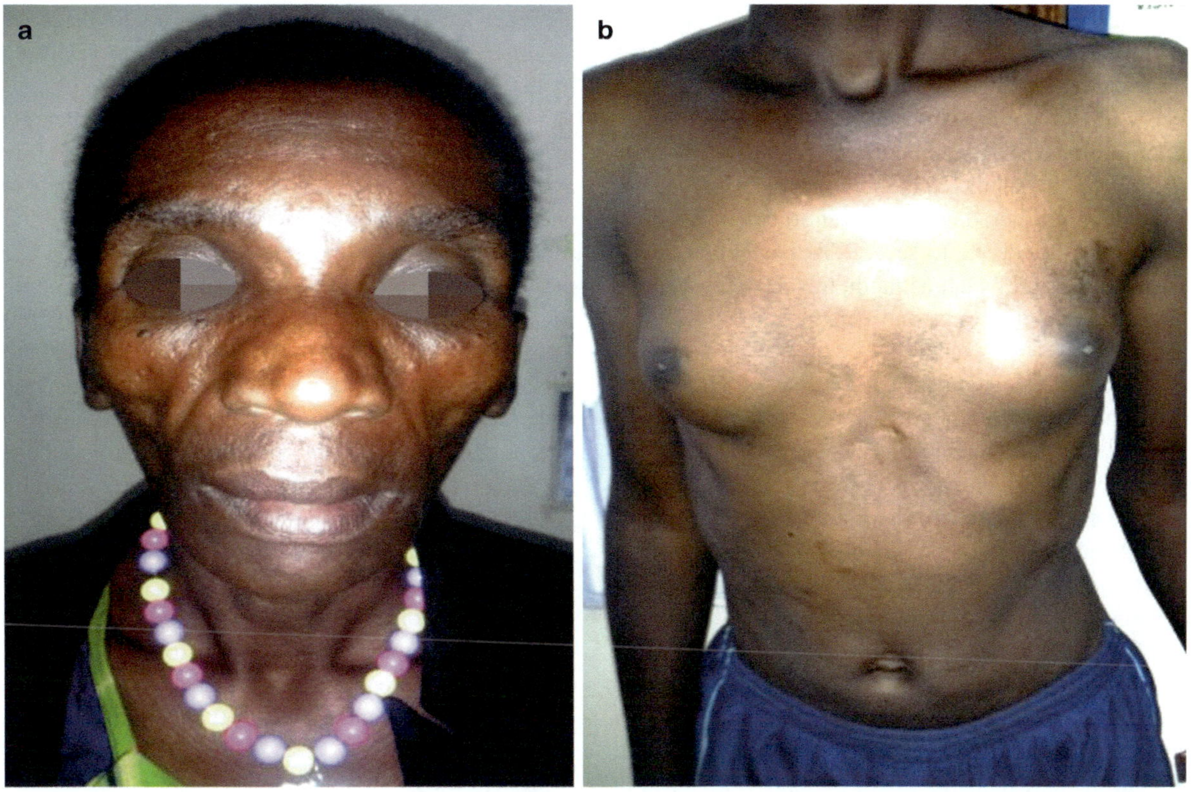

Fig. 37.11 (**a**, **b**) *Facial lipodystrophy* in a patient receiving stavudine and *gynecomastia* in another induced by efavirenz

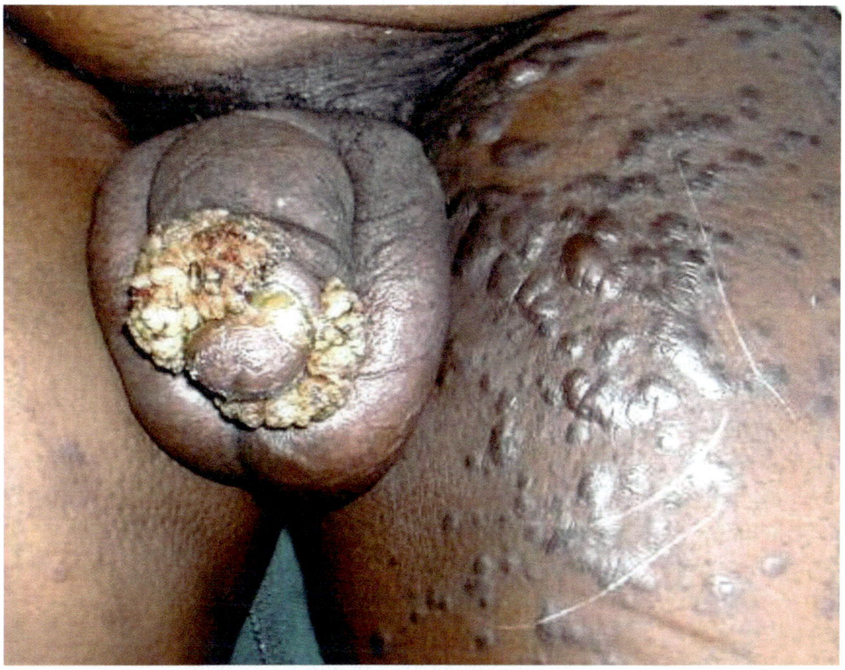

Fig. 37.12 *Squamous cell carcinoma of the penis* in a patient with HIV-associated Kaposi's sarcoma (RDTC, Moshi, Tanzania; courtesy Dr. M. Ketema)

cream. Topical hydrocortisone 1% applied for 1–4 weeks may improve seborrheic dermatitis clinically, but relapses are more frequent than with topical antifungals.

Psoriasis in HIV-infected patients tends to be refractory to treatment; options will depend on the severity of the disease. If the clinical course is mild to moderate, topical approaches are recommended. Phototherapy and antiretrovirals should be considered for moderate to severe disease. When immunosuppressive therapies such as methotrexate are scheduled to be used, the potential risks and benefits should be taken into consideration.

For HPV-associated warts, there is currently no single treatment modality recommended for all patients. Several studies have failed to demonstrate HAART benefit in reducing their prevalence/incidence or severity. Patients may develop widespread lesions years after HAART, as part of IRIS [25]. Available treatments include local application of imiquimod and podophyllotoxin together with cryotherapy and surgical removal [26]. Imiquimod available as 5% cream is applied 3x/week before bed and left to be washed off in the morning, for up to 16 weeks. Patients may use a finger to apply the treatment into the anal canal for treatment of intra-anal warts. In resource-limited areas, imiquimod is not easily available due to its expensive price; podophyllotoxin is an affordable and easily available treatment option. It is applied 2×/day for 3 consecutive days and then 4 days of no management. Application area should not exceed 10 cm^2 with a total volume less than 0.5 ml/day [27]. Surgical excision is the treatment mainstay for patients with both premalignant and malignant lesions. Cryotherapy using liquid nitrogen is applied for 10–20 s. Advantages of cryotherapy include low-cost, easy application, absence of systemic effects, and quick lesion destruction, although some lesions may be elevated and extended. Side effects include pain, erosion, blister formation, and ulceration. In patients with heavily pigmented skin, cryotherapy may result into hypo- or hyperpigmentation which will resolve gradually over time.

The antivirals acyclovir, valaciclovir, and famciclovir are the main drugs for treatment of both primary and recurrent genital herpes. In HIV-infected patients, acyclovir is given orally at a dosage of 400 mg 3×/day or 200 mg 5×/day, while valaciclovir 500 mg 2×/day and fanciclovir 250 mg 2×/day can be given, respectively. Treatment is continued until the lesions are cleared. Occasionally higher doses may be needed to control the disease. For mollusca the use of surgical methods including curettage, cryotherapy, electrodesiccation, and laser surgery is effective. In black skin, cryotherapy may leave disfiguring hypopigmented or depigmented lesions. Cytodestructive treatments include the use of cantharidin, phenol, silver nitrate, and salicylic acid. Chemotherapeutic agents used include cidofovir, alpha-interferon, and imiquimod [28]. Giant mollusca contagiosa were reported to regress after HAART initiation [29].

When antibiotic therapies are necessary for bacterial soft tissue infections, knowledge of their resistance pattern is helpful; methicillin-resistant staphylococci may occur [30]. Bacillary angiomatosis responds remarkably well to antimicrobials, even in patients with very low CD4+ T-cell counts [31]. For HIV-associated visceral leishmaniasis, liposomal amphotericin B and pentavalent antimonials (sodium stibogluconate and meglumine antimoniate) in parenteral form are the most preferred drugs for treatment. The recommended doses are 3-5mg/kg/day for 3-6 days with liposomal amphotericn B, maximum dose 18-21mg/kg/day and for pentavalent antimonials 20mg/kg/day for 28 days. Side effects include hepatotoxicity, nephrotoxicity, and potential fatal cardiac effects [32]. Oral treatment with miltefosine will raise concern on teratogenicity, poor compliance, and drug resistance [33]. PPE can be well controlled by the use of high-dose antihistamines and potent topical corticosteroids. Promethazine at a dose of 25 mg 2×/day was found to be superior to topical corticosteroids [34]. In cases with PPE not responding to conventional treatment, oral thalidomide (100 mg/day) has been used successfully. Due to its teratogenicity, strict contraception is required under management; also, peripheral neuropathy is a potential side effect of thalidomide [11].

Conclusions

Today, there are 36.7 million HIV-infected people worldwide: 25.5 million are living in sub-Saharan Africa, and nearly all of them present with HIV-associated skin disease, with various types of infections and neoplasms. Knowledge of the atypical clinical picture of these entities and their course is mandatory for the physicians and health workers in guiding them to suspect the underlying HIV infection, confirm the diagnosis, and initiate early treatment. Early introduction of ART in asymptomatic or less symptomatic, management-naïve adults gives better outcomes than delayed onset in patients with high viral load and low CD4+ counts [35]. Most HIV-associated skin diseases respond well to ART, despite the fact that in some cases new lesions appear as a sign of immune reconstitution following ART initiation.

References

1. UNAIDS. AIDS by the numbers, AIDS is not over, but it can be. 2016. www.unaids.org
2. Ameen M. Impact of human immunodeficiency virus-related disease on pigmented skin types. Br J Dermatol. 2013;169(suppl 3):11–8.
3. Wernham AG, Vydianath B, Chua SL. Thalidomide-A novel therapeutic approach for pruritic papular eruption of HIV. JAAD Case Rep. 2015;1:109–11.
4. Resneck JS, VanBeek M. Fumanski et al: etiology of pruritic popular eruption with HIV infection in Uganda. JAMA. 2004;292: 2614–21.
5. Chua SL, Amerson EH, Leslie KS, et al. Factors associated with pruritic papular eruption of human immunodeficiency virus infec-

tion in the antiretroviral therapy era. Br J Dermatol. 2014;170: 832–9.
6. Forrestel AK, Kovarick CL, Mosam A, et al. Diffuse HIV-associated seborrheic dermatitis-a case series. Int J STD AIDS. 2016;27: 1342–5.
7. Bilu D, Mamelak AJ, Nguyen RH, et al. Clinical and epidemiologic characterization of photosensitivity in HIV positive individuals. Photodermatol Photoimmunol Photomed. 2004;20:175–83.
8. Anthony FC, Marsden RA. Vitiligo in association with human immunodeficiency virus infection. J Eur Acad Dermatol Venereol. 2003;17:456–8.
9. Mischo M, von Kobyletzki LB, Brundermann E, et al. Similar appearance, different mechanisms: xerosis in HIV, atopic dermatitis and ageing. Exp Dermatol. 2014;23:446–8.
10. Meys R, Gotch FM, Bunker CB. Human papilloma virus in the era of highly antiretroviral therapy for human immunodeficiency virus: an immune reconstitution-associated disease? Br J Dermatol. 2010;162:6–11.
11. Mapesi H, Ramirez A, Tanner M, et al. Immune reconstitution inflammatory syndrome associated with dermatophytes in two HIV-1 positive patients in rural Tanzania: case report. BMC Infect Dis. 2016;16:495.
12. Govender NP, Maphanga TG, Zulu TG, et al. An outbreak of lymphocutaneous sporotrichosis among mine-workers in South Africa. PLoS Negl Trop Dis. 2015;9:e0004096.
13. Bonifaz A, Chang P, Moreno K, et al. Disseminated histoplasmosis in acquired immunodeficiency syndrome: report of 23 cases. Clin Exp Dermatol. 2009;34:481–6.
14. Forrestel AK, Naujokas A, Martin JN, et al. Bacillary angiomatosis masquerading as Kaposi's sarcoma in East Africa. J Int Assoc Provid AIDS Care. 2015;14:21–5.
15. Farhi D, Zizi N, Grange P, et al. The epidemiology and clinical presentation of syphilis in a venereal disease center in Paris, France: a cohort study of 284 consecutive cases over the period of 2000-2007. Eur J Dermatol. 2009;19:484–9.
16. Stevenson J, Health M. Syphilis and HIV infection: an update. Dermatol Clin. 2005;24:497–507.
17. Guarneri C, Tchernev G, Bevelacqua V, et al. The unwelcome trio: HIV plus cutaneous and visceral leishmaniasis. Dermatol Ther. 2016;29(2):88–91. series: Int J STD AIDS 2016; 27: 1342–45.
18. Birbal S, Dheda M, Ojewole E, et al. Adverse drug reactions associated with antiretroviral therapy in South Africa. Afr J AIDS Res. 2016;15:243–8.
19. Stewart A, Lehloenya R, Boulle A, et al. Severe antiretroviral-associated skin reactions in south African patients: a case series and case control analysis. Pharmacoepidemiol Drug Saf. 2016;25:1313–9.
20. Rodriguez O, Kovarick CL. Spectrum and progression of disease from condyloma to aggressive anogenital squamous cell carcinoma in 3-HIV-positive patients. JAAD Case Rep. 2016;2:47–50.
21. Picard A, Badoual C, Hoursean M, et al. Human papilloma virus prevalence in HIV patients with head and neck squamous cell carcinoma. AIDS. 2016;30:1257–66.
22. Thomas JO. Acquired immunodeficiency syndrome-associated cancers in sub-Saharan Africa. Semin Oncol. 2001;28:198–206.
23. Namakoola I, Wakeham K, Parkes-Ratanshi R, et al. Use of nail and oral pigmentation to determine ART eligibility among HIV-infected Ugandan adults. Tropical Med Int Health. 2010;15:259–62.
24. Nikolic DS, Vierro D, Tije VC, et al. Alopecia universalis associated with vitiligo in an 18-year old HIV-positive patient: highly active anti-retroviral therapy as first choice therapy? Acta Derm Venereol. 2014;94:116–7.
25. Price P, Mathiot N, Krueger R, et al. Immune dysfunction and immune restoration disease in HIV patients given highly active antiretroviral therapy. Clin Infect Dis. 2002;34:224–33.
26. Gromley RH, Kovarick CL. Human papillomavirus-related genital disease in the immunocompromised host. J Am Acad Dermatol. 2012;66:867–99.
27. Centers for Disease Control and Prevention, Workworski KA, Berman SM. Sexually transmitted diseases treatment guidelines 2006. MMWR Recomm Rep. 2006;55:62–7.
28. Lohloenya R, Meintjes G. Dermatological manifestations of the immune reconstitution inflammatory syndrome. Dermatol Clin. 2006;24:549–70.
29. Sen S Bhaumik P. Resolution of giant molluscum contagiosum with antiretroviral therapy. Indian J Dermatol Venereol Leprol. 2008;74:267–8.
30. Bar A, Hautschke D, Mirmohammadsadegh A, et al. Spectrum of bacterial isolates in HIV-positive patients with skin and soft tissue infections: emergence of methicillin-resistant staphylococci. AIDS. 2003;17:1253–6.
31. Tappero JW, Perkins BA, Wenger JD, et al. Cutaneous manifestations of opportunistic infections in patients infected with human immunodeficiency virus. Clin Microbiol Rev. 1995;8: 440–50.
32. WHO. Consolidated guidelines on: The Use of Antiretroviral Drugs for Treating and Preventing HIV Infection; recommendations for a public health approach, 2nd edition. 2016. ISBN: 9789241549684.
33. Sundar S, Sinha PK, Rai M, et al. Comparison of short course multidrug treatment with standard therapy for visceral leishmaniasis in India: an open-label, non-inferiority randomized controlled trial. Lancet. 2011;377(9764):477–86.
34. Navarini AA, Stoeckle MM, Navarini S, et al. Antihistamines are superior to topical steroids in managing human immunodeficiency virus (HIV)-associated papular pruritic eruption. Int J Dermatol. 2010;49:83–8.
35. Siegfried N, Uthman OA, Rutherford GW. Optimal time for initiation of antiretroviral therapy in asymptomatic, HIV-infected, treatment-naive adults. Cochrane Database Syst Rev. 2010;3:CD008272.

Kaposi's Sarcoma

38

Alice U. Amani and Constantin E. Orfanos

Kaposi's sarcoma (KS) has been originally described by Kaposi as an idiopathic multiple neoplasm of the skin composed of proliferating vessels and spindle-shaped cells. Its origin has been an issue of debate for long; there is evidence to believe that the tumor is derived from endothelial cells, particularly from lymphatic endothelium. There are four types of KS known today, based on their occurrence and the accompanying clinicopathological data. The classic KS has been first seen and described by Moritz Kaposi in Europe in 1872, an endemic type was recognized in 1960s in sub-Saharan Africa, a KS variant associated with immunosuppressive therapies (iatrogenic) has been reported by various groups in Western countries particularly in organ transplant patients, and the HIV-associated KS type, also called epidemic, first appeared in the United States in 1981. *Human herpesvirus 8* (HHV-8) is considered as an etiological agent for all variants. Primary effusion lymphoma and multicentric Castleman's disease are also linked with this virus.

38.1 Incidence

Kaposi's sarcoma is a relatively rare neoplasm worldwide. GLOBOCAN estimated in 2012 an overall of 44,247 new cases and 26,974 deaths, despite the success of combined antiretroviral therapies [1, 2]. At that time data showed 40,874 of new cases in developing and 3373 new cases in developed countries. The African continent is disproportionately affected; 85% of all cases of the neoplasm occur in Africa. Men are approximately two times more at risk for developing Kaposi's sarcoma than women worldwide.

The global distribution differs: *classic Kaposi's sarcoma* affects elderly, immunocompetent individuals around the Mediterranean area or in Eastern Europe. It is a slowly progressing disease with a relatively benign course. *Endemic or African Kaposi's sarcoma* is common in Central and Eastern Africa and primarily affects adults. *Iatrogenic Kaposi's sarcomas* arise in all continents in patients with compromised immune system, primarily in those who have received organ transplants and immune suppressive therapies. Finally, in HIV-infected individuals, often in men who have sex with men and transmit the virus to each other, an aggressive type of KS develops, due to HIV-induced immunosuppression, the *HIV-associated Kaposi's sarcoma*, also called *epidemic*. In African countries with high rates of HIV infection, KS affects men and women proportionately, and a high incidence was also found in children.

Kaposi's sarcoma (KS) is a multifocal vascular tumor, able to affect virtually any organ, whereby the skin is most frequently involved. It is the most common tumor in HIV-infected individuals in Africa. However, KS was as common in some regions of sub-Saharan Africa as cancer of the colon in much of Western Europe; data from the era of the HIV/AIDS epidemic indicate 20-fold increases in the occurrence of KS in Uganda and Zimbabwe [3]. In South Africa 5 per 100,000 individuals were at risk of developing KS, even before the HIV/AIDS era. The pandemic of HIV infection led the incidence of KS to increase dramatically, particularly in African countries; in some areas it became the most common cancer in men [4]. A study on 1108 cases of KS at the Kenyatta National Hospital, Kenya, showed that mucocutaneous KS had a relative frequency of 2–5%

A. U. Amani
Service de Dermatologie, Centre Hospitalier Universitaire, BP, Kigali, Rwanda
e-mail: chuk.hospital@chuk.rw; amani_alice@ymail.com

C. E. Orfanos, M.D. (✉)
The Free University of Berlin, Medical School Charité, Berlin, Germany
e-mail: corfanos@t-online.de

C. E. Orfanos et al. (eds.), *Pigmented Ethnic Skin and Imported Dermatoses*, https://doi.org/10.1007/978-3-319-69422-1_38

of all malignancies with the male to female ratio declining from 10:1 to 2:1, indicating that the incidence of KS increased considerably among female patients in a dark-skinned population [5].

38.2 Pathogenesis

The pathogenesis of Kaposi's sarcoma has been gradually unraveled using advanced genomic technologies. Tumorigenesis is basically caused by infection with the *HHV-8 virus*, also called *KS-associated herpesvirus* (KSHV). This virus seems to carry oncogenic genes into the endothelial cells of lymphatic and blood vessels, while the opportunistic tumor surfaces under the circumstances of long-term immunosuppression. HHV-8 infection is much more common than KS; most individuals infected do not get KS, and most of them will never show any clinical symptoms. In other words, infection with HHV-8 seems to be needed to cause the tumor, but HHV-8 alone does not necessarily lead to KS [6]. The status of the immune system and its suppression due to older age, drug intake, or HIV infection that reduces the number of CD4+ T-cells are important cofactors for the development of the multifaceted neoplasm.

The percentage of people infected with HHV-8 varies in different countries around the world. In developed Western countries, less than 10% of the overall population is infected with HHV-8; the virus is more common in men who have sex with men than in men who have sex only with women. In African countries HHV-8 infection is widely spread; its mode of transmission is not fully elucidated. In some areas of Africa, more than 90% of the population may show signs of infection. In these areas the virus seems to spread from mother to child. HHV-8 is also found in saliva, which may be one of the ways it is transmitted [7]. In South America (Argentina, Brazil, Chile), the level of seroprevalence was found 3.0–4.3% [8]. High seroprevalence rates of HHV-8 were registered in Amerindians, in contrast to the low rates in the general South American population [9].

38.3 Clinical Picture

The clinical picture of KS differs according to the particular group it belongs:

(a) *Classic Kaposi's sarcoma* typically presents as slowly growing, pink to red-violet macules and papules on the distal lower extremities that may coalesce to form indurate tumor-like plaques. Initially unilateral lesions progress to a more widely disseminated multifocal pattern (Fig. 38.1). Early lesions may regress, while others

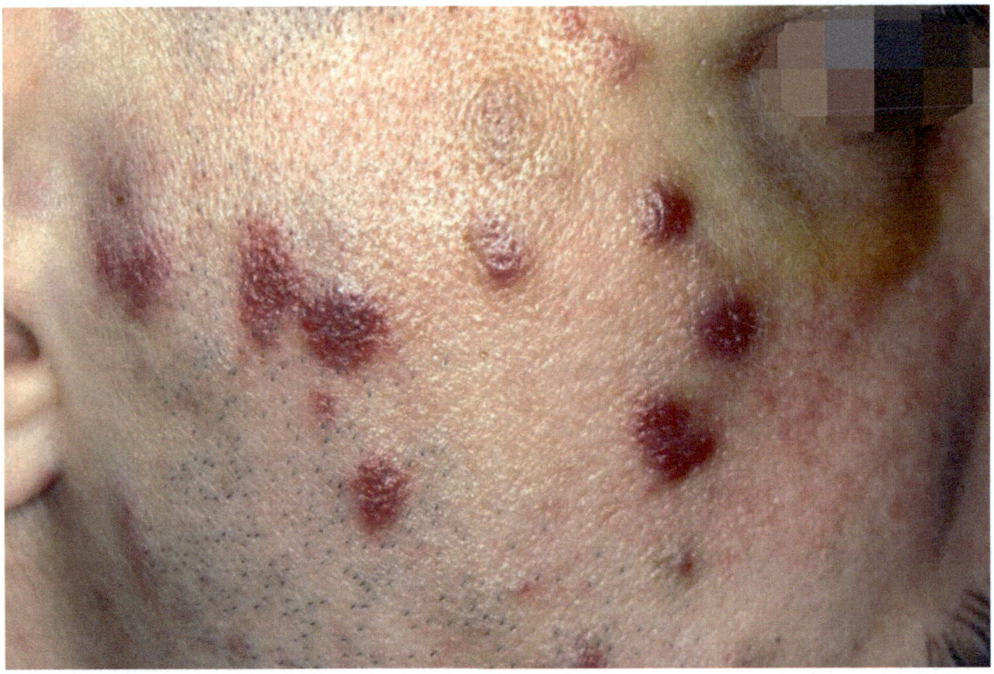

Fig. 38.1 Characteristic macular-papular lesions of Kaposi's sarcoma in a HIV-infected white-skinned Caucasian (Dept. of Dermatology, Berlin, Germany)

evolve, leading to lesions of different stages existing at the same time. Patients with long-standing classic KS may develop lesions in the mouth and the gastrointestinal tract, often asymptomatic.

(b) *African endemic Kaposi's sarcoma* resembles the classic type in appearance and course showing papules, elevated plaques, and nodular lesions, often localized on the lower extremities and the feet (Fig. 38.2). However, florid infiltrative types with nodular lesions may occur, which are more aggressive. A particular lymphadenopathic type is notably different in several regards: it predominantly affects children, and the tumors involve primarily the lymph nodes, although skin and mucosal lesions may also be present. The course is often fulminant and fatal.

(c) *Iatrogenic Kaposi's sarcoma* due to immunosuppression clinically also resembles classic KS. While some patients experience only a single lesion, others have numerous, disseminated. The tumor usually completely resolves after the administered drugs causing immunosuppression are withdrawn. Nevertheless, patients with prolonged high-dose immunosuppression may develop more aggressive posttransplant KS with internal involvement.

(d) The *HIV-associated epidemic Kaposi's sarcoma* most commonly affects infected patients with advanced immune impairment and CD4+ T-cell counts less than 500 cells/μl [10], although immunosuppression is not an unconditioned prerequisite for the development of the neoplasm. Among 130 patients diagnosed during the first two decades of the epidemic, mucosal and visceral involvement was common, and only 10% had a CD4+ count <200/μl at the time of first diagnosis [11].

The clinical features of KS in HIV-infected patients are protean: in most patients multiple disseminated, bluish to violaceous macules and papules are found, often on the trunk; they are oval to lanceolate in shape, arraying along the skin lines of cleavage (Fig. 38.3); occasionally, patients with acrolocalized infiltrative plaques are seen (Fig. 38.4). In other patients infiltrative and indurated plaques intermingled with nodular lesions occur on the lower extremities together with considerable lymphedema (Fig. 38.5).

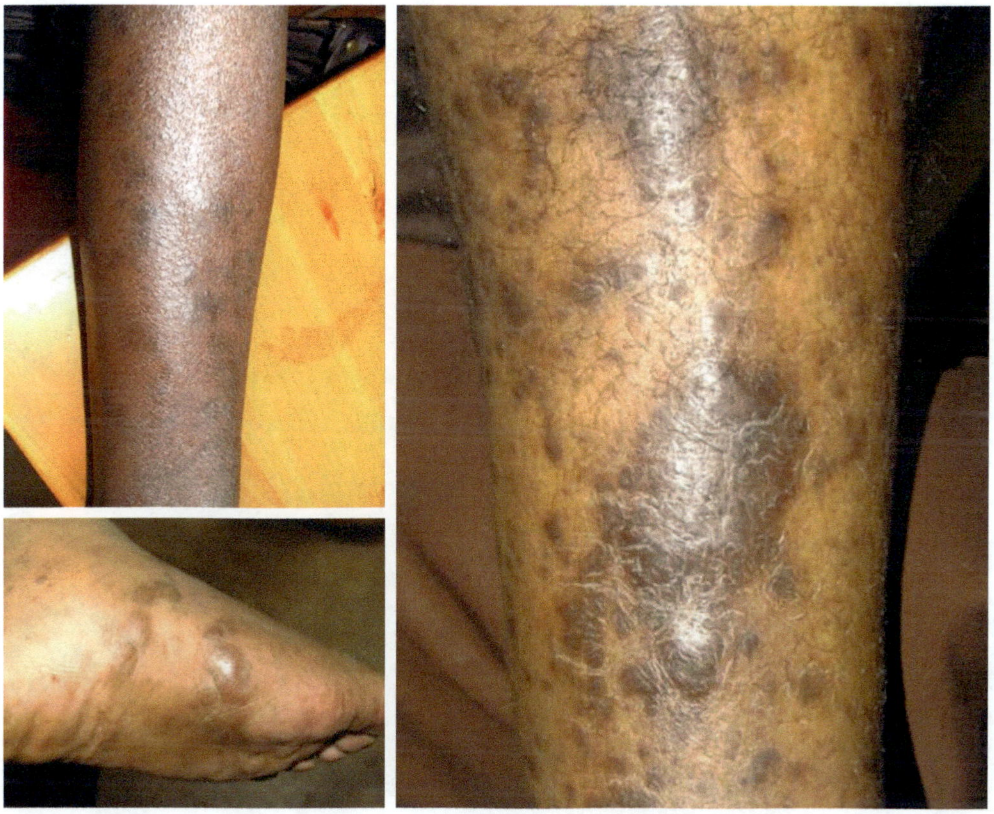

Fig. 38.2 Characteristic lesions of *endemic African KS* in three males in sub-Saharan Africa (Uganda, Tanzania)

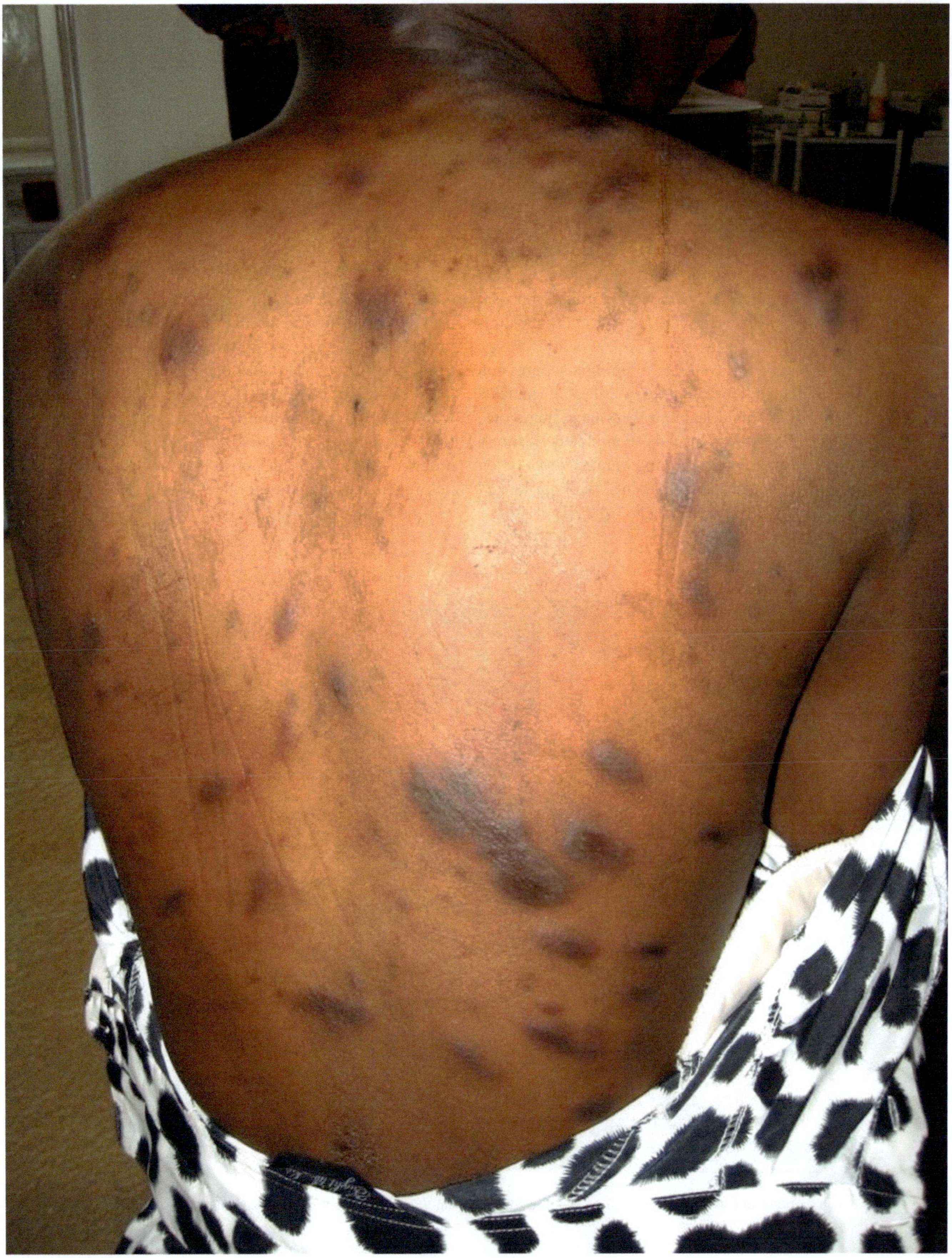

Fig. 38.3 Disseminated lesions of *HIV-associated epidemic KS* on the trunk of a young African male (Rwanda)

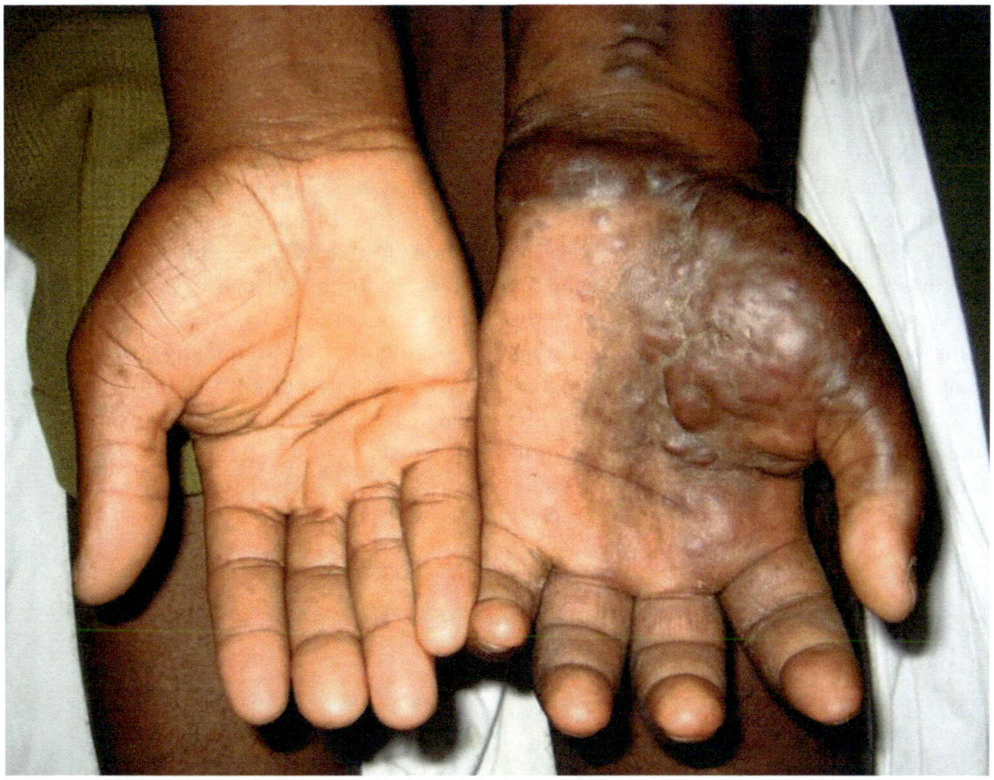

Fig. 38.4 *Acrolocalized HIV-associated Kaposi's sarcoma* (RDTC in Moshi, Tanzania; photo CEO)

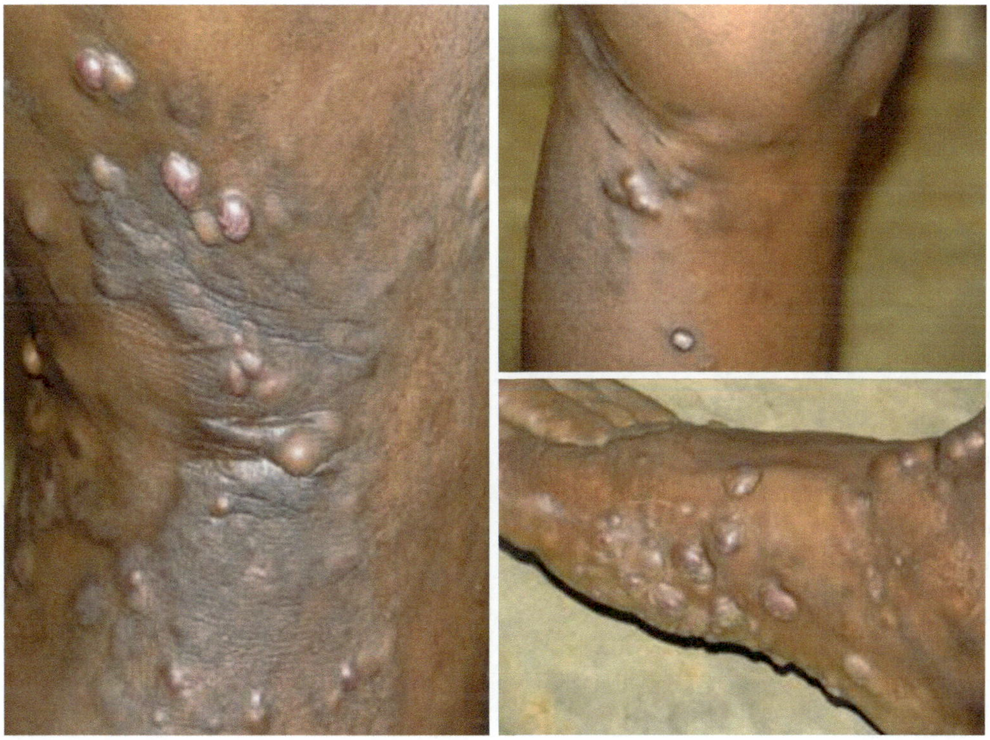

Fig. 38.5 Indurative plaques in *HIV-associated KS* in African males (legs and foot), also showing multiple violaceous nodules. DD: *Bacillary angiomatosis*

HIV-associated KS differs from the African endemic by showing prominent dissemination of lesions, frequent involvement of the craniofacial region and oral mucosa, and more rapid progressive course [12]. No histological differences between the HIV-associated and the non-HIV-associated KS were detected, but densely packed spindle cell infiltrates are more prominent in the latter forming compact nodules (Fig. 38.6).

While any skin surface may be involved, the face and the nose are preferred sites in epidemic KS. Involvement of the oral mucosa is commonly seen in most patients. The lesions may ulcerate at any site and become secondarily infected. In HIV-infected females, facial localization involving the eye and mouth mucosa is regularly found, causing significant distress and disfigurement; also, exophytic cauliflower-like growth of vascular tumors has been seen (Fig. 38.7).

In progressed cases plaques and purple-blackish nodules and multiple, florid nodular tumors are often prevailing in dark-skinned patients; it is a clinical subtype of epidemic KS which is possibly associated with black African ethnicity (Fig. 38.8). In other severely affected patients, coalescing lesions form extensive armor-like constricting plaques in the deeper dermis and cause severe lymphedema of the legs (Figs. 38.9 and 38.10).

Epidemic KS frequently involves the gastrointestinal tract causing recurrent bleeding, and also the lymph nodes and the lung. Pulmonary involvement has an unfavorable prognosis.

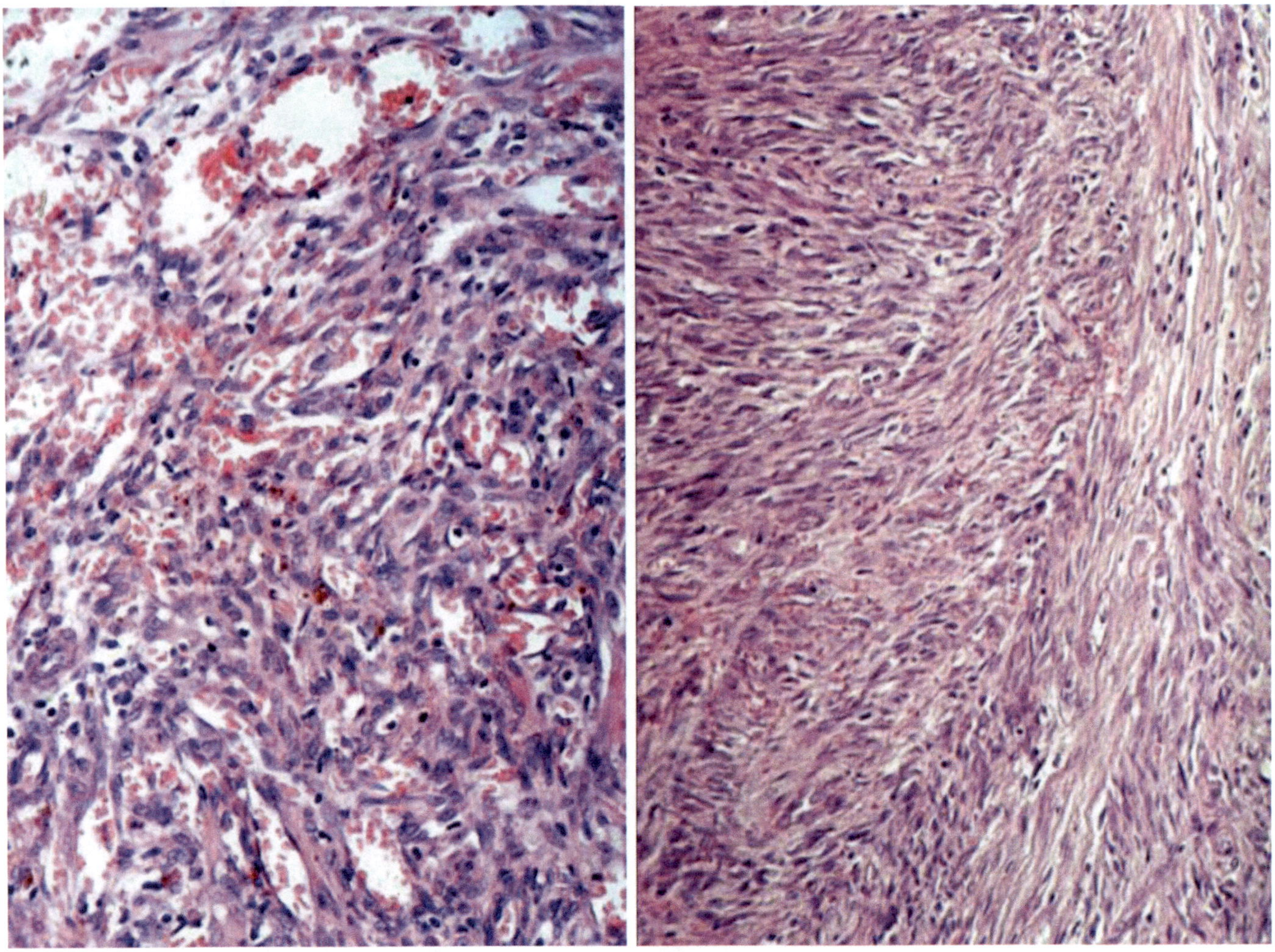

Fig. 38.6 Histological features of HIV-associated KS showing incomplete vascular lumina (left) and, at places, spindle-like cells forming compact nodules (right)

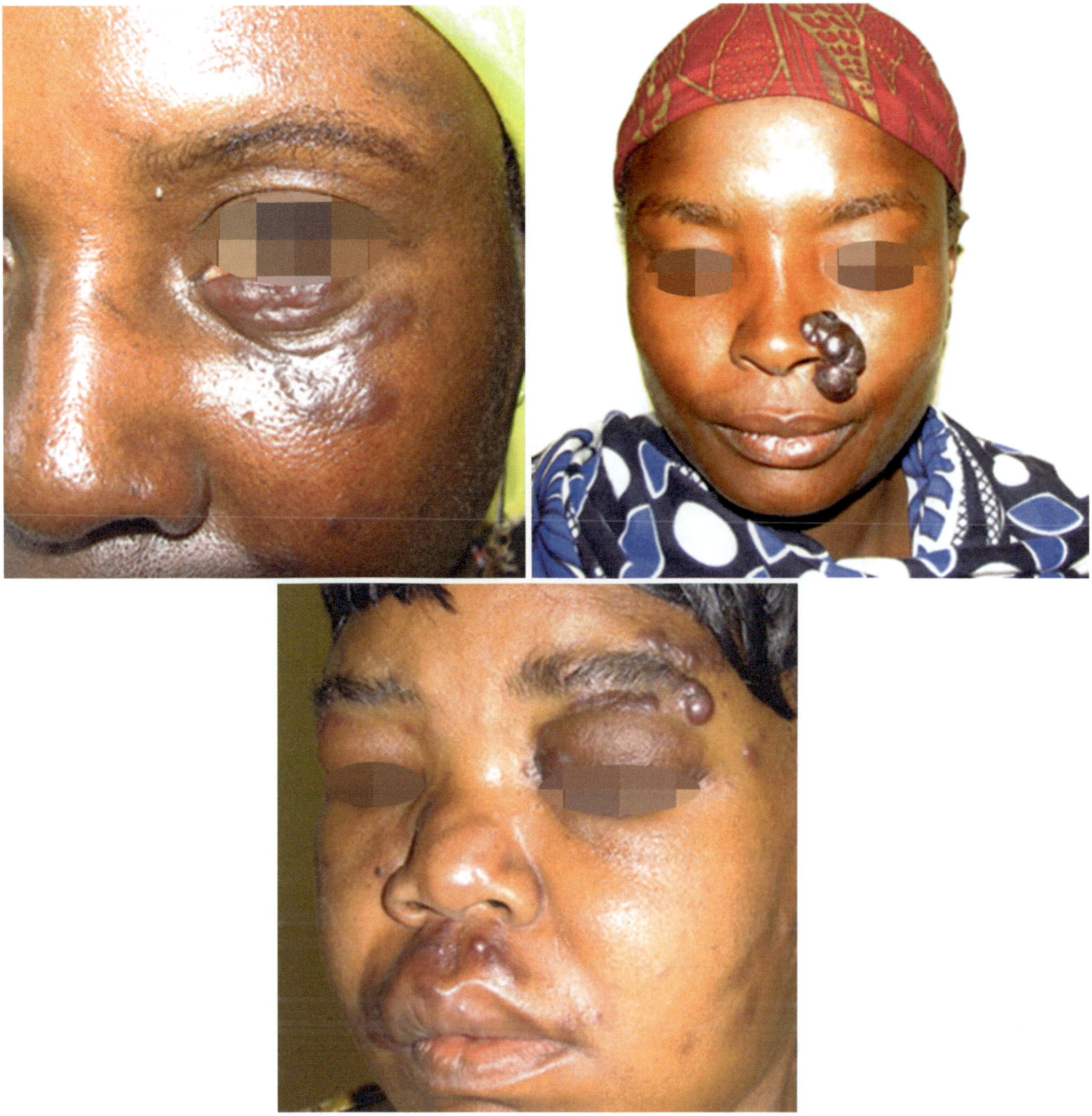

Fig. 38.7 *HIV-associated KS in African females* presenting macular, papular, mucosal, and nodular, partly exophytically growing vascular lesions in different stages of the disease (RDTC Moshi, Tanzania; photos CEO)

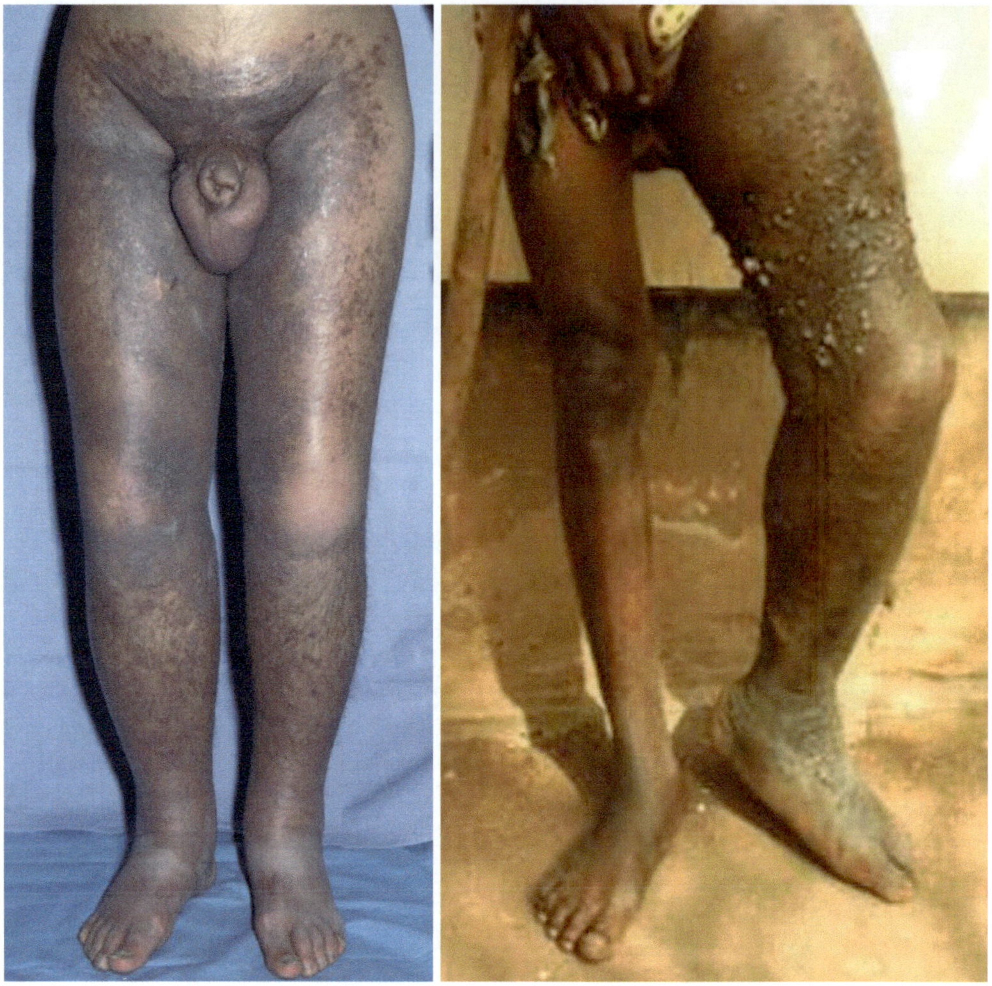

Fig. 38.8 *Left, HIV-associated KS* with severe *lymphedema* of both legs in a male of African descent (Dept. of Dermatology, Berlin, Germany); *Right,* unilateral lymphedematous plaques of *endemic African KS* also showing nodular lesions in a male (Rwanda)

38.4 Management

38.4.1 Local Treatment Modalities

In older immunocompetent patients with stable disease observation, close follow-up is an option. Cryotherapy, laser, or photodynamic therapies and topical alitretinoin can be used to treat superficial KS macules, papules, and plaques. Also 5% imiquimod cream may be an alternative in localized cases. Freezing must usually be sufficiently vigorous to cause superficial necrosis/ulceration, and the resulting scar seems to replace the vascular proliferation of KS. Surgery is only useful for diagnosis and removal of solitary nodular lesions. A complete cure may be an unrealistic expectation in many patients, since recurrence rates are high. Treatment of visible lesions, even in HIV-positive patients with widely disseminated disease, improves the appearance, heightens self-esteem, and provides patients with a sense of control in an otherwise difficult situation.

Radiation is an option for patients presenting multifocal but relatively few localized lesions, mostly on the trunk or the extremities. Application of 8–12 Gy delivered in a single dose or 4 × 3 Gy to an extended field and total body electron beam management (4 Gy) once a week for 6–8 weeks are recommended. Radiation is clearly a practical and effective modality for treatment of localized cutaneous and oral KS, if available, but may have a briefer effect in HIV-associated than in classic KS [13].

For treatment of large or nonresponsive tumors, intralesional injections of vinblastine (0.1 mg/ml) or vincristine (0.001 mg/ml) cause a slow fading of erythema and thickness. High concentrations or volumes of injection may result in ulceration of the overlying epidermis, but lesions still resolve with adequate cosmesis [14].

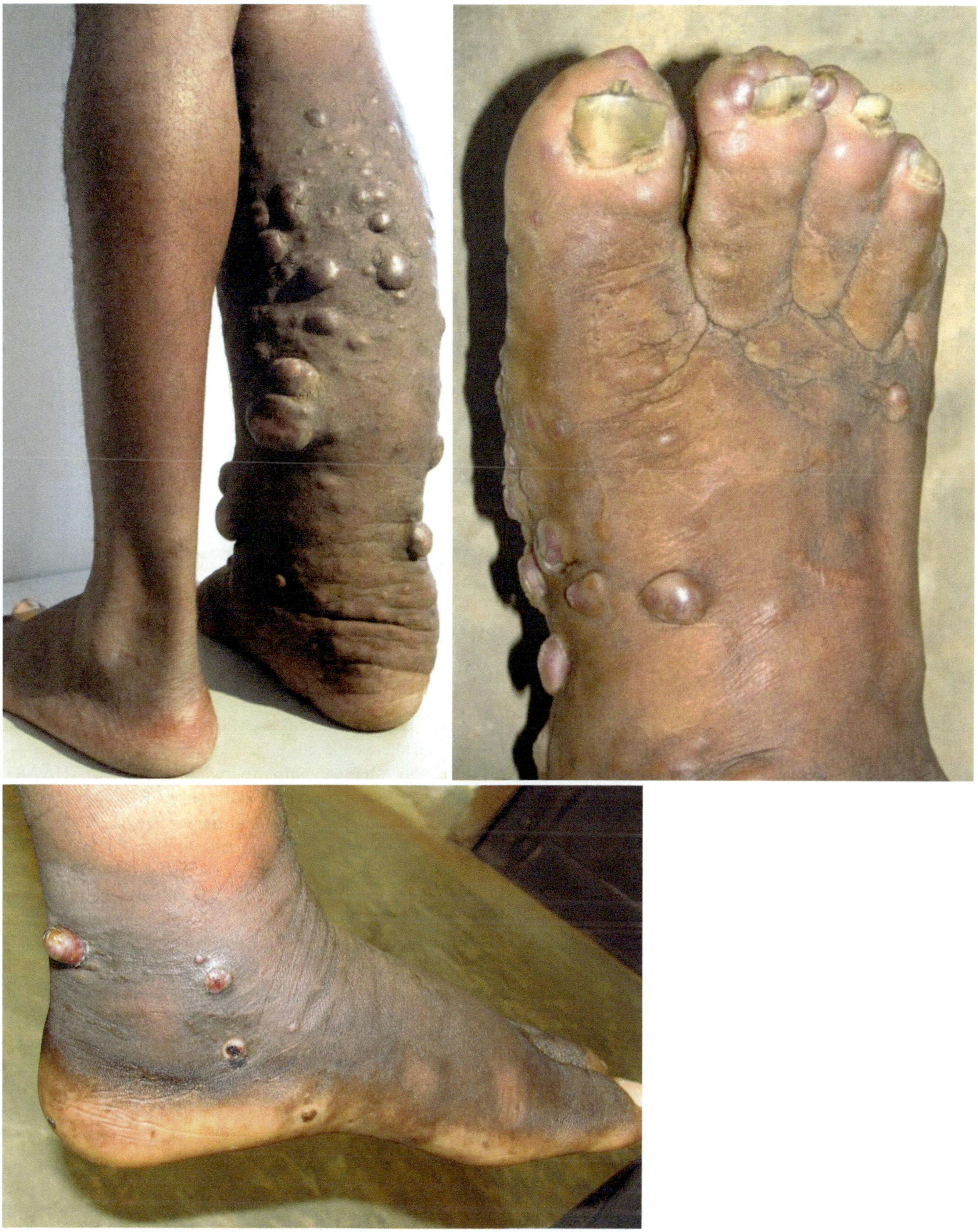

Fig. 38.9 Lymphedematous, nodular type of HIV-associated Kaposi's sarcoma in African males

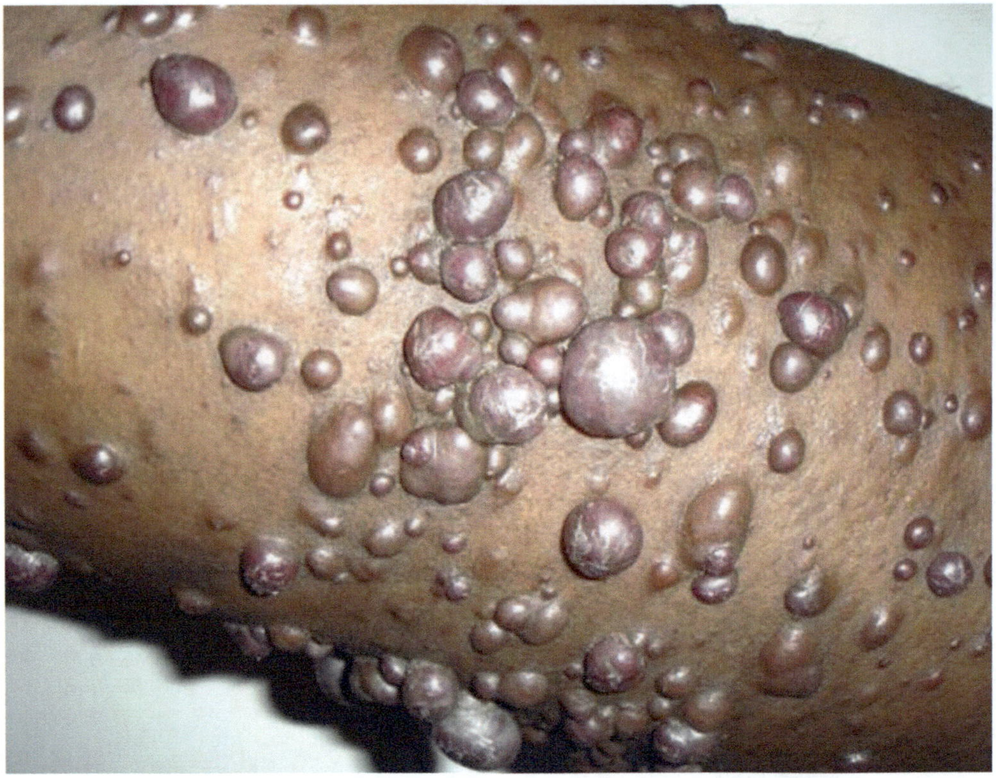

Fig. 38.10 *HIV-associated KS* with severe lymphedema and aggressive course. Multiple florid nodular lesions indicate widespread *bacillary angiomatosis* (RDTC, Moshi, Tanzania; photo CEO)

38.4.2 Systemic Modalities

Systemic *chemotherapy* is the cornerstone of treatment in extensive multifocal KS. Rapidly progressive tumors, defined by the development of ten or more new lesions per month, visceral involvement (gastrointestinal, pulmonary), and prominent lymphedema are indications for systemic chemotherapy. Doxorubicin, vincristine, etoposide, and bleomycin are administered, alone or in combination, partly in liposomal preparations employed to reduce side effects [15, 16]. The taxanes paclitaxel and docetaxel are used for treatment of disseminated KS not responsive to anthracyclines also depending upon the presence concomitant morbidities. Gemcitabine, an analogue of deoxycytidine, has shown some promise in the treatment of classic KS, with limited side effects [17].

Interferon-α is a biological response modifier early introduced in low- and high-dose schedules for KS treatment. 3 or 9–18 million IU s.c. 3×/week alone or in combination with antiretroviral management was effective in all types of the tumor, particularly in cases with mild course. Prolongation of survival was found after such treatment in 30–40% of all treated patients [11]. The lesions regress, while HHV-8 DNA sequences persist in lesional skin [17]. Subcutaneous injections three million IU every second day seemed a standard regimen. Patients will not tolerate the side effects in high-dose levels.

Highly active antiretroviral management (HAART) clearly helps to alleviate AIDS-related KS, most likely by decreasing the viral load and increasing the CD4+ T-cell counts. Under continuing antiretroviral treatment, lesions of HIV-associated KS slow down their progressive course and finally resolve, particularly when protease inhibitors and other new potent compounds are included in the schedule [18]. The HAART regimen has been successful in a large cohort of AIDS/KS patients [19–21]. Potential therapies to emerge may include tyrosine kinase inhibitors (imatinib, sorafenib, gefitinib), pentosan polysulfate, and topical halofuginone [18, 22, 23]. Other systemic modalities that inhibit angiogenesis or target HHV-8 are being investigated.

Organ transplant patients with iatrogenic KS pose a particular therapeutic challenge, balancing the risk of graft rejection with the benefit of improvement in KS. In addition to the reduction of immunosuppression [24], substitution of cyclosporine can lead to clinical improvement of the post-transplant tumor. In 15 renal transplant recipients, substitution with sirolimus led to resolution of all KS lesions in all patients; it seems that sirolimus may inhibit the progression of cutaneous Kaposi's sarcoma in kidney transplant recipients while providing effective immunosuppression [23]. This observation has been independently corroborated by additional studies, albeit not always with equally impressive response rates [25]. Posttransplant KS also responds to conventional local and systemic therapies used in the other forms of the tumor as mentioned above.

Conclusions

Kaposi's sarcoma was first described over a century ago, and new subtypes have been characterized during the last decades, its association with HIV infection in particular. Despite all progress, not all aspects of the pathogenesis and biological behavior of the tumor have been fully clarified. Its occurrence in western countries has been clearly limited after the introduction of HAART, but Kaposi's sarcoma is still one of the most common neoplasms in pigmented and black-skinned African populations. As a cause, HHV-8 has been identified in all subtypes of KS, a virus prevalent in African countries, in Eastern Mediterranean, in Arab populations, and also in some Amerindians. The differences of the geographic distribution and seroprevalence of HHV-8 in various regions may be explanatory, supporting the concept of its role as a universal pathogenetic agent for KS. However, differences in the clinical pictures and courses of the arising tumors are not fully understood. Today, the risk for dark- and black-skinned individuals to develop endemic or HIV-associated KS is still high. Together with methods to enhance immune function, future therapies should be focused for developing drugs to control vascular proliferation and antivirals against HHV-8 in order to broaden our armamentarium against the tumor.

References

1. GLOBOCAN. Estimated cancer incidence, Mortality and Prevalence Worldwide, 2012. www.globocan.iarc.fr. Accessed 5 Nov 2014.
2. Lodi S, Guiguet M, Costagliola D, et al. Kaposi sarcoma incidence and survival among. HIV-infected homosexual men after HIV seroconversion. J Natl Cancer Inst. 2010;102:784–92.
3. Cook-Mozaffari P, Newton R, Baral V, et al. The geographical distribution of Kaposi's sarcoma and of lymphomas in Africa before the AIDS epidemic. Br J Cancer. 1998;78:1521–8.
4. DalMaso L, Serraino D, Franceschi S. Epidemiology of AIDS related tumours in developed and developing countries. Eur J Cancer. 2001;37:1188–201.
5. Onyango JF, Njiru A. Kaposis sarcoma in a Nairobi hospital. East Afr Med J. 2004;81:120–3.
6. Engels EA, Atkinson JO, Graubard BI, et al. Risk factors for human herpes virus 8 infection among adults in the United States and evidence for sexual transmission. J Infect Dis. 2007;196:199–207.
7. Geraminejad P, Memar O, Aronson I, et al. Kaposi's sarcoma and other manifestations of human herpes virus 8. J Am Acad Dermatol. 2002;47:641–55.
8. Pérez C, Tous M, Gallego S, et al. Seroprevalence of human herpesvirus-8 in blood donors from different geographical regions of Argentina, Brazil, and Chile. J Med Virol. 2004;72:661–7.
9. Mohanna S, Maco V, Bravo F, et al. Epidemiology and clinical characteristics of classic Kaposi's sarcoma, seroprevalence, and variants of human herpes virus 8 in South America: a critical review of an old disease. Int J Infect Dis. 2005;9:239–50.
10. Tappero JW, Conant MA, Wolfe SF, et al. Kaposi's sarcoma. Epidemiology, pathogenesis, histology, clinical spectrum, staging criteria and therapy. J Am Acad Dermatol. 1993;28:371–95.
11. Orfanos CE, Husak R, Wölfer U, Garbe C. Kaposi's sarcoma: a reevaluation. Recent Results Cancer Res. 1995;139:275–96.
12. Wamburu G, Masenga EJ, Moshi EZ, et al. HIV-associated and non-HIV associated types of Kaposi's sarcoma in an African population in Tanzania. Status of immune suppression and HHV-8 seroprevalence. Eur J Dermatol. 2006;16:677–82.
13. Antman K, Chang Y. Kaposi's sarcoma. N Engl J Med. 2000;342:1027–38.
14. Brambilla L, Bellinvia A, Tourlaki A, et al. Intralesional vincristine as first-line therapy for nodular lesions in classic Kaposi sarcoma: a prospective study in 151 patients. Br J Dermatol. 2009;162:854–9.
15. Krown SE. Acquired immunodeficiency syndrome associated Kaposi's sarcoma. Biology and management. Med Clin North Am. 1997;81:471–94.
16. Little RF, Aleman K, Kumar P, et al. Phase 2 study of pegylated liposomal doxorubicin in combination with interleukin-12 for AIDS-related Kaposi sarcoma. Blood. 2007;110:4165–71.
17. Pfrommer C, Tebbe B, Tidona CA, et al. Progressive HHV-8-positive classic Kaposi's sarcoma: rapid response to interferon alpha-2a but persistence of HHV-8 DNA sequences in lesional skin. Br J Dermatol. 1998;139:516–9.
18. Vanni T, Sprinz E. Machado MW et al Systemic treatment of AIDS-related Kaposi sarcoma: current status and perspectives. Cancer Treat Rev. 2006;32:445–55.
19. Gascon P, Schwartz RA. Kaposi's sarcoma. New treatment modalities. Dermatol Clin. 2000;18:169–75.
20. Bower M, Weir J, Francis N. The effect of HAART in 254 consecutive patients with AIDS-related Kaposi's sarcoma. AIDS. 2009;23:1701–6.
21. Di Lorenzo G, Konstantinopoulos PA, Pantanowitz L, et al. Management of AIDS-related Kaposi's sarcoma. Lancet Oncol. 2007;8:167–76.
22. Qunibi WY, Barri Y, Alfurayh O, et al. Kaposi's sarcoma in renal transplant recipients: a report on 26 cases from a single institution. Transplant Proc. 1993;25:1402–5.
23. Stallone G, Schena A, Infante B, et al. Sirolimus for Kaposi sarcoma in renal-transplant patients. N Engl J Med. 2005;352:1317–23.
24. Koon HB, Fingleton B, Lee JY, et al. Phase II AIDS malignancy consortium trial of topical halofuginone in AIDS-related Kaposi sarcoma. J Acquir Immune Defic Syndr. 2011;56:64–8.
25. Lebbe C, Euvrard S, Barrou B, et al. Sirolimus conversion for patients with post-transplant Kaposi's sarcoma. Am J Transplant. 2006;6:2164–8.

Epidermolysis Bullosa

39

Mourad Mokni

Hereditary epidermolysis bullosa (HEB) is a group of genetic disorders characterized by fragile skin and mucous membranes with varying degrees of severity. The overall condition is generally classified into three major entities depending on the location of the bulla formation: (a) *EB simplex* (HEBS) which develops intraepidermal blisters at the level of the basal and suprabasal epidermal layers; (b) *junctional EB* (JHEB) developing blisters within the dermoepidermal basement membrane, primarily at the level of lamina lucida; and (c) *dystrophic EB* (DHEB) in which the blisters are located underneath the basement membrane in the upper papillary dermis. In addition, *Kindler syndrome* is considered as a particular subtype of HEB. Further classification of the group continues to evolve based on new criteria and recognition of up to 30 clinical subtypes [1, 2] (Table 39.1).

Recent studies performed in Caucasian families revealed a number of characteristic epidemiological and genetic features offering a broad basis for diagnostic and counseling strategies. However, these may not be applicable to all ethnic populations, possibly because of marked demographic differences, consanguineous marriages, different climatic and environmental conditions, and presence of specialized health facilities.

39.1 Epidemiology

EB occurs in about 1 in 17,000 children born in the UK; in the USA the cumulative prevalence and incidence are 8.2 and 19.6 per 1,000,000 live births, respectively [3]. The disease seems to be rare in the black-skinned population living in the USA, and also in populations of African countries, the incidence of EB is rather low. Nevertheless, it causes several problems related to education, choice of vocation, prospects in marriage, and other social issues. In South Africa, the prevalence of EB is estimated 1 in 354,195 people, with the majority of cases occurring in whites; there is a high death rate among patients with dark pigmented or black skin [4]. In Tunisia the prevalence of EB is estimated 176 per 1,000,000 births with high incidence of recessive cases [5]; this is probably due to the relatively high rate of endogamy and consanguinity [6]. This sociocultural feature is shared by several other countries mainly in North Africa and Middle East [7]. In this geographic area, the rate of EB seems to be low as compared to Western countries; it may be a result of underreporting. Field studies on genodermatoses in Tunisia have shown that less severe EB phenotypes are not referred to the health services.

39.2 Pathogenesis

In patients with EB, mutations have been described in at least 18 different genes, coding for components of the cytoskeleton of epidermal keratinocytes and their adhesion contacts, including the anchoring fibrils [8] (Table 39.2). The molecular aberrations impair the structural and functional integrity of intraepidermal adhesion and dermoepidermal anchoring. The index genes involved are partly expressed also in other epithelia (gastrointestinal, respiratory, urogenital) or mesenchymal organs. This explains the occurrence of extracutaneous manifestations and relevant complications in the group of EB as a multi-system disease with considerable morbidity and mortality.

Blister formation takes place at the level of the dermoepidermal junction depending on which protein is mutated. In *Kindler syndrome* cleavage can occur within the basal keratinocytes at any of those places, being considered as a distinct subtype in the group, caused by mutations in the *FERMT1* gene encoding *kindlin-1* [9].

The molecular epidemiology of hereditary EB in the Middle East differs from that previously delineated in

M. Mokni
Dermatology Department, La Rabta Hospital, Tunis, Tunisia
e-mail: mourad.mokni@rns.tn

C. E. Orfanos et al. (eds.), *Pigmented Ethnic Skin and Imported Dermatoses*, https://doi.org/10.1007/978-3-319-69422-1_39

Table 39.1 Reported clinical variants of the genetic group *epidermolysis bullosa* (adapted from [1])

Epidermolysis bullosa simplex (HEBS)	*Suprabasal bulla formation*	Suprabasal HEBS
	Basal bulla formation	Localized HEBS (type *Weber-Cockayne*)
		Generalized severe HEBS (type *Dowling-Meara*)
		Generalized intermediate HEBS (type *Koebner*)
		HEBS with mottled pigmentation
		HEBS with migratory circinate erythema
		Autosomal recessive HEBS K14
		Trauma-induced skin blistering
		HEBS with muscle dystrophy
		HEBS with pyloric atresia
		HEBS *Ogna* type
		Autosomal recessive HEBS, BP230 deficiency
		Autosomal recessive HEBS, exophilin 5 deficiency
Junctional epidermolysis bullosa (JHEB)	*Generalized bullae*	Generalized severe JHEB (type *Herlitz*)
		Generalized intermediate JHEB (non-Herlitz type)
		JHEB with pyloric atresia
		JHEB, late onset (progressive)
		JHEB with respiratory and renal involvement
	Localized bullae	Localized JHEB (localized JEB, non-Herlitz)
		JHEB inversa
		JHEB, laryngo-onycho-cutaneous syndromes
Dystrophic epidermolysis bullosa (DHEB)	*Dominant*	Generalized DHEB (*Pasini, Cockayne-Touraine*)
		Acral DHEB
		Pretibial DHEB
		DHEB pruriginosa
		DHEB, nails only
		Bullous dermolysis of the newborn
	Recessive	Generalized severe DHEB (type *Hallopeau-Siemens*)
		Generalized intermediate DHEB (non-Hallopeau-Siemens)
		DEB inversa
		Localized DHEB (acral recessive)
		Pretibial DHEB
		DHEB pruriginosa
		DHEB (centripetal variant)
		Bullous dermolysis of the newborn

Europe and the USA [10]. Diagnostic strategies and algorithms based upon molecular epidemiological features determined in populations of Western origin may not be applicable to Middle Eastern populations, possibly due to consanguineous marriages; in addition, the fact that genotype-phenotype correlations firmly established in Western populations are not consistently observed in Middle East suggests the existence of inherited, epigenetic, or environmental modifier traits responsible for modulating the clinical expression of HEB.

39.3 Clinical Pictures

The major clinical feature of all clinical types and subtypes of HEB is the moderate to excessive epithelial fragility in the skin, resulting in blister formation. Secondary lesions such as erosions, ulcerations, and crusts with extensive scarring may result. Others lesions depend on the clinical type of the disease.

1. ***Epidermolysis bullosa simplex:*** Hereditary EBS is usually inherited in an autosomal dominant fashion; it is clearly less common in dark-skinned populations. Onset of the disease is usually at or shortly after birth, although patients may not develop blistering until late childhood or even early adulthood. In a *suprabasal* subtype, intact blisters are hardly ever observed due to the thin blister roofs, but erosions or impaired keratinization with increased desquamation is seen, similar to ichthyoses and palmoplantar keratoses (Fig. 39.1a).

Commonly occurring subtypes are:

(a) The *localized HEBS* (*Weber-Cockayne syndrome*) showing blisters on the extremities, palms, and soles mostly without scarring (Fig. 39.1b), while milia and nail dystrophy are not often seen.
(b) The *generalized intermediate HEBS* with blisters mostly on the hands, feet, and extremities showing lesions healing with atrophy with dyspigmentation (Fig. 39.2a).
(c) The *generalized severe HEBS* (*Dowling-Meara syndrome*) with disseminated, herpetiform lesions on the extremities, neck, and trunk and involvement of the oral mucosa. By late childhood, most patients develop confluent thickening, palmoplantar keratoderma and nail dystrophy (Fig. 39.3a, b). The clinical picture may partially resolve in some patients during midlife to late adulthood. Other rare basal subtypes may present mottled pigmentation and muscular dystrophy. The *Ogna type* is associated with easy bruisability, hemorrhagic blistering, and marked deformities of the nails (onychogryphosis).

Table 39.2 *Epidermolysis bullosa hereditaria* and its molecular heterogeneity (adapted from [8])

Clinical type	Mutated gene	Protein	Inheritance
Epidermolysis bullosa simplex	*KRT5*	Keratin 5	Autosomal dominant (AD)
	KRT14	Keratin 14	AD, semidominant, autosomal recessive (AR)
	DSP	Desmoplakin	AR
	PKP1	Plakophilin-1	
	JUP	Plakoglobin	
	PLEC1	Plectin	AR
	DST	BPAG1	AR
	EXPH5	Exophilin 5	AR
	TGM5	Transglutaminase 5	AR
Junctional epidermolysis bullosa	*LAMA3*	Laminin-332	AR
	LAMB3		AR
	LAMC2		AR
	COL17A1	Collagen XVII	AR
	ITGA6	α6β4 integrin	AR
	ITGB4		AR, AD
	ITGA3	Integrin α3 subunit	AR
Dystrophic epidermolysis bullosa	*COL7A1*	Collagen VII	AR, AD
Kindler syndrome	*FERMT1*	Kindlin-1	

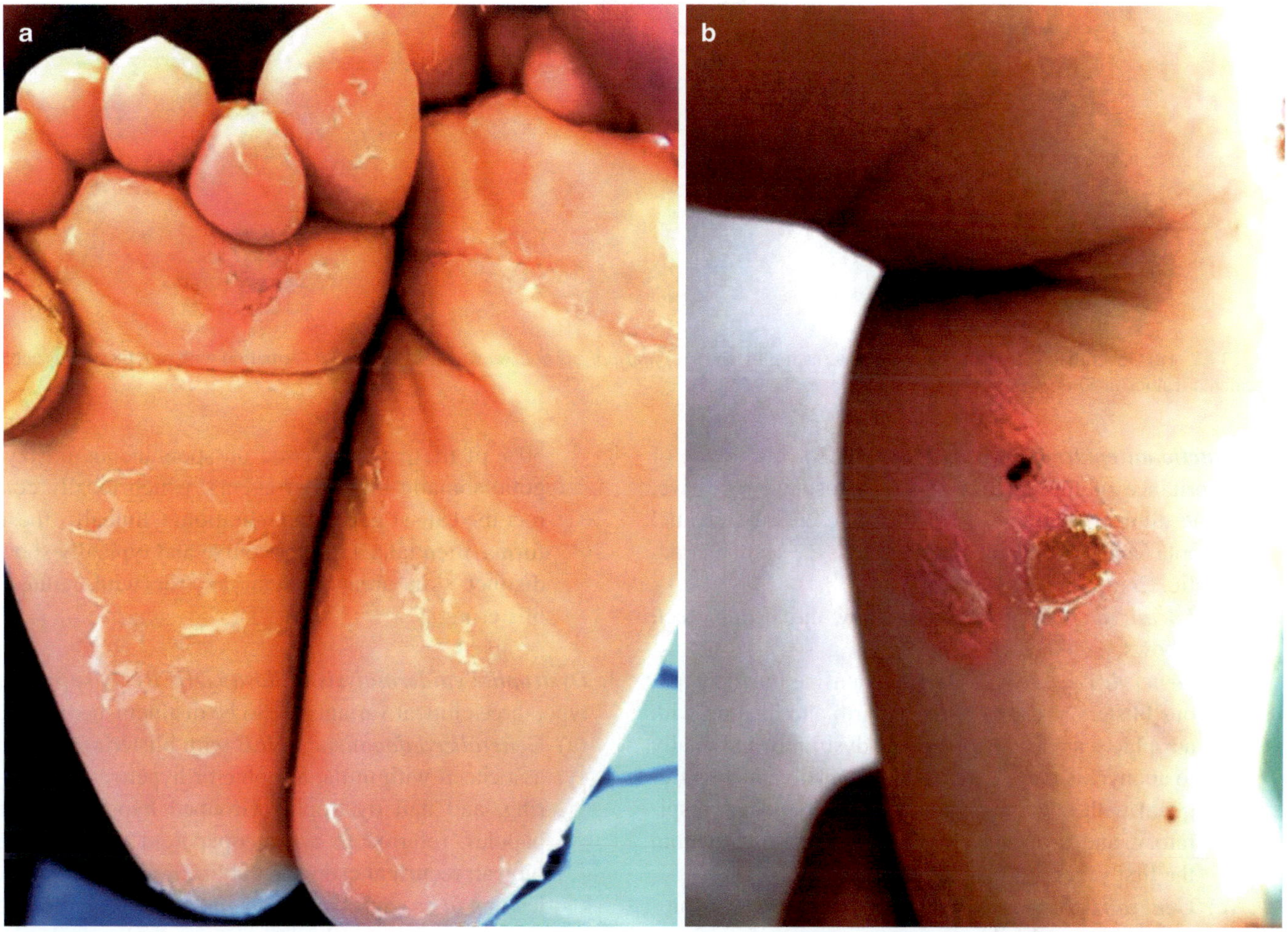

Fig. 39.1 (**a**) Plantar suprabasal desquamation and (**b**) skin fragility with blister formation in *epidermolysis bullosa simplex*

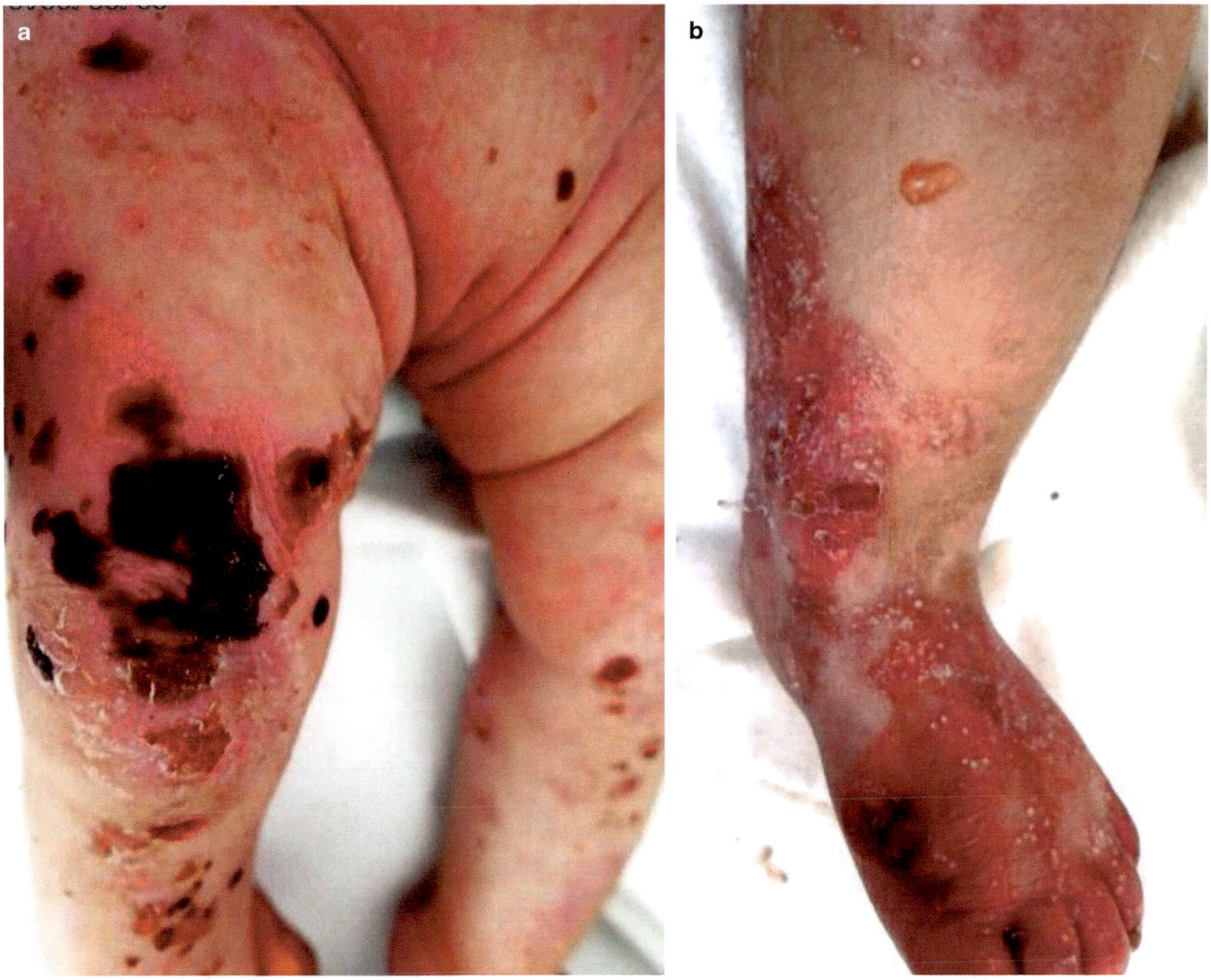

Fig. 39.2 (**a**) Generalized blister formation with crusting in severe *epidermolysis bullosa simplex*. (**b**) Blister formation with polymorphous acro-localized lesions in *Kindler syndrome*

2. ***Junctional epidermolysis bullosa** (JHEB):* The mode of inheritance of this type is mostly autosomal recessive. Some clinical findings such as the presence of enamel hypoplasia and exuberant granulation tissue seem characteristic. Common subtypes are:
   (a) *Localized JEB*, involving mainly the hands, feet, elbows, and knees.
   (b) *Generalized severe JEB* with extensive mucocutaneous blisters already present at birth and healing with atrophic scars leading to onychodystrophy and finally to anonychia (Fig. 39.4). Mucosal involvement is frequent with conjunctival, oral, gastrointestinal, respiratory, and urogenital lesions. The mortality within the first years of life is high.
   (c) *Generalized intermediate JHEB* with similar symptomatology and mild extracutaneous manifestations. Revertant mosaicism is found in approximately 30% of the patients based on spontaneous postzygotic somatic molecular events, which locally correct the causal germ line mutation. Clinically, these forms often take a milder course and typically show distinct skin areas without any or with reduced blistering.

3. ***Dystrophic epidermolysis bullosa** (DHEB):* Also in this type, three clinical variants are to be distinguished:
   (a) *Generalized dominant DHEB* with blistering at birth associated with milia, atrophic or hypertrophic scarring, and nail dystrophy. Grouped hypopigmented papules, referred to as "albopapuloid" lesions, are typical; recurrent esophageal blistering and erosions, leading to progressive dysphagia, rarely occur. In late stages severe mutilations are seen in neglected patients (Fig. 39.5).

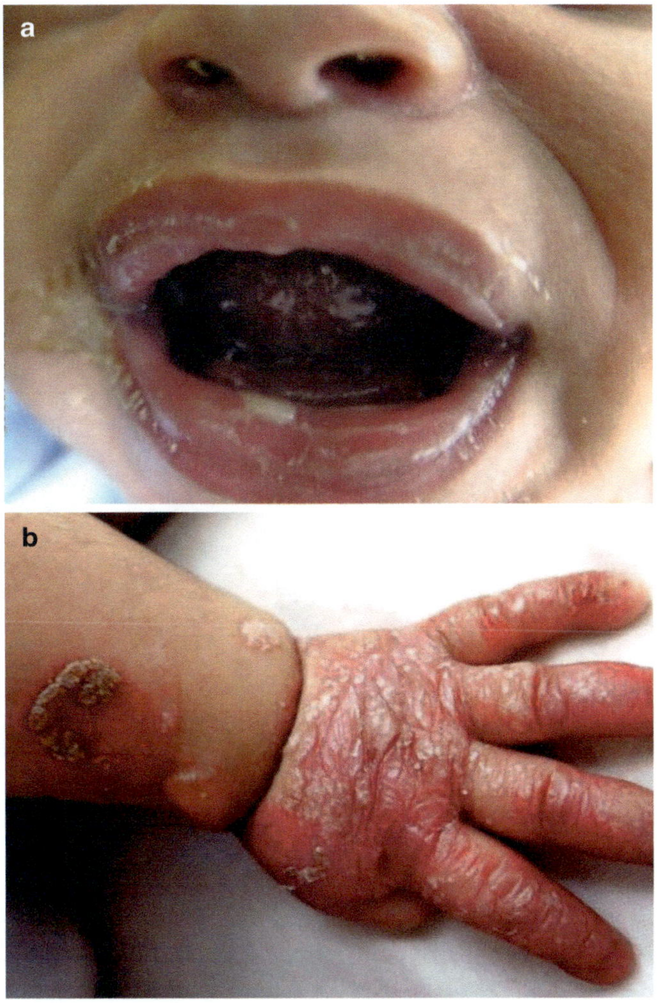

Fig. 39.3 (**a**) Extensive post blistering erosions of the oral (tongue and lip) mucosa in *epidermolysis bullosa* with shedding. (**b**) Blistering associated with milia, atrophic scarring, and nail dystrophy

(b) *Generalized severe recessive DHEB* with similar mucocutaneous presentation but failure to thrive, growth retardation, severe anemia, early infant mortality, and risk of squamous cell carcinoma.

(c) *Generalized intermediate recessive DHEB* with less pronounced symptoms. Mutilating deformations are generally missing, but there are frequent oral and dental manifestations, as well as nail and hair changes with increased risk for developing squamous cell carcinoma.

4. ***Kindler syndrome***: This variant is autosomal recessively inherited, initially characterized by acrolocalized blisters predominantly occurring in childhood (Fig. 39.2b). Photosensitivity and progressive poikiloderma with extensive skin atrophy on UV-exposed areas may come later, in addition. Gingivitis and periodontitis are common; esophageal and urogenital stenoses as well as gastrointestinal symptoms are possible. Patients have an increased risk for developing non-melanocytic skin tumors.

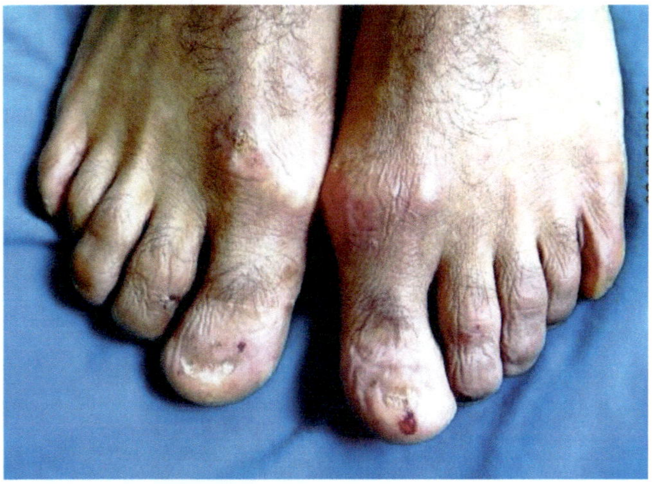

Fig. 39.4 Scarring and late anonychia in an adult with *junctional epidermolysis bullosa (JHEB)*

39.4 Management

There is no effective management for the hereditary epidermolysis bullosa. Major aim of the attending physician is to recognize the condition, problems, and complications as they arise and provide help, in order to reduce painful and disfiguring symptoms, and also to diagnose early life-threatening problems such as various overlapping infections and EB-associated cancer. Patients and their families need lifelong medical supervision together with practical and psychological support. Despite its low incidence, severe EB is a heavy burden for developing countries in Africa. In many of those, dermatology is not established as a specialty in their health services, and the general physicians are challenged [11].

General measures: The general health of the patient must be considered, and supplements may be necessary for those affected by oral ulcerations or strictures in the gastrointestinal tract. Care must be taken to avoid any friction when handling the patient and also briefing the parents on the precautions necessary to avoid further skin damage. Dressings should be nonadherent and carefully cut to the correct size for the coverage required and adhesive tapes be avoided. Clothing must be easy to put on, and turning clothes inside-out can help to reduce the seams rubbing on the skin. Nappies should be lined with a soft material to avoid irritation. Immunization may proceed normally and chickenpox vaccine is also recommended.

Skin and mucosal care: New blisters should be lanced with sterile blade or needle and drained. The blister roof should be left in place to facilitate reepithelialization. When bathing, there are benefits if salt is added to the water to reduce pain and the incidence of infections. Daily use of emollients and moisturizing products is strongly recom-

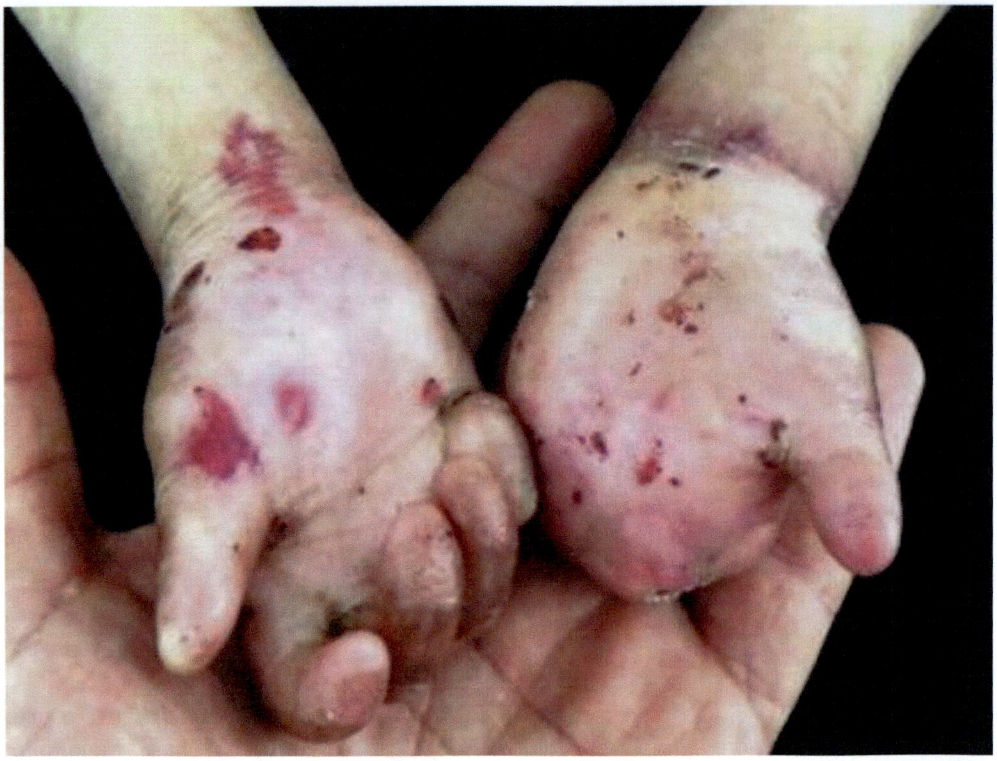

Fig. 39.5 Late stage of *dystrophic epidermolysis bullosa (DHEB)* with severe mutilations

Table 39.3 Major clinical complications in patients with various types of hereditary epidermolysis bullosa

Tissue involved	Major complications
Skin	Chronic/infected wounds, exuberant granulation tissue, atrophic/hypertrophic scars, post-inflammatory pigmentary changes, milia, palmoplantar keratoderma, EB nevi, basal/squamous cell carcinomas
Skin adnexa	Onychodystrophy, shedding or loss of nails, scarring alopecia, hypotrichosis
Oral cavity	Microstomia, ankyloglossia, enamel hypoplasia, multiple caries, periodontitis
External eye	Corneal blepharitis/scarring, symblepharon, ectropion, keratitis, diminished vision
External ear	External auditory canal narrowing
Nose	Nasal narrowing
Gastrointestinal tract	Pyloric atresia, esophageal stenosis, chronic constipation, anal fissures, protein-losing enteropathy
Genitourinary tract	Urethral strictures, vulvovaginal scarring, genitourinary malformations, renal failure
Upper respiratory tract	Tracheolaryngeal stenosis
Musculoskeletal system	Osteopenia and osteoporosis, limb flexion contractures, digit contractures, pseudosyndactyly, mitten deformities, muscular dystrophy
Hematopoietic system	Multifactorial anemia
Heart	Dilated cardiomyopathy
Endocrine	Delayed puberty, amenorrhea

mended for xerotic skin in order to reduce blistering, pain, and itching. Lips, conjunctiva, and nasal mucosa are always vulnerable to damage; regular lubrication with adapted emollients is needed (Table 39.3).

Wound care: Mild antiseptic cleanser should be used for extended and/or infected lesions. Costly advanced dressings (e.g., hydrogels, hydrofibers, and foams) showed only a modest advantage compared to paraffin-impregnated gauzes in accelerating healing of non-EB chronic wounds. Finger and toe dressings should be regularly performed to delay digit fusion and pseudosyndactyly. In case of exuberant granulation tissue, short courses of potent topical corticosteroids are effective in reducing exuberant granulation tissue.

Pain: One of the common complaints of patients with HEB is pain, occurring in blister sites and areas of skin loss. Appropriate analgesia should be performed before bathing or dressing. Topical anesthetics (xylocaine, lidocaine, prilocaine) and paracetamol are recommended before venipuncture and the care of painful tense blisters or wounds. In more severe cases and complex procedures, opioids are indicated, considering their side effects (constipation, pruritus, and rarely respiratory failure). Neuropathic pain components can be managed with pregabalin or gabapentin.

Over the last decade, a number of therapeutic advances have been introduced including gene or cell replacement therapies, protein replacement, treatments with allogeneic fibroblasts, mesenchymal stromal cells, allogeneic bone marrow transplantation, culturing and grafting revertant mosaic keratinocytes, and clinical application of inducible pluripotent stem cells [12]. Although a cure for EB still remains elusive, recent data on animal models and initial clinical trials have raised the expectations of patients, clinicians, and researchers that disease modification and improved quality of life are feasible goals. At present, diagnostic and treatment protocols may provide healthcare professionals with guidance for establishing optimal patient management [13].

39.5 Monitoring and Genetic Counseling

Patients should be regularly monitored and their families must receive continuing support. The disease has a major impact on the quality of life; complications can manifest at every age. Physical and occupational management must be started early in life, particularly in HEBS with muscular dystrophy. Continuing physiotherapy will delay contractures and deformities, improve functional mobility, and enhance patient autonomy and social integration. Also, genetic counseling is mandatory for the attending physician. Prenatal diagnosis offered for pregnant women (chorionic venous sampling at 8–10 weeks or amniocentesis in the second trimester) will indicate if the fetus is affected and termination should be considered. There is a 50% recurrence risk for each pregnancy in autosomal dominant disease and 25% for autosomal recessive disease, with a 50% chance that the offspring will be a carrier and 25% unaffected and not a carrier. However, there are pitfalls in assuming inheritance patterns: if neither parent is affected, a child with EB could have a mild recessive form of EB or a new mutation for a dominant form.

Conclusions

The medical and psychosocial aspects of epidermolysis bullosa as a broad genetic disorder are enormous. Adult patients face problems on issues of social integration, independence, sexuality, marriage, pregnancy, and for finding appropriate clothing and footwear. In the future, educational efforts for family planning and genetic counseling are unconditioned requirements, especially in developing countries with pigmented skin populations. Numerous groups around the globe are doing invaluable efforts to support the individual needs of these patients, their further counseling, and also research on EB. Most of them are from developed countries. A list of these various groups established can be found at the website www.debra-international.org.

References

1. Fine JD, Bruckner-Tuderman L, Eady RA, et al. Inherited epidermolysis bullosa: updated recommendations on diagnosis and classification. J Am Acad Dermatol. 2014;70:1103–26.
2. Laimer M, Prodinger C, Bauer JW. Hereditary epidermolysis bullosa. J Dtsch Dermatol Ges. 2015;13:1125–33.
3. Fine JD. Epidemiology of inherited epidermolysis bullosa based on incidence and prevalence estimates from the National Epidermolysis Bullosa Registry. JAMA Dermatol. 2016;152: 1231–8.
4. Bothwell JE. Lethal epidermolysis bullosa in black South African neonates. Int J Dermatol. 1996;35:422–5.
5. Cherif F, Mnajja N, Feriani S, et al. Hereditary epidermolysis bullosa in Tunisia: an epidemio-clinical and ultrastructural study. Arch Inst Pasteur Tunis. 2005;82:53–8.
6. Ben Halim N, Hsouna S, Lasram K, et al. Differential impact of consanguineous marriages on autosomal recessive diseases in Tunisia. Am J Hum Biol. 2016;28:171–80.
7. Ciubotaru D, Bergman R, Baty D, et al. Epidermolysis bullosa simplex in Israel: clinical and genetic features. Arch Dermatol. 2003;139:498–505.
8. Uitto J, Has C, Vahidnezhad H, et al. Molecular pathology of the basement membrane zone in heritable blistering diseases: the paradigm of epidermolysis bullosa. Matrix Biol. 2016; pii: S0945-053X(16)30112-3. Doi: https://doi.org/10.1016/j.matbio.2016.07.009.
9. Siegel DH, Ashton GH, Penagos HG, et al. Loss of kindlin-1, a human homolog of the Caenorhabditis elegans actin-extracellular-matrix linker protein UNC-112, causes Kindler syndrome. Am J Hum Genet. 2003;73:174–87.
10. Abu Sa'd J, Indelman M, Pfendner E, et al. Molecular epidemiology of hereditary epidermolysis bullosa in a Middle Eastern population. J Invest Dermatol. 2006;126:777–81.
11. George AO. Epidermolysis bullosa, three cases in an African family-medical, social and economic problems in management in a developing country. Trop Geogr Med. 1988;40:171–3.
12. Hsu CK, Wang SP, Lee JY, et al. Treatment of hereditary epidermolysis bullosa: updates and future prospects. Am J Clin Dermatol. 2014;15:1–6.
13. Chiaverini C, Bourrat E, Mazereeuw-Hautier J, et al. Hereditary epidermolysis bullosa: French national guidelines (PNDS) for diagnosis and treatment. Ann Dermatol Venereol. 2017;144:6–35.

40 Inherited Ichthyoses

Mourad Mokni

Inherited ichthyoses are a group of genetic disorders characterized by dry skin, hyperkeratosis, and increased scale desquamation, often associated with erythroderma. The clinical manifestations are due to a series of mutations of genes involved in the development of the stratum corneum and skin barrier formation. The group consists of phenotypic expressions limited only in the skin and its appendages and others with additional extracutaneous involvement. The incidence of ichthyotic conditions in pigmented and black skin ethnic populations is not known. In two reports from the Eastern Province of Saudi Arabia, the incidence of hereditary ichtyosis and non-bullous congenital ichthyosiform erythroderma has been assessed, respectively, 7 per 1000 and 2 per 1000 new patients. These relatively high rates may be attributed to high consanguinity in countries of the Middle East [1, 2]. The commonest type of hereditary ichthyosis was ichthyosis vulgaris followed by non-bullous ichthyosiform erythroderma; 90% of the patients in this group were born with collodion membranes. Also in populations in East Africa, ichthyoses are not rarely seen.

40.1 Pathogenesis

In the process of epidermal differentiation, intermediate keratin filaments responsible for the structural integrity of keratinocytes are among the first proteins to be expressed in a tightly regulated manner. Keratins 5 and 14 are expressed in the basal layers and keratins 1 and 10 in the suprabasal layers. This overall process of differentiation results in the formation of the stratum corneum as a robust barrier composed of keratinocytes and inter-keratinocyte lipids. Mutations in proteins essential for the formation of this barrier, i.e., keratins and enzymes involved in lipid synthesis, lead to the disruption of its integrity resulting in ichthyotic conditions. Mutations in over 50 genes have been reported to cause ichthyoses, affecting a host of cellular functions including DNA repair, lipid biosynthesis, adhesion, and desquamation, as well as other processes. Based on these findings, a recent consensus conference revised the nomenclature and proposed a new clinical classification that distinguishes 36 different types of ichthyosis and 10 related clinical entities [3]. Major consensus was achieved on the proposal to categorize inherited ichthyosis into two types: *Non-syndromic ichthyoses*, in which the phenotypic expression of the underlying genetic defect is only seen in the skin, and *syndromic ichthyoses*, in which the phenotypic expression is also manifested in other organs (Table 40.1).

40.2 Clinical Pictures

Clinical hallmark of all entities is thickening of the cornified layer with visible scaling, often accompanying with features of inflammation presenting as erythroderma. Other symptoms include painful fissuring of the thickened skin, decreased range of motion at joints, decreased tactile sensitivity, hypohidrosis with heat intolerance, and pruritus. In darkly pigmented and black skin, the diagnosis and classification could be challenging because erythroderma is difficult to assess. In addition, patients in tropical countries are faced with challenges of heat intolerance, infections, and social stigma. Families with disfiguring skin diseases usually have difficulties integrating into society, and thus marriage is not encouraged. To safeguard the future of other children, patients with ichthyoses are being isolated and denied further education, thus having no chance for future employment [4].

Non-syndromic ichthyoses include mainly the common ichthyosis vulgaris, a recessive X-linked ichthyosis with delayed onset, the large group of congenital autosomal recessive ichthyotic conditions, and a group of keratinopathic ichthyoses which show flat erosions and bulla formation; the syndromic types are also considered in short.

M. Mokni
Service der Dermatologie, Hopital La Rabta, Tunis, Tunisia
e-mail: mourad.mokni@rns.tn

C. E. Orfanos et al. (eds.), *Pigmented Ethnic Skin and Imported Dermatoses*, https://doi.org/10.1007/978-3-319-69422-1_40

Table 40.1 Classification of major inherited ichthyotic disorders (adapted/modified from [3])

Non-syndromic ichthyoses and genes involved	**Syndromic ichthyosis** and genes involved
DELAYED ONSET	
Ichthyosis vulgaris *FLG* **Recessive X-linked ichthyosis** *STS*	**Refsum syndrome** *PHYH, PAXH*
CONGENITAL	
Autosomal recessive congenital ichthyoses ***Harlequin ichthyosis*** *ABCA12* ***Lamellar ichthyosis*** *TGM1, NIPAL4/ICHTHYIN, ALOX12B, ALOXE3, CYP4F22, ABCA12, PNPLA1, CERS3, LIPN* ***Congenital ichthyosiform erythroderma*** *TGM, NIPAL4/ICHTHYIN, ALOX12B, ALOXE3, CYP4F22, ABCA12, PNPLA1, CERS3, LIPN* ***Self-healing collodion baby*** *TGM1, ALOX12B, ALOXE3* ***Bathing suit ichthyosis*** *TGM1* **Keratinopathic ichthyoses**[a] ***Epidermolytic ichthyosis***[a] *(bullous ichthyosiform erythroderma)* *KRT1, KRT10* ***Superficial epidermolytic ichthyosis***[a] *(bullous type of Siemens)* *KRT2* ***Ichthyosis hystrix*** *(type Curth-Macklin)* *KRT1*	**Netherton syndrome** *SPINKS5* **Sjögren-Larsson syndrome** *ALDH3A2*

[a]New denominations

40.2.1 Non-syndromic Ichthyoses

1. **Ichthyosis Vulgaris**
   Ichthyosis vulgaris is the most common clinical type of ichthyosis, with an overall incidence of 1:250 to 1:1000. It is characterized by xerosis, scaling, pruritus, and eczema, strongly associated with atopic symptoms. The phenotypic manifestations tend to appear from the age of 2 months and often improve in summer. The extensor sides of the lower legs and the back are the most commonly affected location. The chest and the abdomen are often less involved; keratosis pilaris and palmoplantar hyperlinearity are often seen. The discovery of mutations of filaggrin (FLG) as a basic figure of ichthyosis vulgaris led to the insight that the very same loss-of-function mutations confer a strong predisposition to atopic dermatitis [5, 6]. Although the presence of population-specific FLG mutations has been reported in Europeans, Asians, and Africans [7], it is likely that additional factors other than these mutations are involved in African Americans [8] and in Ethiopians [9].

2. **Recessive X-Linked Ichthyosis**
   Recessive X-linked ichthyosis is the second most common ichthyosis with a prevalence of 1:2000 to 1:6000, caused by hereditary deficiency of the steroid sulfatase (STS) enzyme due to mutations of the STS gene. The disease manifests exclusively in males. Cutaneous manifestations are present soon after birth and usually tend not to improve with age. In its clinical expression, X-linked ichthyosis is more severe than ichthyosis vulgaris, as large, dark brown prominent scales form, adhering to the underlying skin and covering the entire body including flexural areas (Fig. 40.1). In mild cases the scaling is less distinguishable but also visible in dark and black skin. Additional features may be present, such as intellectual disability, autism, or attention deficit with hyperactivity, partly influenced by the deletion size of the gene.

3. **Autosomal Recessive Congenital Ichthyoses (Non-bullous)**
   Autosomal recessive congenital ichthyosis (ARCI) is a comprehensive definition term used to represent a generic phenotype of erythrodermic, scaly skin presenting over almost the entire body surface at birth. The ARCI group is clinically divided into three major phenotypes and two subtypes.
   (a) ***Harlequin ichthyosis***
   Harlequin ichthyosis is phenotypically the most severe inherited ichthyosis, occasionally fatal. The clinical features include thick, platelike scales with severe ectropion, eclabium, and flattening of the ears. The diagnosis is clinically not difficult, because of its characteristic phenotype.
   (b) ***Lamellar ichthyosis***
   Lamellar ichthyosis is a major phenotype of autosomal recessive congenital ichthyosis with varying severity (Fig. 40.2a, b), clinically more mild than the harlequin phenotype. The characteristic scales are large, often thickened and dark gray or brown in color, also covering most of the body flexural areas. Palmoplantar keratoderma is frequently seen. A large number of patients who show later in life the classic lamellar phenotype were born as *collodion babies* (Fig. 40.3). In a Moroccan series, 67% of collodion babies evoluted on lamellar ichthyosis and 21% on congenital ichthyosiform erythroderma [10].
   (c) ***Congenital ichthyosiform erythroderma***
   Ichthyosiform erythroderma is another major phenotype of congenital ichthyosis (3b,c); patients are frequently born as collodion babies. After the collodion membrane is dropped, erythroderma and scaling appear. The erythroderma often improves in infancy, but in severe cases the erythrodermic feature becomes persistent. In adults generalized lamellar-type scaling is seen, occasionally with persisting ectropion

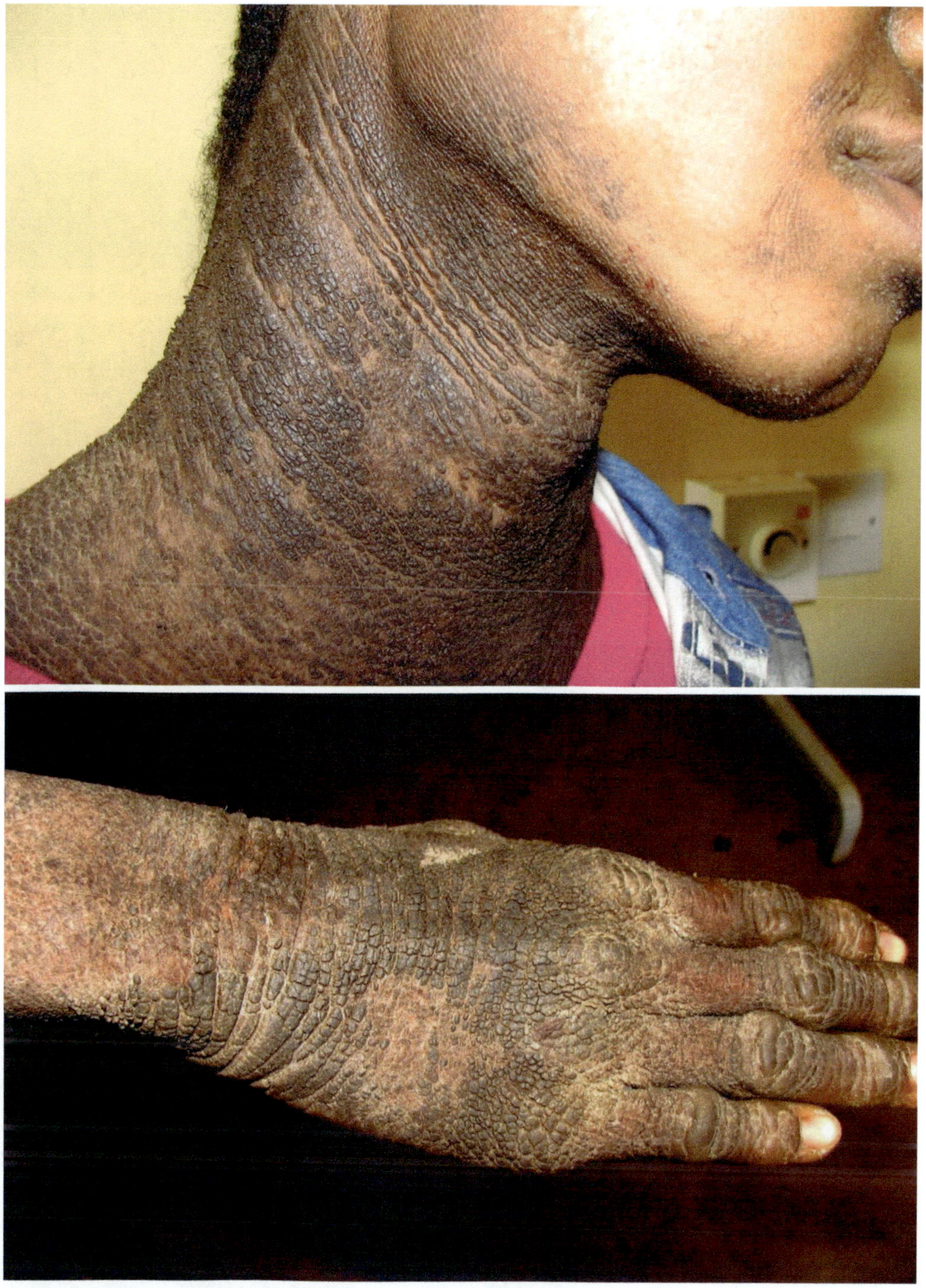

Fig. 40.1 *Severe ichthyosis* showing hystrix type of hyperkeratoses in joints and hands in a young Tanzanian male (most likely autosomal recessive X-chromosomal type)

(Fig. 40.4); in other cases there is prominent dry scaling without erythrodermic features (Fig. 40.5).

(d) ***Self-healing collodion baby***

Collodion babies present at birth with erythroderma and shiny, tight skin resembling parchment covering the neonate's body and may cause ectropion, eclabium, flattening of the ears and nostrils, restricted extension of the digits and extremities, and limitation of chest movement. It spares the mucosal surfaces and stops at the edge of natural orifices and at the cutaneous level of the umbilical cord. Hairs usually penetrate the collodion membrane and nails are exceptionally covered. The membrane gradually peels off during the first 4 weeks, but may not completely disappear until the third month of life usually revealing an ichthyotic phenotype. Hypohidrosis is often associated. Less common features include poor sucking, restricted pulmonary ventilation, digital vascular constriction, and edema of the extremities.

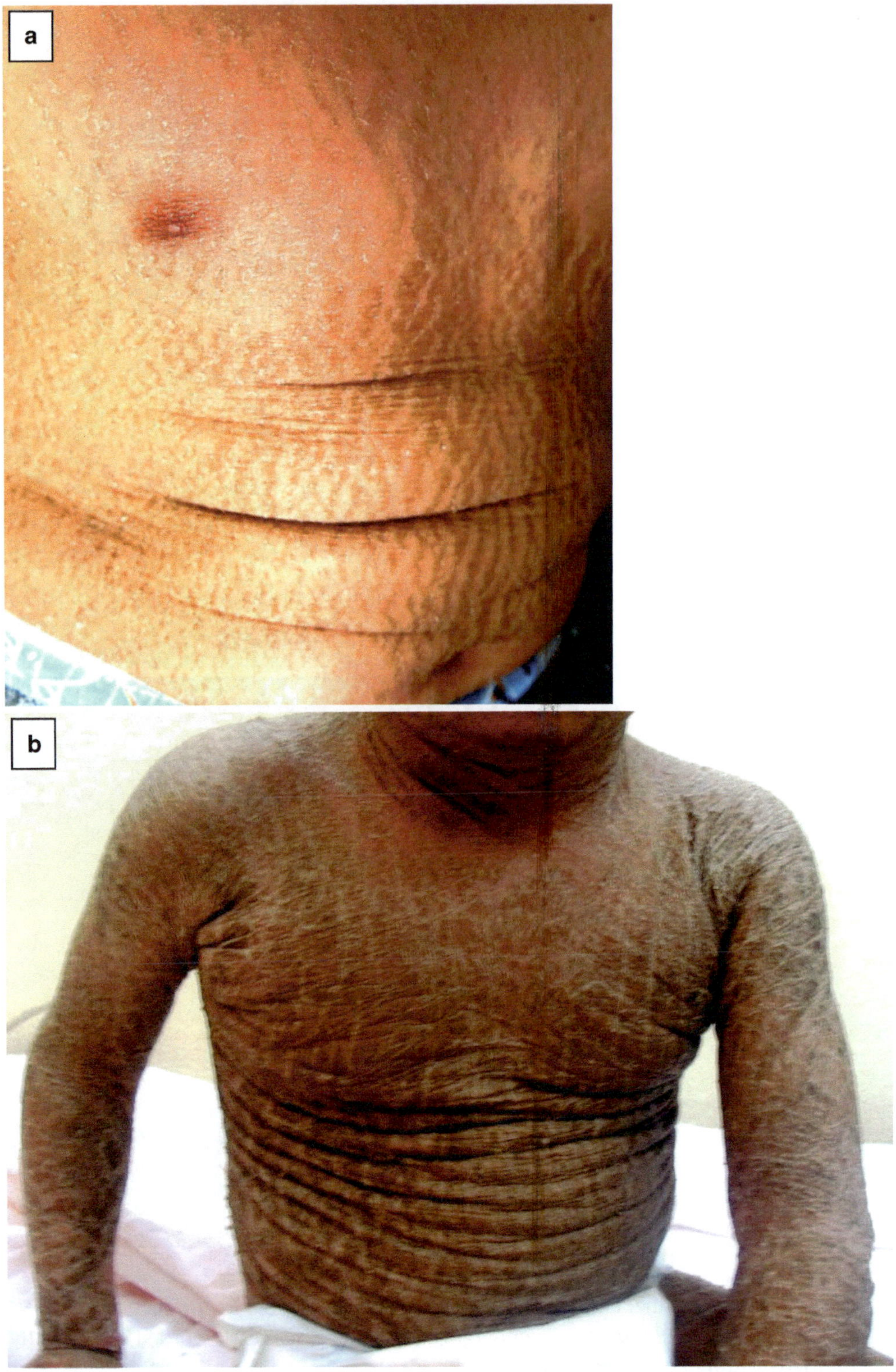

Fig. 40.2 *Lamellar ichthyosis*; (**a**) mild expression of the trunk; (**b**) severe, generalized involvement

(e) ***Bathing suit ichthyosis***

Bathing suit ichthyosis is another minor variant of ARCI, characterized by unique distribution of lesions on the trunk, the most proximal parts of the upper limbs, the scalp, and the neck, but not the central face and the extremities. This unusual phenotype has been first described in a black-skinned population in South Africa [11], and several cases from different ethnic backgrounds were recently reported [12].

4. **Keratinopathic Ichthyoses (bullous)**

The term *keratinopathic ichthyosis* has been proposed as a comprehensive umbrella for patients with ichthyosis presenting epidermolysis often leading to bulla formation; the group includes patients categorized as epidermolytic

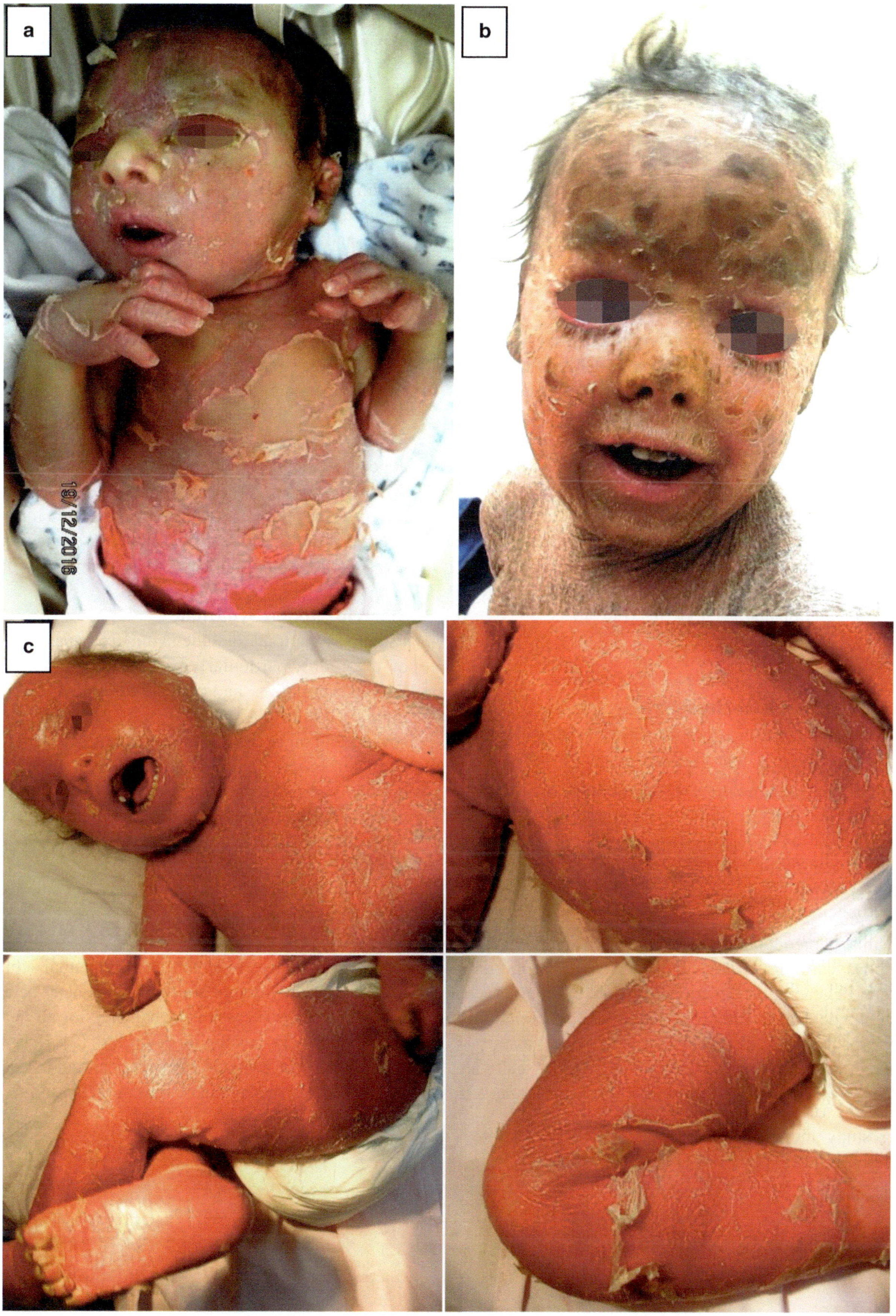

Fig. 40.3 *Collodion babies* (**a**) shortly after birth; (**b**) persisting ectropion in a 4-year-old child; (**c**) *collodion baby* several weeks after birth with severe epidermolytic erythroderma

ichthyosis or superficial epidermolytic ichthyosis and other rare types described such as annular epidermolytic ichthyosis and ichthyosis type Curth-Macklin.

(a) ***Epidermolytic ichthyosis*** *(bullous ichthyosiform erythroderma)*
This subtype is the most prevalent phenotype of keratinopathic ichthyosis characterized by multiple erosions with erythroderma and widespread formation of blisters. The patients show erythema and blistering at birth, diminishing with age, and generalized epidermolytic hyperkeratosis in adulthood (Fig. 40.6).

(b) ***Superficial epidermolytic ichthyosis*** *(bullous ichthyosis of Siemens)*
The term superficial epidermolytic ichthyosis had been proposed to replace the formerly well-defined entity ichthyosis bullosa *Siemens*, which shows a more superficial pattern of epidermolysis and bulla formation. It is clinically characterized by mild epidermal hyperkeratosis over the flexural areas and the development of denuded hyperkeratotic skin with superficial blistering.

(c) ***Ichthyosis hystrix****, type Curth-Macklin*
This is a rare, autosomal dominant disorder characterized by extensive, spiky, or verrucous hyperkeratoses affecting preferably the large joints and the extremities, with or without palmoplantar keratoderma (Fig. 40.7).

40.2.2 Syndromic Ichthyoses

1. **Refsum Syndrome**
Refsum syndrome develops during childhood to adolescence. Most patients show a progressive course, but remission and exacerbation are repeated in some patients. Four of its signs are pigmentous retinitis, peripheral neuritis, cerebellar ataxia, and increased levels of protein in the cerebrospinal fluid. In addition, symptoms, such as anosmia, hemeralopia, vision disorder, cataract, muscular atrophy, cardiomyopathy, bone disorder, progressive myelin degeneration, functional disorder of the nervous system, cochlear hearing loss, ichthyosis, and renal failure, are observed. The skin is dry and cornification is marked, with furfuraceous desquamation. Most scales are brown. Especially in the trunk, cornification is marked. Furthermore, hyperkeratosis is also marked at the olecranon and patella. The diagnosis is verified by the presence of phytanic acid in plasma lipid fractions using gas chromatography.

2. **Netherton Syndrome**
Netherton syndrome is characterized by three main clinical features: (1) a congenital ichthyotic phenotype of varying expression and severity (*ichthyosis linearis circumflexa)*, (2) hair abnormalities, and (3) atopic predisposition and symptoms. Some patients show symmetrical erythematous lesions in various shapes, such as tortuous and double-edged scaling (Fig. 40.8), whereas in other cases generalized dryness and lichenification predominates. Scalp hairs are short, sparse, dry, and not lustrous; under a light microscope, characteristic nodes of the hair shafts are found, also called *bamboo hair*, whereby the distal part of the hair shaft invaginates into the proximal (*trichorrhexis invaginata*). However, bamboo hairs may appear later, and the number and formation of the nodes differ among patients; eyelash or eyebrow defects are also observed in some cases. Chronic hives, bronchial asthma, allergic rhinitis, hay fever, an increase in the serum IgE levels, and eosinophilia have been reported as additional symptoms.

3. **Sjögren-Larsson Syndrome**
Primary symptoms include symmetric spastic paralysis of the limbs, particularly marked in their lower part, mental retardation, and congenital ichthyosiform exanthema (Fig. 40.9). Mental retardation is relatively severe, and more than 50% of patients show an IQ of 50 or lower. In most patients, mental developmental retardation is detected during childhood. Gait disorder is often observed. Convulsion is noted in approximately 40% of the patients.

40.3 Management

There is no definitive treatment for congenital ichthyoses; severe cases usually do not survive the neonatal period. The management of these cases is a challenge for all health services particularly in developing countries [13]. Nevertheless, recent advances in neonatal intensive care and coordinated multidisciplinary management have greatly improved the

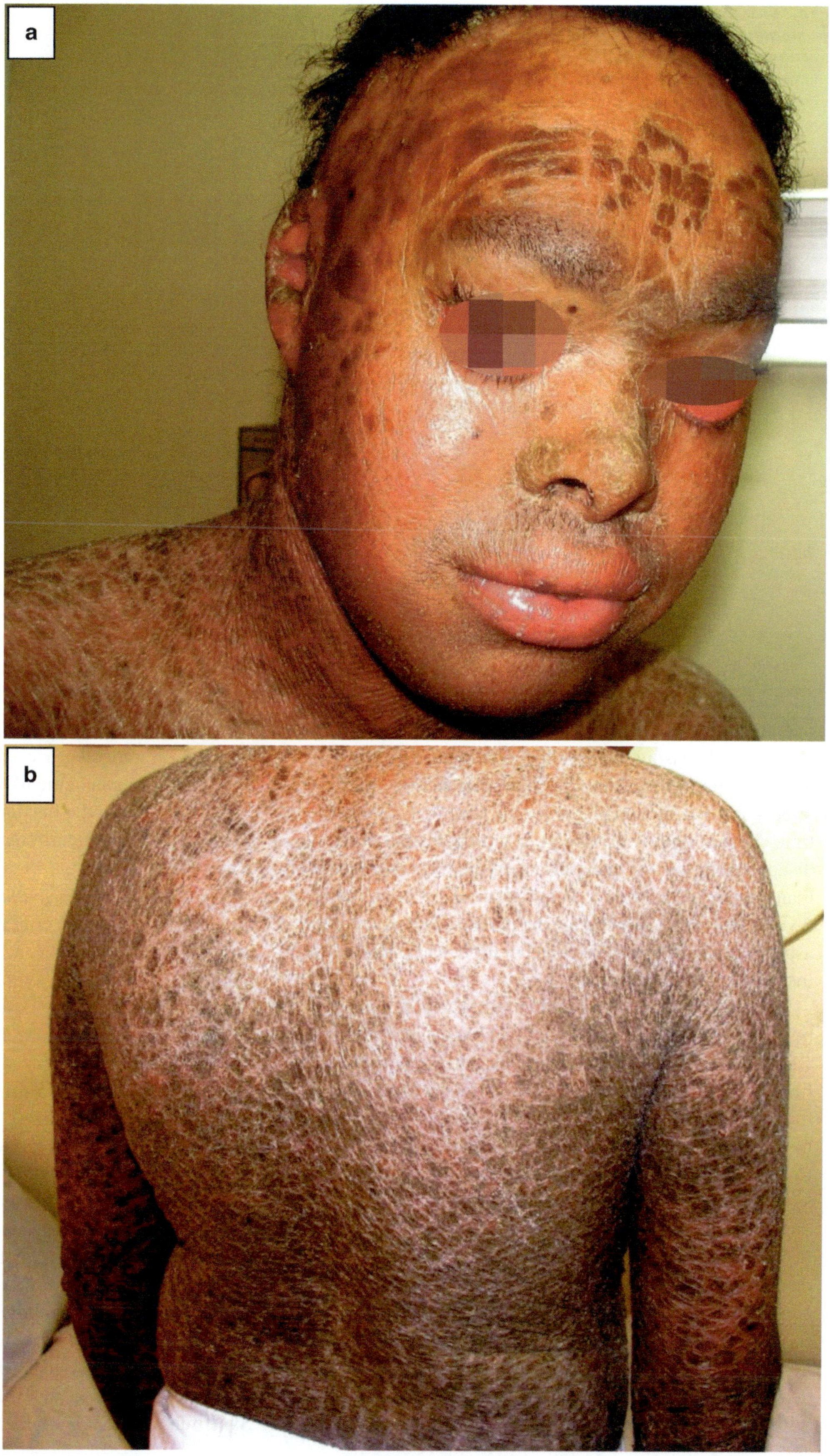

Fig. 40.4 *Congenital ichthyosiform erythroderma* in an adult, (**a**) with persisting ectropion (face treated topically with retinoids); (**b**) severe involvement of the trunk (untreated)

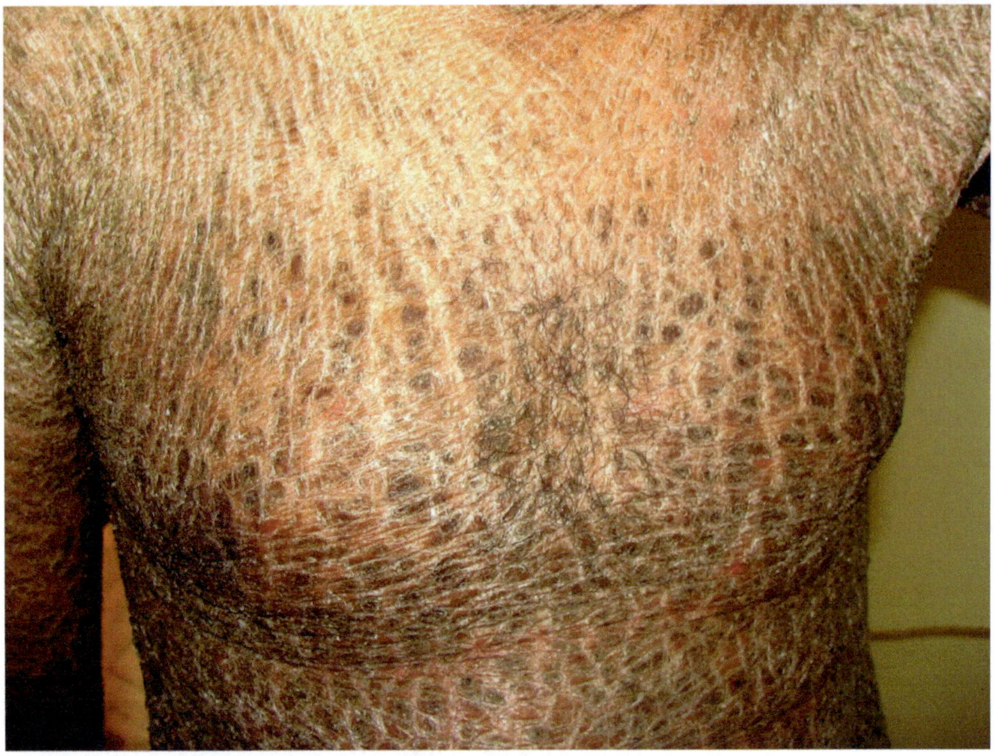

Fig. 40.5 Late stage of *congenital ichthyosiform erythroderma*; non-bullous, lamellar-type scaling without erythrodermic features

overall survival [14]. Although some forms may show spontaneous and seasonal variations, most patients require daily management throughout life. The therapeutic outcome is largely limited by nonadherence, as treatments are not only time consuming and involve greasy products but often show disappointing results and patients frequently withdraw from management. The birth of a child with severe congenital ichthyosis represents a shock for the parents. The psychological aspects must be taken in consideration when dealing with these unfortunate patients.

Neonatal care of severe ichthyosis: The collodion baby is born encased in a transparent, parchment-like membrane, which can interfere with respiration and sucking. Over the first 2 weeks of life, the membrane breaks up and desquamates. During this time, management should include careful monitoring of body temperature, hydration, and blood electrolytes. Management should keep the skin soft and pliable to reduce pain from deep skin fissures and to promote desquamation by using a humidified incubator and application of lubricants. The same basic regimen, although more rigorously exercised, also applies to babies suffering from the harlequin phenotype or epidermolytic hyperkeratosis, two forms of ichthyosis which are potentially lethal in the neonatal period.

Bathing and bath additives: Several years ago, patients with ichthyosis were strongly discouraged from bathing to not affect skin surface pH. Today, we know that ichthyosis patients should take a cleansing bath daily and rub their skin gently to mechanically remove some of their scales. In order to improve the barrier function and facilitate desquamation, sodium bicarbonate could be added to the bath water [15].

Hydration and lubrication: This can be accomplished by creams and ointments containing low concentrations of salt, urea (10%), or glycerol, which increase the water-binding capacity of the horny layer. For ichthyoses with thick scaling and markedly increased stratum corneum thickness, addition of one or more keratolytic agents is needed to decrease corneocyte cohesiveness, promote desquamation, and dissolve keratins and lipids. A wide variety of topical keratolytics can be used, including the α-hydroxy acids (e.g., lactic acid and glycolic acid), salicylic acid, high-dose urea, and propylene glycol. Also 2×/day topical application of 10% N-acetylcysteine as a mucolytic agent in combination with 5% urea in a water-in-oil emulsion showed excellent results in lamellar ichthyosis with no significant side effects [16].

Retinoids are particularly helpful for treatment of ichthyotic and hyperkeratotic conditions [17]. Topically they are used in certain anatomic locations including the face, palms and soles, and also in eyelids for treatment of ectropion. Systemic retinoids are widely administered in severe disease

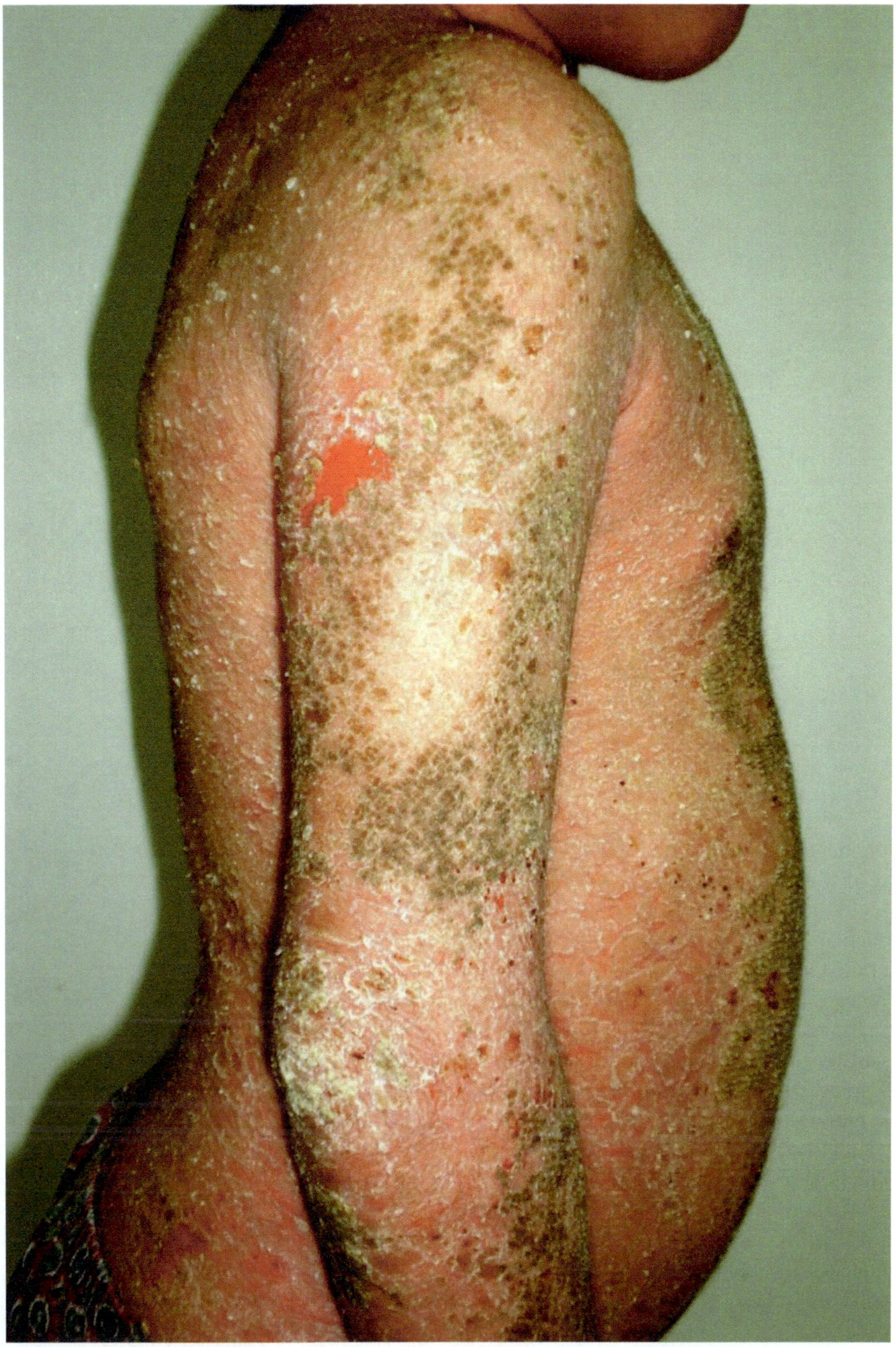

Fig. 40.6 *Epidermolytic ichthyosis* showing flat erosions and superficial blistering

but require close follow-up of patients. Isotretinoin or acitretin 0.5–1.0 mg/kg/day should not be exceeded, and the lowest possible therapeutic dose needs to be titrated. Adverse effects may include mucocutaneous toxicities, hair loss, skeletal hyperostoses, and laboratory abnormalities in blood cell counts and serum lipids. Retinoic acid metabolism blocking agents such as liarozole were shown effective with a favorable tolerability profile [18]; in moderate/severe lamellar ichthyosis, 75–150 mg/day oral liarozole improved scaling and life quality index [19].

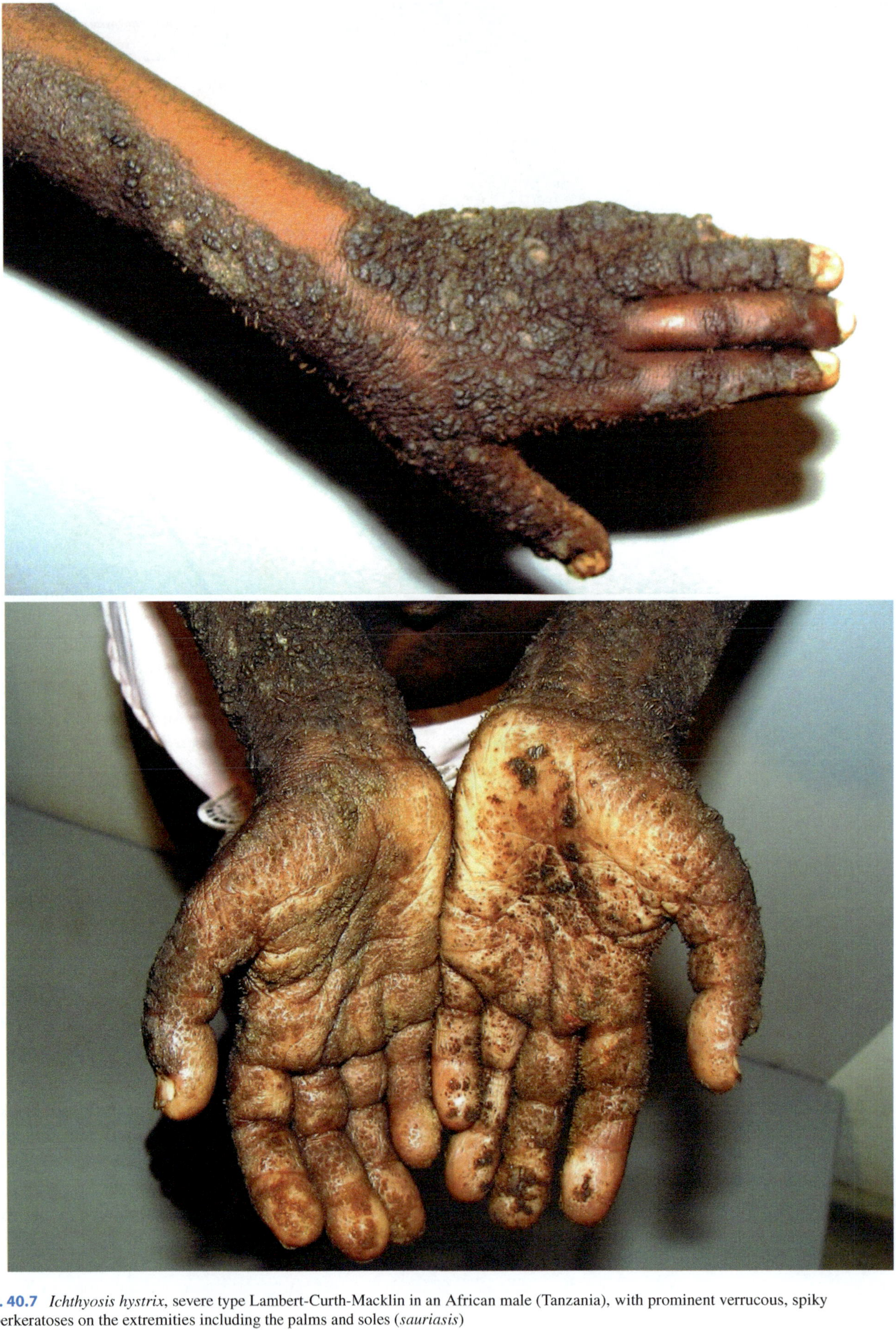

Fig. 40.7 *Ichthyosis hystrix*, severe type Lambert-Curth-Macklin in an African male (Tanzania), with prominent verrucous, spiky hyperkeratoses on the extremities including the palms and soles (*sauriasis*)

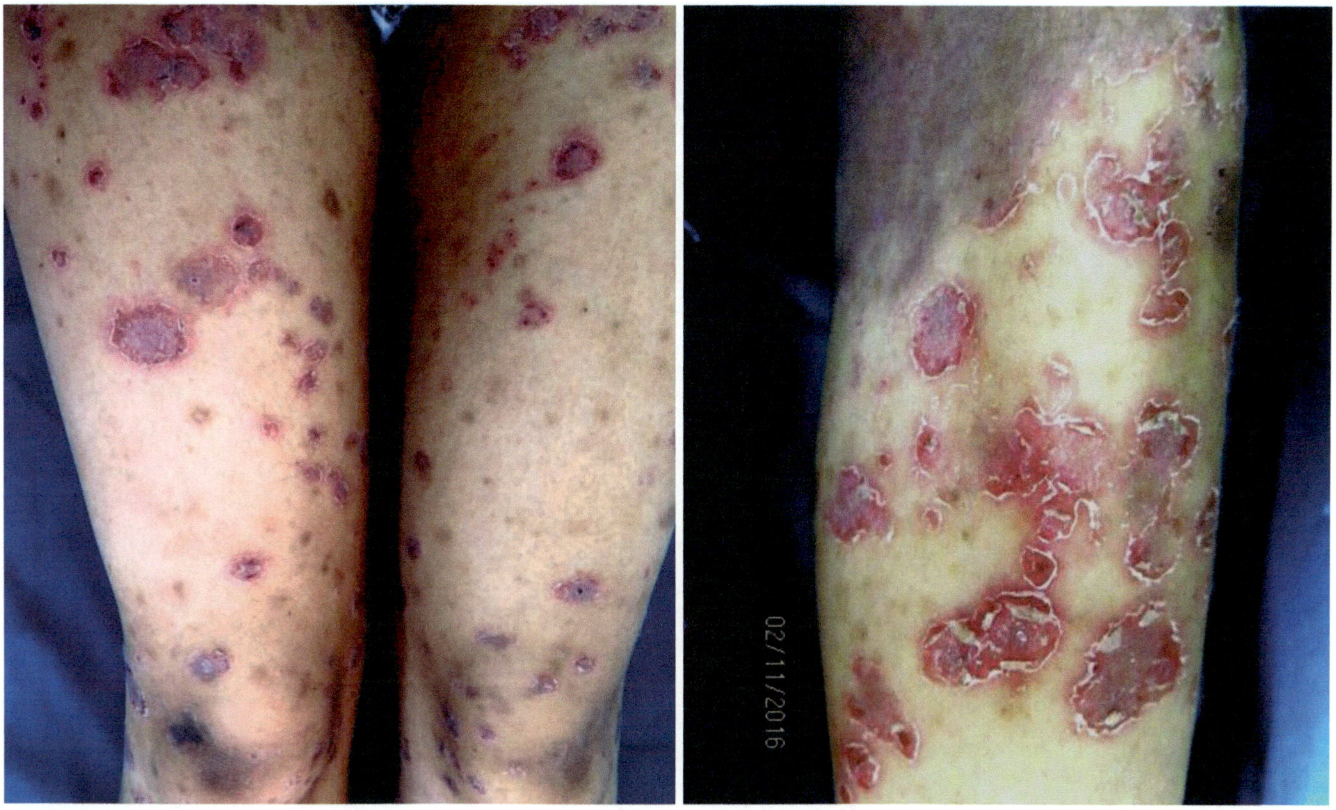

Fig. 40.8 *Netherton syndrome* with dry skin and double edge scaling on the extermities (mutation of *SPINKS5* and bamboo hairs confirmed)

40.4 Course and Further Monitoring

Most patients require lifelong treatment with daily applications of emollients all over the body. They are potential high consumers of such products which are costly, often not reimbursed by health insurances considered as cosmetics. Topical treatment takes time and often has to be repeated many times per day. In children, one should try to convert the therapeutic sessions into something relaxing and positive.

40.5 Prenatal Diagnosis and Genetic Counseling

Parents of children with ichthyosis should be offered appropriate genetic counseling to explain the nature of the disorder, its mode of inheritance, and the probability of future manifestations in the family. In some developed countries, prenatal testing is offered for individuals or couples at risk of having children with severe type of congenital ichthyoses, performed by chorionic villus sampling at 10–12 weeks of

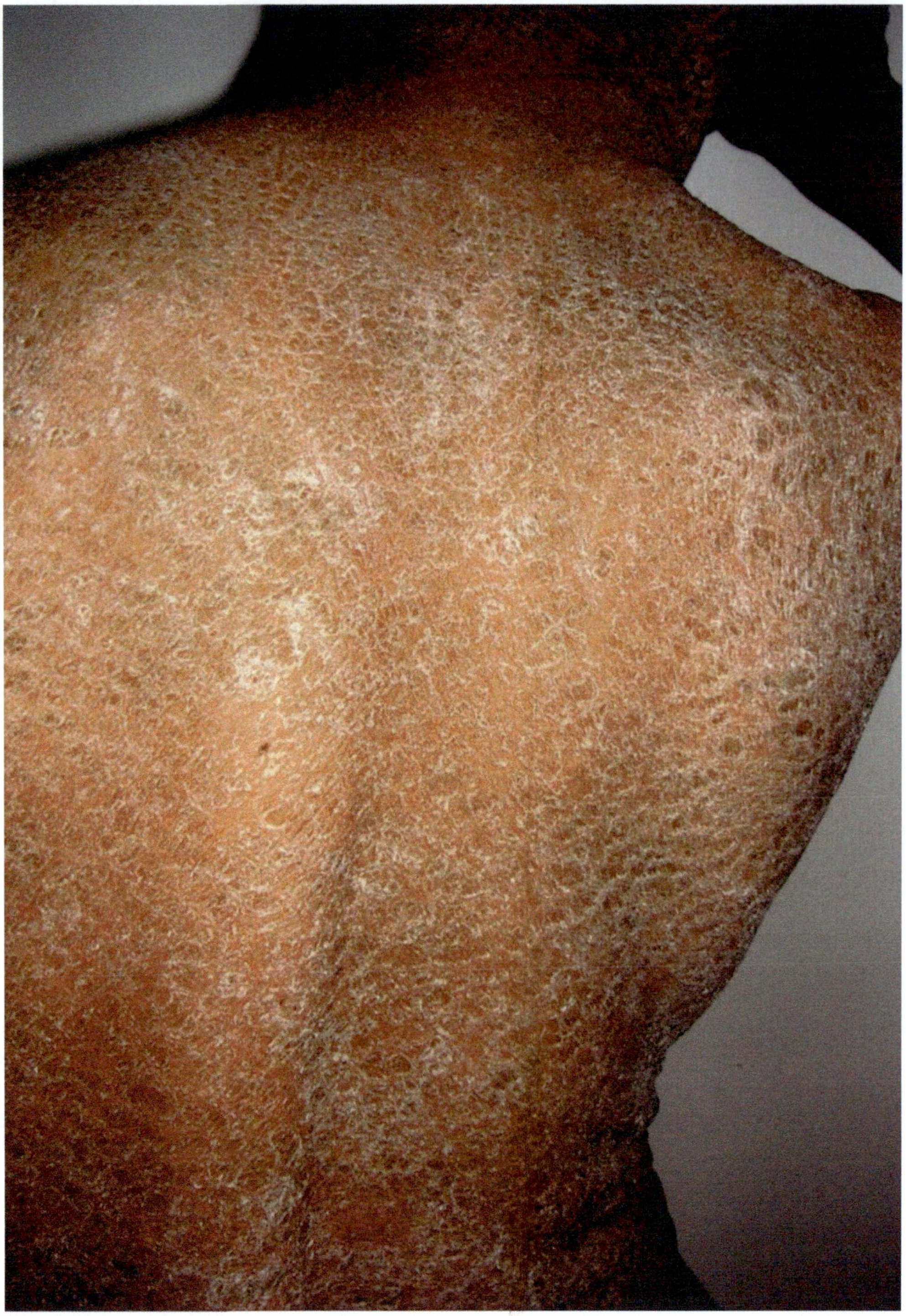

Fig. 40.9 Associated ichthyosis in *Sjögren-Larson syndrome*

gestation. The ethical situation may differ for other types such as moderate lamellar ichthyosis. Helpful contact details can be downloaded from the *Foundation for Ichthyosis and Related Skin Types* (F.I.R.S.T.) and the *Network for Ichthyoses and Related Keratinization disorders* (NIRK). Unfortunately, patient organizations and foundations supporting patients with ichthyosis are almost limited to Western countries.

References

1. Al-Zayir AA, Al-Amro Al-Alakloby OM. Clinico-epidemiological features of primary hereditary ichthyoses in the eastern province of Saudi Arabia. Int J Dermatol. 2006;45:257–64.
2. Al-Amro Al-Akloby OM, Al-Zayir AA. Clinico-epidemiological features of congenital nonbullous ichthyosiform erythroderma in the eastern province of Saudi Arabia. J Eur Acad Dermatol Venereol. 2004;18:659–64.

3. Oji V, Tadini G, Akiyama M, et al. Revised nomenclature and classification of inherited ichthyoses: results of the first Ichthyosis consensus conference in Soreze 2009. J Am Acad Dermatol. 2010;63:607–41.
4. Ibekwe PU, Ogunbiyi AO, Ogun OG, et al. Social stigmatization of two sisters with lamella ichthyosis in Ibadan, Nigeria. Int J Dermatol. 2012;51:67–8.
5. Palmer CN, Irvine AD, Terron-Kwiatkowski A, et al. Common loss-of-function variants of the epidermal barrier protein filaggrin are a major predisposing factor for atopic dermatitis. Nat Genet. 2006;38:441–6.
6. Sandilands A, Terron-Kwiatkowski A, Hull PR, et al. Comprehensive analysis of the gene encoding filaggrin uncovers prevalent and rare mutations in ichthyosis vulgaris and atopic eczema. Nat Genet. 2007;39:650–4.
7. Taylan F, Nilsson D, Asad S, et al. Whole-exome sequencing of Ethiopian patients with ichthyosis vulgaris and atopic dermatitis. J Allergy Clin Immunol. 2015;136:507–9.e519.
8. Polcari I, Becker L, Stein SL, et al. Filaggrin gene mutations in African Americans with both ichthyosis vulgaris and atopic dermatitis. Pediatr Dermatol. 2014;31:489–92.
9. Taylan F, Nilsson D, Asad S, et al. Whole-exome sequencing of Ethiopian patients with ichthyosis vulgaris and atopic dermatitis. J Allergy Clin Immunol. 2015;136:507–9.e19.
10. Khadir K, Benharbit B, Habibeddine S, et al. Treatment outcome for collodion babies: the experience of the dermatology Department of Ibn Rochd Teaching Hospital. Casablanca Ann Dermatol Venereol. 2009;136:731–2.
11. Jacyk WK. Bathing-suit ichthyosis. A peculiar phenotype of lamellar ichthyosis in South African blacks. Eur J Dermatol. 2005;15:433–6.
12. Benmously-Mlika R, Zaouak A, Mrad R, et al. Bathing suit ichthyosis caused by a TGM1 mutation in a Tunisian child. Int J Dermatol. 2014;53:1478–80.
13. Migowa AN, Murungi CW, Gatinu BW, et al. Harlequin ichthyosis in an African child: case report. East Afr Med J. 2010;87:389–92.
14. Glick JB, Craiglow BG, Choate KA, et al. Improved management of harlequin ichthyosis with advances in neonatal intensive care. Pediatrics. 2017;139(1). https://doi.org/10.1542/peds.2016-1003.
15. Traupe H, Burgdorf WHC. Treatment of ichthyosis—there is always something you can do! In memoriam: Wolfgang Küster. J Am Acad Dermatol. 2007;57:542–7.
16. Bassotti A, Moreno S, Criado E. Successful treatment with topical N-acetylcysteine in urea in five children with congenital lamellar ichthyosis. Pediat Dermatol. 2011;28:451–5.
17. Digiovanna JJ, Mauro T, Milstone LM, et al. Systemic retinoids in the management of ichthyoses and related skin types. Dermatol Ther. 2013;26:26–38.
18. van Steensel MA. Emerging drugs for ichthyosis. Expert Opin Emerg Drugs. 2007;12:647–56.
19. Vahlquist A, Blockhuys S, Steijlen P, et al. Oral liarozole in the treatment of patients with moderate/severe lamellar ichthyosis: results of a randomized, double-blind, multinational, placebo-controlled phase II/III trial. Br J Dermatol. 2014;170:173–81.

Oculocutaneous Albinism

41

Constantin E. Orfanos

Albinism is a group of hereditary diseases with varying clinical phenotypes, characterized by disturbances of melanogenesis and reduced amounts or lack of melanin in the skin, the hair, and the eyes (*oculocutaneous*). It involves people of all ethnic backgrounds in all continents, equally affecting both sexes, but is more common in populations with pigmented or black skin in African countries and in Americans of African descent. The worldwide prevalence of various types of oculocutaneous albinism (OCA) has been estimated to be approximately 1:30–40,000, at the average 1:17,000, suggesting that around 1 out of 70 individuals carries a gene for OCA [1]. Large differences of prevalence are seen between geographic regions, urban and rural areas, and ethnic groups, the highest in sub-Saharan countries, 1:5000–10,000 at the average. Rates of albinism as high as 1:1000 have been reported in tribes in Zimbabwe (Tonga), 1:1100 in Nigeria (Ibo), and 1:7900 in Cameroon (Bamileke), also related to the inbreeding tendencies [2].

The obvious lack of melanin in the skin and hair leads to social discrimination and stigmatization of the individuals affected, particularly in geographic areas with dark-skinned populations. Albinos are a most vulnerable social group of people suffering from lack of education and poverty.

41.1 Pathogenesis

The condition results due to the inheritance of various gene mutations, interacting on different levels of expression. Recessive gene alleles control the presence and the activity of tyrosinase, possibly also the maturation and transportation of melanosomes, leading to *syndromic* and *non-syndromic* variants of oculocutaneous albinism (OCA). It seems that four major genes are responsible for the varying phenotypes of the disease: *TYR*, *OCA2*, *TYRP1*, and *SLC45A2* with other candidate genes for the *non-syndromic* [3] and ten further genes for the *syndromic* types [4–6]. Clinical manifestations occur only if the alleles from both parents are inherited, with or without other genetic developmental disorders (Table 41.1). When a dark-skinned father and mother both carry the albino gene, there is a 1:4 chance that their newborn will be albino and be considered as a severe medical and social stigma for a family in sub-Saharan countries. The attending physician is urgently asked to provide genetic counseling, together with medical services (Table 41.2).

Table 41.1 Genetic variations of oculocutaneous albinism (OCA)

I. Non-syndromic variants
Types: OCA1a,b, OCA2, OCA3, OCA4
Various mutational defects, all autosomal recessive; OCA5 and OCA6 types are under discussion
Genes: ***TYR*** (OCA1), ***OCA2*** (OCA2), ***TYRP-1*** (OCA3), ***SLC45A2*** (OCA4) and other candidates
II. Syndromic variants with association to albinism
Genetic: *Hermansky-Pudlak syndrome* (***HPS*** gene; chromosome 10q23)
Chediak-Higashi syndrome (***LYST*** gene; chromosome 1q43)
Developmental: *Klein-Waardenburg syndrome, Waardenburg-Hirschsprung syndrome, Griscelli syndrome, Menkes syndrome, Tietze syndrome* among others

41.2 Clinical Picture and Sociomedical Aspects

The diagnosis of the type of albinism presented is based on the clinical phenotype, i.e., on the degree of pigmentation of skin and hair, together with characteristic ocular or other symptoms of varying severity.

C. E. Orfanos, M.D.
The Free University of Berlin, Medical School Charité, Berlin, Germany
e-mail: corfanos@t-online.de

C. E. Orfanos et al. (eds.), *Pigmented Ethnic Skin and Imported Dermatoses*, https://doi.org/10.1007/978-3-319-69422-1_41

Table 41.2 Genetic counseling: (a) if parents are clinically dark-skinned but both carry the albinism allele, there is a 1:4 risk that one of their children will be an albino; (b) if one of the parents, father or mother, is albino and the other carries the allele, the risk is 1:2

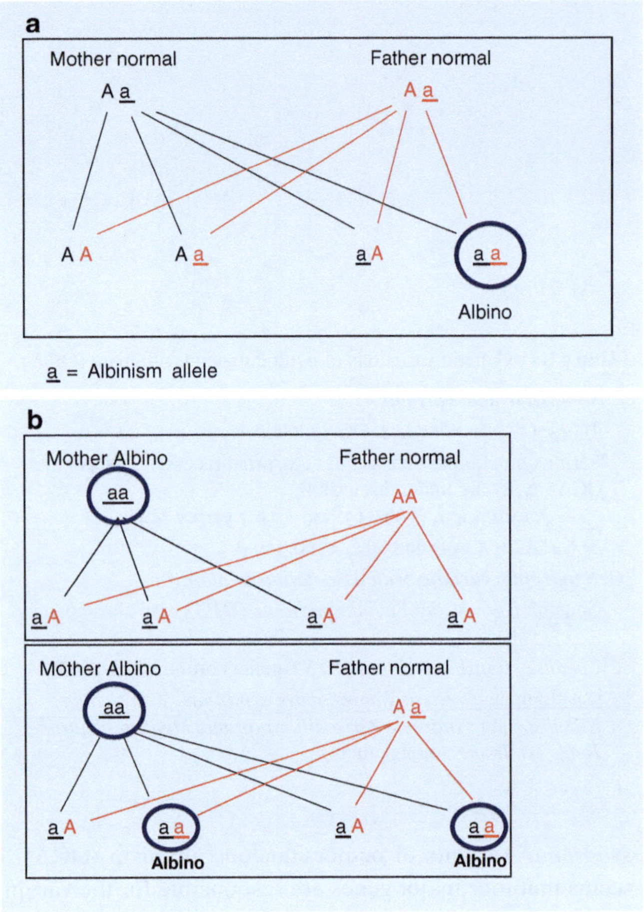

The classical *OCA1a genotype* of albinism is characterized clinically by complete lack of melanin in the skin and eyes, in contrast to patients with *OCA1b* and the other genotypes.

The *OCA2 albinism* is the most common clinical phenotype seen in African countries. Patients present yellowish hair, light blue or brownish eyes, and with or without pigmented freckles on the sun-exposed areas (nevi, ephelides, lentigines).They are similar to irregularly shaped nevi, and their number may increase with increasing age. The iris may be more or less pigmented, with only reduced pigmentation of the retina, and without translucency ("red eye"). In each particular genotype of OCA, the color of hair varies considerably, from white to yellowish brown or reddish (Figs. 41.1, 41.2, 41.3, 41.4, and 41.5). In most OCA2 patients of African descent, a predominant allele mutation occurs.

OCA3 and *OCA4 types* of albinism are also seen in the African continent, having been documented in South Africa, Malawi, and Nigeria [7]. Affected individuals have light-colored skin, beige to light brown hair and blue-green to brown irides with moderate transillumination, reduced retinal pigment, and nystagmus (Table 41.3). Visional problems due to *photophobia*, *strabismus*, *foveal hypoplasia*, and *nystagmus* are common. Involvement of the nervous system, the upper respiratory tract, and the gastrointestinal tract has been documented occasionally; also, hematological alterations may occur.

All clinical phenotypes of the disease are associated with increased vulnerability of the non-melanized skin, being unprotected to sun damage, with early appearance of actinic keratoses and praecanceroses (Fig. 41.6a, b). Later in life bowenoid carcinomas and rapidly growing skin cancers may occur (Figs. 41.7 and 41.8a, b). Black albinos in sub-Saharan Africa are at about a 1000-fold higher risk of developing squamous cell carcinoma of the skin than the general dark-skinned population, and the neoplasms in albinos tend to run an aggressive course [8].

Oculocutaneous albinism causes *social stigmatization* of the newborn and the family in dark-skinned populations. Ocular involvement leads in albino children to early visual handicap and minor school education resulting in lower social status. The majority of children with oculocutaneous albinism have less than 30% vision. In addition, overexposure to sunlight in hot climate zones occurs early in childhood and is lifelong, nearly unavoidable in hot climate zones. Actinic keratoses, praecanceroses, and skin cancer are early induced via outdoor professional activities and prolonged UV exposure. Life expectation is significantly reduced compared to the normal dark-skinned population. Only 10–20% of the albino population becomes older than 30 years of age in Tanzania, in contrast to 30–50% of the normal black population. Intelligence and fertility of the albinos are normal.

Overall, albinism itself does not affect somatic growth and well-being or cause increased mortality; however, life quality and life expectation are strongly reduced in those affected in hot climate zones. High anxiety and depression scores were recorded in African patients using a Hospital Anxiety and Depression Scale [9].

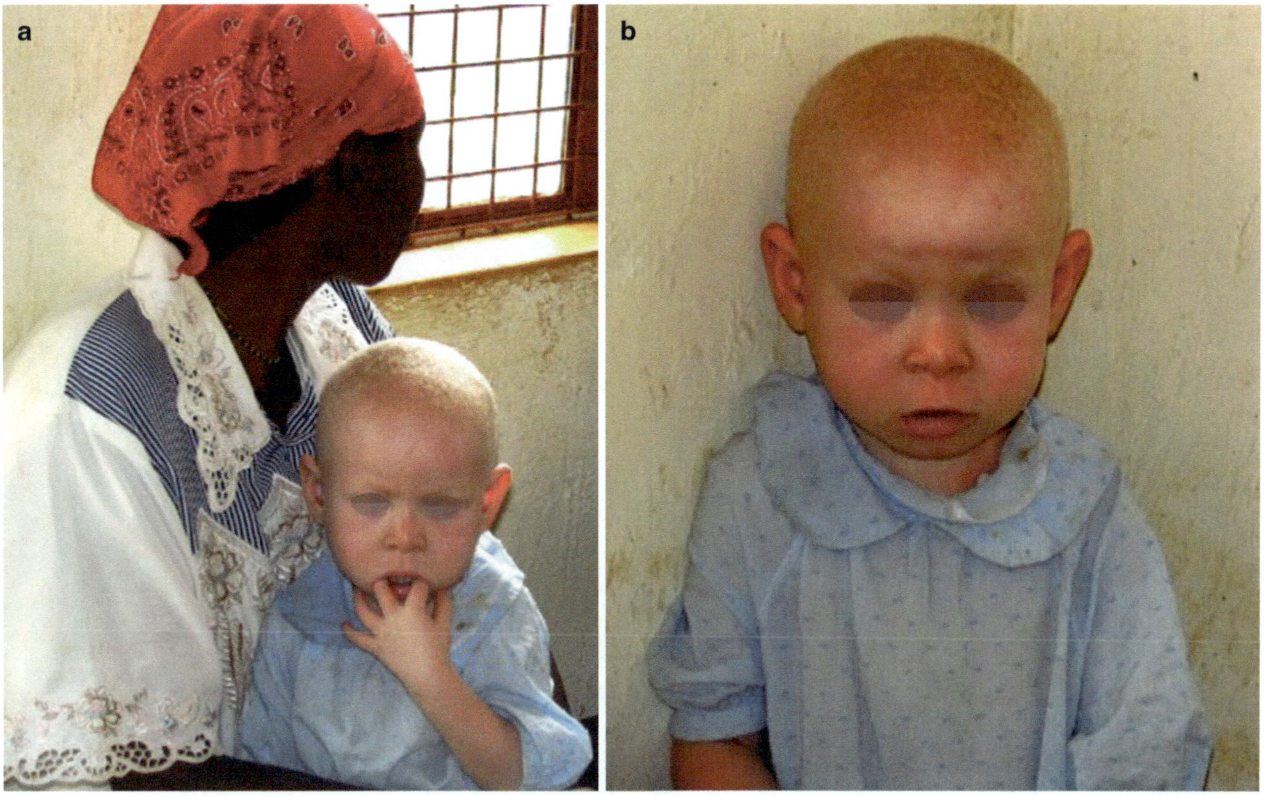

Fig. 41.1 (**a**, **b**) Black-skinned African mother with her with her albino child

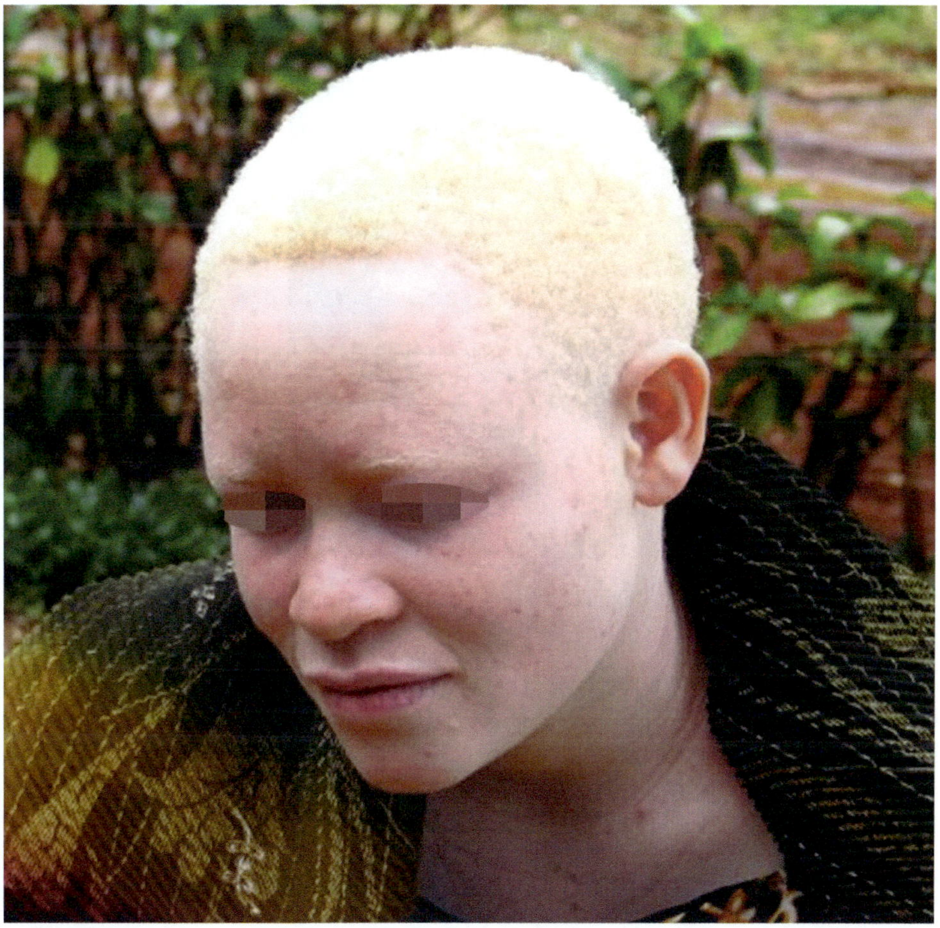

Fig. 41.2 Female African albino, most likely of the *OCA1b* phenotype (yellow albinism)

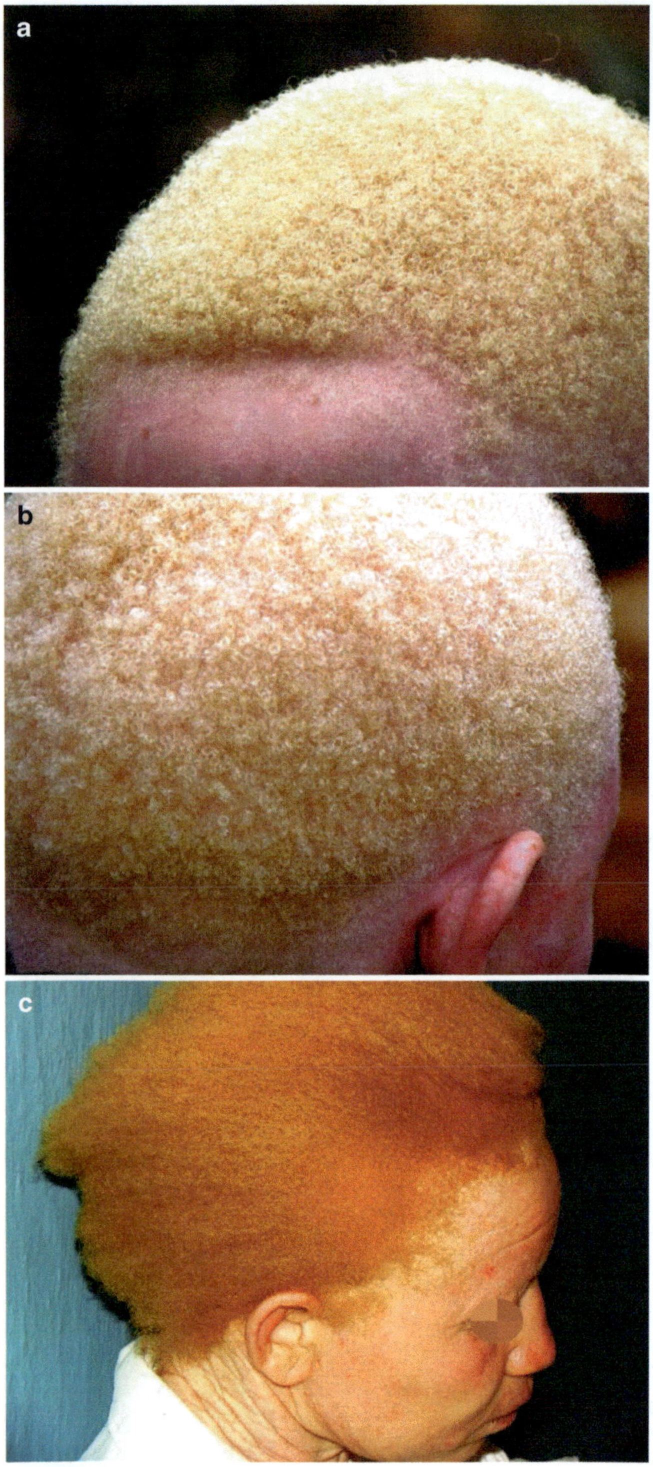

Fig. 41.3 (**a**–**c**) Yellow, yellowish brown, and brown hair color variants in African albinos, corresponding to *OCA1b*, *OCA2*, and *OCA3* phenotypes

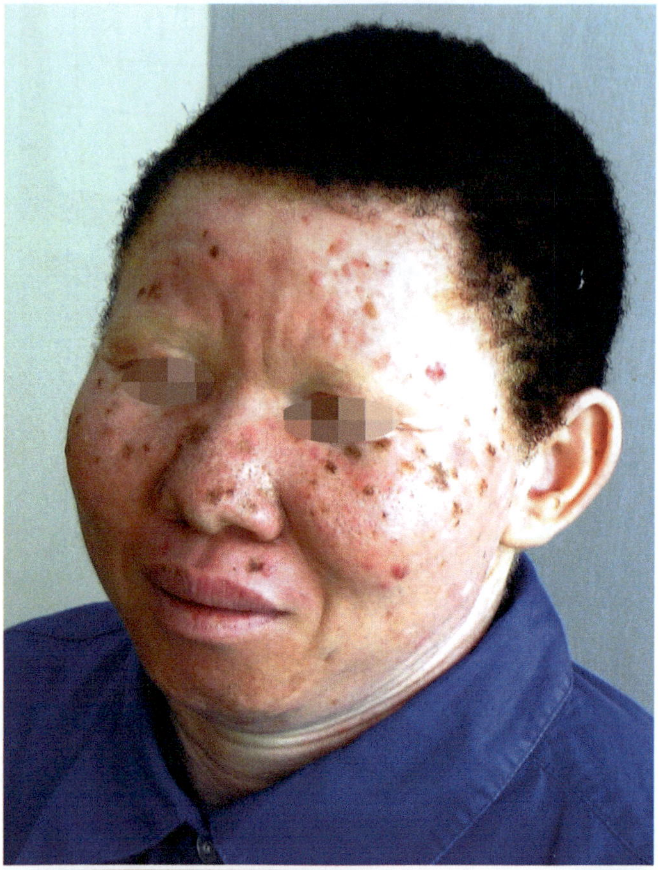

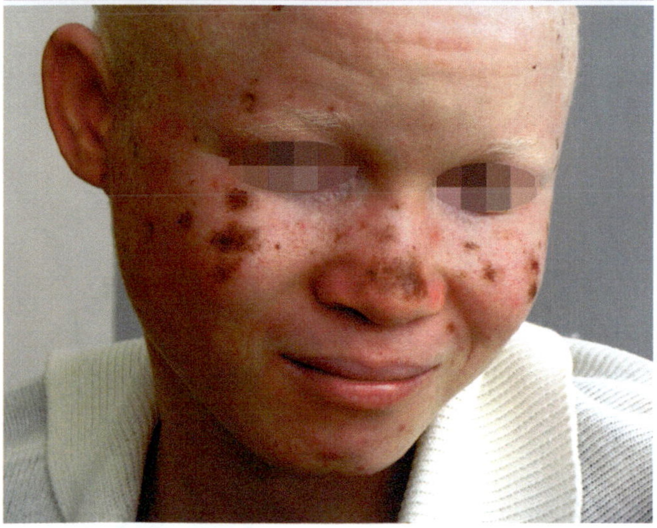

Figs. 41.4 and 41.5 Characteristic African albino with freckles in the sun-exposed face, clinically corresponding to the *OCA2* phenotype

Table 41.3 Genotypes of non-syndromic oculocutaneous albinism (OCA)

OCA1a	
=	Complete loss of tyrosinase activity (nonsense and frameshift mutations), with full clinical expression of the albino clinical phenotype.
OCA1b	
=	Reduced tyrosinase activity causing the so-called yellow albinism with strongly reduced tanning. Some pigment may accumulate in hair and iris with age. Over 50 different mutations occur in the tyrosinase gene (chromosome 11); a major mutational predominance is lacking in Caucasian populations. In cases, only 25% tyrosinase activity is possible at 37 °C, increasing at lower temperature levels (*OCA1-TP*). Clinical manifestation appears only if both alleles of the same mutated gene are inherited. Patients with OCA1 may be heterozygote even for more than two TR mutations.
OCA2	
=	Tyrosinase-positive but variably reduced enzyme activity; several mutations in the p-locus on chromosome 15q, the so-called p-protein. P-protein is a melanocytic-specific membrane-associated protein with 12 potential transmembraneous domains that regulates the transfer and maturation of melanosomes and tyrosine, and is major determinant of brown or blue eye color ("pink-eye dilution gene").
OCA3, OCA4 (*brown albinism*)	
=	Mutational defects in the *TRP-1* and the *SLC45A2* gene leading to deregulation of the tyrosinase enzyme group and synthesis of yellowish or brown melanin.

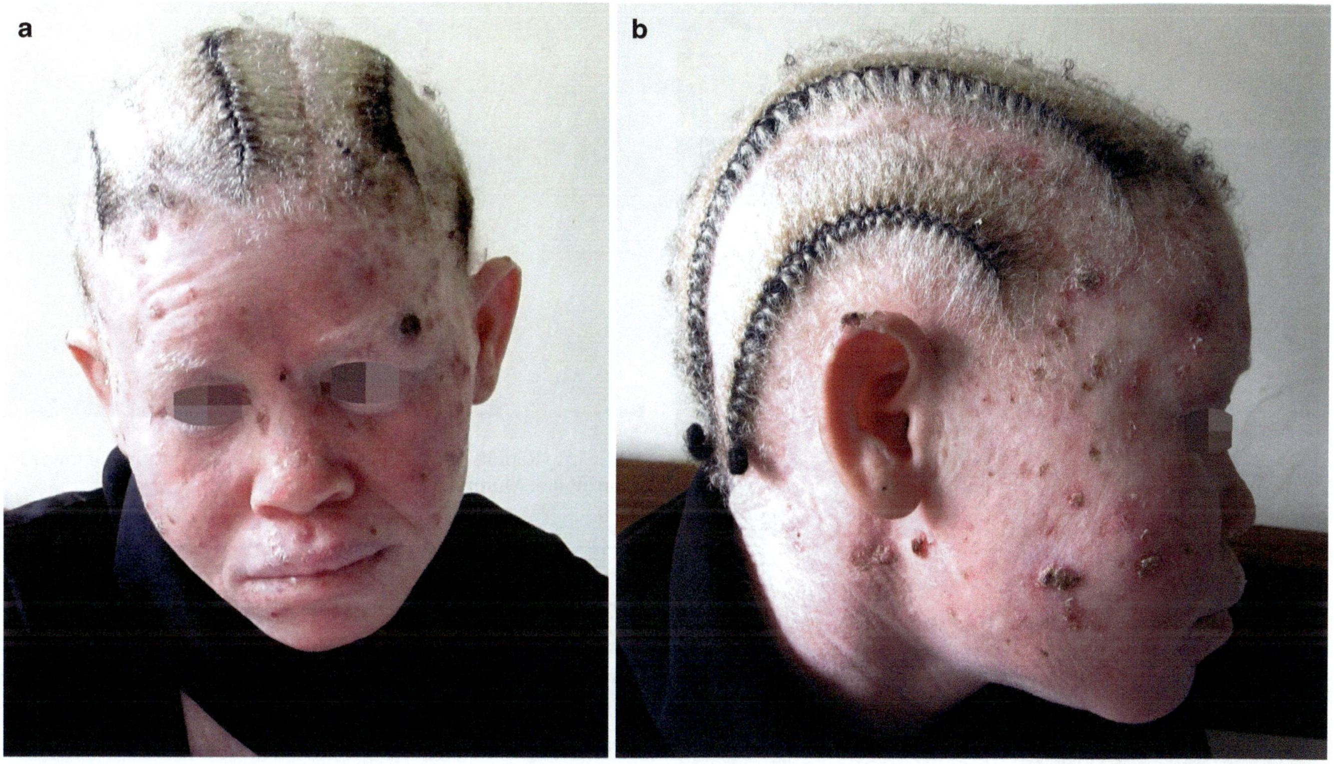

Fig. 41.6 (**a**, **b**) African albino with multiple actinic keratoses and praecanceroses on the face

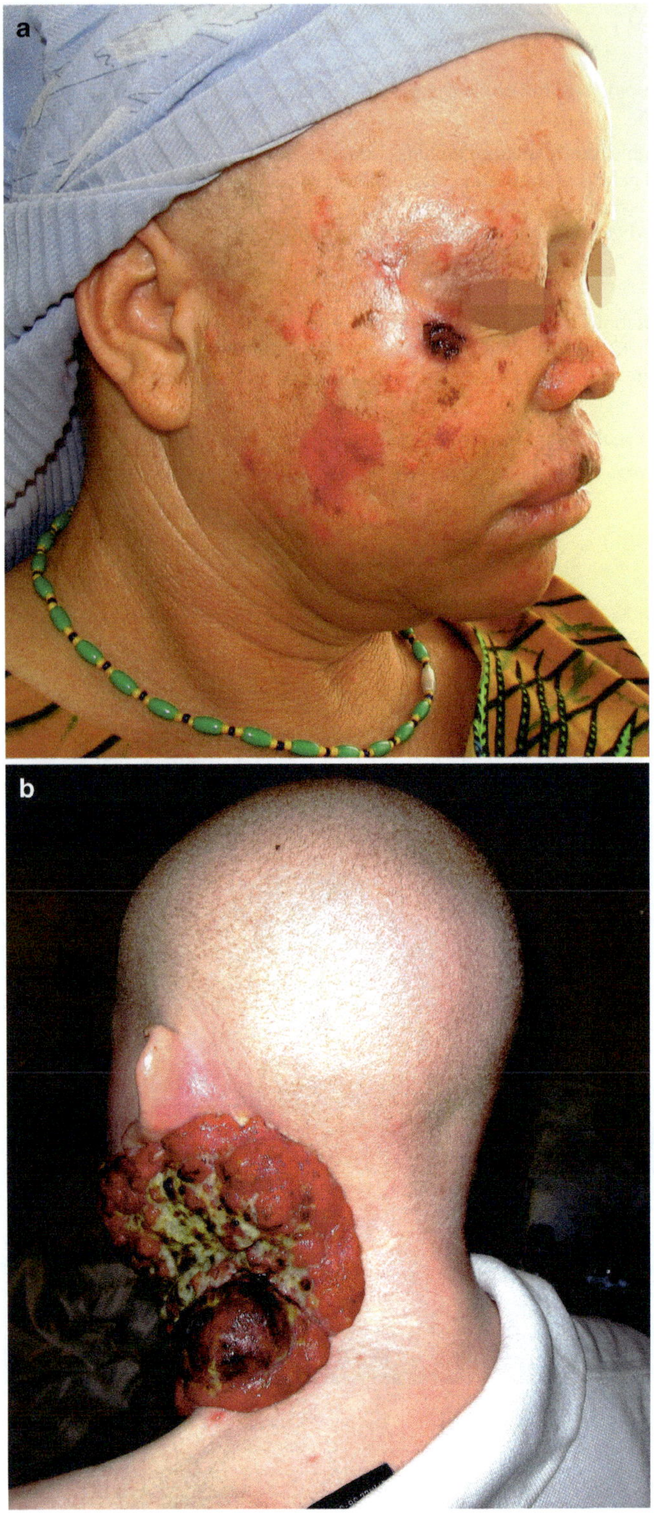

Fig. 41.7 Multiple bowenoid praecanceroses (often treated) in a 42-year-old female (**a**) and rapidly growing, gigantic squamous cell carcinoma (**b**) in a young male albino in Tanzania

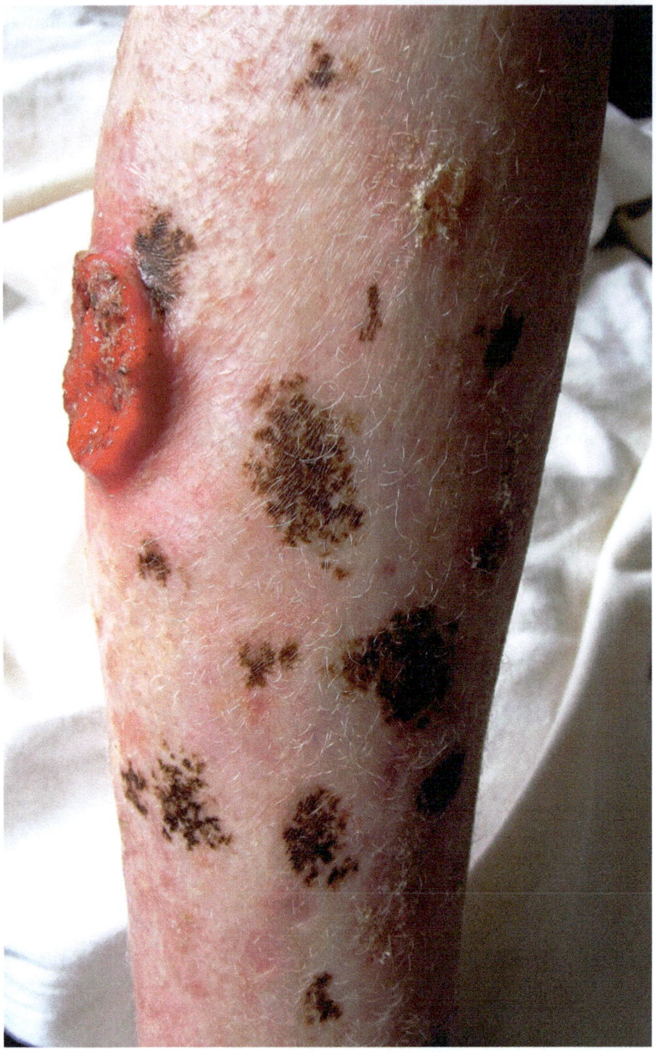

Fig. 41.8 Rapidly growing squamous cell carcinoma in the lower leg of an albino. Multiple nevi-like freckles

41.3 Management

There is no management for the genetic defect of albinism; however, the patients should be checked by the physician in regular intervals (every 3–6 months), and rigorous prophylactic measures should be taken to avoid sun damage. Precancerous lesions should be early diagnosed and be treated early to prevent skin cancer formation. Protection from sunlight through huts, shirts with long sleeves, and long trousers is recommended, together with daily applications of strong sunscreens. In cases with photophobia, dark eyeglasses will be helpful, and any other concomitant ocular problems such as nystagmus, strabismus, reduced visual activity, etc. should be corrected.

Genetic counseling is mandatory, an important task for the attending physician (Table 41.2). Phenotypical diagnosis and *screening of the genetic mutation*, if possible, will help to recognize the carriers of the allele and minimize the incidence of oculocutaneous albinism in future generations [10].

Unfortunately, stigmatization of African albinos is accompanied by various myths, African rituals, and superstition. Kidnappings and killings of albinos, mostly children, by albino hunters still occur today in some sub-Saharan countries, in order to provide albino skin and other body parts to witch doctors. Awareness of the medical community and education of the public is an important goal for the removal of the social stigma and misuse of the people with albinism. It is also the responsibility of the medical community to facilitate their social integration in all areas with high prevalence.

Note: All patients shown in the illustrations were seen and attended in the clinics and the outreach albino program of the RDTC in Moshi, Tanzania, photographed by the author.

References

1. Grønskov K, Ek J, Brondum-Nielsen K. Oculocutaneous albinism. Orphanet J Rare Dis. 2007;2:43.
2. Aquaron R. Oculocutaneous albinism in Cameroun. A 15-year follow-up. Ophthalmic Paediatr Genet. 1990;11:255–63.
3. Wei AH, Zang DJ, Zhang Z, et al. Exome sequencing identifies SLC24A5 as a candidate gene for nonsyndromic oculocutaneous albinism. J Invest Dermatol. 2013;133:1834–40.
4. Wei AH, Zang DJ, Zhang Z, et al. Prenatal genotyping of four common oculocutaneous albinism genes in 51 Chinese families. J Genet Genomics. 2015;42:279–86.
5. DR S, Wang X, Wang C, et al. DNA variations in oculocutaneous albinism: an updated mutation list and current outstanding issues in molecular diagnostics. Hum Mutat. 2013;34:827–35.
6. Mauri L, Barone L, Al Oum M, et al. SLC45A2 mutation frequency in oculocutaneous albinism Italian patients doesn't differ from other European studies. Gene. 2014;533:398–402.
7. Manga P, Kromberg JGR, Turner A, et al. In Southern Africa, brown oculocutaneous Albinism (BOCA) maps to the *OCA2* locus on chromosome 15q: *P*-gene mutations identified. Am J Hum Genet. 2001;68:782–7.
8. Lekalakala PT, Khammissa RA, Kramer B, et al. Oculocutaneous albinism and squamous cell carcinoma of the skin of the head and neck in Sub-Saharan Africa. J Skin Cancer. 2015;2015:167847. https://doi.org/10.1155/2015/167847; Epub 2015 Aug 12.
9. Ajose FOA, Parker RA, Merra LL, et al. Quantification and comparison of psychiatric distress in African patients with albinism and vitiligo: a 5-year prospective study. J Eur Acad Dermatol Venereol. 2014;28:925–32.
10. Renugadevi K, Sil AK, Perumalsamy V, et al. Spectrum of candidate gene mutations associated with Indian familial oculocutaneous and ocular albinism. Mol Vis. 2010;16:1514–24.

42 Scleroderma in Pigmented Skin Populations

Lee Shapiro, Lesley Ann Saketkoo, and Virginia D. Steen

Scleroderma, or more accurately *systemic sclerosis* (SSc), is a multi-organ systemic disease involving inflammation, vascular destruction, and disrepair with collagen deposition and fibrosis. Early recognition leading to timely management positively impacts survival and disease progression.

SSc has an earlier onset and more severe course in African lineages. In much of the world, including sub-Saharan Africa, there can be diagnostic delay due to lack of access to a physician [1]. Even with access to knowledgeable specialists, there are issues that delay recognition and treatment in populations of African descent. In diagnosing SSc, there are two classic early symptoms: Raynaud phenomenon (RP) and skin fibrosis/thickening. Unless there is critical digital ischemia, RP is often underrecognized in pigmented skin by patients and clinicians. Skin fibrosis, although commonly a presenting symptom, often to a severe degree, may not be present in a substantial portion of patients with skin of color and SSc. This makes recognition of SSc, a potentially life-threatening and often disabling disease, particularly in skin of color, challenging even for experienced physicians.

L. Shapiro, M.D. (✉)
Division of Rheumatology, Albany Medical College, Albany, NY, USA

L. A. Saketkoo, M.D., M.P.H.
Clinical Immunology, Allergy and Rheumatology, Pulmonary Diseases, Critical Care and Environmental Medicine, New Orleans Scleroderma and Sarcoidosis Patient Care and Research Center, Tulane University School of Medicine, Tulane Lung Center, New Orleans, LA, USA

V. D. Steen, M.D.
Department of Medicine, Georgetown University Medical Center, Pasquerilla Healthcare Center, Washington, DC, USA
e-mail: steenv@georgetown.edu

42.1 Epidemiology

Scleroderma is an umbrella term that captures two disease entities: *localized scleroderma* which affects isolated and adjacent areas of cutaneous, subcutaneous, and fascial layers and *systemic sclerosis* which involves skin fibrosis and multiple organs throughout the body at any one time. It has been described in patients all over the world with prevalence reports ranging from 50 to 300 per million [2]. Case series of SSc have been reported from Senegal [3], Nigeria [4], Togo [5, 6], and South Africa [7], but these provide insufficient data for comments on prevalence or incidence of the disease. There is much more detailed epidemiologic data on black-skinned populations in the US than in African countries. It seems that individuals with black skin are more likely to develop SSc than white Caucasians and have an earlier age of onset, experience greater morbidity, and have reduced survival. Laing et al. (1997) detected an overall higher incidence of SSc in black-skinned as compared with Caucasian females in Michigan (22.5 vs. 12.8/million/year) and a lower mean age at diagnosis (44.5 vs. 51.5 years, $p < 0.001$). Diffuse skin disease was also more common in African Americans (50 vs. 25%, $p < 0.001$) [8, 9]. In other populations studied, SSc prevalence in black-skinned individuals was significantly higher than in whites (315 vs. 224.7/million) [10, 11]. These findings were consistent with a study investigating US male veterans, which found significantly greater incidence rate (7.1 vs. 1.9/million/year) for non-whites (94% of the patients were black-skinned) (Figs. 42.1 and 42.2) [12].

Clinically well-described large cohorts were reported from other countries with populations with skin of color such as China [13], Thailand [14, 15] and various regions of India [16–22]; however, strong epidemiologic studies are lacking. In New Zealand, no difference in incidence rate between white Caucasians and Polynesians was found [23]. A French multiethnic survey reported prevalence of 140.2/million among Europeans and 210.8/million among non-Europeans (Northern and sub-Saharan African, Asian, and Caribbean). The non-Europeans were significantly more likely to have

C. E. Orfanos et al. (eds.), *Pigmented Ethnic Skin and Imported Dermatoses*, https://doi.org/10.1007/978-3-319-69422-1_42

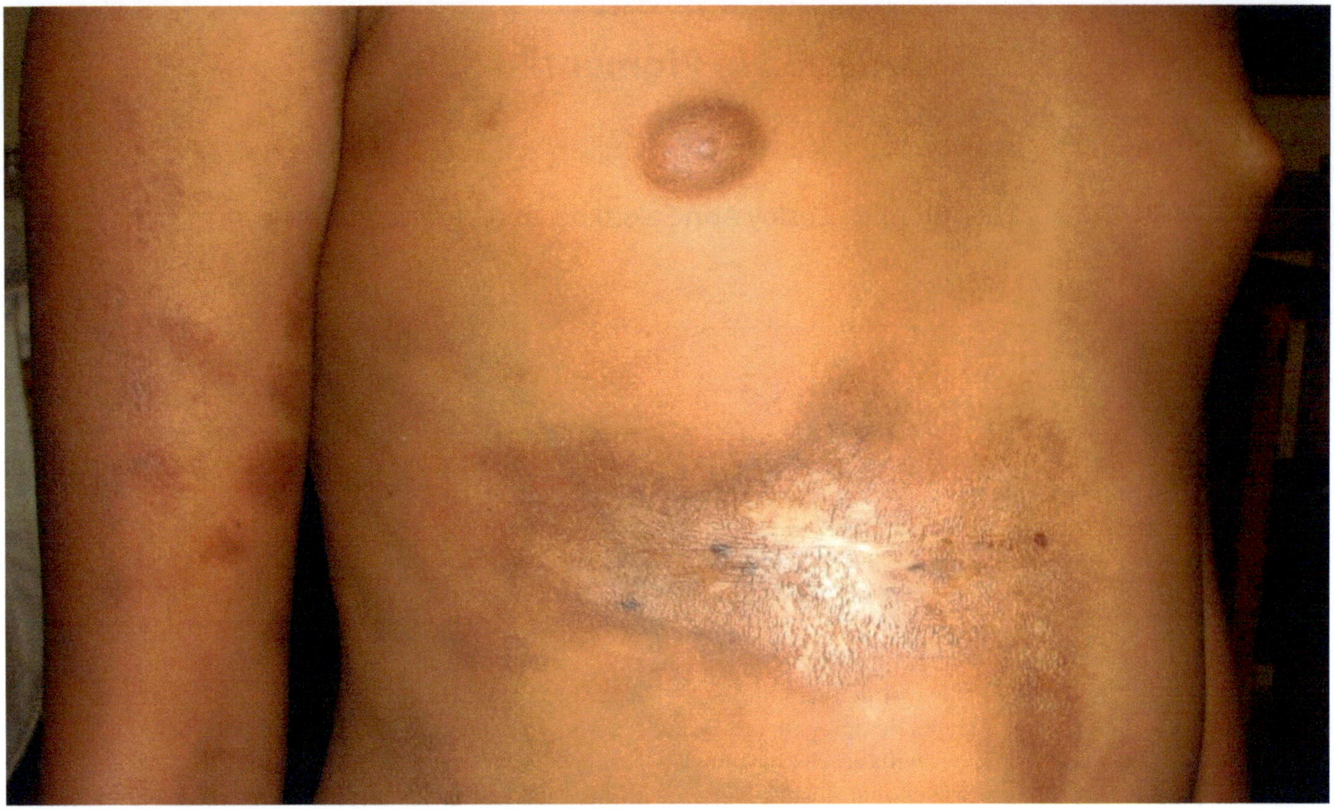

Fig. 42.1 Well-defined *localized scleroderma* of the trunk in a young male of African origin

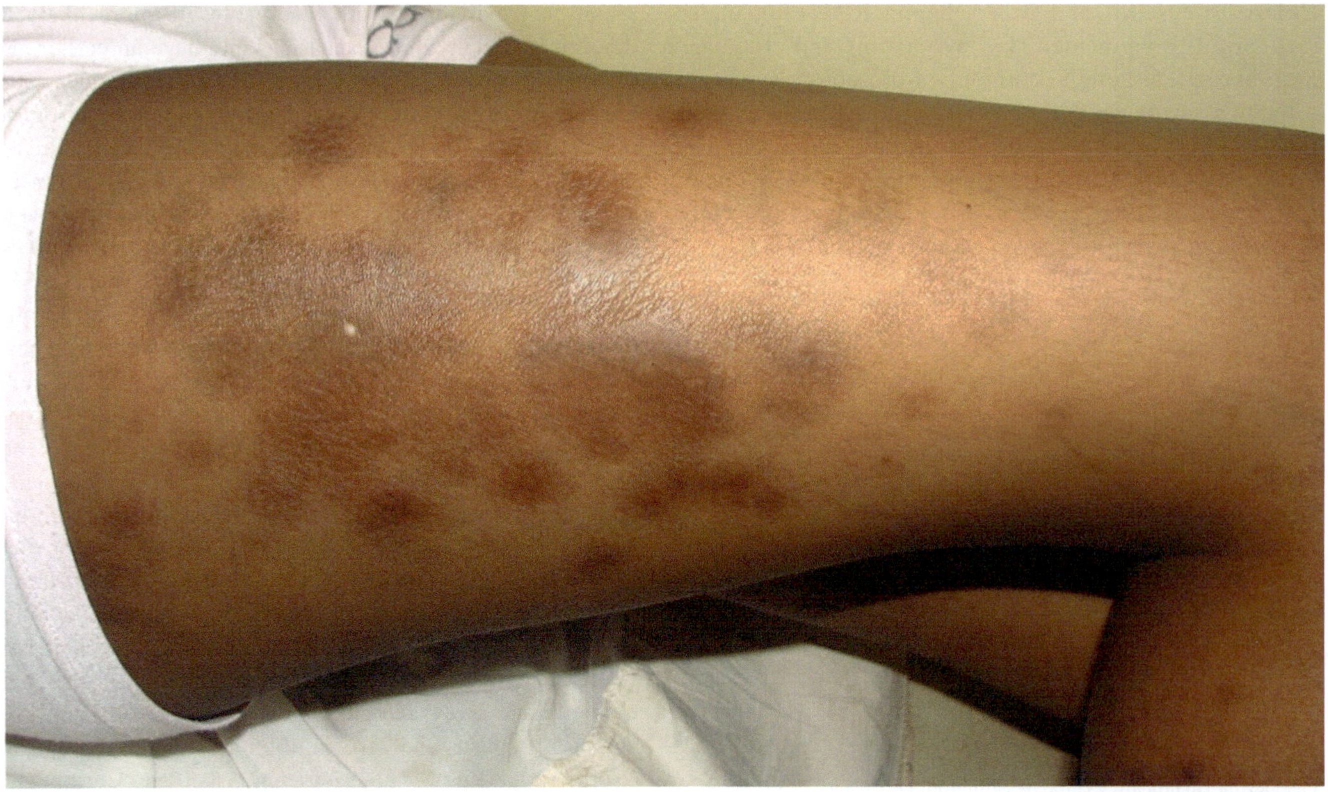

Fig. 42.2 Hyperpigmented patches of *disseminated morphea*, a subtype of limited cutaneous involvement, in a young African female

diffuse disease (34 vs. 17%, $p = 0.04$) and be younger at diagnosis (45.3 ± 14.3 years vs. 52.4 ± 14.5 years, $p = 0.02$) [24]. The National Institutes of Health in the USA is conducting a multicenter genome-wide study. Genome Research in African American Scleroderma Patients (GRASP) study is designed to understand the genetic basis of disease severity in those of African descent and will hopefully provide insight for targeted treatment. An important epidemiologic note is that the diagnosis and treatment of connective tissue disease (CTD) in non-white populations in the USA remains fraught with health disparities that are independent of socioeconomic status [25, 26].

42.2 Etiology/Pathogenesis

Knowledge as to the etiology of SSc is rapidly expanding. Today it is generally recognized that SSc develops in genetically predisposed individuals often associated with exposure to chemical, particulate [27, 28], or microbial [29, 30] triggers over a period of time. Environmental or occupational exposures are reported in localized pockets of higher disease incidence. Though it is challenging to firmly establish causative exposures, there is evidence to support cumulative exposure to crystalline silica and organic solvents as potential triggers of SSc [31, 32]. Furthermore, SSc is considered an occupational disease in South African gold miners with an incidence 25× greater than in railway and harbor workers [33], regardless of their ethnic origin.

Hypotheses regarding pathogenesis generally agree with interplay of inflammation, autoimmunity, fibroblast activation with extracellular matrix deposition, and microvasculopathy. Initially considered as sequential stages, these elements are now recognized as interdependent. Discovery of autoantibodies promoting both vasculopathy and fibrosis as well as transforming vascular cells into myofibroblasts have established the presence of multiple avenues of autoimmunity in SSc progression [34–37]. Regardless of causation, microvascular injury is considered the initial event in a genetically susceptible host. Such an individual has impaired ability to control/repair vascular injury, despite high circulating levels of pro-angiogenic factors [38, 39]. Cellular injury progresses to non-necrotic vascular damage, both inflammatory and autoimmune response and fibroblast activation with abnormal inflammation and collagen deposition. Each of these pathways results in sequential and recurrent injury. This in turn leads to the destruction of normal vessel architecture and neuronal pathways and fibrosis of adjacent tissues with vascular, neural, and parenchymal damage impairing organ function.

Of potential relevance to greater severity and earlier onset in skin of color, it is noted that circulating and organ levels of TGF-β are higher in individuals of African descent. In bronchial fluid analysis, even healthy people of African descent have lower levels of PPAR-γ and matrix metalloproteinase-1 (MMP-1), which is important for parenchymal remodeling and prevention of fixed fibrosis. This has been hypothesized as being responsible for the more severe progression of pulmonary fibrosis in SSc in skin of color [40, 41]. In these populations, overexpression of pro-fibrotic factors TGF-β and IL-6 occurs, with under-expression of anti-fibrotic factors such as caveolin-1, hepatocyte growth factor (HGF) [40], and PPAR-γ. A genetic predisposition to fibrosis may account for much of the ethnic disparity between black-skinned and Caucasian patients with scleroderma [42].

A prototypical example translating pathophysiology into clinical manifestation is the gastrointestinal tract. It may be affected anywhere between the oral aperture and anus and is involved in >90% of patients with SSc. Injury of the GI tract is often multifactorial, resulting from vascular injury/impairment, fibrotic mucosal infiltration, and diminished neurological function. The consequent dysmotility and multilevel sphincter dysfunction lead to the complex spectrum of SSc GI manifestations.

In the skin, multiple factors are responsible for an array of effects. Skin fibrosis and pigmentary changes (spotty depigmentation) are related to fibroblast activation and melanocyte dysfunction. Cutaneous edema, hypersensitivity, and diffuse pruritus are related to a predominately early inflammatory process. Cyanosis, digital ulcers, digital shortening, and telangiectasias are related to vascular impairments (Figs. 42.3 and 42.4).

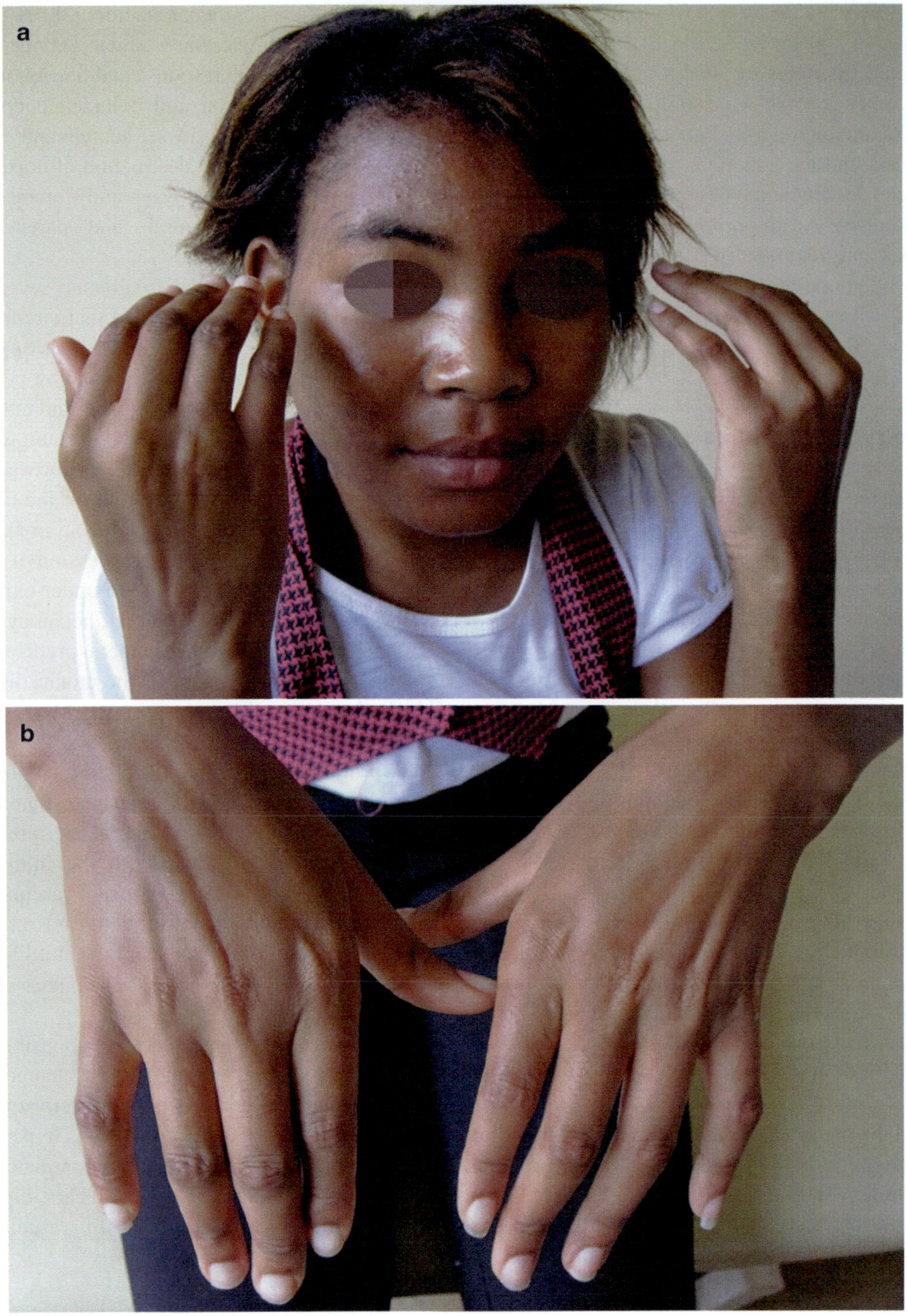

Fig. 42.3 (**a**, **b**) *Early phase of systemic sclerosis* in a young Egyptian female showing involvement of the face, both hands, and the oral mucosa (shortened frenulum linguae)

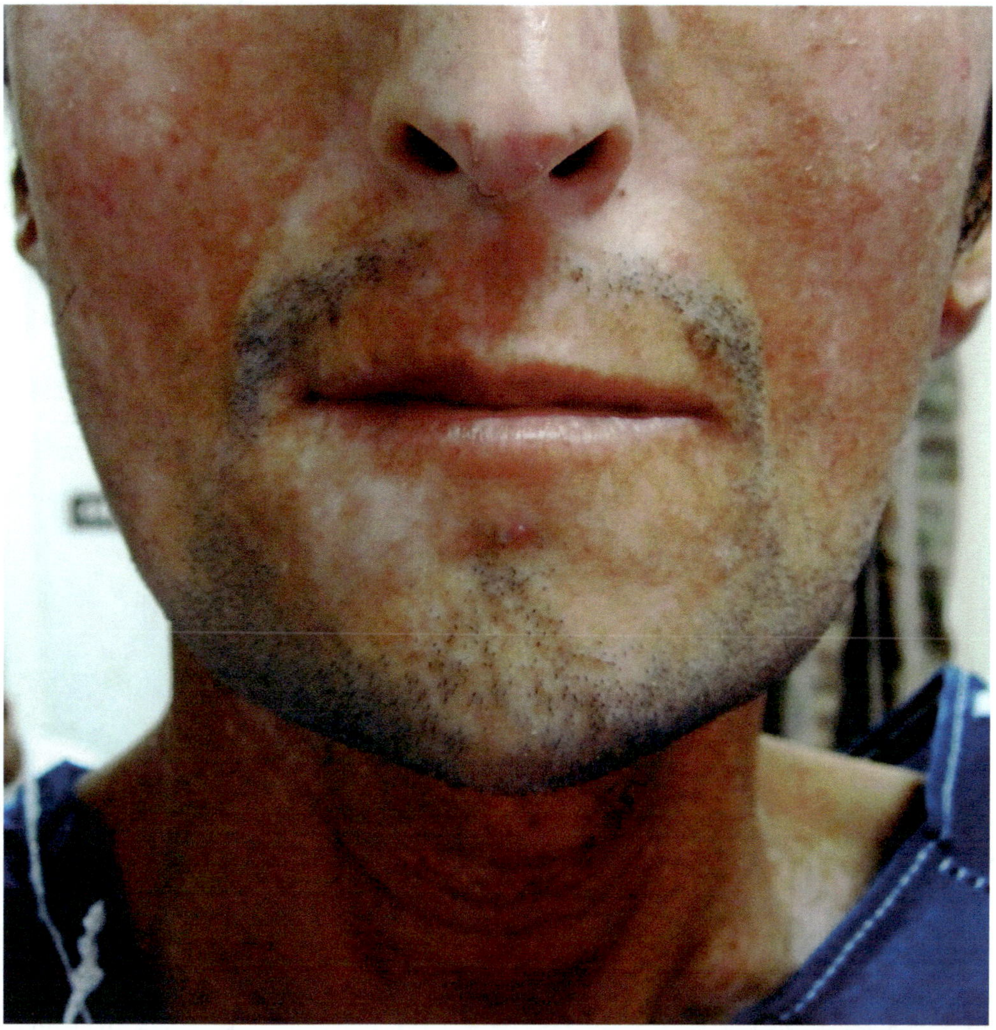

Fig. 42.4 *Progressed stage of systemic sclerosis* in a 38-year-old male Arab patient showing diffuse scarring fibrosis of the face with depigmentation, loss of hair, and microstomia

42.3 Clinical Picture

(a) *Classification*

The clinical picture of scleroderma is heterogeneous. Many subtypes of circumscribed cutaneous sclerodermas have been morphologically described based on the localization, extent, and distribution of skin fibrosis: *scleroderma en coup de sabre*, *hemiatrophia faciei*, *atrophoderma Pasini-Pierini*, *disseminated morphea* (guttate or band-like types), subcutaneous *pansclerotic fasciitis*, and other clinical variants (Fig. 42.5).

Systemic sclerosis (SSc) is a distinct condition subdivided broadly in (a) *limited cutaneous involvement,* whereby the skin of face and areas limited distal to elbows/knees may be involved, (b) *diffuse cutaneous involvement* extending to any area proximal to elbows/knees potentially including the trunk, and (c) cases *sine scleroderma* associated with typical SSc manifestations in the absence of skin fibrosis. Despite the appellations, each of these variants possesses a varying risk of mortality. The pace of progression of skin fibrosis, typically more slowly in those with limited and more variable in those with diffuse disease, is of prognostic importance. It also identifies patients at greatest risk for developing musculoskeletal disability and early internal organ involvement with disease-related mortality. The *2015 ACR/EULAR Classification Criteria* (Table 42.1) outline eight weighted contributory areas with at least 9 points required for the diagnosis of systemic sclerosis. The classic finding and distribution of skin fibrosis alone can establish the diagnosis; however, the new criteria enable SSc to be diagnosed even in the absence of skin lesions when other related manifestations are present. These criteria have been demonstrated to be more sensitive, as well as more specific in distinguishing true SSc from SSc mimics (Figs. 42.6 and 42.7) [43].

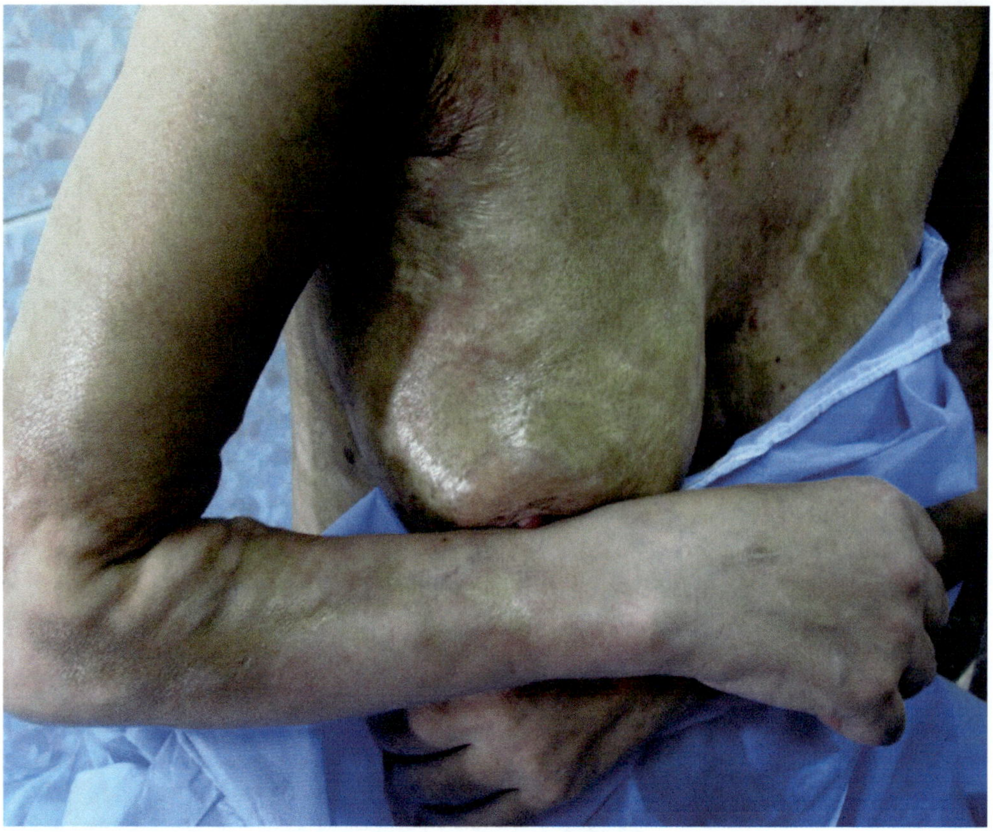

Fig. 42.5 Widespread disseminated skin lesions in progressed *systemic sclerosis*, with subcutaneous fibrotic plaques involving the trunk and the extremities (*pansclerotic subtype*)

Table 42.1 Classification criteria for systemic sclerosis ([43], modified)

Manifestation	Sub-manifestation	Points
Extended skin fibrosis (both hands extending beyond the fingers)		9
Limited skin fibrosis	Puffy fingers	2
	Skin fibrosis on fingers extending between the PIPs and MCPs	4
Fingertip lesions	Ulcers on fingertips	2
	Pitting scars on fingertips	3
Telangiectasias		2
Abnormal nail fold capillaries		2
Lung involvement	Pulmonary arterial hypertension or pulmonary fibrosis	2
Raynaud's phenomenon		2
Presence of antibodies	Centromere, Scl-70, or RNA polymerase	3

There are some challenges with these criteria in pigmented populations, the biggest challenge being the difficulty of early recognition of color changes during Raynaud's episodes. Dark-skinned patients do not experience the same white and purplish colors that occur in white Caucasians [44]. Also, there have been some differences in comparing large cohorts of dark-skinned patients with white Caucasians. In the Pittsburgh SSc cohort seen 1972–2007, the patients with skin of color ($n = 203$) were younger than white Caucasians ($n = 2945$) at disease onset; they were more likely to have diffuse SSc, more severe skeletal muscle involvement, and more frequent and severe pulmonary fibrosis [10]. There was no difference in the frequency of pulmonary hypertension, cardiac, renal, or joint/tendon involvement between the two groups. The Hopkins cohort of 1808 whites and 409 black-skinned patients revealed similar results. Their survival curves estimated for the black-skinned patients were also worse: 66% vs. 75% survival at 5 years and 51% vs. 60% survival at 10 years [45].

(b) *Cutaneous symptomatology*

Besides the presence of characteristic skin lesions with epidermal atrophy, dermal fibrosis, and variable dyspigmentation, *Raynaud's phenomenon* (RP) is the most common first symptom in whites indicating microvasculopathy. However, importantly, only 16% and 28% in large series of SSc patients from Senegal [3] and southern India [8–10] reported RP as the initial symptom. Yet, in the latter study, 58% had digital ulcerations or pitted scars. These near-equatorial climates may lack the necessary thermal trigger

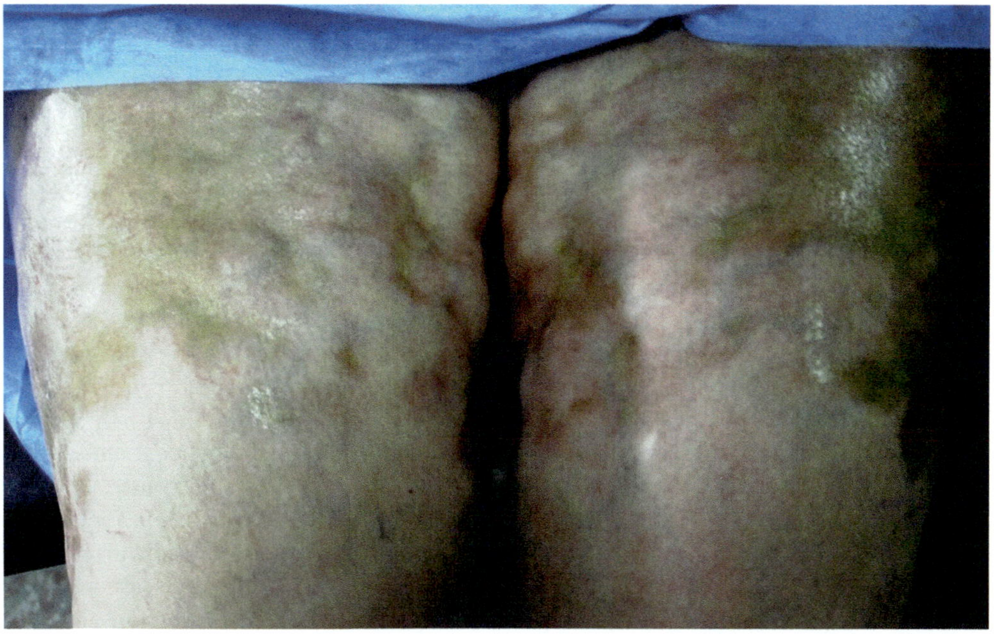

Fig. 42.6 Dyspigmentations in *pansclerotic disseminated morphea*

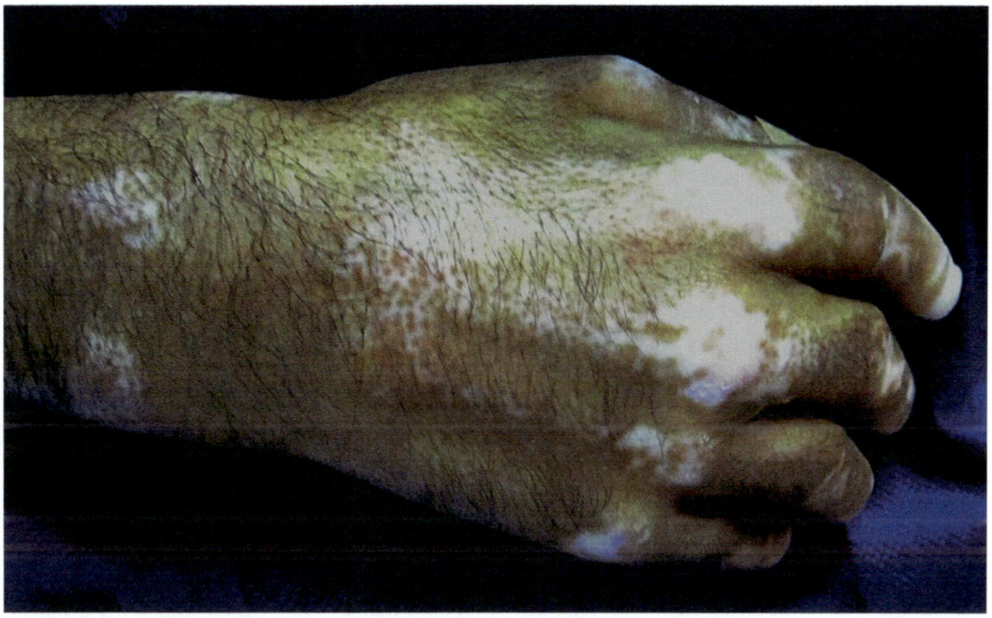

Fig. 42.7 Depigmented sclerotic skin lesions with severe involvement of the hand in *progressed systemic sclerosis*. The follicular openings and hairs are still pigmented

for vasospasm, and episodes of reversible blanching and cyanosis may be less visually apparent in deeply pigmented skin. History-taking strategies have been defined by the account of RP in white populations in which distinct color changes of hypoperfusion (white), cyanosis (blue), and then reperfusion (red) are easily visualized.

Digital ulcers and *pigmentary changes* are the greatest impactors of distress in patients with SSc, whereby pigment changes are an early manifestation and may be the feature that prompts pursuit of medical attention. Black-skinned patients report higher distress than white Caucasians. Body image and digital ulcers are a major source of distress for SSc patients of African descent [46].

Further investigation is needed to determine if this distress stems more from body image perception, more intense pain, more severe hand dysfunction, or more impaired healing processes.

Calcinosis cutis most commonly involves the digits but may occur much more extensively at the elbows, forearms, buttocks, knees, and lower legs. These deposits may be asymptomatic or painful, depending on size and location, and may ulcerate being a locus of secondary infection.

Nodular or keloidal manifestations are seen as a rare clinical presentation of SSc, more common in black-skinned individuals in which plaques or nodules consistent with keloids occur in the setting of other SSc manifestations. The lesions are often hyperpigmented, seen in patients predisposed to keloidal formation in response to diffuse cutaneous inflammatory processes [47].

(c) *Extracutaneous involvement*

Muscle involvement is more severe in patients with skin of color, with proximal weakness as seen in myositis [48]. SSc myopathies may be inflammatory and benefit from immunosuppressive treatment or fibrotic potentially leading to contractures and impaired range of motion. Creatine kinase and aldolase values should be obtained, keeping in mind that normal reference range for creatine kinase is higher in black-skinned populations [49].

Reflux esophagitis was one of the most common extracutaneous presentations noted in a large series of patients from Nigeria [4], despite esophageal reflux being rare in sub-Saharan Africa, probably due to nearly ubiquitous *Helicobacter pylori* infection [50–52]. In addition to esophageal dysmotility, black-skinned patients are more likely to experience other severe gastrointestinal symptoms [51]. Small bowel involvement occurs with higher frequency and may be associated with severe weight loss, nausea, vomiting, early satiety, distension, or diarrhea. Dysmotility can result in bacterial overgrowth and pseudo-obstruction. Anorectal dysfunction may result in fecal leakage or frank incontinence.

Lung involvement with pulmonary fibrosis or pulmonary hypertension (PH) is the leading cause of death in SSc. Severe pulmonary fibrosis with rapid, progressive loss of lung function occurs more commonly in diffuse cutaneous SSc with presence of Scl-70 or nucleolar ANA pattern. Fibrosis is more severe and occurs at earlier age in patients of African descent [53, 54]. If a patient of African descent is suspected to have SSc, it is imperative to obtain pulmonary function testing including lung volumes, spirometry, and diffusion capacity, repeated every 3–6 months. Patients can have considerable reduction of lung volumes and irreversible fibrosis even before patient-reported dyspnea. The most rapid loss of function occurs during the first 2 years, often correlated with high-resolution computed tomography to examine the extent of fibrosis shown to be of prognostic value. Unlike in whites, when PH typically occurs later in the disease process and more frequently in those with limited cutaneous SSc, PH develops at a younger age in patients of African descent with diffuse cutaneous SSc and short duration. The risk of PH is higher when the diffusion capacity declines more rapidly than lung volumes. PH screening is done primarily by echocardiogram or, if possible, by right heart catheterization in specialized units.

Scleroderma renal crisis (*SRC*) is the manifestation requiring the most urgent recognition and intervention. SRC most commonly occurs early in rapidly progressive diffuse cutaneous involvement, especially when associated with RNA polymerase III antibody. High-dose steroid management has been identified as one of the common triggers of renal crisis. Recognition of the onset is frequently delayed; therefore it is important to educate patients in high-risk groups regarding the signs and symptoms of SRC. Since the first usual sign is elevated blood pressure, we encourage high-risk individuals to monitor their blood pressure at home.

(d) *Laboratory markers*

SSc-specific autoantibodies, if present, are an indicator for the course of the disease and the risk of systemic involvement [55, 56]. Anti-topoisomerase I (Scl-70) is associated with a high likelihood of rapid progression of diffuse disease with interstitial lung involvement and is a very common antibody in patients with skin of color. RNA polymerase III with severe diffuse cutaneous disease and 25% risk for developing renal crisis and anti-centromere antibodies with high likelihood of limited cutaneous disease and risk of PH are more common in Caucasian patients. The autoantibody profiles of black and white skin populations are distinctly different; black-skinned patients had significantly higher frequencies of anti-U3 RNP antibody, U1 RNP antibody, and anti-topoisomerase, but lower frequencies of anti-centromere and RNA polymerase III. Of note, U3 RNP antibodies present as a nucleolar pattern of ANA and occur more frequently in people with skin of color, but are not yet part of the diagnostic criteria. The anti-centromere pattern is commonly present only in white Caucasians with SSc. Ethnic differences in severity and age of onset persisted even in subsets of black- and white-skinned patients identified with the same antibody [10]. The presence of anti-topoisomerase I in people of color occurred at significantly younger age (37 vs. 43 years), with greater frequency of pulmonary fibrosis (72% vs. 52%) and with greater severity (44% vs. 18%). Black-skinned patients were 75% more likely to die within 5 years than white Caucasians having the same autoantibody. Though anti-centromere antibodies occur less often, their presence confers a 2× higher risk of mortality in black-skinned patients [29].

42.4 Management

There is no specific treatment for progressive fibrosis of the skin or any other organ. Patients with systemic sclerosis are often treated orally with calcium channel blockers or phosphodiesterase inhibitors to prevent RP flares which worsen severity and frequency of digital ulcers and are encouraged to use gloves and/or hand warmers, if living in cold climate zones. For ulcers occurring at digital pulp as a primary consequence of vasospasm as well as for friction ulcers due to trauma secondary to poor healing, protective dressings are needed together with proper education regarding wound care and signs of infection. Intermittent use of topical lidocaine gel can help alleviate discomfort during wound cleaning or other pain provocative activities. For urgent treatment of severe ulceration, intravenous prostacyclins may be initiated.

Sun protection, protective clothing, etc. are essential particularly in patients with skin of color to prevent further inflammation-driven dyspigmentations. Retinoids have been used to slow down pigmentary changes. Bleaching strategies with hydroquinones have also been used to downregulate tyrosine kinase activity in melanocytes leading to hyperpigmentations.

Counseling patients on range of motion physical exercise is advised as a preventive measure early in the disease course. Patients are also encouraged to notice and report how food selections or restrictions, volumes, and preparations as well as fiber affect any gastrointestinal symptoms. For gastrointestinal involvement, treatment approaches may include rotating antibiotics, motility agents, probiotics, and osmotic laxatives.

Progressive pulmonary fibrosis requires systemic treatment with cyclophosphamide or mycophenolate mofetil. Potential future therapies include nintedanib, tocilizumab, and rituximab for lung, skin, and musculoskeletal efficacy. In black-skinned patients with progressive pulmonary fibrosis, more aggressive therapies may be required than in the white population. Smoking cessation is imperative. Healthy, safe daily exercise is encouraged to optimize respiratory capacity.

Renal recovery requires early recognition and immediate treatment with angiotensin-converting enzyme inhibitors. There is no role for prophylactic treatment with ACE-Is. There does not appear to be a higher incidence of SRC in blacks. Patients should be encouraged to carry a Renal Crisis Prevention Card [57], listing the common presenting symptoms and providing instructions to guide intervention in an urgent care setting.

Conclusions

Scleroderma in pigmented populations differs in many ways from that of white Caucasians. Early recognition is critical for long-term clinical outcomes. In a black-skinned population, this is difficult because of the more aggressive nature of the disease and the earlier incidence of severe pulmonary manifestations. In all pigmented populations with SSc, there is more frequent occurrence of anti-U3 RNP antibody, U1 RNP antibody, anti-topoisomerase, and nucleolar pattern ANA, but lower frequencies of anti-centromere antibody. Because of the effect on body image, concerns regarding pigment changes, pruritus, and digital ulcers are the initial reasons to seek treatment for pigmented populations versus skin thickening and Raynaud's phenomenon as is more common in white populations. Raynaud phenomenon is often not recognized in pigmented populations due to the difficulty in visualizing color changes in heavily pigmented skin.

Acknowledgment The authors wish to gratefully acknowledge the editorial and research contributions of Roberta Lukasiewicz, Heather Sickler, and Tammy Kelly to the development and writing of this chapter.

References

1. Oyoo O, Moots RJ, Ganda B. Stepping into the state of rheumatology in East Africa. Rheumatology (Oxford). 2012;51:1345–6.
2. Chifflot H, Fautrel B, Sordet C, et al. Incidence and prevalence of systemic sclerosis: a systematic literature review. J Semin Arthritis Rheum. 2008;37:223–35.
3. Dia D, Dieng MT, Sy TN, et al. Systemic scleroderma: 92 cases in Dakar. Dakar Med. 2003;48:82–6.
4. Adelowo OO, Oguntona S. Scleroderma (systemic sclerosis) among Nigerians. Clin Rheumatol. 2009;28:1121–5.
5. Mijiyawa M, Amanga K, Oniankitan OI, et al. Connective tissue diseases in the hospital outpatient service in Lomé (Togo). Rev Med Interne. 1999;20:13–7.
6. Pitche P, Amanga Y, Koumouvi K, et al. Scleroderma in a hospital setting in Togo. Med Trop. 1998;58:65–8.
7. Tager RE, Tikly M. Clinical and laboratory manifestations of systemic sclerosis (scleroderma) in Black South Africans. Rheumatology (Oxford). 1999;38:397–400.
8. Steen VD, Oddis CV, Conte CG, Janoski J, Casterline GZ, Medsger TA Jr. Incidence of systemic sclerosis in Allegheny County, Pennsylvania. A twenty-year study of hospital-diagnosed cases, 1963-1982. Arthritis Rheum. 1997;40:441–5. PMID: 90829319.
9. Steen V, Domsic RT, Lucas M, Fertig N, Medsger TA Jr. A clinical and serologic comparison of African American and Caucasian patients with systemic sclerosis. Arthritis Rheum. 2012;64:2986–94. https://doi.org/10.1002/art.34482. PMID: 225766201.
10. Reveille JD, Durban E, Goldstein R, Moreda R, Arnett FC. Racial differences in the frequencies of scleroderma-related autoantibodies. Arthritis Rheum. 1992;35:216–8. PMID: 1734910.
11. Laing TJ, Gillespie BW, Toth MB, et al. Racial differences in scleroderma among women in Michigan. Arthritis Rheum. 1997;40:734–42.
12. Beall AD, Nietert PJ, Taylor MH, et al. Ethnic disparities among patients with pulmonary hypertension associated with systemic sclerosis. J Rheumatol. 2007;34:1277–82.
13. Mayes MD. Scleroderma epidemiology. Rheum Dis Clin N Am. 1996;22:751–64.
14. Mayes MD, Lacey JV Jr, Beebe-Dimmer J, et al. Prevalence, incidence, survival, and disease characteristics of systemic sclerosis in a large US population. Arthritis Rheum. 2003;48:2246–55.
15. Medsger TA Jr, Masi AT. The epidemiology of systemic sclerosis (scleroderma) among male U.S. veterans. J Chronic Dis. 1978;31:73–85.
16. Wang J, Assassi S, Guo G, et al. Clinical and serological features of systemic sclerosis in a Chinese cohort. Clin Rheumatol. 2013;32:617–21.

17. McNeilage LJ, Youngchaiyud U, Whittingham S. Racial differences in antinuclear antibody patterns and clinical manifestations of scleroderma. Arthritis Rheum. 1989;32:54–60.
18. Pakunpanya K, Verasertniyom O, Vanichapuntu M, et al. Incidence and clinical correlation of anticentromere antibody in Thai patients. S Clin Rheumatol. 2006;25:325–8.
19. Krishnamurthy V, Porkodi R, Ramakrishnan S, et al. Progressive systemic sclerosis in south India. J Assoc Physicians India. 1991;39:254–7.
20. Kumar A, Malaviya AN, Tiwari SC, et al. Clinical and laboratory profile of systemic sclerosis in northern India. J Assoc Physicians India. 1990;38:765–8.
21. Pradhan V, Rajadhyaksha A, Nadkar M, et al. Clinical and autoimmune profile of scleroderma patients from Western India. Int J Rheumatol. 2014;2014:983781.
22. Sharma VK, Trilokraj T, Khaitan B, et al. Profile of systemic sclerosis in a tertiary care center in North India. Indian J Dermatol Venereol Leprol. 2006;72:416–20.
23. Eason RJ, Tan PL, Gow PJ. Progressive systemic sclerosis in Auckland: a ten year review with emphasis on prognostic features. Aust NZ J Med. 1981;11:657–62.
24. Le Guern V, Mahr A, Mouthon L, et al. Prevalence of systemic sclerosis in a French multi-ethnic county. Rheumatology (Oxford). 2004;43:1129–37.
25. Kuwana M, Okano Y, Kaburaki J, et al. Racial differences in the distribution of systemic sclerosis-related serum antinuclear antibodies. Arthritis Rheum. 1994;37:902–6.
26. Nietert PJ, Silver RM, Mitchell HC, et al. Demographic and clinical factors associated with in-hospital death among patients with systemic sclerosis. J Rheumatol. 2005;32:1888–92.
27. Rocha LF, Luppino Assad AP, Marangoni RG, et al. Systemic sclerosis and silica exposure: a rare association in a large Brazilian cohort. Rheumatol Int. 2016;36:697–702.
28. Bernatsky S, Smargiassi A, Johnson M, et al. Fine particulate air pollution, nitrogen dioxide, and systemic autoimmune rheumatic disease in Calgary, Alberta. Environ Res. 2015;140:474–8.
29. Jimenez SA, Diaz A, Khalili K. Retroviruses and the pathogenesis of systemic sclerosis. Int Rev Immunol. 1995;12:159–75.
30. Neidhart M, Kuchen S, Distler O, et al. Increased serum levels of antibodies against human cytomegalovirus and prevalence of autoantibodies in systemic sclerosis. Arthritis Rheum. 1999;42:389–92.
31. Marie I, Gehanno JF. Environmental risk factors of systemic sclerosis. Semin Immunopathol. 2015;37:463–73.
32. Maître A, Hours M, Bonneterre V, et al. Systemic sclerosis and occupational risk factors: role of solvents and cleaning products. J Rheumatol. 2004;31:2395–401.
33. Cowie RL, Dansey RD. Features of systemic sclerosis (scleroderma) in South African goldminers. S Afr Med J. 1990;77: 400–2.
34. Del Papa N, Quirici N, Scavullo C, et al. Antiendothelial cell antibodies induce apoptosis of bone marrow endothelial progenitors in systemic sclerosis. J Rheumatol. 2010;37:2053–63.
35. Riemekasten G, Philippe A, Näther M, et al. Involvement of functional autoantibodies against vascular receptors in systemic sclerosis. Ann Rheum Dis. 2011;70:530–6.
36. Baroni SS, Santillo M, Bevilacqua F, et al. Stimulatory autoantibodies to the PDGF receptor in systemic sclerosis. N Engl J Med. 2006;354:2667–76.
37. Riemekasten G, Cabral-Marques O. Antibodies against angiotensin II type 1 receptor (AT1R) and endothelin receptor type A (ETAR) in systemic sclerosis (SSc)-response. Autoimmun Rev. 2016;15:935.
38. Distler JH, Gay S, Distler O. Angiogenesis and vasculogenesis in systemic sclerosis. Rheumatology (Oxford). 2006;45(Suppl 3):iii26–7. Erratum in: Rheumatology (Oxford) 2008;47:234–35.
39. Tsou PS, Rabquer BJ, Ohara RA, et al. Scleroderma dermal microvascular endothelial cells exhibit defective response to pro-angiogenic chemokines. Rheumatology (Oxford). 2016;55:745–54.
40. Bogatkevich GS, Ludwicka-Bradley A, Highland KB, et al. Impairment of the antifibrotic effect of hepatocyte growth factor in lung fibroblasts from African Americans: possible role in systemic sclerosis. Arthritis Rheum. 2007;56:2432–42.
41. Bogatkevich GS, Highland KB, Akter T, et al. The PPARγ agonist rosiglitazone is antifibrotic for scleroderma lung fibroblasts: mechanisms of action and differential racial effects. Pulm Med. 2012;2012:545172.
42. Silver RM, Bogatkevich G, Tourkina E, et al. Racial differences between blacks and whites with systemic sclerosis. Curr Opin Rheumatol. 2012;24:642–8.
43. Van den Hoogen F, Khanna D, Fransen J, et al. 2013 classification criteria for systemic sclerosis: an American college of rheumatology/European league against rheumatism collaborative initiative. Ann Rheum Dis. 2013;72:1747–55.
44. Maricq HR, Weinrich MC. Diagnosis of Raynaud's phenomenon assisted by color charts. J Rheumatol. 1988;15:454–9.
45. Gelber AC, Manno RL, Shah AA, et al. Race and association with disease manifestations and mortality in scleroderma: a 20-year experience at the Johns Hopkins Scleroderma Center and review of the literature. Medicine (Baltimore). 2013;92:191–205.
46. Nusbaum JS, Gordon JK, Steen VD. African American race associated with body image dissatisfaction among patients with systemic sclerosis. Clin Exp Rheumatol. 2016;34 Suppl 100:70–3.
47. Cannick L, Douglas G, Crater S, et al. Nodular scleroderma: case report and literature review. J Rheumatol. 2003;30:2500–2.
48. Ramos PS, Silver RM, Feghali-Bostwick CA. Genetics of systemic sclerosis: recent advances. Curr Opin Rheumatol. 2015;27:521–9.
49. Black HR, Quallich H, Gareleck CB. Racial differences in serum creatine kinase levels. Am J Med. 1986;81:479–87.
50. Spechler SJ, Jain SK, Tendler DA, et al. Racial differences in the frequency of symptoms and complications of gastro-oesophageal reflux disease. Aliment Pharmacol Ther. 2002;16:1795–80.
51. Segal I. The gastro-oesophageal reflux disease complex in sub-Saharan Africa. Eur J Cancer Prev. 2001;10:209–12.
52. Sonnenberg A. Effects of environment and lifestyle on gastroesophageal reflux disease. Dig Dis. 2011;29:229–34.
53. Nietert PJ, Mitchell HC, Bolster MB, et al. Racial variation in clinical and immunological manifestations of systemic sclerosis. J Rheumatol. 2006;33:263–8.
54. McNearney TA, Reveille JD, Fischbach M, et al. Pulmonary involvement in systemic sclerosis: associations with genetic, serologic, sociodemographic, and behavioral factors. Arthritis Rheum. 2007;57:318–26.
55. Greidinger EL, Flaherty KT, White B, et al. African-American race and antibodies to topoisomerase I are associated with increased severity of scleroderma lung disease. Chest. 1998 Sep;114:801–7.
56. Aggarwal R, Lucas M, Fertig N, et al. Anti-U3 RNP autoantibodies in systemic sclerosis. Arthritis Rheum. 2009;60:1112–8.
57. Shapiro LS, Saketkoo L, Farrell JF, et al. Development of a "Renal Crisis Prevention Card" as an educational tool aimed at improving outcomes in high-risk patients with systemic sclerosis. Abstract 2716 ACR/ARHP Annual Meeting, November 2014; Boston, MA.

Dermatoses in Pregnancy

43

Jaheersha Pakran and Anwar Al Hammadi

The hormonal, immunological, and mechanical adaptations that occur during pregnancy to accommodate the growing fetus cause noticeable changes in maternal skin, modulated by various factors. These alterations of skin and its appendages that manifest during pregnancy are considered physiological [1, 2]. As a rule, the majority of pregnant women who experience these changes have a normal healthy pregnancy. However, there are some cutaneous disorders associated with ongoing pregnancy, which can be a harbinger of adverse fetal outcomes and remit postpartum [3]. In addition, when coincidental infections or other skin diseases affect women during pregnancy, their course may be worsened, improved, or unaffected by the pregnancy state (Table 43.1).

Table 43.1 Skin disorders in pregnancy

I.	*Physiologic skin changes*	Pigmentary changes, changes of hair and nails, changes of connective tissue, hormonal and pituitary gland changes, vascular changes
II.	*Specific dermatoses*	1. Polymorphic eruption of pregnancy 2. Pemphigus gestationis 3. Obstetric cholestasis 4. Atopic eruption of pregnancy
III.	*Other skin diseases with special implications in pregnancy*	• *Skin diseases worsening in pregnancy* Impetigo herpetiformis, atopic dermatitis, hereditary angioedema, systemic LE with renal involvement, Hansen's disease, malignant melanoma, neurofibroma, dermatomyositis, eosinophilic granuloma, pemphigus vulgaris, mycosis fungoides, acrodermatitis enteropathica, porphyria cutanea tarda, herpes simplex, varicella, condylomata acuminata, viral exanthemas • *Skin diseases improving in pregnancy* Allergic contact dermatitis, Fox-Fordyce disease, hidradenitis suppurativa, psoriasis (2/3 improve), systemic sclerosis

43.1 Physiological Skin Changes in Pregnancy

Pigmentation: Increased incidence of pigmentary changes is seen in up to 90% of pregnancies; they are triggered by the hormonal changes during pregnancy, exposure to UV light, and genetic predisposition [4]. Melasma occurs in 5–50% of the cases and is more pronounced in darker skin type. Accentuation of pigmented areas such as external genitalia, periumbilical region, inner thighs, areola, and axillae occurs, with darkening of pigmentary demarcation lines. Benign melanocytic nevi may darken and cause alarm to the patient, but pregnancy does not induce specific changes in nevi [5]. It is advisable to defer treatment for excess pigmentation until after delivery; sun protection may be the best strategy for melasma.

Hairs and nails: Hair growth is usually abundant in pregnancy since >85% of scalp hair follicles enter the anagen phase. Body hair in male pattern with frontal thinning can also occur but it slowly reverts to normal postpartum. Observation and reassurance are recommended during pregnancy and lactation. Changes in nails during pregnancy such as transverse line (Beau's line), distal onycholysis, subungual hyperkeratosis, brittleness, and leukonychia have been reported.

Connective tissue: Hormonal changes during pregnancy and mechanical distension lead to striae gravidarum or stretch marks. It affects up to 90% of pregnant women and appears in the second half of pregnancy on the abdomen, breasts, buttocks, hips, or thighs. Initially, they are red to purplish in color, often associated with pruritus or pigmented in darker skin, occasionally hypertrophic (Figs. 43.1 and 43.2). After delivery, the lesions evolve into white atrophic streaks.

J. Pakran (✉)
Department of Dermatology, Hatta Hospital and Rashi Hospital, Dubai Health Authority, Dubai, UAE
e-mail: JPakran@dha.gov.ae

A. Al Hammadi
Department of Dermatology, Dubai Medical Center, Dubai, UAE
e-mail: AnHAlHammadi@dha.gov.ae

C. E. Orfanos et al. (eds.), *Pigmented Ethnic Skin and Imported Dermatoses*, https://doi.org/10.1007/978-3-319-69422-1_43

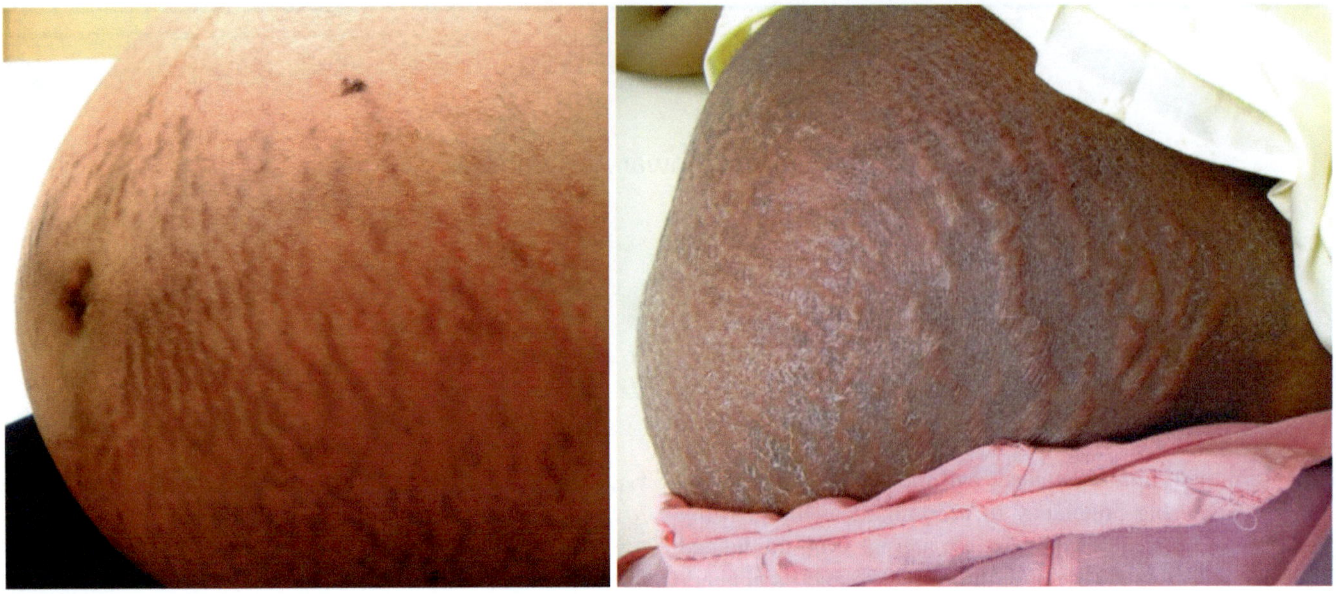

Fig. 43.1 Hyperpigmented and hypertrophic stretch marks in pregnancy (*striae gravidarum*)

Endocrine: Eccrine glands show hyperactivity as pregnancy progresses manifesting as hyperhidrosis, miliaria, and dyshidrotic eczema. Paradoxically, palmar sweating reduces during pregnancy. Apocrine gland activity usually decreases, being clinically manifested as an improvement in Fox-Fordyce disease and hidradenitis suppurativa. Modified sebaceous glands called Montgomery's glands or tubercles on the areola of breast become prominent during pregnancy and lactation period; they secrete an antimicrobial lubricant that protect the nipples from cracking and infections during breastfeeding.

Vascular tissue: Estrogen and angiogenic factors bring about vascular changes in pregnancy critical for maintaining uteroplacental blood flow. They are reflected in skin as palmar erythema, vasomotor instability (flushing or pallor), cutis marmorata, dermographism, varicosities, purpura, and non-pitting edema of face and extremities. Other findings include spider angioma, pyogenic granuloma (gravidarum), hemangiomas, and gingival hyperemia.

Overall, no significant statistical difference was found in the occurrence of these changes between prenatal low- and high-risk pregnancies [2, 6].

43.2 Clinical Entities Associated with Pregnancy

These are four intensely pruritic dermatoses associated with pregnancy, starting usually in the third trimester up to a few days or weeks postpartum [7, 8].

43.2.1 Polymorphic Eruption of Pregnancy

Although papules and plaques are initially the main features of this condition, more than half of the patients develop later polymorphous urticarial, targetoid, and/or eczematous lesions and occasionally vesicles, justifying the term 'polymorphic eruption in pregnancy' in place of the older term of 'pruritic urticarial papules and plaques of pregnancy (PUPPP)', which is also in use.

43.2.1.1 Epidemiology

It occurs in 1/160 to 1/200 of all pregnancies, seen mainly in primiparous women or multiple gestations, rarely recurring.

43.2.1.2 Clinical Features

The rash usually begins in the third trimester or immediately postpartum with a mean onset at 35 weeks of gestation. Initially there are small pruritic urticarial papules on abdominal striae spreading over the body with relative sparing of the periumbilical area, face, palms, and soles (Fig. 43.3). Later the lesions enlarge and form diffuse erythematous plaques. Microvesicles (1–2 mm) may be found over the plaques, but frank bullae never occur. The pruritic lesions may become urticarial and polymorphic; PUPPP can also appear after delivery and disappear after a few weeks (Fig. 43.4). Maternal and fetal prognoses are excellent; spontaneous resolution occurs within 4–6 weeks of onset or 1–2 weeks postpartum. The condition rarely ever recurs in subsequent pregnancies. Pemphigoid gestationis can mimic the early urticarial stage of polymorphic

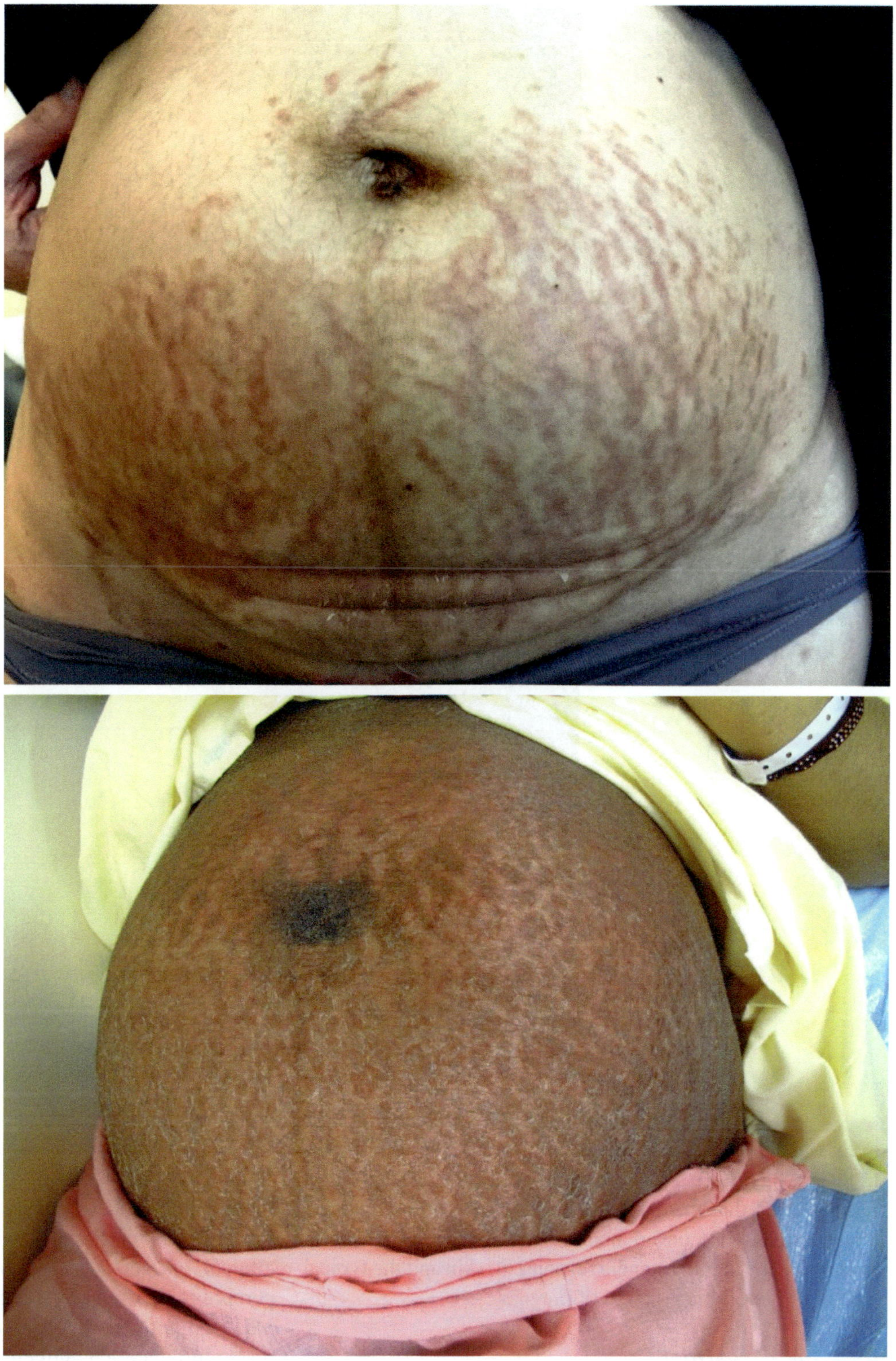

Fig. 43.2 Alterations of abdominal skin in pregnancy (multigravidas, Arab origin)

eruption of pregnancy; direct immune fluorescence is a reliable method for differentiation, since linear depositions of complement are present only in pemphigoid gestationis.

43.2.1.3 Etiology

The cause remains elusive, but hormonal, immunological, and mechanical factors have been implicated in the pathogenesis. Polymorphic eruption of pregnancy is associated with

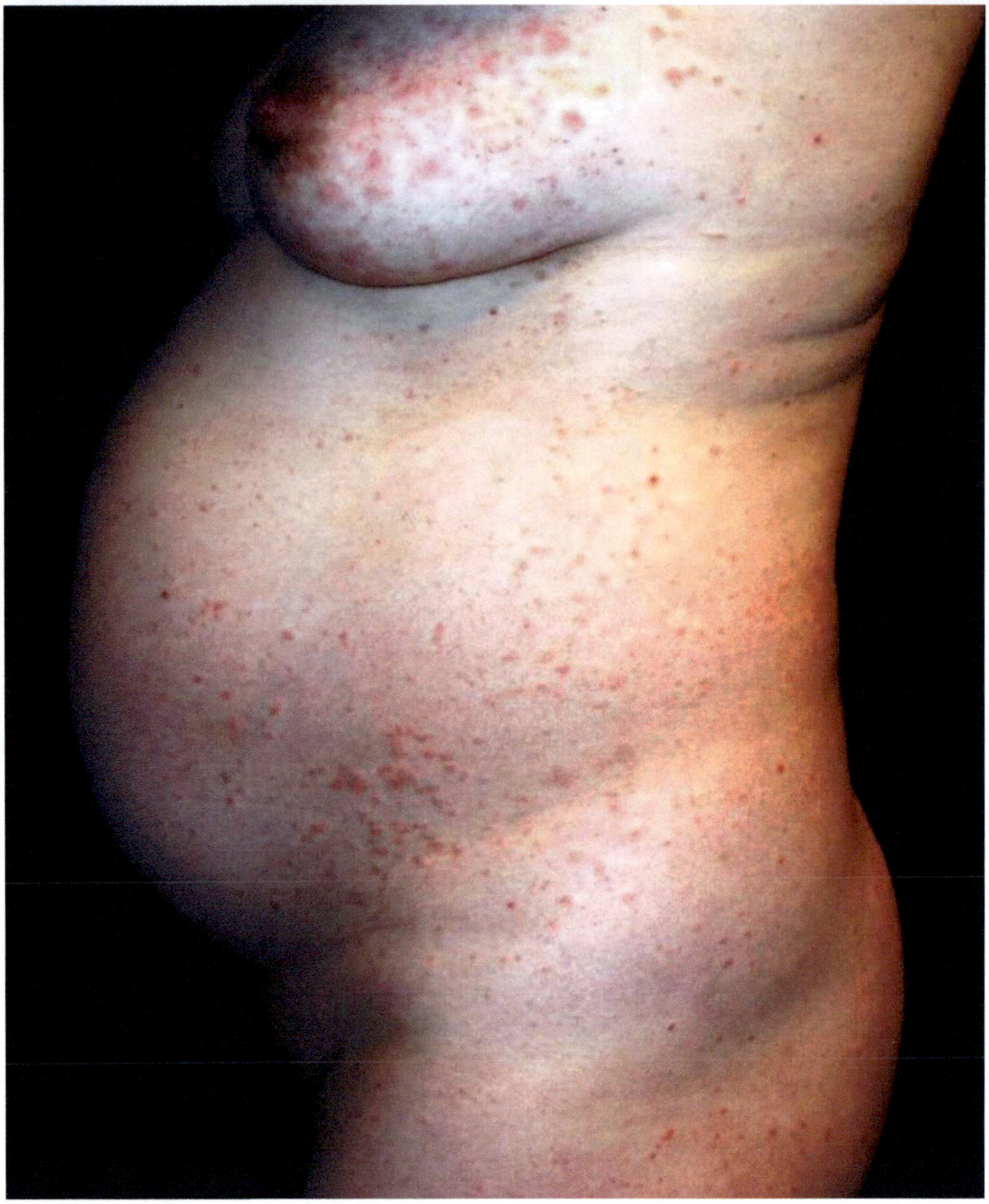

Fig. 43.3 *Polymorphic eruption of pregnancy*, third trimester, strongly pruritic (Asian multigravida)

excess maternal weight gain and multiple gestations, conditions in which excess stretching of skin occurs. Therefore, it is speculated that this stretching may either expose sequestered antigens or convert non-antigenic molecules to antigenic ones leading to immune response to skin and the typical rash of polymorphic eruption of pregnancy.

43.2.1.4 Treatment

Treatment should be tailored to the severity of each case. In women with localized lesions, topical application of mid-strength topical corticosteroids provides symptomatic relief, and oral antihistamines offer some benefit in pruritic patients at bedtime. If severe, a short course of oral prednisolone 20–30 mg/day for 1–2 weeks may be considered.

43.2.2 Pemphigoid Gestationis

Pemphigoid gestationis (PG) is a self-limiting, intensely pruritic bullous disease associated with pregnancy showing clinical, antigenic, and immunologic similarities to bullous pemphigoid. The main difference is that the trigger here is a placental antigen which induces antibodies that later cross-react with maternal antigens.

43.2.2.1 Epidemiology

The condition occurs in approximately 1:50,000 pregnancies. A genetic association with HLA DR3 and HLA DR4 haplotypes is found.

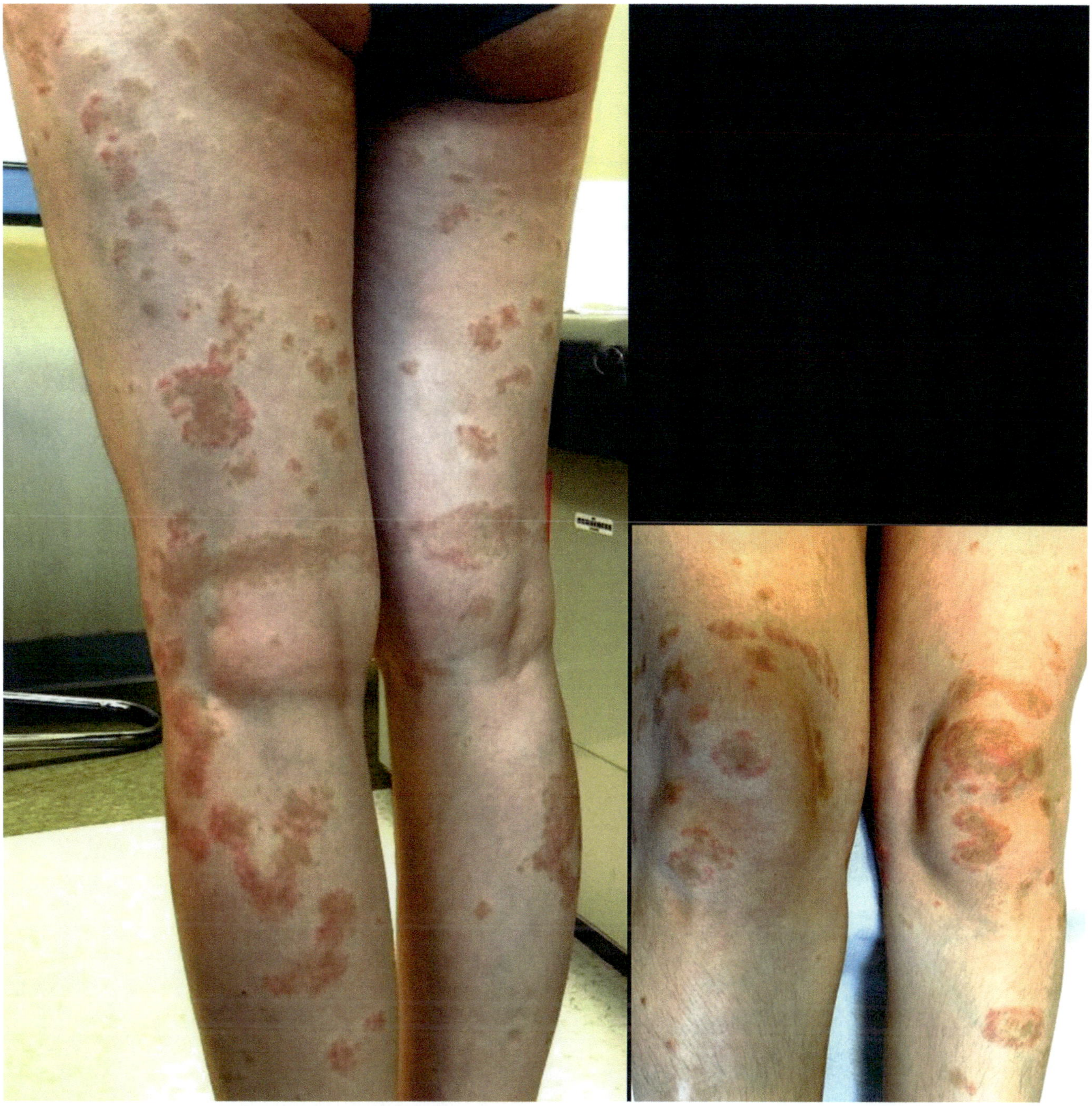

Fig. 43.4 *Polymorphic eruption of pregnancy* (PUPPP) appearing 1 month after delivery (Asian primigravida) spontaneously regressed within 2 months

43.2.2.2 Clinical Features

The disease starts usually during the second and third trimesters, though it may develop anywhere between 1 month of gestation and 1 month postpartum. A short prodromal phase with chills and malaise may occur, followed by a pre-bullous phase characterized by intensely itchy erythematous urticarial papules and plaques in the periumbilical area. The lesions may later generalize; the oral mucosa is affected in only 20% of the cases. After a latent period of 2–4 weeks, the bullous phase appears, and pustules may be seen (Figs. 43.5 and 43.6). Resolution is usually without scarring. In cases with late onset, there may be no bullous phase. The natural course is characterized by exacerbations and remissions throughout pregnancy improving toward term and complete resolution after several months. However, premenstrual flares may occur, also seen under contraceptives (25%) and in

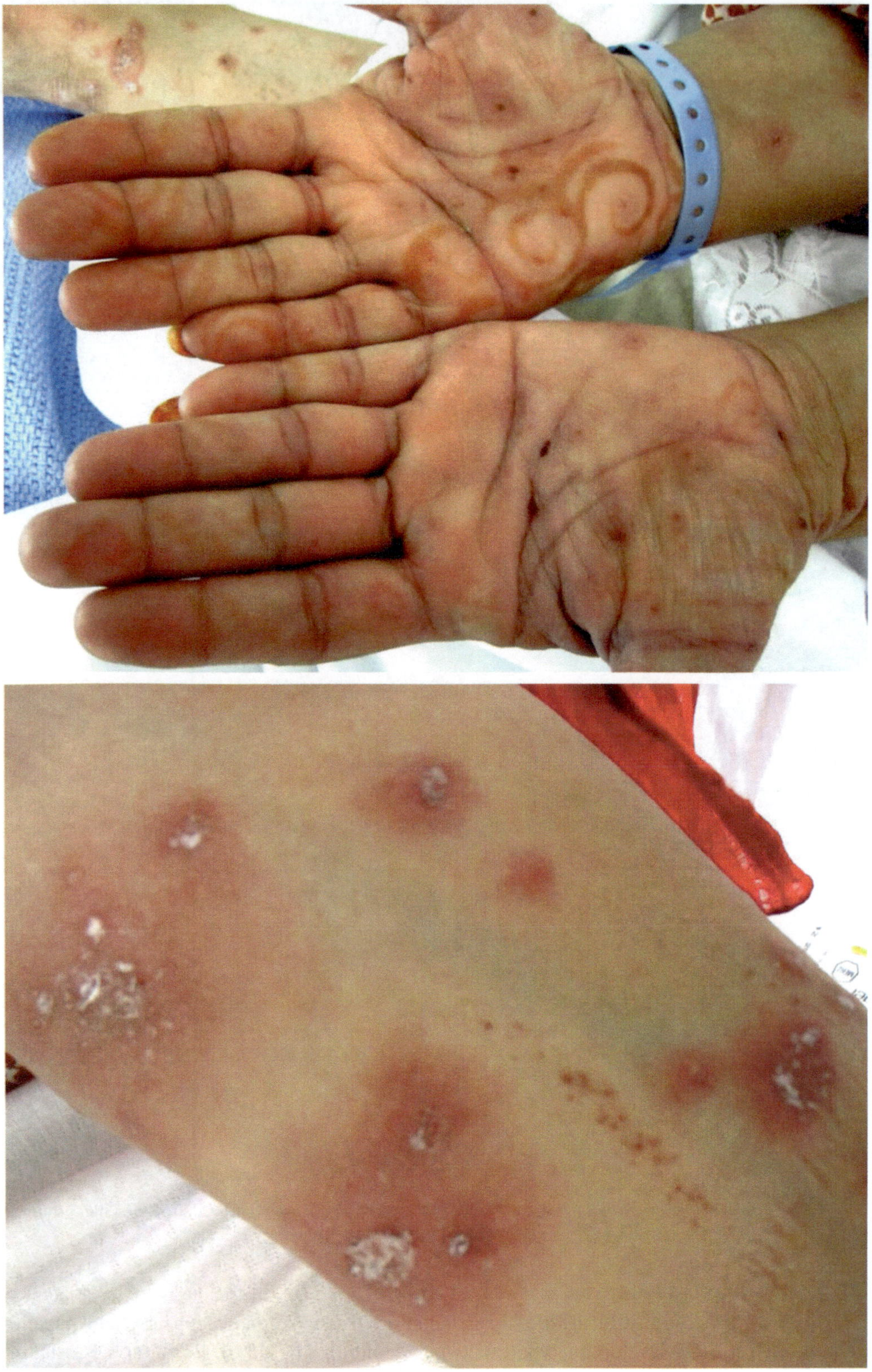

Fig. 43.5 *Pemphigoid gestationis* in the extremities. In the palms rests of cultural paintings with henna are seen among macular and vesicular lesions

subsequent pregnancies. The fetal morbidity correlates with early onset of severe disease and blister formation. There is a risk for premature delivery and for small-for-gestational-age birth weight. Up to 10% of newborns may develop vesiculobullous lesions due to passive transfer of antibodies from mother to fetus. Histology correlates with stage and severity of the disease, showing marked papillary edema, mixed perivascular cell infiltrate, and subepidermal bulla formation with eosinophils. Direct immunofluorescence of perilesional skin is the gold standard for diagnosis, showing linear C3

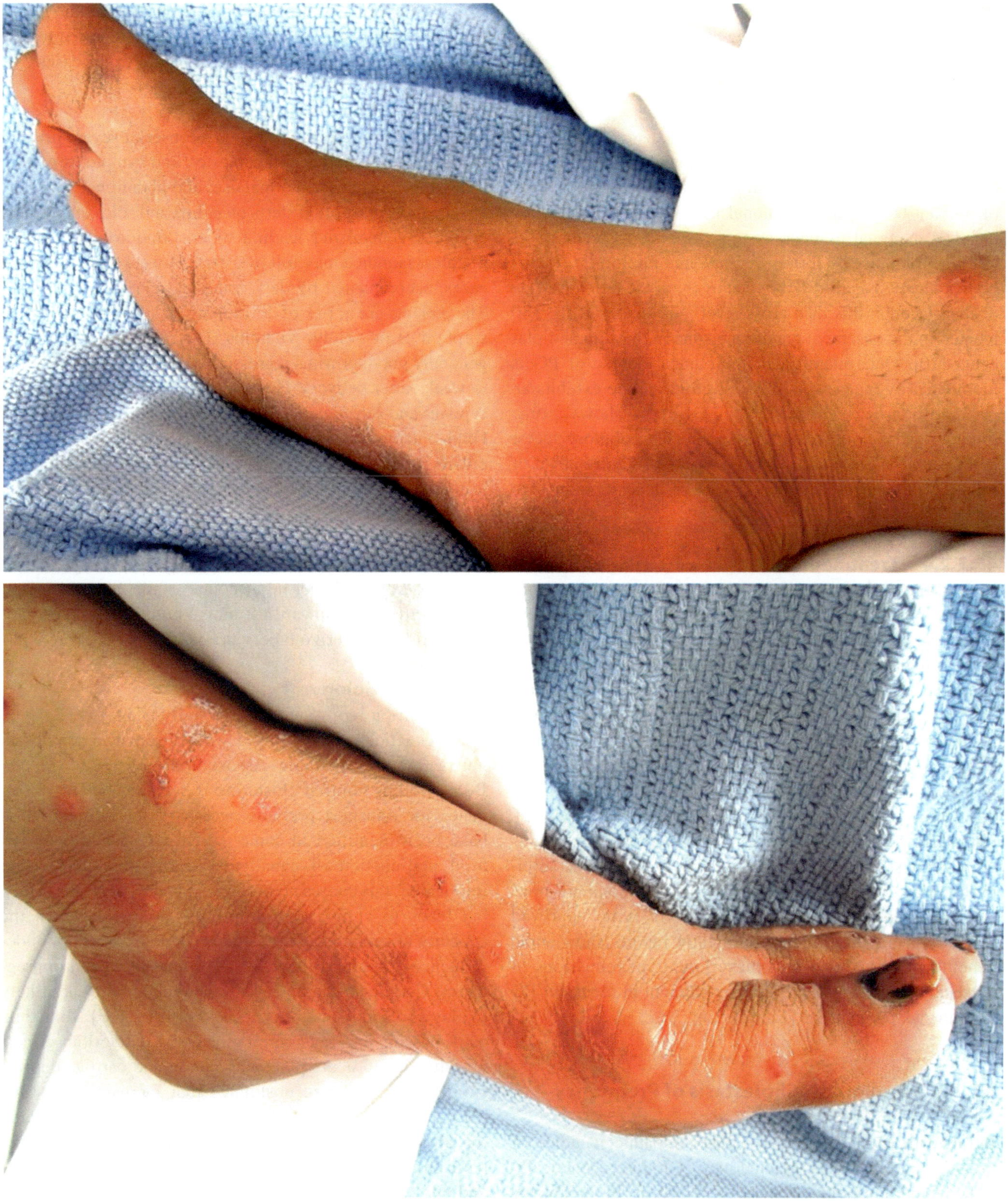

Fig. 43.6 *Pemphigoid gestationis* with EM-like lesions on both feet, partly in bullous stage (second trimester, para 7, similar eruption during the last two pregnancies)

deposition along the dermo-epidermal junction in 100% of cases, often associated with IgG deposition. Circulating IgG antibodies are found in patient's serum in more than 30% of the cases; their levels correlate with disease activity. An emerging strategy for diagnosis of PG is the immunohistochemical detection of C4d which is a stable product of complement activation and thus can be identified in formalin fixed tissue specimen, eliminating the need for special media and processing required for direct immunofluorescence testing.

43.2.2.3 Etiology

Pathogenetically, it seems that three major pathogenic factors may lead to PG: loss of immune privilege, development of autoantibodies, and hormonal modulation in pregnancy [9]. The maternal immune system responds to break of its immune tolerance by forming complement fixing IgG1 antibodies directed against BP-180 antigen on the amniotic side of the placenta; this then cross-react with maternal BP-180 located in the basement membrane zone in the skin and placenta [10]. Once manifested, the clinical course of PG is modulated by maternal hormones; progesterone exhibits an immunosuppressive effect, and estrogen shows some immune-enhancing properties. Another contributory factor is a C4 null allele mutation that may impair the removal of immune complexes and facilitate their deposition in skin tissue.

43.2.2.4 Treatment

In mild pre-bullous stages, topical use of potent corticosteroids combined with oral antihistamines may be sufficient. However, 80% of the patients require systemic corticosteroids (prednisolone 0.25–0.5 mg/kg tapered down to low maintenance with 5–10 mg/day) during pregnancy. It is prudent to step up the steroid dose before the exacerbation anticipated immediately after delivery and later taper it off over several weeks or months according to clinical activity in the post-partum period. In severe cases, plasmapheresis or high-dose intravenous immunoglobulins can provide temporary improvement. In non-breastfeeding mothers, agents such as tetracyclines, nicotinamide, dapsone, pyridoxine, and sulfapyridine are other options. Neonatal skin lesions are transient and require no management. There is no approved medication for prevention; preliminary reports show some benefit with rituximab to achieve long-term remissions in persistent PG and as a preventive treatment in recurrent PG of high-risk pregnancies [11, 12].

43.2.3 Intrahepatic Cholestasis of Pregnancy

Intrahepatic cholestasis, also called idiopathic jaundice of pregnancy or pruritus gravidarum, is a rare, genetically linked, and hormone-dependent cholestasis in pregnancy with or without jaundice [13]. The condition shows no primary skin lesions but causes intractable pruritus [14].

43.2.3.1 Epidemiology

Incidence of 0.1–1.5% has been described for Europe and North America; highest rates were observed in Chile and Bolivia, particularly among women of Araucanian Indian descent. Hepatitis C seropositivity has been reported to be a risk factor. Family history is present in half of the cases.

43.2.3.2 Clinical Features

The condition presents with sudden onset of severe pruritus any time in second or third trimester, and symptoms of cholestasis such as anorexia, malaise, and abdominal pain may also be present. It often starts on palms and soles and rapidly becomes generalized leading to excoriations and prurigo nodules. Jaundice may follow after 2–4 weeks in 10–50% of cases, accompanied by dark urine and clay-colored stools. The patients are at risk of developing steatorrhea and malabsorption of fat-soluble vitamins. The maternal prognosis is generally good; pruritus regresses spontaneously within days to weeks after delivery. However, it recurs with oral contraceptives and subsequent pregnancies in 60–70% of the cases. Fetal outcome is affected; there are several adverse fetal effects with a three- to fivefold increased risk for fetal death in utero. The most sensitive indicator for diagnosis is elevated level of bile acids in blood with levels beyond 11 μmol/L, especially above 40 μmol/L, being associated with higher risk of adverse fetal outcome. Elevated liver enzymes are found later in the course of the disease.

The differential toward the atopic eruption in pregnancy, in particular its prurigo type, can be clinically challenging.

43.2.3.3 Etiology

The condition represents a hormonally triggered cholestasis in genetically predisposed women; environmental and gut factors are debatable. Association with HLA A31 and B8 as well as familial clustering is seen, and mutations of genes for transport proteins necessary for bile excretion have been identified in some patients. Genetically linked mild malfunction of canalicular transporters have been implicated; this causes no problems in non-pregnant women but leads to clinical symptoms of cholestasis when the capacity to secrete substrates is exceeded, as occurs under influence of high levels of sex hormones produced in pregnancy. Certain sulfated progesterone metabolites are likely to play a role in the pathogenesis of pruritus [13]. Toxic bile acids passing into fetal circulation cause deleterious effects on fetus due to acute placental anoxia and cardiac depression. It has been also postulated that increased intestinal permeability ("leaky gut") may play a role by enhancing the absorption of bacterial endotoxins and the enterohepatic circulation of cholestatic metabolites of sex hormones and bile salts.

43.2.3.4 Treatment

Early diagnosis, prompt measures to reduce serum bile acids, and active fetal management are cornerstones of treatment, requiring an interdisciplinary approach of dermatologists, gynecologists, gastroenterologist, and neonatologists.

Ursodeoxycholic acid, a naturally occurring hydrophilic bile acid, is the treatment of choice with 15 mg/kg/day or 1 g daily, either as single dose or divided in 2–3 doses until delivery. It stimulates the excretion of hydrophobic and potentially hepatotoxic bile acids thereby correcting the leakage to the fetoplacental unit and reducing the risk of premature delivery. With exception of occasional mild diarrhea, there are no adverse effects. Steatorrhea may respond to treatment with pancreatic enzymes, and vitamin K intramuscular injections are given in prolonged cases as prophylaxis for postpartum hemorrhage.

43.2.4 Atopic Eruption of Pregnancy

Historical terms of pruritic disorders associated with pregnancy such as Besnier's prurigo, prurigo and pruritic folliculitis of pregnancy, eczema in pregnancy, etc. have been currently grouped into a single umbrella entity called atopic eruption of pregnancy [7].

43.2.4.1 Epidemiology

As a group, the condition is the most common skin disorder accounting for 50% of all dermatoses seen in pregnant women [15]. The estimated incidence accounts 1 per 300–450 pregnancies.

43.2.4.2 Clinical Features

The main characteristics of the condition are its onset before the third trimester (in 75% of cases), the presence of an atopic background of the patient or her family, and recurrence in subsequent pregnancies. Serum total IgE elevations may aid but are not essential for diagnosis. Depending on the morphology of the lesions, the eruption is subclassified into an eczematous E-type, present in two- thirds of the cases and a papular/prurigo P-type, encountered in the rest. Their coexistence occurs relatively often. The eczematous lesions are located in typical atopic sites, whereas prurigo nodules and pruritic folliculitis appear as grouped, discrete erythematous papulonodules especially over the extensor surfaces of the extremities (Fig. 43.2). Generalization of the lesions can occur. The lesions tend to persist throughout gestation but usually resolve in the early postpartum period. Post-inflammatory hyperpigmentation or scarring may occur, especially in skin of color.

There are no specific tests available to confirm the clinical diagnosis. Histopathology of skin lesions is nonspecific, and serum IgE levels and eosinophil counts are elevated in only 20–70% of the cases. Examination of serum bile acid levels to exclude obstetric cholestasis is mandatory. The patient should be reassured that the maternal and fetal prognosis is excellent. The risk of infantile atopic dermatitis is related to the atopic background of the mother. However, recurrences can occur in subsequent pregnancies.

43.2.4.3 Etiology

Clinically, it may correspond to an intrinsic type of atopic dermatitis triggered in pregnancy without elevation of IgE levels or allergies to aeroallergens and/or food; however, its pathogenesis and classification are not fully clarified [16]. The physiologic switch from cell-mediated to humoral immunity (Th1 to Th2 shift) during gestation to prevent rejection of fetus by the maternal immune system is speculated to play a pathogenetic role.

43.2.4.4 Treatment

Patients with mild involvement are treated with emollients (urea 3–10%) or topical medications such as calamine lotion, camphor (1–2%), and menthol (1–2%) considered safe in pregnancy; however their effect is modest. Mid- or high- potency non-halogenated topical corticosteroids can lead to rapid improvement. Oral antihistamines can provide relief of symptoms; diphenhydramine or chlorpheniramine is safe in gestation and preferred. In resistant cases, a short course of low-dose prednisolone 20–30 mg/day for 1–2 weeks followed by tapering and maintenance with topical medication is recommended. Phototherapy with narrowband UVB is a safe additional tool. Topical and intralesional corticosteroid steroids can be beneficial. Narrowband UVB therapy (20–30 sessions) has been reported successful.

43.3 Other Entities with Special Implications in Pregnancy

43.3.1 Impetigo Herpetiformis

Impetigo herpetiformis is a rare life-threatening pustular skin eruption in pregnant women. It is generally considered a variant of pustular psoriasis occurring during pregnancy [17, 18]. However, there are advocates for classifying the disease as a separate entity. Clinically the patient usually present in the third trimester an acute pustular rash on erythematous base, often associated with fever, malaise, and chills. The lesions spread peripherally and heal centrally with hyperpigmentation and/or crusting. Painful oral erosions and onycholysis may accompany the rash. The condition persists until delivery and it rarely continues in the postpartum period. There is an increased risk of morbidity and mortality for the mother from sepsis, renal, or cardiac failure and risk of stillbirth and neonatal death for the fetus. Pathogenetically, a link to hypocalcemia and hypoparathyroidism has been presumed. Blood and pus cultures are negative. The mainstay of treatment is oral prednisolone 1 mg/kg/day, tapered after delivery; cyclosporin [19] have been also successfully administered, alone or combined with prednisolone. New biologicals may become an alternative for treatment; uneventful pregnancy has been reported under ustekinumab [20, 21]. In life-threatening cases, expedite delivery should be considered preferably as soon as lung maturity of fetus is anticipated. There is a risk of recurrence with subsequent pregnancies and on use of oral contraceptives.

43.3.1.1 Psoriasis

Pregnancy has a variable effect on patients with psoriasis. Although common plaque psoriasis improves in pregnancy, the skin involvement may worsen in around 10–20% of the pregnant females and pustular eruptions develop (Fig. 43.7), which may often generalize. A safe option for patients with limited disease is topical therapy, including moisturizers and mild topical corticosteroids as well as UVB phototherapy.

43.3.1.2 Varicella Zoster Virus Infection

Viral infections of the skin may have serious consequences for the mother and the offspring [22]. Chicken pox in mother places fetus at risk from fetal varicella syndrome and neonatal viral pneumonia and encephalitis in 1–2% of cases; recently, precise recommendations for prevention and management were given by Canadian Maternal Fetal Medicine Committee [23]. Passive immunization can protect or ameliorate the disease if given within 72 h of contact. Oral or i.v. acyclovir should be given to mother and affected neonate depending on the severity. A planned delivery should be avoided for at least 7 days after the onset of the maternal rash to allow the passive transfer of protective antibodies from mother to child, if continuing the pregnancy does not pose any additional risks.

43.3.2 Herpes Simplex Virus Infection

Primary HSV infection may lead to severe illness in pregnancy and may be associated with transplacental virus transmission and fetal infection [24]. Herpes genitalis is seen in around 2% of pregnancies. Aim of treatment is not just symptomatic relief to mother but also to prevent perinatal transmission, which can result in neonatal morbidity and mortality. The treatment is the same as for non-pregnant state with acyclovir 400 mg TID for 5–7 days. The neonatal risk is highest for primary infection acquired in pregnancy or recurrent HS infection during the last 6 weeks of pregnancy. For such cases, a suppressive management is warranted with oral acyclovir at dose of 400 mg TID or valaciclovir 500 mg BD, starting from 36 weeks of pregnancy until delivery. In addition, caesarean

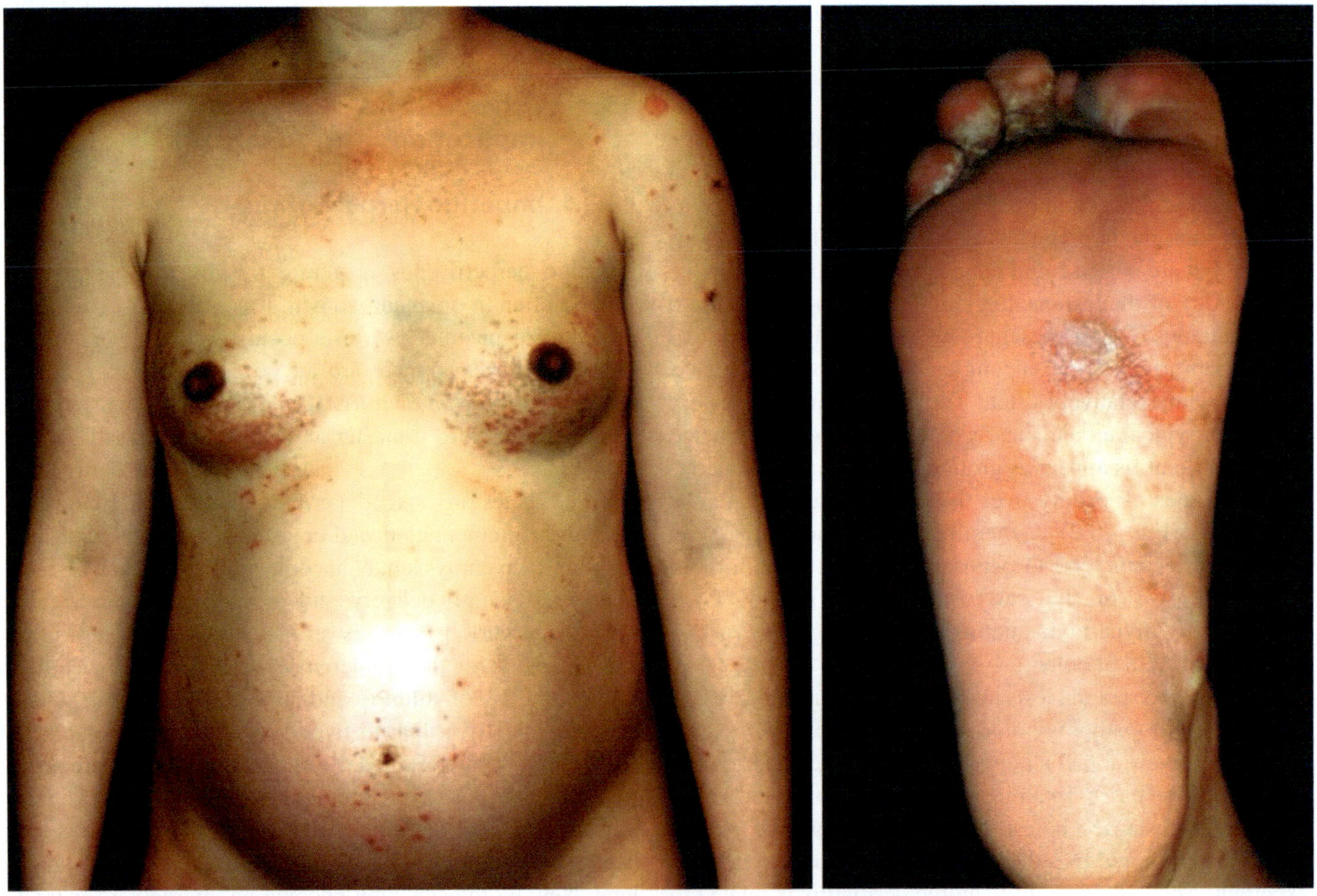

Fig. 43.7 Pustular rash with peripheral pustules and plantar involvement mimicking pustular psoriasis

section should be recommended to women presenting with primary episode genital herpes lesions at the time of delivery, or within 6 weeks of the expected date of delivery, in order to reduce exposure of the fetus to the virus that may be present in maternal genital fluids.

43.3.3 Pityriasis Rosea

Studies have shown that pityriasis rosea, a viral infection caused by HHV-6 and HHV-7 may cause premature delivery with neonatal hypotonia and even fetal demise especially if it develops within first 15 weeks' gestation [25]. Apart from topical emollients, topical corticosteroids, and oral antihistamines, the patient and gynecologist must be informed about the fetal risks.

43.3.4 Autoimmune Disorders

Systemic lupus erythematosus flares in 60% of patients in pregnancy, associated with maternal and fetal morbidity and mortality. Those with Sjogren's syndrome and SCLE often have circulating anti-Ro antibodies as a marker for possible congenital heart block in 2–3% of neonates. Cardiac screening of fetus from 16 weeks' gestation and maternal treatment with i.v. immunoglobulin has been useful in some high-risk cases.

43.4 Pruritus in Pregnancy

A major concern in pregnancy is how to control pruritus that is a predominant symptom in up to a quarter of all pregnancies. Pruritus in pregnancy is often associated with xerosis, especially of the legs, and with the stretching of the skin on the abdomen and breasts. However, when primary skin lesions are absent, the clinician should rule out cholestasis of pregnancy along with other internal pruritogenic causes such as liver or renal disease, thyroid disorders, drug-induced itch, parasitic infestation, malignancy, etc. A detailed history and workup together with an appropriate panel of laboratory investigations is warranted before initiating any treatment.

43.5 Drug Use During Pregnancy

Corticosteroids and antihistamines are generally safe in pregnancy and lactation [26, 27]; however, any drug used in pregnancy carries a basic risk for adverse effects; careful risk/benefit assessment should be carried out (Table 43.2). Phototherapies are generally regarded safe in pregnancy. For scabies permethrin 5% cream is considered the drug of choice in pregnant women, since its systemic absorption after topical application is poor. Chemical topical UV filters have been reported to have the ability to cause endocrine and reproductive impairments [28] and cannot be recommended until further clarification.

Table 43.2 Antipruritic modalities used in pregnancy

Drug class	1st line	Comments	2nd line	Comments
Antihistamines	Chlorpheniramine maleate, dexchlorpheniramine	First-generation antihistamines are relatively safe in pregnancy	Loratadine, cetirizine	Less effect on quality of life, less sedation; to be used with caution after the first trimester
Topical corticosteroids	Betamethasone, mometasone, methylprednisolone	Relatively safe in pregnancy, no teratogenic effects	Clobetasol propionate cream	Limit usage to small areas and short duration
Systemic corticosteroids	Prednisolone, methylprednisolone	Low doses (<7.5 mg/day) are safe; teratogenic risk for orofacial clefts exists when used in first trimester	Cortisone, hydrocortisone, betamethasone, dexamethasone,	Better avoided as they readily cross the placenta and has teratogenic risks
Sunscreens	Physical modalities like clothing, sunglasses; sun avoidance	Chemical UV filters have potential endocrine effects	Physical sunscreens	Physical sunscreens (zinc oxide, titanium dioxide) appear safe and do not penetrate intact skin; if disrupted penetration is unpredictable
Narrowband UVB phototherapy	Considered safe in pregnancy, better to supplement folic acid as Rx has been associated with low levels of maternal serum folate			

References

1. Kar S, Krishnan A, Shivkumar PV. Pregnancy and skin. J Obstet Gynaecol India. 2012;62:268–75.
2. Hassan I, Bashir S, Taing S. A clinical study of the skin changes in pregnancy in Kashmir valley of north India: a hospital based study. Indian J Dermatol. 2015;60:28–322.
3. Panicker VV, Riyaz N, Balachandran PK. A clinical study of cutaneous changes in pregnancy. J Epidemiol Glob Health. 2017;7:63–70.
4. Bieber AK, Martires KJ, Stein JA, et al. Pigmentation and pregnancy: knowing what is normal. Obstet Gynecol. 2017;129:168–73.
5. Bieber AK, Martires KJ, Driscoll MS, et al. Nevi and pregnancy. J Am Acad Dermatol. 2016;75:661–6.
6. Fernandes LB, Amaral WN. Clinical study of skin changes in low and high risk pregnant women. An Bras Dermatol. 2015;90:822–6.
7. Sävervall C, Sand FL, Thomsen SF. Dermatological diseases associated with pregnancy: pemphigoid gestationis, polymorphic eruption of pregnancy, intrahepatic cholestasis of pregnancy, and atopic eruption of pregnancy. Dermatol Res Pract. 2015;2015:979635.
8. Ambros-Rudolph CM, Sticherling M. Specific dermatoses of pregnancy. Hautarzt. 2017;68:87–94.
9. Semkova K, Black M. Pemphigoid gestationis: current insights into pathogenesis and treatment. Eur J Obstet Gynecol Reprod Biol. 2009;145:138–44.
10. Sadik CD, Lima AL, Zillikens D. Pemphigoid gestationis: toward a better understanding of the etiopathogenesis. Clin Dermatol. 2016;34:378–82.
11. Cianchini G, Masini C, Lupi F, et al. Severe persistent pemphigoid gestationis: long-term remission with rituximab. Br J Dermatol. 2007;157:388–9.
12. Tourte M, Brunet-Possenti F, Mignot S, et al. Pemphigoid gestationis: a successful preventive treatment by rituximab. J Eur Acad Dermatol Venereol. 2017;31:e206–7. https://doi.org/10.1111/jdv.13962.
13. Kremer AE, Wolf K, Ständer S. Intrahepatic cholestasis of pregnancy: rare but important. Hautarzt. 2017;68:95–102.
14. Kenyon AP, Tribe RM, Nelson-Piercy C, et al. Pruritus in pregnancy: a study of anatomical distribution and prevalence in relation to the development of obstetric cholestasis. Obstet Med. 2010;3:25–295.
15. Masood S, Rizvi DA, Tabassum S, et al. Frequency and clinical variants of specific dermatoses in third trimester of pregnancy: a study from a tertiary care centre. J Pak Med Assoc. 2012;62:244–88.
16. Roth MM, Cristodor P, Kroumpouzos G. Prurigo, pruritic folliculitis, and atopic eruption of pregnancy: facts and controversies. Clin Dermatol. 2016;34:392–400.
17. Wolf Y, Groutz A, Walman I. Impetigo herpetiformis during pregnancy: case report and review of the literature. Acta Obstet Gynecol Scand. 1995;74:229–32.
18. Kondo RN, Araújo FM, Pereira AM. Pustular psoriasis of pregnancy (impetigo herpetiformis)-case report. An Bras Dermatol. 2013;88(suppl 1):186–9.
19. Gao QQ, Xi MR, Yao Q. Impetigo herpetiformis during pregnancy: a case report and literature review. Dermatology. 2013;226:35–40.
20. Mervic L. Management of moderate to severe plaque psoriasis in pregnancy and lactation in the era of biologics. Acta Dermatovenerol Alp Pannonica Adriat. 2014;23:27–31.
21. Alsenaid A, Prinz JC. Inadvertent pregnancy during ustekinumab therapy in a patient with plaque psoriasis and impetigo herpetiformis. J Eur Acad Dermatol Venereol. 2016;30:488–90.
22. Müllegger RR, Häring NS, Glatz M. Skin infections in pregnancy. Clin Dermatol. 2016;34:368–77.
23. Shrim A, Koren G, Yudin MH, et al. Management of varicella infection (chickenpox) in pregnancy. J Obstet Gynaecol Can. 2012; 34:287–92.
24. Sauerbrei A, Wutzler P. Herpes simplex and varicella-zoster virus infections during pregnancy: current concepts of prevention, diagnosis and therapy. Part 1: herpes simplex virus infections. Med Microbiol Immunol. 2007;196:89–94.
25. Drago F, Broccolo F, Zaccaria E, et al. Pregnancy outcome in patients with pityriasis rosea. J Am Acad Dermatol. 2008; 58(suppl 1):S78–83.
26. Chi CC, Wang SH, Wojnarowska F, et al. Safety of topical corticosteroids in pregnancy. Cochrane Database Syst Rev. 2015;(10):CD007346.
27. Schatz M. H1-antihistamines in pregnancy and lactation. Clin Allergy Immunol. 2002;17:421–36.
28. Maipas S, Nicolopoulou-Stamati P. Sun lotion chemicals as endocrine disruptors. Hormones (Athens). 2015;14:32–46.

Use and Misuse of Cosmeceuticals and Cosmetic Procedures in Pigmented Ethnic Skin

44

Medhat Abdelmalek

Incidence, clinical presentation, and treatment of skin disorders show prominent differences in individuals with pigmented ethnic skin compared to Caucasians with white skin. This is primarily due to decisive differences in the cutaneous structure and function of the skin and hair. For example, the use of pore-clogging substances by Caucasians may result in predominant clinical inflammation with papules and pustules that develop over a period of 2–3 weeks. On the other hand, non-Caucasian skin responds by rupturing the follicular wall early in the process [1]. Moreover, patients with pigmented or black skin have unique cosmetic concerns and necessitate particular consideration when it comes to apply cosmeceuticals and/or receive aesthetic procedures, such as laser and chemical peels. Ethnic skin individuals are easily susceptible to trauma which can lead to permanent pigmentary changes. Recent advances in this area resulted in the development of safer technologies and products.

There is an increased demand in the number of patients requesting cosmetic procedures to attain even skin color, reduce the signs of aging, and remove unwanted hair [2]. Dermatologists are required to administer cosmeceuticals in their biologically active form to the skin and ensure the use of sufficient amounts of the appropriate agent in order to obtain desirable effects.

44.1 The Pigmented Ethnic Skin

Pigmented ethnic skin is considered to be more prone to irritation from topical agents as compared to Caucasian skin. This is due to a less skin barrier strength and higher level of skin sensitivity compared to other skin types.

Studies showed that most common skin conditions in ethnic skin populations are acne vulgaris, hypertrophic scars, keloid, melasma, and other pigmentary disorders. It has been observed that the large number and the labile response of cutaneous melanocytes make pigmented skin prone to disfiguring pigmentary changes. Hence, dermatologists have the responsibility to discuss best treatment options and related cosmetic complications, such as post-inflammatory pigment alterations [3].

UV and long-wave visible light induce pigmentation in skin types IV and VI [4]. Therefore, it is crucial to spot the light on the importance of using sunscreens to shield against ultraviolet exposure [5]. Unfortunately, a considerable number of people in the Middle East are not aware of the importance of applying sunscreens to protect their skin from sun-induced damage.

Acquired hyperpigmentations affect different skin types. However, pigmentary lesions are more noticeable in pigmented ethnic skin and more resistant to treatment; management is still challenging (Fig. 44.1). Hyperpigmentation treatment in ethnic skin could be supported by using sunscreens, chemical peels, and microdermabrasion, together with topical melanocytotoxic agents and tyrosinase inhibitors [2].

Several patients may insist on the use of lasers and chemical peels. However, this may worsen their condition (Fig. 44.2). Therefore, it is the responsibility of the physician to explain that many dermatologic conditions take time to improve or fully resolve. For example, patients suffering from melasma should understand that their condition is recurrent chronic, difficult to treat and manage. It is also important to clarify that the use of sun protection with broad spectrum sunscreens is the mainstay of management [6].

Furthermore, the manifestation of photoaging is less severe in pigmented ethnic skin and starts to appear 10–20 years later compared to white Caucasian skin, as compared in aged-matched groups [2]. In fact, research showed that the major manifestation of photoaging in ethnic skin is associated with pigmentary changes; The higher melanin content provides long-term photo protection. Also, the aging pattern of ethnic skin presents fewer wrinkles compared to white skin individuals [7].

M. Abdelmalek, MD
Consultant Dermatologist and Venereologist,
Amman, Jordan

C. E. Orfanos et al. (eds.), *Pigmented Ethnic Skin and Imported Dermatoses*, https://doi.org/10.1007/978-3-319-69422-1_44

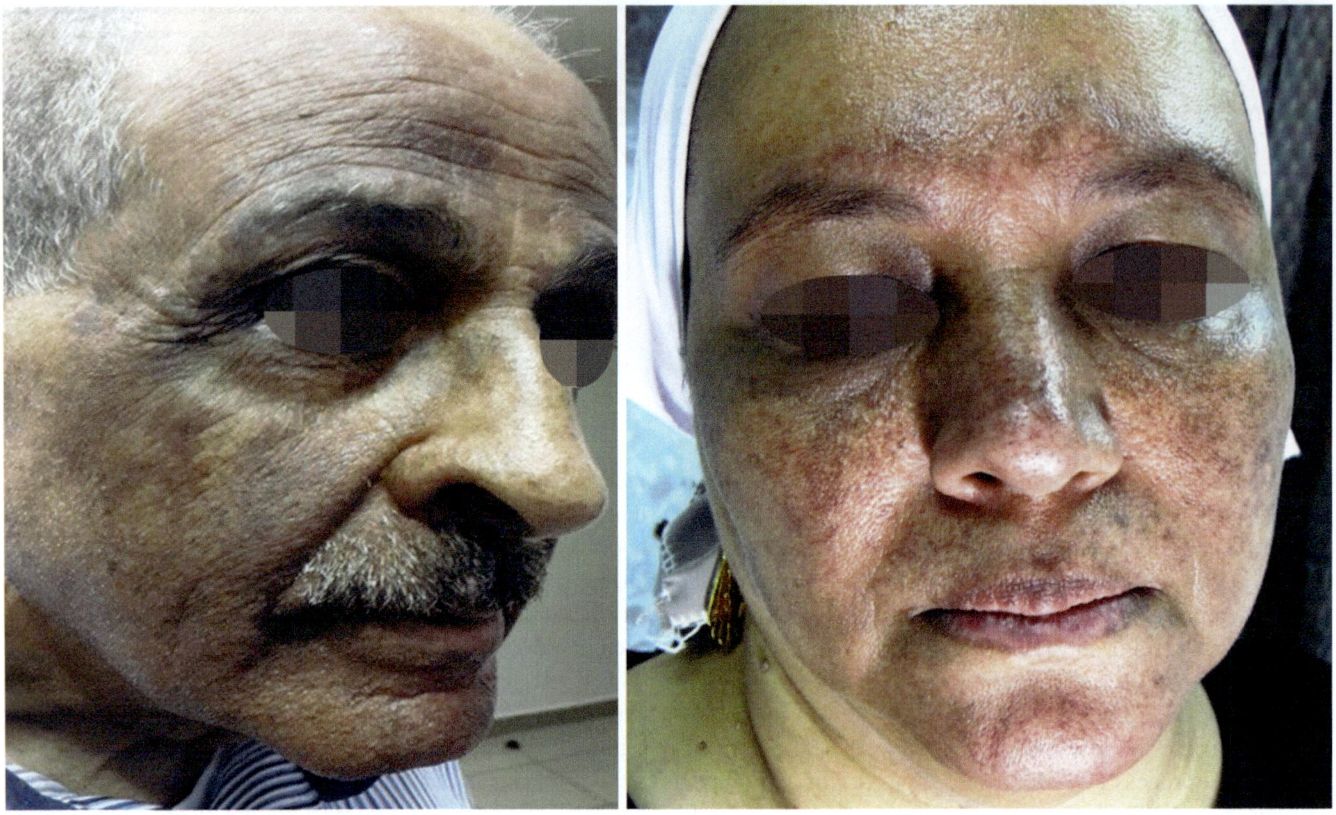

Fig. 44.1 Left: Grayish hyperpigmentation of the face after chronic sun exposure. DD: *lichen pigmentosus*. Right: *periorbital melanosis* with spotted facial hyperpigmentations, sun-induced

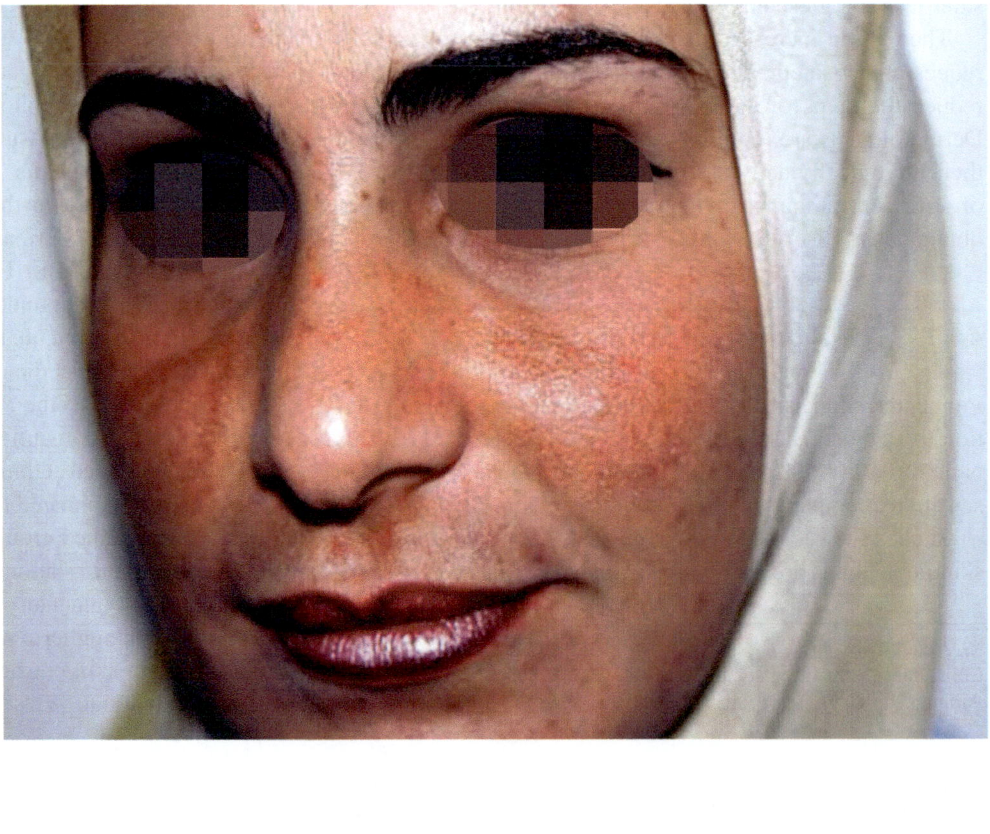

Fig. 44.2 *Melasma* induced by intense pulsed light laser

44.2 Cosmeceutical Products and Procedures

44.2.1 Facial Cleansers

Facial cleansers are used in combination with other dermatocosmetics as a part of skin care regimens to clear the skin from dirt, bacteria, dead skin, makeup, etc. Acne patients are recommended to use lipid-free cleansers, exfoliants, synthetic detergents (syndets) and astringents. It has been observed that using facial cleansers twice a day reduces the level of inflammatory and non-inflammatory lesions. Scrubs are useful to exfoliate skin; however, they might be not beneficial for patients with sensitive skin susceptible to develop toxic or allergic contact dermatitis. We recommend mild, nonabrasive, and alcohol-free cleansers with neutral or slightly acidic pH. Some of these agents may contain low concentrations of salicylic acid or benzoyl peroxide [8].

44.2.2 Dermatocosmetics for Acne: Moisturizers and Corneolytics/Comedolytics

Most dermatocosmetics for acne are composed of components that particularly target the inflammatory process, seborrhea, uneven skin texture, and photoaging. Dermatologists who treat acne in patients with pigmented ethnic skin must consider the high risk for developing post-inflammatory hyperpigmentation (Fig. 44.3) and keloidal scarring. This imposes more challenge to take all measures to limit possible cutaneous injury [9]. Moisturizers for acne have to be compatible with treatment regimens. It is important to prescribe moisturizers that are noncomedogenic, non-acnegenic, non-irritating, and hypoallergenic. Patients are usually recommended to apply moisturizers before other topical agents to reduce the stinging and drying effect of acne treatments [8]. Multiple studies on ethnic skin patients showed that topical corneolytics are beneficial and safe for the treatment of post-inflammatory changes, active lesions, and acne scars. However, there is still lacking evidence on the effect of cosmeceuticals containing corneolytics in different Asian skin types [8].

44.2.3 Fillers

Fillers are considered to be an option targeting overall enhancement and rejuvenation [10]. It is an effective method for augmenting soft tissue redistribution and reducing volume loss. The thinning of collagen bundles and elastic tissue is less in individuals with pigmented ethnic skin than in Caucasian skin. This makes the efficacy of fillers that stimulate collagen production more effective for the non-Caucasian population.

Several types of fillers can be used alone or in combination [11]. The most common is hyaluronic acid which rarely causes hypersensitivity reactions and has better longevity than collagen fillers. Superficial fillers are used for the treatment of fine wrinkles; deep fillers are injected for the treatment of deep grooves. Shetty [10] showed that in Indians fillers administered on the outer zones of the face rather than on the inner zone give better aesthetic results. However, it has been observed that hyaluronic acid may accumulate over repeated sessions. Possible complications are bruising, inflammation, tenderness, pruritus, pain, granulomas, infection, hypersensitivity reactions, and skin necrosis.

Ethnic skin is more likely to develop erythema after filler injection compared to Caucasian skin. This can be minimized by the number of skin punctures, using fanning techniques or linear threading. Filler migration from injection sites and filler misplacement may also occur [12].

44.2.4 Botulinum Toxin

Botulinum toxin A is commonly used as a minimal invasive aesthetic procedure for improving glabellar rhytides, eyebrow elevation, horizontal forehead lines, and asymmetry. Many studies confirmed its efficacy and safety in pigmented skin individuals. Some mild to transient undesired effects have been also reported. This includes local local bruising, local swelling, headache [13], flu-like symptoms, and migration of botulinum toxin from the injection site leading to inappropriate muscle paralysis. This may cause eyelid ptosis, brow ptosis, and ectropion [13]. It is pivotal to educate clinicians on the proper patient selection, appropriate injection techniques, and possible side effects.

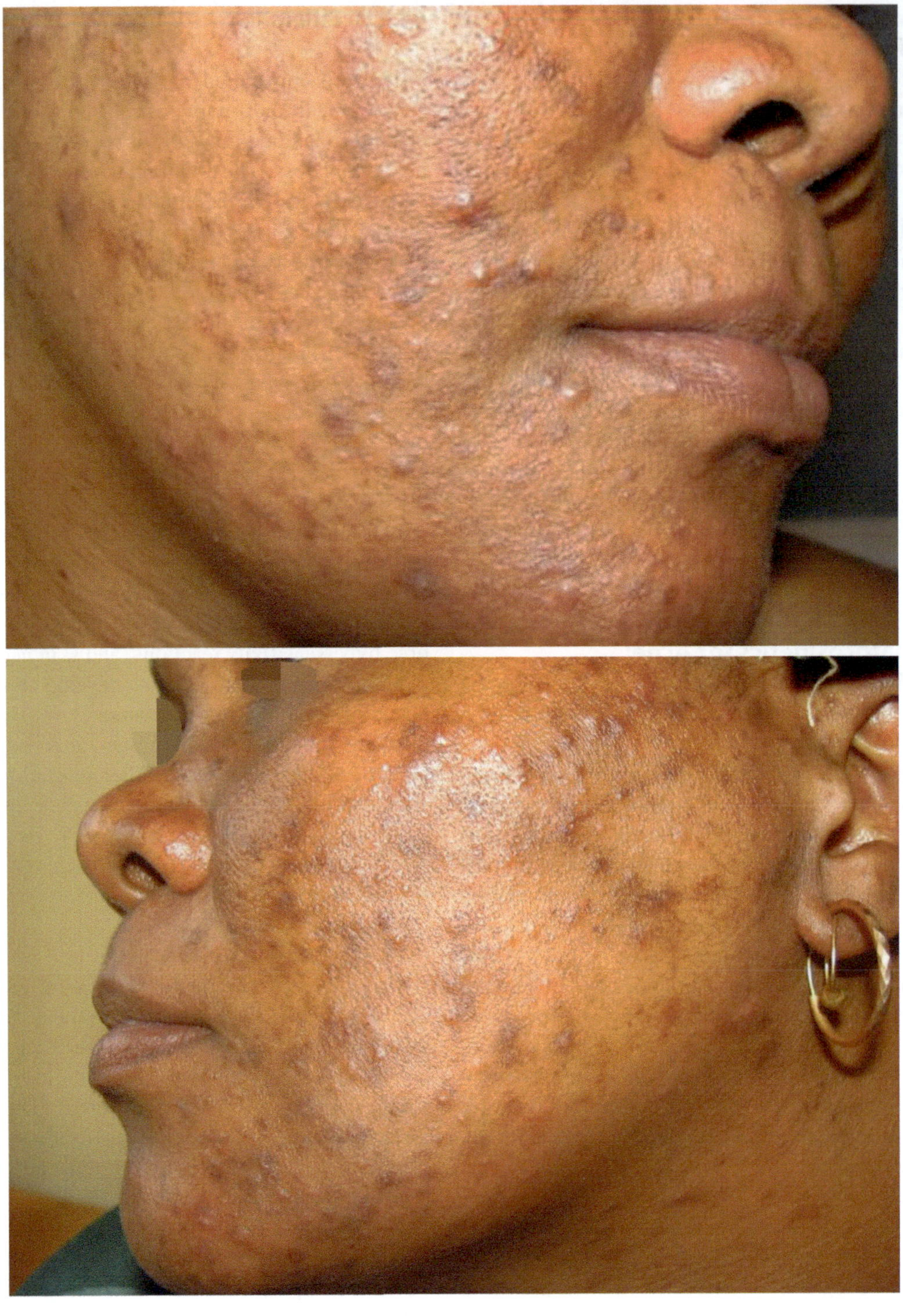

Fig. 44.3 *Acne* in pigmented ethnic skin. Note persisting spotted hyperpigmentations

44.2.5 Lipolysis

Lipolysis with energy-based devices is a new, effective, and safe body contouring technique. It avoids epidermal melanin induction as a result of its deep penetration. High-intensity focused ultrasound (HIFU) is also used to percutaneously disrupt adipocytes. This method does not cause skin damage because the ultrasound energy intensity applied at the skin surface is low; pigmentary changes are not likely to occur. These techniques may be efficacious in reducing the level of unwanted fat in pigmented skin patients; however, more research is needed to further clarify and prove the safety profile of such novel technologies [2].

44.2.6 Lasers

There is an increasing demand for lasers, light, and energy-based procedures among the non-Caucasian populations. Available cosmetic procedures with lasers include skin tightening, hair removal, lipolysis, and procedures with nonabrasive lasers [2]. Special consideration is required when treating ethnic skin patients with such procedures because any significant trauma may result in temporary or permanent scarring and/or pigmentary changes. One should stress on the importance of applying sunscreens to minimize the risk and prevent the recurrence of post-inflammatory hyperpigmentation. A study on Korean volunteers with skin types II–IV using bipolar radiofrequency combined with diode laser or infrared light for skin rejuvenation showed that both methods are effective and safe for treating facial wrinkles and skin laxity [14]. Radiofrequency is an effective method to induce dermal heating, collagen denaturation, and collagen remodeling; it is frequently used to improve skin laxity appearance [15].

44.3 Common Complications with Laser Techniques

Hair removal: Highest risk tends to occur in pigmented ethnic skin when using intense pulsed light (IPL) and Alexandrite laser. IPL is considered to be the least desired hair removal method for pigmented skin patients; the energies required are risky technologies [2]. Modified light and heat energy systems may lead to erythema, dyschromias, and posttreatment burn with crusting. Some patients may also develop persistent hypopigmentation and paradoxical hypertrichosis. Complications associated with super long-pulsed 810 nm diode laser on pigmented skin patients includes erythema, purpura, epidermal whitening, blistering, hyper- and hypopigmentation, Nikolsky sign, and pain [16]. It seems that the use of Nd:YAG laser may be the safest option for hair removal in pigmented skin.

Treatment of melasma: The response of melasma to lasers in patients with pigmented ethnic skin is variable. Frequent complications include lack of response, dyschromias, and recurrences. In addition, melasma-like hyperpigmentations may be induced by IPL (Fig. 44.3). This modality should be used with caution for skin type IV and be avoided for skin types V and VI.

Removal of tattoos: Several wavelengths may be used to remove multiple tattoo pigments. The high content of epidermal melanin in pigmented skin and its ability to absorb laser energy makes tattoo removal a challenging process. It is recommended to apply minimum fluence techniques since high fluences may cause pinpoint bleeding, tissue splattering, transient hyperpigmentation, permanent hypopigmentation, and scarring. Caution is necessary when using Q-switched Nd:YAG for tattoo removal in pigmented skin individuals [2].

Removal of vascular lesions: For treating port-wine stains, facial telangiectasias, and haemangiomas, 585 nm PDL is considered to be the most effective and safe laser technique. In patients with pigmented skin, dyschromias may occur; the risk could be reduced by using skin-cooling techniques [17].

Treatment of acne: Acne scars are often seen in pigmented skin individuals. In Asian countries, ablative lasers are commonly used for treatment of post-acne scars. Complications associated with ablative laser resurfacing on pigmented skin include erythema, post-inflammatory hyperpigmentation, persistent hypopigmentation, secondary bacterial and herpes simplex infection, and scarring. In a study from Singapore, the authors concluded that post-inflammatory hyperpigmentation from laser resurfacing in an ethnic skin population is not as common as expected. However, dyspigmentations may be severe in individuals that are already affected. Laser-induced hyperpigmentations gradually disappear 6–12 months after treatment [6].

44.4 Chemical Peels

Chemical peels are resurfacing techniques, used for the treatment of skin aging, photodamage, pigmentation abnormalities, and textural concerns such as enlarged pores, scarring secondary to acne, and roughness. This process results in the generation of new epidermis and dermal collagen remodel-

Table 44.1 Chemical peels

Type	Contents	Indications	Comments
Superficial light peel Target: Str. corneum, Str. spinosum	Glycolic acid (20–50%) Salicylic acid (20–30%)	Melasma and solar lentigines	Safe and effective. Occasionally transient erythema and scaling. Rarely PIH[a] may develop
Superficial deeper peel Target: All epidermal strata	TCA (10–30%)[b] Jessner's solution, 70% glycolic acid	Solar lentigines and actinic keratoses	In pigmented and black skin higher risk for developing dyschromias. Caution
Medium-depth peel Target: Upper dermis	35–40% TCA 88% phenol solid CO_2 + TCA Jessner's + 35% TCA 70% glycolic acid + 35% TCA	Moderate skin damage due to photoaging, melasma, and scars	Transient erythema and scaling. Not recommendable for skin type VI. Hydroquinone could be used for treating PIH
Deep peel Target: Middermis	Baker-Gordon phenol peel	Dermal-type melasma and severely photoaged skin	Used for skin types I–II only. Not effective for eradicating wrinkles at vermillion border. Risk of transient or prolonged erythema/scaling and prolonged hypopigmentation. Lines of demarcation may be seen

[a]*PIH* post-inflammatory hyperpigmentation
[b]*TCA* trichloroacetic acid

ing [3]. The products are classified based on the targeted skin depth (Table 44.1). Superficial peels are generally tolerated in all skin types, with mild improvement and minor side effects. If medium-depth peels are used in skin types IV and V, the risk of inducing post-peel pigmentary alterations is high. Patients are asked to apply topically hydroquinone 4% plus retinol 2×/day for 6 weeks after the chemical injury heals, or only once, also using a strong sunscreen (SPF 50) several times during the day. Deep peels are not recommended for pigmented ethnic skin due to unacceptable dyschromias. Posttreatment monitoring after peeling sessions is mandatory, a few days up to several weeks after treatment. Subsequent long-term complications could be reduced by using topical corticosteroids. Also, creams with 2–5% hydroquinone are administered by some clinicians before or after the peel to minimize the post-inflammatory hyperpigmentation risk.

44.5 Skin Bleaching Products

Bleaching products are available as cream or lotion-based formulations to be applied 1–2×/day to lighten the skin color. Hydroquinone-based products frequently in concentrations above 5% are administered together with potent corticosteroids (0.05% clobetasol propionate). Their long-term use may cause steroid-induced acne (Fig. 44.4). A combination of hydroquinone 4%, tretinoin 0.05%, and fluocinolone 0.01% is recommended. Mercurial compounds, salicylic acid preparation, and lemon juice are also in use [18]. The phototoxic effect of hydroquinone may lead to periorbital hyperpigmentation, whereas its long-term use may result in *exogenous ochronosis*, i.e., accumulation of homogentisic acid in the connective tissue caused by the topical administration of hydroquinone and other phenol complexes. The condition is clinically characterized by discolorations presented in malar areas, chin, upper limb, upper back, and neck reversible after withdrawing the compound (Fig. 44.5). Other side effects include irritant or allergic contact dermatitis, cutaneous squamous cell carcinomas, and cutaneous neoplasms. Long-term use of mercurial products may induce glomerulonephritis and neurological disorders. The long-term side effects of corticosteroids are well known, topical, and systemic. Physicians are urged to encourage their patients to stop using skin lightening products; the desire to minimize skin pigmentation, however, is still dominating people's perspective on beauty.

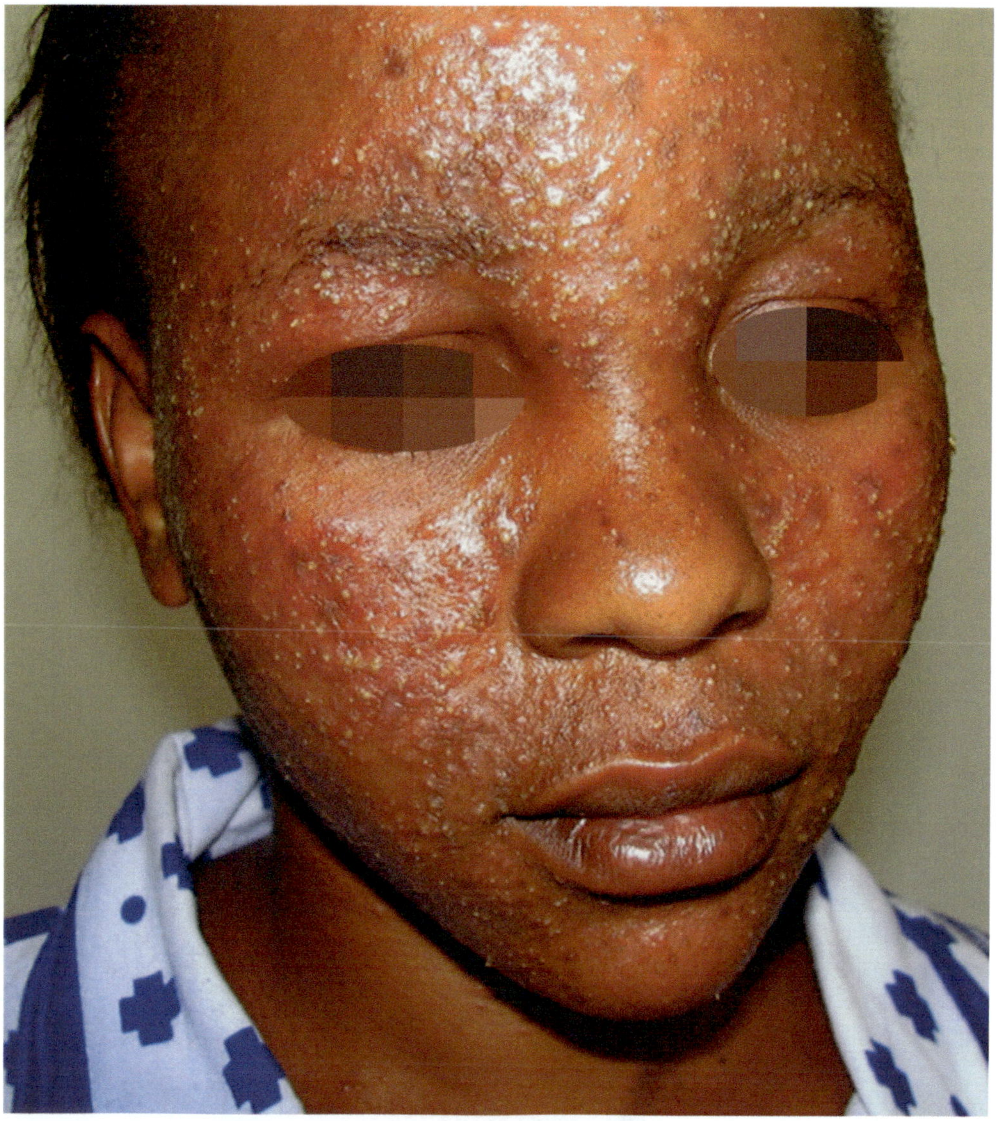

Fig. 44.4 *Steroid-induced acne* after repeated use of potent fluorinated corticosteroids for skin bleaching

Conclusions

Pigmented ethnic skin varies in tone and texture and responds differently to dermatocosmetics. This should be considered before prescribing products to patients. In addition, it is pivotal to educate the patients on their use. This will allow dark-skinned individuals to benefit from the offered cosmetic procedures while minimizing any side effects. For reducing the high risk of dyspigmentation, which is a major concern among most ethnic skin populations, it is important to raise awareness and stress on the importance of applying sunscreens on a daily basis.

Features of skin aging are displayed in Caucasian skin differently compared to those in non-Caucasian skin. Ethnic skin shows intrinsic facial aging, whereas white skin primarily shows extrinsic changes. Common cosmetic procedures can be used in both; nevertheless, the differences in skin types and aging patterns should be recognized and considered before deciding on the procedure to follow. More aggressive techniques such as chemical peeling and laser resurfacing are clearly beneficial to patients. However, it is necessary that physicians consider the high risk of dyschromias in pigmented ethnic skin.

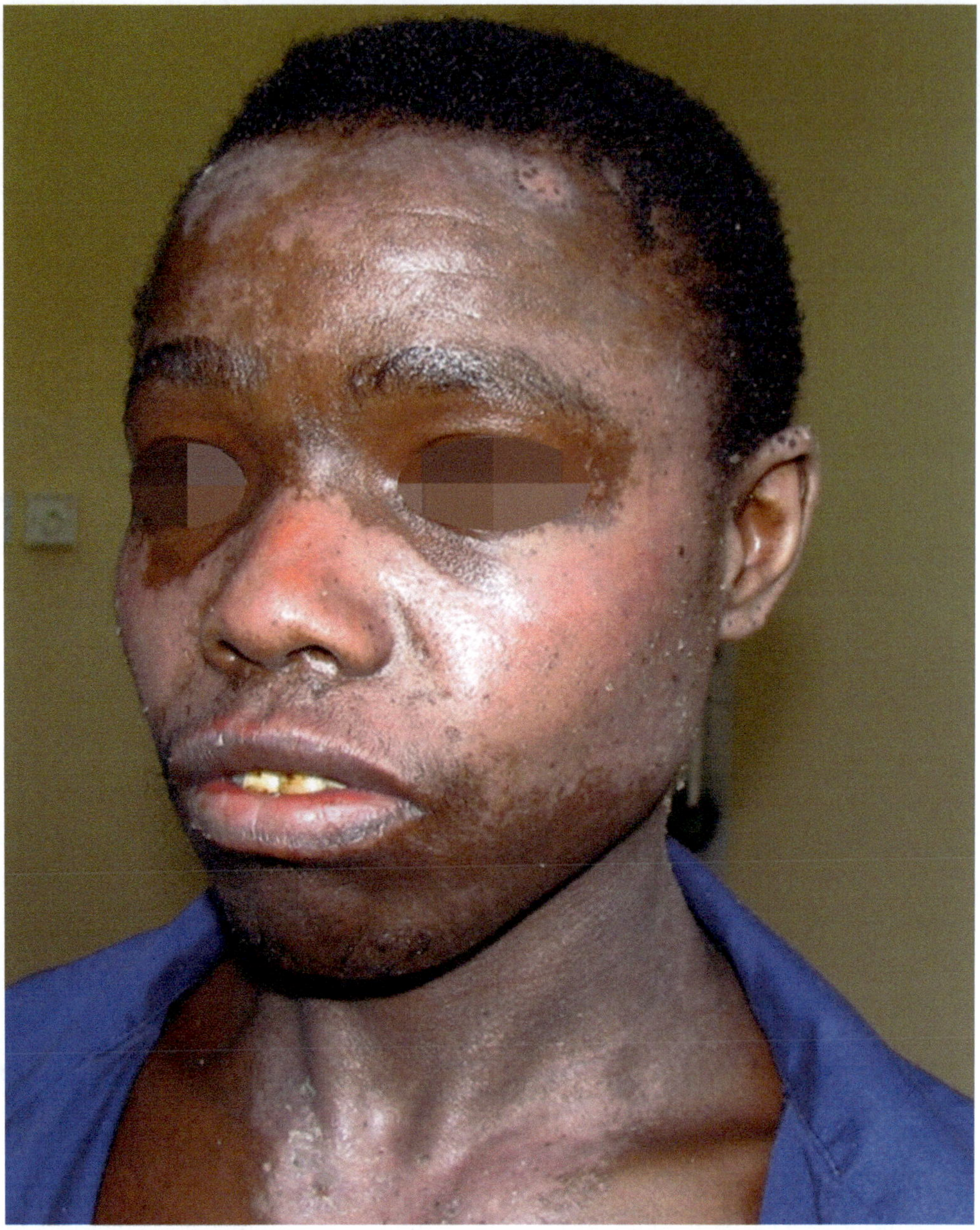

Fig. 44.5 H*ydroquinone-induced discoloration* of face and neck with periocular hyperpigmentation due to uncontrolled topical application of bleaching preparations. DD: *Exogenous ochronosis* (Photo: CEO)

References

1. Draelos ZD. Cosmeceuticals. Philadelphia: Elsevier; 2005.
2. Woolery-Lloyd H, Kammer J. Overview of cosmetic concerns in skin of color. In: Alexis A, Barbosa V, editors. Skin of color: a practical guide to dermatologic diagnosis and treatment. New York: Springer; 2013. p. 221–36.
3. Ferguson L, Rossi A, Alexis A, et al. Cosmetic dermatology in ethnic skin. In: Dadzie OE, Petit A, Alexis A, editors. Ethnic dermatology: principles and practice. Chichester: Wiley; 2013. p. 273–86.
4. Mahmoud B, Hexsel C, Hamzavi I, et al. Effects of visible light on the skin. Photochem Photobiol. 2008;84:450–62.
5. Grimes P. Management of hyperpigmentation in darker racial ethnic groups. Semin Cutan Med Surg. 2009;28:77–85.
6. Tay Y. Treatment of pigmented lesions in the Asian skin. In: Tay YK, Chan YC, editors. Textbook of laser and light dermatology in the Asian skin. Singapore: World Scientific Publishing; 2011. p. 37–58.
7. Vashi N, Maymone M, Kundu R. Aging differences in ethnic skin. J Clin Aesthet Dermatol. 2016;9:31–8.
8. Goh C, Noppakun N, Micali G, et al. Meeting the challenges of acne treatment in Asian patients: a review on the role of dermocosmetics as adjunctive therapy. J Cutan Aesthet Surg. 2016;9:85–92.
9. Shah S, Alexis A. Acne and rosacea in skin of color. In: Alexis A, Barbosa V, editors. Skin of color: a practical guide to dermatologic diagnosis and treatment. New York: Springer; 2012. p. 21–36.
10. Shetty R. Outer circle versus inner circle: special considerations while rejuvenating an Indian face using fillers. J Cutan Aesthet Surg. 2015;8:169–72.
11. Burgees C. Fillers in ethnic skin. In: Alexis A, Barbosa V, editors. Skin of color: a practical guide to dermatologic diagnosis and treatment. New York: Springer; 2012. p. 247–62.
12. Abduljabbar M, Basendwh MA. Complications of hyaluronic acid fillers and there managements. J Dermatol Dermatol Surg. 2016;20:100–6.

13. Small R. Botulinum toxin injection for facial wrinkles. Am Fam Physician. 2014;90:168–75.
14. Choi Y, Lee J, Ahn J. The safety and efficacy of a combined diode laser and bipolar radiofrequency compared with combined infrared light and bipolar radiofrequency for skin rejuvenation. Indian J Dermatol Venereol Leprol. 2012;78:146–52.
15. Gold M. The increasing use of nonablative radiofrequency in the rejuvenation of the skin. Exp Rev Dermatol. 2011;6:139–43.
16. Rogachefsky A, Silapunt S, Goldberg J. Evaluation of a new super-long pulsed 810 NM diode laser for the removal of unwanted hair: the concept of thermal damage time. Dermatol Surg. 2002;28:410–4.
17. Chiu C, Chan H, Ho W. Prospective study of pulsed dye laser in conjunction with cryogen spray cooling for treatment of port-wine stains in Chinese patients. Dermatol Surg. 2003;29:909–15.
18. Mahe A. Cosmetic use of skin lightning products. In: Dadzie OE, Petit A, Alexis AF, editors. Ethnic dermatology: principles and practice. Chichester: Wiley; 2012. p. 287–92.

Steroid-Modified Dermatophytosis: A Potential Epidemic in Developing Countries

45

Shyam B. Verma and Anupam Das

Superficial dermatophytoses constitute a large proportion of skin diseases seen by dermatologists in tropical countries. Their prevalence in hot climate zones has always been high since hot and humid weather favors their acquisition and perpetuation. However, in the Indian subcontinent superficial dermatophytoses have become infamous for being the commonest infective dermatosis.

Especially *tinea corporis* and *tinea cruris* show a hyperendemic or epidemic distribution [1] and have attained the status of a public health problem with confusing presentation and often unpredictable outcome [2].

45.1 Pathogenetic Considerations

The large majority of dermatophytoses is caused by *Trichophyton (T.) rubrum* [3]. Widespread cases have been often described as *T. rubrum syndrome* or *tinea corporis generalisata* characterized by involvement of at least four body sites such as the feet, hands, nails, as well as another site with the exclusion of the inguinal area [4]. These patients have a *T. rubrum*-related functional deficiency of phagocytosis; *T. rubrum* escapes the immune system of the host as a spore till it finds a warm and moist area of skin, where it starts colonizing [5]. The arthroconidia adhere to the keratinocytes and invade the epidermis, penetrate the epidermal layers, and grow further; arthroconidia germinate to produce radially expanding hyphae [6]. The penetration of the stratum corneum is aided by fungal proteases, which allows rapid expansion of the fungus. The clearance of the organism largely depends on host cell-mediated immunity (CMI) and is Th1-/Th17-dependent [7]. Acute dermatophytosis is associated with Th1 response, whereas cases of chronic dermatophytosis are related to Th2 response with high levels of IgE and IgG4 antibodies. Individuals with defective tilt of immunity toward Th2 cytokines are likely to be more predisposed to chronic dermatophytic infection. However, the exact mechanism involved in this defective shift of immunity and selective absence of CMI with respect to dermatophytosis is still poorly understood. In patients with chronic dermatophytosis, defective phagocytosis of the fungal hyphae has been observed. Mannans produced by *T. rubrum* work by inhibiting the critical steps in antigen processing and presentation. The free radicals and nitric oxide release have been found to be 20–30% lower than that of controls in patients of chronic dermatophytosis, indicating a defective killing mechanism as well. The downregulation of toll-like receptor 4 by *T. rubrum* further decreases the inflammatory response by decreasing pro-inflammatory cytokine production and recruitment of neutrophils [8]. The combination of ineffective phagocytosis of the hyphae in the presence of an anti-inflammatory milieu leads to chronicity. This may also explain why the lesions keep spreading centrifugally as expected but do not clear in the center. The erratic application may switch on and switch off the inflammation induced by the causative agent and lead to partial clearance, bizarre shapes such as *tinea pseudoimbricata* and eczematous areas within the lesions. This is further aggravated in patients with immunocompromised status and diabetes mellitus and in those receiving systemic corticosteroids. The chronicity of recurrent cases could be attributed to host, agent, environmental, or pharmacological factors.

45.2 Steroid-Modified Dermatophytosis

Recently, iatrogenically perpetuated, *steroid-modified dermatophytosis* has emerged as a bothersome entity, showing an altered morphological picture and course. The factors

S. B. Verma, M.B.B.S., D.V.D., F.A.A.D., F.R.C.P. (✉)
Nirvana Skin Clinic, Vadodara, Gujarat, India

A. Das
Department of Dermatology, KPC Medical College and Hospital, Kolkata, West Bengal, India

C. E. Orfanos et al. (eds.), *Pigmented Ethnic Skin and Imported Dermatoses*, https://doi.org/10.1007/978-3-319-69422-1_45

which have led to their development include erratic use of topical and oral antifungal drugs, rising prevalence of inflammatory dermatophytoses caused by *T. mentagrophytes*, growing resistance to antifungal drugs, and, most importantly, the menace of using creams containing a steroid, antifungal, and antibacterial compound, often with three to five molecules in the product [1, 9, 10]. Topical antifungal drugs are often applied combined with potent molecules such as clobetasol propionate available as over-the-counter medications and are grossly abused. Patients may buy these formulations and apply them for weeks, months, or even years [9–14].

In developing countries, pharmaceutical companies may employ various means to overcome laws that prevent manufacture and sale of topical steroid-containing creams with antifungals and antibacterials. The drug regulatory authorities seem to be in a slumber as far as permissions to manufacture and sell such formulations are concerned. Permissions are given to ludicrous combinations that defy science and logic. Licenses to manufacture and market these products in developing countries may be obtained in the absence of sufficient safety or efficacy data [9, 10].

45.3 Clinical Presentation

Topical application of potent corticosteroids, alone or together with antifungals, often leads to a wide array of variations in the morphological patterns of dermatophytoses. A series of clinical presentations have been observed to occur in patients after applying creams containing topical steroids erratically:

(a) Appearance of *Tinea pseudoimbricata* characterized by multiple concentric rings or "rings within rings" occurring in patients with immune suppression and those receiving systemic corticosteroids leading to partial clearance of the fungus with waxing and waning of inflammation within the lesions (Fig. 45.1); the concentric rings found in *Tinea imbricata* due to *T. concentricum* are not always seen [15–17]. Some lesions show pustular borders or pustular lesions, attributed to an increased virulence of the organism or increased inflammatory response.
(b) Large-sized, multiple lesions in more than one anatomical location, often with absence of central clearing and eczematization of the center; arciform types and dumbbell-shaped tinea are seen (Fig. 45.2).
(c) Hardly recognizable tinea faciei occurs (Fig. 45.3); almost all patients have a coexisting tinea corporis and/or cruris. This is often accompanied by the involvement of the auricular pinna of the affected side, being referred to as "ear sign" [18].
(d) Increasing number of inflammatory tinea with pustules, also in females and obese children due to overcrowding and sharing of bed linen and towels (Fig. 45.4).
(e) Cases of genital tinea are often seen; they are more common in males and more on the penis rather than the scrotum, with classic active borders on the penis shaft (Figs. 45.5 and 45.6); ill-defined scaly lesions and powdery scaling are also encountered [12].
(f) Erythrodermic variants of tinea corporis may arise characterized by widespread involvement of the body surface with variable erythema and profuse scaling.

All steroid-modified tinea is accompanied by the presence of cutaneous side effects of application of topical corticosteroids like atrophy, striae, dyspigmentation, and telangiectasias.

45.4 Management

The therapeutic options found to give good clinical outcomes in such cases are itraconazole 200 mg/day for 3–4 weeks or fluconazole 150 mg thrice weekly for 8 weeks. Griseofulvin 500 mg 2×/day for 6 weeks is also effective. In contrast, topical antifungals like clotrimazole and miconazole were found ineffective. Newer azoles, such as eberconazole and sertaconazole, with documented anti-inflammatory effects are popular in India. Luliconazole and amorolfine have also emerged as excellent options. However, the most important strategy in combating this challenge lies in proper counseling of the patients regarding the perils of using triple and quadruple drug combinations containing topical steroids, especially without a prescription. Scrupulously ruling out the infection in other family members is a challenging task and is identified as a significant cause for recalcitrance of the infection.

In addition, we suggest strict avoidance of any preparations containing steroids and meticulous explanation of the side effects of applying steroids stressing on the importance of regularity of medication and adherence to the prescription. The topicals should be applied 2 cm beyond the margin of the lesion for at least 2 weeks beyond clinical resolution. We advise our patients against wearing tight clothing promoting the use of loose, cotton garments. We discourage sharing of bed linen, towels, and clothes and taking regular showers and recommend wearing clothes only after thoroughly drying the body and washing the clothes and bed linen in hot water and then sunning them; infected clothes should be washed separately. The patients with tinea cruris should preferably wear "boxer shorts" instead of the tight fitting ones. We also instruct all affected families to wet mopping or vacuuming the house followed by cleaning with detergent, in order to reduce the spore load in the immediate environment.

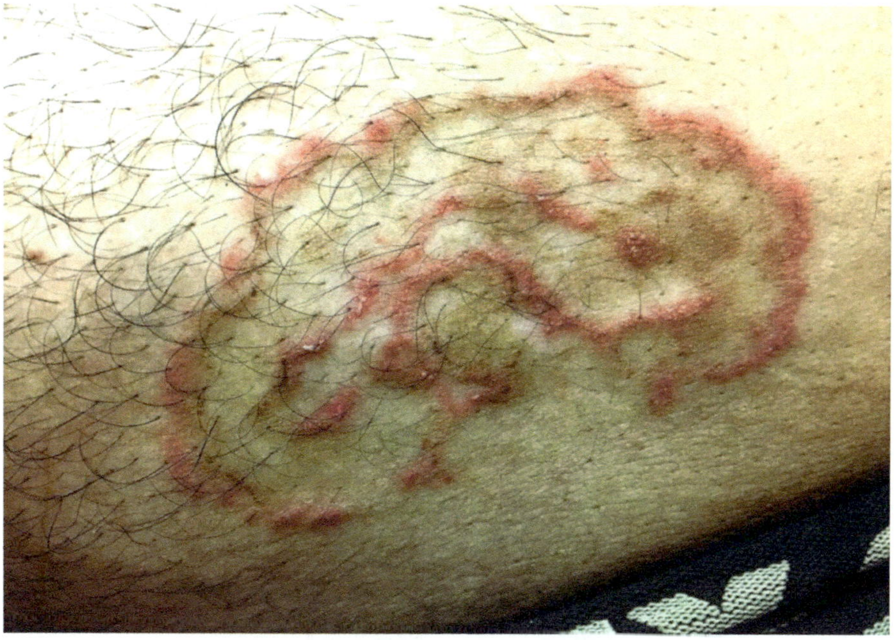

Fig. 45.1 *Tinea pseudoimbricata*, characterized by multiple concentric rings or "rings within rings"

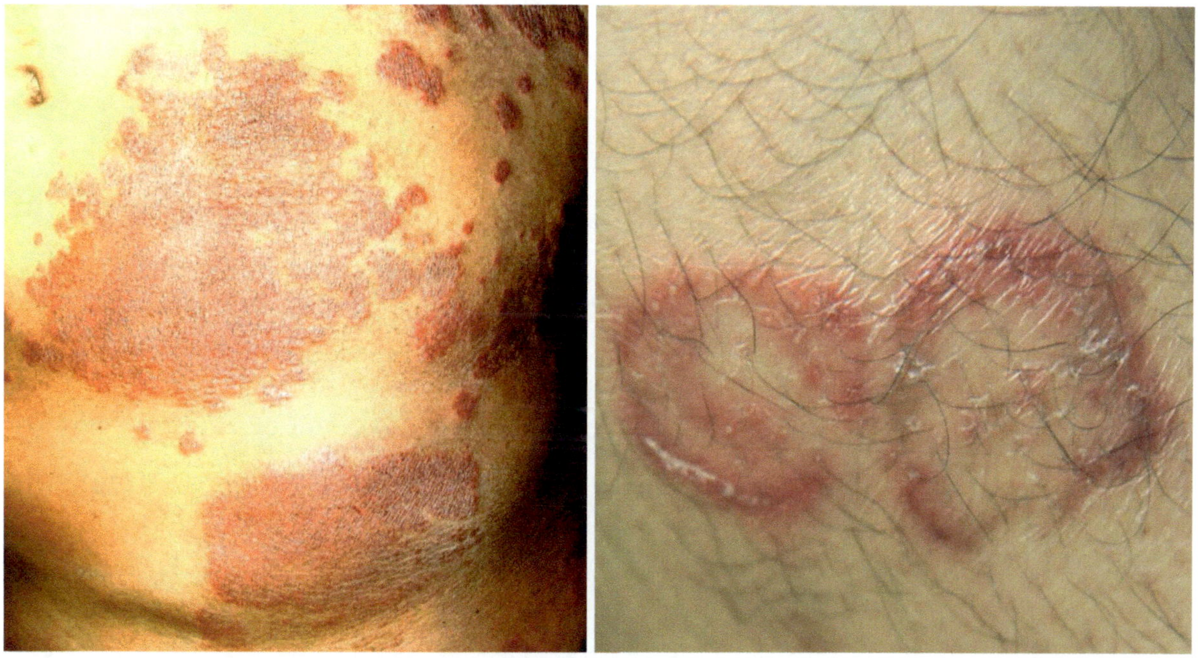

Fig. 45.2 *Steroid-modified dermatophytosis*. Absence of central clearing with eczematization of the lesions and dumbbell-shaped formation

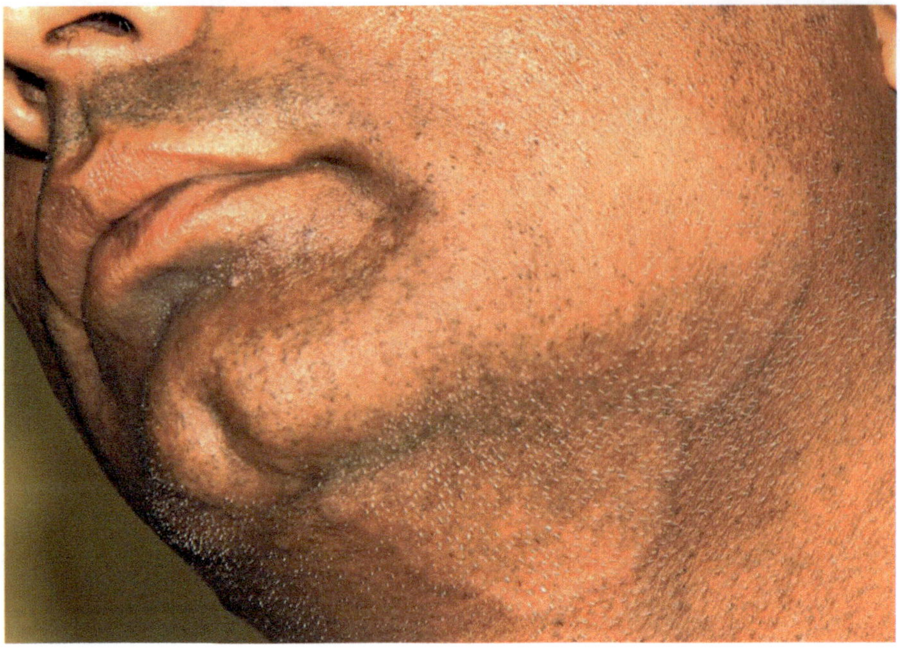

Fig. 45.3 Steroid-modified, hardly recognizable tinea faciei

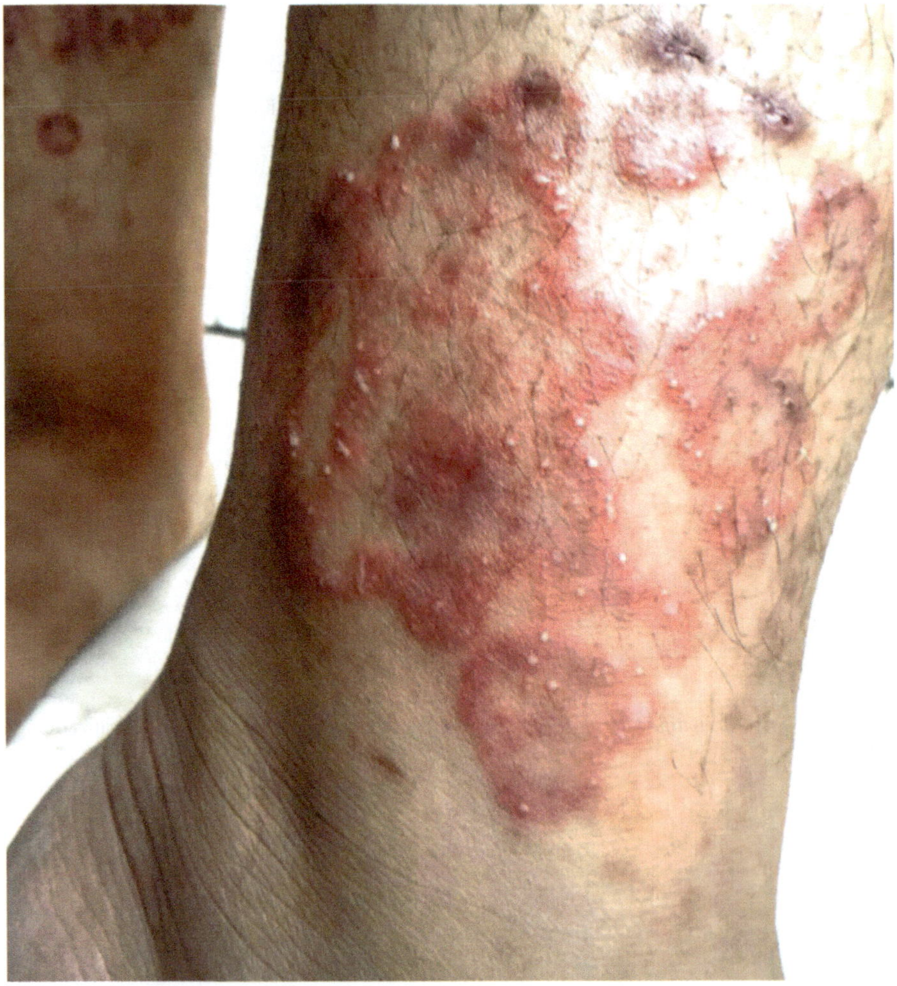

Fig. 45.4 Steroid-modified tinea with pustular borders attributed to an increased virulence of the organism or increased inflammatory response

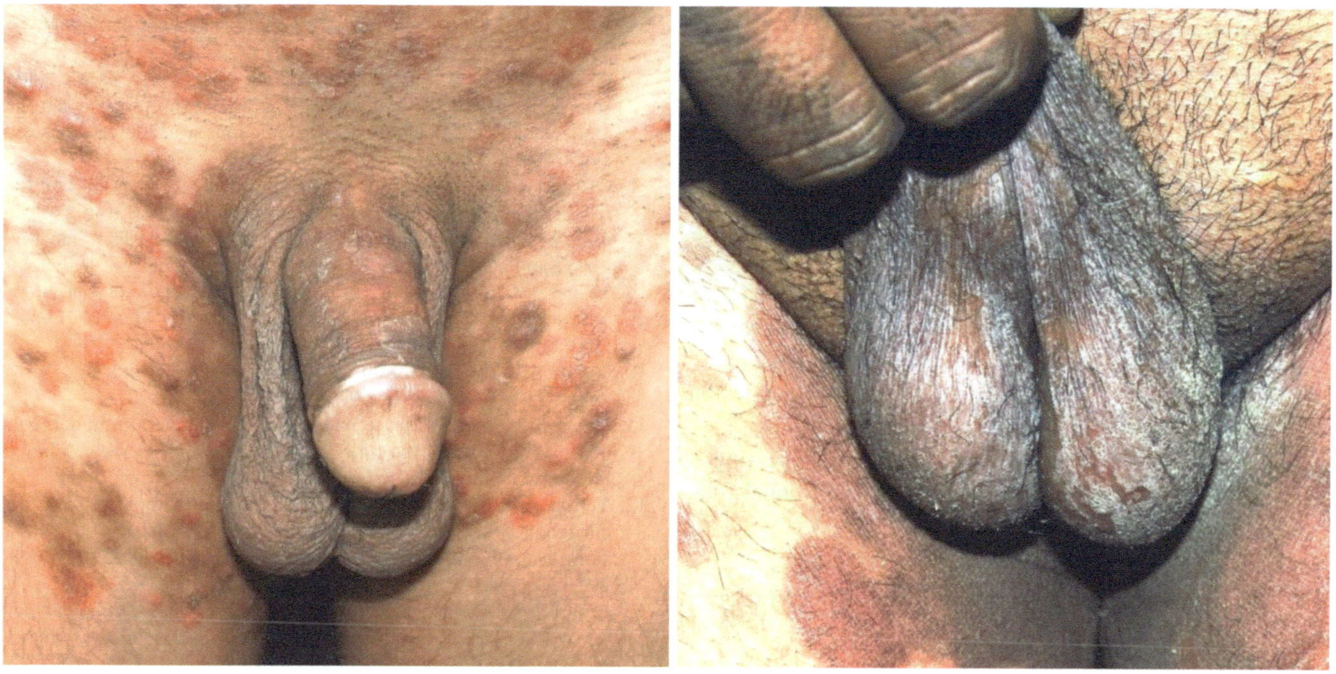

Fig. 45.5 Steroid-modified genital tinea

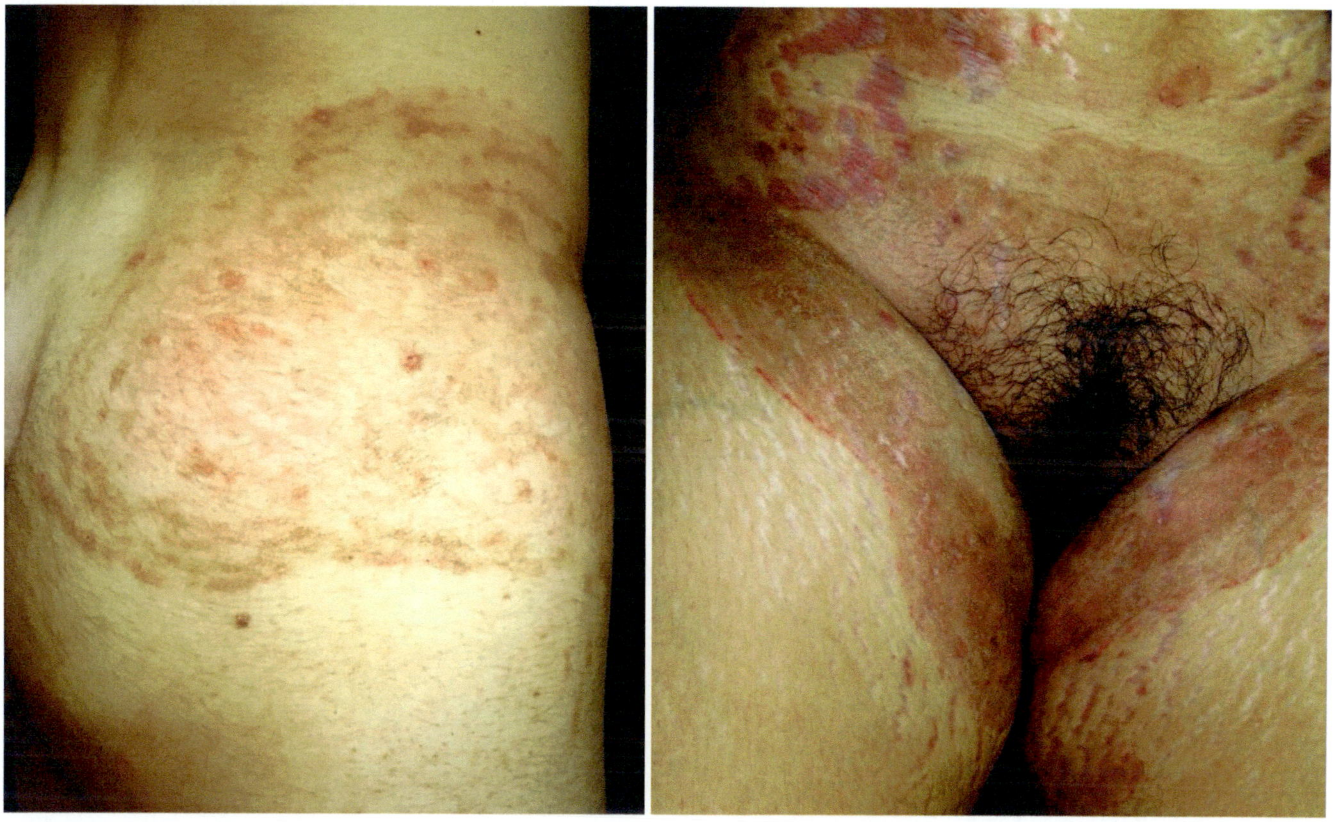

Fig. 45.6 Steroid-modified tinea corporis in females

Conclusions

Chronic dermatophytosis is a complex and vexing problem for the physician in developing countries which seems to be defying recommendations for treatment of superficial tinea; patients should discontinue the use of topical corticosteroids and be discouraged to further apply steroid-laden formulations for dermatophytosis. Well-designed studies to document the prevalence of steroid-modified tinea as well as the best possible modalities for tackling the menace are missing, and no accepted guidelines exist. Topical antifungal creams and oral antifungals need to be administered for a longer duration. The reappearance of preexisting lesions after discontinuing any oral or topical management, the so-called breakthrough lesions or even lesions appearing de novo in other areas despite an ongoing antifungal treatment, complicates the management.

References

1. Verma S, Madhu R. The great Indian epidemic of superficial dermatophytosis: an appraisal. Indian J Dermatol. 2017;62:227–36.
2. Verma S. Topical corticosteroid modified superficial dermatophytosis: morphological patterns. In: Lahiri K, editor. A treatise on topical corticosteroids in dermatology. Singapore: Springer; 2017. p. 151–8.
3. Kaaman T. The clinical significance of cutaneous reactions to trichophyton in dermatophytosis. Acta Derm Venereol. 1978;58: 139–43.
4. Piñeiro L, Larruskain J, Idigoras P, et al. Trichophyton rubrum syndrome: the tip of the iceberg and a preventable outcome. Mycoses. 2010;53:186.
5. Dahl MV, Grando SA. Chronic dermatophytosis: what is special about Trichophyton rubrum? Adv Dermatol. 1994;9:97–109.
6. Vermout S, Tabart J, Baldo A, et al. Pathogenesis of dermatophytosis. Mycopathologia. 2008;166:267–75.
7. de Sousa Mda G, Santana GB, Criado PR, et al. Chronic widespread dermatophytosis due to Trichophyton rubrum: a syndrome associated with a Trichophyton-specific functional defect of phagocytes. Front Microbiol. 2015;6:801.
8. Oliveira CB, Vasconcellos C, Sakai-Valente NY, et al. Toll-like receptors (TLR) 2 and 4 expression of keratinocytes from patients with localized and disseminated dermatophytosis. Rev Inst Med Trop Sao Paulo. 2015;57:57–61.
9. Verma SB. Sales, status, prescriptions and regulatory problems with topical steroids in India. Indian J Dermatol Venereol Leprol. 2014;80:201–3.
10. Verma SB. Topical steroid misuse in India is harmful and out of control. BMJ. 2015;351:h6079.
11. Dogra S, Uprety S. The menace of chronic and recurrent dermatophytosis in India: is the problem deeper than we perceive? Indian Dermatol Online J. 2016;7:73–6.
12. Verma SB, Vasani R. Male genital dermatophytosis—clinical features and the effects of the misuse of topical steroids and steroid combinations—an alarming problem in India. Mycoses. 2016;59:606–14.
13. Rathi SK, D'Souza P. Rational and ethical use of topical corticosteroids based on safety and efficacy. Indian J Dermatol. 2012;57:251–9.
14. Kumar S, Goyal A, Gupta YK. Abuse of topical corticosteroids in India: concerns and the way forward. J Pharmacol Pharmacother. 2016;7:7–15.
15. Verma S, Hay RJ. Topical steroid-induced tinea pseudoimbricata: a striking form of tinea incognito. Int J Dermatol. 2015;54:e192–3.
16. Lim SP, Smith AG. "Tinea pseudoimbricata": tinea corporis in a renal transplant recipient mimicking the concentric rings of tinea imbricata. Clin Exp Dermatol. 2003;28:332–3.
17. Verma SB. A closer look at the term 'Tinea incognito'—a factual as well as grammatical inaccuracy. Indian J Dermatol. 2017;62:219.
18. Agarwal US, Mathur D, Mathur D, et al. Ear sign. Indian Dermatol Online J. 2014;5:105–6.

Cutaneous Manifestations of Torture and Intentional Abuse

46

Coleen Kivlahan, Jan Gutermuth, and Karlijn Clarysse

In 1984, Article 1 of the United Nations Convention Against Torture and Other Cruel, Inhuman or Degrading Treatment or Punishment [1] (UNCAT) defines torture as:

> *...any act by which severe pain or suffering, whether physical or mental, is intentionally inflicted on a person for such purposes as obtaining from him or a third person information or a confession, punishing him for an act he or a third person has committed or is suspected of having committed, or intimidating or coercing him or a third person, or for any reason based on discrimination of any kind, when such pain or suffering is inflicted by or at the instigation of or with the consent or acquiescence of a public official or other person acting in an official capacity. It does not include pain or suffering arising only from, inherent in or incidental to lawful sanctions.*

It is impossible to ascertain the precise number of people experiencing torture annually. Torture is frequently underreported. Reasons for failure to report include detention of victims, paucity of attorneys and physician experts to support documentation, and threats from perpetrators and death due to torture or its sequelae. Amnesty International documented torture in 141 countries [2] over the last 5 years. The International Rehabilitation Council for Torture Victims (IRCT 2010) estimated that there are about 400,000 victims of torture living in the EU and a similar number in the USA [3]. No one is immune from the risk of torture, and reported cases include teachers, politicians, journalists, health professionals, human rights defenders, people in detention or prison, members of ethnic minorities, and student leaders [4].

46.1 Political Asylum Status

Political asylum may be sought by people who have suffered persecution, torture, or fear due to race, religion, nationality, membership in a particular social group, and political opinion. In most cases, people are fleeing from armed conflicts in politically unstable countries of origin [5]. Fifty percent more applications for asylum or refugee status were submitted to 174 countries in 2015 than in 2014. 172,700 asylum seekers submitted a claim to the USA for protection, while 441,900 applicants sought protection in Germany in 2015 alone. Over 600,000 asylum claims were received in the EU in 2014 [6].

Physicians play an important role in assuring the health of refugees and asylees from all over the world, as well as identifying and documenting evidence of torture. The Manual on the Effective Investigation and Documentation of Torture and Other Cruel, Inhuman or Degrading Treatment or Punishment (the Istanbul Protocol) was developed as an international guideline for the assessment of persons who allege torture and ill-treatment [7]. Doctors must consider the possibility of torture as a potential etiology and screen for intentional injuries using a few simple questions [8] such as: "Some people in your situation have experienced difficult conditions in their countries; did anything like this happen for you? If so, what happened" and "While in captivity, did you ever experience mental or physical suffering that was inflicted by another person?". Physicians may engage in the forensic medical documentation of physical findings of torture. Ninety percent of asylum seekers with medical documentation of past torture are granted asylum compared to 37% of those lacking medical support, which emphasizes the role of the physician in this process [9].

People of color are at greater risk for torture. Torture mostly occurs in political unstable countries where victims are often held in detention or custody. Torture rates are highest in people seeking political asylum, and countries with the highest number of claims are those with high rates of poverty, civil wars, and dark-skinned populations. Twenty to forty

C. Kivlahan, M.D., M.S.P.H.
Department of Family and Community Medicine, Primary Care Services, UCSF School of Medicine, San Francisco, CA, USA

J. Gutermuth (✉) • K. Clarysse
Department of Dermatology, Universitair Ziekenhuis Brussel, Vrije Universiteit Brussel, Brussels, Belgium
e-mail: Jan.Gutermuth@uzbrussel.be

C. E. Orfanos et al. (eds.), *Pigmented Ethnic Skin and Imported Dermatoses*, https://doi.org/10.1007/978-3-319-69422-1_46

percent of asylum-seeking refugees from Somalia, Ethiopia, Eritrea, Senegal, Sierra Leone, Tibet, and Bhutan report being tortured [8].

46.2 Etiology and Mechanisms of Injury

Dermatology and forensics use different taxonomies to describe skin lesions and have different purposes for their description. Dermatologists characterize skin findings using the physical and anatomic descriptors of the lesion such as macule, papule, vesicle, and plaque for the purposes of diagnosis and treatment. Forensic science often combines dermatologic descriptions with mechanisms of injury such as laceration, abrasion, or contusion in order to reflect the relationship between the physical finding and the associated type of injury for the purpose of medical conclusions and legal documentation.

In order to document skin lesions for forensic purposes, a comprehensive physical examination is necessary in order to identify injury sequelae that may appear in multiple locations on the body. This practice stands in contrast to a routine dermatological evaluation that often focuses on a limited area of the skin. The standard of care for evaluating intentional injury is a full physical examination from head to toe. While many scars are nonspecific, their patterns, atypical shapes, unusual and multiple locations, etc. can help to support a history of torture [10]. Findings consistent with inflicted injuries often include lack of symmetry, patterned or linear lesions in irregular configurations, circumferential injuries around an extremity, and areas of hyperpigmentation or hypertrophy surrounding a scar. None of these findings are diagnostic; evaluations must be accompanied by a comprehensive history of torture-related events. Special attention during the physical examination should be paid to the high-risk, but often neglected, areas of the ears, mouth, teeth, bottoms of feet, and genitalia. In addition to the physical examination, a detailed history of the alleged torture, related events, and symptoms will help the physician develop conclusions about the significance of skin findings, both torture and non-torture-related lesions. Clinicians examining patients claiming injuries as a result of torture generally have advanced training in medical forensic documentation of skins, signs of intentional injury, as well as the knowledge and experience within their own medical specialty and expertise in tortured patterns across the world.

46.3 Forensic Documentation

Documenting medical findings can provide important evidence for torture victims. The UN General Assembly states that "All States have a clear obligation to investigate acts of torture and other cruel, inhuman or degrading treatment or punishment (other ill-treatment)… Effective medical and forensic documentation can provide evidence of torture and other ill-treatment to light, so that perpetrators may be held accountable. Forensic specialists provide expert analysis of whether there is a correlation between the medical evidence and the allegations." Medical documentation, using medical records, photographs, and expert reports, can overcome the lack of objective evidence faced by survivors of torture since torture usually occurs without witnesses [11]. Article 19 of the UN Convention Against Torture and Other Cruel, Inhuman or Degrading Treatment or Punishment of 2013 [12] sets out the right to consultation with a physician for the purposes of medical documentation of any torture or intentional injury.

46.4 Types of Skin Injuries

Intentional injuries as a result of torture may be seen in both their acute and chronic phases, medically evaluated days to years after the event. Torture-related lesions may directly result from physical injuries or skin conditions in association with detention (scabies), as well as those induced by physical conditions or psychological trauma (cutting). There are several approaches to classify wounds resulting from intentional trauma. One common forensic approach is categorization by the type of force used to inflict the injury such as blunt force wounds, sharp force wounds, and non-kinetic injuries. Blunt force wounds include lacerations, abrasions, and contusions. Sharp force wounds include incisions, stab, and chop wounds. Thermal, chemical, and electrical injuries are considered non-kinetic wounds [13]. The main types of mechanical injuries (blunt or sharp trauma) associated with torture include lacerations, abrasions, contusions, and avulsions. The mechanisms of those injuries vary widely [14].

Lacerations are injuries in which the skin or tissue is cut or torn, usually resulting in full thickness skin penetration. Lacerations typically result from blunt impact causing compression or stretching, and usually the resulting injury does not reproduce the shape of the weapon. They most commonly occur when force is exerted between the skin and underlying solid tissue on the head, lower legs, shoulders, or face. Lacerations often appear with other injury types such as abrasions, crush, and contusions. Kicking by boots, for example, may cause an abrasion, contusion, or laceration, and multiple scars can result (Fig. 46.1). Other scars may result from burns with cigarettes (Fig. 46.2).

Avulsions are a type of laceration in which sections of tissue are torn, partially or completely. Avulsions are caused by a shearing force that detaches a portion of skin surface from its underlying attachment. The skin, muscles, organs, and bones may be crushed or fractured. Avulsions often occur with abrasions or lacerations.

Abrasions (scratches, brushes) are superficial injuries, in which the epidermis is not fully penetrated. Abrasions may

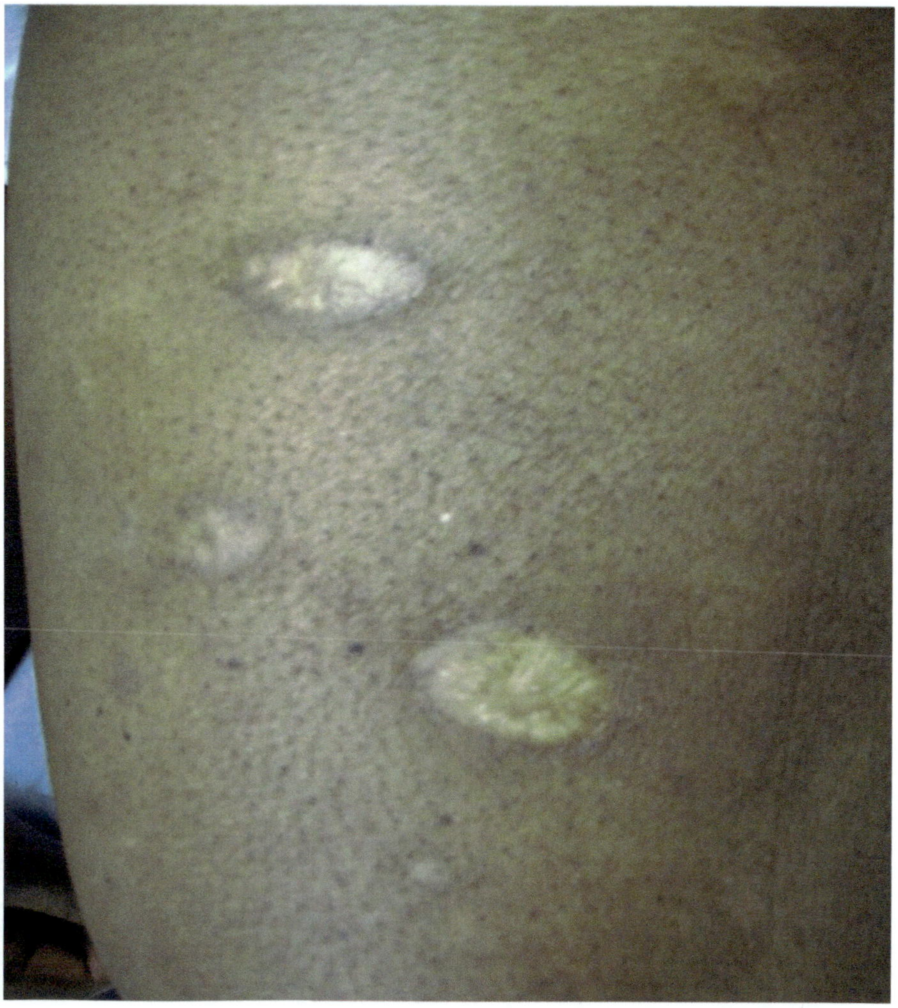

Fig. 46.1 Atrophic scars on the upper thigh due to repeated kicking with steel-toed boots

be caused by falls, dragging over rough surfaces (Fig. 46.3), or skin compression from fingernails, hands, feet, whip, or baton. They are usually caused by tangential motion to the skin. The direction of the force frequently can be identified by observing the pattern or shape of epidermal fragments at the end of the lesion where contact with the object stopped. The injury direction may also be vertical to the skin, which usually results in a crush injury, and the weapon pattern may be seen.

Contusions (can induce bruises or ecchymoses) are caused by a forceful blow or blunt trauma, in which the epidermis is usually intact. Patterns may or may not be visible on the skin based on the amount of force used and site of injury. The appearance of a contusion depends upon the skin color, the intensity of the force, the space within and resilience of the underlying tissue, the age of the victim, comorbid medical conditions, and medications. Contusions may show patterns such as fingerprint bruises, bite marks, round or patterned contusions from kicks, and blunt trauma from whips, rods, or batons. Scars can reflect the type of inflicting weapon, such as a baton or stick, resulting in hyperpigmented parallel linear scars, commonly known as tramline patterns (Figs. 46.4 and 46.5).

Incisions typically have sharp edges in which the tissue strands in the wound are severed; while in the laceration, the fascia, vessels, and other tissue strands may be intact. There is usually little bruising or crushing of the wound margins. The term "incised wound" usually includes stabbing or puncturing injuries from a knife, sword, razor, glass, or an axe, but some authors describe stab wounds as a separate group and incisions as injuries that are longer than they are deep [14].

Thermal, chemical, electrical, and firearm injuries. Thermal injuries include those due to cold, cold immersion, and hypothermia, as well as those related to heat and electrical injuries such as electrocution, radiation, exposure to heat, and burns, including from cigarettes (Figs. 46.3 and 46.6). Immersion injuries may include suffocation, water immersion, and drowning. Chemical injuries include exposure to acids or alkalis and skin exposure to pepper, salt, and toxic agents. Some scars may itch, become hypertrophic, or form

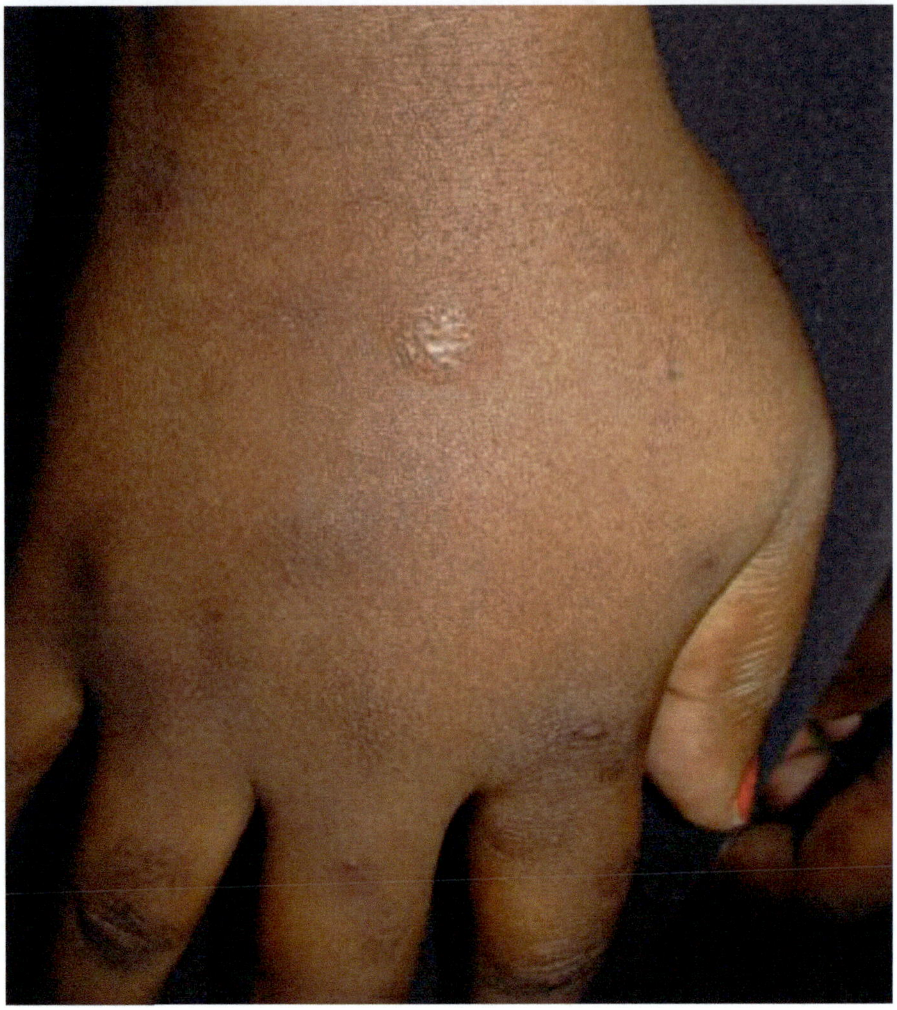

Fig. 46.2 Scar on the dorsum of the right hand from cigarette burn

keloids. Infected wounds may become thickened, puckered, atrophic, or hyperpigmented.

46.5 Types of Torture

Human torture appears in an almost endless variety. The type of implement used influences the nature of the scar. All weapons should be described including their color, shape, material, and dimensions. Types of torture and the weapons/devices commonly used include examples such as:

- Blunt trauma such as punch, kick, slap, whip, and falls, with devices/weapons including human hands and feet, batons, sticks, whips, wires, hammers, and other tools.
- Burns using cigarettes, heated metal rods and instruments, electrocution, hot water.
- Head trauma such as contusions, bleeding, loss of consciousness, vision and hearing changes due to the use of blunt or sharp trauma, and penetrating trauma such as gunshots or screwdrivers.
- Forced positional torture such as squatting, prolonged standing, hanging, suspension, stretching, and constraint of movement, using chains, pulleys, restraints, or confinement in small spaces.
- Asphyxiation using wet or dry means, smothering with tape or cloth, choking, and ingestion of liquids, powders, or chemicals.
- Penetrating injuries including stabbing, punctures, gunshot, and wire/needle insertion.
- Crush injuries involving hand or leg cuffs or restraints, nail injuries, strangling, and rolling pins.
- Chemical exposure including acids/alkalis, gasoline, salt, chili, and toxins.
- Avulsions or amputations of limbs, nails, and digits using knives, pliers, saws, or deep bites.
- Forced ingestion of medications, toxic substances, or injections.
- Attacks by other detainees or interrogators, insects or animals such as rats, dogs, etc.
- Sexual violence including threats, touching, forced nudity, mutilation, virginity testing, electrocution, abor-

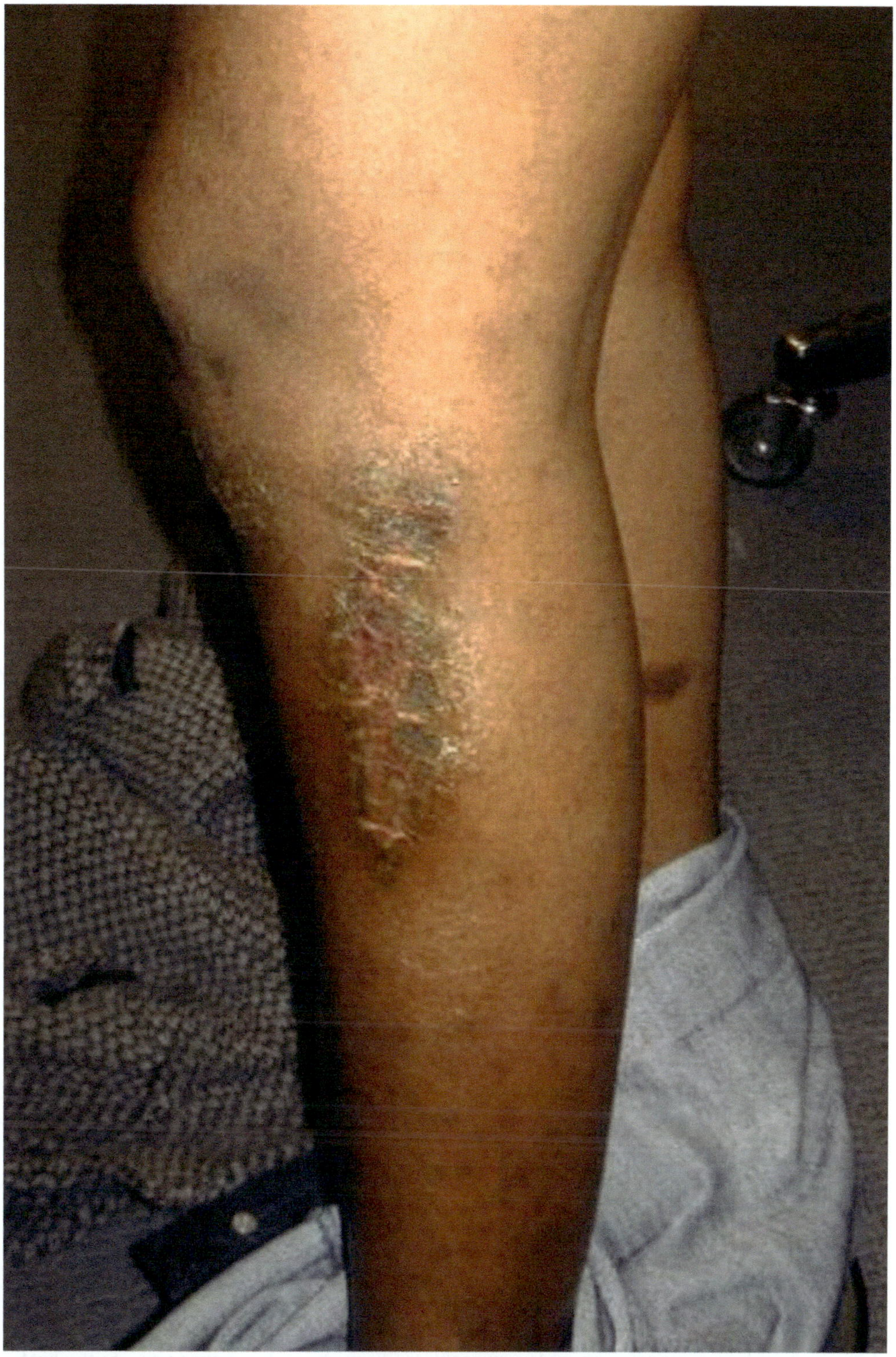

Fig. 46.3 Irregular atrophic abrasion scars from being dragged over dirt road

tion, sexual slavery, forced marriage, and penetration of mouth, vagina, or rectum.
- Psychological trauma including threats, witness to trauma of others, forced participation in torture of others, isolation, sleep deprivation, and use of noise/light exposure.

46.6 Appearance of Healed Injuries

The method of torture, force, duration, age, underlying conditions, and skin type will determine the appearance of older healed scars seen in victims of torture [15]. Examples include the following: (a) handcuffing, ligatures, or suspen-

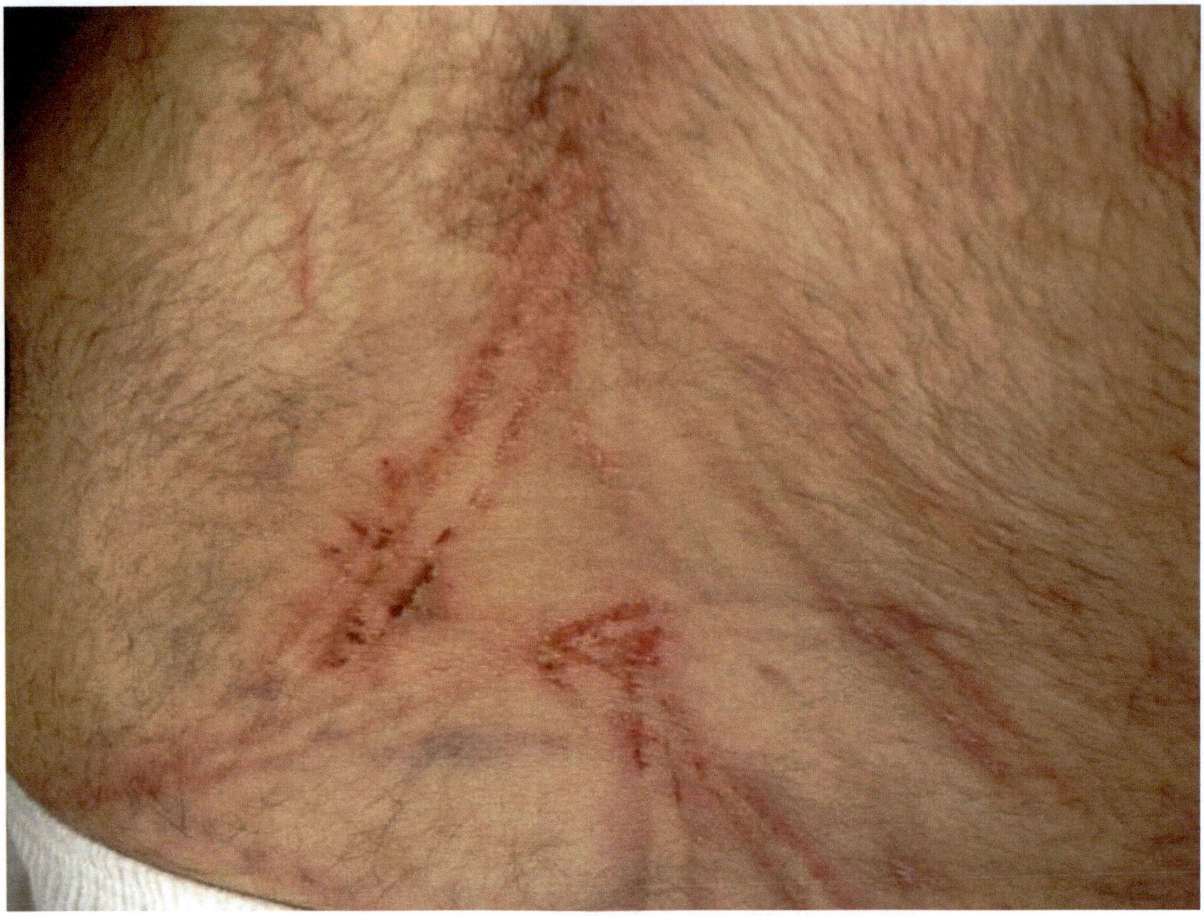

Fig. 46.4 Acute tramline abrasions and contusions on the back due to repeated blunt force whipping with electrical cords

sion which may appear as circumferential scars or linear patches of scarring alopecia at the wrist; (b) beating or whipping as permanent hyperpigmented tramline scars; (c) falanga (beating of the feet) as scarring and flattening of the soles; (d) bayonet or knife injuries as teardrop-shaped scars; (e) electrical injuries as small raised scars symmetrically around the earlobes, nipples, or genitalia; and (f) deep abrasions and wounds appearing as patterned scars (Fig. 46.7).

46.7 Differentiation of Signs of Torture from Other Conditions

Refugees and immigrants may also present with many other findings such as pruritus, pain, scars, pigmentary changes, infectious diseases, systemic illnesses, and injuries from self-harm or self-treatment. Populations with dark skin present more often with keloid scars, nail pigmentation, pigmentary demarcation lines, post-inflammatory pigmentation changes, discoid lupus erythematosus, cutaneous sarcoidosis, traction alopecia, acne keloidalis nuchae, dermatosis papulosa nigra, and pseudofolliculitis barbae. Conditions with higher prevalence in dark skin should be considered when evaluating for signs of torture [16]. Thus, the medical evaluation of torture survivors must consider differential diagnoses including incidental findings, unrelated skin conditions, scars from accidental injury, and culturally specific and self-inflicted injuries. Scars resulting from work, sport, or accidents are typically found in exposed body parts like hands, bony prominences on the scalp, face, lower arms, knees, or lower legs. The pattern and appearance of accidental injuries are usually quite typical.

Incidental findings such as striae may appear on the shoulders/upper arms, buttocks, hips, and lower back and are generally of uniform size and bilateral in a symmetrical pattern. Acne may produce scars on the back and face. Infected insect bites or chickenpox may leave scars anywhere on the body and resemble cigarette burns in the healed state. Immunization or injection scars can be found on the arms or buttocks. Tribal markings are typically in parallel lines or patterns and bilaterally symmetrical. Other traditional healing practices can result

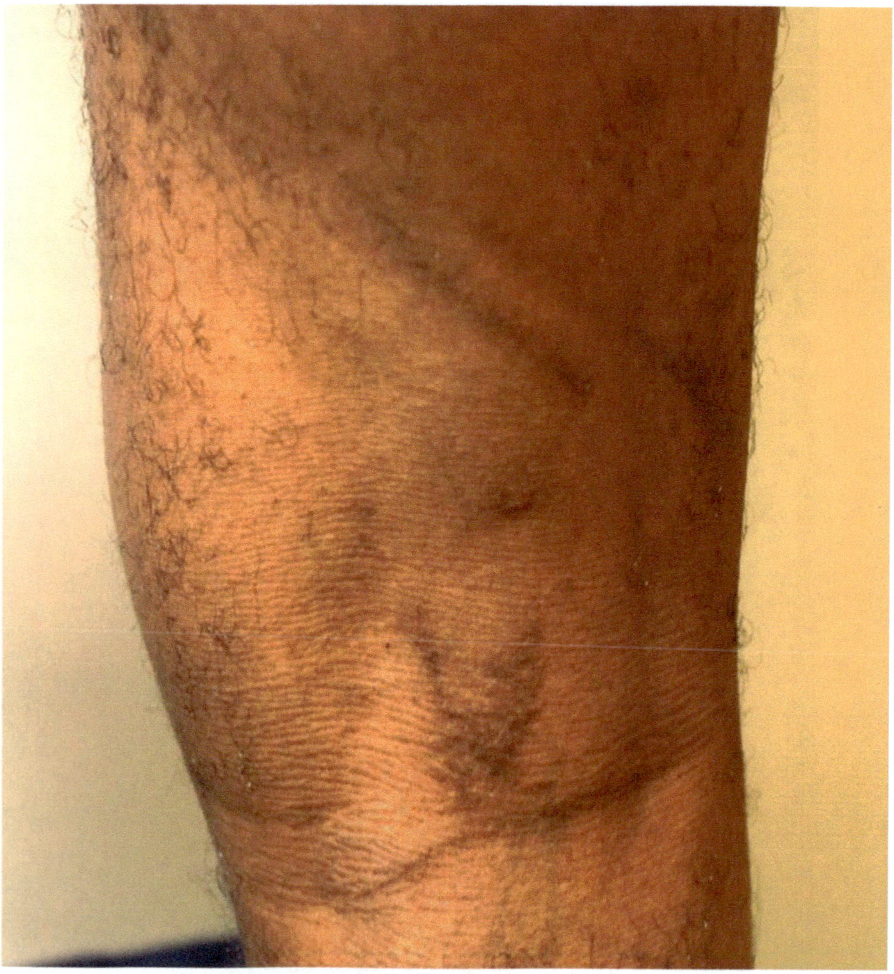

Fig. 46.5 Hyperpigmented scarring lesions on the posterior right knee with tramline pattern due to blunt force trauma

in scars from knives, razor blades, cupping, or burning. Cultural and religious practices may result in whipping or cutting injuries such as ritual self-flagellation or *hejamat* (bloodletting). Generally, self-inflicted scars appear on accessible areas such as the wrists and forearms, trunk, or upper back and are multiple and superficial. Self-inflicted injuries can also occur during detention due to prolonged isolation or serious trauma such as sexual violence [17].

46.8 Management

Torture victims present to medical facilities in a variety of ways. Most come to the attention of physicians in the usual course of a medical examination for an unrelated medical or psychological problem. Some present to the emergency room for an acute condition and others to primary care for typical outpatient concerns. Underrecognition of torture survivors by healthcare workers is the norm [4], and disclosure occurs in only a minority of cases and rarely at the first meeting [18]. While the physician is caring for skin lesions, injuries to other parts of the body may be noted which create suspicion for torture [8]. Physicians trained in forensic evaluation of torture may seek informed consent for documentation in any of these settings. The standard evaluation includes comprehensive history, physical examination, photographs, body diagrams, basic psychological evaluation, and medical documentation using international guidelines.

Treatment of acute lesions does not differ from standard wound care. Healed lesions can present as esthetic challenges for the patient, can create psychological distress, and may have resulted in keloid or hypertrophic scar formation. There are some acute injuries that may demand immediate treatment, such as eye or head injuries, suspension torture with plexus injuries, and compartment syndromes resulting from recurrent beating [18]. It should be remembered that some forms of torture leave no or minimal physical findings, such as electrical injury or kicking in the abdomen [16].

Hyperpigmented scars can be treated by using topical bleaching agents, peelings, or laser therapies. These should be done carefully as there is a greater risk of hyper- or hypopigmentation posttreatment in patients with skin phototypes IV–VI compared to III or lower. Topical application of

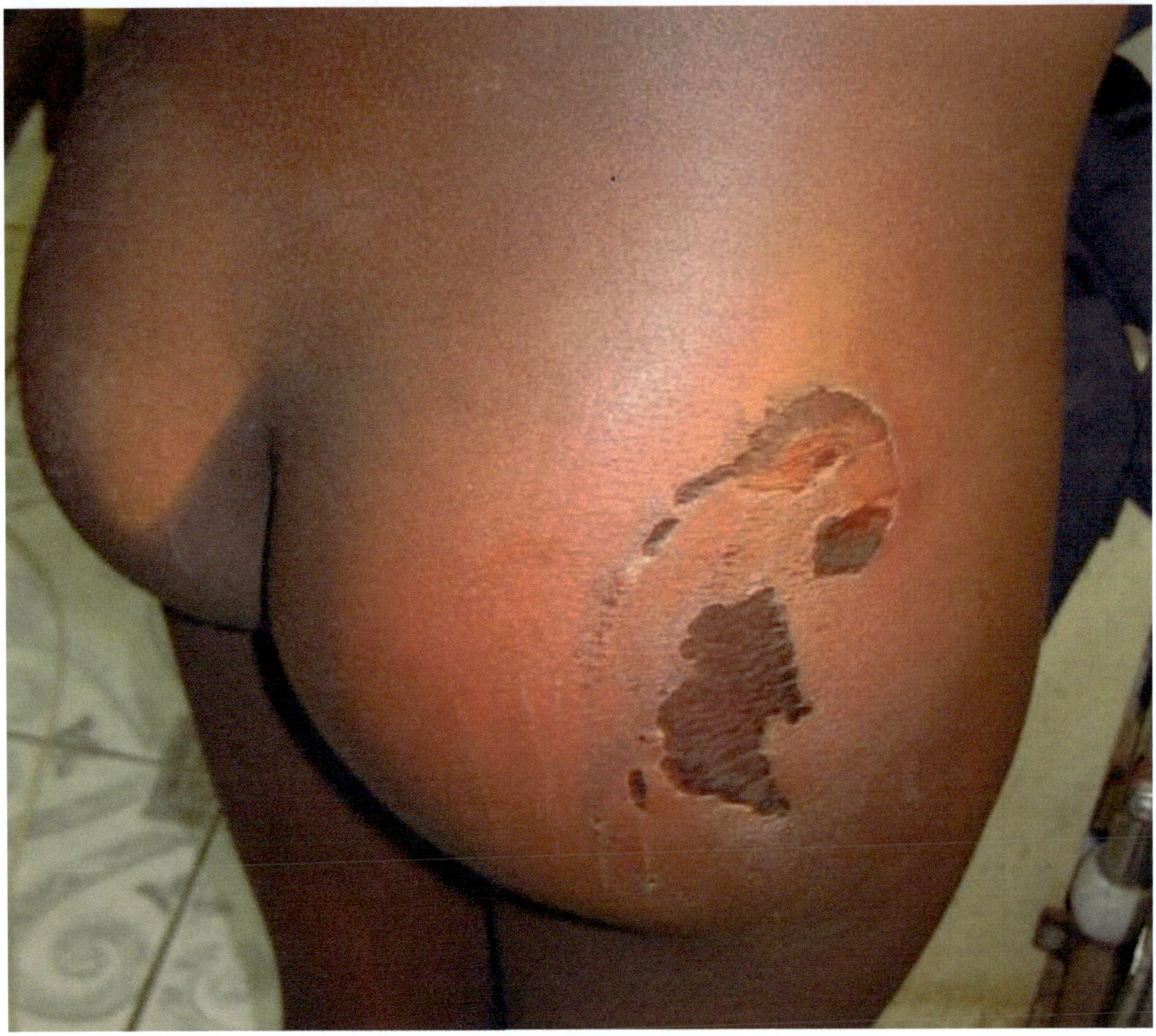

Fig. 46.6 Acute erythema and patterned scars from burn on buttock after being forced to sit on a hot log in the fire

hydroquinone 2–5% represents best practice and can be safely used in dark skin types. The combination of hydroquinone 4%, tretinoin 0.05%, and hydrocortisone acetate 1% also known as "Kligman formula" has proven to be most effective. Other topical agents are kojic acid and arbutin, which have a similar working mechanism as hydroquinone. Ascorbic acid and alpha-tocopherol are also widely used, as antioxidants that inhibit some oxidative steps in melanin formation [19].

Chemical peels are aimed at destruction of the epidermis, leading to exfoliation and regeneration of new skin. However, medium to deep peels are contraindicated in skin types IV–VI because of the increased risk of post-inflammatory hyperpigmentation. Trichloroacetic acid, commonly used in lighter skin, should be avoided in dark-skinned individuals due to the risk of dyschromias. Frosting can be difficult to evaluate in dark skin and lead to overtreatment. Glycolic acid (GA) can be safely used for peelings in dark skin types. Several GA peelings may be necessary with a 2–3-week interval. Gradual augmentation in GA concentration is recommended to avoid adverse events. Priming the skin with the Kligman formula 2 weeks prior to peeling may enhance the effect of the GA peeling and reduce post-inflammatory hyperpigmentation. The following agents can be used safely for superficial peels in dark skin types [20]: glycolic acid solution 30–70%, salicylic acid 20–30%, Jessner's solution (resorcinol, salicylic acid, and lactic acid), or tretinoin 1–5%. The use of ablative CO2 and Er:Yag lasers for resurfacing are contra-indicated in dark skin types due to high risk of pigmentary abnormalities. Non-ablative and fractional lasers, which mainly cause dermal injury, are recommended; however, a more conservative approach of treatment is necessary compared to skin types I–III [21, 22].

Dark skin types are predisposed to keloidal scars as compared to fair skin. Keloids are hard, raised, and outgrow the original wound margins. Despite multiple treat-

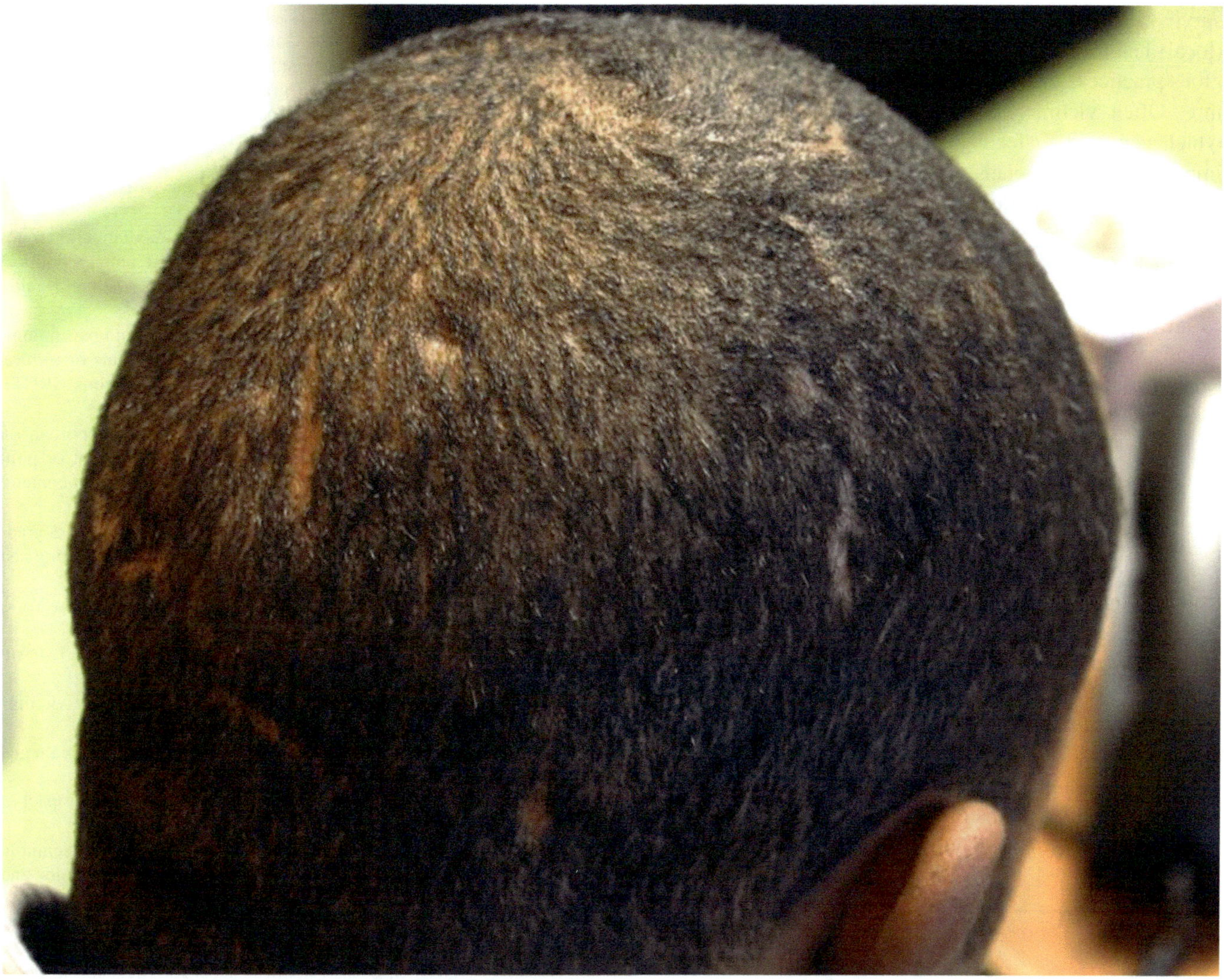

Fig. 46.7 Multiple scars on the scalp after blunt force trauma with a baseball bat studded with embedded nails

ment regimens, recurrences often occur [23]. Intralesional steroids such as triamcinolone acetonide are considered a first line of treatment for keloids. Pretreatment with pulse dye lasers can reduce the firmness and edema of the scar and facilitate the injection. Pulse dye laser can be used in dark skin types to reduce the vascularity in keloids and thereby inhibit fibroblast growth [24]. 5-Fluorouracil should be avoided in dark skin due to the risk of post-inflammatory hyperpigmentation; cryotherapy is effective, but also bears the same risk.

46.9 Impact of Torture

The most important physical consequence of torture is chronic pain. This frequently presents as headaches and back, abdominal, or extremity pain. The appearance of healed scars is dependent on skin type and factors related to the mechanism of injury. In people of color, scars that remind the patient of torture events and pigment inhomogeneity can be highly distressing. Other serious physical consequences of torture can include nerve plexus injuries, amputations, and sexual dysfunction [15]. In addition to chronic pain, symptoms related to depression, anxiety, post-traumatic stress disorder, and separation from family and country can lead to serious and persistent distress for victims. People may develop disabilities or restricted function due to torture injuries and have multiple, complex health problems, complicated by their assimilation into a new country or environment. However, cognitive behavioral management and narrative exposure management have been shown to be effective in reducing trauma symptoms [17]. Physicians must assume a humble, empathic, and open, curious attitude rather than one of rapid-fire, closed questions and a rush to diagnoses and treatment. The psychological care of survivors of torture should involve healthcare providers with (local) language proficiency, knowledge of cultural and religious practices, and experience with a variety of forms of torture. Often victims have being humiliated during torture, which can lead to feelings of worthlessness or guilt. It is important for physicians to avoid the re-experience of the trauma by the victim during medical evaluations.

Conclusions

Torture occurs worldwide, and dark-skinned populations are at greater risk of experiencing physical and psychological torture due to conditions in their countries of origin such as extreme poverty, conflicts, and unstable governments. Perpetrators of torture use an endless array of techniques, leading to injuries such as lacerations, avulsions, contusions, and neuromuscular injuries and damage to internal organs. These inhumane crimes frequently leave lasting scars on the body and psychological trauma. Victims may seek safety in other countries as refugees and asylum applicants. Dermatologists, as well as other primary care and specialist physicians, have a duty to provide their clinical expertise to augment the forensic documentation of torture and its impact, seeking advanced training in order to better recognize acute and chronic sequelae of torture. Doctors have a unique role in garnering trust, in reporting and documenting cases of torture, and in reducing impunity by developing their forensic skills as one type of powerful evidence against the perpetrators of these crimes.

References

1. Convention against torture and other cruel, inhuman or degrading treatment or punishment. United Nations of Human Rights. 1987. www.ohchr.org/EN/ProfessionalInterest/Pages/CAT.aspx.
2. Amnesty International. Overview torture. www.amnesty.org/en/what-we-do/torture/.
3. Convention Against Torture Initiative (CTI). http://cti2024.org/content/images/CTI%20seminar%20on%20rehabiliation%20%20discussion%20paper.pdff.
4. International Rehabilitation Council for Torture Victims (IRCT). Defining torture. www.irct.org/what-is-torture/defining-torture.aspx.
5. U.S. Citizenship and Immigration Services. Asylum Division Affirmative Asylum Scheduling Bulletin. https://www.uscis.gov/humanitarian/refugees-asylum/asylum.
6. The UN Refugee Agency. Facts and figures about refugees. http://www.unhcr.ie/about-unhcr/facts-and-figures-about-refugees.
7. Manual on the effective investigation and documentation of torture and other cruel, inhuman or degrading treatment or punishment, Istanbul Protocol (IP), Professional Training Series No.8/Rev.1, UNHCHR, 2004. http://www.ohchr.org/Documents/Publications/training8Rev1en.pdf.
8. Miles SH, Garcia-Peltoniemi RE. Torture survivors: what to ask, how to document. J Fam Pract. 2012;61:E1–5.
9. Lustig SL, Kureshi S, Delucchi KL, et al. Asylum grant rates following medical evaluations of maltreatment among political asylum applicants in the United States. J Immigr Minor Health. 2008;10:7–15.
10. Peel M, Hinshelwood G, Forrest D. The physical and psychological findings following the late examination of victims of torture. International Rehabilitation Council for Torture Victims (IRCT). Torture. 2000;10:12–5.
11. UN general assembly Interim report of the Special Rapporteur on torture and other cruel, inhuman or degrading treatment or punishment, 23 September 2014. http://antitorture.org/wp-content/uploads/2014/10/Forensics_Report_SRT.pdf.
12. Convention against torture and other cruel, inhuman or degrading treatment or punishment. http://www.ohchr.org/EN/ProfessionalInterest/Pages/CAT.aspx.
13. Saukko P, Knight B. Knight's forensic pathology. 4th ed. New York: CRC Press; 2016.
14. Reddy K, Lowenstein EJ. Forensics in dermatology: part I. J Am Acad Dermatol. 2011;64:801–8.
15. Carinci AJ, Mehta P, Christo PJ. Chronic pain in torture victims. Curr Pain Headache Rep. 2010;14:73–9.
16. Danielsen L, Rasmussen OV. Dermatological findings after alleged torture. Torture. 2006;16:108–27.
17. C de C Williams A, van der Merwe J. The psychological impact of torture. Br J Pain. 2013;7:101–6.
18. Torp-Pedersen S, Amris K, et al. Vascular response to ischemia in the feet of falanga torture victims and normal controls-color and spectral Doppler findings. Torture. 2009;19:12–8.
19. Sarkar R, Arora P, et al. Cosmeceuticals for hyperpigmentation: what is available? J Cutan Aesthet Surg. 2013;6:4–11.
20. Sarkar R, Bansal S, et al. Chemical peels for Melasma in dark-skinned patients. J Cutan Aesthet Surg. 2012;5:247–53.
21. Gold M. Update on fractional laser technology. J Clin Aesthet Dermatol. 2010;3:42–50.
22. Alexis AF. Lasers and light-based therapies in ethnic skin: treatment options and recommendations for Fitzpatrick skin types V and VI. Br J Dermatol. 2013;169(suppl 3):91–7.
23. Cole P, Hatef D. Laser therapy in ethnic populations. Semin Plast Surg. 2009;23:173–7.
24. Ud-Din S, Bayat A. Strategic management of keloid disease in ethnic skin: a structured approach supported by the emerging literature. Br J Dermatol. 2013;169(suppl 3):71–81.

47 Lasers in Pigmented Skin

Luis Torezan

47.1 Introduction

The wide absorption spectrum of melanin (250–1200 nm) and the increased epidermal melanin content and melanosome density account for most of the increased risks of lasers in darker skin types. However, while melanin's absorption is broad, it is not the same across the spectrum (peaks in the ultraviolet and declines as wavelengths get longer) [1, 2].

Considering melanin as a chromophore, there is a greater absorption of energy in the epidermis when treating pigmented skin. Therefore, more side effects and thermal damage to surrounding tissues are expected, if one uses higher fluencies during a laser procedure. Also, the more melanin there is, the greater is the likelihood that melanin will absorb the energy and compete with other chromophores, thereby reducing the efficacy of the treatment [3].

Highly melanized skin absorbs electromagnetic energy much more efficiently than fair skin. For instance, epidermal melanin absorbs approximately 4× as much energy when irradiated by 694 nm ruby laser when compared to the longer wavelength 1064 nm Nd:YAG laser, allowing high tissue penetration [2, 4].

In general, the majority of lasers used to safely treat darker skin types use longer wavelengths and longer pulse durations. Melanin absorption and epidermal thermal heating contribute to thermal damage, especially in darker phototypes. In addition, effectively cooling the skin surface (cold air, cooled gel, ice packs, or inherent cooling of the laser system) is also essential to minimize erythema, edema, and pain during treatment [1].

New lasers which use longer wavelengths with increased pulse durations, expanded range of treatment fluencies, and more efficient cooling devices are now available in most laser technologies, decreasing the likelihood of adverse events while effectively treating darker skin types.

47.2 Light-Tissue Interaction

When a laser is used on the skin, the light may be absorbed, reflected, transmitted, or scattered. The amount of absorption is determined by the chromophore present in the skin and whether a wavelength that corresponds to the absorptive characteristics of that chromophore is used. The main endogenous chromophores of the skin are water, melanin, and haemoglobin [3, 5, 6]. Tattoo ink is an example of an exogenous chromophore. Once laser energy is absorbed in the skin, five effects are possible: *photothermal*, when a chromophore absorbs the corresponding wavelength of energy and destruction of the target results from the conversion of absorbed energy into heat; *photochemical,* photosensitizer-related reactions that serve as the basis of photodynamic management; *photomechanical*, when extremely rapid thermal expansion leads to acoustic waves and subsequent photomechanical destruction of the absorbing tissue; *photobiomodulation*, when light is used to modulate intra- and intercellular activities; and *selective photothermolysis*, when a targeted lesion is destructed without significant thermal damage to surrounding normal tissue by a wavelength that is absorbed preferentially by the intended tissue target or chromophore [5, 6]. To limit the amount of thermal energy deposited within the skin, the exposure duration of the tissue to light (pulse duration) must be shorter than the chromophore's thermal relaxation time, defined as the time required for the targeted site to cool to one half of its peak temperature immediately after laser irradiation [3]. In order to achieve the correct pulse duration, we need to observe the TRT (thermal relaxation time) of the target tissue.

The depth of penetration of laser energy into the skin is dependent upon absorption and scattering. Although scattering is minimal in the epidermis, it is greater in the dermis as a result of the presence of collagen fibers [3]. The amount of

L. Torezan
Laser and Nonmelanoma Skin Cancer Divisions,
Hospital das Clínicas, University of Sao Paulo Medical School,
São Paulo, Brazil
e-mail: torezanluis@uol.com.br

C. E. Orfanos et al. (eds.), *Pigmented Ethnic Skin and Imported Dermatoses*, https://doi.org/10.1007/978-3-319-69422-1_47

scattering of laser energy is inversely proportional to the wavelength of incident light. In general, the depth of penetration of laser energy increases with wavelength until the mid-infrared region of the electromagnetic spectrum [3, 5]. Penetration of 300–400 nm is limited by strong scattering of the beam, whereas scattering is minimal at longer wavelengths (1000–1200 nm), allowing greater penetration into the skin. However, wavelengths in the mid- to upper-infrared range of the electromagnetic spectrum penetrate superficially as a result of high absorption by tissue water. Another concept is the fluency or energy density delivered by the laser which must be sufficient to achieve destruction of the target within the allotted time [5].

The main characteristics to consider when performing laser procedure in dark-skinned population are increased epidermal melanin, larger melanosomes widely distributed within epidermal keratinocytes, labile melanocyte responses, and reactive fibroblasts [1, 2, 7]. Increased melanin content, packaging, and epidermal distribution lead to a greater protection against deleterious effects of ultraviolet radiation, and therefore, signs of photoaging tend to be less marked and delayed in lighter skin types. Labile melanocyte responses contribute to an increased prevalence of pigmentary disorders in nonwhite populations. Of particular relevance to laser or light procedures, the tendency for injury or inflammation to incite alterations in pigment production is associated with a greater risk for post-procedure hyper- or hypopigmentation in dark-skinned individuals [2, 4, 7].

Racial differences exist in the frequency of keloids, with the highest prevalence being observed in populations of African origin or ancestry. This is probably due to genetic factors that contribute to increased fibroblast reactivity among individuals at risk. Therefore, a greater overall risk of keloids and hypertrophic scars associated with iatrogenic dermal injury is observed in nonwhite populations [4].

From what is discussed above, the basic principles of selective photohermolysis are [5, 7]:

(a) ***Ideal wavelength*** that is absorbed only by the target tissue or chromophore
(b) ***Ideal pulse duration*** that should be sufficient to produce the desired effect on any target tissue, but fast enough to cause minimal effect on the surrounding tissues, i.e., confining the energy in the chromophore
(c) ***Energy*** enough to reach the treatment effect

47.3 Hair Removal

Common dermatologic conditions in dark skin types are pseudofolliculitis and hirsutism. Hair and epidermal melanin have similar absorption spectra, increasing the potential for depigmentation disorders after laser- or light-based hair removal. The use of longer wavelengths as well as longer pulse durations such as diode (810 nm) and Nd:YAG (1064 nm) increases the efficacy with fewer side effects. The use of epidermal cooling devices and longer pulse durations is considered of extreme importance [7, 8]. The goal is to effectively target the melanin in the hair follicle and surrounding stem cells and minimize the epidermal thermal damage. The long-pulsed 1064 nm Nd:YAG laser is considered the safest laser for hair removal for dark-skinned patients [4, 7, 8]. Pulse durations in the 30–40 ms range (or even higher) provide a safety profile to treat skin phototypes V and VI. Also, using long-pulse diode laser (810 nm) with pulse durations of 100 ms or higher has shown to decrease the incidence of thermal injury while providing good efficacy for hair removal.

The most common adverse events with lasers for hair removal are secondary to epidermal thermal damage. Erythema, edema, blisters, and ablation may occur and evolve to depigmentation and scarring of the skin. These side effects may be delayed by up to 24–48 h. Test spots may also be necessary for some patients in order to better evaluate the potential risks and benefits of the laser treatment (Figs. 47.1 and 47.2) [9].

47.4 Lasers for Pigmented Benign Lesions and Tattoos

Despite being one of the most frequent dermatological concerns among dark-skinned patient populations, there is a paucity of studies investigating the safety and efficacy of lasers in the treatment of pigmentary disorders in this specific population.

Epidermal and dermal-pigmented lesions, such as *melasma*, *lentigines*, *naevus of Ota and Hori*, and *post-inflammatory hyperpigmentation* (PIH), are common complaints and difficult to treat. PIH is considered one of the most frequent complications of lasers [4]. Quality-switched lasers produce very short pulses in nano- or picosecond domains, shorter than the thermal relaxation time of melanosomes. The QS systems currently available are Nd:YAG (532 and 1064 nm), alexandrite (755 nm), and ruby (694 nm) [6, 7, 10]. The absorption peaks of melanin lie in the UV range and decrease at the longest wavelengths. Moreover, shorter wavelengths (e.g., 532 nm) are highly absorbed by epidermal melanin. Thus, longer wavelengths are preferable and lead to more effective treatment of pigmented dermal lesions and hair follicles. Also, longer pulse durations and noncoherent systems (intense pulsed light) have shown good clinical results, although IPL with shorter cutoff filters may cause dyschromia and should be avoided in dark-skinned population. Targeting any pigmented lesion should always come

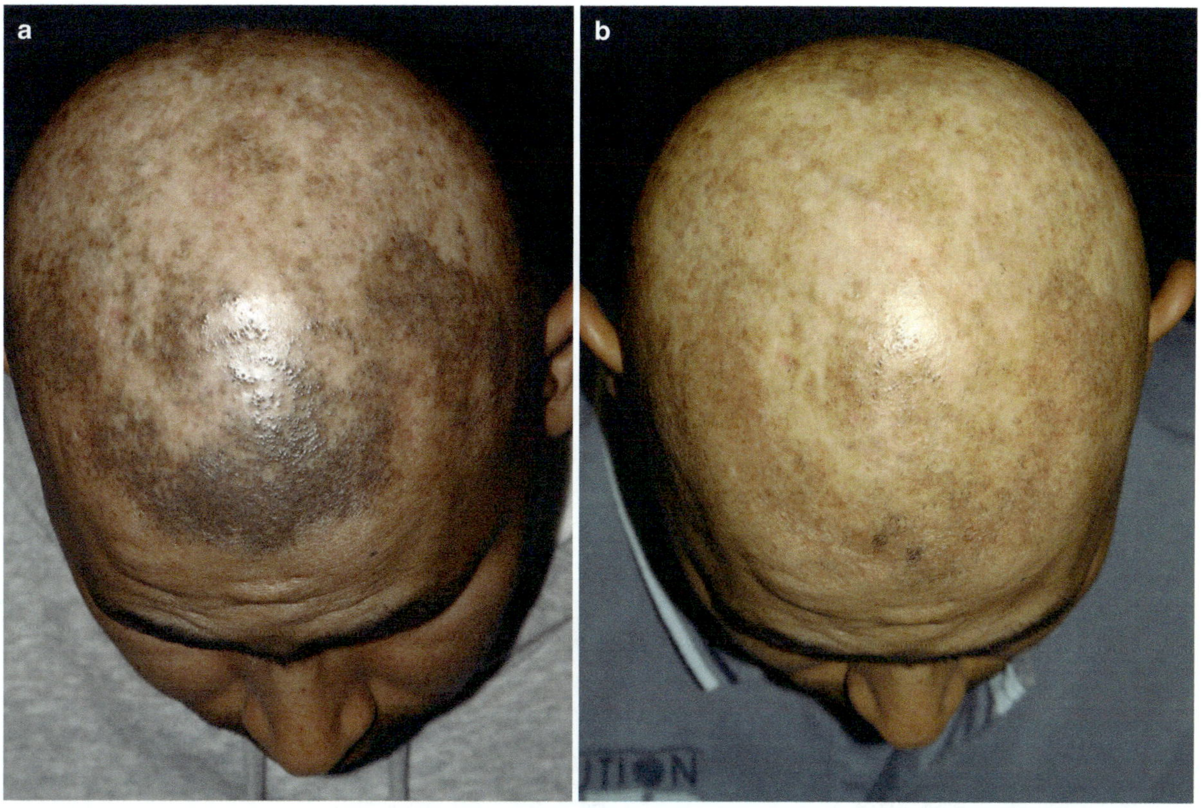

Fig. 47.1 (**a**) Hair removal in a patient with folliculitis capitis abscedens et suffodiens before treatment. (**b**) After long-pulsed 1064 Nd:YAG laser (six sessions)

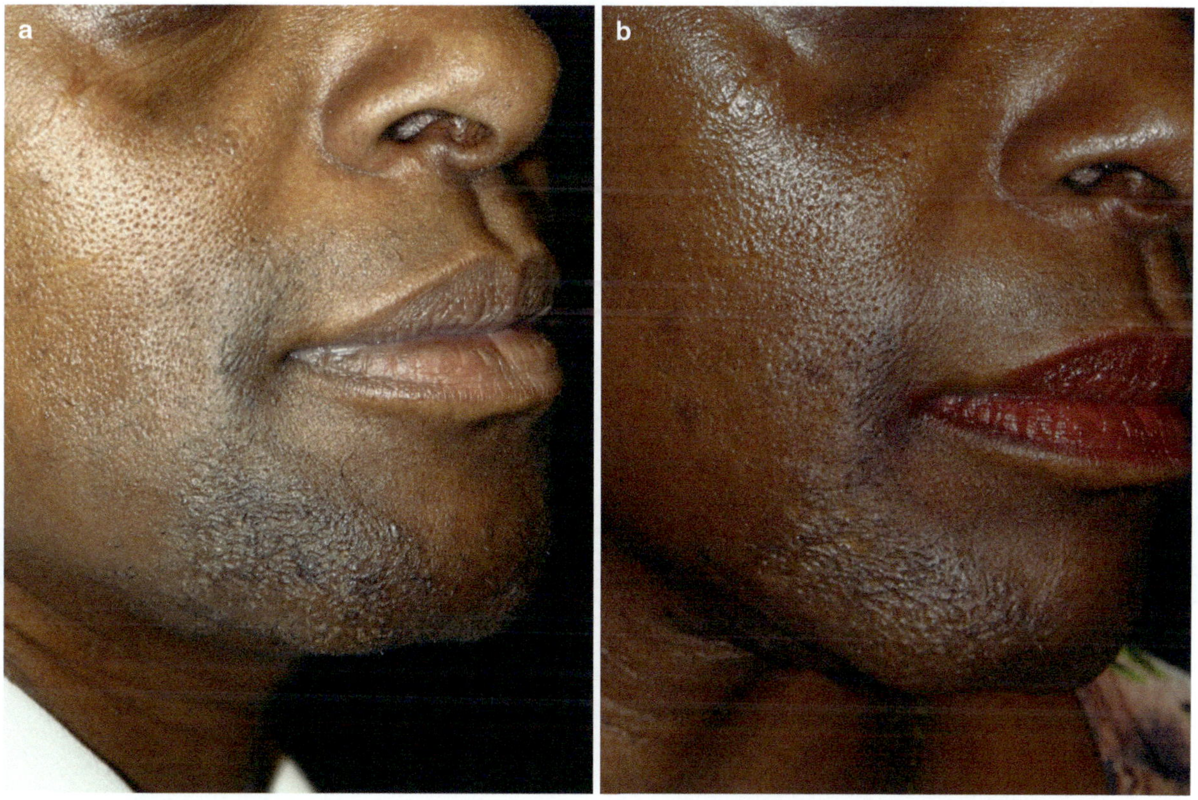

Fig. 47.2 (**a**, **b**) Hirsutism before and after hair removal with long-pulsed 1064 Nd:YAG laser

with caution; the dermatologist should initiate the treatment at threshold fluency. High fluencies may lead to epidermal exfoliation, blistering, and bulk heating, increasing the likelihood of skin textural changes and scarring.

Melasma still remains very difficult to treat in dark-skinned populations. The use of any pigment-specific laser is highly unpredictable and increased chances of worsening of melasma and PIH. Recently, the use of low-fluence QS Nd:YAG 1064 nm laser has shown more predictable results with fewer side effects, although recurrences are expected in longer follow-ups [11].

Tattoos may respond unpredictably to laser treatments. The exogenous pigments are highly variable and are placed deep into the dermis, and epidermal melanin may offer a barrier to laser penetration resulting in long-lasting or even permanent dyschromia. The QS ruby and alexandrite lasers are highly efficacious in removing black, green, and blue inks. QS ND:YAG 1064 nm laser may be considered a better choice since it is less absorbed by epidermal melanin and offers high efficacy for black and blue pigment removal. Shorter wavelengths, such as 532 nm, should be avoided due to high incidence of dyschromia. Given the higher risk of pigmentary complications in phototypes V and VI (especially when treating complex or multicolored tattoos), test treatments are recommended. The use of the lowest effective fluency is also a preferred approach to minimize laser-induced dyschromia (Figs. 47.3, 47.4, and 47.5) [3, 6, 9, 10].

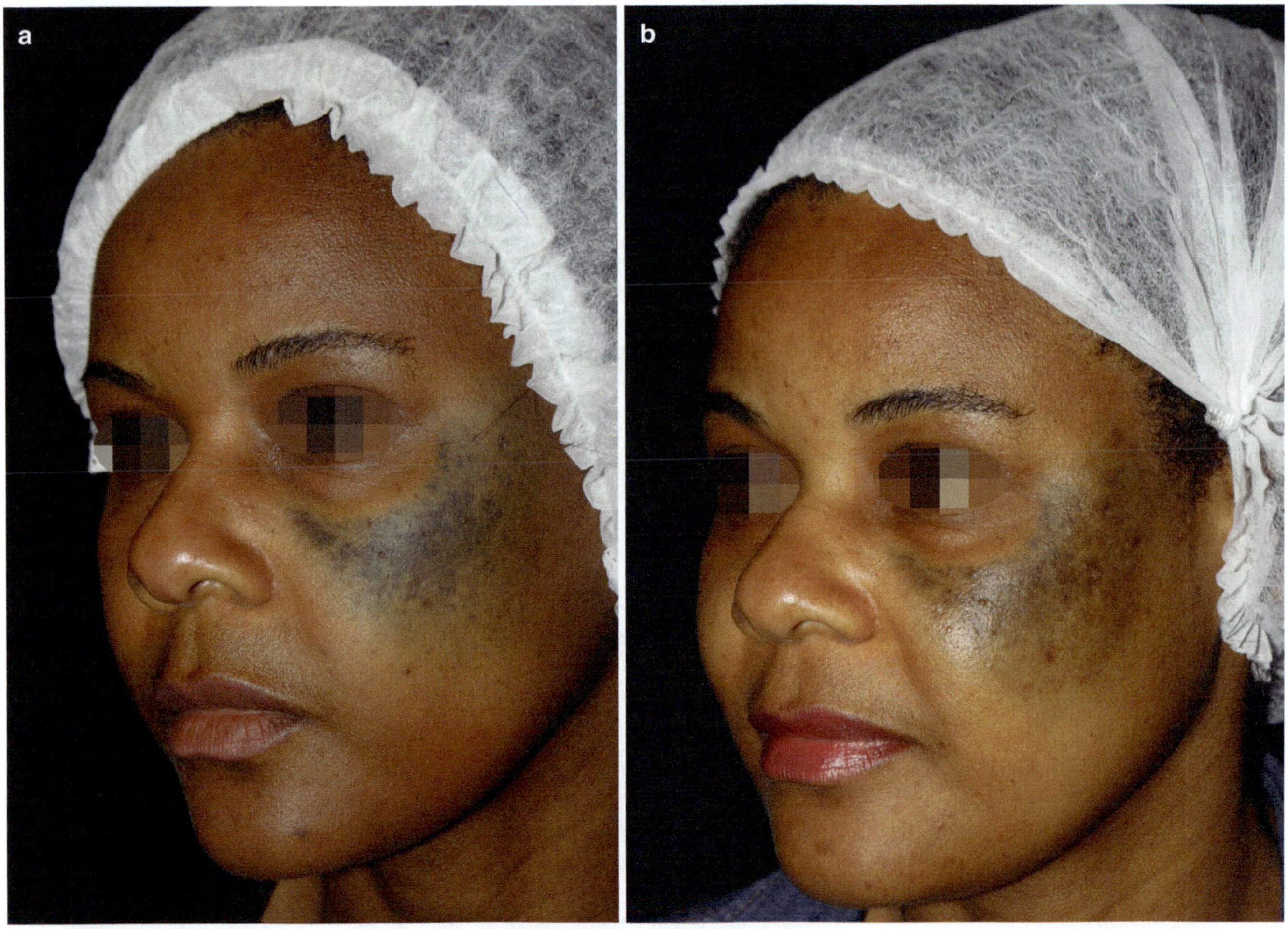

Fig. 47.3 (**a**) Naevus Ota before treatment. (**b**) Naevus Ota after QS Nd:YAG 1064 nm laser (four sessions)

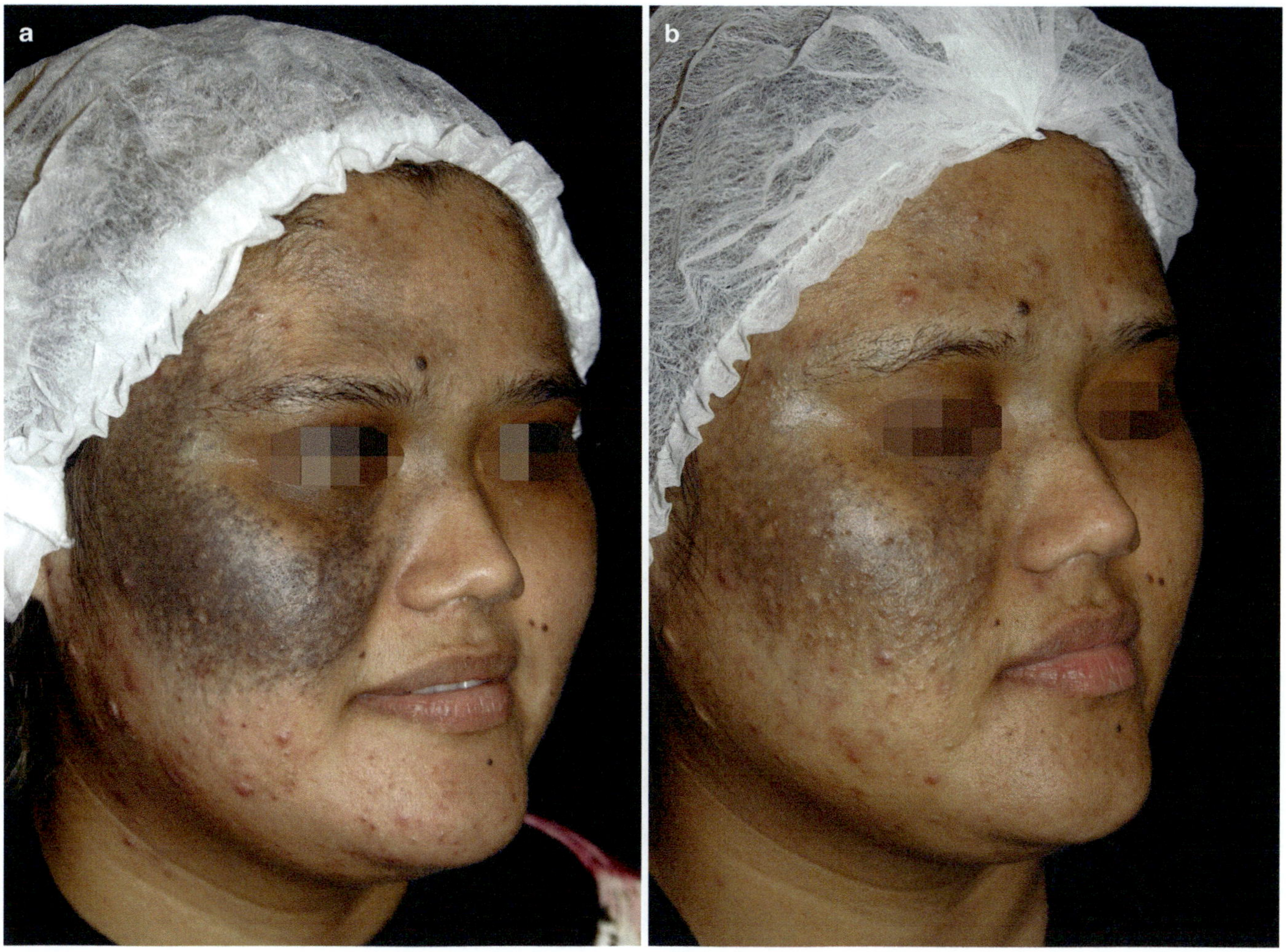

Fig. 47.4 (**a**) Naevus Ota before. (**b**) Naevus Ota after QS Nd:YAG 1064 nm laser (eight sessions)

47.5 Photoaging

Skin rejuvenation mainly includes collagen remodeling and stimulation in order to improve the texture, decrease pore size, and tighten skin laxity. Dermal heating with lasers can induce collagen stimulation and remodeling. Traditional laser resurfacing with ablative CO_2 or Er:YAG lasers is associated with high rates of severe pigmentary abnormalities and scarring in dark-skinned patients [3, 6, 7]. Delayed onset of hypopigmentation and hyperpigmentation and transient erythema are common side effects of skin resurfacing. Therefore, patients with phototypes V and VI were generally excluded from having such procedures due to the unfavorable risk to benefit ratio [7, 9].

The development of non-ablative and fractional lasers has provided safe and effective treatment options for patients with darkly pigmented skin [4, 12].

Non-ablative technologies (laser, light-based, or radiofrequency devices) are considered safer and more efficacious in dark-skinned patients. A series of monthly treatments is delivered so that thermal injury is mostly delivered in the dermis, avoiding epidermal damage. Radiofrequency (RF) devices, unlike lasers, deliver an electric current which nonselectively generates heat by the tissue's resistance to the flow of ions (Ohm's Law). Thus, RF can be safely applied regardless of the skin type, because it is not absorbed by melanin [4].

Non-ablative fractional lasers which operate in the 1550 nm are more appropriate to treat photoaging skin

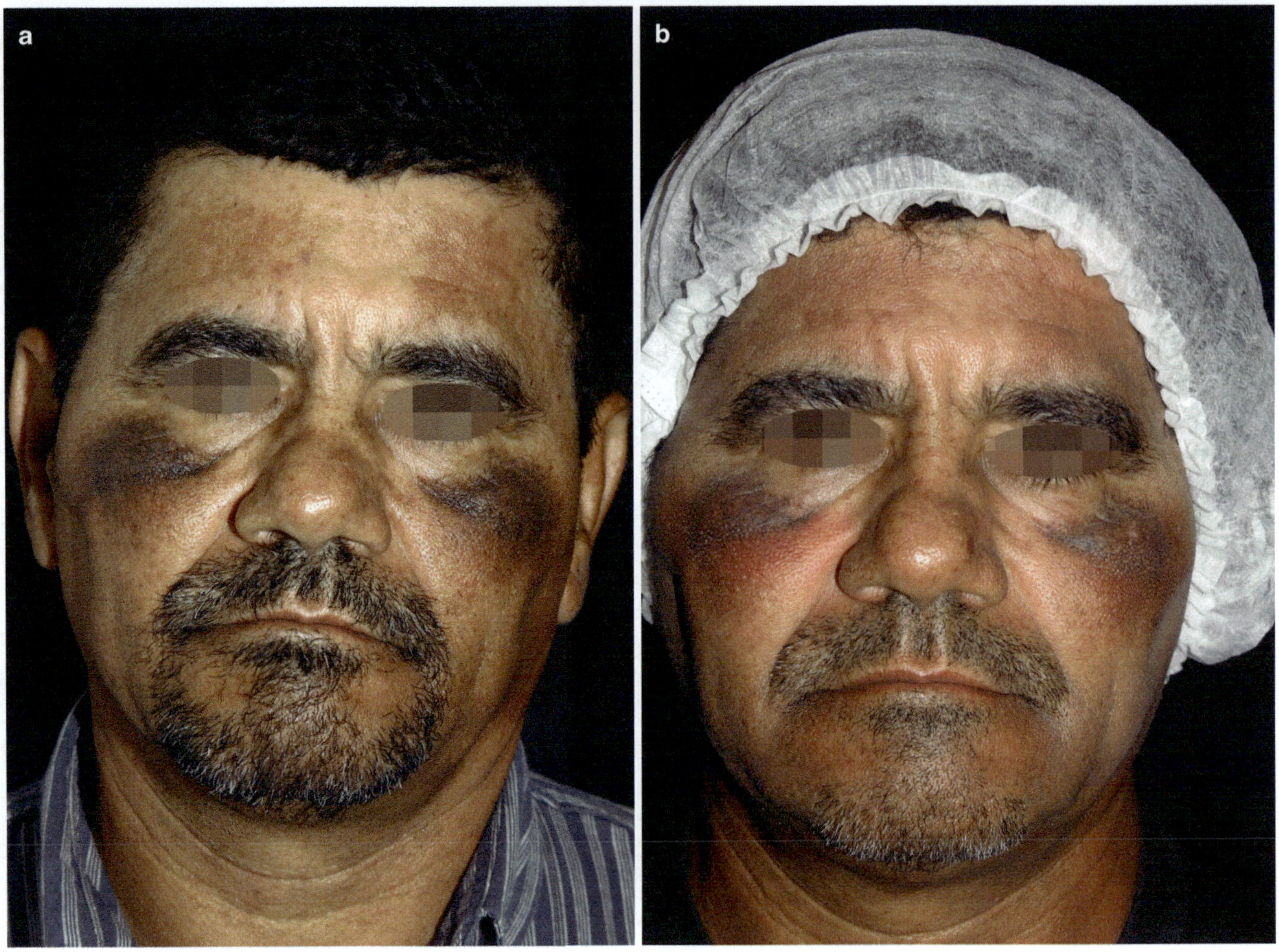

Fig. 47.5 (**a**) Exogenous ochronosis before treatment. (**b**) Exogenous ochronosis after treatment with IPL (ten sessions)

and acne scarring of phototypes higher than IV. It is absorbed by water but in a lesser extent than CO_2 or Er:YAG lasers [12]. Thus, the result is a deeper penetration in the skin with very little interaction with epidermis. Also, being a fractionated laser, microscopic treatment zones of denatured tissue surrounded by normal tissue provide rapid wound healing. It has been applied to successfully improve *wrinkles*, *atrophic scars*, *dyschromia*, and *striae distensae*. Despite the minimal side effects and relatively short recovery period, the results are not as pronounced as ablative fractional resurfacing [9, 12] (Figs. 47.6 and 47.7).

47.6 Vascular Lesions

The major absorption peak of oxyhemoglobin in the 577 nm range is what makes the pulsed dye laser (585–600 nm) the most specific laser to target these chromophores. The best clinical results for hemangiomas, port-wine stains, and facial telangiectasias are achieved with the PDL, regardless of patient phototype [3–6].

The presence of increased epidermal pigment in patients with darker skin phototypes interferes with the targeted hemoglobin's absorption of the laser energy. However, darker-skinned patients can be treated safely and effectively with theses lasers [2]. Oxyhemoglobin can be targeted by different wavelengths: 532, 577, 585, and 595. However, the shorter the wavelength, the shallower the penetration, which means that long-pulsed 532 nm KTP laser may cause more epidermal injury in these patients. A longer wavelength such as 1064 nm (Nd:YAG long-pulsed lasers) is currently used to target violaceous telangiectasias of the leg and larger reticular veins [4, 7]. Once there is a deeper penetration and less interaction with epidermal melanin, these lasers offer a valuable treatment option for vascular birthmarks and telangiectasias for dark-skinned people. The long-pulsed 755 nm alexandrite laser can also target hemoglobin and be used to treat hemangiomas and port-wine stains. However, there is more absorption by epidermal melanin and should be used

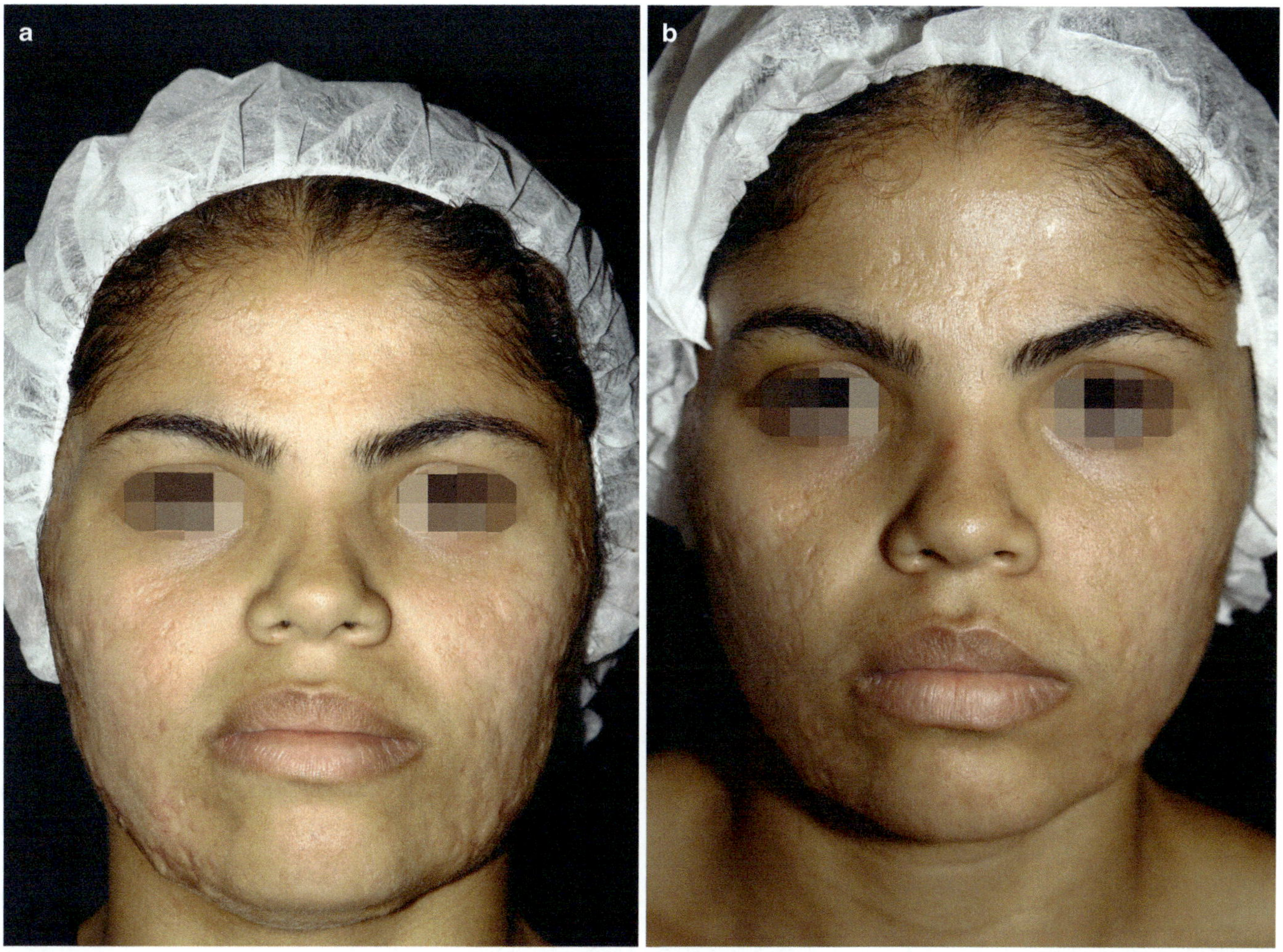

Fig. 47.6 (**a**) Acne scars before laser treatment. (**b**) Acne scars after fractional non-ablative 1550 nm (five sessions)

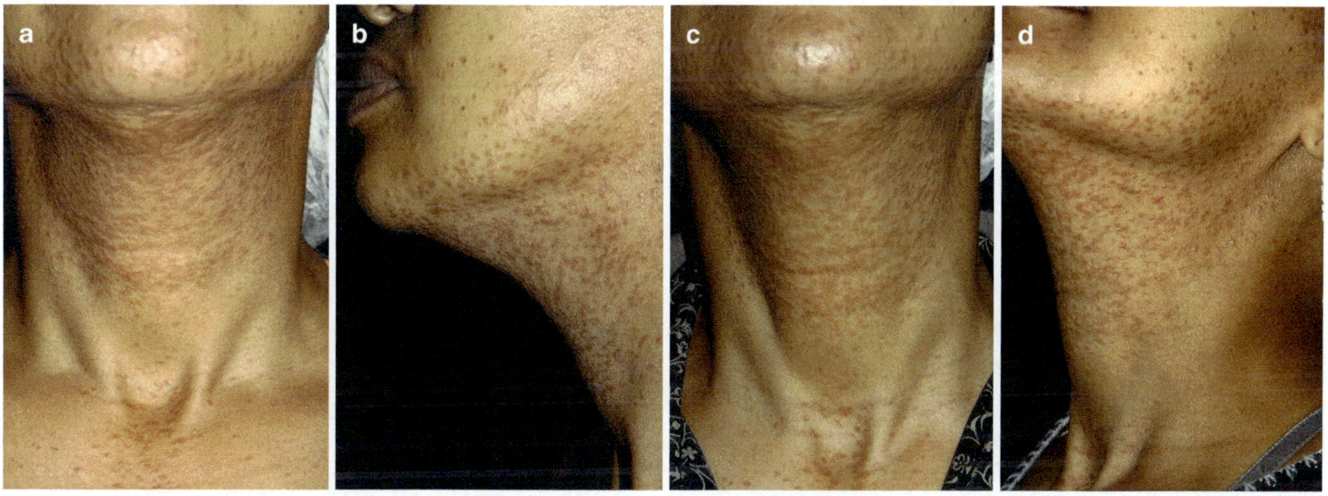

Fig. 47.7 (**a**, **c**) Eruptive syringomas before treatment. (**b**, **d**) Eruptive syringomas after treatment with fractional CO_2 laser (two sessions)

with caution, because it can lead to more depigmentation of the skin [6, 8, 9].

IPL systems with short cutoff filters target oxyhemoglobin and epidermal melanin. Although very efficacious in treating facial telangiectasias, the side effects from nonspecific epidermal injury are more common and should be avoided for patients with suntanned skin and phototypes higher than IV. Longer cutoff filters may be used more safely, although less efficacy is generally observed (Figs. 47.8 and 47.9) [2, 6, 9].

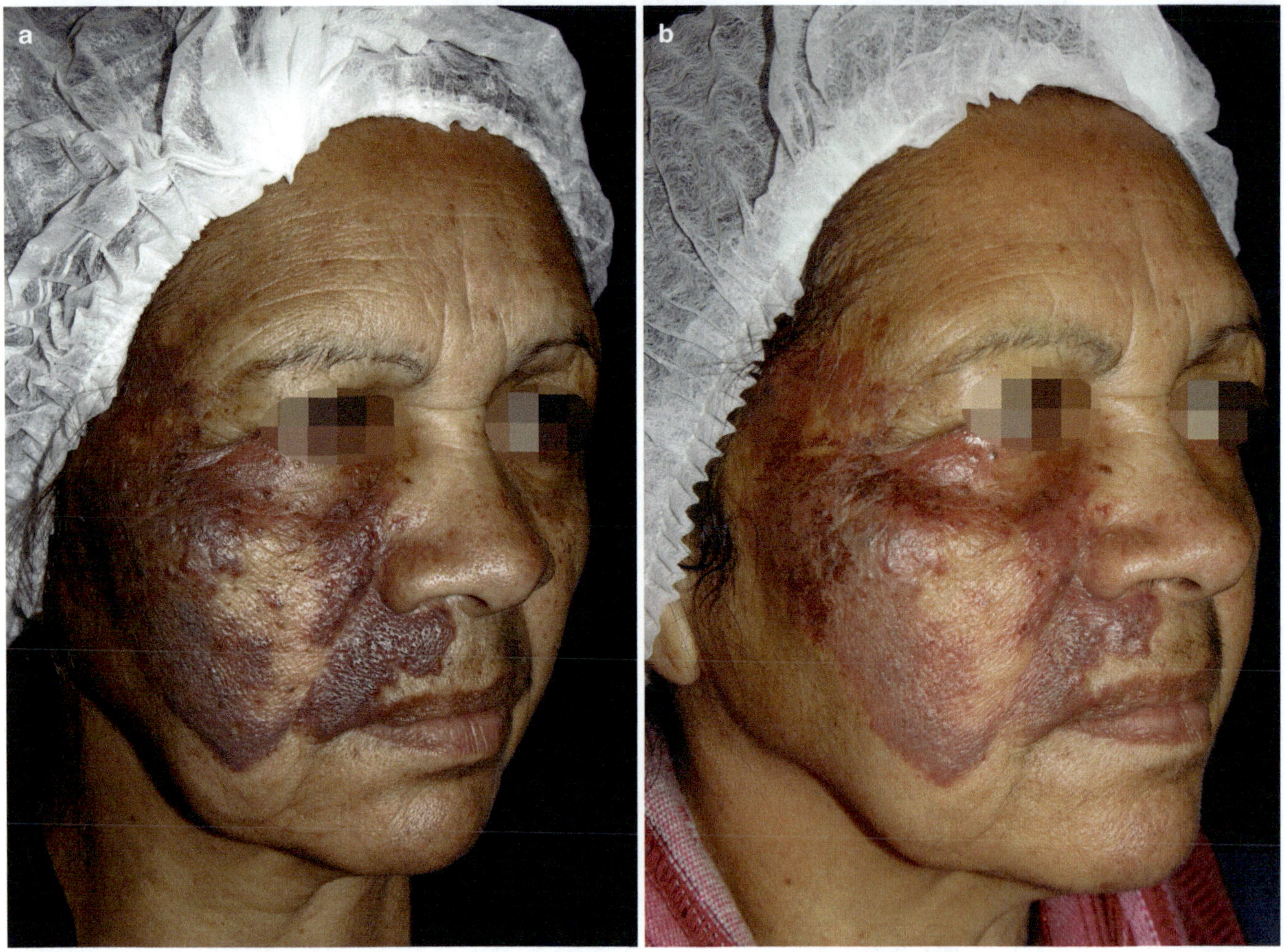

Fig. 47.8 (**a**) Port-wine stain before treatment. (**b**) Port-wine stain after IPL treatment (ten sessions)

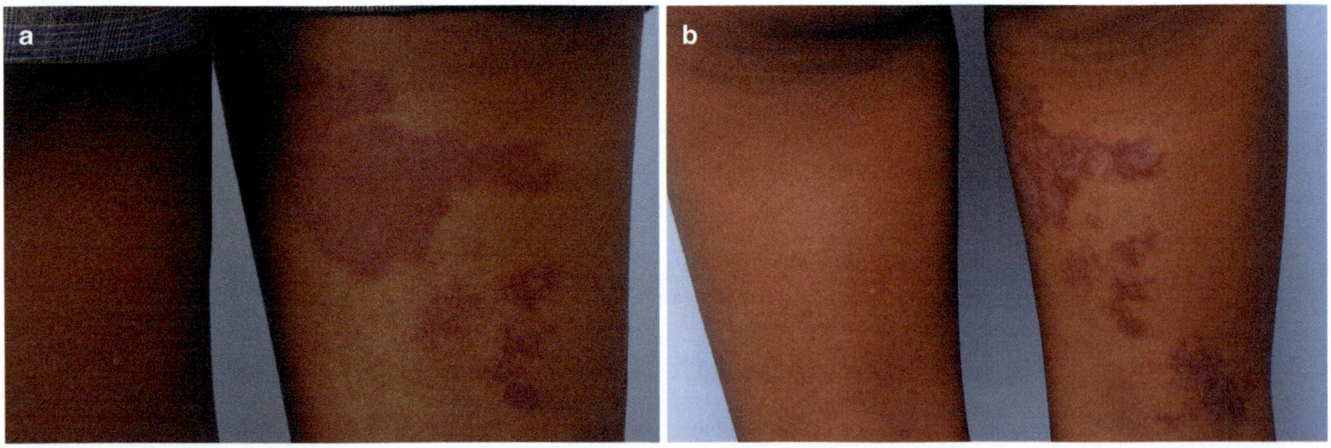

Fig. 47.9 (**a**) Port-wine stain before treatment. (**b**) Port-wine stain with long-pulsed alexandrite laser test spots

References

1. Van Buren N, Alster T. Laser treatment of dark skin: a review and update. J Drugs Dermatol. 2009;8:821–7.
2. Battle EF Jr. Cosmetic laser treatment for skin of color: a focus on safety and efficacy. J Drugs Dermatol. 2011;10:35–8.
3. Tanzi EL, Lupton JR, Alster TS. Lasers in dermatology: four decades of progress. J Am Acad Dermatol. 2003;49:1–31.
4. Alexis AF. Lasers and light-based therapies in ethnic skin: treatment options and recommendations for Fitzpatrick skin types V and VI. Br J Dermatol. 2013;169:91–7.
5. Stewart N, Lim AC, Lowe PM, et al. Lasers and laser-like devices: part one. Australas J Dermatol. 2013;54:173–83.
6. Sebaratnam DF, Lim AC, Lowe PM, et al. Lasers and laser-like devices: part two. Australas J Dermatol. 2014;55:1–14.
7. Battle EF Jr, Soden CE. The use of lasers in darker skin types. Semin Cutan Med Surg. 2009;28:130–40.
8. Woolery-Lloyd H, Viera MH, Valins W. Laser therapy in black skin. Facial Plast Surg Clin North Am. 2011;19:405–16.
9. Alam M, Warycha M. Complications of lasers and light treatments. Dermatol Ther. 2011;24:571–80.
10. Ibrahimi OA, Sakamoto FH, Anderson RR. Picosecond laser pulses for tattoo removal: a good, old idea. JAMA Dermatol. 2013;149:241.
11. Hofbauer-Parra CA, Careta MF, Valente NY, et al. Clinical and histopathologic assessment of facial melasma after low-fluence Q-switched neodymium-doped yttrium aluminium garnet laser. Dermatol Surg. 2016;42:507–12.
12. Manstein D, Laubach HJ. Fractional photothermolysis. In: Nouri K, editor. Lasers in dermatology and medicine. London: Springer; 2011. p. 123–47.

GPSR Compliance

The European Union's (EU) General Product Safety Regulation (GPSR) is a set of rules that requires consumer products to be safe and our obligations to ensure this.

If you have any concerns about our products, you can contact us on ProductSafety@springernature.com

In case Publisher is established outside the EU, the EU authorized representative is:

Springer Nature Customer Service Center GmbH
Europaplatz 3
69115 Heidelberg, Germany

Batch number: 10762486

Printed by Printforce, the Netherlands